7TH EDITION VILLAGE MEDICAL MANUAL

A Guide to Health Care in Developing Countries

VOLUME 2 SYMPTOMS, ILLNESSES, TREATMENTS

MARY VANDERKOOI M.D., D.T.M.& H.

Correspondence with the author may be addressed to:
vanderkooim@gmail.com
maryalicevanderkooi@yahoo.com
www.villagemedicalmanual.org

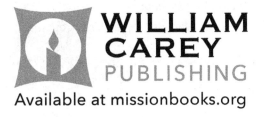

WILLIAM CAREY PUBLISHING

Available at missionbooks.org

Village Medical Manual: A Guide to Health Care in Developing Countries
Volume 1: Principles, Procedures, and Injuries
Volume 2: Symptoms, Illnesses, and Treatment

Previous three editions published by:
William Carey Library
1605 East Elizabeth St.
Pasadena, CA 91114 USA

Published by William Carey Publishing
10 W. Dry Creek Cir
Littleton, CO 80120 USA
publishing@wclbooks.com | missionbooks.org | williamcarey.com

William Carey Publishing is a ministry of Frontier Ventures
Pasadena, CA 91104 | www.frontierventures.org

DG Wynn, managing editor
Melissa Hicks, copyeditor
Mike Riester, cover design
Mary Vanderkooi and Mike Riester, interior design
Otis Wilson (OW), illustrator
Angela Baird (AB), illustrator
Katie McGaffey, production coordinator

Printed in the United States of America

23 22 21 20 19   1 2 3 4 5   IN1500

ISBNs: 978-0-87808-060-1 (paperback), 978-0-87808-062-5 (fixed-page epub)

Library of Congress Cataloging-in-Publication Data

Names: Vanderkooi, Mary, author.

Title: Village medical manual: a guide to health care in developing countries / Mary Vanderkooi.

Description: Seventh edition. | Littleton, CO: William Carey Publishing, [2019] | Includes indexes.

Identifiers: LCCN 2018031832 (print) | LCCN 2018032118 (ebook) | ISBN 9780878080625 (epub) | ISBN 9780878080601 (pbk.)

Subjects: | MESH: Rural Health | Community Health Workers | Developing Countries | Medicine | Pharmaceutical Preparations | Popular Works

Classification: LCC RC81 (ebook) | LCC RC81 (print) | NLM WA 395 | DDC 362.109172/4—dc23

LC record available at https://lccn.loc.gov/2018031832

IMPORTANT NOTICE AND DISCLAIMER

This book is intended for use only by those who are forced by location and circumstances to render medical care for which they are not professionally trained. It does not reflect the state of medical art in Western countries, and it is not to be used as a substitute for professional medical care. Please take note of the following:

1. Medicine is not an exact science. Diagnosis is largely an art learned by experience and training.

2. To the best of the author's knowledge, only conditions that are common in some parts of the developing world are included in this book.

3. Only the most common and constant symptoms are listed for each condition.

4. Only the most common diseases are listed for each symptom. Diseases that are not treatable in developing areas are not listed or not emphasized. The emphasis is almost entirely on infectious and nutritional diseases. These are most common in developing areas and are treatable in that context.

5. Descriptions given for diseases will in general be correct, but they may not be true in certain areas of the world. Diseases manifest differently according to the particular strain of the infecting organism, the environment, and the age and genetic heritage of the patient. For example, the symptoms of typhoid fever in India may be quite different from those in South America.

6. Only the most common, the safest and lowest cost drugs are listed. More effective alternatives may be available. Every effort has been made to check and double-check the recommended doses, but it is essential that doses of unfamiliar drugs be checked against another reference.

7. Only the most important precautions about drug use and possible side-effects are listed. It is essential, before using drugs, to check recent information regarding safety, precautions and side-effects. This information changes frequently. The following web addresses are useful: www.drugs.com; www.webmd.com; www.rxlist.com; www.medicinenet.com

8. Verbal descriptions and illustrations give only a very rough approximation of how to do procedures and physical examination. They do not adequately substitute for hands-on training and experience.

9. The assumption is made that only minimal drugs and equipment are available. There are frequently better treatments where there are better facilities. More accurate diagnosis will be available in locations where there are laboratory and imaging facilities.

10. Only the common and less serious injuries are addressed in the injury section. If an injury does not match a description, studying the principles and following those is usually more reliable than following specific directions for an injury that is similar but not the same.

11. Recommendations for evacuation are made on the assumption that sending out would entail a considerable amount of time, expense and difficulty. For situations in which professional medical help is readily available, it should be used in all cases.

12. Maps are unreliable. Lack of shading indicates both absence of the disease in question and absence of any data regarding that disease. The two are not equivalent. Sometimes data is absent because intelligent people know enough not to enter the area.

13. Maps are unreliable. To make them, educated people must do surveys. This requires at a minimum
    a.) The absence of local armed conflict;
    b.) A functional infrastructure, including roads;
    c.) Creature comforts such as hotels, food and water
    d.) Friendly nationals who will cooperate.
    Where any of these amenities is lacking, maps are unreliable. Grant money is awarded for disease elimination, so results of surveys may be modified accordingly. Disease distributions change rapidly, especially with migration, flooding or drought. Be particularly sceptical of shading that ends at political borders. Germs don't respect border controls. On the other hand, if the nearest shading to your location is 1000 miles away, you will not likely see the disease except in travelers. Maps can be helpful to illustrate generalities; however, the borders of areas indicated are constantly in flux in the real world.

14. The protocols in this manual were developed for use in medcical scenarios where Western medical care is not readibly available. **Do not try to use these protocols to bypass licensed medical care in the West**, as the spectrum of disease in the West is different from that in developing areas.

15. In particular, the assumption of the book is that the presenting complaint of the patient has only one explanatory diagnosis. This, in some cases, may not be true. If a patient comes down with malaria and hepatitis at the same time, the protocols will be entirely misleading. Only Western-type medical care can help.

TOC

SYMPTOMS

DIFFERENTIALS

CONDITIONS

DRUG INDEX

REGIONAL NOTES

INX

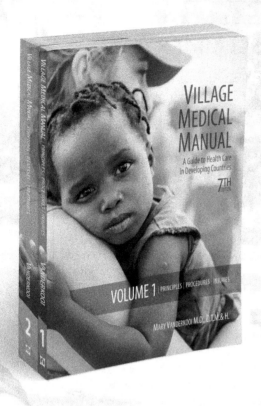

THE VILLAGE MEDICAL MANUAL IS THE PERFECT RESOURCE FOR TEACHING THE ABILITY TO DELIVER REASONABLE AND COMPETENT HEALTHCARE IN AREAS WHERE PROFESSIONAL CARE IS UNLIKELY/ UNAVAILABLE. THE MANUAL'S DIAGNOSTIC PROTOCOLS AND EXTENSIVE INFORMATION ON TROPICAL DISEASES ARE INCOMPARABLE. I HIGHLY RECOMMEND THESE BOOKS TO ANYONE INTERESTED IN DELIVERING EFFECTIVE HEALTHCARE TO CULTURES REMOTE FROM REALISTIC MEDICAL CARE.

—FREDERICK "BO" KAIL R.N., MSN
PROFESSOR AND PRACTITIONER OF TRANSCULTURAL NURSING

IT IS A VALUABLE RESOURCE FOR PRIMARY CARE PROVIDERS IN DEVELOPING COUNTRY SETTINGS EVERYWHERE—CONSIDERABLY MORE USEFUL AND COMPREHENSIVE THAN OTHER INTRODUCTORY HEALTHCARE MANUALS.

—GEOFF PROTHEROE, M.D., MSc
HEALTH CONSULTANT, AIM INTERNATIONAL

VOLUME 2 CONTENTS

VOLUME 1 CONTENTS

TOC

SYMPTOMS

DIFFERENTIALS

CONDITIONS

DRUG INDEX

REGIONAL NOTES

INX

TOC

SYMPTOMS

DIFFERENTIALS

CONDITIONS

DRUG INDEX

REGIONAL NOTES

INX

ABOUT THE AUTHOR

Mary Vanderkooi (b. 1941; nee Rooze) obtained her undergraduate education from Calvin College and the University of Rochester, receiving a B.S. degree in Chemistry from the latter institution. This was followed by an M.S. degree in Medical Physiology, also from the University of Rochester. She received the M.D. degree from the University of Wisconsin-Madison in 1975. Following residency training in Internal Medicine at Hines Veterans Administration Hospital, she worked in emergency care facilities at several hospitals in northern Illinois. During 1987 she studied at the Bangkok School of Tropical Medicine, Mahidol University and was awarded the Diploma in Tropical Medicine and Hygiene (D.T.M.& H.). She has had a long-standing interest in the medical problems of Third-World countries. During the 1980's she made several trips to Africa and Southeast Asia to do medical work. In 1994 she and her husband took early retirement and moved to Ethiopia, where they continue to live. They are doing medical and educational work in and around Soddo-Wolaitta. She teaches medical courses when given opportunity.

ACKNOWLEDGMENTS

Many people have contributed to the composition of this book, for which I am deeply grateful. James Padron did some of the art early on. Several of his pictures are still included. Kim and Dan Hardy introduced me to artist Otis Wilson and hosted the two of us in their home for a total of 17 days, so we could work together. Angela Baird drew most of the pictures for the second volume; Otis Wilson drew the rest. James Padron drew some of the pictures for the first volume, with contributions from Darwin Dunham and Garret Vanderkooi. Mary Modderman tutored me (pseudonym Alex Rhoods, AR) in drawing. Steven Gardner provided input on faithfulness-based HIV counseling. Several medical professionals helped with the early editions; these included particularly Neva Abbott, M.D. Janet Fraker, a dietitian, educated me on nutrition and also furnished the data upon which Chapter 5 is based. Lawrence Ahrens did all the art work for the early editions, using his extebded family as models; the present art is based on their work. Lois Ingels and Linda Sanford provided English grammar input.early on. My sister, Ruth Salomons, advised me concerning remaining gramatical questions. Denise Wynn and Melissa Hicks both of William Carey Publishing were of great assistance.

DEDICATION

To James R. Jacobs of Eau Claire, Wisconsin.

He was the agent through whom

my life was redeemed from

destruction and crowned

with tender mercies.

PREFACE TO THE SEVENTH EDITION

This book is intended for use by Western-educated expatriates living in isolated locations who, by necessity, must sometimes function as physicians. The intention is to provide such people with a reference book, using a vocabulary which they can understand, to treat the medical problems they are forced to treat and to intelligently refer those that can be referred.

This book is considerably more advanced than the widely used books *Where There Is No Doctor* and *Primary Child Care*, but it is not as advanced as standard medical reference works. The latter texts presuppose a medical education, use technical jargon and assume the availability of high-tech medical facilities. This book uses ordinary English to make the text understandable to anyone with a Western education. In the author's experience, people who have received their primary and secondary education in developing nations cannot follow the logic used in this work.

There is a strong emphasis on the problems of the tropical Third-World, but the scope of the book is not limited to the tropics. There are regional notes for Central Asia and the Arctic. Many non-tropical diseases are also covered, and the injury section is generally applicable.

This book is not intended to supplant the role of the physician. The treatments described were chosen on the basis of low cost, low-tech, wide availability and safety; there are better options when medical expertise is available. The reality of life in developing countries is such that even radio contact with a nurse may be a luxury. The book deals with this by attempting to indicate the degree of urgency of acquiring advanced care for a patient with a given set of symptoms.

The diagnostic protocols were written on the assumption that laboratory and imaging facilities are minimal or non-existent. Diagnosis is mainly by history and physical examination. Some useful low-tech laboratory procedures which require a minimum of equipment are described in Appendix 2. Diagnosis is confirmed by a positive response to treatment. **When and if advanced diagnostic facilities are available, they should be utilized.**

The recommended treatments are reasonably current, considering the constraints of a Third-World environment. They presuppose the absence of specialized equipment or expensive drugs. Oral medications in the Third-World are usually better than injectable, both for safety and cost. Amongst oral medications, the older, cheaper drugs are preferable to the newer ones, unless free samples are available. Western medical doctors who are used to high-tech facilities, and who are pursuing service in the tropics for the first time, may find this text useful, along with the cases in the Village Medical Tutorial.

Medical personnel will note that diseases are lumped into groups. For example, *acute abdomen* is a single diagnosis. A surgeon needs to know the precise problem, but a non-professional only needs to send the patient to a surgeon. Any attempt to make finer distinctions would only confuse the lay reader. *Cancer* is described briefly and as a single entity, because more detail would lead to confusion without enhancing early diagnosis and treatment. Western expatriates can travel to expert medical care. Cancer in the absence of Western-type medical care is generally diagnosed late and uniformly fatal.

Any lay person expecting to use this book **must** take time to read (at a minimum) the first 5 chapters of Volume 1, *before* a crisis arises. He, or she should also become acquainted with the contents of the rest of both volumes. A helpful exercise is to look up how you would deal with the following problems: breech childbirth; a sprained ankle; a 50 y.o. woman who fell and then had shoulder pain on the side of her left shoulder; a sore throat with a low fever and large red tonsils; bloody diarrhea with a high fever in a 1 y.o. child; a red, swollen, extremely painful great toe with no prior injury, in a 60 y.o. man.

Changes in the Seventh Edition:

- The first chapter has been revised and expanded.

- The orthopedic section is expanded to facilitate diagnosis and treatment without x-rays.

- Otis Wilson, Angela Baird and James Padron prepared illustrations, replacing Lawrence Ahrens who died after a long illness.

- The Symptom Index now breaks down long lists of differential diagnoses into shorter lists.

- Descriptions from clinically oriented old medical texts have modified the Condition Index, particularly the syphilis entry.

- The Differential Diagnosis Index has been changed to a more user-friendly format. Protocols for symptomatic, generic treatments have been added.

- Regional Notes have been added for the Arctic and the Central Asian Republics.

- In response to feedback from users, there is now a lot of information about when, where and how to refer for higher-level medical care.

- The book is cross-referenced to the Village Medical Tutorial.

Contact the author:

Mary Vanderkooi Box 131; Wolaitta-Soddo, Ethiopia
vanderkooim@gmail.com
maryalicevanderkooi@yahoo.com
www.villagemedicalmanual.org

TOC

SYMPTOMS

DIFFERENTIALS

CONDITIONS

DRUG INDEX

REGIONAL NOTES

INX

DRUG INTERACTIONS

> ⚠ **PRECAUTION:**
> The following list of drugs can alter electrical activity in the heart which might cause sudden death.
> Thus they should not be combined with any other drug on this list.

Azithromycin	Fluconazole	Ketoconazole	Quinidine
Chloroquine	Halofantrine	Levofloxacin	Quinine
Clarithromycin	Itraconazole	Mefloquine	Stibogluconate
Erythromycin			

HOW TO USE THESE MANUALS

1—BEFORE A CRISIS

Any lay person expecting to use this book **must** take time to read (at a minimum) the first 5 chapters of Volume 1, *before* a crisis arises. He or she should also become acquainted with the contents of the rest of both volumes. A helpful exercise is to look up how you would deal with the following problems: breech childbirth; a sprained ankle; a 50 y.o. woman who fell and then had shoulder pain on the side of her left shoulder; a sore throat with a low fever and large, red tonsils; bloody diarrhea with a high fever in a 1 y.o. child; a red, swollen, extremely painful great toe with no prior injury, in a 60 y.o. man.

2—DEFINING THE PROBLEM

INJURY—VOLUME 1 | NON-INJURY—VOLUME 2

Chief complaint: What bothers the patient the most?

POISONING	SOFT TISSUE	BONE, LIGAMENT, JOINT	NON-INJURY	WHOLE-BODY ILLNESS	BODY PART(S)
Venomous bite or sting > Chapter 9	Non-laceration > Chapter 9 Laceration > Chapter 10	Principles > Chapter 11 Upper body > Chapter 12 Lower body > Chapter 13	Skin wound or rash > Protocols A.14–18	Whole body pain > Protocol B.2 Abnormal vital signs: > Protocols A.1–4 Disorders of: • alertness • emotion • movement • food intake • sensation • growth • miscellaneous > Protocols A.5–13	Head Neck Shoulders Upper limbs Chest Abdomen Pelvis/rectum Lower limbs Back > Protocols A.19-64

3—READING IT RIGHT

Within Volume 2 you'll notice some conditions and drugs are written in ALL CAPS. When you see **ALL CAPS** it means that these conditions or drugs are the titles of entries in the condition or drug index. Thus OLD AGE is listed as one cause of visual loss.

When the same word (e.g. condition) is in **lower case** or merely **Captitalized** it means that the word or words should be understood with their usual meaning in English. Old age is one cause of decreased immunity to infectious diseases.

4—FINDING THE ANSWERS

A full index of both volumes is located at the back of each volume.

SYMPTOM INDEX

TOC

SYMPTOMS

DIFFERENTIALS

CONDITIONS

DRUG INDEX

REGIONAL NOTES

INX

TOC

SYMPTOMS

DIFFERENTIALS

CONDITIONS

DRUG INDEX

REGIONAL NOTES

INX

TOC

SYMPTOMS

DIFFERENTIALS

CONDITIONS

DRUG INDEX

REGIONAL NOTES

INX

NORMAL VITAL SIGNS: QUICK REFERENCE

Normal corrected temperatures

1 month to 5 years	36.6°–37.2°C	98.0°–99.5°F
6 years to adult	36.4°–37.1°C	97.5°–99.0°F

Normal pulse pressure

The difference between the two blood pressure numbers should be between 20 and 80.

Normal respirations/minute at rest

Newborn	30–60
1 year	20–40
2–3 years	20–30
5 years	20–25
10 years	17–22
Adult	12–20

Normal arm circumference in centimeters

Age	Minimum	Danger
1 month	9.0	6.7
3 months	10.6	8.0
6 months	11.5	8.6
9 months	12.2	9.2
1-5 years	14.0	12.5
8 years	18.4	14.6
11 years	20.4	16.3
14 years	23.2	18.6
Adult	26.0	22.0

Normal blood pressures

Adult Westerners	90/50—140/90
Non-Western adults	80/40—130/80
Children 8–12	110/70—120/80
Children 3–6	104/63—116/74

Normal oxygen saturation

95% or more at sea level
93% or more at 6000 feet or 1800 meters

Normal pulse/minute at rest

Newborn	100–180
1–6 months	90–140
7–18 months	90–130
2–6 years	80–120
7–10 years	70–110
Adults	60–100
Athletes	36–70

TOC

SYMPTOMS

DIFFERENTIALS

CONDITIONS

DRUG INDEX

REGIONAL NOTES

INX

CALCULATING THE CORRECTED TEMPERATURE

In the past the standard for core body temperature was the rectal temperature, taken with a mercury thermometer. Oral temperatures read a degree Fahrenheit (0.5°C) lower than rectal. Armpit temperatures read 2° Fahrenheit (1.0°C) below rectal. Armpit temperatures tend to be inaccurate unless special care is taken to have the patient hold his arm tightly against his chest. With some reasonable precautions these temperatures were easy and safe to determine. An alcohol or iodine wipe between uses prevented transmission of infection from one patient to another.

Environmental and safety enthusiasts decided that mercury thermometers are unacceptable. Small, plastic, inexpensive digital thermometers became popular. However, these are not accurate. For most purposes they are fine, but for couples using morning temperatures as a means of birth control, they are unreliable. Digital thermometers vary in accuracy. The longer it takes to register the temperature, the more accurate they are. Thirty seconds is a reasonable, minimal time. The same corrections for oral and armpit temperatures must be made with these digital devises.

Then LED thermometers were invented. They are currently all the rage in spite of the fact that they usually read low. There are, at present, three types: ear thermometers, forehead thermometers and no-touch thermometers. These only measure surface temperature, not core temperature. They have been shown to be dangerously unreliable in the context of heat stroke; hence they should not be used when heat illness is a concern: athletes, miners and foundry workers. In the low-altitude tropics they should not be used at all; heat illness is always a concern there.

Reportedly forehead LED thermometers measure the temperature of an artery on the side of the head and this correlates well with the core temperature. However, if this is so, it implies absolutely perfect technique, something not attainable in any Third-World clinic.

My own experience with ear LED thermometers in an emergency department in the States was that in January no one had fevers, and in August everyone had fevers. This was true even on busy days, when patients sat around for a couple hours before being seen. In my current context (Ethiopia) the output from my ear thermometer seems to be totally random. There is no correlation whatsoever with mercury or forehead thermometer readings nor with clinical impression.

In writing this edition of the book, my first inclination was to recommend just not using these LEDs at all. Then I realized this is not realistic. Rather than giving them up completely, it is feasible to correct the displayed temperature for the built-in error.

In the environment where you work, measure the body temperatures of about 100 people who are not complaining of illness. Tally the number of people who register each temperature, to 0.1°C or 0.2°F. Most likely the temperature registered for the largest number of people will be the normal for that ethnic group, location and situation. Then, when you take subsequent temperatures, add the difference between that value and 36.9°C which is the average, normal, true body temperature.

Here is an example: in the case of a clinic forehead thermometer, the most common value was 36.4°. Hence, the temperature correction with this device was 0.5°C or 0.9°F more than the number displayed.
37.5° becomes a corrected temperature of 38.0° and so forth. It is essential to use the corrected temperature, not the displayed temperature, when determining if your patient has a fever. An accurate value is also essential if you are considering whether the patient has a slow pulse for his fever. Be sure to also use a mercury or non-LED digital thermometer if and when you are considering the condition of heat illness or heat stroke. In that case simply correcting an LED reading is not adequate.

TOC

SYMPTOMS

DIFFERENTIALS

CONDITIONS

DRUG INDEX

REGIONAL NOTES

INX

I—ABNORMAL VITAL SIGNS

PROTOCOL A.1—ABNORMAL TEMPERATURE

First consider this!

Before addressing abnormal temperatures, read page A-5 as well as the section on thermometers in Volume 1, Chapter 1. In all cases, use the corrected temperature to determine if your patient has a normal or an abnormal temperature. The corrected temperature is the displayed number plus the estimate of how much your device reads low.

If the armpit temperature or a rapid electronic thermometer indicates a fever, then the patient has a fever. However, he may still have a fever if the reading is normal. Only a mercury or a slow electronic thermometer, used rectally, can rule out a fever.

A.1.A—Low body temperature

A.1.B–1.D General notes on fevers

A.1.B—Mild fevers

A.1.C—Episodic fevers

A.1.D—Sustained high fever

Protocol A.1.A—Low corrected body temperature below 36.4°C or 97.5°F[1]

Be sure you are using the corrected temperature; see page A-5

Before proceeding with this protocol, cover the patient with warm blankets or have someone lie next to him.

Is the patient malnourished, an infant or elderly, or does he have HEART FAILURE?

NO	YES to one or more
|	Check after warming the patient; he probably has trouble controlling his body temperature.
|	Also consider SEPSIS.

Has the patient been wet and poorly covered, exposed to cold weather or both?

NO	YES
|	**Consider** HYPOTHERMIA; **treat immediately**.

Has the patient had prior fever, chills or both?

NO	YES
|	**Consider** MALARIA, RELAPSING FEVER[2] or SEPSIS.
|	

LOW TEMPERATURE, NO COLD EXPOSURE, NO PRIOR FEVER, NOT MALNOURISHED, INFANT OR ELDERLY

Dying patient	Blood pressure drops also; patient usually unconscious
THYROID TROUBLE	Low-thyroid: low temperature continually, always sleepy, slow onset and chronic
SEPSIS	Newborn, new mother, recent injury or infection
CHOLERA	Severe watery diarrhea, possibly vomiting also, muscle cramps
PLANT POISONING	Ackee: ate unripe fruit, sweaty, lethargic or unconscious; West Africa and West Indies
ENTERIC FEVER	ENTERIC FEVER plus ASPIRIN can cause a subnormal temperature.

---

1 *That is, the minimum acceptable temperature is 0.6 °C or 1.3 °F less than the mean displayed value for healthy people in your environment. A body temperature significantly less than this merits your working through this protocol if the patient appears ill.*

2 *Relapsing fever: present in tropical and high altitude areas but not in the islands of SEA or the South Pacific.*

General notes on fevers for Protocols A.1.B–1.D

*If you are using an LED thermometer, forehead, ear or no-touch, first determine the corrected temperature: page A-5

For fevers with other symptoms use the following B Protocols:

- B.2—fever plus headache and body pains
- B.3—fever plus anemia
- B.5—fever plus jaundice
- B.9—fever plus abdominal pain
- B.10—fever plus lethargy
- B.13—fever plus back pain

Fever pattern is defined as how the body temperature changes with time. This pattern can often be used to help diagnose the problem.

- When trying to determine the fever pattern, do not give anti-fever medications or antibiotics which confuse the results. Take the patient's temperature every 4–6 hours, around the clock and write it down, together with the time and date. Do this for at least 3 days in order to find the fever pattern.

- Determining the fever pattern is particularly valuable when there are several people who have the same undiagnosed illness. Doing this with a few patients will enable you to better treat all the patients who have similar symptoms.

- Listed below are various fever patterns and the most common diseases which cause them. Do not take these suggested diagnoses as absolute!

- Understand that your patient will have chills when his temperature rises and sweats as it falls. Have the patient report both chills and sweats, and take the temperature at those times in addition to regularly scheduled times.

Definitions of fever patterns: each of these fever patterns is either acute (lasting less than 2 weeks) or chronic (lasting more than 2 weeks).

Sustained fever is a fever which does not vary by more than 2.0°F (1.0°C), any one day and does not return to normal daily: BRUCELLOSIS, SPOTTED FEVER,[7] SCARLET FEVER, ENTERIC FEVER, DRUG ERUPTION, SERUM SICKNESS, RELAPSING FEVER.[1]

Episodic, intermittent fever is a fever which commonly returns to normal:

with one daily return to normal: ABSCESS, MALARIA, SEPSIS.

with two daily returns to normal: VISCERAL LEISHMANIASIS[4] and some rare infections.

> ⚠ **EMERGENCY**
>
> **FEVER EMERGENCIES**
> Stiff neck
> Lethargic
> Weak
> Severe abdominal pain
> Respiratory distress
> Recent-onset craziness
> Related to anesthesia or anti-vomiting medicine, with stiffness[8]

Episodic, remittent fever is a fever which varies by more than 2.0°F (1°C), and does not return to normal daily: falciparum MALARIA, TUBERCULOSIS, VISCERAL LEISHMANIASIS.[4] If the remittent fever is chronic (lasting more than 2 weeks) the diagnosis is probably TUBERCULOSIS, ENTERIC FEVER, ABSCESS, LARVA MIGRANS, HIV INFECTION, SEPSIS, AMEBIASIS, TRICHINOSIS or MONONUCLEOSIS.

Episodic, relapsing fever[1] might have any of these patterns, but then the fever goes away for a matter of days before it returns.

One relapse only: DENGUE FEVER,[2] LEPTOSPIROSIS, YELLOW FEVER,[3] POLIO, ARBOVIRAL FEVER.

More than one relapse, illness lasting less than 2 weeks: RELAPSING FEVER,[1] YELLOW FEVER,[3] BRUCELLOSIS, DENGUE FEVER,[2] MALARIA, RAT BITE FEVER, DRUG ERUPTION, SERUM SICKNESS, LEPTOSPIROSIS.

Chronic relapsing fever, illness lasting more than 2 weeks: VISCERAL LEISHMANIASIS,[4] AFRICAN SLEEPING SICKNESS,[5] CHAGA'S DISEASE,[6] RELAPSING FEVER,[1] BRUCELLOSIS, LYME DISEASE, LEPTOSPIROSIS.

---

1 *Relapsing fever: it is important to distinguish the symptom relapsing fever from the disease RELAPSING FEVER. The symptom is defined above. The disease was named for its most prominent symptom before the advent of the antibiotic era. Now it is a misnomer. Of all diseases with fever, it has the most sustained fever. If the disease runs its course without treatment, then the fever suddenly drops after 5–10 days; then it relapses. When and where antibiotics are available, it is inevitable that someone will treat the patient with some antibiotic, not allowing the disease to run its normal course. With antibiotic the sudden drop in fever and subsequent relapse is altered or abolished.*
2 *Dengue fever: in the Americas only near or north of the equator. In Africa, east coastal, south and west. Prevalent in India, Southeast Asia and the Pacific. Occasionally found in the Mediterranean area. The disease may spread.*
3 *Yellow fever: South America north of Sao Paolo, central and western Africa and the Sudan.*
4 *Visceral Leishmaniasis: found in scattered areas of Central and South America, (mainly eastern) Africa north of the equator, the Mediterranean area, the Indian subcontinent, eastern Europe, central Asia and mainland China.*
5 *African sleeping sickness: scattered areas of Africa, south of Bamako, Mali and Lake Chad; north of Lusaka, Zambia.*
6 *Chaga's disease: found in scattered areas in the Americas.*
7 *Spotted fever: worldwide including the Arctic, but not in the islands of Southeast Asia.*
8 *See NEUROLEPTIC MALIGNANT SYNDROME.*

TOC
SYMPTOMS
DIFFERENTIALS
CONDITIONS
DRUG INDEX
REGIONAL NOTES
INX

Protocol A.1.B—Mild fever

Be sure you are using corrected temperatures: see page A-5.

Definition: Mild fevers in temperate climates are corrected temperatures of less than 38.5°C/101.3°F. In the hot tropics, corrected temperatures up to 100°F [38°C] are considered normal.

Fevers are a common problem in the hot (low elevation) tropics; it is more efficient to look up another symptom, if there is one, than to use this protocol. This protocol does not list all causes of fevers, but only those that commonly occur with fever as the main or only symptom. See also page A-9 regarding fevers in general.

Is the patient malnourished, an infant or elderly, or does he have HEART FAILURE?

NO	YES
	In a hot environment, try cooling the person first; he may have trouble controlling his body temperature. Also consider causes of high fevers in these patients.
	Otherwise follow the "NO" arm for this question.
	Consider KIDNEY INFECTION in anyone; EAR INFECTION in infants.

Does the patient have a dry mouth?

NO	YES
	Consider severe DEHYDRATION; also consider drugs and PLANT POISONING with effects like the drug ATROPINE.

Is the patient extremely ill?

NO	YES
	Consider DIPHTHERIA, TETANUS, RABIES, SEPSIS or use Protocol A.1.D.

Has the patient been ill for less than 5 days?

NO	YES
	Consider an early stage of an illness which will cause a high fever.

Has the patient had weight loss, cough or both for a month or more?

NO to all	YES to any
	Consider TUBERCULOSIS, HIV INFECTION, VISCERAL LEISHMANIASIS,[1] BRUCELLOSIS, HEPATITIS, CANCER.

Does the patient have loss of appetite, yellow eyes or both?

NO to both	YES, one or the other or both
	Consider these with localized pain: MALARIA (head), BRUCELLOSIS (back), HEPATITIS or LIVER FLUKE (upper right abdomen), KIDNEY INFECTION (flank[s]), SYPHILIS (headache), AMEBIASIS (abdomen), MUMPS (face/ear/jaw), LEAD POISONING (headache), CANCER (anywhere).
See the table below.	**Consider these with generalized pain or no pain:** ADDICTION to uppers, HEAT ILLNESS, INFLUENZA, BRUCELLOSIS.

---

1 *Visceral Leishmaniasis: found in scattered areas of Central and South America, Africa north of the equator, the Mediterranean area, the Indian subcontinent, eastern Europe, central Asia and mainland China. Not present south of the equator.*

MILD FEVER, NO DRY MOUTH, ILL FOR >5 DAYS, NO WEIGHT LOSS, COUGH OR YELLOW EYES

Related to an environmental exposure	
DRUG ERUPTION	First dose or after a week on a drug; skin condition
SERUM SICKNESS	Rapid onset after a bite, sting or injection; or early stage of some diseases, such as SCHISTOSOMIASIS (especially Japonicum), URINARY INFECTION, HIV INFECTION, LIVER FLUKE, HEPATITIS, MALARIA, LARVA MIGRANS, STREP INFECTION
PLANT POISONING	Argemone oil; bad cooking oil

No prominent localized pain in one body part

MONONUCLEOSIS Also very tired, large neck lymph nodes, big, red tonsils, maybe sore throat.

CHICKEN POX Older children, fever before rash, not very ill.

TOXOPLASMOSIS Also large neck lymph nodes, normal throat, fatigue.

Prominent localized pain in one body part, likely the trunk

MASTITIS Nursing mother; sore **breast(s)** also.

URINARY INFECTION Cloudy urine, possibly **abdominal, flank** or **urination** pains.

BRUCELLOSIS Exposure to animals, feeling awful, low **back** pain most common.

Prominent localized pain in body part(s), likely the limb(s)

FILARIASIS Also some body swelling along with the fever.

PYOMYOSITIS Also swelling and tenderness of muscles, usually one hip or thigh.

BRUCELLOSIS Exposure to animals, lower limb joint pains that may migrate, complaining a lot.

Protocol A.1.C—Episodic fevers

Be sure you are using corrected temperatures: see Page A-5. Check your thermometer to be sure it works right.

Definition: episodic fevers are fevers which vary by more than 2.0°F (1.0°C). The temperature may or may not return to normal daily. Using this protocol assumes that there has been at least one fall in temperature with a second rise. Use this protocol if a fever has been sustained, but others with a similar illness have varying temperatures. Fevers are a common problem in the tropics. Not all causes of fevers are listed in this protocol, but only those that commonly present with fever as the main or only symptom. For fevers with other symptoms, consider the following Index B Protocols: B.2, B.3, B.5, B.9, B.10, B.13.

Does the patient have shaking chills and drenching sweats?

NO **YES**

| **Regular timing:** MALARIA

| **Irregular timing, no prominent skin problem**: MALARIA, LEPTOSPIROSIS, AMEBIASIS,
| VISCERAL LEISHMANIASIS,[1] BARTONELLOSIS.[2]

| **Irregular timing, likely prominent skin problem:** RELAPSING FEVER,[8] SPOTTED FEVER,[3]
| KATAYAMA DISEASE, RAT BITE FEVER,[4] rarely early AFRICAN SLEEPING SICKNESS.[5]

Does the patient have pain in his upper abdomen?

NO **YES**

| **Consider** MALARIA, AMEBIASIS, YELLOW FEVER,[6] FAMILIAL MEDITERRANEAN FEVER,[7]
| VISCERAL LEISHMANIASIS.[1]

Does the patient have at least two of these: cough, weight loss, diarrhea?

NO, one or none **YES at least two**

See table on next page. **Consider**: TUBERCULOSIS, HIV INFECTION, DYSENTERY, AMEBIASIS.

---

1 *Visceral Leishmaniasis: found in scattered areas of Central and South America, (mainly eastern) Africa north of the equator, the Mediterranean area, the Indian subcontinent, eastern Europe, central Asia and mainland China.*

2 *Bartonellosis: scattered areas in Peru and adjacent countries.*

3 *Only the kind of spotted fever that occurs in the Americas.*

4 *Rat bite fever: there is history of an animal bite. The fever is sustained for days and then goes away by itself and recurs. Therefore, depending on when you see the patient, it may be sustained or up and down. This disease is rare outside of Asia.*

5 *African sleeping sickness: scattered areas of Africa, south of Bamako, Mali and Lake Chad; north of Lusaka, Zambia.*

6 *Yellow fever: South America north of Sao Paolo, central and western Africa and the Sudan.*

7 *Familial Mediterranean fever: this affects persons of Mediterranean genetic heritage: Jews, Arabs, Turks and Armenians.*

8 *Relapsing fever: tropical and high altitude areas, but not in the islands of SEA or the South Pacific*

TOC   SYMPTOMS   DIFFERENTIALS   CONDITIONS   DRUG INDEX   REGIONAL NOTES   INX

EPISODIC FEVERS, NO CHILLS/SWEATS, NO ABDOMINAL PAIN, NO COUGH/WEIGHT LOSS/DIARRHEA

Onset over hours, generalized body pains

DENGUE FEVER	Severe bone and muscle pains and pains behind eyes; epidemics.
RELAPSING FEVER	Sustained fever for days until crisis; tropical, high altitude and camping contexts.
LEPTOSPIROSIS	Totally erratic fevers; red eyes, muscle pains or both; ground water exposure context.

Onset over days to weeks, generalized body pains

TRICHINOSIS	Ate poorly cooked meat within the past month.

Onset over weeks to months, generalized body pains

BRUCELLOSIS	Slow onset; joint pains, **leg or back pains**, maybe headache.

Prominent[1] localized body pain other than headache

FILARIASIS	Young or recently arrived in the area; **limb(s) or breast.**
TRENCH FEVER	Urban homeless or refugee contexts, body lice, headache, **shin pain;** temperate.

Minimal body pain other than headache

VISCERAL LEISHMANIASIS[2]	Evening fevers; large spleen, large liver after third month.
AFRICAN SLEEPING SICKNESS[3]	Fevers erratic; has been in an affected area.
SERUM SICKNESS	Fevers, HIVES, headache, fatigue intermittently.
DRUG ERUPTION	First dose or else after a week; also may have a skin rash.
THALLASEMIA	Hereditary; infants; not nursing well, positive family history.
TULAREMIA	Exposed to small animals or their insects; temperate areas.

---

1 *A prominent pain is a pain that interrupts sleep in spite of non-narcotic medication.*

2 *Visceral Leishmaniasis: found in scattered areas of Central and South America, (mainly eastern) Africa north of the equator, the Mediterranean area, the Indian subcontinent, eastern Europe, central Asia and mainland China.*

3 *African sleeping sickness: found only in scattered locations in sub-Saharan Africa. See Regional Notes F.*

Protocol A.1.D—Sustained high fever

Be sure you are using corrected temperatures: see Page A-5.

Definition: a sustained fever may or may not relapse. The patient has a corrected body temperature over 38°C/100.4°F, and it is usually over 38.5°C/101.3°F; it may rise and fall by 2.0°F or less, but it never returns to normal and then becomes high again within a day. One cannot be certain that a fever is sustained unless it has been present for 10 days or more. If it has been less than 10 days and others with similar illnesses have up and down fevers, then See Protocol A.1.C.

▷TREATMENT

Treatment for any high fever

Unclothe the person; put cool, damp cloths over him, fanning if possible. Give an anti-fever medication: ACETAMINOPHEN, IBUPROFEN or ASPIRIN. Do not use ASPIRIN in children with viral infections.

Is the patient a baby who is fussy but too young to say where he has pain?

NO	YES
	Consider KIDNEY INFECTION, EAR INFECTION, ROSEOLA, ENTERIC FEVER, MALARIA,
Continued on the next page.	MEASLES, SICKLE CELL DISEASE,[1] /// PYOMYOSITIS, OSTEOMYELITIS, MENINGITIS.

---

1 *Sickle cell disease: this affects those of African genetic origin, mainly in western Africa and the Americas. Some Indians and Arabs are also affected.*

Is the patient very ill with a severe headache, SEIZURE or an abnormal mental state?

NO	YES
	Consider FEBRILE SEIZURE, cerebral MALARIA, ENTERIC FEVER, MEASLES, /// ENCEPHALITIS, MENINGITIS, SEPSIS, TYPHUS, HEAT ILLNESS (stroke), TULAREMIA,[1] SPOTTED FEVER,[2] RAT BITE FEVER.

Does the patient have pain along with redness and swelling in the same area?

NO	YES
	Skin: CELLULITIS, DRUG ERUPTION, TULAREMIA, LEPROSY reaction, FAMILIAL MEDITERRANEAN FEVER.[3]
	Throat: STREP INFECTION, DIPHTHERIA, ANTHRAX, MONONUCLEOSIS, TULAREMIA.[1]
	Breast: MASTITIS.
See table below	**Muscles/bones/joints**: PYOMYOSITIS, OSTEOMYELITIS, RHEUMATIC FEVER.
	Wound: CELLULITIS, ANTHRAX, RAT BITE FEVER, OSTEOMYELITIS.

1 *Tularemia: North America, central Asia, Europe, Far East, the north coast of Africa; exposure to small animals.*
2 *Spotted fever: worldwide including the Arctic, but not in the islands of Southeast Asia.*
3 *Familial Mediterranean fever: this affects persons of Mediterranean genetic heritage, mainly Jews, Arabs, Turks and Armenians.*

SUSTAINED HIGH FEVER, NOT A BABY, NO HEAD PROBLEM, NO REDNESS & SWELLING

Prominent rash always

CHICKEN POX	Child, not very ill, blistery rash on upper back and face, spreads.
MEASLES	Child, very ill, red eyes, cough, rash onset about day 3.
MONKEYPOX	Humid areas, central and west Africa; blistered rash by day four.

Prominent rash on non-black skin

SPOTTED FEVER[3]	From ticks, fleas or bad food.
TYPHUS	Bitten by flea or body louse; general aching, very ill.
SCRUB TYPHUS[1]	Bitten by a mite, gradual fever onset, light avoidance.
EBOLA VIRUS DISEASE	Exposure to a known or likely case, epidemic setting in Africa.

Rash unlikely, prominent localized pain likely

PNEUMONIA	Chest pain or shoulder pain, cough, maybe short of breath.
URINARY INFECTION	Urinary or back pain; urine dipstick shows leukocytes.

Rash unlikely, prominent whole-body pain

ENTERIC FEVER	Lethargic; abdominal pain, cough; constipation, diarrhea, or headache.
YELLOW FEVER[2]	Not immunized against this; upper right abdominal pains.
LASSA FEVER	Humid areas of West Africa; chest pains also.

Rash unlikely, no prominent pain

PNEUMONIA	Fever, cough, rapid respirations, abnormal lung sounds.
ROSEOLA	Children, fever unresponsive to usual cooling devices.

Rash unlikely, long-term or recurrent ill health

THYROID TROUBLE	High-thyroid: also nervous, fast pulse, big appetite, weight loss.
SICKLE CELL DISEASE[4]	Abdominal or bone pains usual; pale or yellow.
IRIS	Simultaneous treatment for TB and HIV, usually.

1 *Scrub typhus: Asia and Pacific areas; always fever, eye symptoms, headache, constipation.*
2 *Yellow fever: South America north of Sao Paolo, Central and western Africa and the Sudan.*
3 *Spotted fever: worldwide including the Arctic but not in the islands of Southeast Asia.*
4 *Sickle cell disease: an inherited condition affecting mostly Africans, sometimes Arabs, Indians and Greeks.*

SYMPTOMS DIFFERENTIALS CONDITIONS DRUG INDEX REGIONAL NOTES INX

PROTOCOL A.2—BLOOD PRESSURE ABNORMAL

A.2.A—High blood pressure
A.2.B—Low pulse pressure

A.2.C—High pulse pressure
A.2.D—Low blood pressure

Protocol A.2.A—High blood pressure

Definition: the blood pressure is equal to or greater than 130/86 in someone from a Western country; greater than 120/80 in someone from a developing country. If the measured pressure is high, first check the size of the cuff; a regular cuff on an obese patient will give a falsely high blood pressure reading; add 10 points to the permissible pressure if this is the case.

Is the patient a female who is 6 months or more pregnant?

NO	YES
	Consider TOXEMIA.

Is the patient fearful, upset or both?

NO	YES
	Ignore the problem for now if the pressure is less than 180/100; recheck when calm. Give a small dose of DIAZEPAM if necessary.

HIGH BLOOD PRESSURE, NOT FEARFUL OR UPSET, NOT MORE THAN 24 WEEKS PREGNANT

Most common

HYPERTENSION	Usually no other symptoms or just headache.
HEART FAILURE[1]	Short of breath, fatigued, swollen ankles or any combination.

Moderately common

KIDNEY DISEASE	Abnormal, little or no urine; dry, flaky skin, fatigue.
ADDICTION, uppers	History of taking some substance that keeps the patient awake.
PLANT POISONING, ephedra	History of taking this herbal remedy; also fast pulse.
THYROID TROUBLE	Also a rapid pulse, insomnia, maybe weak legs.

Very rare, very distinctive specific symptoms

TETANUS	Severe muscle spasms and wild swings in blood pressure.
RABIES	Cannot swallow water or paralyzed or cannot tolerate a breeze.

---

1 *If the heart failure is the result of the hypertension, merely treat hypertension.*

Protocol A.2.B—Low pulse pressure

Definition: difference between blood pressure numbers is less than 15, for example a pressure of 120/112.
May be normal if there is a very rapid pulse; check Protocol A.3 if the pulse is rapid.
May be normal if there is fluid in the abdomen; check Protocol A.46 A if the abdomen is swollen.

HEART FAILURE	Valvular or restrictive type: short of breath or swollen ankles and feet.
TUBERCULOSIS	This is one cause of PERICARDITIS.
PERICARDITIS	Swollen neck veins, fatigue.
LASSA FEVER	High fever, severe headache and chest pains, West Africa.

Protocol A.2.C—High pulse pressure

Definition: difference between blood pressure numbers is over 60, for example, 90/10. This is normal with emotional upset, fevers or pregnancy. It may be due to old age in a Westerner. It is also normal anytime that the pulse is slow; if the pulse is slow, ignore the high pulse pressure, and pursue diagnosis for the slow pulse.

ANEMIA	Pale inside lower eyelid, mouth or fingernails.
SYPHILIS, tertiary/congenital	Patient, partner or parent was exposed.
BERIBERI	Also weakness with walking, swollen ankles, malnourished.
HEART FAILURE, valvular	History of RHEUMATIC FEVER; usually abnormal heart sounds.
EXFOLIATIVE DERMATITIS	Skin peeling off in sheets.

Protocol A.2.D—Low blood pressure

Definition: the blood pressure is less than 90/60 in someone from a Western country; it is less than 80/50 in someone from a developing country. Low pressures should be ignored if the patient feels healthy. Some ethnic groups normally have low pressures. Check the pressures of presumably healthy persons of the same age range and ethnic origin. A common cause of low blood pressure is a blood pressure cuff that is too large for the patient; standard Western adult cuffs are made for those 50 kg or over. A standard cuff on a petite person will give a pressure that is low by 10–20 points.

Is the patient sweating, with poor skin color, and/or very lethargic or unconscious?

NO	YES
|	First arrange transport to a hospital.
|	**Consider** SHOCK,[1] HYPOTHERMIA, HEAT ILLNESS, TYPHUS, SEPSIS, NECROTIZING FASCIITIS,
|	MALARIA or that the patient is dying.

Is there facial swelling, shortness of breath, itching, any two or all of these?

NO	YES
|	Treat with EPINEPHRINE (see the Drug Index).
|	**Consider** ANAPHYLAXIS, ALLERGY. Rarely, consider AFRICAN SLEEPING SICKNESS.[2]

Is the patient's mouth dry?

NO	YES
|	Give the person water to drink. **Consider** DEHYDRATION, DIABETES.

Is the patient taking medication for high blood pressure?

NO	YES
|	Reduce the dose, recheck in one or two days.

Is the patient very ill or does he have wildly varying vital signs?

NO	YES to either or both
|	**Consider** DIPHTHERIA, PLANT POISONING due to botulism, RABIES, TETANUS, NECROTIZING
Table on the next page.	FASCIITIS, EBOLA VIRUS DISEASE (Africa).

---

1 SHOCK is an emergency. Consider the following as possible causes: ANAPHYLAXIS, CHOLERA, HEART ATTACK, HEMORRHAGIC FEVER, TUBAL PREGNANCY, ACUTE ABDOMEN, RELAPSING FEVER; in West Africa consider LASSA FEVER, EBOLA VIRUS DISEASE.

2 African sleeping sickness: scattered areas of Africa, south of Bamako, Mali and Lake Chad; north of Lusaka, Zambia. Low blood pressure is especially common in the East African form.

LOW BLOOD PRESSURE, NO SHOCK, NO ALLERGY, MOUTH NOT DRY, NO BLOOD PRESSURE MEDS, NOT VERY ILL

Most common, check these first	
MALARIA	Patient has been ill with this for some time; severe falciparum.
HEART FAILURE	Short of breath, fatigued, swollen ankles or any combination.
Less common than previous two conditions	
NECROTIZING FASCIITIS	Extreme localized pain, rapid onset, decreased urine production.
ADDICTION, downers	History of taking some substance that causes sedation or sleep.
PLANT POISONING	Cassava or claviceps; history of eating this.
Spinal cord injury	Blood pressure is commonly low right after such an injury.
SEPSIS	History of a previous infection of some sort, now the patient became worse.

Unusual causes are related to hormone deficiencies. Sometimes a high salt intake is helpful either as highly salted food or as ingestion of salt tablets or capsules.

PROTOCOL A.3—PULSE ABNORMAL

A.3.A—Slow pulse without fever
A.3.B—Slow pulse relative to fever
A.3.C—Rapid pulse relative to a fever

A.3.D—Rapid pulse, no fever
A.3.E—Irregular pulse

Use a corrected temperature for A.3.A–A.3 C.

Normal pulse rate by age

Age	Normal pulse rate
Newborn	100–180
1–6 months	90–140
7–18 months	90–130
2–6 years	80–120
7–10 years	70–110
Adults	60–100
Athletes	36–70

Protocol A.3.A—Slow pulse without fever

Definition: pulse is slower than the normal range

By far most common

HEART FAILURE   Short of breath or fatigued or both; intolerant of exercise.

Rapid-onset fatigue

HEART ATTACK   Patient ate a Western diet; chest, jaw or arm pain; sweating.

Related to environment or ingestion

PLANT POISONING   Muscarine, claviceps.

DIGITALIS (drug)   Drug effect; ignore if slightly low, decrease dosage if very slow.

PROPRANOLOL (drug)   Drug effect; ignore if slightly low, decrease dosage if very slow.

ADDICTION   Downers; these are also sedative; the patient will be lethargic.

HYPOTHERMIA   Patient was exposed to cold environment, low body temperature.

Slow-onset fatigue

THYROID TROUBLE   Usually low body temperature, chronic fatigue

CHAGA'S DISEASE   Fatigued, swollen ankles, large liver or spleen, Americas only

Protocol A.3.B—Slow pulse relative to a fever[1]

Definition: a fever normally makes the pulse more rapid. The normal range for adults will increase by about 15–18 beats for every degree Celsius above 37° or 8–10 beats for every degree Fahrenheit above 99°. The increased pulse relative to a fever does not begin until a child is 2 years old. In older children the rise is 21–27 beats per degree Celsius or 12–15 beats per degree Fahrenheit. The conditions listed below cause the patient's pulse to be slow relative to his fever. In an athletic person, calculate the expected pulse relative to the patient's usual pulse, not the normals for his age, since athletes' pulses normally run slow at rest. There are quite a few heart medications that will slow the pulse. These do not cause fevers.

USUAL PULSE RELATIVE TO A FEVER: NORMALS VS FEVER AND AGE RANGE[2]

	37.5°/99.5°	38°/100.4°	38.5°/101.3°	39°/102.2°	39.5°/103.1°	40°/104°	40.5°/104.9°
2–6 y.o.	93–133	106–146	119–159	132–172	145–185	158–198	173–213
7–10 y.o.	81–121	92–132	103–143	114–154	125–165	136–176	147–187
>10 y.o.	68–108	76–116	84–124	92–132	100–140	108–148	116–156

---

1 *Be sure you are using a corrected temperature. See page A-5.*

2 *Do not read this chart too carefully; a pulse rate anywhere in the neighborhood of the normal range should be considered normal. But be aware that high altitude, anemia and pain will accelerate the pulse.*

TOC

SYMPTOMS

DIFFERENTIALS

CONDITIONS

DRUG INDEX

REGIONAL NOTES

INX

Common drug effect to consider first

DIGITALIS (drug)	A slow pulse is an effect of this drug, even with normal doses.
PROPRANOLOL (drug)	A slow pulse is an effect of this drug, even with normal doses.

Mentally abnormal, whole-body pain, onset over 3+ days

ENTERIC FEVER	Lethargic; headache or abdominal pain.
TYPHUS	Severe headache, mentally abnormal; history of flea or louse bite.

Mentally normal, whole-body pain, onset over <3 days

EBOLA VIRUS DISEASE	Vomiting, diarrhea, chills, dizzy, aching all over, epidemic setting in Africa.
DENGUE FEVER[6]	Onset over hours, severe bone pain, maybe depressed.
SPOTTED FEVER[1]	Sudden onset high fever, headache, red eyes, rash.
SCRUB TYPHUS[2]	Scab from tick bite; rash begins on the face, seventh day.
YELLOW FEVER[3]	Not immunized; general aching, maybe yellow whites of eyes.
ARBOVIRAL FEVER	CCHF;[4] animal contact, healthcare worker or exposure to ticks.
DIPHTHERIA	Fever, if any, is not high; there is a wound on the skin or in the throat.
LASSA FEVER[5]	Sudden onset headache, fever and chest pains; epidemic setting.

1 *Spotted fever: worldwide including the Arctic, but not in the islands of Southeast Asia.*
2 *Scrub typhus: Indian subcontinent, Southeast Asia, central Asia and Pacific areas.*
3 *Yellow fever: South America north of Sao Paolo, Central and western Africa and the Sudan.*
4 *Crimean-Congo hemorrhagic fever: occurs in Africa and in western and southern Asia; there is potential of its spreading.*
5 *Lassa fever: occurs in epidemics in West Africa.*
6 *Dengue fever: in the Americas only near or north of the equator. In Africa, east coastal, south and west. Prevalent in India, Southeast Asia and the Pacific. Occasionally found in the Mediterranean area. The disease may spread.*

Protocol A.3.C—Rapid pulse relative to a fever

Some infections cause a pulse that is rapid relative to the fever: SMALLPOX, RELAPSING FEVER, PLAGUE, DIPHTHERIA, MALARIA, SEPSIS, AFRICAN SLEEPING SICKNESS, RHEUMATIC FEVER. This may also be the effect of certain drugs such as ATROPINE and EPINEPHRINE.

Protocol A.3.D—Rapid pulse, no fever

Definition: the pulse is more rapid than the normal ranges given in Protocol A.3.A, for a patient at rest. If the patient is in pain or upset do not use this protocol; emotion is probably making the pulse faster.

Is the patient pale and sweaty and either unconscious or ready to faint?

NO	YES to all
|	Arrange transportation to the nearest hospital. **Consider** SHOCK,[1] MALARIA, HYPOGLYCEMIA,
|	SEPSIS, HEART ATTACK, RELAPSING FEVER.[2]

Is or was (recently) the patient very short of breath?

NO	YES
|	See Protocol A.36 first. Use no DIAZEPAM. Then follow the "NO" arm for this question.

Is the patient upset or frightened or in pain?

NO	YES
|	Recheck when calm. Use DIAZEPAM if no shortness of breath.

Continued on next page.

1 *In the absence of trauma, consider the following as possible causes of SHOCK: ANAPHYLAXIS (emergency), CHOLERA, HEART ATTACK, HEMORRHAGIC FEVER, TUBAL PREGNANCY, ACUTE ABDOMEN, RELAPSING FEVER*
2 *Relapsing fever: present in tropical and high altitude areas, but not in the islands of SEA and the Pacific.*

Is the patient's mouth dry?

NO	YES
|	Give the patient water to drink. **Consider** DEHYDRATION or DIABETES, PLANT POISONING due to datura or jimson weed. Also some drugs can do this, those used for allergy or abdominal pains.

Is the patient pale (check for paleness inside lower eyelids, in mouth and fingernails)?

NO	Yes
|	**Consider** ANEMIA along with its causative diseases, TUBERCULOSIS, MALNUTRITION, rarely AFRICAN SLEEPING SICKNESS.[3]

RAPID PULSE; NOT PALE, NOT UPSET, NOT THIRSTY

Most common causes of a rapid pulse

HEART FAILURE   Cannot tolerate exertion, short of breath when lying flat or swollen ankles.

Related to some ingestion

PLANT POISONING   Cassava, khat,[1] ephedra.

ADDICTION   Due to uppers or withdrawal from downers.

Onset likely over less than 2 weeks

YELLOW FEVER[2]   Not immunized; general aching, maybe yellow eyes.

DIPHTHERIA   The patient's pulse varies greatly from very slow to very fast.

Onset likely over more than 2 weeks

THYROID TROUBLE   High-thyroid; also insomnia, nervousness.

TROPICAL SPLENOMEGALY   Very large spleen, highly malarious area.

Geographically confined conditions

AFRICAN SLEEPING SICNESS[3]   Fevers and headache early; incoordination later.

CHAGA'S DISEASE[4]   Also fatigued; swollen ankles, liver or spleen.

---

1   *This is a stimulant drug, used in the Middle East and Northeastern Africa.*
2   *Yellow fever: South America north of Sao Paolo, Central and Western Africa and the Sudan.*
3   *African sleeping sickness: scattered areas of Africa, south of Bamako, Mali and Lake Chad; north of Lusaka, Zambia*
4   *Chaga's disease: found only in scattered areas of the Americas.*

Protocol A.3.E—Irregular pulse

Definition: it is impossible to predict the next beat when you feel or listen while trying to keep time by tapping a foot or finger.

An irregular pulse may be normal in children; pulse rate usually varies with respiration. It may also be a normal (not significant) effect of caffeine and other stimulants.

TOC

SYMPTOMS

DIFFERENTIALS

CONDITIONS

DRUG INDEX

REGIONAL NOTES

INX

Most common causes

HEART FAILURE	Short of breath on exertion; fatigue or swollen ankles.
SCURVY	Diet devoid of fresh fruits and vegetables; swollen gums.
DIGITALIS (drug)	Excess drug; stop the drug for a while.

Related to a recent-onset illness

RHEUMATIC FEVER	History of red, swollen joints on both sides; maybe heart murmur.
DIPHTHERIA	Also sharp pains, very swollen neck, very ill.
SEPSIS	Extremely ill; history of a recent infection.
HEART ATTACK	Western diet; chest, arm or jaw pain, sweaty.

Chronic or recurrent illness, prominent respiratory symptoms

RESPIRATORY INFECTION	Coughing for months or years; short of breath.
ASTHMA	Wheezing episodes come and go, gets better and worse over years.

Chronic or recurrent illness, prominent bone or chest symptoms

SYPHILIS, tertiary/congenital	Patient, partner or parent was exposed.
BRUCELLOSIS	Fevers off and on; joint pains or backache.

Geographically very confined

AFRICAN SLEEPING SICKNESS	Fevers and headache early; incoordination later; scattered areas of Africa south of the Sahara and north of South Africa.
CHAGA'S DISEASE	Also other symptoms of HEART FAILURE; Americas only.

PROTOCOL A.4—RESPIRATION ABNORMAL

A.4.A—Slow respiration   A.4.B—Irregular respiration   A.4.C—Rapid respiration

Normal respiratory rates

Age	Normals	Age	Normals
Newborn	30–50	5 y.o.	20–25
1 y.o.	20–40	10 y.o.	17–22
2–3 y.o.	20–30	Adults	12–20

Protocol A.4.A—Slow respiration

▷ **SYMPTOMATIC TREATMENT**   Withdraw any sedative medication.

Is there weakness or paralysis of one or more limbs or a drooping face?

NO	YES
	Consider STROKE, DIPHTHERIA, TICK PARALYSIS or POLIO, rarely PLANT POISONING due to botulism: these are emergencies; also consider RABIES, not an emergency.

Is there a lot of swelling of the face, throat or neck?

NO	YES
	Consider ANTHRAX, ALLERGY, GOITER. These are emergencies.

Does the patient have general body spasms?

NO	YES
	First arrange transport to the nearest hospital. Consider TETANUS, SEIZURES, rarely PLANT POISONING due to strychnine.

Continued on next page.

Protocol A.4 continued | *Village Medical Manual 7th Edition Volume 2* | **A-19**
CHAPTER PAGE

TOC

SYMPTOMS

DIFFERENTIALS

CONDITIONS

DRUG INDEX

REGIONAL NOTES

INX

Is the patient obviously laboring hard to breathe or is he unconscious?

NO	YES to either or both
|	**Consider** ASTHMA, RESPIRATORY FAILURE.

Does the patient have sharp chest pain that is worse with breathing?

NO	YES
|	See Protocol A.35.B. Use IBUPROFEN to treat the pain.

Consider ADDICTION or drug usage of downers without addiction.

Protocol A.4.B—Irregular respiration

Does the patient have pain aggravated by breathing?

NO	YES
|	Due to the pain; diagnose the cause from Protocol A.35 or treat the pain with IBUPROFEN.

Does the patient sigh frequently?

NO	YES
|	**Consider** DEPRESSION, STRESS.

Is the patient very ill or does he have prominent mental abnormalities?

NO	YES to either or both
|	First arrange transport to the nearest hospital, if possible.
|	**Consider** cerebral MALARIA, BRAIN DAMAGE, HEART FAILURE, MENINGITIS, ENCEPHALITIS, STROKE, head injury, ALTITUDE SICKNESS, SEPSIS. The patient may be dying.
See table below	

IRREGULAR RESPIRATION, NO BREATHING PAIN, NO SIGHING, NOT MENTALLY ABNORMAL

More likely	
HEART FAILURE	Alternate fast and absent respiration in severe cases only.
STROKE	Like HEART FAILURE; usually paralysis also.
Less likely	
KIDNEY DISEASE	Like HEART FAILURE and urine tests are abnormal.
DIPHTHERIA	The patient's pulse also varies greatly from slow to fast.

This may also be due to poisons or drugs, especially those having the side effect of drowsiness.

Protocol A.4.C—Rapid respiration

See SHORTNESS OF BREATH: Protocol A.36 and also Protocol B.4: Shortness of breath.

Frightened, upset or sexually aroused: rapid respiration is normal.

Peculiar body odor: KIDNEY DISEASE (like urine); DIABETES (fruity).

Paleness inside lower eyelids or tongue or fingernails: ANEMIA and its causative diseases.

Hot environment: HEAT ILLNESS.

History of recreational drug usage: ADDICTION to uppers or withdrawal from downers.

II—WHOLE-BODY PROBLEMS

PROTOCOL A.5—DISORDERS OF ALERTNESS

A.5.A—Lethargy, apathy, excessive sleep

A.5.B—Sustained unconsciousness or coma

A.5.C—Fainting, loss of consciousness

A.5.D—Day and night reversal

A.5.E—Hyperactivity, insomnia, irritability

A.5.F—Confusion, decreased mental functioning

Protocol A.5.A—Lethargy,[1] apathy, excessive sleep

Definition: the patient sleeps excessively, but he can be awakened. He can object to or resist treatment. Chronic conditions such as OLD AGE, HEART FAILURE, KIDNEY DISEASE, TUBERCULOSIS, VISCERAL LEISHMANIASIS[2] and THYROID TROUBLE, can cause these symptoms when death is near. (Also see Index B, Protocols B.3, B.10)

Is the patient pale and sweaty?

NO	YES
|	Give sugar immediately. Check HYPOGLYCEMIA, SHOCK.

Does the patient have DIABETES or [fast respiration, DEHYDRATION and vomiting]?

NO	YES
|	Give sugar to a diabetic who is being medicated. Send others to a hospital.

Is the entire mouth dry, both on top of and below the tongue and inside the cheek?

NO	YES
|	Give the patient fluids to drink if he is alert enough to swallow. Otherwise give him
|	fluids by stomach tube, rectum or intraperitoneal.

Has part of the body been rhythmically jerking or twitching?

NO	YES
|	SEIZURE. Lethargy is normal for an hour after a seizure. See Protocol A.7.A.

Is the problem of sudden onset and related to some injury or spontaneous pain?

NO	YES
|	Send the patient out.
|	**Consider** SHOCK; NECROTIZING FASCIITIS if there is extreme pain.

Is the patient's pulse or respiration grossly abnormal?

NO	YES
|	Pursue diagnosis by checking the appropriate Protocol (A.3 or A.4). Lethargy is probably
|	related to the abnormal vital sign(s).

Has the patient either recently taken sedative drugs, or is he depressed?

NO	YES
|	Withdraw drug(s) or See Protocol A.6.C.

Does the patient have a corrected temperature over 38.5°/101.3°, or did he have one recently?

NO	YES
|	See Protocol B.10.A.

Does the patient have general weakness or fatigue?

NO	YES
|	See Protocol A.8.A without weight loss, Protocol A.9.A with weight loss.

See the table on the next page.

---

1 *Lethargy means that the person is not normally aware of his environment.*

2 *Visceral Leishmaniasis: found in scattered areas of Central and South America, Africa north of the equator, the Mediterranean area, the Indian subcontinent, eastern Europe, central Asia and mainland China.*

TOC

SYMPTOMS

DIFFERENTIALS

CONDITIONS

DRUG INDEX

REGIONAL NOTES

INX

CAUSES OF LETHARGY WITHOUT WEAKNESS OR A VITAL SIGN EXPLANATION;
* THIS INDICATES MAYBE SUSTAINED LOSS OF CONSCIOUSNESS.

Condition	Fever	Onset	Other characteristics
MALARIA (PMNS)	Had one	Unknown	Within 2 months after severe malaria.
KATAYAMA DISEASE[1]	Episodic	Recurrent[1]	ALLERGY with fevers.
LEPTOSPIROSIS[2]	Episodic	Rapid	Red eyes, sore muscles or both.
*STROKE	Unusual	Rapid	Weak or paralyzed.
Related to food and water intake			
DEHYDRATION	Maybe	Variable	Very dry mouth.
ZINC DEFICIENCY	No	Days/weeks	Hot and dry climate or sweating.
MALNUTRITION	No	Days/weeks	Skinny upper arms, thin hair.
PELLAGRA	No	Weeks/months	Burning pain with swallowing, poor diet.
Related to a long-term illness; slow onset likely, positive urine bilirubin			
LIVER DISEASE	Unusual	Days/weeks	Yellow eyes, big belly or both.
SCHISTOSOMIASIS JAPONICUM[3]	Unusual	Months/years	Exposed to water with snails, Asia/Pacific.
Decreasing mental capacity without vocal complaints likely			
*AFRICAN SLEEPING SICKNESS[7]	Maybe	Over weeks	Clumsy, or HEART FAILURE.
TUBERCULOSIS	Common	Weeks, months	Sweating and loss of appetite.
Decreasing mental capacity with vocal complaints likely.			
LEPROSY	Unusual	Very slow	Changes in the skin.
*RESPIRATORY FAILURE	Maybe	Variable	Patient blue, breathing poorly, shortness of breath.
BRUCELLOSIS	Maybe	Variable	Pastoral area, joint pains.
Toxic or environmental exposure			
DEMONIZATION	No	Variable	A curse was put on the patient.
*CARBON MONOXIDE POISONING	No	Minutes to hours	Exposure to fumes.
PLANT POISONING	No	Minutes to hours	Ackee,[4] cassava, claviceps, datura, lolism,[5] margosa oil,[6] nicotine, valerian.
*HYPOTHERMIA	No	Over hours	Exposure to cold or wet.
ADDICTION	No	Weeks/years	History of drug use or abuse.
RADIATION ILLNESS	No	Variable	History of radiation exposure.

1 *Katayama disease: each episode can come on fast, over hours to a day. There is usually an interval of days to weeks between episodes, with each episode lasting for days. The time pattern may, however, vary.*
2 *Lethargy in a patient with leptospirosis indicates a poor prognosis.*
3 *Schistosomiasis Japonicum: in areas of mainland China, the Philippines, parts of the Celebes, the upper Mekong and the Thai-Malaysia border.*
4 *Plant poisoning, ackee: found in scattered areas of western Africa and the West Indies.*
5 *Plant poisoning: lolism: found only in the African, Mediterranean and Middle Eastern areas.*
6 *Plant poisoning: margosa oil; a yellow oil used as an ethnic medicine worldwide, by persons from the Indian subcontinent.*
7 *African sleeping sickness: scattered areas in Africa south of the Sahara and north of South Africa.*

Protocol A.5.B—Sustained unconsciousness or coma

Anything that can cause lethargy, apathy and excessive sleeping as described in Protocol 5 A can also cause sustained unconsciousness (coma). Those diseases listed in Protocol A.5.A with an asterisk (*) are the most likely causes.

Also see Protocols B.10.A: fever plus Lethargy or B.10.B: Lethargy or Confusion Without a Fever.

SYMPTOMS
DIFFERENTIALS
CONDITIONS
DRUG INDEX
REGIONAL NOTES
INX

TOC

SYMPTOMS

DIFFERENTIALS

CONDITIONS

DRUG INDEX

REGIONAL NOTES

INX

Protocol A.5.C—Fainting, loss of consciousness

▷ SYMPTOMATIC TREATMENT | Have the patient lie down. Then check his vital signs.

Did the patient experience an injection or an insect sting within the last hour?

NO	YES
|	**Consider** ANAPHYLAXIS, ALLERGY; treat immediately!

Is the patient pale and sweaty even when lying down?

NO	YES
|	Give sugar to the patient if his blood pressure is normal or high.
|	Treat for SHOCK if his blood pressure is low. Consider HEAT ILLNESS.

Is the patient emotionally upset or has he been standing for a long time?

NO to both	YES to either
|	Have the patient lie down; he'll likely be fine.

Did the fainting occur after coughing or urinating with a very full bladder?

NO	YES
|	Have the patient lie down; he'll likely be fine.

Are the patient's hands cramped but not jerking or twitching?

NO	YES
|	**Consider** HYPERVENTILATION, rarely TETANUS, PLANT POISONING due to strychnine.

Is any part of the patient's body jerking or twitching?

NO	YES
|	SEIZURE. See Protocol A.7.A.

Is the patient very ill, or has he wildly varying vital signs?

NO to both	YES to either or both
|	**Consider** DIPHTHERIA, BRUCELLOSIS, PLANT POISONING due to botulism, RABIES, TETANUS,
|	NECROTIZING FASCIITIS.

FAINTING, FOR NO OBVIOUS REASON, NOT SWEATY, OKAY VITAL SIGNS, NO JERKING OR CRAMPING

ANEMIA	Pale inside lower eyelid or inside mouth or fingernails, rapid pulse.
DEHYDRATION	The patient is thirsty, his tongue is dry or both.
HEAT ILLNESS	Infant, elderly or exercising while not acclimatized, hot environment.
Head injury	Should be obvious from history or looking at the patient's head.
ALTITUDE SICKNESS	Recent ascent, also headache, short of breath or both.
HEART FAILURE	Patient is short of breath with exertion; swollen ankles or short of breath lying down.
STROKE	Weak in one or more limbs or has trouble talking.

Protocol A.5.D—Day and night reversal

Definition: the patient sleeps excessively during the day and is awake at night. There is no obvious cause like night-shift work.

	Vital signs likely grossly abnormal
AFRICAN SLEEPING SICKNESS[1]	Headaches, itching rash or large nodes, maybe HEART FAILURE.
TYPHUS	Fevers also and quite sick; bitten by flea or louse.

	Vital signs likely grossly normal; mood changes prominent
STRESS	Trouble falling asleep or like DEPRESSION.
DEPRESSION	Falls asleep okay, awakens early and cannot sleep again.
DEMONIZATION	Occult experience or someone put a curse on the patient.
FIBROMYALGIA	Sore muscles with tender spots; symmetrical right and left.
SYPHILIS, tertiary/congenital	Patient, partner or parent was exposed, mental changes.
ATTENTION DEFICIT DISORDER	Since childhood brain hyperactive, maybe body also.

	Vital signs likely grossly normal; no prominent mood changes
OLD AGE	Awakens early, frequently naps.
JET LAG	After an east or west flight over six or more time zones.

---

1 African sleeping sickness: *scattered areas of Africa, south of Bamako, Mali and Lake Chad and north of Lusaka, Zambia.*

Protocol A.5.E—Hyperactivity, insomnia, irritability

Definition: the patient is awake more than is normal; he sleeps very little if at all. This Protocol assumes no day and night reversal (see preceding protocol). See Protocol A.6.B if there is nervousness or Protocol A.6.A for bizarre behavior.

Is the patient six months or more pregnant?

NO	YES
|	**Consider** TOXEMIA.

Is the patient very ill with a corrected temperature over 38.5°/101.3°?

NO	YES
|	**Consider** MALARIA, HEAT ILLNESS (stroke), ///TYPHUS, BRUCELLOSIS, THYROID
|	TROUBLE, BARTONELLOSIS,[1] ENCEPHALITIS, MENINGITIS, PLAGUE, RABIES.

Is the patient going through emotional turmoil?

NO	YES
|	**Consider** STRESS, DEPRESSION, ATTENTION DEFICIT DISORDER, DEMONIZATION.

See the table on the next page.

---

1 Bartonellosis: *scattered areas in Peru and adjacent countries.*

HYPERACTIVE, NOT ADVANCED PREGNANCY, NO HIGH FEVER, NOT EMOTIONALLY STRESSED

Life-long, recurrent problem, onset in childhood

ATTENTION DEFICIT DISORDER[1]	Adjustment or academic problems since childhood.

Onset recent, rapid or both

HEAT ILLNESS (exhaustion)	Very old or very young or exercising and not acclimatized, hot environment.
ENTEROBIASIS	Insomnia or irritability because of an itchy rectum at night.

Significant pain also likely

PELLAGRA	Prominent **abdominal pain**; poor diet.
RABIES	Pain **swallowing** or in muscles; headache.
THYROID TROUBLE	**Leg pain**; weakness walking up stairs also, high-thyroid.
AFRICAN SLEEPING SICKNESS[4]	Uncoordinated or history of the disease, previously treated; variable pain; usually history of a **headache.**

Toxic exposure history likely

ALCOHOLISM	History of heavy or regular drinking, now withdrawing.
ADDICTION	Withdrawal from downers, drug effect of uppers.
Drug side effect	Stimulants or uppers in most; sedatives in the hyperactive.[1]
PLANT POISONING	Margosa oil,[2] khat,[3] mushrooms.
RADIATION ILLNESS	History of recent radiation exposure.

---

1 *People who have attention deficit disorder sometimes become hyperactive with sedative drugs.*
2 *Margosa oil: this is a yellow oil, used as an ethnic medicine worldwide, by persons from the Indian subcontinent.*
3 *Khat: this is a stimulant, used in the Middle East and eastern Africa.*
4 *African sleeping sickness: scattered areas in African south of the Sahara and north of South Africa.*

Protocol A.5.F—Confusion, decreased mental function

Definition: one might think of this as recent-onset stupidity whereby a normally intelligent person suddenly cannot remember recent events, and does not seem to understand simple concepts although he appears to be wide awake (not lethargic or unconscious). He is walking, talking and caring for himself normally. Usually recent memory is the first to lapse; the person knows his childhood address but doesn't remember what he ate for breakfast that morning. Then a sense of time goes—he doesn't know the date—then place—he doesn't know where he is—and finally he does not recognize persons.

Decreased mental functioning: see Protocol B.10.

This may arise from Alzheimer disease. It can arise from any illness that affects the brain such as CANCER originating elsewhere in the body. It is a common complication of ENCEPHALITIS. It is common with any infection in the elderly.

PROTOCOL A.6—DISORDERED EMOTIONS AND BEHAVIOR

6.A Bizarre behavior   6.B Nervousness   6.C Depression

Definition: the patient's behavior is abnormal by the standards of his own culture. Only someone from the same culture can make the judgment. DEMONIZATION is a medical/mental overlap diagnosis.

Mental vs. medical causes of emotional symptoms: behavioral problems that start for the very first time in a person who is 30 or more and who has had a previous good adjustment are almost always medical (or demonic) in origin. New-onset incontinence indicates a medical origin. A medical cause will manifest with all three of these elements: 1. He cannot pay attention; 2. Either the onset was rapid or the symptoms change over hours to days; 3. The patient doesn't make sense when he talks, he is lethargic, or he is hyperactive.

Protocol A.6.A—Bizarre behavior

Behavior is bizarre if it cannot be classified as simple lethargy or hyperactivity. An example would be talking to a parking meter. See Protocol A.5.A or A.5.E if the behavior is also either lethargic or hyperactive.

Is the patient 6 months or more pregnant or delivered within the past week?

NO	YES
|	**Consider** TOXEMIA if there is no fever.

Does the patient eat a poor or unbalanced diet?

NO	YES
|	**Consider** BERIBERI, PELLAGRA, ALCOHOLISM, LIVER FAILURE, CIRRHOSIS, COBALAMIN[1]
|	DEFICIENCY.

Does the patient have a fever, a headache or both?

NO to both   **YES to either or both**

|	**Sustained, corrected temperature over 38.5°/101.3° + headache**: cerebral MALARIA, TYPHUS, HEAT ILLNESS, MENINGITIS, ENCEPHALITIS.
|	**Previous ill health**: HIV INFECTION, SYPHILIS (tertiary/congenital), IRIS.
|	**Distinctive symptoms:** TYPHUS (other symptoms before the fever), PLAGUE (swollen blackened lymph nodes), BARTONELLOSIS (Peru area only), RABIES (paralyzed or won't swallow water), AFRICAN SLEEPING SICKNESS[2] (sleep disturbance).

Does the patient have joint or back pains, slow onset or recurrent?

NO	YES
|	**Consider** HIV INFECTION, BRUCELLOSIS, SYPHILIS (tertiary/congenital).

BIZARRE BEHAVIOR, NOT ADVANCED PREGNANCY, NO HIGH FEVER, OKAY DIET, NO JOINT OR BACK PAINS

Conditions	Fever	Other characteristics
Easily diagnosed from characteristics		
ZINC DEFICIENCY	No	Sweating or hot, dry climate; not acclimatized.
DEPRESSION	No	Suicidal speech is common.
DEMONIZATION	No	Varies; blasphemous and; foul speech common.

Table continues next page.

---

1   Cobalamin is VITAMIN B$_{12}$. It is found in animal products such as milk, meat, eggs.
2   African sleeping sickness: scattered areas of Africa, south of Bamako, Mali and Lake Chad and north of Lusaka, Zambia.

Condition	Fever	Other characteristics
Rapid onset is likely (hours to days)		
ENCEPHALITIS	Maybe	Severe headache; usually some weakness also.
PLANT POISONING	No	Claviceps, jimson weed, margosa oil,[1] mushrooms.
ALTITUDE SICKNESS	No	Recent ascent, high altitude, severe headache.
IRIS	Usual	Simultaneous treatment for TB and HIV.
RABIES	Maybe	Muscle spasms with breeze or swallowing liquid.
Slow onset is likely (weeks or longer)		
SYPHILIS, tertiary/congenital	Rare/No	Patient, partner or parent was exposed.
MENTAL ILLNESS	No	Recurrent, first time under age 25.
ADDICTION: Alcohol, Outers	No	ALCOHOLISM or withdrawal; hallucinogen drugs.
Slow onset and prior prominent ill health		
HIV INFECTION	Usual	Weight loss, diarrhea, other similar cases.
LIVER FAILURE	Maybe	Positive urine bilirubin; urine foams with shaking.
AFRICAN SLEEPING SICKNESS[2]	Maybe	Large nodes in back of neck, or HEART FAILURE.
SCHISTOSOMIASIS JAPONICUM[3]	No	Also a large liver and distended abdomen.

---

3 *Planst poisoning: margosa oil: this is a yellow oil used as a folk medicine by Indians (from India) worldwide.*

4 *African sleeping sickness: scattered areas of Africa, south of Bamako, Mali and Lake Chad and north of Lusaka, Zambia.*

5 *Schistosomiasis Japonicum: found in areas of mainland China, the Philippines, parts of the Celebes, the upper Mekong and the Thai-Malaysia border.*

Protocol A.6.B—Nervousness

Definition: the patient appears to be continually in a heightened state of awareness or fear, as if he, or she were in a threatening situation when there is no threat.

STRESS can cause this. Also ALCOHOLISM, ADDICTION: uppers (stimulants) or withdrawal from downers, THYROID TROUBLE, LIVER FAILURE. This often accompanies ATTENTION DEFICIT DISORDER, which is common in Westerners. If the patient has a corrected temperature over 38.5°/101.3°, consider PLAGUE (rare). See Protocol A.5.E.

This is common in people who sense that they are dying; spiritual counseling is appropriate. Patients commonly sense they are dying before their physicians are aware of the seriousness of their conditions.

Protocol A.6.C—Depression

Definition: the patient appears to be sad or grieving out of proportion to any recent losses in his life.

With **recent travel,** consider culture shock or JET LAG. If the patient is **not otherwise ill**, see DEMONIZATION or DEPRESSION. With a **slow pulse or low blood pressure**, consider THYROID TROUBLE, ADDICTION. Depression with a **fever or a history of fever,** consider HIV INFECTION, DENGUE FEVER,[4] TUBERCULOSIS, BRUCELLOSIS, ENTERIC FEVER, TYPHUS, SAND FLY FEVER. Depression with a **rash or history thereof:** PELLAGRA, DENGUE FEVER.[1] Depression with **diarrhea:** HIV INFECTION, PELLAGRA or SPRUE.[2] Consider ALCOHOLISM in someone who drinks regularly or in binges.

---

1 *Depression can last for years with dengue fever. Dengue is found in the Americas only near or north of the Equator. In Africa it is east coastal, south and west. It is prevalent in India, Southeast Asia and the Pacific. It is occasionally found in the Mediterranean. It may spread since the mosquitoes that carry it are all over.*

2 *Sprue: in the Americas only near or north of the equator. In Africa only Nigeria and southern Africa. Prevalent in India and Southeast Asia. It is occasionally found in the Mediterranean area.*

TOC

SYMPTOMS

DIFFERENTIALS

CONDITIONS

DRUG INDEX

REGIONAL NOTES

INX

PROTOCOL A.7—DISORDERS OF BODY MOVEMENT

A.7.A—Seizures   A.7.C—Gait disorders   A.7.E—Incoordination

A.7.B—Spasms, jerking, twitching   A.7.D—Trembling

DIFFERENTIATING SEIZURES AND CHILLS

Seizures	Chills
Usually lasts only a few minutes	Lasts a half-hour or more
Does not speak words	Able to speak words
Likely incontinent	Not incontinent
May hurt himself	Never hurts himself
If not feverish at first, does not become feverish	Develops a fever during the chills.

DIFFERENTIATING VARIOUS KINDS OF REPETITIVE ABNORMAL MOVEMENTS

	Movement	Rhythm	Force
Trembling	Fine	Regular	Not forceful
Seizures	Coarse	Regular	Forceful
Twitches	Either	Irregular	Either

Protocol A.7.A—Seizures

Definition: the patient has rhythmic, jerky movement of his whole-body or one or more limbs. Either his eyes are rolled back, and he is unconscious or else the abnormal movement starts in one hand or foot and progresses up that limb and possibly crosses to the other side. If the patient is conscious and the seizure does not have a progressive pattern, see Protocol A.7.B

▷ SYMPTOMATIC SEIZURE TREATMENT

Keep the patient from hurting himself.
Do not put your fingers in his mouth.
Time the seizures with a watch.
Cool him if he has a fever.

Is the patient a newborn?

NO	YES
	It is likely that the seizures are due to some birth injury.
	Consider HYPOGLYCEMIA, TETANUS, MENINGITIS or jaundice of the newborn, Chapter 7, Volume 1.
	Send the patient to a hospital, but first give sugar.

Is the patient being treated for DIABETES or is he sweaty or both?

NO to all	YES to any
	Give him sugar immediately; treat other disease(s) if necessary. See HYPOGLYCEMIA.

Is the patient supposed to be taking medication for EPILEPSY?

NO	YES
	Give him more. He probably forgot to take it or gained weight without increasing the dose, or he has STRESS. His drug supply may be substandard or fake, especially if he started a new bottle.

Is the patient very ill with a corrected temperature over 38.5°/101.3°?

NO	YES
	Consider MALARIA, HEAT ILLNESS, FEBRILE SEIZURE, ///MENINGITIS, ENCEPHALITIS, SEPSIS, RABIES.

Is the patient 6 months or more pregnant or recently delivered?

NO	YES
	Consider TOXEMIA

See table on next page.

NOT A NEWBORN, NO DIABETES, NO MEDICATION FOR EPILEPSY, NO HIGH FEVER, NOT ADVANCED PREGNANCY

Conditions	Fever	Other characteristics
Probably healthy-appearing before the seizure		
MALARIA/ PMNS	Not now	About 2 months after severe malaria.
DEMONIZATION	No	Foul/blasphemous speech or disrupts worship.
STROKE	No	Some weakness or paralysis also.
HYPERVENTILATION	No	Rapid breathing; numb, cramped hands.
CYSTICERCOSIS	No	Ate insufficiently cooked pork.
Related to environment or ingestion		
Injury	No	Head injury, any loss of consciousness; refer the patient.
PLANT POISONING	No or low	Ackee,[1] margosa oil,[2] claviceps, cassava, water hemlock
ADDICTION	No	Withdrawal from downers (sedatives.)
ALCOHOLISM	No	Withdrawing after drinking heavily or regularly.
RADIATION ILLNESS	No	History of radiation exposure.
Long-term, whole-body illness before the seizure		
SCHISTOSOMIASIS JAPONICUM[3]	No	Swollen abdomen, large liver; Asia.
LIVER FAILURE	Unusual	Abnormal bleeding, maybe fluid in abdomen.
SYPHILIS, tertiary/congenital	No	Patient, partner or parent was exposed.
Short-term, whole-body illness before seizure		
RABIES	Maybe	Either paralysis or spasms with swallowing.
PERTUSSIS	No	Patient has severe, persistent coughing.

1 Plant poisoning: ackee: found in scattered areas of western Africa and the West Indies.
2 Plant poisoning: margosa oil; a yellow oil used by persons from the Indian subcontinent, worldwide.
3 Schistosomiasis Japonicum: in areas of mainland China, the Philippines, parts of the Celebes, the upper Mekong and the Thai-Malaysian border.

There may be no discernible reason for the seizure; it may be new-onset EPILEPSY. Rarely may be due to AMEBIASIS, PARAGONIMIASIS (mainly Asia), BRUCELLOSIS or LARVA MIGRANS in adults, RICKETS in babies. This can also be caused by head injury, electric shock and by any condition in which the brain is deprived of oxygen, such as near-drowning. See BRAIN DAMAGE.

Protocol A.7.B—Spasms, jerking, twitching

Definition: Irregular, sudden muscle contractions that appear to be involuntary. Distinguish this from trembling and from seizures. Trembling is regularly rhythmic, fine, not forceful, whereas twitching and jerking are irregular in rhythm. Seizures are rhythmic and forceful.

Does the patient jerk only when falling asleep?

NO   **YES**

| This is normal.

Does the patient have hiccups?

NO   **YES**

| See the box at right.

▷ SYMPTOMATIC TREATMENT FOR HICCUPS

The drug CHLORPROMAZINE might work if home remedies don't work.

Is the patient unconscious?

NO   **YES**

| *See* Protocol A.7.A.

See the table on the next page.

TOC

SYMPTOMS

DIFFERENTIALS

CONDITIONS

DRUG INDEX

REGIONAL NOTES

INX

SPASMS OR JERKING, NOT WHEN FALLING ASLEEP, NOT HICCUPS, THE PATIENT IS NOT UNCONSCIOUS

Most common	
Vomiting	Late consequence, if severe and persistent. See Protocol A.47.
Diarrhea	Severe watery diarrhea with DEHYDRATION. See Protocol A.56.
Rapid onset without a whole-body illness	
HYPERVENTILATION	Feels short of breath or a history of rapid breathing.
DEMONIZATION	No fever; occult activity, patient or in his culture.
Night cramps[1]	Painful spasms of calf muscles, relieved by standing.
Result of thyroid surgery	Painful spasms of hands and other muscles; treat with CALCIUM.
During a whole-body illness, likely ill for more than a month	
KIDNEY DISEASE	Urine too much or too little or abnormal dipstick.
LIVER FAILURE	Hands flap when arms are held out with fingers spread wide.
BERIBERI	Poor diet; difficulty walking, weak legs.
RICKETS	History of deficient exposure to direct sunlight.
Spinal cord injury	Spasms occur during the transition from floppy to stiff weakness.
BRAIN DAMAGE	Spasms occur during the transition from floppy to stiff weakness.
During a whole-body illness, likely ill for less than a month	
TYPHUS	Other symptoms before fever; severe headache, general pains.
TRENCH FEVER	Fever, headache, eye pain, shin pain, sudden onset; body lice.
POLIO	Cold or diarrhea followed by muscle spasms and weakness.
RABIES	Throat spasms with drinking or with a breeze on the face.
TETANUS	All muscles contracted, hard, very visible.
Related to an ingestion	
CHLORPROMAZINE or METACLOPRAMIDE	These drugs cause spasms of facial muscles, maybe neck muscles. If there is no fever with this, it is not a problem; it will wear off.
ANTACID overdose	Large amounts for a long time; like HYPERVENTILATION.
PLANT POISONING	Due to strychnine (homicidal) or to lathyrism.[2]

---

1 *Low doses of QUININE at bedtime can be quite helpful if the patient is not pregnant.*
2 *Plant poisoning, lathyrism: found in East Africa, the Indian area and the Mediterranean area.*

TOC

SYMPTOMS

DIFFERENTIALS

CONDITIONS

DRUG INDEX

REGIONAL NOTES

INX

TOC

SYMPTOMS

DIFFERENTIALS

CONDITIONS

DRUG INDEX

REGIONAL NOTES

INX

Protocol A.7.C—Gait disorders

If the patient has back or leg pain (Protocols A.63 or A.60) or weakness (Protocols A.64 or A.62), then his gait will necessarily be abnormal.

Limping may be caused by pain in hips, legs or feet. If there is no obvious cause for the pain from the history or examination, consider birth injury, PYOMYOSITIS, OSTEOMYELITIS or bone TUBERCULOSIS in children. SLIPPED DISC or ARTHRITIS of one hip is more likely in adults. Also consider BRUCELLOSIS, especially in older men.

Dragging one foot may be due to STROKE, an old head injury, BRAIN DAMAGE or a complication of POLIO, DIPHTHERIA or AFRICAN SLEEPING SICKNESS.[1]

Waddling may be due to pregnancy, fluid in the abdomen, overweight, RICKETS in adults. Many hip problems which cause limping, if present on both sides, will cause waddling. Waddling is frequently related to weakness; this may occur with normal body weight and relatively weak legs or with normal legs and excessive body weight.

Foot slapping with a wide-based gait: Due to SYPHILIS (tertiary) or COBALAMIN DEFICIENCY.

Wide-based gaits are caused by BERIBERI, any muscular weakness (Protocols A.62 & A.64), SYPHILIS (tertiary), spinal TUBERCULOSIS, DEMONIZATION. Incoordination causes a wide-based gait.

Stiff, spastic walking is from old paralysis or from BERIBERI, CRETINISM, TROPICAL SPASTIC PARAPARESIS, SPINAL NEUROPATHY or PLANT POISONING: cassava, lathyrism.

Staggering, lurching, twisting gaits with gross incoordination:

with a fever: ENTERIC FEVER, AFRICAN SLEEPING SICKNESS,[1] (rarely) PLAGUE.

recent onset: alcohol intoxication, PLANT POISONING: datura, lolism,[2] ADDICTION, CANCER.

long-lasting: BRAIN DAMAGE from any cause, SYPHILIS (tertiary), BERIBERI, AFRICAN SLEEPING SICKNESS,[1] CEREBRAL PALSY.

Crab walk is walking purposely bow-legged on the sides of the feet. This is caused by YAWS or any pain in the big toe side of the feet.

High-stepping gaits are from LEPROSY, BERIBERI, SYPHILIS (tertiary) or ANEMIA (nutritional). This is normal when learning or relearning to walk. It can also be caused by injury (to the mother) during hard labor and childbirth.[3] It may be due to a nerve injury from trauma to the leg or pelvis on one side.

Shuffling is from PARKINSON'S DISEASE or long use of major tranquillizers. If there is a fever, consider ENTERIC FEVER. It may also be a natural response to fear of falling on a slippery surface.

Labored walking is from heavy, usually swollen legs. See Protocol A.61.

---

1 African sleeping sickness: scattered areas of Africa, south of Bamako, Mali and Lake Chad and north of Lusaka, Zambia.

2 Plant poisoning, lolism: found only in the African, Mediterranean and Middle Eastern areas.

3 In this case, the nerve that works the muscles to hold the foot out straight is damaged. As a result the foot drops down and the patient must lift the leg high to avoid hurting her toes.

Protocol A.7.D—Trembling

Definition: Regular, fine, rhythmic involuntary muscle movements. This refers to physical trembling, not just a manifestation of nervousness (Protocol A.6.B). Distinguish trembling (fine, rhythmic) from spasms, jerking and twitching which are coarse, non-rhythmic or both (Protocol A.7.B). If the patient is sweaty, give him sugar to eat; then pursue diagnosis. See HYPOGLYCEMIA. If the patient is having shaking chills, see Protocol A.13. Many different kinds of poisonings can cause tremors; if the patient has consumed a poison or some tainted food, make him vomit if he is alert.

There are three kinds of tremors:

- PARKINSON'S DISEASE causes trembling at rest which **decreases with intentional movement**; AFRICAN SLEEPING SICKNESS[1] and some drugs may also cause this. The patient appears to be rolling pills between his fingers with his hands on his lap.

- Some BRAIN DAMAGE causes tremor when the patient tries to do something, as well as gross incoordination. The trembling **increases with intentional movement.**

- Causes of action tremors (all other causes) are listed below: in this case there is trembling only when the hand is held out straight, not when it is resting. The trembling **increases with intentional movement.**

TREMBLING THAT IS WORSE WHEN THE PATIENT TRIES TO USE HIS HAND

STRESS	Person is nervous or angry.
OLD AGE	A certain amount of trembling develops with advanced age.

Arising during a long-term illness, usually no or low fever

SYPHILIS, tertiary/congenital	Patient, partner or parent was exposed.
LIVER FAILURE	Hands flap with arms held out with fingers up and spread out.
AFRICAN SLEEPING SICKNESS[3]	Also abnormal sleep patterns, possibly HEART FAILURE also.
KIDNEY DISEASE	Abnormal amount of urine, abnormal urinalysis or both.
PELLAGRA	Pain with swallowing; poor diet, rough skin, maybe craziness.

Related to an illness with a sustained, fever

ENTERIC FEVER	High fever, appears withdrawn, onset is several days, abdominal pains or cough.
TYPHUS	Headache and body pains present before fever; appears withdrawn.

Related to an ingestion

ADDICTION	Due to either uppers effect or downers withdrawal.
ALCOHOLISM	History of heavy or regular drinking; withdrawing now.
PLANT POISONING	Ackee,[2] ephedra, lolism;[3] history of eating an affected plant product.

_____

1 *African sleeping sickness is found in some scattered areas of sub-Saharan Africa north of South Africa.*
2 *Plant poisoning, Ackee: found in Africa and the Americas only.*
3 *Plant poisoning: lolism: found in the African, Mediterranean and Middle Eastern areas.*

Protocol A.7.E—Incoordination

Definition: the patient cannot make his hand(s) or foot/feet do what he wants them to do. Aside from innate clumsiness, the most common causes are ALCOHOLISM and ADDICTION. If the patient is also weak, see Protocols A.8.B and A.8.C. See Protocol A.7.C if the problem is specifically with walking. See Protocol A.20 if the patient complains of dizziness. Other causes are listed below:

Most common

ATTENTION DEFICIT DISORDER	Hyperactive or else under-active body with a racing brain.
BRAIN DAMAGE	CEREBRAL PALSY or a consequence of some diseases.
STROKE	Appears uncoordinated because of specific weakness, rapid onset.

Related to a condition with little or no fever at present

MALARIA (PMNS)	Within 2 months after treated severe malaria.
DIPHTHERIA	Unimmunized; wound or sore throat and scum on tonsils.
RADIATION ILLNESS	History of recent exposure to radiation.
Injury	A head or spinal cord injury can cause incoordination.

Related to a long-term, chronic illness, maybe fevers, maybe not

AFRICAN SLEEPING SICKNESS[1]	Abnormal sleep pattern, maybe craziness, or HEART FAILURE.
SYPHILIS, tertiary/congenital	Patient, partner or parent was exposed.
PARKINSON'S DISEASE	An early symptom, initially one limb, slow onset, before trembling starts.
COBALAMIN DEFICIENCY	Elderly patient of a European genetic heritage.

Related to a poor diet

BERIBERI	Eats only carbohydrates; weak limbs, lower more than upper.
COBALAMIN DEFICIENCY	Diet devoid of animal products.

Related to an illness with a corrected temperature over 38.5°/101.3° at least sometimes

BRUCELLOSIS	Whole-body illness, some numbness or weakness also.
ENTERIC FEVER	Withdrawn ("not there"), headache, abdominal pains or cough.
PLAGUE	Sudden onset; mental changes; very ill; large, black lymph nodes.
HIV INFECTION	Weight loss, diarrhea or both.

Related to an ingestion

PLANT POISONING	Due to datura; large pupils, rapid pulse, nausea.
PLANT POISONING	Due to kava-kava; history of taking plant substance.

---

1 *African sleeping sickness: scattered areas of Africa, south of Bamako, Mali and Lake Chad; north of Lusaka, Zambia*

PROTOCOL A.8—WEAKNESS, PARALYSIS, FATIGUE

A.8.A—Fatigue, no weight loss or lethargy
A.8.B—Floppy weakness of body part(s); paralysis
A.8.C—Stiff weakness of body part(s); paralysis

Definitions

Weakness means that the person cannot exert muscle power at any time.

Paralysis is weakness that is severe enough that the person is not able to voluntarily move the body part at all. Paralysis and weakness may be either stiff or floppy. With stiff paralysis it is hard for another person to move the limb; with floppy, it is easy.

Fatigue means that he can exert muscle power after he has rested a while but cannot sustain physical activity for a long time. Weakness and fatigue involve the limbs; lethargy is mental fatigue. This is the usual consequence of any severe disease; it may also result from a viral illness that has otherwise healed. It is common in old age.

Protocol A.8.A—Fatigue, no weight loss or lethargy

If there is weight loss, then See Protocol A.9.

▽ BEFORE PROCEEDING WITH THIS PROTOCOL:

Entirely undress the patient and look at every bit of skin to find a tick, especially the scalp. Some ticks cause paralysis. See TICK PARALYSIS in the Condition Index. If you find one and remove it, don't fail to look for another. The one you removed is not necessarily the one causing the weakness or paralysis.

This protocol presupposes that the problem affects the whole-body and that it is a major symptom of the disease. If it is mainly or only in a specific limb or muscle group, then See Protocol A.8 B or A.8.C.

TOC

SYMPTOMS

DIFFERENTIALS

CONDITIONS

DRUG INDEX

REGIONAL NOTES

INX

Has the patient lost body fluid from vomiting, diarrhea or a hot environment?

NO

YES

Give the patient water and ORS to drink. See Protocol A.47 or A.56.

Consider HEAT ILLNESS; ZINC DEFICIENCY; HEPATITIS; SPRUE;[11] MALABSORPTION; SCHISTOSOMIASIS MANSONI;[1] PELLAGRA; PLANT POISONING, water hemlock.

Does the patient have a fever or a recent history of fevers?

NO

YES

ADDITIONAL SYMPTOMS; READ FROM TOP TO BOTTOM:

WITH PROMINENT PAIN:

SEVERE CHEST OR ABDOMINAL PAINS

AMEBIASIS; pain on right side, near waist.

LASSA FEVER:[2] chest pains: center front, center back.

BARTONELLOSIS:[3] fatigue occurs before the fever.

JOINT, BONE, MUSCLE PAINS, PROMINENT RASH NOT LIKELY

BRUCELLOSIS: back, joint pains; sweats or chills, feels awful.

RHEUMATIC FEVER: red, swollen joints, symmetrical.

LEPTOSPIROSIS: ground water contact; muscle and eye pains.

TRENCH FEVER: refugee or homeless: body lice, shin pain, temperate.

JOINT, BONE, MUSCLE PAINS, PROMINENT RASH LIKELY

DENGUE FEVER: sudden onset, severe bone pains.

SPOTTED FEVER:[4] headache; small scab(s).

RAT BITE FEVER: open wound, or healed wound plus rash.

LYME DISEASE: rash, red circles or targets, temperate areas.

TULAREMIA:[5] contacted small animal(s) or their insects.

SEVERE HEADACHE

MALARIA: chills, waist pain, shoulder pain.

RELAPSING FEVER:[6] onset minutes to hours.

NO PROMINENT PAIN: also see Protocols B.3: and/or B.10.A:

FATIGUE WITHOUT SEVERE PAIN

MONONUCLEOSIS: large neck lymph nodes, sleeps a lot.

TOXOPLASMOSIS: fatigued; lamb meat or cat exposure likely.

SYPHILIS, secondary: sexual exposure or patient is an infant.

UP AND DOWN FEVERS

VISCERAL LEISHMANIASIS:[7] huge spleen, large liver.

KATAYAMA DISEASE: itchy skin rash; skin is swollen.

TULAREMIA:[5] scab and nearby redness.

SEPSIS: a previous infection became much worse.

Is the problem of sudden onset (over minutes to a day) and with no fever?

NO

See the table following.

Footnotes are on the next page.

YES

Check vital signs; consider SHOCK and see appropriate protocols. Recheck the patient for ticks. **Consider** DEMONIZATION, ALTITUDE SICKNESS, PLANT POISONING due to argemone oil, water hemlock or botulism,[9] DIPHTHERIA, poisonous bite,[10] HYPOGLYCEMIA, HEART ATTACK.

1 *Schistosomiasis Mansoni: scattered areas within Africa, the Arabian Peninsula, the Caribbean and parts of eastern South America.*

2 *Lassa fever: only in Africa, mainly west and central, usually in outbreaks.*

3 *Bartonellosis: occurs only in Peru and adjacent countries.*

4 *Spotted fever: not in the islands of Southeast Asia.*

5 *Tularemia: North America, central Asia, Europe, Far East, the north coast of Africa; exposure to small animals.*

6 *Relapsing fever: tropical and high altitude, but not in the islands of SEA and the Pacific.*

7 *Visceral Leishmaniasis: found in scattered areas of Central and South America, Africa north of the equator, the Mediterranean area, the Indian subcontinent, eastern Europe, central Asia and mainland China.*

8 *Tularemia: North America, central Asia, Europe, Far East, the north coast of Africa; exposure to small animals.*

9 *With botulism, the weakness starts with the head and moves down. It is symmetrical. There are no mental changes. Constipation and inability to urinate are common. With other paralysis, the problem is asymmetric, there are mental changes or the weakness ascends upward from the lower body.*

10 *Occasionally a scorpion or fish bite, as well as a snake bite, may cause a similar effect. See Volume 1, Chapter 8.*

11 *Sprue: in the Americas only near and north of the equator. In Africa only Nigeria and southern Africa. Prevalent in India and Southeast Asia. It is occasionally found in the Mediterranean are.*

FATIGUE WITHOUT LETHARGY, NO FEVER, GRADUAL ONSET, NO FLUID LOSS

Abnormal vital signs likely

ANEMIA[1]	Fast pulse or pale fingernails or pale mouth.
HEART FAILURE	Short of breath with exertion, maybe with lying down.
KIDNEY DISEASE	Maybe dry, flaky skin; blood pressure high or urine abnormal.
THYROID TROUBLE	Low-thyroid; slow pulse, brittle hair, low body temperature.
PLANT POISONING, water hemlock	Abdominal pain, large pupils, nausea or vomiting, difficulty breathing.

Significant pain likely

AMEBIASIS	Burning or pain, upper right abdomen or lower right chest.
SCURVY	Abnormal bruising; bone pains; swollen gums.
LIVER FLUKE[2]	Also a large, tender liver; living in an affected area.
PELLAGRA	Digestive complaints, burning pains, rough skin rash.
FIBROMYALGIA	Insomnia and symmetrical muscular pains, adults, chronic.

Neither abnormal vital signs nor significant pain likely

DEMONIZATION	Caused by a curse by someone involved in witchcraft.
DEPRESSION	Early morning awakening, can't sleep again.
AFRICAN SLEEPING SICKNESS[3]	Also large nodes in back of neck, or HEART FAILURE.
SYPHILIS, tertiary/congenital	Patient, partner or parent was exposed.
SCHISTOSOMIASIS MANSONI[4]	Bloody diarrhea or JAUNDICE or a distended abdomen.

1 *Also consider the diseases that cause anemia.*

2 *Liver fluke: found worldwide, especially in Southeast Asia and the Far East.*

3 *African sleeping sickness: scattered areas of Africa, south of Bamako, Mali and Lake Chad and north of Lusaka, Zambia.*

4 *Schistosomiasis Mansoni: scattered areas within Africa, the Arabian Peninsula, the Caribbean and parts of eastern South America.*

Protocol A.8.B—Floppy weakness of body part(s); paralysis

Definition: the patient cannot easily move his body part(s) but someone else can move them easily since they are floppy. It is paralysis if the patient cannot move the body part(s) at all.

Arm weakness will be floppy with a spinal cord problem in the lower neck/upper back. Arm weakness will be stiff (possibly after an initial floppy interval) if the problem is above there. Leg weakness will be floppy with a spinal cord problem in the mid-back, below the level of the shoulder blades. It will be stiff if the problem is above that area.

▽ BEFORE PROCEEDING WITH THIS PROTOCOL:

Entirely undress the patient and look at every bit of skin to find a tick, especially on the scalp. Some ticks cause paralysis. See TICK PARALYSIS in the Condition Index. If you find one and remove it, don't fail to look for another. The one you removed is not necessarily the one causing the weakness or paralysis. Recovery will be rapid in the Northern Hemisphere; it may be delayed in the Southern Hemisphere.

Did the weakness develop within the past days, less than two weeks in all?

NO	YES
|	**Consider:** head injury, STROKE, BRAIN DAMAGE, MENINGITIS, ENCEPHALITITS,
|	MALARIA (cerebral or PMNS), PLANT POISONING due to ginger-jake.

Did the weakness develop during or after a severe or feverish illness?

NO	YES
|	**Consider** POLIO, /// DIPHTHERIA, BRUCELLOSIS, RABIES, RELAPSING FEVER[1], SPINAL NEUROPATHY,
|	MALARIA (PMNS), ENCEPHALITIS, TUBERCULOSIS.

See table below.

---

1 *Relapsing fever: tropical and high altitude, but not in the islands of SEA and the Pacific.*

FLOPPY WEAKNESS OF BODY PART(S), NOT RELATED TO A SEVERE ILLNESS

Condition	Onset	Characteristics
Likely no significant pain		
THYROID TROUBLE	Weeks	Always sleepy or trouble walking up stairs.
DEMONIZATION	Variable	Due to a curse or involvement in witchcraft.
COBALAMIN DEFICIENCY	Very slow	Older Westerner or diet devoid of animal products.
Likely significant pain in the center line of the back or neck		
TUBERCULOSIS	Weeks–months	Tenderness with tapping on the back bone.
FLUOROSIS	Unknown	Neck pain, discolored teeth.
SPINAL NEUROPATHY	Varies	Also numbness, tingling, bladder or bowel problems.
Likely significant pain in limb(s), may be symmetrical		
RICKETS	Weeks	Deficient sun exposure; lack of vitamin D.
SYPHILIS, congenital or tertiary	From birth	Refusal to move limb; pain; maybe brittle bones, newborn.
BERIBERI	Weeks–months	Very poor diet (maybe rice only) or alcoholic.
Likely significant pain in limb(s), not likely symmetrical		
POLIO	Days, weeks	Onset after a fever plus "cold," or "flu".
LEPROSY	Weeks–months	Skin changes, shooting pains, numbness.
CARPAL TUNNEL SYNDROME	Weeks	Arm and hand only; worse at night, dominant side first.

Continued on the next page.

TOC

SYMPTOMS

Related to an ingestion or event

PLANT POISONING	Variable	Ginger-jake, botulism,[1] manicheel,[2] tobacco-cow's urine,[3] water hemlock. History of the patient exposed to the plant.
LEAD POISONING	Slow	ANEMIA, headache, history of exposure.
TICK PARALYSIS	Sudden	Tick on skin; removal is curative.
Spinal cord injury	Variable	History of neck injury or back injury.
Snake bite	Sudden	Report of an encounter with a snake.
IMMERSION FOOT	Unknown	Due to cold and/or wet feet; skin changes.

1 With botulism, the weakness starts with the head and moves down. It is symmetrical. There are no mental changes. Constipation and inability to urinate are common. With other paralysis, the problem is asymmetric or there are mental changes or the weakness ascends upward from the lower body.

2 Plant poisoning: manicheel: found in the Americas only.

3 This is an ethnic medicine found in some parts of Africa.

Protocol A.8.C—Stiff weakness of body part(s); paralysis

Definition: the patient cannot move his own limbs well nor can someone else, since they are stiff. This is **paralysis** if the patient cannot move the body part(s) at all. The most common cause is BRAIN DAMAGE. There are two kinds of stiff weakness. One is that due to floppy weakness after which no one moved the patient's limbs regularly, so they became stiff from scaring of the joints and shortening of the ligaments and tendon. They never jerk involuntarily. The second kind of stiff weakness is from damage to the nerves higher in the body than the weak limb. In this case, although the patient cannot move the limb himself, if you tap below his knee or on the back of his ankle (the Achilles tendon), his limb will jerk involuntarily. This means the problem is in the mid-to-upper neck or the brain if the arms are involved; it is above the center-back of the chest if the legs are involved.

Did the stiff weakness develop gradually from a weakness that was first floppy?

NO	YES
|	**Consider** MENINGITIS, ENCEPHALITIS, TUBERCULOSIS of the spine, PLANT POISONING due to ginger-jake.
STIFF WEAKNESS, NOT INITIALLY FLOPPY	

Condition	Onset	Characteristics
Emergency condition, very sudden onset		
NEUROLEPTIC MALIGNANT SYNDROME	Seconds-Minutes	Always in the context of getting some medication: anesthesia, anti-vomiting or for emotional upset; high fever.
Not related to diet; likely to be others similarly affected, no fever		
RICKETS	Weeks	Curved limbs in infants, mother lacks sun exposure.
PLANT POISONING, cassava	Slow	Ordinary cassava not properly processed.
PLANT POISONING, strychnine	Very rapid	Immediately after eating or drinking; homicidal, always fatal.
Related to diet; likely to be others similarly affected.		
PELLAGRA	Weeks-months	Maybe a rash, burning with swallowing, no fever.
SCURVY	Unknown	Bleeding gums, doesn't eat fruits and vegetables, no fever.
TRICHINOSIS	Days	Very sore and swollen muscles, fever.
Unlikely to be others similarly affected		
SYPHILIS, tertiary/congenital	Variable	Patient, partner or parent was exposed.
BRAIN DAMAGE	Variable	Usually problems with speech or thinking also.
TETANUS	Hours-days	Peculiar, pinched smile, jaw tightly shut.
Prominent bowel and bladder problems		
TROPICAL SPASTIC PARAPARESIS	Gradual	Adults, symmetrical, little or no numbness.
SPINAL NEUROPATHY	Varies	Numbness and tingling, usually.

DIFFERENTIALS CONDITIONS DRUG INDEX REGIONAL NOTES INX

TOC

SYMPTOMS

DIFFERENTIALS

CONDITIONS

DRUG INDEX

REGIONAL NOTES

INX

PROTOCOL A.9—DISORDERS OF FOOD INTAKE AND WEIGHT CHANGE

A.9.A. Loss of appetite with weight loss

A.9.B. Cravings

A.9.C. Weight loss with a good appetite

A.9.D. Excessive appetite with constant or increased weight

First check for DEHYDRATION; if present, treat that while pursing further diagnosis. Confirm that the patient is not eating by checking a urine dipstick. If he truly is not eating, his urine will be positive for ketones.

INSTRUCTIONS FOR DEALING WITH AN INFANT TOO WEAK TO SUCK

Add sugar if you are using formula, then try the following in order:

1. Carefully enlarge the nipple hole if he is being bottle-fed.
2. For a breast-fed baby, have the mother exchange babies, just for a few minutes with a mother who has a healthy hungry baby. The little one gets an easy feed and the vigorous sucking of the healthy baby makes the milk come better.
3. Use an eyedropper to feed the child, giving just one or two drops every 5 minutes, almost continually.
4. If the child is not short of breath or vomiting, then use a stomach tube. See Volume 1, Appendix 1.

Protocol A.9.A—Loss of appetite with weight loss

First check the patient's vital signs: pulse, temperature and respiratory rate.
Are these reasonably normal or are they grossly abnormal?

Normal or nearly so	**Grossly abnormal**
|	Make every effort to send the patient out. If this is not possible, then pursue a diagnosis according to other symptoms. Do not use a stomach tube or try to feed the patient. If he is dehydrated, then IV, rectal or intraperitoneal fluids are acceptable.

Is the patient a very small or premature newborn or very malnourished and under 3 months old?

NO	**YES**
|	The patient is probably too weak to suck; see the instructions above for dealing with this. Then pursue diagnosis down the "No" arm. Also consider SYPHILIS, TUBERCULOSIS, RICKETS, SCURVY, looking for evidence in the breast-feeding mother. Give MULTIVITAMINS.

Is this a child who plays and responds normally?

NO	**YES, he plays and responds**
|	**Consider** that some children just decide not to eat for a while for no good reason; just watch him.

Is this a child whose illness started more than a week ago?

NO	**YES**
|	**Consider:** SYPHILIS (congenital), RICKETS, SCURVY, HIV INFECTION,[1] TUBERCULOSIS.

See the following eight tables.

- Quick and easy diagnoses with specific characteristics
- Referrals to other A._ protocols
- Loss of appetite and fatigue only
- Loss of appetite with fever for more than a week
- Loss of appetite with anemia
- Loss of appetite with diarrhea
- Loss of appetite with jaundice or swollen abdomen
- Loss of appetite with mental symptoms

---

1 *Check the child's skin and mouth. If he has no rash and no mouth sores, HIV infection is unlikely. If his mother gets sun exposure and eats a balanced diet, then rickets and scurvy are unlikely.*

QUICK AND EASY DIAGNOSES BECAUSE OF SPECIFIC CHARACTERISTICS

DIABETES	Drinks and urinates excessively; urine positive for glucose, possibly ketones also.
ADDICTION, uppers	The patient ingests khat or some other stimulant which decreases appetite.
SPRUE	Current or recent tropical residence, mainly Asia; sore mouth and severe diarrhea.
MALABSORPTION	Prompt diarrhea, eliminating food just eaten, right after eating.
BERIBERI	Also burning pains in feet and leg weakness; diet of white rice or carbohydrates only.
ENTEROBIASIS	Adults feel worms by anus, itching; small children may be irritable and have insomnia.
RADIATION ILLNESS	Early effect (within hours) of large-dose radiation exposure.
SYPHILIS, congenital	Failure to thrive; mother exposed or had been; not necessarily ill since birth.

LOSS OF APPETITE PLUS SPECIFIC OTHER SYMPTOMS

Additional symptom	Applicable protocol
Mouth or throat pain	Protocol A.29
Shortness of breath	Protocol A.36 & Protocol B.4.
Difficulty swallowing	Protocol A.30.D
Abdominal pain	Protocols A.39–45
Diarrhea	Protocol A.56
Fatigue	Protocol A.8.A
Early satiety[1]	Protocol A.46

---

1 *The patient feels hungry and tries to eat but becomes full after a couple bites. This may be due to a large spleen or liver which pushes on the stomach. It might also be due to CANCER.*

LOSS OF APPETITE AND FATIGUE ONLY; FEW OR NO OTHER SYMPTOMS

Likely a normal mental state, considering the circumstances

MALNUTRITION	Not enough food available; at some point these patients also lose appetite.
HEAT ILLNESS	Very hot environment and not acclimatized; infant, elderly, exercising.
TUBERCULOSIS	Night sweats are common; TB exposure, maybe some indigestion.
CANCER	Increasing fatigue, usually slowly, over weeks and months.

Likely a lethargic or sad mental state

DEPRESSION	Genetically thin patient, recent loss; may or may not be crying a lot.

Likely bizarre behavior

DEMONIZATION	Curse or else occult involvement; may be triggered by drugs.
ADDICTION	Use of uppers or outers: amphetamine, khat, etc.

May be normal, sad or bizarre, depending on the individual

STRESS	Genetically thin patient, recent stress; may or may not be nervous.
PELLAGRA	Poor diet and carbohydrate only; abdominal pains.
BERIBERI	ALCOHOLISM or a diet of white rice or carbohydrates only.
SYPHILIS, tertiary/congenital	Patient, partner or parents were exposed.

LOSS OF APPETITE PLUS FEVER MORE THAN A WEEK

Corrected body temperature not likely to be high

HEPATITIS	History of liver-toxic drugs or a tender liver.
TUBERCULOSIS	Chronic cough or large neck lymph nodes.
CANCER	Lump somewhere or large lymph nodes or other symptoms.
VISCERAL LEISHMANIASIS[1]	Very large spleen; geographically confined.

Corrected body temperature likely is high off and on or continually, over 38.5°/101.3°

MALARIA	Large spleen, waist pain, shoulder pain, headache, joint pains.
HIV INFECTION	Frequent infections, sexual or blood exposure.
TYPHUS	Illness before the fever; body lice or exposure to fleas.
LEPTOSPIROSIS	Red eyes, severe muscle pains or both; fevers erratic over hours.
BRUCELLOSIS	Fevers come and go over days, pains in lower body, fatigue.

LOSS OF APPETITE PLUS ANEMIA

Most common, check these first

MALNUTRITION	Food availability problem or patient eats just one kind of food.
HOOKWORM	Areas with sandy soil; stool tests positive for blood.
TUBERCULOSIS	Cough or large neck lymph nodes or history of TB exposure.
HIV INFECTION	Frequent infections; may look just like TB.

Pain likely a major complaint

LEAD POISONING	**Head**: lead exposure from paints, herbs or metal work.
BRUCELLOSIS	**Back pain**: slow onset of whole-body misery.
CANCER	Localized **anywhere,** possibly a rotten-meat body odor.

Pain not likely a major complaint

VISCERAL LEISHMANIASIS[1]	Huge spleen, large liver, fevers off and on.
AFRICAN SLEEPING SICKNESS[2]	Headaches early on, fevers, abnormal sleep, falls asleep eating.
KIDNEY DISEASE	Urine-like body odor, nauseated, flaky skin.

---

1 *Visceral Leishmaniasis: found in scattered areas of Central and South America, Africa north of the equator, the Mediterranean area, the Indian subcontinent, eastern Europe, central Asia and mainland China.*
2 *African sleeping sickness: scattered areas of Africa, south of Bamako, Mali and Lake Chad and north of Lusaka, Zambia.*

LOSS OF APPETITE PLUS DIARRHEA

Most common, check these first

HIV INFECTION	Frequent infections, sexually active, blood exposure or ill parents.
MALABSORPTION	Prompt diarrhea, maybe recognizable food, right after eating.
TUBERCULOSIS	Drank raw milk or exposed to someone with lung TB.

Likely an expatriate

GIARDIASIS	Watery diarrhea, much gas, maybe vomiting.
SPRUE[1]	Rumbling, gassy abdomen; sore mouth.

Related to unsanitary or unhealthy diet; usually a national

PELLAGRA	Poor diet; maybe rash or burning with swallowing.
CAPILLARIASIS[2]	History of eating raw fish, usually Southeast Asia.
INTESTINAL FLUKE[3]	History of eating raw or rare fish or water plants.

1 Sprue: in the Americas only near or north of the equator. In Africa only Nigeria and southern Africa. Prevalent in India and Southeast Asia. It is occasionally found in the Mediterranean area.
2 Capillariasis: Philippines mainly; rarely Thailand, found in Egypt with potential of spreading.
3 Intestinal fluke: not in Africa south of the Sahara or Eastern Europe. In the Americas, only in Guyana.

LOSS OF APPETITE PLUS JAUNDICE OR ABDOMINAL SWELLING:

Jaundice before swollen abdomen likely; fever or history of fever

HEPATITIS	Liver is tender and may be enlarged; joint pains common.
LEPTOSPIROSIS	Sudden-onset erratic fevers; red eyes, muscle pains or both.

Jaundice before swollen abdomen likely; maybe fever or history of fever

LIVER FLUKE[5]	History of eating raw or pickled fish; upper abdominal pains.
CANCER	Abnormal lump or wound; maybe rotten-meat body odor.

Jaundice before swollen abdomen likely; fever or a history of fever unlikely

LIVER FAILURE	Yellow eyes, swollen abdomen, bilirubin in the urine.
MALNUTRITION	Abnormal hair, abnormal skin color, poor diet, skinny upper arms.
SPRUE[1]	Severe diarrhea, rumbling, gassy abdomen; sore mouth.

Indeterminate: either jaundice or swelling might occur first

AMEBIASIS	Dysentery; burning pains in right upper abdomen.

Swollen abdomen only or swollen abdomen before jaundice

MALNUTRITION	Thin upper arm circumference; roughened skin.
TUBERCULOSIS	Cough or large neck lymph nodes; abdomen feels like bread dough.
SCHISTOSOMIASIS MANSONI[2]	History of DYSENTERY common; check geography.
SCHISTOSOMIASIS JAPONICUM[3]	Swollen abdomen, maybe also mental symptoms, check geography.
KIDNEY DISEASE	Urine abnormal in quantity or urinalysis; urine-like body odor.
VISCERAL LEISHMANIASIS[4]	Huge spleen, large liver, fevers off and on.

1 Sprue: in the Americas only near or north of the equator. In Africa only Nigeria and southern Africa. Prevalent in India and Southeast Asia. It is occasionally found in the Mediterranean area.
2 Schistosomiasis Mansoni: scattered areas within Africa, the Arabian peninsula, the Caribbean and parts of eastern South America.
3 Schistosomiasis Japonicum: in areas of mainland China, the Philippines, parts of the Celebes, the upper Mekong and the Thai-Malaysia border.
4 Visceral Leishmaniasis: found in scattered areas of Central and South America, Africa north of the equator, the Mediterranean area, the Indian subcontinent, eastern Europe, central Asia and mainland China. Not present south of the equator.
5 Liver fluke is found worldwide; it is especially common in Southeast Asia and the Far East.

LOSS OF APPETITE WITH MENTAL SYMPTOMS:

Almost exclusively expatriate teens

Anorexia nervosa — Female with teen adjustment issues; Western parents.

Depression with a fever

ENTERIC FEVER — Onset over days, withdrawn; headache or abdominal pain common.

DENGUE FEVER[2] — Onset over hours, severe headache, very severe bone and joint pain.

Depression prominent, no fever

DEPRESSION — Abnormal sleep pattern; patient genetically thin.

SPRUE[3] — Severe watery diarrhea, sore mouth, bizarre behavior possible also.

Either depression or craziness, maybe fever

HEAT ILLNESS — Exposure to hot climates without prior acclimatization.

CANCER — Lump or open wound somewhere, or headaches.

HIV INFECTION — Frequent infections, diarrhea.

BRUCELLOSIS — Headache; fevers, chills or sweats off and on; animal exposure.

Bizarre behavior likely prominent with a fever or history of fever

MALARIA — Commonly fevers, chills and headache, but symptoms vary between people.

Bizarre behavior likely prominent, no fever

DEMONIZATION — Due to a curse on the patient or patient involved in witchcraft.

ADDICTION, uppers — Stimulants decrease appetite and make the patient hyperactive.

General incompetence likely prominent, maybe an element of craziness

SYPHILIS, tertiary/congenital — Grandiose or acts stupid; patient, partner or parent was exposed.

PELLAGRA — Mainly corn diet; roughened sun-exposed skin; bowel trouble.

BERIBERI — Alcoholic or poor diet; pains and weakness in legs.

AFRICAN SLEEPING SICKNESS[1] — Abnormal sleep patterns, headache, fever or history of fever.

1 African sleeping sickness: scattered areas of Africa, south of Bamako, Mali and Lake Chad and north of Lusaka, Zambia.
2 Dengue fever: in the Americas only near or north of the equator. In Africa, east coastal, south and west. Prevalent in India, Southeast Asia and the Pacific. Occasionally found in the Mediterranean area. The disease may spread.
3 Sprue: in the Americas only near or north of the equator. In Africa only Nigeria and southern Africa. Prevalent in India and Southeast Asia. It is occasionally found in the Mediterranean area.

Protocol A.9.B—Cravings

Definition: the patient eats non-food substances or else excessive and unusual amounts of food stuffs (e.g. emptying a salt shaker into his coffee and then drinking it). Usually due to pregnancy in pregnant females; Also consider ASCARIASIS, TRICHURIASIS, HOOKWORM. Salt craving requires higher level care. Meantime encourage salt consumption.

Protocol A.9.C—Weight loss with a good appetite

Consider bulimia in a young Western female. Weight loss with a good appetite is common in those who first arrive in the tropics; this does not need treatment but check a urine dipstick to make sure the patient does not have DIABETES or LIVER DISEASE. It takes time to locate, buy and figure out how to cook palatable food. Meantime, the person will lose weight. It may be due to an otherwise-thin mother trying to breast feed a large infant or twins; she cannot consume enough calories to support both herself and the child. Other causes are listed below:

Most likely	
ASCARIASIS	Belly pains, constipation, may pass worms
TAPEWORM[1]	History of eating raw or rare meats
DIABETES	Also excessive thirst and excessive urination
ADDICTION	Patient has access to and is taking uppers.
Less likely than the conditions above	
THYROID TROUBLE	High-thyroid; insomnia, a rapid pulse and nervousness
VISCERAL LEISHMANIASIS[2]	Large spleen, left upper belly pains, fevers

---

1 *Tapeworm may occur even in babies who are exclusively breastfed, because sibling fingers might transmit the worm eggs.*
2 *Visceral Leishmaniasis: found in scattered areas of Central and South America, Africa north of the equator, the Mediterranean area, the Indian subcontinent, eastern Europe, central Asia and mainland China. Not present south of the equator.*

Protocol A.9.D—Excessive appetite with constant or increased weight

Normal in growing children and teenagers. Otherwise most frequently due to STRESS or DEPRESSION in those prone to overweight; to pregnancy; or to THYROID TROUBLE (low-thyroid). It is normal in children who were starved and now have food available and in diabetics who recently started treatment. It may be due to steroid drugs.

PROTOCOL A.10—DISORDERS OF FEELING AND SENSATION

A.10.A—Numbness and tingling
A.10.B—Sharp, shooting pains
A.10.C—Aching all over

A.10.D—Total body itching
A.10.E—Other sensation problems

Protocol A.10.A—Numbness and tingling

Is the numbness/tingling in a stocking-glove distribution (similar on the thumb/big toe side of the hand/foot as on the little finger/little toe side?

YES

See the table beginning on the bottom of the next page.

NO

See the table beginning at the top of the following page.

NUMBNESS AND TINGLING, NOT IN A STOCKING/GLOVE DISTRIBUTION

Condition	Body part(s)	Characteristics
Related to a prominent skin condition		
SHINGLES	One side only	Blistery rash on skin, a band on the trunk, an area on the face
LEPROSY	Cool body parts	Skin bumps or color changes
Recurrent problem, not related to whole-body illness		
CARPAL TUNNEL SYNDROME	Hand, dominant first	Pain with numbness and tingling, palm-thumb side of hand
Likely related to a whole-body illness, slow-onset or long-lasting		
BRUCELLOSIS	Lower limbs	Also some floppy weakness, maybe incoordination
CANCER	Anywhere	Weight loss; symptoms constant or worsening
TUBERCULOSIS, bone	Backbone	Pain and tenderness in the backbone
SPINAL NEUROPATHY	Genital/saddle area	Maybe problems with passing urine or stool
TROPICAL SPASTIC PARAPARESIS	Lower limbs, maybe upper also.	Burning pains also, stiffness of legs, adults only, bowel/bladder problems, numbness is minimal
Likely related to a whole-body illness, onset over hours to days in previously healthy patient		
DIPHTHERIA	Variable	Also weakness of some muscles, especially head
RABIES	Area bitten	Not symmetrical; also paralysis or throat spasms
LOIASIS	Anywhere	Local swelling on the same side, maybe itchy; humid central Africa
NECROTIZING FASCIITIS	Muscles or genital	Seemingly minor infection with inordinately severe pain
Likely onset over seconds to hours, no fever, no whole-body illness		
HYPERVENTILATION	Around lips	Short of breath, cramped hands, rapid onset
SLIPPED DISC	Limbs	Back pain with leg(s) or neck pain with arm(s)
STROKE	Right or left side	Usually weakness also, older patient or prior ill health
TICK PARALYSIS	Anywhere	History of outdoor activity; search for a tick, including in hair
Related to an ingestion; variable onset from minutes to years		
ISONIAZID (drug)	Limbs, symmetrical	Patient taking drugs for TB, onset over weeks usually
ARSENIC POISONING	Hands/feet	Burning, skin changes
PLANT POISONING	Hands/feet	Due to ergot; chest pain is common also
FOOD POISONING	Anywhere	Also vomiting, diarrhea; due to fish; Pacific area

NUMBNESS AND TINGLING LIKELY IN A STOCKING/GLOVE DISTRIBUTION, DISEASES AND CONDITIONS

Disease/condition	Weakness also?	Other characteristics
COBALAMIN DEFICIENCY	Yes	Vegan diet or European genetic heritage probably
MALABSORPTION	Maybe	Severe diarrhea; see Protocol B.24
DEMONIZATION	Maybe	Occult environment, due to a curse
HIV INFECTION	Little	Weight loss, diarrhea, frequent infections
LYME DISEASE	Maybe	Temperate climate disease; tick exposure
DIPHTHERIA	Yes!!	Painful wound or sore throat with scum on tonsils
BERIBERI	Yes	Diet deficient in B vitamins; alcoholics.

TOC

SYMPTOMS

DIFFERENTIALS

CONDITIONS

DRUG INDEX

REGIONAL NOTES

INX

NUMBNESS AND TINGLING IN A STOCKING/GLOVE DISTRIBUTION: DRUGS AND TOXINS

Drug or toxin problem	Weakness also?	Other characteristics
ISONIAZID	Maybe	TB medication; treat with vitamin B$_6$
HAART (HIV drugs)	Little if any	Patient is on HIV drugs
ARSENIC POISONING	Yes	Homicide, industrial or ethnic remedies
INSECTICIDE POISONING	Yes	Homicide or environmental exposure
LEAD POISONING	Yes	Industrial toxins or ethnic remedies

Protocol A.10.B—Sharp, shooting pains

Definition: the patient has pains that rapidly travel away from the trunk. Most of the diseases of A.10.A can also cause sharp, shooting pains. The following are causes of sharp, shooting pains possibly WITHOUT numbness and tingling.

Likely related to a slow onset (over a month or more) illness

TUBERCULOSIS	Also neck or back pain with tenderness; fevers common
LEPROSY	Also skin bumps or color changes; maybe swollen nerves like strings under the skin
SYPHILIS, tertiary/congenital	Patient, partner or parent was exposed. Mostly adults
BRUCELLOSIS	Episodic fevers, back pain, joint pains, lower body

Related to an environmental exposure

FLUOROSIS	Pains in the arms; neck pains also; related to water supply
IMMERSION FOOT	Cold or water exposure; skin changes

Likely related to a rapid-onset (over less than a week) illness

SLIPPED DISC	Low back pain also if leg pain; neck pain if arm pain
LOIASIS	Also swellings that come and go; only rural, humid tropical Africa

TOC
SYMPTOMS
DIFFERENTIALS
CONDITIONS
DRUG INDEX
REGIONAL NOTES
INX

Protocol A.10.C—Aching all over

▷ SYMPTOMATIC TREATMENT

Use IBUPROFEN or ACETAMINOPHEN for pain control. ASPIRIN is okay for adults if there are no contraindications to its use.

Does the patient have a corrected temperature over 38.5°/101.3°, or did he within the past few days?

NO to both

YES to either

See Protocol B.2 also. Consider these from the top down.

Chest pain worse than other pain

ARBOVIRAL FEVER: also headache; seek local lore.

BARTONELLOSIS:[1] JAUNDICE; ANEMIA also.

LASSA FEVER:[2] cough also; occurs in epidemics.

Headache worse than other pain

SPOTTED FEVER:[3] rash begins on limbs, moves to trunk.

RELAPSING FEVER:[4] chills, sweats, sustained fever.

MALARIA: chills; erratic fever becomes regular over time.

YELLOW FEVER:[5] not immunized; abnormal urinalysis.

RAT BITE FEVER; history of an animal bite.

TULAREMIA: exposed to small animals or their insects.

TYPHUS: exposed to body lice or fleas; headache before fever.

Other pain worse than headache[6]

DENGUE FEVER:[8] severe **bone/joint and eye** pains.

LYME DISEASE: temperate climate; **joints, commonly knee**.

ENTERIC FEVER: patient withdrawn; **abdominal pain**.

LEPTOSPIROSIS: red eyes and headache; **muscle pain**.

TRICHINOSIS: also very swollen and painful **muscles**.

TULAREMIA:[7] **muscle** pains.

TYPHUS: mentally abnormal, **shin** pain, body lice, epidemics.

TRENCH FEVER: **shin** pain, had body lice, urban homeless.

BRUCELLOSIS: fatigue, **lower back** pain

INFLUENZA: epidemic context, headache, cough, congestion

Table below

---

1 *Bartonellosis: only occurs in Peru and adjacent countries.*
2 *Lassa fever is present in scattered areas of western and central Africa.*
3 *Spotted fever: not in the islands of Southeast Asia.*
4 *Relapsing fever: tropical and high altitude, but not in the islands of SEA and the Pacific.*
5 *Yellow fever: South America north of Sao Paolo, Central and western Africa and the Sudan.*
6 *The bold-face type identifies the most prominent pain with each of these entries.*
7 *Tularemia: in eastern Europe, persons exposed to small animals or their insects.*
8 *Dengue fever: in the Americas only near or north of the equator. In Africa, east coastal, south and west. Prevalent in India, Southeast Asia and the Pacific. Occasionally found in the Mediterranean area. The disease may spread.*

ACHING PAIN WITHOUT A CURRENT OR RECENT HIGH FEVER

Conditions	Fever	Characteristics
Healthy presently or within the past 2 days, no or slight fever		
HEAT ILLNESS	Maybe	Hot environment and not acclimatized to heat
MUSCLE STRAIN	No	Recent unaccustomed exercise
HANGOVER	No	The morning after alcohol ingestion
LICE	No	"Flu" after having body lice some time before

Conditions	Fever	Characteristics
Likely bedridden or would like to be; rapid onset, less than a week.		
POLIO	Usual	Weakness of limb(s), usually legs
RUBELLA	Low	Rash, usually children and adolescents
TETANUS	Maybe	Muscle spasms, back and jaws
CHOLERA	No/slight	Severe watery diarrhea, sudden onset
RABIES	Maybe	Paralyzed or throat spasms or both
Likely bedridden or would like to be; slow onset, more than 2 weeks.		
BRUCELLOSIS	Episodic	Back pain and joint pains; complaining loudly
LIVER FLUKE	No	Liver is large, tender or both.
CHAGA'S DISEASE	Usual	Current or recent bug bite with swelling; Americas only

Protocol A.10.D—Total body itching

▷ SYMPTOMATIC TREATMENT

Try soothing skin creams for dry skin; try COLESTYRAMINE for the itching of LIVER DISEASE, SICKLE CELL DISEASE and KIDNEY DISEASE. VITAMIN B_6 may also be helpful.

The most common cause in almost all cultures is SCABIES; in this case there are visible itchy spots.

Visible rash: (apart from scratch marks) but it is not scabies, then see Protocol A.15.A; if there are swollen areas on the skin, consider ALLERGY, SERUM SICKNESS, CHIKUNGUNYA FEVER, KATAYAMA DISEASE, CONTACT DERMATITIS.

Deep itching with no visible rash aside from scratch marks: the problem is probably some sort of liver disease; see JAUNDICE in the Condition Index. Also consider ONCHOCERCIASIS,[3] KIDNEY DISEASE, ANEMIA due to iron deficiency, DIABETES, THYROID TROUBLE (low or high), BIRTH CONTROL PILLS, withdrawal from alcohol or drugs A relatively rare cause in all cultures is lymphoma, a type of CANCER. In this case there is also weight loss, fatigue and night sweats.

Skin itching with no visible rash aside from scratch marks: consider ASCARIASIS, BERIBERI, ONCHOCERCIASIS,[3] SCABIES, body LICE, CHLOROQUINE (drug for MALARIA), CANCER, MALARIA (in patients with African genetic heritage), LIVER FAILURE, GALLBLADDER DISEASE, KATAYAMA DISEASE, ALLERGY, CONTACT DERMATITIS (especially caused by an allergy to soap).

Protocol A.10.E—Other sensation problems

Common

SYPHILIS, tertiary/congenital	Cannot tell where a limb is in space without looking; incoordination in the dark worse than light; maybe also mental changes.
TYPHUS	High fever, severe headache, a variety of painful sensations; mainly louse-borne
COBALAMIN DEFICIENCY	Similar to SYPHILIS; mainly elderly of European heritage, malnourished and vegans
LARVA MIGRANS	Patient feels a worm crawling beneath the skin, maybe a visible line.
BERIBERI	Patient feels as if there are insects crawling over or in the skin.
DEMONIZATION	Like BERIBERI or other strange manifestations

Less common in general, but may be locally common

AFRICAN SLEEPING SICKNESS[1]	A tap on the shin produces severe pain after several seconds.
LOIASIS[2]	Patient feels a worm crawling beneath his skin.
ONCHOCERCIASIS[3]	Patient feels a tingling, creeping sensation in his skin.
PELLAGRA	Burning pains; diarrhea; rough, dry rash; mental changes
TROPICAL SPASTIC PARAPARESIS	Burning pains along with stiffness of the lower limbs

1 *African sleeping sickness: scattered areas of Africa, south of Bamako, Mali and Lake Chad and north of Lusaka, Zambia.*
2 *Loiasis: scattered areas in rural, humid, western and central Africa.*
3 *Onchocerciasis: present in scattered area in Africa, in the Americas north of the Amazon, in Yemen and Saudi Arabia.*

PROTOCOL A.11—POISONING

First, if applicable, see FOOD POISONING if the problem is a person's eating spoiled food containing meat. See PLANT POISONING for poisoning from plant foods or ethnic medicines. See ARSENIC POISONING,[1] LEAD POISONING,[2] INSECTICIDE POISONING or FLUOROSIS (from bad water) if applicable.

Was the poison a corrosive such as a strong acid or base (e.g. lye) or else gasoline—kerosene type or does the patient have mouth burns (chalk-white or black patches on the pink parts of his mouth)?

NO to all	YES to either
| | |	Use no stomach tube, no IPECAC. Give PROMETHAZINE by injection. Give large amounts of milk or water if the patient is conscious. If he is not conscious, see paragraph 2 below. Send the patient out or call for help.

Note: in Western countries the standard poisoning protocol has changed from what it used to be, on account of technological advances. Since Western technology is not available to those who legitimately use this book, the procedures given here are based on the old methods. If the patient is alert, use paragraph 1 (as follows). If not alert, see the instructions in paragraph 2.

1. If and only if he is alert:

Option 1 (preferable): have the patient drink a large amount of activated charcoal.

Option 2: have him drink syrup of IPECAC or put down a stomach tube and pour the syrup down the tube. Follow this with warm water in either case. This will make him vomit.

2. Lethargic or unconscious patient:

Send to a hospital promptly. If the patient is unconscious because of the poison; he will probably die. Be sure to position the patient head down, so if he vomits on his own, the vomit will run out rather than down his lungs. Either place a plastic airway in his mouth or stay with him to protect his airway (see Chapter 4 in Volume 1).

3. Antidotes:

These are generally not available or useful. Exception: for IODINE poisoning give a suspension of any kind of starch (e.g. flour or cornstarch in water or mashed potatoes). It will turn the iodine blue and render it harmless. For wood alcohol (methanol) give the person potable alcoholic beverage or IV ALCOHOL, keeping him thoroughly intoxicated for 3 days; calculate the dose from the Drug Index. Large amounts of baking soda are also helpful. The pH of the urine will rise with baking soda. Check it with a urine dipstick. Keep the pH at 8 or above. Major hospitals have other antidotes sometimes.

OVERDOSE CALCULATIONS: for the following medications, these are the amounts that may be lethal for an average adult. Keep in mind that an average Western adult weighs considerably more than an average Third-World adult.

CHLOROQUINE: 2500 mg (2.5 grams)   ASPIRIN: 10,000 mg (10 grams)
ACETAMINOPHEN: 7500 mg (7.5 grams)   IRON (Ferrous sulfate): 37,500 mg (37.5 grams)

The maximum amount possibly taken (in milligrams) can be estimated as follows:

Mg possibly taken = (Maximum number of tablets missing from bottle) x (mg per tablet)

If the **mg possibly taken** is equal to or greater than the number above, the patient must be transported to a hospital while being treated with ACTIVATED CHARCOAL (preferable) or else IPECAC.

If the patient took less than the potentially lethal amount given above, then also calculate the **"mg/kg dose possibly taken":**

"mg/kg dose possibly taken" = (mg possibly taken) divided by (body weight in kilograms)

Compare the mg/kg possibly taken to the numbers below (This calculation takes account of body size):

CHLOROQUINE: 50 mg/kg;   ACETAMINOPHEN: 140 mg/kg;
ASPIRIN: 150 mg/kg;   IRON (as ferrous sulfate) 750 mg/kg

---

1 *Arsenic poisoning may be suicide/homicide, but some very old antibiotics contain it. These might still be available in developing countries. Arsenic is commonly present in herbal remedies and is sometimes used in cancer chemotherapy.*

2 *Lead poisoning is usually from paints, traditional medicines, cosmetics or metal work. It is commonly present in ethnic cosmetics and in herbal remedies.*

PROTOCOL A.12—DISORDERS OF GROWTH OR DEVELOPMENT

A.12.A—Poor growth
A.12-B—Excessive growth

A.12.C—Abnormal sexual development
A.12.D—Delayed mental development

Protocol A.12.A—Poor growth

Does the patient have loss of appetite?

NO	YES
	Go to Protocol A-9 first, then check the "no" arm also.

Does the patient have a large spleen[1]?

NO	YES
	Consider TROPICAL SPLENOMEGALY,[1] SCHISTOSOMIASIS MANSONI,[2] SICKLE CELL DISEASE,[3] SCHISTOSOMIASIS JAPONICUM,[4] THALLASEMIA, VISCERAL LEISHMANIASIS,[5] congenital SYPHILIS.

Does the patient have diarrhea, constipation or abdominal pains?

NO	YES
	Consider GIARDIASIS, PELLAGRA, ASCARIASIS, TAPEWORM, SCHISTOSOMIASIS MANSONI,[2] SPRUE,[6] TUBERCULOSIS, HIV INFECTION, MALABSORPTION

Is the patient an infant?

NO	YES
See table below	**Consider** RICKETS, SCURVY, TUBERCULOSIS, KIDNEY INFECTION, congenital SYPHILIS, CRETINISM (check the mother.)

POOR GROWTH, NOT AN INFANT, SPLEEN NOT LARGE, NO ABDOMINAL SYMPTOMS

Common in expatriates

GIARDIASIS[7]	Without symptoms or might have gas, diarrhea or vomiting.
ZINC DEFICIENCY	Hot weather, night blindness, fatigue, not acclimatized.

Not common in expatriates

MALNUTRITION	Poor or unbalanced diet, particularly a diet lacking in protein.
TUBERCULOSIS	Cough or night sweats or child living in home with TB patient.
TAPEWORM	Consumed raw or rare meats; maybe infants with older siblings.
SYPHILIS, congenital	Parent(s) are or have been exposed to venereal syphilis.

Likely a whole-body illness

HIV INFECTION	MALNUTRITION even though good food is available.
SCHISTOSOMIASIS HEMATOBIUM[8]	Bloody urine, now or previously; problem in the community.
SCHISTOSOMIASIS MANSONI[2]	Large spleen, large liver or bloody diarrhea; big belly.
SCHISTOSOMIASIS JAPONICUM[4]	Distended abdomen, possibly diarrhea or DYSENTERY.
RADIATION ILLNESS	Infants of mothers irradiated at or after 2 months pregnant.
SICKLE CELL DISEASE	Family history of ill health in someone of African heritage, maybe Arab or Indian.

---

1 *The large spleen presses on the stomach, making it difficult to eat sufficient food to sustain life.*
2 *Schistosomiasis Mansoni: scattered areas within Africa, the Arabian peninsula, the Caribbean and parts of eastern South America.*
3 *Sickle cell disease: this affects those of African genetic origin, mainly in West Africa and the Americas. Some Indians and Arabs are also affected.*
4 *Schistosomiasis Japonicum: in areas of mainland China, the Philippines, parts of the Celebes, the upper Mekong and the Thai-Malaysia border.*
5 *Visceral Leishmaniasis: found in scattered areas of Central and South America, Africa north of the equator, the Mediterranean area, the Indian subcontinent, eastern Europe, central Asia and mainland China.*
6 *Sprue: in the Americas only near or north of the equator. In Africa only Nigeria and southern Africa. Prevalent in India and Southeast Asia. It is occasionally found in the Mediterranean area.*
7 *This is a common cause of failure to thrive in expatriate children without other symptoms. It should be treated on mere suspicion, since it is so common and the treatment is benign.*
8 *Schistosomiasis hematobium: found in areas of Africa and the Middle East.*

TOC SYMPTOMS DIFFERENTIALS CONDITIONS DRUG INDEX REGIONAL NOTES INX

Protocol A.12.B—Excessive growth

See swelling if applicable (Protocols A.34.B, A.46.B, A.61.D, A.13.B). Women who have DIABETES during pregnancy are likely to have very big babies. Rarely there may be a genetic defect causing giantism.

ACROMEGALY	Very coarse facial features, large bony structure.
MYCETOMA	Large foot with sores on it; awkwardness is more troublesome than pain.
MOSSY FOOT	Swollen foot or feet with thick, rough skin; awkwardness is more troublesome than pain.
FILARIASIS	Initially swelling comes and goes; geographically confined.

Protocol A.12.C—Abnormal sexual development

Definitions: early sexual development, before age nine, is a serious problem that must be referred to a major medical center within a couple of weeks. Delayed sexual development may be caused by any chronic disease such as HEART FAILURE, VISCERAL LEISHMANIASIS, TUBERCULOSIS, MALNUTRITION. Also, see the list below.

THALLASEMIA	Large spleen, ANEMIA.
LEPROSY	Skin is bumpy on much of the body, including ear lobes.
ZINC DEFICIENCY	Delayed growth, night blindness, fatigue.
SICKLE CELL DISEASE[1]	Recurrent chest, abdominal or bone pains; family history.
SCHISTOSOMIASIS MANSONI[2]	Also a swollen abdomen and poor general growth.
AFRICAN SLEEPING SICKNESS[3]	Large neck lymph nodes, incoordination, or HEART FAILURE.
SCHISTOSOMIASIS JAPONICUM[4]	Distended abdomen, possibly diarrhea or DYSENTERY.

---

1 *Sickle cell disease: this affects those of African genetic origin, mainly in West Africa and the Americas. Some Indians and Arabs are also affected.*
2 *Schistosomiasis Mansoni: scattered areas within Africa, the Arabian Peninsula, the Caribbean and parts of eastern South America.*
3 *African sleeping sickness: scattered areas of Africa, south of Bamako, Mali and Lake Chad and north of Lusaka, Zambia.*
4 *Schistosomiasis Japonicum: in areas of mainland China, the Philippines, parts of the Celebes, the upper Mekong and the Thai-Malaysia border.*

Protocol A.12.D—Delayed mental development

First check for deafness and CEREBRAL PALSY as these are easily mistaken for mental retardation.
Most often retardation has an obscure cause, not one listed below.

Does the patient have a history of some illness that left him/her bedridden for weeks or months?

NO	YES
See the table below	**Consider** cerebral MALARIA, MENINGITIS, ENCEPHALITIS, AFRICAN SLEEPING SICKNESS.

NO HISTORY OF AN ILLNESS INVOLVING BEING BEDRIDDEN

MALNUTRITION	History of deficient food intake.
SYPHILIS, congenital	Parent(s) were exposed; maybe rash, bone swelling.
DOWN SYNDROME	Wide set eyes, maybe palm crease uninterrupted.
BRAIN DAMAGE	Due to any event affecting the brain, be it injury or illness.
PELLAGRA	Rash, diarrhea; usually a poor diet.
CRETINISM	Low body temperature, lethargic, overweight.
RADIATION ILLNESS	Infant of a mother irradiated at or after 2 months pregnant.

TOC
SYMPTOMS
DIFFERENTIALS
CONDITIONS
DRUG INDEX
REGIONAL NOTES
INX

PROTOCOL A.13—MISCELLANEOUS WHOLE-BODY PROBLEMS

A.13.A—Odor
A.13.B—Whole-body swelling
A.13.C—Drenching sweats

A.13.D—Chills
A.13.E—Generalized bleeding

Protocol A.13.A—Odor

MUSTY, ROTTEN ODORS

Moldy leather odor	TYPHUS, sometimes LIVER FAILURE, some SEPSIS, some CANCER
Fishy musty odor	VAGINITIS; CHOLERA (odor of the diarrhea).
Putrid sweet	SCURVY, DIPHTHERIA.
Foul, rotten odor	Poor dental hygiene, sores in mouth or throat, STREP THROAT, RESPIRATORY INFECTION due to sinusitis, ABSCESS (possibly in the lung), SEXUALLY TRANSMITTED DISEASE, CANCRUM ORIS, RHINITIS, severe PNEUMONIA, CANCER, GANGRENE, VINCENT STOMATITIS. Pus with a foul, rotten odor should be drained and the patient given METRONIDAZOLE.

FOOD AND DRINK-LIKE ODORS

Stale beer	TUBERCULOSIS involving the lymph nodes, if there are breaks in the skin.
Fresh baked bread	ENTERIC FEVER
Garlic	ARSENIC POISONING, garlic ingestion
Butcher shop	YELLOW FEVER
Sweet	DIPHTHERIA

CHEMICAL/CLEANING/SOLVENT-LIKE ODOR

Medicinal odor	PARALDEHYDE (a seizure medication)
Bleach-like odor	human semen
Glue, solvent odor	MALNUTRITION, DIABETES, some SEPSIS

OTHER ODORS:

Ammonia or urine smell:	KIDNEY DISEASE or spilled urine which was not washed off.
Fresh feathers:	RUBELLA.

Protocol A.13.B—Whole-body swelling

See Protocol B.15.

Protocol A.13.C—Drenching sweats

May be normal in children at night or menopausal women at any time of day. If the patient has DIABETES or an abnormal mental state, give him sugar immediately. With RICKETS, excessive sweating is confined to the head. Any disease that causes a sudden drop of a high fever will also cause sweats. Except for the sweats associated with MENOPAUSE, it is important to find the fever pattern, if any, before starting symptomatic treatment. Take the patient's temperature every 2 hours around the clock for several days, noting on the record sheet when he has chills and/or sweats.

DRENCHING SWEATS: start at the top and read down.

Condition	Fevers	Other Characteristics
Most common, consider these first		
MENOPAUSE	No	45–60 yo female
ALCOHOLISM	No	Withdrawal after heavy drinking
HYPOGLYCEMIA	No	Also trembling and mental symptoms or hungry
HIV INFECTION	Usual	Exposure within the past 4 weeks, an infecting contact
TUBERCULOSIS	Usual	Also chronic cough, weight loss, maybe large neck nodes

Condition	Fever	Other characteristics
Patient is very ill, bedridden		
LEPTOSPIROSIS	Erratic	Muscle pains, red eyes or both; treat promptly
MALARIA	Yes	Chills, headache; see HYPOGLYCEMIA
DIPHTHERIA	Unusual	Sore throat, trouble with eyes/throat
RELAPSING FEVER	Yes	Body LICE or a history of camping or poor housing; tropical and high altitude
DENGUE FEVER	Yes	Rapid-onset, severe bone and muscle and eye pains; mainly Asia
RABIES	Maybe	Limb paralysis or muscle spasms with swallowing
Likely prominent pain in back and limbs, maybe fever		
BRUCELLOSIS	Off /On	Back pains, joint pains, fatigue, night sweats
KIDNEY STONES	Unlikely	Very sudden onset flank and/or genital pain
FILARIASIS	Off /On	Some neighbors have very swollen limb(s).
TETANUS	Off /On	Severe muscle spasms, variable pulse rate
Likely prominent pain in trunk (chest/abdomen)		
AMEBIASIS	Usual	Pain, right upper abdomen
HEART ATTACK	No	Chest pain, left arm pain or short of breath
Likely no prominent pain but other symptoms involving the trunk		
VISCERAL LEISHMANIASIS[1]	Off /On	Very large spleen, liver large after the third month
PNEUMONIA	Usual	Also a cough and quite ill, rapid onset
TUBERCULOSIS	Usual	Cough, weight loss or both, slow onset
CANCER (lymphoma)	Maybe	Large lymph nodes, ANEMIA, weight loss
Related to an ingestion or exposure		
PLANT POISONING	No	Ackee, botulism, muscarine, nicotine
INSECTICIDE POISONING	No	Heavy exposure or sensitive patient

Protocol A.13.D—Chills

Definition: the patient shivers and complains of being cold when the environment is not cold. Any disease that causes sudden onset of high fevers will also cause chills. Chills are most frequent when the body temperature rises quickly from normal to very high. They also occur with MENOPAUSE in which case there usually is no fever. Except for the chills associated with MENOPAUSE, it is important to find the fever pattern, if any, before starting symptomatic treatment. Take the patient's temperature every 2 hours around the clock for at least 3 days, noting on the record sheet when he has chills and/or sweats. VISCERAL LEISHMANIASIS[5] might cause daily chills in spite of the fever never being really high.

Protocol A.13.E—Generalized bleeding

Definition: the patient has nosebleeds, persistent bleeding from minor injuries, bleeding gums, excessive menstrual bleeding and positive tests for blood in stool and urine.

With a recent onset fever, consider HEMORRHAGIC FEVER, EBOLA VIRUS DISEASE; see Protocol B.2. Other causes with a recent-onset fever are DENGUE FEVER, TYPHUS, RELAPSING FEVER and LEPTOSPIROSIS. With a distended abdomen, consider LIVER FAILURE. This may be due to a genetic defect in an infant or preschooler. Consider CANCER. With a poor diet, consider SCURVY; in Africa south of the equator, consider ONYALAI.

---

1 *Visceral Leishmaniasis: found in scattered areas of Central and South America, Africa north of the equator, the Mediterranean area, the Indian subcontinent, eastern Europe, central Asia and mainland China.*

III—SKIN PROBLEMS

VOCABULARY OF SKIN PROBLEMS: ENGLISH VS. MEDICAL TERMINOLOGY

English	Medicalese	Protocol	Definition
Spot	Macule	A.14	A portion of skin that is a different color from the surrounding skin, less than 5 mm in diameter on the average. They are seen but can't be felt.
Spot	Maculopapule	A.14	Skin that is a different color and raised above the level of normal skin, less than 5 mm in diameter on the average, both seen and felt.
Bump	Papule	A.14	A bit of skin that is raised up from the surrounding skin, less than 1 cm in diameter; one can feel that it is different than normal skin, felt more than seen.
Lump	Nodule	A.14	Raised up, more than 1 cm diameter, the skin on top is intact.
Cyst	Cyst	A.14	Like a lump/nodule but one can feel a firm sphere beneath the skin.
Blob	——	A.14	A raised area, more than 1 cm diameter, bumpy on top but with a smooth, not rough, surface texture, like a bit of mashed potato on the skin.
Wart	Plaque	A.15	Raised up, flat and rough on top, possibly with scales.
Hive[1]	Wheal	A.15	Raised up; relatively flat and smooth skin on top; itchy.
Small blister	Vesicle	A.15	Raised and watery inside, less than 5 mm diameter.
Big blister	Bulla	A.15	Raised and watery inside, more than 5 mm diameter.
Scale	Scale	A.15	Dried, attached little pieces of dead skin.
Crust	Crust	A.15	Dried secretions (gunk) on the skin, some yellowish color.
Patch	Macule	A.16	A portion of skin that is a different color from the surrounding skin, more than 5 mm in diameter on the average; one cannot feel it.
Bruise, purple	Purpura	A.16	Bleeding into the skin, purplish at first, then changes colors.
Red	Erythema	A.16	In non-black skin, color change; in black skin, warmth.
Scab	Eschar	A.17	A black crust like one that forms on a wound before healing with a halo.
Ulcer	Ulcer	A.17	A crater with the skin surface absent and a raw center.

1 Hive implies that the problem is due to allergy and that it is itchy. If something looks like hives but is not due to allergy and is not itchy, it will be called hive-like in this manual.

PROTOCOL A.14—SKIN SPOTS, BUMPS AND LUMPS

A.14.A—Red spots with a fever

A.14.B—Red rashes, lumps and bumps; no fever

A.14.C—Skin bumps, not red, fever present

A.14.D—Skin bumps, not red, maybe fever

A.14.E—Skin bumps, not red, no fever

Protocol A.14.A—Red spots with a fever

Red spots, not bumpy; fever plus measles-type red rash: quick differential.[1]

- *Rash affects the palms and soles:* spotted fever, typhus, syphilis (secondary).
- *Fever and feeling ill* before the rash: typhus, enteric fever, spotted fever, fifth disease, dengue fever, measles, rubella (older children and adults), tularemia, chikungunya fever, arboviral fever.
- *Fever and rash appear together*: rubella (small children), meningitis.
- *First "flu" symptoms*, then fever, then rash: typhus; maybe enteric fever.
- *Mental changes*: spotted fever, meningitis, enteric fever, typhus, arboviral fever (some kinds), dengue fever (depression).
- *Rash is itchy*: swimmer's itch and seabather's eruption (very itchy); dengue fever; typhus (after a while); syphilis, secondary (African genetic heritage); chikungunya fever; any rash that peels is likely to be itchy at that time.
- *Body odor*: enteric fever (baked bread), typhus (musty), rubella (feathers).

Codes used in the following table

Sickness designation (How ill?): N = not sick; S = slightly sick (less active than usual); M = moderately sick; V = very sick.

Rash designation: B = begins; S = spreads from there to—; H = heaviest; L = lightest, there are parts of the body not affected or lightly affected; M = maybe.

RED SPOTTED RASH WITH A FEVER: THE SPOTS, SMALLER THAN PIMPLES, ARE ALL SIMILAR IN APPEARANCE.

Condition How ill	Rash	Who	History	Specific[1] symptoms
Likely to be multiple cases				
STREP INFECTION S To M	B: neck; S: trunk and limbs; H: skin folds; L: around mouth	Anyone, more children than adults.	Sore throat only or belly pain; tongue rash, red & white.	Red tonsils or a tender abdomen; redness disappears with pressure at first.
MEASLES M to V	B: head; S: trunk and limbs; starts day 3	Unimmunized children.	Sore eyes, cough, runny nose first.	Spots coalesce. There are spots in the mouth.
CHIKUNGUNYA M to V	Measles-like	Worldwide tropical.	Epidemics	Severe joint pains, headache.
MENINGITIS M to V	B: pressure points S: everywhere, sizes vary; red, blistery, bluish	Anyone, mainly young, in epidemics.	Sudden onset, severe headache; children vomit.	Unconscious, stiff neck or both, maybe seizures; vomiting is invariable in children.
Multiple cases unlikely				
SYPHILIS (secondary) N to S	B: trunk and face; S: limbs; M: palms soles symmetrical	Mostly sexually mature.	Incubation 2–24 weeks; maybe "flu" symptoms.	Variable; maybe moist "warts", maybe hair loss, fatigue and joint pains.
SYPHILIS (congenital) N to S	Varies; symmetry usual; involves palms and soles	Birth to 2 years.	One or both parents unfaithful; likely miscarried sibling(s).	Variable; maybe like secondary above; maybe blistery or peeling.
MONONUCLEOSIS S to M	Unknown symmetrical	Mostly children and teenagers.	Patient had a fever and severe fatigue.	Swollen tonsils with white on them; swollen lymph nodes or spleen.

Table continues on the next page.

---

1 *In this listing conditions are not in upper case and there are no geographic footnotes. Otherwise the formatting would have been impossible.*

RED SPOTTED RASH WITH A FEVER CONTINUED

Condition How ill	Rash	Who	History	Specific[1] symptoms
History of outdoor activity				
SPOTTED FEVER (Americas) M To V	B: ankles, forearms, day 1–5; S: trunk, palms, soles	Outdoor activity; ticks.	Fever for 1-5 days before the rash.	Maybe a little scab; spleen large and firm.
SPOTTED FEVER (Eastern Hemisphere) M To V	B: limbs day 4 or 5; H: wrists and ankles, M: palms & soles	Outdoor activity.	Tick bite, muscle pains, vomiting, mental changes.	One or more little scab(s).
TULAREMIA M To V	B: site of insect bite; S: red lumps spread to trunk;	Children, hunters.	Small mammal contact, temperate areas.	Small scab with a red ring around it; large lymph nodes.
Peculiar body odor				
RUBELLA N to M	B: face/trunk; S: face/trunk clear; H: on limbs	Infants: rash and fever together.[2]	Joint pains in older patients; aching all over.	Body odor like feathers.
ENTERIC FEVER M to V	White skin only; few; trunk only; "freckles"	Anyone; poor sanitation, not immunized.	Onset over days; belly pain; headache.	Acts withdrawn, abdomen tender and quiet, body odor is like fresh bread.
TYPHUS M to V	B: waist and armpits, 3rd to 7th day; S: trunk and limbs; L: face	Anyone, especially the poor.	Mental symptoms, headache, constipated.	Musty body odor; can't stick out tongue.

1 These symptoms are not necessarily sensitive; not finding them does not eliminate the diagnosis.
2 Older children and adults feel ill and have a fever before the rash breaks out. For all ages the rash lasts for 3 days—hence the name, "three-day measles".

RED SKIN CONDITIONS WITH FEVERS: LUMPS, BUMPS, AREAS, WHITE-ON-RED

Condition How ill	Rash	Who	History	Specific[3] symptoms
DENGUE FEVER M to V	Unknown but affects the forearms; begins days 8–11.	Mostly children & expatriates; epidemics; tropical areas.	Severe bone pains, high fever drops, then rises.	Previous rashes; this rash in fair skin is red with white dots on it.
ERYTHEMA NODOSUM[1] S to V	Lower legs, maybe the arms, tender to touch, color changes.	Mostly young females.	History of some other infection or medication.	Multiple red lumps, tender, under the skin of the shins.
ERYTHEMA MULTIFORME S to V	B: limbs, symmetrical S; anywhere, may be near large joints.	Anyone.	History of infection, taking some drug or toxin exposure.	Some target-like red areas, lasts at least 7 days.
SERUM SICKNESS S to V	Anywhere or everywhere.	Mostly Whites; from some diseases or drugs.[2]	Fever plus an itchy rash resembling hives.	Areas of skin are red and swollen or very pale; this may cause arthritis.
TULAREMIA M to V	B: site of bite; S: red lumps between bite and trunk; no general rash.	Children, hunters.	Small mammal contact, temperate areas.	Small scab with a red ring around it; large lymph nodes.

1 This is medicalese for red lumps. They are usually 1 cm or more in diameter.
2 Katayama disease is a kind that comes from exposure to schistosomes. Sulfa drugs are the main offenders drug-wise.
3 These symptoms are not necessarily sensitive; not finding them does not eliminate the diagnosis.

SYMPTOMS

DIFFERENTIALS

CONDITIONS

DRUG INDEX

REGIONAL NOTES

INX

TOC

RED RASHES: CIRCLES, TARGETS OR IRREGULAR RED PATCHES ON NON-BLACK SKIN; MAYBE FEVER

Condition	Characteristics	Who gets it	History	Exam
No whole-body illness likely at this time				
AFRICAN SLEEPING SICKNESS[1]	Raised, red, painful skin area.	East Africa: game parks; West Africa.	Bite of a dive-bombing fly.	Maybe large lymph nodes.
LEPROSY	Mostly limbs and head/neck.	Residence in an affected area.	Sharp-shooting pains and maybe weakness.	Loss of sensation (cold/hot and light touch).
CELLULITIS	Red only, smooth, irregular area, maybe swelling.	Anyone, esp. those with poor immunity.	Maybe a minor injury.	Area tender; large lymph nodes, maybe fever.
General, whole-body illness is likely, along with the rash				
LYME DISEASE	B: site of bite; red spot expands to become a doughnut or target more than 1 cm in diameter.	Those outdoors in temperate climates, from tick bites.	Most forget tick bite but there is a history of outdoor activity.	Initially not sick; most often thigh, groin or trunk; sick later on.
TUBERCULOSIS	Rough and crusty.	Exposure to a coughing adult.	Active tuberculosis or exposure to TB.	May find evidence of active TB.
RHEUMATIC FEVER	Circles and rings, raised up above skin surface, on trunk and upper limbs., Changes over hours.	Those with untreated strep infection.	Sore throat, abdominal pain or a fine red rash with a fever.	Possibly arthritis, a heart murmur or little lumps under the skin.
SYPHILIS (congenital)	Bright red, slightly raised, spots or circles.	Less than 2 years old.	History of parental syphilis, miscarriages or infant deaths.	Usually large liver/spleen, not healthy.
DRUG ERUPTION	Trunk and limbs, symmetrical, very itchy, changes in size and location.	Those taking phenytoin, dapsone, allopurinol, sulfa, anti-HIV drugs.	Patient began the drug 2 days to 8 weeks previously.	Maybe fever, facial swelling and large tender lymph nodes.

1 *African sleeping sickness occurs in sub-Saharan African, in scattered areas, north of Lusaka, Zambia.*

Protocol A.14.B—Red spots, lumps and bumps; no fever

Also consider conditions listed as being with a fever if the patient is elderly, malnourished or has waning immunity from HIV infection or cancer. He may not show a fever when he should.

Condition	Itch Where	Who/Characteristics
Patient is otherwise ill but without a fever		
LIVER FAILURE	Not usually. Trunk.	Red spots with wiggly lines radiating out—appear like tiny red spiders.
ONCHOCERCIASIS[1]	Yes! Unknown.	Fair skin only; also back and joint pains; maybe eye symptoms. History of being in an affected area.
SYPHILIS congenital	No. Whole-body.	Infants of syphilitic mother; large liver/spleen, maybe "cold" symptoms, limb problems, misshapen skull, other ill health.

Table continues on the next page.

1 *Onchocerciasis: present in scattered area in Africa, in the Americas north of the Amazon, in Yemen and Saudi Arabia.*

RED SPOTS, LUMPS AND BUMPS, NO FEVER, CONTINUED

Condition	Itches where	Characteristics
Immediately after swimming, very sudden onset over minutes to an hour or two; otherwise healthy		
SWIMMER'S ITCH	Whole-body, itches much.	After swimming in fresh water where there are water birds, bird schistosomes (worm larvae) burrow into the skin.
SEABATHER'S ERUPTION	Whole-body, itches much.	After swimming in salt water, there is an immediate very itchy red rash, mainly on clothing pressure points.
Onset less than a day, otherwise healthy		
SCABIES	Itches, first fingers, toes, waist.	Itching before any red spots; B: web spaces, waist, joints; S: all over; L: face; Ink rubbed on and then wiped off shows little lines between the spots.
CONTACT DERMATITIS	Yes, area touched by something.	Spots and roughening of the skin in an area that touched some liquid or solid to which the person is allergic; people who have other allergies are vulnerable.
Bedbug bites See Volume 1, Appy 10	Maybe itches.	Bedbugs are usually not seen. If many, the room may have an acrid odor. The red spots appear upon arising and then fade during the day.
Flea bites See Volume 1, Appy 10	Maybe itches, anywhere.	Small, black, jumping creatures are seen occasionally. Fleas like some people and not others.
HOOKWORM & LARVA MIGRANS	Itches, skin that touched soil.	There are raised spots or lines in part(s) of the body that touched soil, usually the toe web-spaces—areas where there is poor sanitation.
STRONGYLOIDIASIS	Itching by anus.	Red, wiggly lines are under the skin, near the anus or on the buttocks.
MYIASIS	May itch. Exposed skin.	A countable number of discrete, large spots, maybe itch or painful, places touched by damp cloth where a fly laid its egg; the larvae burrowed into the skin.
Onset more than a day, otherwise healthy		
CANDIDIASIS	Itches; sweaty areas.	Below breasts, groin, armpits. An area of red, spotted, swollen skin has satellite red dots around it.
CUTANEOUS LEISHMANIASIS	Minimal itching if any, exposed skin.	Slow-onset, over weeks, skin may itch or hurt but not intensely; does not change rapidly over days, only over weeks. Appearance varies; may be bumps or open sores. Present in scattered tropical and subtropical areas north of the equator.
DONOVANOSIS	No itching.	Genital area; beefy-red cauliflower-like surfaces.

Protocol A.14.C—Skin bumps, not-red, fever

Condition	Itch/Pain Body part	Color	Other characteristics
RHEUMATIC FEVER	Neither By joints	Skin.	Pea-sized; recent history of symmetrical, red swollen joints; maybe a heart murmur.
AIDS/CANCER	No Anywhere	Blue/black/ red/skin	A CANCER associated with HIV; commonly a cauliflower-type surface, 1–3 bumps only.
RAT BITE FEVER	Neither Chest/arms	Purple	Look like warts; mainly Asia; maybe a history of a rat bite which may have healed initially.

Protocol A.14.D—Skin bumps, not-red, maybe fever

Condition	Itch/Pain Body part	Color	Other characteristics Size relative to ordinary pimples (medium)
ABSCESS	Pain Anywhere	Skin or reddish	Swollen area, tender to touch; changes slowly over days, becoming softer; more than 1 cm diameter; 1–2 bumps only.
RHEUMATOID ARTHRITIS	Neither Limbs	Skin	Not tender, no discoloration, intact normal skin; large; the size of cherry or apricot pits.

Table continues on the next page.

SKIN BUMPS, NOT-RED, MAYBE FEVER, CONTINUED

Condition	Itch/Pain Body part	Color	Other characteristics
LEPROSY	Neither Cool parts[1]	Skin or slightly reddish	Develop slowly; innumerable bumps resembling cobblestones or bunches of tiny grapes; small to large; roughly symmetrical.
PKDL	Neither Anywhere	Skin reddish or pale	Same as leprosy, indistinguishable, but the patient was treated for visceral Leishmaniasis; small to large; mainly face and genitals.
HIV INFECTION	Itch Forearms[2]	Skin greyish	About 2–4 mm across, watery inside, look like small warts or molluscum contagiosum; discreet and countable; medium size.
ERYTHEMA MULTIFORME	Unknown; usually limbs first; spreads.	Purple outer ring of target areas.	Develops over hours to days, resolves over weeks; much larger than ordinary pimples—coin-sized.
BARTONELLOSIS	Unknown Face/limbs	Purple	Only Peru and adjacent countries; also severe joint pains; patient had a fever which dropped; skin bumps the size of pimples or larger.
YAWS	Neither Exposed skin	Off-white	Humid tropics only; cauliflower-type surface; at first one sore which heals and then many break out; large, some raised, some craters.
BRUCELLOSIS	Unknown Unknown	Skin or purplish	Gradual-onset general body pains and feeling awful; episodic fevers.
AFRICAN SLEEPING SICKNESS[3]	Maybe pain at the site of fly bite, 1–6 weeks after.[2]	Dark halo, skin-color swelling.	Swelling or target areas of various configurations; flies that transmit this are dive-bombers.

1 *The skin bumps themselves are not painful, but the patient may have sharp, shooting pains in the general area. The outer ears are almost always affected; hands and feet are commonly affected; genitals almost never are affected.*

2 *Perhaps pain elsewhere also*

3 *African sleeping sickness occurs in sub-Saharan African, in scattered areas, north of Lusaka, Zambia.*

Protocol A.14.E—Skin bumps, not-red, no fever

Condition	Itch/pain Body part	Color	Other characteristics/size relative to pimples
Wart-like, tiny, cylindrical blobs or plaques on top of the skin			
WARTS	Neither Face/limbs	Skin or greyish	Rough top; hard and dry-looking; no center hole; number varies; medium-large.
MOLLUSCUM CONTAGIOSUM	Neither Face/limbs	Skin or greyish	Just like warts but there is a center hole in some; number varies/medium-large; insides cheesy.
TREPONARID	Itch? Exposed skin	Skin or whitish	Look like moist warts; small to large; arid tropics only, with poor sanitation.
SYPHILIS tertiary/congenital	Neither Varies	Skin	Slow-growing lumps under the skin; mostly sexually mature; incubation 10+ years; may break open to become ulcer(s).
Long and wiggly, under the skin			
VARICOSE VEINS	Neither Legs	Bluish	Soft lumpy lines, more than 2 mm in diameter, under the skin; disappear with raising the legs; diameter like licorice sticks; legs ache.
LARVA MIGRANS	Itch Soil exposed	Varies; maybe red	Diameter 2 mm or less; does not disappear with elevation; end moves slowly; mark with a pen and recheck in 2 hours.

Table continues on the next page.

TOC

SYMPTOMS

DIFFERENTIALS

CONDITIONS

DRUG INDEX

REGIONAL NOTES

INX

SKIN BUMPS, NOT-RED, NO FEVER, CONTINUED

Condition	Itch/Pain Body part	Color	Other characteristics
Blobs or lumps, irregular surfaces; some small coin-size or larger			
DONOVANOSIS	Neither Sexual contact	Varies	1-2 areas; scar tissue; large; mainly found in ports, along transport routes; prevalent in the Pacific area.
KELOID	Neither Scar	Skin +/−	Hard, lumpy, excessive scar tissue at the site of any old injury, even very minor; size varies but may be large.
MYCETOMA	Unknown Feet	Skin; black or colored grains.	Slow-onset of swelling; large; looks bad but pain is minimal; arid areas only; history of a thorn injury is common.
PLANT POISONING, argemone oil	Unknown Unknown	Bluish	Coin-shaped and sized; bleed readily when disturbed.
CUTANEOUS LEISHMANIASIS[1]	Either[2] Exposed skin	Varies	One or few spots or areas, usually large, maybe an satellite spots; maybe like warts; geographically confined.
CANCER skin type, melanoma	Neither initially Anywhere	Varies	Slow-onset, usually over weeks to months, commonly with loss of appetite; commonly the color is dark or mixed colors.
Blobs, bumps or lumps, irregular surfaces, smaller than coin-size			
TUNGIASIS	Both Nails/webs	Black/white	Small, spherical pea-size bumps burrow under nails; small-medium.
Skin surface smooth, not discolored or disrupted			
ONCHOCERCIASIS[3]	Neither Head/trunk	Skin	Peaked bumps; countable; insides feel lumpy; skin is rough and itchy. The peaked lumps don't especially itch.
CYSTICERCOSIS	Neither Under skin	Skin	Firm, small pea-size under the skin; small to medium; history of consuming pork or having a pork-consuming kitchen maid.
LOIASIS	Pain? Anywhere	Skin	Large swellings come and go; humid central and western Africa, may be itchy.
HYDATID DISEASE	Neither Under skin	Skin	Lump feels like a water balloon; comes and stays; large; arid tropics with dogs or northern, temperate forested areas.
LIPOMA	Anywhere	Skin	Slow onset, fatty, very soft, totally non-painful and non-tender; definite margins, size from a cherry to an apple.

1 Cutaneous Leishmaniasis: not in Southeast Asia or Pacific area; elsewhere present in scattered areas only, only north of the equator.

2 They might itch or hurt but neither the itching nor hurting is intense; it is more just irritation.

3 Onchocerciasis: present in scattered area in Africa, in the Americas north of the Amazon, in Yemen and Saudi Arabia.

PROTOCOL A.15 BLISTERING, ROUGH, SCALING, PEELING SKIN

15.A—Severe Itching; rough, scaling, peeling   15.B—Rough, scaling, peeling, mild or no itching

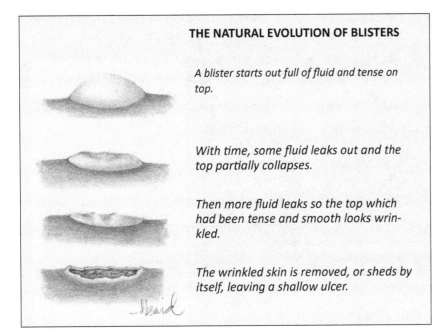

THE NATURAL EVOLUTION OF BLISTERS

A blister starts out full of fluid and tense on top.

With time, some fluid leaks out and the top partially collapses.

Then more fluid leaks so the top which had been tense and smooth looks wrinkled.

The wrinkled skin is removed, or sheds by itself, leaving a shallow ulcer.

⚠ EMERGENCY

BLISTER EMERGENCIES

Blood blisters: consider CELLULITIS, ONYALAI (southern Africa), HEMORRHAGIC FEVER

Sudden onset of huge blisters with peeling skin: consider SEPSIS, DRUG ERUPTION, MENINGITIS

Sudden onset of an uncountable number of blisters with fever and body pain: consider SMALLPOX, MONKEYPOX (central Africa)

Protocol A.15.A—Severe Itching[1]; rough, scaling, peeling

▷ SYMPTOMATIC TREATMENT

Calamine lotion helps but for just a little while. Try very warm water which will increase the itching—then rub the affected area vigorously with a rough Turkish towel. Thereafter put cold packs on the area. The itching will be relieved for a matter of a couple of hours. Reportedly alternatives are oatmeal baths, hydrocortisone cream or chlorpromazine (by mouth).

Abbreviations: E = early in the course of the illness. L = later in the course of the illness

Condition	Blisters	Flaking	Swelling	Other
Probably no whole-body illness				
SCABIES	No	Maybe	No	Very itchy; E web spaces; never face.
CANDIDIASIS	No	Maybe	Some	Sweaty skin; red center with red spots around.
Burns	E Yes	Usual	Usual	Itching with healing; history of a burn.
TINEA	No	Yes	Maybe	Round/oval areas or mottled.
CONTACT DERMATITIS	Maybe	Unusual	Usual	A defined area that touched something.
ECZEMA	No	Yes	Maybe	Usually hands or face; allergy in family, affluent.
ONCHOCERCIASIS[2]	No	Yes	Maybe	Bumps under skin; hilly areas near streams, tropical.
PINTA	No	Yes	Some	Americas only; rare; appearance variable.
SEABATHER'S ERUPTION	Maybe	Maybe	Yes	Immediately after salt water swimming.
SHINGLES	Yes	No	No	Also painful. maybe itchy, in a band if on the trunk.

Table continues on the next page.

---

1 *The amount of itching varies between people. Generally black skin is more itchy than fair skin, but there is a lot of individual variation.*

2 *Onchocerciasis: present in scattered area in Africa, in the Americas north of the Amazon, in Yemen and Saudi Arabia.*

TOC

SYMPTOMS

DIFFERENTIALS

CONDITIONS

DRUG INDEX

REGIONAL NOTES

INX

Condition	Blisters	Flaking	Swelling	Other
Has a whole-body illness, recent onset				
CHICKEN POX	Yes	Late	No	Fever; epidemics; E trunk; some heal while others start.
MONKEYPOX	Yes! E	Late	Some	Fever; only humid central and western Africa.
DENGUE FEVER[4]	No	Yes	Maybe	Sudden onset; severe bone pains; tropics only.
PLANT POISONING, atriplicism	Yes	Late	Maybe	Fingers turn pale and ache; Chinese traditional medicine.
CHIKUNGUNYA FEVER	Maybe	Maybe	Yes	Severe joint pains; epidemic context; worldwide.
Has a whole-body illness, probably remote and/or gradual onset				
KIDNEY DISEASE	No	Yes	No[1]	High blood pressure or abnormal urine dipstick.
LIVER FAILURE	No	Yes	No[2]	Swollen abdomen or yellowish eyes.
AFRICAN SLEEPING SICKNESS[3]	No	Yes	No	Abnormal sleep pattern; weight loss; headaches.

1 *The skin is not swollen but the face, legs and feet are.*
2 *No swelling of the skin but there is general body swelling, especially the abdomen.*
3 *African sleeping sickness: scattered areas in Africa between 15° north and 20° south.*
4 *Dengue fever: in the Americas only near or north of the equator. In Africa, east coastal, south and west. Prevalent in India, Southeast Asia and the Pacific. Occasionally found in the Mediterranean area. The disease may spread.*

Protocol A.15.B—Rough, scaling, peeling, mild or no itching

Abbreviations: E = early in the course of the illness. L = later in the course of the illness

Condition	Blisters	Flaking	Swelling	Other
Maybe blisters				
STD	Maybe	Maybe	Occasional	HERPES, LYMPHOGRANULOMA VENEREUM.
IMPETIGO	Maybe	Yes	Some	Irregular areas, some yellowish crusts.
MEASLES	Rare	Much	Some	Dark skin peels.
GANGRENE	Maybe	Late	Usual	Skin cool, looks dead.
REITER SYNDROME	Maybe	No	Yes	Palms, soles, scalp, other.
HEAT ILLNESS	Maybe	No	Little	General, sand-papery rash; sweaty body parts.
SYPHILIS, congenital	Maybe	Yes	Maybe	Babies born to syphilitic mothers.
MALNUTRITION	Unusual	Yes	Usual	Skin like peeling paint.
HAND-FOOT-MOUTH DISEASE	Yes	Unknown	Unknown	Hairy side of hand, tender, red halos, resolves by itself within a week.
Rough only, no blisters; likely no whole-body illness				
TINEA	No	Yes	Maybe	Round or oval areas; patient is not sick.
FILARIASIS	No	Maybe	Yes!	Onset slow, over months; locally common.
CUTANEOUS LEISHMANIASIS[1]	No	Yes	Maybe	Unclothed skin only; usually discolored.
DONOVANOSIS	No	No	Yes	Rough swollen area, sexually ransmitted.
MOSSY FOOT	No	Maybe	Yes!	Patient walked barefoot over reddish clay soil.
YAWS, tertiary	No	Yes	Yes!	Palms/soles skin very thick and splits open.
LEPROSY, tuberculoid	No	Yes	Maybe	Numbness, sharp pains.
PINTA	No	Yes	Some	Americas only.
ECZEMA	No	Yes	Maybe	Family history of allergy; relatively affluent.

1 *Cutaneous Leishmaniasis: tropical and subtropical north of the equator, but not present in Southeast Asia or the Pacific areas.*

Condition		Blisters	Flaking	Swelling	Other
Blisters, likely significant whole-body illness					
SPOTTED FEVER	Rickettsial pox	Yes	??	??	Blisters are a countable number, not innumerable.
	MENINGITIS	Maybe	Yes	Maybe	Bisters large, patient very ill.
	MONKEYPOX	Yes!	Yes	Yes	Many blisters, central African context.
	HERPES	Yes	Yes	Probably	Very painful, probably genital.
	GONORRHEA	Yes	??	??	Relatively few; history of sexual risk factor(s).
No blisters; likely there is a whole-body illness					
	ARSENIC POISONING	No	Yes	Maybe	Dry, scaly, flaky skin.
	EXFOLIATIVE DERMATITIS	No	Yes!	Maybe	Skin peels off in large amounts.
	PELLAGRA	No	Yes!	Maybe	Symmetrical; sun-exposed, malnourished.
	SCURVY	No	Yes	No	Dry, rough skin with dark spots on it.
	KIDNEY DISEASE	No	Yes	Face and lower limbs	High blood pressure and/or abnormal urine dipstick.

PROTOCOL A.16—SKIN COLOR CHANGES

16.A—Skin color fairer than normal

16.B—Skin color darker than normal

16.C—Reddish skin

16.D—Other skin color changes

Protocol A.16.A—Skin color fairer than normal

The most common cause is scar on naturally dark skin. Examples would be burns or diaper rash. The skin will heal lighter than normal; it may darken over time. Some lighter patches of skin in the center line of the body are normal in those of African and Latino genetic heritage. A person who is generally pale without being cool and sweaty is likely to have ANEMIA, TUBERCULOSIS or MALNUTRITION. If the skin is pale and cool and (maybe) sweaty, see SHOCK, HEART ATTACK, PLANT POISONING due to claviceps or ergot. If the problem is confined to the limb(s), see FROSTBITE, GANGRENE.

PATCHES OF SKIN ARE PALE:

Condition	Itchy	Shape	Distinct[1]	Other
TINEA	Yes	Round or oval	Fairly distinct	Gradual onset, maybe slightly roughened.
VITILIGO	No	Very irregular	Very distinct	Symmetrical on neck and below;[2] like normal fair skin.
LEPROSY tuberculoid	No	Round or irregular	Varies	Can't feel touch or can't distinguish cold & hot on the pale patches.
ONCHOCERCIASIS[3]	Yes	Irregular	Yes	Whole-body itchy; maybe eye trouble; hilly areas.
PKDL	No	Unknown	Unknown	After treatment for VISCERAL LEISHMANIASIS; especially face and genitals.
Scar	Not much	Variable	Yes	Normally dark skin temporarily turns fair with scarring.

1 That is, the transition from normally colored skin to discolored skin is at a definite line so that two observers would agree where it is.

2 It is not necessarily symmetrical on the face.

3 Onchocerciasis: present in scattered area in Africa, in the Americas north of the Amazon, in Yemen and Saudi Arabia.

PALE BODY PARTS OR WHOLE BODY PALE

ANEMIA	Pale tongue and fingernails; either from poor diet or else from abnormal blood loss (menstruation, stool or injury); rapid pulse.
TUBERCULOSIS	Slow-onset; yellowish tinge to the skin; weight loss; frequently a chronic cough.
MALNUTRITION	Poor diet, weight loss; overlaps with TB and ANEMIA. Only dark skin becomes light; fair skin becomes dark with malnutrition.
HEMOSIDEROSIS	Greyish skin color, hereditary or from iron pots; due to excess iron.
IMMERSION FOOT	Limb(s) exposed to cold and/or wet; pain or numbness.

Protocol A.16.B—Skin color darker than normal

Dark colored nails, either lines on the nails or entire nails, is common in those of African genetic heritage.

Usually no fever

MONGOLIAN SPOT	Healthy child; buttocks and back of some brown-skinned people—looks like bruising but symmetrical and doesn't change over time.
MALABSORPTION	Causes MALNUTRITION and therefore darkening of fair skin.
ONCHOCERCIASIS[1]	In Arabs with medium-dark skin; not in black skin. There is whole-body itching.
CHAGA'S DISEASE	Scattered areas in the Americas; a swollen area of the body has a bruised appearance.
CANCER (skin)	Black or multicolored discoloration, mostly in fair skin; slow onset.
VISCERAL LEISHMANIASIS,[2] PKDL	After treatment for VL, nationals develop darkening of the skin, mostly on the face.

Related to an ingestion, no fever

PLANT POISONING	Argemone oil; dark spots on the skin , especially south Asians; these spots bleed easily. There is swelling and maybe a fever.
ARSENIC POISONING	Also numbness, tingling and weakness of limbs; homicidal, occupational or from ethnic remedies.

Related to a poor diet, no fever

ANEMIA	Anemia due to vitamin deficiency, either FOLIC ACID or VITAMIN B_{12}, may cause skin darkening.
COBALAMIN DEFICIENCY	Patient is vegan (eats no animal products), or European genetic heritage and has been for the past three years.
SCURVY	Diet devoid of fresh fruits and vegetables; bleeding into the skin and also bleeding gums with loose teeth.
MALNUTRITION	Generally darkening in fair skin.
PELLAGRA	Dark discoloration with a bit of roughening; usually poor diet.

Fever is present, and the patient is very ill

PLAGUE	Dark discoloration over firm, enlarged, very tender lymph nodes.
HEMORRHAGIC FEVER	Very ill; spontaneous bruising; may be small or large areas.
GANGRENE[3]	Usually fingers or toes; skin appears dry, dark and dead.
MENINGITIS	Very ill; bleeding into skin which may form blisters and peel.
RELAPSING FEVER	Tiny black and blue marks; fevers last for a matter of days and then disappear.

---

1 *Onchocerciasis: present in scattered area in Africa, in the Americas north of the Amazon, in Yemen and Saudi Arabia.*

2 *Visceral Leishmaniasis: found in scattered areas of Central and South America, (mainly eastern) Africa north of the equator, the Mediterranean area, the Indian subcontinent, eastern Europe, central Asia and mainland China.*

3 *The patient may not be very ill if only a small portion of his body, like a finger tip, has gangrene.*

TOC

SYMPTOMS

DIFFERENTIALS

CONDITIONS

DRUG INDEX

REGIONAL NOTES

INX

Protocol A.16 continued | *Village Medical Manual 7th Edition Volume 2* | **A-63**
CHAPTER PAGE

SYMPTOMS

TOC

DIFFERENTIALS

CONDITIONS

DRUG INDEX

REGIONAL NOTES

INX

Protocol A.16.C—Reddish skin

If the skin is fair or brown, then red is usually visible. If it is dark black, then red is not visible, but the area may be warm to the touch. This protocol focuses on red skin over large areas, not just a spot or two. If the red area consists of many fine spots that merge, see Protocol A.14. Also see Protocol A.21.E if the face is involved. For red areas of skin or red rings with pale centers, see Protocol A.14.A.

Condition	Fever	Characteristics
Previously healthy, recent-onset illness		
ABSCESS	Maybe	Redness over a swollen, tender area below.
Sunburn	Unusual	History of sun exposure.
CELLULITIS	Maybe	Red area, warm, maybe with red streaks, large nodes.
STREP INFECTION	Usually	Fine spotty red rash; pale around lips and eyes.
ROSEOLA	Had one	Fine rash with a drop in fever.
FIFTH DISEASE	Had one	Facial redness develops with a drop in fever; maybe sore joints; children.
DENGUE FEVER[1]	Yes	Early: red rash on white skin; Late: white spots on red skin.
ANTHRAX	Usual	Also extraordinary swelling; possibly a wound.
CARBON MONOXIDE POISON	No	Exposed to exhaust or fire; headache and nausea or vomiting.
EXFOLIATIVE DERMATITIS	Maybe	Initially looks like sunburn before flaking and peeling.
Remote onset or recurrent illness		
PELLAGRA	No	Behind ears and sun-exposed areas of skin; malnourished.
LEPROSY	Maybe	Leprosy reaction during treatment or early leprosy in fair skin.
IMMERSION FOOT	No	Previously white, cold, numb foot becomes red & hot.
FAMILIAL MEDITERRANEAN FEVER[2]	Yes	Skin also swollen and painful, mainly or only below the knees; hereditary in people of Mediterranean genetic heritage.

1 *Dengue fever: in the Americas only near or north of the equator. In Africa, east coastal, south and west. Prevalent in India, Southeast Asia and the Pacific. Occasionally found in the Mediterranean area. The disease may spread.*

2 *Familial Mediterranean fever: this affects persons of Mediterranean genetic heritage such as Jews, Arabs, Turks and Armenians.*

Protocol A.16.D—Other skin color changes

Purple-black areas on the skin; the skin looks dry and dead, or it oozes water: this is a form of GANGRENE that is almost universally fatal unless the patient can be transported to a major hospital promptly.

Purplish areas on the skin, does not look dead: consider NECROTIZING FASCIITIS if there is severe pain and the patient is very sick with a fast-onset illness. Consider that the patient may have abnormal bleeding: Protocol A.13.E.

Purplish, can feel the abnormality without looking: MENINGITIS, GONORRHEA, SPOTTED FEVER (Rocky Mountain, only the Americas), ERYTHEMA MULTIFORME, SMALLPOX, abnormal bleeding: Protocol A.13.E.

Purplish, cannot feel the abnormality without looking. SEPSIS, LIVER FAILURE, SCURVY, recent injury.

Bluish skin color: RESPIRATORY FAILURE, IMMERSION FOOT, some poisonings, METHYLENE BLUE (drug).

Yellow skin color: from some liver or blood problem. See JAUNDICE. Sometimes TUBERCULOSIS can cause this without causing bilirubin in the urine.

Abnormally shiny skin: from BERIBERI or some rare diseases.

A-64
CHAPTER PAGE

Village Medical Manual 7th Edition Volume 2

TOC

SYMPTOMS

DIFFERENTIALS

CONDITIONS

DRUG INDEX

REGIONAL NOTES

INX

PROTOCOL A.17—SKIN BROKEN OPEN

A.17.A—Many small holes or raw skin   A.17.B—One or few skin openings

Abbreviations for the tables below

Fever	M = maybe	Y! = high	Y = yes	U = usually		
Itch/pain	F = at first	L = later	M = maybe	Y = yes	N = no	U = usually
Onset	H = hours	D = days	W = weeks	M = months	Y = years	? = unknown

Protocol A.17.A—Many small holes or raw skin

Condition	Part[1]	Fever	Itch	Pain	Onset	Characteristics
IMPETIGO	Face, Legs	N	N	Sl	H–W	Roughened, scabbed, yellowish crusts.
TUNGIASIS	Digits	No	?	Yes	H–D	White and/or black spots by nails.
MYCETOMA	Feet	N	N	L	W–Y	White, black or colored dry grains visible; area generally swollen.
TUBERCULOSIS	Neck, face, chest	U	N	N	W–M	Lumps or raw areas; lumps may break open. skin drains fluid which crusts.
MYIASIS	Wounds	M	?	U	H–D	Maggots (short, fat 'worms') visible.
YAWS, secondary	Anywhere	N	N	Y	Unknown	Multiple ulcers with pus.
YAWS, tertiary	Feet	N	N	Y	W–M	Thick, cracking skin on soles; hard to walk.

1 That is, the usual body part that is affected; there will be exceptions.

Protocol A.17.B—One or few skin openings

BODY PARTS WITH SEXUAL CONTACT, RECENTLY OR PREVIOUSLY[1]

Condition	Fever	Itch	Pain	Onset	Characteristics
SYPHILIS Primary, genital area	N	N	N	D–W	Round or oval ulcer with swelling below; rolled edges, does not bleed easily.
SYPHILIS Primary, non-genital area	N	N	Usual	D–W	Usually no swelling below; edges may be flat; occurs on hands, lips, etc.
CHANCROID	N	N	Y	D?	Large groin lymph nodes; round or oval ulcer is tender to touch; maybe a red halo.
DONOVANOSIS	N	N	L	W–M	Ragged edges, may smell bad, irregular shape, bleeds easily.
LYMPHOGRANULOMA VENEREUM (LGV), primary/secondary	N	N	M	H–D	Maybe a small ulcer; large groin nodes with a groove down the center along the leg crease(s).
AMEBIC SKIN ULCER	M	N	Y	H–D	Lower trunk or genitals, anus, progresses rapidly.
LYMPHOGRANULOMA VENEREUM tertiary	M	N	Y!	D–W	Painful abnormal holes in genitals and/or lower abdomen.
GONORRHEA	M	N	Y	W–Y	Painful abnormal holes in genitals; history of painful urination.

1 A person engaging in sexual relations is most likely to develop a sore on his, or her genitals. However, usually the mouth, hands and breasts are also involved in such a relationship. These body parts can develop the sores of sexually transmitted diseases. The basic elements in choosing this part of the protocol are the types(s) of sexual activity and the exposure of the body part to human secretions. Consider the time interval between that activity and the appearance of the ulcer vs. the incubation period of the disease. One can have a syphilis ulcer on the lips or gonorrhea infecting the hand.

BODY PARTS WITHOUT SEXUAL CONTACT:

Condition	Part[1]	Itch	Pain	Onset	Characteristics
No fever likely					
TROPICAL ULCER	Legs/ feet	N	U	D–W	Crater, round or oval, sharp edges.
ZINC DEFICIENCY	Old injury	M	M	D–W	Non-healing old injury.
MYIASIS	Old injury	M	Y	H–D	Maggot(s) present.
TUNGIASIS[2]	Nails	M	Y	H	Black/white split peas; skin touched the soil.
AMEBIC SKIN ULCER	Pelvis	N	Y	D–W	Lower trunk and/or genitals; has a discharge.
TUBERCULOSIS, skin	Chest, neck	M	N	W–M	Usually with lung TB; maybe crusts or bumps.
BURULI ULCER	Limbs	M	N	W	Ragged edges which overhang an ulcer crater; swampy tropical areas only.
YAWS	Palms, soles	N	Y	M?	Humid tropics, mostly children; prior history of blobs and ulcers.
GUINEA WORM[9]	Water contact	?	Y!	D–W	Blister which breaks open revealing the end of a very long, skinny worm.
CUTANEOUS LEISHMANIASIS[3]	Exposed	Sl	Sl	W	Unclothed areas of the body; slowly developing bump, ulcer or roughened area.
Maybe fever; maybe whole-body illness					
ABSCESS	Old injury	N	Y	D–W	Initially warm, swollen, firm; then broke open.
YAWS primary/secondary	Trunk/limbs	N	N	D–W	Off-white pus present, some blobs and some ulcers.
DIPHTHERIA	Anywhere	N	Y	?	Blister first; opens to become a skin ulcer; patient ill.
Fever and whole-body illness					
SCRUB TYPHUS[5]	Any	N	M	D	1–3 small black scabs; very ill.
ANTHRAX	Upper body	F	N	H–D	Black center; swelling around.
TULAREMIA[6]	Bitten part	N	N	D	Tiny black scab by insect bite.
SPOTTED FEVER[7]	?	N	N	D	Black scab(s); maybe red halo(s).
CANCRUM ORIS	Face finger	N	Y	H–D	Cheek, chin or sucked digit; black flesh, foul odor; malnourished.
PLAGUE[8]	Anywhere	?	Severe	D	Small scab(s) large, tender lymph nodes with black skin over top; may break open.

1 That is, the part of the body that is usually affected; there are exceptions.
2 Tungiasis: parts of Africa, the Americas and India only.
3 Cutaneous Leishmaniasis: not in Southeast Asia or Pacific area; scattered areas north of the equator elsewhere.
5 Scrub typhus: Indian Subcontinent, Southeast Asia, central Asia and the Pacific areas.
6 Tularemia: temperate areas; persons exposed to small animals or their insects.
7 Spotted fever: in the Americas there is likely to be one scab; in Africa and the Mediterranean areas there are likely to be multiple scabs.
   Spotted fever in these two locations are very different diseases.
8 Plague: those exposed to rodents or their fleas.
9 Guinea worm: scattered within Africa and the Middle East only; where there are wells into which people step to draw water.

TOC
SYMPTOMS
DIFFERENTIALS
CONDITIONS
DRUG INDEX
REGIONAL NOTES
INX

PROTOCOL A.18—CREATURES IN, ON, OR UNDER THE SKIN

Condition	Size/Shape	Where	Characteristics
Itchy, no movement felt, no creature visible			
SCABIES	Microscopic; ovals with legs.	First web spaces or other soft skin.	Red, itchy spots; ink rubbed on & off leaves lines.
Itchy, visible creature seen and felt moving on the skin, not under			
LICE	Small commas.	Hairs, head or body; seams of clothing.	Small but visible; may be seen moving; eggs attached to hairs.
ENTEROBIASIS	Around 0.5 cm like tiny pieces of thread.	Rectum, vagina.	White color; seen moving at night or on awakening.
MYIASIS	Under 0.5 cm usually, many are worm-shape.[1]	Injuries and pink, moist parts.	Look like short, fat "worms", might be seen moving.
TRICHURIASIS	Coiled with tail; visible, partly a spiral.	Near the rectum.	Coiled, whitish worms on the pink, moist surface.
TAPEWORM	Size of holes from a paper punch but squarish.	Near rectum.	Small, whitish rectangles like confetti visible; nothing that looks wormy.
Not itchy; white, red or dark creatures on the skin visible with magnification			
TUNGIASIS	Tiny split peas, the size of small pin heads.	Nails that touched soil.	Black outside; white insides under or near nails.
Ticks	Oval; size varies.	Attached to skin.	Head attached to skin; oval shape.
Fleas	Black dots that jump.	Anywhere.	Walk and then jump.
LICE	Small commas.	Hairs, head or body; seams of clothing.	Small but visible; may be seen moving; eggs attached to hairs.
ENTEROBIASIS	Around 0.5 cm like tiny pieces of thread.	Rectum, vagina.	White color; seen moving at night or on awakening.
Creatures under the skin, movement felt, painful or itchy			
LARVA MIGRANS	Wiggly line the diameter of thin spaghetti.	Under skin that touched sand or soil.	Itchy; red, line under the skin; a pen mark will show that it moves slowly.
STRONGYLOIDIASIS	Less than 10 cm; wiggly line.	Buttocks, near the rectum.	Like larva migrans; lasts hours to days, then disappear and recur later on.
LOIASIS[3]	Like a small bird's egg.	Under skin, anywhere.	Lumps arise under the skin, then disappear and arise elsewhere.
GUINEA WORM[2]	Long thread, around 100 cm.	Legs; initially under skin.	Blister which breaks open and reveals the end of a very long, skinny worm.
None of the above			
BERIBERI	No creatures, maybe a rash.	Anywhere or everywhere.	The patient says there are moving insects, but there are none.
Leeches	Less than 5 cm, like flattened worms.	Skin or mouth and throat.	Long, narrow wormy creatures attach and then swell, suck blood.

1 *The size and shape varies greatly from one kind to the other; see the regional notes for your area.*
2 *Guinea worm: scattered within Africa and the Middle East only; where there are wells into which people step to draw water.*
3 *Loiasis: humid central and western Africa only.*

IV—HEAD PROBLEMS

PROTOCOL A.19—HEADACHE

A.19.A—Headache with a fever   Also see Protocol A.21.G—Face Pain, if appropriate.

A.19.B—Headache without fever

▷ SYMPTOMATIC TREATMENT
Headache without fever
ACETAMINOPHEN or IBUPROFEN. Do not use ASPIRIN or narcotics.

⚠ EMERGENCY	▽ NON-EMERGENCY
HEADACHE EMERGENCIES	**Non-emergency conditions originating elsewhere**
Instantaneous-onset or worst-ever headache.	Upper neck problems in back can cause headache.
Increasing severity and frequency.	Check the patient's vision; occasionally this is a cause.
Vomiting without nausea.	Check for facial tenderness; consider RESPIRATORY INFECTION (sinusitis).
Mental changes: lethargy or confusion.	Check for scalp tenderness; may or may not be serious.
Stiff neck or abnormal limb motion.	

Protocol A.19.A—Headache with a fever (corrected temperature over 38°/100.4°

Did the patient change from healthy to very ill[1] in less than a week?

NO   YES

| *Does the patient have moderate to severe pain other than headache?*

| NO   YES

| **Consider**: [MALARIA, HEAT ILLNESS,
| MENINGITIS, ENCEPHALITIS],[2] ARBOVIRAL
| FEVER, ENTERIC FEVER, RELAPSING FEVER[3]

| **General pain:** Protocol B.2
| **Specific pains**

         Lymph nodes very painful: PLAGUE

         Abdominal pains: ENTERIC FEVER

         Face pain: RESPIRATORY INFECTION, INFECTION, INFLUENZA

         Shin pain: TRENCH FEVER, TYPHUS

         Back pain: TYPHUS

         Limb pain: FILARIASIS, DENGUE FEVER,[6] ARBOVIRAL FEVERS,
                            SPOTTED FEVER[5]

         Joint pain: CHIKUNGUNYA, DENGUE FEVER[6,] ARBOVIRAL FEVER,

Has the patient been ill for two weeks or more?

NO   YES

| **Consider**: MALARIA, RESPIRATORY INFECTION, SYPHILIS, KATAYAMA DISEASE, AFRICAN
| SLEEPING SICKNESS,[4] BRUCELLOSIS, AMEBIASIS.

See table on the next page.

---

1 *Very ill means that the patient cannot attend to his own needs. He needs help with toilet duties.*

2 *These 4 conditions are indistinguishable; if you consider any of them, you should treat for all of them.*

3 *Relapsing fever: tropical and high altitude, but not in the islands of SEA and the Pacific.*

4 *African sleeping sickness: scattered areas of Africa, south of Bamako, Mali and Lake Chad and north of Lusaka, Zambia.*

5 *Spotted fever: worldwide including the tropics but not in the islands of Southeast Asia.*

6 *Dengue fever: in the Americas only near or north of the equator. In Africa, east coastal, south and west. Prevalent in India, Southeast Asia and the Pacific. Occasionally found in the Mediterranean area. The disease may spread.*

TOC SYMPTOMS DIFFERENTIALS CONDITIONS DRUG INDEX REGIONAL NOTES INX

FEVER, HEADACHE ALONE, ONSET LESS THAN A WEEK, DURATION LESS THAN 2 WEEKS

Condition	Fever pattern	Other
By far most common		
MALARIA	Varies	History of chills; patient will tell you the diagnosis.
INFLUENZA	Low usually	Recent onset, generally achy, other cases also.
Mental symptoms are likely		
ENTERIC FEVER	Sustained high	Apathy; may have abdominal pains or a cough.
Prominent rash likely		
SPOTTED FEVER[2]	Variable	Maybe scab from insect bite; prominent rash starts on limbs.
ARBOVIRAL FEVER	High	Aching muscles; epidemic context; seek local lore.
MONKEYPOX[1]	High	Blister-rash, humid areas only, monkey contact.
Prominent swollen groin lymph nodes likely		
LYMPHOGRANULOMA VENEREUM	Variable	Large nodes in the groin; tender, maybe a genital sore.

1 *Monkeypox: northern D. R. Congo and adjacent Central African Republic; rarely found in western Africa.*
2 *Spotted fever: worldwide including the Arctic but not in the islands of Southeast Asia.*

Protocol A.19.B—Headache without a fever

Has the patient had a head injury?

NO   **YES**
|
| Expect a headache for months, send out if he was unconscious for more than 30 minutes.

Is the patient at a high altitude, exposed to fire or near exhaust fumes?

NO to all   **YES to any**
|
| **Consider** ALTITUDE SICKNESS, CARBON MONOXIDE POISONING.

Does the patient have high blood pressure?

No   **Yes**
|
| **Consider** TOXEMIA, HYPERTENSION, KIDNEY FAILURE

Is the pain continual or almost continual over weeks or more?

NO   **YES**
|
| **Related to an ingestion**: LEAD POISONING, CYSTICERCOSIS, TRICHINOSIS
| **Mental changes likely**: DEMONIZATION, PELLAGRA, STRESS
| **Long-term ill health likely**: CANCER, KIDNEY DISEASE, DIABETES, BRUCELLOSIS.
|

Is the headache recurrent: the same headache comes and goes with pain-free intervals?

NO   **YES**
|
| **Consider** MIGRAINE, HYPERTENSION, MALARIA, CANCER, PELLAGRA, SCURVY,
See table on the next page.   PLANT POISONING, FOOD POISONING

SINGLE EPISODE HEADACHE, NO FEVER NOW OR RECENTLY

Conditions	Pain Pattern	Other
INFLUENZA	Variable	Also general muscle aching.
HANGOVER	Variable	Morning after intoxication.
DEMONIZATION	Variable	Occult involvement or due to a curse.
HEAT ILLNESS	Generalized, dull	Very hot environment, patient weak, has nausea.

PROTOCOL A.20—DIZZINESS

⚠ EMERGENCY	⚠ EMERGENCY
Emergencies with spinning/tilting-type dizziness	**Emergencies with off-balance-type dizziness**
Dizziness begins immediately after changing head position to the problematic position. *Dizziness doesn't lessen with maintaining the head position.* *Dizziness happens predictably any time the head is put into the problematic position.* *Dizziness is mild, not severe.* *The patient has grossly abnormal vital signs.*	*Staggering* *Garbled speech* *Numbness* *Double vision* *No different with eyes closed or open.*

Also see Protocol A.7.E if the patient is uncoordinated; it is easy to confuse incoordination and dizziness; they commonly occur together.

Is the patient sweaty, shaky and pale?

NO	YES
|	**Immediately give him sugar; consider HYPOGLYCEMIA.**
|	

Does the patient have low blood pressure, a slow pulse or abnormal respirations?

NO	YES
|	See Protocols A.2 and A.3.

Is the patient very ill with a corrected temperature over 38.5°/101.3°?

NO	YES
|	**Prominent ear pain**: EAR INFECTION
|	**Prominent headache**: MALARIA, ENTERIC FEVER, MENINGITIS, ENCEPHALITIS, ARBOVIRAL FEVER, RELAPSING FEVER,[1] TYPHUS, SPOTTED FEVER.[2]
|	**Prominent limb pain**: DENGUE FEVER,[3] TRENCH FEVER. ARBOVIRAL FEVER, TYPHUS.

Did this develop rapidly after the person took some food, drink or medicine?

NO	YES
|	**Consider** ALCOHOL or STREPTOMYCIN (drug) side effect, PLANT POISONING: lolism,[4]
See table on the next page	cassava, nicotine.

1 *Relapsing fever: tropical and high altitude, but not in the islands of SEA and the Pacific.*
2 *Spotted fever: worldwide, but not in the islands of Southeast Asia.*
3 *Dengue fever: in the Americas only near or north of the equator. In Africa, east coastal, south and west. Prevalent in India, Southeast Asia and the Pacific. Occasionally found in the Mediterranean area. It can spread.*
4 *Plant poisoning, lolism: found in the Mediterranean and Middle Eastern areas.*

DIZZY WITH NO OR LOW FEVER, NO INGESTION, ORDERED ACCORDING TO TYPE OF DIZZINESS

Conditions	Type	Fever	Other
ANEMIA	Weak/faint.	Rare	Pale inside eyelids, mouth or nails.
Menstruation	Weak/faint.	No	Use IBUPROFEN (drug) to treat it.
HEAT ILLNESS	Weak/faint.	Maybe	Hot weather, nauseated, headache.
HEART FAILURE	Faint.	Maybe	Irregular pulse or low blood pressure.
DEHYDRATION	Faint.	No	Dry mouth, thirsty, fast pulse.
HYPERVENTILATION	Faint.	No	Numb by mouth, short of breath.
COBALAMIN DEFICIENCY[1]	Off-balance.	Rare	Worse with eyes closed than open.
SYPHILIS, tertiary/congenital	Off balance.	No	Worse with eyes closed than open.
AFRICAN SLEEPING SICKNESS[2]	Off balance.	No/low	Lumps on back of neck, or HEART FAILURE.
EAR INFECTION	Spinning or tilting.	Usual	Red ear drum(s) or pus visible.
Wax in ears	Spinning or tilting.	No	Can see the wax; remove it carefully.
SYPHILIS, congenital	Spinning or tilting.	No	Age 5–30; developing deafness.
BRAIN DAMAGE	Unsteady.	Maybe	Worse with eyes open than closed.
TUBERCULOSIS	Variable.	Maybe	Draining ear, antibiotics don't work.
STROKE	Variable.	No	Weakness or paralysis, maybe high BP.
DIABETES	Variable.	No	History of diabetes or dehydrated.

1 This is a vitamin B_{12} deficiency, commonly in elderly expatriates and anyone malnourished.
2 African sleeping sickness: scattered areas of Africa, south of Bamako, Mali and Lake Chad; north of Lusaka, Zambia.

PROTOCOL A.21—OTHER HEAD PROBLEMS

A.21.A—Hair problems   A.21.B—Mongoloid face   A.21.C—Facial swelling   A.21.D—Skull misshapen; bossing
A.21.E—Flushed face   A.21.F—Drooping face   A.21.G—Face pain   A.21.H—Other face and head problems

Protocol A.21.A—Hair problems

Condition	Hair Problem	Other Characteristics
Most common; check these first		
Childbirth and OLD AGE	Hair thinning and loss.	Common after childbirth, will regrow; old age, will not regrow.
Lice	Creatures and eggs.	Lice visible; patient itching behind ears.
MALNUTRITION	Color change,[1] thin.	Weight loss, thin arms, thinning of hair.
CHLOROQUINE(drug)	Premature greying.	Drug for prevention of MALARIA or treatment thereof.
Hair loss, probably generalized, thinning; not in patches		
THYROID TROUBLE	Hair thin, brittle.	Tired and constipated, weight gain.
ZINC DEFICIENCY	Variable hair loss.	Very hot or dry climate, not acclimatized.
TYPHUS	Loss after illness.	Fever, sick for weeks; from fleas or lice.
VISCERAL LEISHMANIASIS[2]	Thinning, loss.	Large spleen, weight loss.
PREDNISONE (drug)	Thinning, loss.	Fat face, weight gain.
LEPROSY, lepromatous	Loss of hair, rare.	Europeans and Japanese-bumpy skin.
LEPROSY, lepromatous	Loss of eyebrows common.	Bumpy skin usually; numb fingers/toes.
RADIATION ILLNESS	Hair loss.	Onset about 10 days post exposure.
LASSA FEVER[3]	Hair loss.	High fever, severe pains, sudden onset.

Hair loss, probably in patches		
FAVUS[4]	Bald patches	Yellow crusts after a time.
SYPHILIS, secondary	Loss in patches, no thinning	Skin in bald spots looks normal; present or recent history of a fever; "flu", but not extremely ill.
TINEA	Loss in patches	Dry, scaly rash on bald spot.

1 Normally black hair becomes reddish or blond. In some ethnic groups, curly hair becomes straight and brittle, breaking off so it looks like a short crew cut. Normally blond hair turns darker with malnutrition.
2 Visceral Leishmaniasis: found in scattered areas of Central and South America, Africa north of the equator, the Mediterranean area, the Indian subcontinent, eastern Europe, central Asia and mainland China.
3 Lassa fever: found in West Africa, and occurs mostly in epidemics.
4 Favus: this occurs in the Middle East/ Mediterranean area only; see R regional notes.

Protocol A.21.B—Mongoloid face

Definition: low bridge of the nose, eyes set wide apart and sloping down toward the nose, face abnormally rounded, maybe tongue large and may protrude; possibly appearance of retardation.

Mentally retarded	
DOWN SYNDROME	Retarded, maybe a continuous horizontal crease on palm.
CRETINISM	Retarded, very big tongue, mother had GOITER during pregnancy.
Patient is not retarded, may appear to be	
SYPHILIS	Depressed bridge of the nose, not present since birth.
THALLASEMIA	Hereditary, large spleen, ANEMIA, family history of ill health.

Protocol A.21.C—Facial swelling

Is the patient a child who is otherwise fine, and has one swollen eyelid without bruising?

NO	YES
	This is from an insect bite; it should disappear in a day or two; otherwise consider CHAGA'S DISEASE

Is the swelling of sudden onset after an injection, insect bite or eating something?

NO	YES
	Consider ANAPHYLAXIS; treatment is EPINEPHINE (drug). CHAGA'S DISEASE.[1]

Is the patient short of breath?

NO	YES
	Consider ALLERGY, BERIBERI, KIDNEY DISEASE, ANTHRAX, PERTUSSIS,[5] rarely HEART FAILURE, very rarely CANCER.

Is the patient very ill with a corrected temperature over 38.5°/101.3°?

NO	YES
	With a skin condition consider CELLULITIS, TYPHUS, ANTHRAX, MONKEYPOX,[3] HEMORRHAGIC FEVER, KATAYAMA DISEASE, SERUM SICKNESS, SCRUB TYPHUS.
	Without a skin condition consider KIDNEY DISEASE, TYPHUS, YELLOW FEVER,[2] LASSA FEVER,[4] TRICHINOSIS, SERUM SICKNESS, SCRUB TYPHUS.[6]

See the table on the following page.

1 Chaga's disease: found in scattered areas of Central and South America.
2 Yellow fever: South America north of Sao Paolo, central and western Africa and the Sudan.
3 Monkeypox: northern D. R. Congo and adjacent Central African Republic; rarely in western Africa.
4 Lassa fever: found in West Africa and occurs mostly in epidemics.
5 Pertussis causes severe coughing spells which may result in swollen eyelids and the whites of the eyes becoming red.
6 Scrub typhus: Asia/Pacific area, always headache, fever, eye symptoms, constipation.

Swelling, likely eye(s) only

EYE INFECTION	Also pain, bloodshot or visible pus.
NAIROBI EYE[1]	Lid(s) only, eyeball is perfectly fine; black/orange insects.
CHAGA'S DISEASE[2]	One eye swollen shut; swelling lasts a week or more, feels firm.
LOIASIS[3]	Sudden onset of severe pain in eye; like LARVA MIGRANS.
THYROID TROUBLE	Patient fatigued, low body corrected temperature, always sleepy.
LARVA MIGRANS	Patient feels something moving in his eye(s).

Maybe, eye(s) only, maybe eye(s) and face

CELLULITIS[4]	Indistinct borders to swelling, warm to touch, maybe fever.
ANTHRAX	Sore or scab present on or near the swollen area.

Swelling likely the eye(s) and face

PERTUSSIS	Child also has a severe coughing spasms with vomiting.
PLANT POISONING	Manicheel[5] or atriplicism.[6]
KIDNEY DISEASE, nephrotic	Protein in the urine, swelling worse in the morning.
AFRICAN SLEEPING SICKNESS[7]	Headaches, abnormal sleep pattern, maybe HEART FAILURE.

Swelling of the face in general, not the eyes in particular

MUMPS	Swelling by the ears and jaw, mildly ill, mostly children.
MALNUTRITION	Swelling by the ears, maybe associated with ALCOHOLISM.
PREDNISONE (drug)	Symmetrical, history of taking the drug for more than a week.
YAWS	Hard swelling over the bridge of the nose.
HIV INFECTION	Infants; history of risky parental behavior or blood transfusion.
LEPROSY, lepromatous	Face is cobblestoned; symmetrical; bumps on outer ears.
CANCER	Slow-onset, progressive swelling, not symmetrical, adults usually.
BURKITT LYMPHOMA	Children, humid tropics, rapidly progressive.

Swelling whole body

KIDNEY DISEASE	Abnormal urinalysis; eyelids swollen, soft, especially mornings.
TRICHINOSIS	Also swollen, sore muscles, aching all over, fevers.

---

1 Nairobi eye is caused by insects which are found in East Africa; they are brown and orange, flying and tend to occur in large numbers at certain times of the year.

2 Chaga's disease: scattered areas in the Americas.

3 Loiasis: humid, rural western and central Africa.

4 Cellulitis of the tissues around the eye can be an emergency. Seek higher level care promptly.

5 Plant poisoning, manicheel: Americas only.

6 Plant poisoning, atriplicism: Chinese and in the Far East.

7 African sleeping sickness: scattered areas of Africa, south of Bamako, Mali and Lake Chad and north of Lusaka, Zambia.

TOC
SYMPTOMS
DIFFERENTIALS
CONDITIONS
DRUG INDEX
REGIONAL NOTES
INX

Protocol A.21.D—Skull misshapen; bossing

In infants, most commonly due to the birth process; usually will correct itself. See below for bossing.

Definition: rather than being regularly rounded, the skull is a funny shape, sticking out more on the forehead and on both sides above the ears; the shape is slightly like a clover leaf if viewed directly from the front. The following can cause bossing: this may also be simply a family trait.

RICKETS	Top of the head may be flat.
RICKETS	Legs are bowed in or out, result of inadequate sunlight.
SYPHILIS, congenital	Patient 30 yo or less; parent(s) exposed or they had been.
SICKLE CELL DISEASE[1]	Pain episodes which begin before age 2; pale, jaundiced or both.
THALLASEMIA	Family history, large spleen, ANEMIA.
ACROMEGALY	Large, coarse features, with large hands and feet.

1 *Sickle cell disease: this affects those of African genetic origin, mainly in West Africa and the Americas. Some Indians and Arabs are also affected.*

Protocol A.21.E—Flushed face

Definition: Black skin does not flush; being warm to the touch is equivalent to flushing. Fair or light tan skin appears abnormally reddish. This may be caused by sunburn or any fever, especially TYPHUS, or by the following:

FIFTH DISEASE	A fever which drops as a "slapped cheek" rash breaks out.
DENGUE FEVER[1]	Sudden onset, high fever, severe bone pains.
PLANT POISONING: cassava	From improperly processed cassava or from cassava water.
PLANT POISONING: betel nut	Asian women, red and black around the mouth.
ALCOHOLISM	Nose particularly red; currently or habitually intoxicated.
CARBON MONOXIDE POISONING	Exposed to fumes from fire or an engine; headache & nausea.
STREP INFECTION	Sore throat or belly pain; face red except pale around the lips.

1 *Dengue fever: in the Americas only near or north of the equator. In Africa, east coastal, south and west. Prevalent in India, Southeast Asia and the Pacific. Occasionally found in the Mediterranean area. The disease may spread.*

Protocol A.21.F—Drooping face

Definition: When the patient smiles one side of his mouth is markedly different than the other, or he cannot close one or both eye(s) completely OR his whole face droops, both sides. May be from BRAIN DAMAGE from any cause.

Is this the consequence of a severe illness with a corrected temperature over 38.5°/101.3°?

NO	YES
	Consider EAR INFECTION, DIPHTHERIA, MENINGITIS, ENCEPHALITIS, BELL'S PALSY

DROOPING FACE, NO HIGH FEVER

BELL'S PALSY	Adults; sudden onset, maybe no reason or associated with an infection such as LEPROSY
STROKE	Also some other weakness or disability; adults; rarely children
EAR INFECTION	History of ear pain or ear discharge
PARKINSON'S DISEASE	Expressionless symmetrical face, trembling at rest which lessens with intended motion
BRAIN DAMAGE	Any cause of brain damage might make the face droop.
POLIO	History of a flu-type recent illness; usually other paralysis also
LEPROSY	Skin color changes and loss of a sense of touch on the skin so affected.
DIPHTHERIA	Painful, open spontaneous skin ulcer or swollen tonsils with white or gray scum.

Any facial swelling, if severe, can press on the nerve that controls the face, causing drooping; see Protocol A.21.B.

Protocol A.21.G—Face pain

No visible skin abnormality likely

RESPIRATORY INFECTION	History of a stuffy nose; upper back teeth all hurt.
Dental problems	Check for tenderness, swollen gums and broken or decayed teeth.
ANGINA	Jaw pain; possibly chest pain also, maybe pale and sweaty and faint.
BRUCELLOSIS	Slow onset, up and down fevers, pain in front of ears with chewing.

Visible skin abnormality

CELLULITIS	Redness and swelling along with a fever; maybe prior injury.
SHINGLES	Burning or shooting pain, then a blistery rash.
CANCRUM ORIS	A spontaneous wound on the lower face; malnourished child.

Protocol A.21.H—Other face and head problems

Any of the problems listed under Protocol A.21.F may occasionally affect both sides of the face. A visual problem may cause an abnormal head posture in an older child or an adult.

TOXEMIA	Six months or more pregnant; itching of the face.
PARKINSON DISEASE	Expressionless, symmetrically drooping face; peculiar, falling gait.
ALLERGY	Sneezing; itchy, runny nose; itchy eyes.
SYPHILIS, tertiary/congenital	Swelling or holes; patient, partner or parent exposed.
RESPIRATORY FAILURE	Patient nods with each breath; obviously very short of breath.
TETANUS	Tight smile due to spasms of the facial muscles.
MASTOIDITIS	Red, swollen bump(s) behind the ear(s); fever.
RICKETS (children)	Head very sweaty.
RICKETS (infants)	Open soft spot well past 18 months of age.
SYPHILIS, congenital	Open soft spot well past 18 months of age or middle face looks pushed in.
HIV INFECTION (infants)	Open soft spot well past 18 months of age.

PROTOCOL A.22—EYE PAIN

A.22.A—Eye pain with no or low fever

A.22.B—Eye pain maybe with a fever

A.22.C—Eye pain with fever

A.22.D—Itching eyes

▷ SYMPTOMATIC TREATMENT	⚠EMERGENCY	
EYE PAIN ACETAMINOPHEN or IBUPROFEN is appropriate. Stronger pain medications may be used after diagnosis. Do not use eye anesthetic drops repeatedly to relieve pain since they will permanently blind the patient.	**EYE EMERGENCIES** If there is a sensation of moving foreign body(s) in the eye, then check with a magnifier. If you see moving creatures, send the patient out for immediate care. Larvae must be removed with forceps under local anesthetic—they will not wash out with saline. They must be removed to prevent penetration into the eye and possibly total blindness in both eyes.	**In a Western adult**, sudden onset of eye pain and visual loss, the pain aggravated by eye movement warrants evacuation to at least a level 3 medical facility.

See the table at the beginning of Protocol A.23 also.

Protocol A.22.A—Eye pain with no or low fever

**If the eyes are both painful and red, then see Protocol B.8.

Types of pain designations

FB = "foreign body"; pain like something stuck in the eye.

Irritated = not really pain, just an annoying, scratchy feeling.

Eye motion = pain is worse when moving the eyes.

Does the patient say it feels as if something is in the eye?

NO	YES
|	Check the section on eye injuries, Chapter 9 of Volume 1.
|	**Consider** KERATITIS, TRACHOMA, MYIASIS, LARVA MIGRANS, LOIASIS.[3]

Is there much tearing and the pain worse in light?

NO	YES
|	**Consider** XEROPHTHALMIA, LEPROSY, IRITIS, KERATITIS, PLANT POISONING due to
|	jimson weed, SYPHILIS, congenital.

EYE PAIN, NO FOREIGN BODY SENSATION, PAIN NOT MUCH WORSE IN LIGHT, NO OR LOW FEVER

Conditions	Pain Type	Red?	Other Characteristics
Patient likely at least moderately ill; in bed or wants to be			
MALARIA	Aching	No	Fevers, chills, headaches, waist pain, shoulder pain.
MIGRAINE	Throbbing	No	Headache, maybe one-sided; nausea.
GLAUCOMA	Variable	Yes	Hard eyeball; nausea if rapid onset.
BERIBERI	Unknown	No	Mist over the central visual field, both eyes.
Patient likely doing his usual, without decreased stamina			
EYE INFECTION	Irritated / burn	Yes	Pain rarely severe; more irritation.
OLD AGE	Irritated	Maybe	Relieved by closing eyes; use artificial tears.
Eye strain	Burning	Maybe	Using eyes in poor light.
PINGUECULA	Irritated	Maybe	White growth, irritated with lid movement.
TRACHOMA	Irritated or FB	Yes	Lids misshapen or bubbles under the lid.
Patient likely up and around but attending to his eyes, not working as usual			
NAIROBI EYE[1]	Burning eyelids	Lids only	Brown and orange insects seen in the environment.[1]
ONCHOCERCIASIS[2]	Variable	Maybe	Itching skin also; skin bumps.
LOIASIS[3]	Punch in eye	Probably	May see worm, swollen eye.
LARVA MIGRANS	Punch in eye	Probably	Swollen eye

1 *The Nairobi eye insects are prevalent in East Africa.*

2 *Onchocerciasis: scattered areas in Africa, the Middle East, Central America and northern South America.*

3 *Loiasis: found in humid west and central Africa only*

Protocol A.22.B—Eye pain maybe with a fever

Condition	Pain Type	Red?	Other Characteristics
Mainly eye symptoms likely			
IRITIS	IRITIS[3]	Yes	Pupil not round; key hole shape.
CHAGA'S DISEASE[1]	Unknown	Unknown	Swelling, one side only, from insect bite.
Maybe prominent eye symptoms			
CELLULITIS	Burning	No[2]	Red and/or warm to touch.
TUBERCULOSIS	IRITIS[3]	Yes	Painful bump on cornea-white border.
LOIASIS[4]	Punch-like	Yes	Swelling, may see worm or his track.
Prominent non-eye symptoms likely, maybe whole-body illness			
SHINGLES	Burning	Maybe	Blister-type skin rash, one side only.
SYPHILIS, tertiary/congenital	IRITIS[3]	Yes	Aching or sees flashing lights.
Moderate to severe whole-body illness likely			
REITER SYNDROME	Burning	Yes	Adult, tears, avoids light, also joint pain.
DIPHTHERIA	With light	Unknown	Sore throat or wound; very ill.
BRUCELLOSIS	Eye motion	Unknown	Slow onset, joint pains, fevers episodic.
RABIES	With light	Unknown	Paralyzed or won't drink water.

1 Chaga's disease: scattered areas in the Americas.
2 Usually the whites are not red, but the lids are.
3 Pain is worse in the light and there is excessive tearing. Light shown into the other eye (provided that eye is not blind) will cause pain in the affected eye. The pain of iritis is worse when the patient attempts to change from near to far vision.
4 Loiasis: only in humid, west or central Africa.

Protocol A.22.C—Eye pain with fever

Condition	Pain Type	Fever	Other
Rash unlikely, variable onset			
MALARIA	Aching	Yes	Headache, chills, sweats.
Maybe rash, variable onset			
LEPTOSPIROSIS	Aching	Erratic	Muscle pains, very red eyes, fevers very erratic.
MENINGITIS	With light	High	Severe headache, stiff neck, very ill.
TYPHUS, murine	Eye motion	Yes	Headache, muscle pains.
ARBOVIRAL FEVER	Variable	High	Aching all over.
Rash likely, onset over days			
MEASLES	Aching	Yes	Rash spotted or sand-papery, prominent.
SCRUB TYPHUS[1]	Aching	High	Large spleen, constipated, rash 7th day or after.
SPOTTED FEVER[2]	Throbbing	High	Pain worse with light; rash starts on limbs, prominent.
Rash likely, very rapid onset, less than 12 hours			
RELAPSING FEVER[3]	With light	Up/down	A kind of IRITIS; non-round pupils.
DENGUE FEVER[4]	Eye motion	High	Severe bone and joint pains, rash prominent.

1 Scrub typhus: Asia and Pacific areas only; always fever, eye symptoms, headache, constipation.
2 Spotted fever: not in the islands of Southeast Asia.
3 Relapsing fever: tropical and high altitude, but not in the islands of SEA and the Pacific.
4 Dengue fever: in the Americas only near or north of the equator. In Africa, east coastal, south and west. Prevalent in India, Southeast Asia and the Pacific. Occasionally found in the Mediterranean area. The disease may spread.

TOC

SYMPTOMS

DIFFERENTIALS

CONDITIONS

DRUG INDEX

REGIONAL NOTES

INX

Protocol A.22.D—Itching eyes

ALLERGY	No fever; either a hot climate or other allergies.
LARVA MIGRANS	Patient feels movement or a worm is visible.
KATAYAMA DISEASE	Also fever, hives, loss of appetite.
LOIASIS[1]	Itching becomes pain; visible worm or its track.

> **▷ SYMPTOMATIC TREATMENT**
>
> Rinse the eyes with water or artificial tears. Do not use steroid eye drops or ointment until they are prescribed by a physician for this patient on this occasion.

1 *Loiasis: humid areas of west and central Africa only.*

PROTOCOL A.23—ABNORMAL EYE APPEARANCE

A.23.A—Red eyes with a fever, now or recently
A.23.B—Red eyes, possible fever
A.23.C—Red eyes without fever
A.23.D—Yellow eyes, jaundice

A.23.E—Swollen eye(s)
A.23.F—Abnormal whites and corneas
A.23.G—Abnormal pupils
A.23.H—Other eye abnormalities

Table of various eye problem characteristics

	Pupil	Pain	Vision	Cornea	Secretions	Eyeball
CONJUNCTIVITIS	Normal	Little/ none	Normal	Clear	Milky	Normal
IRITIS	Small	Moderate	Decreased	Spots	Watery	Normal
GLAUCOMA	Large	Severe	V poor	Cloudy	Watery	Hard
KERATITIS	Varies	Severe	Varies	Irregular	Watery	Normal

Protocol A.23.A—Red eyes with a fever, now or recently

**If the eyes are both painful and red, then see Protocol B.8.

Maybe rash

LEPTOSPIROSIS	Very red; erratic fever, muscle aching all over; history of ground water exposure.
ARBOVIRAL FEVER	Aching all over; headache, other symptoms variable, usually multiple cases.
TYPHUS	Fleas or body lice; fever & rash start day 3 or 4, after other symptoms.
HEMORRHAGIC FEVER	Whites of eyes may have bright red blood; may be other abnormal bleeding.
SPOTTED FEVER[1]	Very ill, severe headache, eye pain worse with light.
SCRUB TYPHUS[2]	Gradual onset of fever, large spleen, constipation, rash begins around 7th day.

Prominent rash

DENGUE FEVER[3]	Severe joint and bone pains, onset over a few hours, fever may drop and relapse.
MEASLES	Cough, spotty or sand papery rash by day three, usually multiple cases.

1 *Spotted fever: not in the islands of Southeast Asia. The rash may be invisible in very dark skin. Occasionally it does not occur in fair skin.*

2 *Scrub typhus: Asia and Pacific areas only; always fever, eye symptoms, headache, constipation.*

3 *Dengue fever: in the Americas only near or north of the equator. In Africa, east coastal, south and west. Prevalent in India, Southeast Asia. and the Pacific. Occasionally found in the Mediterranean area. The disease may spread.*

TOC   SYMPTOMS   DIFFERENTIALS   CONDITIONS   DRUG INDEX   REGIONAL NOTES   INX

Protocol A.23.B—Red eyes, possible fever

**If the eyes are both painful and red, then see Protocol B.8.

CELLULITIS	Redness is on lids and face; local swelling present.
GONORRHEA	Sexually active or child of an infected adult; much pus.
IRITIS	Pupil not round; key hole shape or scalloped.
GLAUCOMA	Cornea is cloudy, vision very poor.

Protocol A.23.C—Red eyes without a fever

This is commonly due to old age. Use artificial tears. If the eyes are both painful and red, then see Protocol B.8.
**Blood-red spot(s) on whites, painless, sudden onset, no illness, will resolve on their own.

ALCOHOL effect	Patient acts intoxicated or has a hangover; alcoholic beverage odor.

Prominent respiratory symptoms

RESPIRATORY INFECTION	Patient is congested, with an obvious cold.
PERTUSSIS	Severe cough, blood-red spots on whites of eyes.
ALLERGY	Eyes itchy, also runny nose.

Isolated eye symptoms

EYE INFECTION	Pus or watery discharge; eyes may be stuck shut in the morning.
KERATITIS	Severe eye pain; feels as if there is something in the eye.
TRACHOMA	Bubbles underneath lids early; poor vision later.

Prominent skin symptoms

ONCHOCERCIASIS[1]	Also very itchy skin; blindness common locally.

Prominent mouth symptoms

ARSENIC POISONING	Also numbness, tingling, burning of palms and soles.
SCURVY	Blood-red spots on whites of eyes; gums bleeding also.

1 Onchocerciasis: scattered areas in Africa, the Middle East, Central America and northern South America.

Protocol A.23.D—Yellow eyes, jaundice

Definition: the whites of the patient's eyes are uniformly yellow. A little yellow along the edges of the whites are normal. After you have worked through this protocol, then also see Protocol B.5.

Is the patient taking a medication that affects the liver?[1]

NO	YES
	Stop the medication immediately.

Is the patient a newborn (less than 4 weeks old)?

NO	YES
	If the yellow is intense or the patient acts ill, send him to a hospital or see Volume 1, Chapter 7. **Consider** SEPSIS, KIDNEY INFECTION, congenital SYPHILIS.

Is the problem of recent[2] onset, with a corrected temperature over 38.5°/101.3°, in a patient in prior good health?

NO to any	YES to all
Continued on the next page.	**Consider** MALARIA, SEPSIS, PNEUMONIA,[3] LEPTOSPIROSIS, GALLBLADDER DISEASE, BARTONELLOSIS.[4]

Footnotes are on the next page.

Does the patient, with previously good health, have pain by his right lower chest/upper abdomen area but not the left?

NO	YES
|	**Consider** HEPATITIS, AMEBIASIS, PNEUMONIA,[5] LEPTOSPIROSIS, YELLOW FEVER,[6]
|	LIVER FLUKE,[7] GALLBLADDER DISEASE, CANCER.

Has the person been ill over two weeks, either this time or recurrently?

NO
YES

See Protocol B.7 if there is bilirubin in the urine. The diseases listed below likely have excessive urine urobilinogen[8] but negative bilirubin.

AFRICAN SLEEPING SICKNESS:[9] abnormal sleep pattern.

Family history of large spleen and ANEMIA

SICKLE CELL DISEASE:[10] recurrent bone pains; early deaths in family.

THALLASEMIA: Mediterranean or southern Asian genetic heritage.

OVALOCYTOSIS: European or New Guinea genetic heritage.

Enormous spleen

VISCERAL LEISHMANIASIS:[11] large liver also after 3 months.

TROPICAL SPLENOMEGALY: normal-size liver.

JAUNDICE, NO MEDICATION, NOT A NEWBORN, NO LIVER PAIN, INTERMEDIATE DURATION

Consider	Fever	Other
HEPATITIS	Low if any	Nausea, fatigue improved with jaundice.
AMEBIASIS	Maybe	Burning abdominal pain, worse with walking.
GALLBLADDER DISEASE	Unusual	Light-colored stools; general itching.
MALARIA	Usually high	Headaches, chills are common.

1 Instructions are to reduce the dose in liver disease or with a side effect of LIVER FAILURE.
2 That is, onset within the past two weeks.
3 Those of Mediterranean and African genetic origin only.
4 Bartonellosis: only in Peru and adjacent countries.
5 Those of Mediterranean and African genetic origin only.
6 Yellow fever: South America north of Sao Paolo, central and western Africa and the Sudan.
7 Liver fluke: present worldwide, including temperate climates; common in Southeast Asia and the Orient.

8 Many normal people have some urobilinogen; only 2+ to 4+ are abnormal.
9 African sleeping sickness: scattered areas of Africa, south of Bamako, Mali and Lake Chad and north of Lusaka, Zambia.
10 Sickle cell disease: this affects those of African genetic origin, mainly in West Africa and the Americas. Some Greeks, Indians and Arabs are also affected.
11 Visceral Leishmaniasis: found in scattered areas of Central and South America, Africa north of the equator, the Mediterranean area, the Indian subcontinent, eastern Europe, central Asia and mainland China.

Protocol A.23.E—Swollen eye(s)

Is the patient a child who may have been bitten by an insect but is not ill?

NO	YES
|	In the Americas consider CHAGA'S DISEASE; in Africa it may be NAIROBI EYE; otherwise
|	this is common and most often trivial.

Are the eyes very itchy and tearing?

NO	YES
|	**Consider** ALLERGY, LOIASIS (humid tropical Africa), KATAYAMA DISEASE, TRACHOMA.

Does the patient have a rash involving much or all of his body?

NO	YES
|	**Consider** KIDNEY DISEASE, MONKEYPOX (central Africa), MALNUTRITION.

Are the eyeballs swollen so they appear to pop out at you, pushing the eyelids out?

NO	YES
See table on next page.	**Consider** THYROID TROUBLE, CELLULITIS, CANCER (babies), rarely ABSCESS.

TOC SYMPTOMS DIFFERENTIALS CONDITIONS DRUG INDEX REGIONAL NOTES INX

EYE(S) SWOLLEN, NOT ITCHY AND TEARING, NO PROMINENT RASH, EYEBALLS NOT SWOLLEN

Swelling likely eye(s) only

EYE INFECTION	Also pain or red or visible pus.
NAIROBI EYE[1]	Lid(s) only, eyeball is perfectly fine; black/orange insects.
CHAGA'S DISEASE[2]	One eye swollen shut; swelling lasts a week or more, feels firm.
LOIASIS[3]	Sudden onset of severe pain in eye; like LARVA MIGRANS.
THYROID TROUBLE	Patient fatigued, low body temperature, always sleepy.
LARVA MIGRANS	Patient feels something moving in his eye(s).
SCRUB TYPHUS	Fever illness, nasal congestion, Asia/Pacific area only.

Maybe eye(s) only, maybe eye(s) and face

CELLULITIS[4]	Indistinct borders to swelling, warm to touch, maybe fever.
ANTHRAX	Sore or scab present on or near the swollen area.
PERTUSSIS	Child also has severe coughing spasms with vomiting.

Swelling likely the eye(s) and face

PLANT POISONING	Manicheel[5] or atriplicism.[6]
AFRICAN SLEEPING SICKNESS[7]	Headaches, abnormal sleep pattern, maybe HEART FAILURE.

Swelling face and elsewhere on the body

KIDNEY DISEASE	Abnormal urinalysis; eyelids swollen, soft, especially mornings.
TRICHINOSIS	Also swollen, sore muscles, aching all over, fevers.

---

1 *Nairobi eye is caused by insects which are found in East Africa; they are brown and orange, flying and tend to occur in large numbers at certain times of the year.*
2 *Chaga's disease: scattered areas in the Americas.*
3 *Loiasis: humid, rural western and central Africa.*
4 *Cellulitis of the tissues around the eye can be an emergency. Seek higher level care promptly.*
5 *Plant poisoning, manicheel: Americas only.*
6 *Plant poisoning, atriplicism: Chinese and in the Far East.*
7 *African sleeping sickness: scattered areas of Africa, south of Bamako, Mali and Lake Chad and north of Lusaka, Zambia.*

Protocol A.23.F—Abnormal whites and corneas

See Protocol A.23.A–D for reddish or yellowish whites.

Is the patient of African genetic heritage, with greyish whites or brownish spots on the whites?

NO	YES
	Probably normal but check XEROPHTHALMIA, PELLAGRA.

Does the patient have a skin condition affecting large areas of skin?

NO	YES
	Consider LEPROSY, ONCHOCERCIASIS,[1] CHICKEN POX, PELLAGRA.

Does the patient have white growing over the cornea?

NO	YES
See table below.	**Consider** TRACHOMA,[2] ONCHOCERCIASIS,[1] LEPROSY, PTERYGIUM, SYPHILIS (congenital).

---

1 *Onchocerciasis: scattered areas in Africa, the Middle East, Central America and northern South America.*
2 *The white of trachoma starts at the top of the cornea, usually. Onchocerciasis is like snowflakes. Leprosy can be any pattern. Pterygium is a thick white wedge, like a pie slice, growing from the side. Syphilis is usually in older children and teens, a smeared out, irregular white, stringy, opacity within the cornea, not on the surface.*

ABNORMAL APPEARANCE, NOT BROWN SPOTS, NO WHITE OVERGROWTH, NO SKIN CONDITION

Isolated eye problem; severe eye pain

KERATITIS	Severe eye pain, corneal surface not totally smooth.
GLAUCOMA	The whites of the eyes may be bluish; there is pain.
LOIASIS[1]	Worm seen crawling, or track where it had been.

Isolated eye problem; likely no generalized body illness

XEROPHTHALMIA	Cornea dry, maybe the white is brownish or wrinkled, maybe "soapsuds" on the eyelids.
PINGUECULA	White bump on the white, near the corneal edge.

This is likely part of a whole-body illness.

ANEMIA	Whites look bluish.
TUBERCULOSIS	Bump at the white--cornea border; painful.

1 Loiasis: humid, rural western and central Africa.

Protocol A.23.G—Abnormal pupils

Definition: the pupils are not black, round and rapidly responsive to light. The color, shape or behavior is abnormal.

Most common problem worldwide

CATARACT	Cloudy or white pupils, mostly old people.

Either too large or too small pupils

BRAIN DAMAGE	Likely other disorders of movement of the face and structures of the head.
ENCEPHALITIS	Fever and other symptoms of BRAIN DAMAGE.
MENINGITIS	Likely unconscious; pupils may not be round.
DIPHTHERIA	Pupils will not change size.

Small pupils

PLANT POISONING	Small pupils due to strychnine or muscarine.
INSECTICIDE POISON	Small pupils, round, also much tears, much saliva, diarrhea.
IRITIS	Small pupils, not exactly round, light-sensitive.

Large pupils

QUININE (drug) toxicity	Large pupils that do not respond to light.
PELLAGRA	Large pupils, light avoidance; abdominal symptoms, rough skin rash.
PLANT POISONING	Large pupils due to cassava, datura, water hemlock or jimson weed.

Other pupil problems

XEROPHTHALMIA	Irregularly shaped pupils quite late in the disease.
SYPHILIS, tertiary/congenital	Pupils which do not respond to light, or unequal pupils.
GLAUCOMA	Pupil(s) hazy, may not be round.

TOC   SYMPTOMS   DIFFERENTIALS   CONDITIONS   DRUG INDEX   REGIONAL NOTES   INX

SYMPTOMS

DIFFERENTIALS

CONDITIONS

DRUG INDEX

REGIONAL NOTES

INX

Protocol A.23.H—Other eye abnormalities

If tears spray in an infant rather than running down the cheek, the problem may correct itself, or it is correctable at a modern hospital.

	Dry eyes
OLD AGE	Burning pain; treat with artificial tears.
LEPROSY	Skin bumps, rash, sharp shooting pains or any combination.
DEHYDRATION	Mouth is also dry and skin hangs loosely on the body.
XEROPHTHALMIA	Wrinkles on the white of the eyes; corneas look dry.
	Excessive tearing
ALLERGY	This is the most common cause; also itching and runny nose.
XEROPHTHALMIA	Light avoidance, maybe wrinkled whites.
EYE INFECTION	Eye pain also; if due to a virus, causes tears rather than pus.
PLANT POISONING	Due to muscarine; atriplicism in a Chinese cultural setting.
INSECTICIDE POISONING	Recent exposure; also cough, runny nose.
LEPROSY	Also some skin problems and thin or absent eyebrows.
	Eyelid(s) rolled in or out
TRACHOMA	Some clouding of the cornea starting on top; eyes painful.
LEPROSY	Also some skin problems and thin or absent eyebrows.
	Abnormal eye movements, likely not recent onset
Infancy	Crossed eyes are common in babies, some need care, some correct themselves.
BRAIN DAMAGE	Patient has some other problem in moving or feeling.
CRETINISM	Mentally retarded; either short or deformed limbs; onset in infancy.
SYPHILIS, congenital	Eyes crossed; onset before age 30.
SEIZURES	Eyes are rolled back and there is some jerking of the limbs.
	Abnormal eye movements, likely recent onset
LYME DISEASE	Temperate areas, history of ARTHRITIS.
DIPHTHERIA	Quite ill for weeks; sore throat or skin infection.
FOOD POISONING	Botulism; recently ate tainted food, meat or vegetables.
	Abnormality of eye closing
BELL'S PALSY	Cannot close one eye, sudden onset, face droops on one side.
LEPROSY	Like BELL'S PALSY but very gradual onset.
THYROID TROUBLE	Eyes always at least half closed or else seem to bulge out.
DIPHTHERIA	Quite ill for weeks; sore throat or skin infection.
	Eyes set wide apart and prominent forehead
DOWN SYNDROME	Mentally retarded, large tongue, crease entirely across the palm.
THALLASEMIA	Family history of anemia and ill health, not mentally retarded.
CRETINISM	Mentally retarded; patient is either short, or he has deformed limbs; onset in infancy.
	Bleeding from the eyes
HEMORRHAGIC FEVER	Also other abnormal bleeding; EBOLA VIRUS DISEASE is one kind.
	Eyebrows thin or absent
SYPHILIS, secondary	Also a generalized rash, fever and aching all over.
LEPROSY	Also a bumpy face and/or ear lobes or a skin rash with numbness.
THYROID TROUBLE	Due to low-thyroid, loss of outer 2/3 of eyebrows only.

Abnormal substance in the eye(s)

EYE INFECTION	Some pus in the eyes which are stuck shut in the morning.
GONORRHEA	Much pus coming from eyes which look bloodshot.
MYIASIS	Maggots in the eyes; patient feels movement.
XEROPHTHALMIA	White foam on the eyelids, whites of the eyes may look wrinkled.

PROTOCOL A.24—LOSS OF VISION

A.24.A—Vision loss with normal eye appearance   A.24.C—Distorted vision

A.24.B—Vision loss with abnormal eye appearance

Protocol A.24.A—Vision loss with normal eye appearance

This is usually due to the normal effects of heredity and age; however, check below:

Has the patient consumed homemade beverage or wood alcohol within the past six hours?

NO   **YES**

| The loss of vision is due to wood alcohol (methanol). See Protocol A.11 in this index.

Did the vision loss start while the patient took ETHAMBUTOL, QUININE or CHLOROQUINE (drugs)?

NO   **YES**

| Side effect of the drug; stop the drug!

Is the vision loss mainly or only in dim light (night blindness)?

NO   **YES**

| **Consider** ZINC DEFICIENCY and XEROPHTHALMIA if the patient is not generally ill; consider
| DIPHTHERIA, PLANT POISONING due to botulism; if the patient is quite ill, RABIES or TETANUS.

Did the problem begin with a severe illness with a fever, over 38.5°/101.3°?

NO   **YES**

| **Consider** all causes of BRAIN DAMAGE with fever, both in the Condition Index and in your Regional
| Notes. Also consider MEASLES, ARBOVIRAL FEVER,[1] EBOLA VIRUS DISEASE, SCRUB TYPHUS.[2]
| May be due to QUININE or CHLOROQUINE (drugs for MALARIA).

Does the person also have a skin condition covering a large portion of his body?

NO   **YES**

See table below   **Consider** LEPROSY, ONCHOCERCIASIS.[3]

1 *Rift Valley fever, which occurs in central and eastern Africa.*
2 *Scrub typhus: Asia and the Pacific; always fever, eye symptoms, headache, constipation.*
3 *Onchocerciasis: scattered areas in Africa, the Middle East, Central America and northern South America.*

LOSS OF VISION, NO HIGH FEVER, NO MAJOR SKIN CONDITION, NO DRUG OR ALCOHOL INGESTION

SYPHILIS, tertiary/congenital	Sees or saw flashing lights and vision is distorted; maybe pain.
DIABETES	The patient is a known diabetic, or he has sugar in his urine.
TOXEMIA	6 months or more pregnant; high blood pressure; swollen ankles.
GLAUCOMA	Eyeball(s) feel(s) rock hard (feel them through eyelid.)
LARVA MIGRANS	History of sudden onset of pain, feels movement in the eye.
PLANT POISONING	Nicotine, cassava or tobacco/cow's urine.
RADIATION ILLNESS	Infant of a mother who was irradiated after 8 weeks of pregnancy.

TOC   SYMPTOMS   DIFFERENTIALS   CONDITIONS   DRUG INDEX   REGIONAL NOTES   INX

Protocol A.24.B—Vision loss with abnormal eye appearance

The most common cause is an old injury. If the eye is shrivelled, consider XEROPHTHALMIA also.

Cornea likely looks abnormal, skin condition unlikely

TRACHOMA	Eye lid(s) turn inward and scratch cornea; painful.
KERATITIS	Bloodshot; some opacities on the cornea.
GLAUCOMA	Eyeballs are hard and cornea is hazy.
PTERYGIUM	Fleshy, white growth over the cornea.

Cornea likely looks abnormal, prominent skin problem likely

LEPROSY	Numbness somewhere on the face, slow onset.
HERPES	Eye pain and not-totally smooth surface of the cornea.
ONCHOCERCIASIS[1]	Itchy skin rash, bumps on the skin; blindness common locally.

Pupil likely looks abnormal

QUININE (drug) toxicity	Pupils large, don't respond to light; patient is blind.
CATARACT	The pupil (normally black part) looks white or cloudy.
PLANT POISONING, water hemlock	Large pupils; severe vomiting, maybe seizures, weakness, shortness of breath.

Whites likely look abnormal

XEROPHTHALMIA	Cornea dry, whites maybe look wrinkled, "soap suds" on lids.
LOIASIS[2]	Worm visible in the eye or a track where he had been.
IRITIS	Redness around the cornea and irregular shape to the pupil.
PLANT POISONING	Due to nicotine or muscarine.

1 Onchocerciasis: scattered areas in Africa, the Middle East, Central America and northern South America.
2 Loiasis: humid, rural west and central Africa.

Protocol A.24.C—Distorted vision

Halos or rainbows around white lights

GLAUCOMA	Also eye pain and eyeball(s) is/are very hard.
CATARACT	The patient complains of cloudy vision.
LEPROSY	There are also skin bumps or rash or areas of numbness.
SYPHILIS, tertiary/congenital	Patient, partner or parent was exposed.
ONCHOCERCIASIS[1]	Some distortion of the cornea, "snowflakes" or lower opacities.
CHLOROQUINE (drug)	Toxicity after taking this for MALARIA prevention for years.

Seeing flashing lights

BERIBERI	Also leg weakness, poor diet, mist in central visual field.
SYPHILIS, tertiary	Also other eye symptoms, usually 35-55 yo, common with HIV INFECTION.

Vision blurred

IRITIS	Problem has lasted a long time, with frequent eye pains.
PLANT POISONING	Due to muscarine (a substance in mushrooms) or jimson weed.
FOOD POISONING	Botulism, from sausage or tainted vegetables; rare manifestation.
DIPHTHERIA	Pupils don't change size readily; neck swelling or facial weakness.

Cloudy vision

CATARACT	Pupil appears greyish or whitish rather than black.
TRACHOMA	Whitish scarring on the cornea, starts at the top.

Footnote on the next page at the end of this table.

Difficulty seeing in bright lights	
KERATITIS	Eye pain like a foreign body stuck in the eye.
LEPROSY	Also skin bumps or a rash or numbness somewhere.
SYPHILIS, tertiary/congenital	Patient, partner or parent was exposed.
ONCHOCERCIASIS[1]	Some distortion of the cornea, "snowflakes" or lower corneal opacities.

1 *Onchocerciasis: present in scattered area in Africa, in the Americas north of the Amazon, in Yemen and Saudi Arabia.*

PROTOCOL A.25—HEARING LOSS

Hearing loss due to most problems cannot be treated except in a major medical center. In the absence of drug ingestion, head injury or ear pain, SYPHILIS is by far the most common cause of ringing in the ears followed by increasing deafness. It starts on one side and spreads to the other. It may be due to congenital SYPHILIS with onset ages 2–30; after age 30, it is due to personally acquired SYPHILIS. Complete treatment prevents disastrous consequences, even if hearing is not restored.

Does deafness run in the patient's family?

NO	YES
|	There is probably not much to do about it, but check SYPHILIS.

Does or did the patient have ringing in his ears?

NO	YES
|	**Consider** a side effect of QUININE or ASPIRIN (drugs); may be due to a head injury,
|	EAR INFECTION, SYPHILIS[1] or wax in the ear canals. This may be due to OLD AGE.

Is the patient taking STREPTOMYCIN or another similar injectable antibiotic?

NO	YES
|	Stop the drug (preferably) or reduce the dose.

Does the patient have either pain or a plugged feeling in his ears?

NO	YES
|	**Consider** ear wax, EAR INFECTION, RESPIRATORY INFECTION, MYIASIS. See Protocol A.26
|	for ear pain.

Did the hearing loss begin with an illness with a corrected temperature over 38.5°/101.3°?

NO	YES
|	**Consider** MEASLES*, LASSA FEVER*,[2] TYPHUS*, EAR INFECTION, SICKLE CELL DISEASE,[3]
|	MENINGITIS*, ENCEPHALITIS*, SCRUB TYPHUS,[4] TRICHINOSIS.
See table on the next page.	* = Hearing is not usually recovered.

1 *This is most often due to congenital SYPHILIS, onset in older children or young adults, first ringing in the ears, then deafness, usually starts on one side but eventually affects both sides. Hearing may be recovered if it is treated early. Even if hearing is not recovered, the treatment will prevent other disastrous consequences.*
2 *Lassa fever: found in West Africa.*
3 *Sickle cell disease: this affects those of African genetic origin, mainly in West Africa and the Americas. Some Greeks, Indians and Arabs are also affected.*
4 *Scrub typhus: Asia and Pacific Areas; always fever, eye symptoms, headache, constipation.*

LOSS OF HEARING, NO RINGING, NO DRUG INGESTION, NO PLUGGING, NO HIGH FEVER

Consider	Fever	Other
Onset likely recent		
PLANT POISONING	No	Due to nicotine, cassava, tobacco/cow's urine (Africa).
Onset indeterminate		
Ear wax	No	Tan or dark brown wax in canals.[1]
BRAIN DAMAGE*	Maybe	Hearing loss may be a consequence of any cause of this.
SYPHILIS, tertiary/congenital	No	Patient, partner or parent was exposed.
Onset probably from birth or in infancy		
SICKLE CELL DISEASE	Maybe	Belly and limb pains, began in infancy; family history of early deaths.
CRETINISM*	No	Also poor growth, mentally retarded.
RADIATION ILLNESS*	No	Infant of a mother irradiated after 8 weeks of pregnancy.

* = Hearing is likely not recovered.

PROTOCOL A.26—EAR PAIN

⊳ SYMPTOMATIC TREATMENT

ACETAMINOPHEN or IBUPROFEN is always appropriate. ASPIRIN is usually appropriate but should not be given until you have reached a diagnosis.

Any injury can affect the outer ears or the ear canals. See Chapter 9, Volume 1.

Condition	Fever	Other Characteristics
By far the most common everywhere		
EAR INFECTION, MIDDLE	Usual	No change in pain with pulling on the outer ear; maybe a red or opaque ear drum.
Dental problem	Unusual	A molar tooth hurts or ear pain worse with tapping on the tooth.
General, whole-body illness, nothing abnormal visible in ear or throat		
MUMPS	Maybe	Swelling of face, maybe neck also, one or both sides.
TUBERCULOSIS	Usual	Hoarse, pain with swallowing or draining ear; almost always a cough also.
TYPHUS	High	Severe body aching, mentally abnormal, other symptoms before fever.
BRUCELLOSIS	Erratic	Pain in the jaw joints in front of the ears; lower limb or back pain likely.
Visible problem in ear		
Wax in ears	No	Ear canals are packed with wax which varies from tan to dark brown.
MYIASIS	Rare	Maggots, resembling short, fat "worms" in the ear.
EAR INFECTION, EXTERNAL	Rare	Increased pain with pulling on the ear; history of recent swimming or scratch.
Insect in ear	No	Patient will tell you the diagnosis.[1]
HEMORRHAGIC FEVER	Yes	Bleeding from the ear with a severe whole-body illness.
Visible problem in mouth or throat		
STREP THROAT	Usual	Ears look normal; throat is red.
Tooth problem	Maybe	Obvious decay in a molar on the affected side.
DIPHTHERIA	Low	Patient quite ill; leathery scum on the throat.

---

1 *The treatment is to drown the insect with cooking oil as long as the ear drum is not broken (the patient can hear on that side). These creatures tend to get stuck in ear wax, which acts like fly paper. As they struggle to free themselves, legs and wings tend to hit against the ear drum, causing severe pain and loud (to the patient) noise. Once the creature is dead, the normal outward flow of the ear wax will remove him from the canal. Do not try to dig the insect out yourself, though a physician who knows what he is doing might be able to do so.*

PROTOCOL A.27—OTHER EAR PROBLEMS

Swelling in front of ears: ABSCESS, TYPHUS, MUMPS, LIVER DISEASE, CIRRHOSIS, CHAGA'S DISEASE,[1] HIV INFECTION in infants.

Swelling behind ear(s): MASTOIDITIS, large lymph nodes.

Bumps on outer ears: if firm (like the outer ear), due to LEPROSY; if hard (like pebbles), due to GOUT, maybe scar or KELOIDS due to an old injury.

Acquired thick earlobes: normal in those overweight; may be a late consequence of ear piercing, especially in patients prone to KELOIDS; consider LEPROSY.

Ears itching: ALLERGY, CANDIDIASIS, CONTACT DERMATITIS, occasionally EAR INFECTION.

Maggots in ears: MYIASIS.

Rash on skin of outer ears: ears can have the same problems as skin elsewhere; see Protocols A.14–A.18.

Strange-looking ears at birth: congenital SYPHILIS or else needs a major medical center or live with it.

Ringing in the ears: OLD AGE is most common; Also consider ear wax; ASPIRIN overdose (first symptom); possibly QUININE (drug) side effect; EAR INFECTION, MIDDLE; TUBERCULOSIS; SYPHILIS; common after head injury. If it is on one side only it may be due to CANCER.

Ears feel plugged: either due to wax or else RESPIRATORY INFECTION (a cold). Wax must be cleaned out by someone who has the use of an otoscope; wax softeners may be helpful.

Pus running out of ears: EAR INFECTION, middle or external, TUBERCULOSIS in children.

Cold, white outer ears: FROSTBITE.

Bleeding from the ears: EAR INFECTION; EBOLA VIRUS DISEASE, or HEMORRHAGIC FEVER if quite ill.

PROTOCOL A.28—NOSE PROBLEMS

Bloody nose: see the procedure described in Volume 1, Appendix 1 to stop bleeding. Check out Protocol B.7 if this is one manifestation of a generalized bleeding problem. Otherwise this is most likely due to dry air or nose picking.

> **If it is a small amount**, less than a cup of blood, it may be due to a local nose problem or a general illness such as DIPHTHERIA, SYPHILIS, LEPROSY, TUBERCULOSIS, CUTANEOUS LEISHMANIASIS.[2]

> **Recently ill with a corrected temperature over 38.5°/101.3°:** DENGUE FEVER,[8] HEMORRHAGIC FEVER, TYPHUS, RELAPSING FEVER,[3] SAND FLY FEVER.

> **Recently ill, no fever:** may be due to some poisons.

> **Ill for quite a while, family history of ill health or no fever:** if there is bilirubin in the urine, see Protocol B.7. Also consider SCURVY, VISCERAL LEISHMANIASIS,[4] SICKLE CELL DISEASE,[5] THALLASEMIA, TROPICAL SPLENOMEGALY, ONYALAI.[6]

Sneezing: ALLERGY, early MEASLES, may be due to any irritation of the nose by dust.

Loss of smell: this may occur for no reason at all or from a RESPIRATORY INFECTION or prior injury or surgery. Otherwise ZINC DEFICIENCY, ALLERGY, DIABETES, /// LEPROSY, BRAIN TUMOR, BRAIN DAMAGE, ENCEPHALITIS, some poisons. This may be the side effect of some medications for lowering blood pressure.

Runny nose (watery): RESPIRATORY INFECTION (cold), ALLERGY, MEASLES, rarely head injury (serious if due to this; send out). If the patient is quite ill, possibly DIPHTHERIA. Common in SYPHILIS (congenital, infants). Consider INSECTICIDE POISONING and PLANT POISONING. May be due to a foreign body in the nose, particularly in preschool children.

Runny nose (pus): RESPIRATORY INFECTION (sinusitis); MENINGITIS. Occasionally LEPROSY, CUTANEOUS LEISHMANIASIS.[7]

Low bridge of nose: may be a family trait; otherwise, if present from infancy, DOWN SYNDROME, CRETINISM, THALLASEMIA, congenital SYPHILIS. If acquired later in life, may be due to LEPROSY, YAWS or tertiary (acquired) SYPHILIS.

Wormy creature(s) in the nose: MYIASIS, ASCARIASIS; may be a leech (see Volume 1, Chapter 9).

---

1 *Chaga's disease: found in scattered areas of Central and South America.*

2 *Cutaneous Leishmaniasis: scattered areas in the Americas, Africa, the Mediterranean, Europe, central Asia, the Middle East and the Indian subcontinent.*

3 *Relapsing fever: tropical and high altitude, but not in the islands of SEA and the Pacific.*

4 *Visceral Leishmaniasis: found in scattered areas of Central and South America, Africa north of the equator, the Mediterranean area, the Indian subcontinent, eastern Europe, central Asia and mainland China.*

5 *Sickle cell disease: this affects those of African genetic origin, mainly in West Africa and the Americas. Some Indians and Arabs are also affected.*

6 *Onyalai: only in certain parts of southern Africa.*

7 *Cutaneous Leishmaniasis: scattered areas in the Americas, Africa, the Mediterranean, Europe, central Asia, the Middle East and the Indian subcontinent.*

8 *Dengue fever: in the Americas only near or north of the equator. In Africa, east coastal, south and west. Prevalent in India, Southeast Asia and the Pacific. Occasionally found in the Mediterranean area. The disease may spread.*

Bumpy or misshapen nose: LEPROSY, YAWS, ALCOHOLISM, CUTANEOUS LEISHMANIASIS,[2] family trait, middle age changes. SYPHILIS if the patient, partner or parent is or was exposed.

Ulcers or boils: SYPHILIS, YAWS, TREPONARID, MYCETOMA, LEPROSY, CUTANEOUS LEISHMANIASIS,[2] CANCER, CANCRUM ORIS.

Holes in the center divider of the nose: SYPHILIS, congenital or acquired; old injury.

Food regurgitation through the nose: SYPHILIS, DIPHTHERIA, RABIES, POLIO, STROKE, any paralysis of the face.

Congestion/stuffy nose: RESPIRATORY INFECTION, ALLERGY, sometimes a drug side effect or INSECTICIDE POISONING; rarely DIPHTHERIA, MEASLES or SCRUB TYPHUS[1] if the patient is very ill. In an epidemic context, consider INFLUENZA.

Blood blisters in the mouth: ONYALAI, southern Africa only; see Regional Notes F.

1 *Scrub typhus: in northern Australia and throughout the Eastern Hemisphere north of there and east of Afghanistan, as far north as Mongolia.*
2 *Cutaneous Leishmaniasis: tropical and subtropical north of the equator, but not present in Southeast Asia or the Pacific areas.*

PROTOCOL A.29—MOUTH AND THROAT DISORDERS

A.29.A—Sore throat   A.29.B—Sore mouth   A.29.C—Other mouth/throat problems:

A.29.C 1—Throat	A.29.C 4—Lips	A.29.C 7—Voice
A.29.C 2—Tongue	A.29.C 5—Teeth	
A.29.C 3—Mouth	A.29.C 6—Jaw	

⚠ EMERGENCY	▷ SYMPTOMATIC TREATMENT
EMERGENCIES OF THE MOUTH AND THROAT Inability to swallow—drooling Noisy breathing in Abscess in the throat Shortness of breath Major swelling.	**SORE THROAT** Gargling with salt water (a teaspoon in a glass) will remarkably relieve pain. Sometimes sitting up to sleep at night will help. ACETAMINOPHEN or IBUPROFEN is always appropriate; ASPIRIN may be appropriate in adults, but it should not be given until you have reached a diagnosis.

Protocol A.29.A—Sore throat

Sore throat plus diarrhea should be treated like STREP INFECTION but with ERYTHROMYCIN rather than PENICILLIN.

Condition	Fever	Other Characteristics
Most common, check these first		
RESPIRATORY INFECTION	Low if any	Stuffy or runny nose or cough, common cold.
MUMPS	Maybe	Swelling of face, pain with swallowing.
HERPES	Probably	Blisters or ulcers visible; common in HIV+ patients.
Prominent large lymph nodes in the neck, previously healthy, recent onset		
STREP INFECTION	Yes	Big red tonsils with pus, big lymph nodes, no runny nose.
HIV INFECTION, sero conversion	Probably	Flu-like illness, measles-type rash, exposure within the last 4 months.
DIPHTHERIA	Low if any	Gray/white throat scum extends rapidly; very ill.
MONKEYPOX[1]	Yes	Also a blistered rash that breaks out all at once.
TOXOPLASMOSIS	Maybe	History of cat exposure or rare meat.
MONONUCLEOSIS	Yes	Large tonsils, very tired, large neck lymph nodes.
No prominent lymph nodes, previously healthy, recent onset		
DENGUE FEVER[2]	High	Also severe bone and joint pains, fevers.
PLANT POISONING	No	Botulism usually from sausage or tainted vegetables.
LASSA FEVER[3]	Yes	Headache, cough, chest pain; very ill.
RABIES	Maybe	Painful spasms of throat; cannot swallow liquids.
EBOLA VIRUS DISEASE	Yes	Also abdominal pains, vomiting, profound fatigue, Africa only.

Footnotes on the next page at the end of this table.

Associated with severe fatigue

Condition	Fever	Other Characteristics
MONONUCLEOSIS	Yes	Large tonsils, very tired, large neck lymph nodes.
TOXOPLASMOSIS	Maybe	History of cat exposure or rare meat.

Geographically very confined

Condition	Fever	Other Characteristics
TREPONARID[4]	Maybe	White patches on pink inside the mouth.
FAMILIAL MEDITERRANEAN FEVER[5]	Maybe	Hereditary, recurrent, also abdominal or joint pains.
Leech	No	Visible leech in throat (See Volume 1, Chapter 9.)

Slow-onset burning pain

Condition	Fever	Other Characteristics
TUBERCULOSIS	Usual	Pain with swallowing over months; night sweats.
ARSENIC POISONING	No	Abdominal pain, numb, tingling, weak, skin changes.
PELLAGRA	No	Burning pain with swallowing; poor diet, skin changes.

1 Monkeypox: found in northern D. R. Congo and adjacent areas of Central African Republic. It is rare in West Africa.
2 Dengue fever: in the Americas only near or north of the equator. In Africa, east coastal, south and west. Prevalent in India, Southeast Asia and the Pacific. Occasionally found in the Mediterranean area. The disease may spread.
3 Lassa fever: found in West Africa where it usually occurs in epidemics.
4 Treponarid: arid portions of Africa, Asia, the Middle East and the Pacific area.
5 Familial Mediterranean fever affects Sephardic Jews, Arabs, Greeks, Italians, Spaniards. Because of migrations, consider Hispanics and Irish also.

Protocol A.29.B—Sore mouth

▷ SYMPTOMATIC TREATMENT

ACETAMINOPHEN or IBUPROFEN is always appropriate; ASPIRIN may be appropriate in adults but should not be given until you have reached a diagnosis. See Protocol A.29.C also.

Condition	Fever	Other Characteristics
Blisters or ulcers, likely localized to the face or mouth		
HERPES	Maybe	White blisters on red base, very tender.
APHTHOUS STOMATITIS	No	Painful ulcers, red around the edges.
SHINGLES	Maybe	Blister-type rash, right or left only.
CANCRUM ORIS	Maybe	Malnutrition, hole into the mouth.
TUBERCULOSIS	Maybe	Painful small ulcer(s), tip or sides of the tongue.
MALABSORPTION, SPRUE[1]	No	Severe diarrhea, gassy abdomen.
White scum in the mouth with reddening underneath		
CANDIDIASIS	No	Occurs in those who took antibiotics and in those with poor immunity.
Rash, blisters or ulcers likely not exclusively on the face		
REITER SYNDROME	Usual	Painful or painless ulcers; also ARTHRITIS.
TYPHUS	High	Sores inside mouth; very ill, musty body odor.
MEASLES	High	White spots on red base, also cough and red eyes.
ONYALAI	Unknown	Southern Africa only.
Swelling with disruption of the gum surface		
VINCENT STOMATITIS	Maybe	Red, swollen gums with black, dead tissue.
DONOVANOSIS	No	History of oral sex; Pacific, ports, transport corridors.
CUTANEOUS LEISHMANIASIS[2]	No	Also facial skin disrupted; mainly the Americas.

1 Sprue: in the Americas only near or north of the equator. In Africa only Nigeria and southern Africa. Prevalent in India and Southeast Asia. It is occasionally found in the Mediterranean area.
2 Cutaneous Leishmaniasis: tropical and subtropical north of the equator, but not present in Southeast Asia or the Pacific areas.

TOC · SYMPTOMS · DIFFERENTIALS · CONDITIONS · DRUG INDEX · REGIONAL NOTES · INX

TOC

SYMPTOMS

DIFFERENTIALS

CONDITIONS

DRUG INDEX

REGIONAL NOTES

INX

Protocol A.29.C—Other mouth and throat problems

29.C1—THROAT

Very large tonsils: normal in preschoolers; if red, see Protocol A.29.A.

Swelling of throat: ALLERGY, ANAPHYLAXIS, ABSCESS; rarely ANTHRAX, DIPHTHERIA, MONONUCLEOSIS, /TUBERCULOSIS.

Itchy throat: ALLERGY.

Hoarseness: may be due to OLD AGE or occupational in speakers. Common with RESPIRATORY INFECTION (croup), LARYNGITIS. Also may be due to GOITER, THYROID TROUBLE, TUBERCULOSIS, LEPROSY, DIPHTHERIA, SYPHILIS in infants, PLANT POISONING due to botulism.

Whisper voice, soft voice: patient either has a very sore throat, is near death or is trying to act ill, though TUBERCULOSIS may occasionally cause this. Distinguish this from laryngitis when a person chooses to whisper rather than talk in a hoarse voice or cause himself pain. May sometimes be due to GOITER, DIPHTHERIA, PLANT POISONING due to botulism or CANCER.

29.C2—TONGUE

Lengthwise cracks on tongue: SYPHILIS (tertiary/congenital), TUBERCULOSIS, CANCER.

Abnormal tongue color:

white patches: CANDIDIASIS.

pale: ANEMIA; check out the causative diseases of anemia also.

bluish: RESPIRATORY FAILURE, some kinds of HEART FAILURE.

deep red: MALNUTRITION, PELLAGRA, SCARLET FEVER, ENTERIC FEVER third week, CARBON MONOXIDE POISONING, SPRUE.[2]

brown: KIDNEY DISEASE, MEASLES at the beginning.

gray patches, symmetrical, not furry: normal in persons of African genetic heritage.

yellowish scum: ENTERIC FEVER, TYPHUS, many severe illnesses with high fevers.

black, furry: smokers and after a person takes some antibiotics; do not treat this.

gray-white furry coating: ENTERIC FEVER during the first week, TYPHUS, SCARLET FEVER, some other illnesses with fevers.

strawberry tongue (red and white): STREP THROAT.

purplish tongue: PELLAGRA

Sore tongue: STREP THROAT, PELLAGRA, ALCOHOLISM, SPRUE,[2] MALNUTRITION, MALABSORPTION, CANDIDIASIS, ANEMIA due to lack of IRON.

Tongue ulcers: advanced TUBERCULOSIS (small, crater-like), REITER SYNDROME, some SEXUALLY TRANSMITTED DISEASEs.

Large tongue: ALLERGY, SCURVY, ANTHRAX, CRETINISM, DOWN SYNDROME, ACROMEGALY.

Cannot stick out tongue: TYPHUS, sometimes CANCER or an ABSCESS under the tongue.

Black on tongue and inside the mouth: may be normal with dark skin or due to PLANT POISONING: betel nut. Also consider ANEMIA, VINCENT ANGINA, CANCRUM ORIS or antibiotic side effect. If very ill, tongue dry and black, consider TYPHUS.

29.C3—MOUTH

Thirst and dry mouth: DEHYDRATION; DIABETES; BRUCELLOSIS; PLANT POISONING: botulism, coral plant,[1] jimson weed; side effect of some drugs. A patient might experience a dry mouth as thirst. If so, consider DIPHTHERIA, TETANUS, RABIES. A patient who has diarrhea from any cause will be thirsty since his bowel is not absorbing water as it should.

Dark pigmented patches on pink surfaces: normal if symmetrical in persons of African genetic heritage; if asymmetrical, it may be caused by CANCER.

Strange taste in the mouth: RESPIRATORY INFECTION (sinusitis), DENGUE FEVER,[3] ARSENIC POISONING, LEAD POISONING, HEARTBURN, pregnancy, side effect of some medications (most commonly METRONIDAZOLE); may be due to a dental infection.

Cannot taste: check ZINC DEFICIENCY, LEPROSY, PELLAGRA, KIDNEY DISEASE. Check if the problem is really with the sense of smell.

Rash in mouth: HERPES, RUBELLA, SPRUE, MEASLES, SHINGLES, CHICKEN POX, LEPTOSPIROSIS, SYPHILIS, YAWS, DIPHTHERIA, CANDIDIASIS, MONONUCLEOSIS, PELLAGRA, LASSA FEVER (Africa).

---

1 Plant poisoning, coral plant: African and Middle Eastern areas.

2 Sprue: in the Americas only near or north of the equator. In Africa only Nigeria and southern Africa. Prevalent in India and Southeast Asia. It is occasionally found in the Mediterranean area.

3 Dengue fever: in the Americas only near or north of the equator. In Africa, east coastal, south and west. Prevalent in India, Southeast Asia and the Pacific. Occasionally found in the Mediterranean area. The disease may spread.

Painless ulcers: REITER SYNDROME, SYPHILIS, DONOVANOSIS, CANCER, other causes.

Painful ulcers: VINCENT STOMATITIS, HERPES, DONOVANOSIS with secondary infection.

Difficulty chewing: DIPHTHERIA, MUMPS, any mouth or tooth pain, any general weakness, any BRAIN DAMAGE.

Excessive saliva: TETANUS, PLANT POISONING: nicotine, muscarine; INSECTICIDE POISONING, ADDICTION (narcotic withdrawal), PELLAGRA. If there is a severe cough, consider PERTUSSIS.

Worm crawling up into the mouth: ASCARIASIS.

Swelling between teeth and cheek: ACTINOMYCOSIS, ABSCESS (tender), early CANCRUM ORIS.

Bleeding from mouth: injury and infection, poor dental hygiene, consider DONOVANOSIS, HEMORRHAGIC FEVER. Check out Protocols A.13.E and B.7 if this is one manifestation of generalized easy bleeding.

Hole in the roof of the mouth: birth defect, YAWS,[3] SYPHILIS (congenital or acquired), CANCRUM ORIS, CANCER.

29.C4—LIPS

Chapped lips: may be due to vitamin deficiency. Try MULTIVITAMIN tablets. The problem responds slowly, over weeks.

Vertical cracks: SPRUE,[2] MALNUTRITION, overdose of VITAMIN A.

Horizontal cracks: CANDIDIASIS, SYPHILIS, TREPONARID, YAWS,[3] any vitamin deficiency.

Rash on lip: DIPHTHERIA, IMPETIGO, HERPES, vitamin deficiency.

Blue around lips: RESPIRATORY FAILURE, HEART FAILURE, ANAPHYLAXIS, ALTITUDE SICKNESS.

Black and red around lips: PLANT POISONING due to betel nut.

Splits on sides of lips: SYPHILIS, YAWS,[3] TREPONARID, PELLAGRA, vitamin deficiency.

Shrivelled lips: PELLAGRA.

Sore on lip: SEXUALLY TRANSMITTED DISEASE, TREPONARID (arid areas), DIPHTHERIA, HERPES, IMPETIGO.

Swollen lips: tertiary YAWS, ALLERGY.

29.C5—TEETH AND GUMS

Toothache alone, upper teeth, no redness or swelling: RESPIRATORY INFECTION (sinusitis). Molar pain may be due to EAR INFECTION, middle.

Secondary front teeth have single notches on their cutting edges: congenital SYPHILIS.

Teeth have serrated cutting edges: normal variant.

Toothache with redness and swelling: use PENICILLIN or ERYTHROMYCIN for any tooth but the last molars. For the last molars, use METRONIDAZOLE. It may be necessary to pull the tooth.

Gums red and swollen with black crud on them: VINCENT STOMATITIS.

Teeth falling out: poor dental hygiene, DONOVANOSIS, congenital SYPHILIS.

Malformed teeth: CRETINISM; THALLASEMIA; SYPHILIS if there are single notches in upper two front permanent teeth.

Delayed teething: may be normal, RICKETS, HIV INFECTION, SYPHILIS, congenital.

Bleeding gums: mouth infection (Gram-positive), SCURVY, PELLAGRA; poor dental hygiene, HEMORRHAGIC FEVER, VISCERAL LEISHMANIASIS,[1] LIVER FAILURE of any kind, ARSENIC POISONING, LEAD POISONING, DONOVANOSIS. See Protocols A.13.E and B.7 if this is part of a general bleeding problem. See protocol B.2 for a recent-onset whole-body illness.

Green teeth: late consequence of JAUNDICE in a newborn.

Swollen gums: PHENYTOIN (drug), SCURVY, PELLAGRA, SYPHILIS, tooth ABSCESS, DONOVANOSIS.

Dark discoloration of teeth: side effect of childhood or prenatal TETRACYCLINE (drug); FLUOROSIS.

Blue line on gums: LEAD POISONING.

---

1 *Visceral Leishmaniasis: found in scattered areas of Central and South America, Africa north of the equator, the Mediterranean area, the Indian subcontinent, eastern Europe, central Asia and mainland China.*

2 *Sprue: in the Americas only near or north of the equator. In Africa only Nigeria and southern Africa. Prevalent in India and Southeast Asia. It is occasionally found in the Mediterranean area.*

3 *Yaws: only in the humid tropics.*

TOC

SYMPTOMS

DIFFERENTIALS

CONDITIONS

DRUG INDEX · REGIONAL NOTES · INX

29.C6—JAW

Swollen jaw: MUMPS, ABSCESS in a tooth, injury, BURKITT LYMPHOMA, jaw bone OSTEOMYELITIS, CANCER, CANCRUM ORIS, VINCENT STOMATITIS, ACTINOMYCOSIS.

Cannot open mouth: face injury (see Volume 1, Chapter 9), TETANUS if there are muscle spasms, tooth problem, PLANT POISONING due to strychnine.

Cannot close mouth: if the jaw locks in the open position, see Volume 1, Chapter 12.

Difficulty chewing: DIPHTHERIA, BRUCELLOSIS, TRICHINOSIS, POLIO, not enough teeth.

Jaw pain: dental problem, GALLBLADDER DISEASE, HEART ATTACK, HEART FAILURE. Jaw pain can be caused by jaw problems but also by disease elsewhere in the body. In this case the jaw is painful but not tender. The nerves are wired up so that disease in one area can cause pain in another area. This is called referred pain. In the case of the jaw pain, the heart is the structure most commonly responsible for referred pain.

29.C7—VOICE PROBLEMS

Difficulty talking; any very ill patient; DIPHTHERIA, MUMPS, POLIO, any weakness, RESPIRATORY FAILURE

Grunting with each breath: RESPIRATORY FAILURE.

Whispering or hoarseness: many respiratory illnesses; DIPHTHERIA, lung TUBERCULOSIS, congenital SYPHILIS in an infant, common when a patient is near death.

Staccato or slurred speech, nasal speech, a growling tone or new-onset stammering: brain problems (head injury, STROKE, ENCEPHALITIS, etc.) may cause this.

Slurred speech, no fever: ALCOHOL effect, other drug side effects, head injury, snake bite, ALTITUDE SICKNESS, STROKE, AFRICAN SLEEPING SICKNESS,[1] PLANT POISONING: cassava or lolism,[2] SYPHILIS, tertiary/congenital, BRAIN DAMAGE, ADDICTION to downers, PLANT POISONING due to botulism, any severe weakness.

Slurred speech with a fever: DENGUE FEVER,[3] cerebral MALARIA, TYPHUS, AFRICAN SLEEPING SICKNESS,[1] RHEUMATIC FEVER, DIPHTHERIA, rarely due to PLAGUE.

---

1 *African sleeping sickness: scattered areas of Africa, south of Bamako, Mali and Lake Chad and north of Lusaka, Zambia.*

2 *Plant poisoning, lolism: found in the African, Mediterranean and Middle Eastern areas.*

3 *Dengue fever: in the Americas only near or north of the equator. In Africa, east coastal, south and west. Prevalent in India, Southeast Asia and the Pacific. Occasionally found in the Mediterranean area. The disease may spread.*

Village Medical Manual 7th Edition Volume 2

A-93
CHAPTER PAGE

TOC

SYMPTOMS

DIFFERENTIALS

CONDITIONS

DRUG INDEX

REGIONAL NOTES

INX

V—NECK PROBLEMS

PROTOCOL A.30—NECK PAIN

A.30.A—Pain with forward motion only

A.30.B—Pain with motion sideways

A.30.C—Pain in one or two areas of the neck

A.30.D—Pain with swallowing

⚠ NECK PAIN / INJURIES	▷ SYMPTOMATIC TREATMENT
Neck pain along with fever, headache, vomiting, mental changes; also pain with recent-onset numbness, tingling, sharp-shooting pains, heaviness, weakness or paralysis. For pain that is the result of injury, see Neck Injury in Volume 1, Chapter 4 (major), Chapter 9 and Chapter 12 (minor).	Use ACETAMINOPHEN or IBUPROFEN, not ASPIRIN.

Protocol A.30.A—Pain with forward motion only in a moderately to very sick patient

Definition: the patient cannot comfortably put his chin on his chest, but he can turn his head from side to side, and he can throw his head back.

Problem	Sensitive (negative eliminates the diagnosis)	Specific (positive makes it likely)
Sustained fever (unless an infant, elderly or malnourished)		
MALARIA, cerebral	Severe headache, mental changes, vomiting.	Recent history of malaria.
SPOTTED FEVER[1]	Severe muscle aching; rash by day 4 or 5.	Tiny black scab or scabs.
MENINGITIS	High fever; headache (adults), vomiting (children), very ill (both), mental changes.	Rash: black-and-blue or large blisters.
ENCEPHALITIS	High fever; headache (adults), vomiting (children).	Nothing specific.
Erratic, mild or no fever		
POLIO	Muscle spasms, back pains also, weak limb(s).	Asymmetrical, prior "cold" or "flu".
HERPES	Skin rash consisting of painful tiny blisters.	Sensitive is also specific.
STROKE	Instantaneous onset of a severe headache initially.	Numbness, weakness or both.
RABIES	Spasms with a breeze or swallowing liquids.	At first swallows solids easier than liquids.
LEPTOSPIROSIS	Erratic fever, ill for days, sore eyes or muscles.	Rash on roof of mouth, pain in calves & back.

1 *Spotted fever: worldwide including the Arctic, except not in the islands of Southeast Asia.*

Protocol A.30.B—Not very sick, pain is aggravated with any neck motion, or both

Problem	Fever	Other Characteristics
Symptoms likely localized to the neck and maybe the arm on one side		
MUSCLE STRAIN	No	History of unusual exercise or a minor accident.
TORTICOLIS	No	Not ill, head tilted sideways, sudden onset, no injury.
SLIPPED DISC	No	Pain also on the thumb or little finger side of the hand,[1] better with arms raised.
RADICULOPATHY	Unusual	Arm heavy, numb or weak, improved with arms raised.
OSTEOMYELITIS	Usual	Very localized bony pain and tenderness with warmth, maybe visible swelling also.
Maybe localized, maybe a whole-body illness		
TUBERCULOSIS	Maybe	Pain is worse with turning the head sideways; slow onset, maybe a bulge in back.
ARTHRITIS	Maybe	Back of neck, warm and tender; maybe other joints also.

1 *Pain that affects all fingers equally is not likely due to slipped disc. Frequently the arms feel heavy. Radiculopathy is one consequence of slipped disc, so distinguishing the two conditions is not necessary.*

Protocol A.30.C—Pain confined to one or two areas of the neck

Problem	Fever	Other Characteristics
STRESS	No	Headache in back of the head or in a band around; affects the upper neck in back.
LEPROSY	Rare	Shooting pains up and down neck, along nerves which may be swollen and tender, usually not symmetrical.
ANGINA	No	Pressure-type pain also in chest and/or left arm, jaw, not localized in one spot

Protocol A.30.D—Swallowing pain or difficulty swallowing without pain

Definition: Either the patient complains of pain with swallowing, or he says that his food gets stuck (usually temporarily) somewhere between his throat and stomach. He may have both pain and a sticking sensation.

See Protocol 29.A—Sore Throat if this is applicable; otherwise proceed.

The most common cause is something swallowed that got stuck or scratched the patient on its way down. Have the patient sit up for 24 hours and give him generous doses of crushed or injectable pain medication and tranquillizer. Send out if the problem persists after 24 hours. Don't let him swallow anything else meanwhile. Give him a bowl to spit his saliva into. If this is due to a throat problem, see Protocol A.29. If leeches are common in your area, consider a leech swallowed with drinking water. See Volume 1, Chapter 9.

What happened first?

- If **liquids** were first difficult before solids, then the problem probably has to do with the nervous system: liquids come out of the nose with attempts to swallow. Consider POLIO, DIPHTHERIA, RABIES, STROKE, BRAIN DAMAGE, PLANT POISONING due to botulism, SYPHILIS.
- If **solids** were a problem before liquids, then the problem is more likely an obstruction.

Has the patient been ill more than a month, and he coughs up sputum that has a foul, rotten odor?

NO to either	YES to both
	May be due to a lung abscess: requires surgical care.

Is the patient at risk for SYPHILIS, either tertiary or congenital?

NO	YES
	He may have a heart problem from the SYPHILIS. There is nothing you can do short of a level 4 or 5 hospital.

Does the patient have visible swelling on his, or her neck?

NO	YES
	Consider GOITER, CANCER, TUBERCULOSIS, ANTHRAX, DIPHTHERIA, TRICHINOSIS, VINCENT STOMATITIS

See the table on next page.

SWALLOWING PAIN OR DIFFICULTY SWALLOWING WITHOUT PAIN

Level refers to where the problem is. H is high, above the collar bones; M is medium, between the collar bones and the middle of the breast bone; L is low, below the middle of the breast bone; A is anywhere. Patients can usually localize the problem accurately.

Problem	Fever	Level	Other Characteristics
Prominent pain; visible skin or mouth manifestations likely			
PELLAGRA	No	A	Burning pain, sore mouth, skin rash.
CANDIDIASIS	No	A	White scum visible in the mouth.
HERPES	Maybe	H	Blisters in the mouth or around the mouth.
HIV INFECTION	Usual	A	Frequently associated with CANDIDIASIS, or HERPES.
Prominent pain; neither visible skin nor mouth manifestations likely			
PERICARDITIS	Maybe	L	Pain worse lying, relieved by sitting, leaning forward.
RABIES	Maybe	H	Rapid onset; liquids are a problem before solids.
TRICHINOSIS	Yes	A	Ate raw or rare pork or game within the past month.
Maybe pain, no muscle weakness likely; solids first			
CANCER	Maybe	A	Slow-onset; painless at first, painful after a while.
MUMPS	Maybe	H	Swelling of the jaw, one side or both.
ANTHRAX	Yes	A	Sore with a black scab; large amount of swelling.
Maybe pain; likely prominent muscle weakness; likely liquids first			
POLIO	Usual	A	Other weakness after an initial "cold" or "flu".
DIPHTHERIA	Maybe	A	Vision problems; sore throat or wound infection.
RABIES	Maybe	A	Swallowing water difficult before swallowing food.
Likely without prominent pain, no other bodily weakness; solids first			
GOITER	No	H	Choking sensation, lower front neck swelling.
Likely without prominent pain, likely has other bodily weakness; liquids first			
STROKE	No	A	Sudden or stuttering onset, other weakness.
BRAIN DAMAGE	Unusual	A	Mental changes, other weakness or numbness.
PLANT POISONING (botulism)	No	A	From tainted food, beans or sausage commonly; symptoms start on the head, travel down.
Likely a distended abdomen			
TROPICAL SPLENOMEGALY	Unusual	L	Huge spleen; malarious area, spleen not tender usually; it is firm, not soft or hard; liver normal size.
VISCERAL LEISHMANIASIS[2]	Maybe	L	Huge spleen, large liver after month 3, very slow onset, geographically confined.
LIVER FAILURE	Maybe	L	Also swollen belly with big veins on the skin.
CHAGA'S DISEASE[1]	No	A	Also constipation, maybe HEART FAILURE.

1 *Chaga's disease: found in scattered areas in the Americas.*

2 *Visceral Leishmaniasis: found in scattered areas of Central and South America, (mainly eastern) Africa north of the equator, the Mediterranean area, the Indian subcontinent, eastern Europe, central Asia and mainland China.*

TOC

SYMPTOMS

DIFFERENTIALS

CONDITIONS

DRUG INDEX

REGIONAL NOTES

INX

PROTOCOL A.31—OTHER NECK PROBLEMS

A.31. A—Swollen neck

A.31.B—Miscellaneous neck problems

⚠ EMERGENCY

EMERGENCY CONDITION: Neck swelling accompanied by shortness of breath.

Protocol A.31.A—Swollen neck

Is the swelling mainly lower center front, right above the breastbone?

NO	YES
	Consider: GOITER—there may be one or multiple swellings.

Is the swelling discreet, lump(s) or is it over an area? Discreet means it is evident where the lump starts and stops.

Discreet lumps	**Over an area**
	Consider: GOITER, ABSCESS, ANTHRAX, MUMPS, CANCER, rarely BURKITT LYMPHOMA.

Is the swelling visible from the front or only from the back?

Visible from the front	**Visible only from the back**
	Consider: AFRICAN SLEEPING SICKNESS,[1] LICE (head lice), RUBELLA, EAR INFECTION, IMPETIGO of the scalp, MONONUCLEOSIS, SYPHILIS, CANCER.

Is the throat obviously abnormal—swollen, red tonsils, maybe with gray or white scum on them?

NO	YES
	Consider: STREP THROAT, DIPHTHERIA, MONONUCLEOSIS, TULAREMIA, ANTHRAX.

Has the patient had ear pain, pus coming out of his ear or little white spots on his head hair?

NO	YES
See table below.	**Consider:** EAR INFECTION, MUMPS, tooth ABSCESS,[2] or head LICE.

1 African sleeping sickness: scattered areas of Africa, south of Bamako, Mali and Lake Chad; north of Lusaka, Zambia.
2 There will not be pus from the ear, but if the tooth is a molar, the patient likely has ear pain.

NECK SWELLING, LUMPY, VISIBLE FROM THE FRONT, NO THROAT OR EAR PROBLEM

Problem	Other large nodes[1]	Other symptoms
Most likely possibilities; consider these first		
MUMPS	No	Likely an unimmunized child; not very ill, swelling in front of ears
TUBERCULOSIS	Probably	Multiple lumps, stuck together, maybe open skin, maybe stale-beer odor
HIV INFECTION	Probably	History of positive blood test or exposure
CANCER	Maybe	Slow-onset, initially painless, usually older folk
Fever but no skin abnormality likely		
TOXOPLASMOSIS	Maybe	Extreme fatigue, large spleen, lamb meat or cat poop exposure
RHEUMATIC FEVER	Maybe	Heart murmur, joint pains or both
HIV INFECTION, sero conversion	Maybe	Exposure within 4 weeks, flu-like illness
IRIS	Probably	Respiratory distress is likely; treatment for both HIV and (TB or LEPROSY)
BARTONELLOSIS[2]	Maybe	Oroya type; ANEMIA, jaundice, chest pains and joint pains

Footnotes at end of the table.

Fever plus skin abnormality likely		
LEPROSY reaction	Yes	Patient taking medication for leprosy; red, warm, swollen skim.
SCRUB TYPHUS[3]	Usual	Also eye pain in light, constipation, quite ill.
PLAGUE	Maybe	Extremely tender nodes with blackened skin, mental changes, very ill.
TULAREMIA[4]	Maybe	Flu-like illness; rodent or rabbit contact.
MONKEYPOX[5]	Yes	Dense, sudden, prominent blister-type rash; patient very ill.
Maybe fever, maybe skin abnormal		
CELLULITIS	No	Red or warm area of skin, head or neck; probably a history of a wound.
SYPHILIS, secondary	Maybe	Likely history of an open wound a spontaneous open wound on the lips or in the mouth.
HERPES	Maybe	Blistered or rough area of skin, head or neck.
IRIS	Maybe	Treatment for AIDS and (TB or LEPROSY) at the same time.
No fever		
SCURVY	No	Bleeding gums; bruising; diet without fresh fruit
CHAGA'S DISEASE[6]	Maybe	Usually swelling of one eye also, now or previously
COCCIDIOMYCOSIS[7]	Maybe	Also cough, chest pain

1 These may be found in the armpits, in the groins (leg creases), on the side of the elbows and behind the knees.
2 Bartonellosis: occurs only in Peru and adjacent countries.
3 Scrub typhus: Asia and the Pacific area; always fever, eye symptoms, headache, constipation.
4 Tularemia: temperate climates, people exposed to small animals or their insects.
5 Monkeypox: northern D.R. Congo and adjacent border area in Central African Republic; rarely West Africa.
6 Chaga's disease: found in scattered areas in the Americas.
7 Coccidiomycosis: in the arid areas of Central and South America.

Protocol A.31.B—Miscellaneous neck problems

Weakness; anything that can cause upper limb weakness can also cause neck weakness; see Protocols A.8.B and A.8.C.

Difficulty swallowing: see Protocol A.30.D.

Stiffness: OLD AGE, previous injury or some types of ARTHRITIS. If there is pain: see Protocol A.30.A or B.

Neck arched back: see Protocol A.30.A.

Swelling center front lower neck: probably GOITER or ABSCESS; rarely ANTHRAX, CANCER.

VI—UPPER LIMB PROBLEMS

PROTOCOL A.32—SHOULDER PROBLEMS

A.32.A—Shoulder pain   A.32.B—Other shoulder problems

▽ NON-EMERGENCY	⚠ EMERGENCY
Injury: see Volume 1, Chapter 12. Neck injury can cause shoulder pain. Hand and arm problems (illness or injury) can also cause shoulder pain; the listing for hand and arm pain is more complete.	**SHOULDER EMERGENCIES**
	Fast onset, extreme pain with tenderness, rapid progression: NECROTIZING FASCIITIS.
	Any exercise (even leg exercise) aggravates the pain, but it is relieved by rest: ANGINA, SYPHILIS (tertiary), RHEUMATIC FEVER, HEART ATTACK, HEART FAILURE.
Skin problems: treat like skin problems elsewhere.	Shoulder pain with a tender spleen after an abdominal injury: SPLENIC CRISIS.
Abdominal pain also: be aware that upper abdominal problems will manifest with shoulder pain. In this case the pain in the shoulder(s) will not increase with pushing on the painful shoulder area. The shoulder pain will likely increase with your pushing on the abdomen.	Shoulder pain with sweating, chest pain, arm pain and (maybe) jaw pain may indicate a HEART ATTACK.
	In the presence of abdominal pain, consider ACUTE ABDOMEN, SPLENIC CRISIS, GALLBLADDER DISEASE.

Protocol A.32.A—Shoulder pain

Fevers and aching all across shoulders in back:[1] MALARIA (left or both sides), AMEBIASIS (right side usually); SPLENIC CRISIS (left side only).

With movement mainly, but it also hurts when the patient relaxes his shoulders and you move them:

without fever: SICKLE CELL DISEASE,[2] MUSCLE STRAIN, ARTHRITIS,

with fever: DENGUE FEVER,[3] RHEUMATIC FEVER, BRUCELLOSIS, OSTEOMYELITIS, BARTONELLOSIS,[4] sometimes ARTHRITIS, SICKLE CELL DISEASE,[2] FAMILIAL MEDITERRANEAN FEVER.[5]

Specific points very tender: BURSITIS, TENDINITIS, OSTEOMYELITIS, some ARTHRITIS, FIBROMYALGIA; see Volume 1 Chapter 9.

Breathing aggravates pain: PNEUMONIA, TUBERCULOSIS, AMEBIASIS, GALLBLADDER DISEASE; may be due to excessive gas.

Any exercise (even leg exercise) aggravates the pain, but it is relieved by rest: ANGINA, SYPHILIS (tertiary), RHEUMATIC FEVER, HEART FAILURE.

Pain in a band that comes from the neck in back and goes down the arm: SHINGLES, ARTHRITIS of the spine, SLIPPED DISC, RADICULOPATHY, any injury to the neck, BRUCELLOSIS, LEPROSY or TUBERCULOSIS of the spine, rarely FLUOROSIS, CANCER, SPINAL NEUROPATHY. Also see Volume 1 Chapters 9 and 11.

Pain worse with arms up; patient cannot raise his arm to the side, but he tolerates your moving it well: probably due to a tendon injury in the shoulder; see Chapters 9, 11 and 12 in Volume 1.

Muscle pains in shoulders: MUSCLE STRAIN, TENDINITIS, TUBERCULOSIS, TRICHINOSIS, CYSTICERCOSIS. See Protocol A.10.C.

---

1 *Shoulders sometimes hurt, not because of a shoulder problem but because of a problem elsewhere in the body. The nerves are wired up so that pain in one part of the body is felt in another part. This is called referred pain. In the case of pain in the shoulders, the heart, the liver, the spleen, the gallbladder, the lower parts of the lungs and the diaphragms are likely to cause referred pain.*

2 *Sickle cell disease: this affects those of African genetic origin, mainly in West Africa and the Americas. Some Indians and Arabs are also affected.*

3 *Dengue fever: in the Americas only near or north of the equator. In Africa, east coastal, south and west. Prevalent in India, Southeast Asia and the Pacific. Occasionally found in the Mediterranean area. The disease may spread.*

4 *Bartonellosis: occurs only in Peru and adjacent countries.*

5 *Familial Mediterranean fever: this affects persons of Mediterranean genetic heritage such as Jews, Arabs, Turks and Armenians.*

TOC

SYMPTOMS

DIFFERENTIALS

CONDITIONS

DRUG INDEX

REGIONAL NOTES

INX

Protocol A.32.B—Other shoulder problems

One shoulder higher than the other: SCOLIOSIS (backbone is curved to one side).

Swollen collar bone(s), painless: SYPHILIS (congenital, onset in older children, young adults.)

Large lymph nodes in arm pits with prominent skin condition likely: CELLULITIS (red), ABSCESS, LEPROSY reaction (red), TULAREMIA or secondary SYPHILIS (open sores), PLAGUE[1] (black), TYPHUS (maybe rash in fair skin).

Large lymph nodes in arm pits with prominent arm swelling likely: ANTHRAX, FILARIASIS[2] (Brugian, Asia), CANCER.

Large lymph nodes in arm pits, other: SYPHILIS,[3] IRIS, ENTERIC FEVER, TUBERCULOSIS, CANCER, PLAGUE[1] (extreme pain and tenderness). See Protocol A.31.A for instructions on evaluating lymph nodes. Also See Volume 1 Chapter 1 and Protocol B.12 which deal with large lymph nodes generally.

Weak shoulders: TUBERCULOSIS of the neck bones; HIV INFECTION; PLANT POISONING: botulism; TICK PARALYSIS, RADICULOPATHY, POLIO, THYROID TROUBLE; anything that can cause weak arms; see Protocol A.8.

Stiff shoulders: ARTHRITIS; also check similar diseases.

Shoulder joint swelling: ARTHRITIS, CANCER, previous injury, CELLULITIS, OSTEOMYELITIS, PYOMYOSITIS.

Shoulder joint won't move: due to a previous problem. If a shoulder is held immobile for a period of time, it will freeze, so it never moves again. There is nothing you can do about it.

---

1 *Plague: present in Vietnam, Madagascar, and occasionally other areas. It can happen anywhere.*
2 *The kind of filariasis affecting the arms and breasts is found only in scattered areas of Southeast Asia, not east of Sulawesi. It is also found in Bangalore, India and west of that location as far as the coast.*
3 *This may be secondary syphilis in which case the patient will have used his hands for a sexual relationship, handled an infant with a congenital syphilis rash, or shook hands with someone with secondary syphilis. Syphilis spirochetes do not enter intact skin, but nobody knows that his or her skin is totally intact.*

PROTOCOL A.33—ARM AND HAND PAIN

A.33.A—Muscular, crampy pains

A.33.B—Neuritis in arms or hands

A.33.C—Bone and joint pains

A.33.D—Other kinds of problems

▽ NON-EMERGENCY	⚠ EMERGENCY
If the patient injured his head or neck, see Head and Neck Injury, either in Chapter 4 of Volume 1 if the injury is major or in Chapter 12 if it is minor. If pain is due to an arm or hand injury, see Chapter 12 of Volume 1. Treat skin problems like skin problems elsewhere. See Wound Infection section in Chapter 10 of Volume 1 if applicable. Pain after unaccustomed exercise is addressed in Chapter 9 H, Volume 1.	**ARM EMERGENCIES** Fast onset, extreme pain with tenderness, skin discoloration, rapid progression: NECROTIZING FASCIITIS. Any exercise (even leg exercise) aggravates the pain, but it is relieved by rest: ANGINA, SYPHILIS (tertiary), RHEUMATIC FEVER, HEART ATTACK, HEART FAILURE. Arm pain with a cold, dusky-colored hand which is numb and tingling and/or difficult to use: this requires immediate surgical care in order to save the limb.

TOC

SYMPTOMS

DIFFERENTIALS

CONDITIONS

DRUG INDEX

REGIONAL NOTES

INX

Protocol A.33.A—Muscular, crampy pains

See Protocol A.10.C for general aching if the patient has general body pain; or Protocol 33.D for aching that is not due to muscle cramps. See Protocol B.2 if the pain is part of an illness with fever, headache and general body pains.

Problem probably confined to one or both arms; no generalized illness

MUSCLE STRAIN	Tight, aching pain, usually after unaccustomed exercise.
TENDINITIS	Pain and tenderness adjacent to a joint after repetitive joint usage.
FILARIASIS[1]	Episodes of fever and swelling; large lymph nodes.
GANGRENE	Black or white, dead-looking, cool skin; swelling; maybe blisters.

Problem part of a whole-body illness

FIBROMYALGIA	Morning stiffness, sleep disturbances, muscle pains worse with exercise.
POLIO	Also fevers; limb weakness develops during and after aching.
TETANUS	General, whole-body muscle spasms, back more than arms.
CHOLERA	Muscle cramps after severe watery diarrhea with DEHYDRATION.
TRICHINOSIS	Also muscle swelling; the patient looks muscular.

1 *The kind of filariasis affecting the arms and breasts is found only in scattered areas of Southeast Asia, not east of Sulawesi. It is also found in Bangalore, India and west of that location as far as the coast.*

Protocol A.33.B—Neuritis in arms or hands

Definition: Neuritis is nerve inflammation, causing pain that is usually sharp and shooting, though it may be burning or aching. It moves from the neck or shoulder to the arm or hand, usually favoring either the thumb side or little finger side. There may be muscle cramps, weakness, numbness, tingling. This may be caused by injury; see Volume 1, Chapters 4 and 11-13. If it is the result of a neck problem, then there will also be pain and stiffness in the neck.

Is the patient taking medication for TUBERCULOSIS, eating a poor diet or both?

NO to both	YES to either or both
	Consider ISONIAZID (drug) side effect, BERIBERI, PELLAGRA.

Does the patient have a fever or is he very ill or both?

NO	YES
See table below.	**Consider** TYPHUS, BRUCELLOSIS, DENGUE FEVER[1], RABIES, TUBERCULOSIS.

1 *Dengue fever: in the Americas only near or north of the equator. In Africa, east coastal, south and west. Prevalent in India, Southeast Asia and the Pacific. Occasionally found in the Mediterranean area. The disease may spread. It might spread.*

NEURITIS, DIET OKAY, NO TB MEDS, NO FEVER, NOT VERY ILL

Likely no visible skin changes

CARPAL TUNNEL SYNDROME	Numbness, tingling starts dominant hand, from repetitive motion, middle age or older
SYPHILIS, tertiary/congenital	Patient, partner or parent was exposed
SLIPPED DISC	Usually only right or left or worse on one side than the other; weakness common
BRUCELLOSIS	Off-and-on fevers, fatigue, other joint or low back pains, night sweats, miserable

Likely visible changes on the skin

ARSENIC POISONING	Also weakness; homicide, vocational exposure or ethnic medicine, flaky skin
LEPROSY	Skin changes may be a color change, a rough, scaly area or bumps
LOIASIS[1]	Swollen areas on arm or shoulder, come and go

1 *Loiasis: humid, rural central and western Africa only.*

Protocol A.33.C—Bone and joint pains

Definition: there is a deep, throbbing pain that is worse at night. It is also worse with movement regardless of whether the patient himself moves or if someone else moves the limb for him.

Has the patient had an injury?

NO	YES
	Go to the injury section, Chapters 9, 11, 12 in Volume 1.

Is the problem brittle bones that break easily?

NO	YES
	Consider SYPHILIS (congenital), RICKETS, THALLASEMIA, HYDATID DISEASE,[1] OLD AGE,
	any paralysis or immobilization that lasted a long time.

Does the problem run in a family or does it involve ANEMIA or both?

NO to both	YES to either or both
	Consider SICKLE CELL DISEASE,[2] THALLASEMIA, BARTONELLOSIS,[3] FAMILIAL MEDITERRANEAN
	FEVER.[7]

Is there only pain without swelling?

NO	YES
	Without a fever consider: MANSONELLOSIS PERSTANS,[4] RICKETS.
	With fever consider: ARBOVIRAL FEVER, HEPATITIS, MANSONELLOSIS PERSTANS,[4] DENGUE
	FEVER,[8] RELAPSING FEVER,[5] YELLOW FEVER,[6] RUBELLA, CHIKUNGUNYA FEVER, FILARIASIS.

The patient has both pain and swelling. Did the problem start only or mainly over a joint?

NO to both	YES
See Protocol B.6.B	See Protocol B.6.A

---

1 Hydatid disease: there are two kinds: one is in cattle-raising areas of the tropics where there are dogs that live close to people. The other kind is in temperate, rural areas where there are wild animals and people eat gathered, wild plant life that might be contaminated with the stool of animals.

2 Sickle cell disease: this affects those of African genetic origin, mainly in West Africa and the Americas. Some Indians and Arabs are also affected.

3 Bartonellosis: only in Peru and adjacent countries.

4 Mansonellosis perstans is present in Africa between 20 degrees north and 15 degrees south, west of 35 degrees longitude. It occurs additionally in Tanzania and in northern Mozambique. It also occurs in northern Argentina and north of there.

5 Relapsing fever: tropical and high altitude.

6 Yellow fever: scattered areas in Africa south of the Sahara and in the Americas.

7 Familial Mediterranean fever: this affects persons of Mediterranean genetic heritage such as Jews, Arabs, Turks and Armenians.

8 Dengue fever: in the Americas only near or north of the equator. In Africa, east coastal, south and west. Prevalent in India, Southeast Asia and the Pacific. Occasionally found in the Mediterranean area. The disease may spread.

Protocol A.33.D—Other kinds of pains

Burning pain in someone eating a poor diet: PELLAGRA, BERIBERI, MALNUTRITION, COBALAMIN DEFICIENCY.

Burning pain without a poor diet: ARSENIC POISONING, TYPHUS, COBALAMIN DEFICIENCY.

Deep, aching pain as with a blood pressure cuff left on too long: ANGINA, GANGRENE, TYPHUS, PLANT POISONING due to claviceps or ergot.

Pain that is markedly worse after rest; one point very tender: FIBROSITIS.

A small area of tenderness: BURSITIS, TENDINITIS; see Volume 1, Chapters 9 and 11.

Pain in the area of the hands normally covered with gloves: HIV INFECTION, LYME DISEASE.

Skin pain: CELLULITIS.

Sharp pains in someone with swelling on or around the shoulder: due to the shoulder problem; deal with that.

TOC SYMPTOMS DIFFERENTIALS CONDITIONS DRUG INDEX REGIONAL NOTES INX

TOC

SYMPTOMS

DIFFERENTIALS

CONDITIONS

DRUG INDEX

REGIONAL NOTES

INX

PROTOCOL A.34—OTHER ARM AND HAND PROBLEMS

A.34.A—Abnormal shape of hands or arms

A.34.B—Swelling of arms, hands and fingers

A.34.C—Abnormal fingernail appearance

A.34.D—Abnormal feeling and function, arms and hands

A.34.E—Other abnormal appearance—hands and fingers

Protocol A.34.A—Abnormal shape of hands or arms

Broad hands with very short fingers: CRETINISM, DOWN SYNDROME, genetic trait in some families.

Hand like a claw: injury to shoulder, arm or neck; may be due to LEPROSY or BRAIN DAMAGE.

Wrist bent, cannot straighten: LEPROSY; injury to shoulder, arm or neck; BRAIN DAMAGE.

Crooked limbs: long-standing ARTHRITIS, old injury, birth defect, TREPONARID, congenital SYPHILIS.

Missing limbs: old injury, birth defect, OSTEOMYELITIS,[1] LEPROSY.

Hands cramped: HYPERVENTILATION; injury; TETANUS; PLANT POISONING, strychnine; neck TB.

Protocol A.34.B—Swelling of arms, hands and fingers

See Protocol B.6 for help in distinguishing the various causes of limb swelling.

Muscle swelling and soreness: CELLULITIS, ABSCESS TRICHINOSIS, CYSTICERCOSIS, PYOMYOSITIS.

Swelling with thickened, roughened skin: TREPONARID; FILARIASIS, (Asia only); rarely MYCETOMA.

Swollen joints: ARTHRITIS, BURSITIS, tertiary or congenital SYPHILIS,[2] SCURVY, RICKETS, ARBOVIRAL FEVER, SICKLE CELL DISEASE,[8] CHIKUNGUNYA FEVER, RHEUMATIC FEVER.

Swelling of all fingers in a child: SICKLE CELL DISEASE, (painful but not red or hot, maybe toes also), SYPHILIS (painful, may also involve long bones); TUBERCULOSIS (painless, does not involve the toes).

Swollen lymph nodes by elbows: CELLULITIS, ABSCESS, HIV INFECTION, FILARIASIS (Asia only), ENTERIC FEVER, TUBERCULOSIS, /// TYPHUS, AFRICAN SLEEPING SICKNESS,[3] LEPROSY reaction, ANTHRAX, rarely TULAREMIA,[4] RAT BITE FEVER, PLAGUE,[5] CANCER, BARTONELLOSIS.[6]

Swollen finger tips (clubbing): This may be hereditary; first check family members.

severe: HIV INFECTION (infants), HEART FAILURE, TRICHURIASIS, CANCER, SEPSIS, RESPIRATORY INFECTION that has lasted for a long time, PARAGONIMIASIS,[7] FELON.

mild: early in the course of one of the diseases above; also consider LIVER FAILURE, LIVER DISEASE or MALABSORPTION.

Slow-growing, hard, tender swellings in hands: TUBERCULOSIS (Africa only).

Swelling generally: injury or infection, SICKLE CELL DISEASE,[8] KIDNEY DISEASE, LEPROSY reaction, LOIASIS,[9] FILARIASIS (Asia only), GANGRENE, ARSENIC POISONING, RAT BITE FEVER, MALNUTRITION, LARVA MIGRANS.

---

1 *This is a bone infection which may cause a limb to fall off.*

2 *Swelling of the hands and close portion of the fingers, with sparing of the end joints of the fingers.*

3 *African sleeping sickness: scattered areas of Africa, south of Bamako, Mali and Lake Chad and north of Lusaka, Zambia.*

4 *Tularemia: North America, central Asia, Europe, Far East, the north coast of Africa; exposure to small animals flu-like symptoms and fevers.*

5 *The nodes are very painful and tender to touch. The skin over top may be black. The patient is very ill.*

6 *Bartonellosis: occurs only in Peru and adjacent countries.*

7 *Paragonimiasis: occurs in parts of Asia and the Pacific area, rarely in Africa, India and the Americas.*

8 *Sickle cell disease: this affects those of African genetic origin, mainly in West Africa and the Americas. Some Indians and Arabs are also affected.*

9 *Loiasis: humid, rural west and central Africa.*

Protocol A.34.C—Abnormal fingernail appearance

Mottled and rough fingernails: FUNGUS INFECTION; do not treat this.

Very pale: ANEMIA.

Dark stripes or patches or totally dark: normal with dark skin.

Scooped out: in infants, ANEMIA due to iron deficiency; maybe RHEUMATIC FEVER.

Yellow: with large lymph nodes in the armpits, the fingernails may turn yellow before swelling of the arm occurs. Most common in FILARIASIS (Asia only). Also due to smoking.

Shaped like an upside-down saucer: see swollen fingertips, Protocol A.34.B.

3/4 white, pink tips: LIVER FAILURE, CIRRHOSIS, LIVER DISEASE (bilirubin in the urine).

Have little bits of blood beneath: usually due to injury; otherwise SEPSIS, TRICHINOSIS, HEMORRHAGIC FEVER, HEART FAILURE due to bad valves.

White horizontal lines: any prior illness, ARSENIC POISONING.

Protocol A.34.D—Abnormal feeling and function, arms and hands

Numbness, tingling, weakness and/or paralysis: see Protocols A.8 and A.10.

Itching palms: ALLERGY; maybe FOOD POISONING due to fish in the Pacific area.

Burning palms: PELLAGRA, TYPHUS.

Abnormal joint motion: SYPHILIS, tertiary; sometimes due to heredity.

Brittle bones, break easily: OLD AGE, paralyzed limbs, SYPHILIS in infants, THALLASEMIA, maybe birth defect.

Stiff limbs:[10] ARTHRITIS, CRETINISM, PLANT POISONING due to cassava, TROPICAL SPASTIC PARAPARESIS, FIBROMYALGIA, LEPROSY, SCURVY, any paralysis that has lasted for long.

Spasms or cramps:[11] HYPERVENTILATION (see the illustration in Volume 1, Chapter 4) severe diarrhea, any head or neck injury, POLIO, TETANUS, TROPICAL SPASTIC PARAPARESIS, RABIES (rare).

Arms feel heavy: RADICULOPATHY, FLUOROSIS, SLIPPED DISC; see Volume 1 Chapter 9.

Weakness; any disease that can cause neuritis-type pain (Protocol A.33.B); PLANT POISONING: botulism; ginger-jake; snake bite; TICK PARALYSIS, RADICULOPATHY; SLIPPED DISC; ARSENIC POISONING; STROKE; DIPHTHERIA; CARPAL TUNNEL SYNDROME; POLIO; sometimes side effects of drugs; diseases listed in Protocol A.8; pain in the hands and arms will cause the patient to refuse to use them and appear to be weakness.

Trembling or incoordination: see Protocol A.7.C, D or E; also consider causes of weakness as listed above. If some muscles are weak, then the patient will be uncoordinated.

Hands very cold: exposure to cold, GANGRENE, FROSTBITE, prior injury, SHOCK, TYPHUS, OLD AGE (Europeans).

Protocol A.34.E—Other abnormal appearance - hands and fingers

Fingers rotting: CANCRUM ORIS, GANGRENE, OSTEOMYELITIS, TYPHUS, SPOTTED FEVER.[12]

"Split peas" by finger joints: RHEUMATIC FEVER, TUBERCULOSIS, TREPONARID, YAWS.

Dark palm creases: ANEMIA, some kinds.

Dark patches of skin on the palms: normal in those of African genetic heritage.

Pale, cool fingers: PLANT POISONING, claviceps or atriplicism,[13] GANGRENE, TYPHUS.

Peeling skin of palms: SYPHILIS in infants, ECZEMA, sometimes TYPHUS; see Protocol A.15.

---

10 *Stiff limbs implies that the person has been this way for at least two months.*

11 *Spasms or cramps implies that the problem has been of more recent onset, less than the past 2 months. In the case of hyperventilation (and perhaps diarrhea) the onset is over hours.*

12 *Particularly Queensland tick typhus, listed under SPOTTED FEVER, not separately.*

13 *Plant poisoning, atriplicism: occurs among the Chinese in the Far East.*

VII—CHEST PROBLEMS

PROTOCOL A.35—CHEST PAIN

A.35.A—Heavy or burning chest pain

A.35.B—Sharp chest pain, worse with breathing

A.35.C—Chest pain with swallowing

A.35.D—Chest wall pain

A.35.E—Breast, other chest pain

See Chapter 4, Volume 1 if pain is due to an accident. If the patient has abdominal pain, tenderness or both, see Protocol A.39; the chest pain may be referred pain from the abdomen.

> ⚠️ **EMERGENCY**
>
> **CHEST PAIN EMERGENCIES**
>
> Severe heaviness, burning or aching in the center front chest, along with sweating, jaw or arm pain, and/or a sense of doom.
>
> Inordinately severe center-front chest pain radiating to the back in a >40 y.o. Westerner or someone with SYPHILIS.
>
> Any pain accompanied by shortness of breath and bluish skin color (check the color of the tongue in patients with dark skin).

Protocol A.35.A—Heavy or burning chest pain

Definition: chest pain that is heavy, burning or aching, frequently also felt in the jaw, the shoulder or the arm, frequently accompanied by paleness and sweating. It is usually made worse with exercise, sometimes helped with rest. It is not aggravated by deep breathing, coughing or pressure on the chest wall. It is felt mainly in the front of the chest rather than the sides or back.

Is the patient also short of breath, more so lying than sitting?

NO	YES
|	**Consider** ANGINA; HEART ATTACK; HEART FAILURE; ALTITUDE SICKNESS; SYPHILIS, tertiary;
|	RHEUMATIC FEVER; PULMONARY EMBOLISM; CHAGA'S DISEASE.[1]

Did extreme fatigue begin with the chest pain?

NO	YES
|	**Consider** HEART ATTACK, HEART FAILURE, RHEUMATIC FEVER, PERICARDITIS, LASSA FEVER.[2]
|	

Was or is the chest pain associated with a corrected temperature over 38.5°/101.3°?

NO	YES
|	**Consider** RHEUMATIC FEVER, LASSA FEVER,[2] RELAPSING FEVER,[3]
|	BARTONELLOSIS,[4] maybe PERICARDITIS.

Continued on table, next page.

---

1 *Chaga's disease: scattered areas within Central and South America.*

2 *Lassa fever: found in West Africa; occurs in epidemics.*

3 *Relapsing fever: throughout the tropcs and high altitudes, but not in the islands of Southeast Asia or the Pacific.*

4 *Bartonellosis is found only in Peru and adjacent countries.*

PROMINENT CHEST PAIN, NOT SHORT OF BREATH, NO HIGH FEVER, NO EXCESSIVE FATIGUE

Most common; check these out first.

RESPIRATORY INFECTION	Coughing or congestion, with production of sputum.
GALLBLADDER DISEASE	Recurrent after meals; usually the right side; also in shoulder or back.
HEART FAILURE	Short of breath with exertion; maybe swollen ankles, murmur.
SYPHILIS, tertiary/congenital	Patient, partner or parent was exposed.
PERICARDITIS	Pain goes to back; sitting and leaning forward decreases the pain.

Associated with emotional issues

DEPRESSION	Sighing, insomnia, changes in appetite.
STRESS	Sighing, insomnia, changes in appetite.

Associated with just having swallowed something

Stomach acid	Usually from lying down right after eating; treat with ANTACID.
Swallowed foreign body[1]	Anything stuck may cause symptoms like a HEART ATTACK.
MIGRAINE	Medications used for migraine can cause this kind of pain.
PLANT POISONING	Claviceps or ergot; similar to ANGINA or a HEART ATTACK.

1 *Send the patient to a hospital. Do not have him swallow anything else.*

Protocol A.35.B—Sharp chest pain, worse with breathing

Definition; pain is usually felt in the sides, upper front or back of the chest, increased with deep breathing. The pain is sharp. It is not aggravated by touching the chest or pushing on it. A patient may take short, shallow breaths to avoid pain. He may hold his chest or bandage it tightly for pain relief. If the pain is on the lower right, check the patient for a tender liver; check Protocol A.40 or A.41 if you find one. If the pain is on the lower left, check for a tender spleen (Protocol A.41.B).

SHARP CHEST PAIN, WORSE WITH BREATHING

Condition	Fever	Onset	Other characteristics
Variable, recurrent and unknown onsets			
RESPIRATORY INFECTION	Low if any	Varies recurs	Cough, sometimes congestion or cold symptoms
SICKLE CELL DISEASE[1]	Probably	Recurs	Ill off and on since infancy/preschool; family history
FAMILIAL MEDITERRANEAN FEVER[7]	Yes	Recurs	Hereditary, recurrent, abdominal or joint pains common
COCCIDIOMYCOSIS[2]	Yes	Varies	Cough, fatigue; may have large neck lymph nodes

Footnotes at the end of the table, next page.

TOC

SYMPTOMS

DIFFERENTIALS

CONDITIONS

DRUG INDEX

REGIONAL NOTES

INX

Condition	Fever	Onset	Other characteristics
Ordered by onset, from most rapid to most slow			
PNEUMOTHORAX	No[3]	Instant	Instantaneous onset of pain and shortness of breath, commonly after some chest trauma.
PULMONARY EMBOLISM	Unusual	Sec–min	Sedentary or Westerners; short of breath; no prior respiratory symptoms before the pain onset.
PERICARDITIS	Maybe	Min–Hrs	Leaning forward minimizes the pain.
RELAPSING FEVER[4]	High	Hrs–D	Fevers, sweats, headaches; body lice or tick bite.
PLEURISY	Low if any	Hrs–D	Few or no other symptoms, usually, not short of breath.
PNEUMONIA	Yes	Hrs–D	Cough, short of breath, rapid respiration.
LASSA FEVER[5]	High	Hrs–D	Like PERICARDITIS; epidemics in West Africa.
PARAGONIMIASIS[6]	Maybe	Days	Cough, worse mornings, brownish or reddish sputum.
AMEBIASIS	Usual	D–Wks	Lower right side, cough and sweating, fatigued.
TUBERCULOSIS	Maybe	Mo	Cough, night sweats, loss of appetite, slow onset.
HYDATID DISEASE	Unusual	Yrs	Tropical areas with dogs or northern temperate forest.

1 *This is an inherited condition affecting mainly those of African genetic heritage.*
2 *Coccidiomycosis: found in arid areas of the Americas only.*
3 *There is no fever unless the underlying disease that caused the pneumothorax also caused a fever. Usually a pneumothorax occurs for no good reason, or it is the result of chest trauma.*
4 *Relapsing fever: tropical and high altitude, but not in the islands of SEA and the Pacific.*
5 *Lassa fever: only in Africa, mainly west and central, usually in outbreaks.*
6 *Paragonimiasis: found in the Indian subcontinent, Asia and the Pacific; rarely in Africa and the Americas.*
7 *This is an inherited condition affecting Sephardic Jews, Spaniards, Italians, Greeks, Turks, and Arabs.*

Protocol A.35.C—Chest pain with swallowing

This is most frequently due to something swallowed that scratched the patient on its way down. If this is the case, it will usually heal within 24 hours. Also see Protocol A.30.D and check PERICARDITIS.

Protocol A.35.D—Chest wall pain

Definition: Chest pain that may be of any quality (sharp, dull, burning, aching), but it is always aggravated by one of the following: deep breathing, twisting, raising the arms or pushing on the chest. Sores on the skin are treated like any skin problem. Treat injuries. Breast pain is addressed in Protocol A.35.E.

Is the patient's corrected temperature normal; he has no fever?

NO	YES, fever absent
	Consider COSTAL CHONDRITIS, MUSCLE STRAIN, ARTHRITIS, SHINGLES, maybe bruised or broken rib, tertiary SYPHILIS, RICKETS, RESPIRATORY INFECTION.

CHEST WALL PAIN WITH A CORRECTED TEMPERATURE, OVER 37.5°/99.5°

Pain in a band around the chest, higher in back than in front

SHINGLES	Blistery rash by day 4; burning and sharp shooting pains.
TRENCH FEVER	Body lice, headache, severe shin pain, urban homeless.

Pain in muscles

TRICHINOSIS[1]	History of eating raw or rare meat in the last month, muscles swollen.
TYPHUS	Body louse or flea bites; headache; pains in back and/or shins; first ill then fevers.
LEPTOSPIROSIS	General muscle pains, red eyes, erratic fevers; context of ground water exposure.

Footnotes at the end of the table, next page.

Family history of ill health and early deaths

SICKLE CELL DISEASE[2]   History of ill health; repeated crises with shortness of breath.

Pain in joints of ribs/spine and ribs/breast bone

COSTAL CHONDRITIS   Tenderness along the edge(s) of the breast bone.

ARTHRITIS   Pain in spine or rib joints, front or back.

Localized pain, one location on the chest

AMEBIASIS   Tenderness present between the lower right ribs.

BARTONELLOSIS[3]   Severe pains in breast bone in front; fatigue occurs before fever.

---

1 *Trichinosis: the patient ate rare or raw pork or wild game within the past month.*
2 *Sickle cell disease: this affects those of African genetic origin, mainly in West Africa and the Americas. Some Indians and Arabs are also affected.*
3 *Bartonellosis: occurs only in Peru and adjacent countries.*

Protocol A.35.E—Breast, other chest pain

This is normal during adolescence and milk production. Otherwise check MASTITIS, CELLULITIS, ABSCESS, TUBERCULOSIS, FILARIASIS[4] and (rarely) CANCER.

---

4 *The kind of filariasis affecting the arms and breasts is found only in scattered areas of South Asia, not east of Sulawesi. It is also found in Bangalore, India and west of that location as far as the coast.*

PROTOCOL A.36—SHORTNESS OF BREATH

A.36.A—Shortness of breath: adults and children over three years old
A.36.B—Shortness of breath: children under three years old
Also see Protocol B.4 for help in distinguishing the various causes of shortness of breath.

⚠ EMERGENCY

SHORTNESS OF BREATH EMERGENCIES
- Food or a foreign object is stuck in the throat; see Volume 1, Chapter 4, Heimlich maneuver.
- Sudden-onset shortness of breath with a bluish discoloration of the tongue.
- Shortness of breath with noisy inspiration.
- Shortness of breath with muscle weakness that is getting worse.
- Shortness of breath related time-wise to neck or facial swelling.

Protocol A.36.A—Shortness of breath, adults and children over three years old

▷ SYMPTOMATIC TREATMENT

Try having the patient breathe near a cool mist vaporizer or steam. Have the patient sleep sitting up; a bean bag chair or lazy boy chair is best. A non-drying COUGH SYRUP may be helpful.

Is the problem of sudden onset (over less than 10 minutes)?

NO	YES
	ANAPHYLAXIS, HEART ATTACK, ALLERGY, ASTHMA, /// PULMONARY EMBOLISM, PNEUMOTHORAX, inhaling a foreign body: treat immediately! Rarely, ANTHRAX, PLANT POISONING due to botulism or water hemlock.

Is the patient less short of breath sitting than lying flat?

NO	YES
 Continued on next page.	**Consider**: HEART FAILURE, KIDNEY DISEASE, RESPIRATORY FAILURE, IRIS, LIVER FAILURE (distended abdomen); at high altitudes consider ALTITUDE SICKNESS.

TOC

SYMPTOMS

DIFFERENTIALS

CONDITIONS

DRUG INDEX

REGIONAL NOTES

INX

Is the patient pale inside his lower eyelids, on his tongue, on his fingernails?

NO | **YES**

| **Consider** ANEMIA and the diseases associated with it, as well as conditions causing it. The most common worldwide are: pregnancy, MALNUTRITION, blood loss from any cause, HOOKWORM, KIDNEY DISEASE, THALLASEMIA, SICKLE CELL DISEASE,[2] VISCERAL LEISHMANIASIS.[3]

Is the patient breathing fast without really feeling short of breath?

NO | **YES**

| **Consider** ANEMIA, DEHYDRATION, SEPSIS, STRESS, /// SHOCK, KIDNEY DISEASE, ADDICTION (uppers) or DIABETES. This may be a normal effect of high altitude.

Does the patient have a corrected temperature more than 38.5°/101.3°?

NO | **YES**

| Most likely PNEUMONIA; less likely MALARIA,[1] ENTERIC FEVER, SICKLE CELL DISEASE,[2] TYPHUS, ANTHRAX, HIV INFECTION, DIPHTHERIA, FAMILIAL MEDITERRANEAN FEVER,[4] rarely PLAGUE or TRICHINOSIS.

Does the patient have weak muscles; he has trouble moving arms and legs as well as breathing?

NO | **YES**

See table below. | See Protocol A.8

---

1 The kind of malaria that is common in SEA, especially Borneo and Malaysia, tends to present this way. It can be rapidly fatal. It responds to CHLOROQUINE. The name is Plasmodium Knowlesi. Falciparum malaria may also cause this.

2 Sickle cell disease: this affects those of African genetic origin, mainly in West Africa and the Americas. Some Greeks, Indians and Arabs are also affected.

3 Visceral Leishmaniasis: found in scattered areas of Central and South America, (mainly eastern) Africa north of the equator, the Mediterranean area, the Indian subcontinent, eastern Europe, central Asia and mainland China.

4 Familial Mediterranean fever: this affects persons of Mediterranean genetic heritage such as Jews, Arabs, Turks and Armenians.

SHORT OF BREATH, NO HIGH FEVER, NOT PALE, NOT SUDDEN ONSET, NOT MUCH BETTER SITTING

Consider	Fever	Other Characteristics
Most common; check these first		
PNEUMONIA	Usual	Cough, chest pains, chills, sweats or all of these.
MALARIA	Usual	History of shaking chills, drenching sweats and headaches.
RESPIRATORY INFECTION	Maybe	Sick a long time, big neck muscles from breathing.
Environmental problems		
ALTITUDE SICKNESS	No	Coughing, headache, worse lying down; over 2000 m altitude.
SMOKE INHALATION	No	History of being by a fire.
CARBON MONOXIDE POISONING	No	History of being by a fire or an engine; headache also.
PLANT POISONING	No	Muscarine, botulism or nicotine.
INSECTICIDE POISONING	No	Much saliva, tears, diarrhea.
Likely slow onset over days or weeks		
ANEMIA	Maybe	Pale inside lower eyelids, mouth or fingernails.
TUBERCULOSIS	Usual	Long-lasting cough with weight loss; gradual onset.
HEART FAILURE	Maybe	Intolerance of exercise, swollen ankles or fatigue.
Abdomen distended	Maybe	Gas, fluids or pregnancy hinders breathing.
MANSONELLOSIS PERSTANS[1]	No	Also general bone and joint pains; slow onset.
CANCER	Maybe	Weight loss; lump somewhere; fatigued.
IRIS	Maybe	Simultaneous treatment for HIV and TB.

---

1 Mansonellosis perstans: only in Africa (west and central) and in South America (northern Argentina and north of there).

TOC SYMPTOMS DIFFERENTIALS CONDITIONS DRUG INDEX REGIONAL NOTES INX

Protocol A.36.B—Shortness of breath children under three years old

Newborns may have no fever with diseases that usually cause fever. Babies may have grunting, or head nodding synchronized with each breath. Their chests or upper abdomens may pull in also. The following problems are most frequent; also consider the problems listed for older persons.

SHORTNESS OF BREATH, CHILDREN UNDER 3 YEARS OLD

Problem	Onset	Fever	Other Characteristics
Dry mouth			
DEHYDRATION	Hrs–D	Maybe	Tongue, mouth or both are dry.
Likely previous good health			
Stuffy nose	Hrs–D	Low if any	Clean the nose or use drops.
RESPIRATORY INFECTION	Hrs–D	Usual	Stuffy or runny nose or a barking cough.
PERTUSSIS	D–Wk	Low	Coughing spells with noisy gasping, vomiting.
PNEUMONIA	Hrs–D	Usual	Moist-sounding cough; fever if over one year old.
Moderately to very ill			
MEASLES	D–Wk	High	Red eyes; very ill; spots in the mouth or rash.
HEART FAILURE	Wk–Mo	Maybe	Short of breath with exercising; difficulty nursing.
SEPSIS	Varies	Usual	Very ill, usually unconscious; won't nurse.
Pale tongue and fingernails			
SICKLE CELL DISEASE[1]	D–Wk	Usual	ANEMIA, family history of ill health.
ANEMIA	Wk–Mo	Maybe	Pale inside lower eyelids, mouth or fingernails.

1 *Sickle cell disease: this affects those of African genetic origin, mainly in West Africa and the Americas. Some Greeks, Indians and Arabs are also affected.*

PROTOCOL A.37—COUGH

A.37.A—Dry cough or with white sputum

A.37.B—Cough with green or yellow sputum

A.37.C—Cough with blood, bloody or brownish sputum

Protocol A.37.A—Dry cough or with white sputum

Is the patient's sputum frothy?

NO
|
|
Continued on the next page.

YES

Consider: ALTITUDE SICKNESS, HEART FAILURE, rarely PLAGUE. If the patient is not short of breath, frothy sputum is saliva from the mouth, not sputum from the lungs.

TOC

SYMPTOMS

DIFFERENTIALS

CONDITIONS

DRUG INDEX

REGIONAL NOTES

INX

Has the cough been continual or recurrent and present for over a month with weight loss?

NO to either   **YES to both**

Very specific symptoms

ASTHMA: harder to breathe out than to breathe in; wheezes at times.

HEART FAILURE: shortness of breath with exertion, maybe wheezing.

PERTUSSIS: coughing spells, with choking, vomiting, gasping.

Fever likely, at least off and on, probably not high

RESPIRATORY INFECTION: barrel chest, wheezing, usually smoker.

TUBERCULOSIS: night sweats, loss of appetite with weight loss.

AMEBIASIS: pain in upper right or central abdomen.

Likely large spleen and/or lymph nodes

TROPICAL SPLENOMEGALY: malarious area; large spleens common.

HIV INFECTION: multiple infections, diarrhea, severe weight loss.

VISCERAL LEISHMANIASIS:[1] huge spleen, large liver.

Is there a corrected temperature over 38.5°/101.3°?

NO   **YES**

See table below.   **Probably** PNEUMONIA, MEASLES, ENTERIC FEVER, AMEBIASIS, IRIS; rarely LASSA FEVER,[2] COCCIDIOMYCOSIS,[3] PLAGUE. In an epidemic context consider INFLUENZA.

---

1 *Visceral Leishmaniasis: found in scattered areas of Central and South America, Africa north of the equator, the Mediterranean area, the Indian subcontinent, eastern Europe, central Asia and mainland China.*

2 *Lassa fever: occurs in epidemics in west Africa.*

3 *Coccidiomycosis: arid parts of the Americas only.*

COUGH WITH NO OR LOW FEVER, PRESENT FOR LESS THAN A MONTH.

Consider	Fever	Other Characteristics
Most common		
PNEUMONIA	Usual	Sudden onset, usually after a cold; fast respiration.
RESPIRATORY INFECTION	Low if any	Not very ill unless chronic or the patient is an infant, malnourished, or elderly.
ASTHMA	No	Prolonged expiration, tight cough, maybe wheezing, history of the same.
HEART FAILURE	No	Shortness of breath with exertion; abnormal breath sounds or swollen ankles.
PERTUSSIS	Maybe	Much white mucus, coughing spells with gasps, maybe vomiting.
Temperate forest with raw wild plants or arid rural tropics with dogs		
HYDATID DISEASE[1]	No	Sudden onset of coughing up salty fluid.
Simultaneous treatment for HIV and (TB or LEPROSY).		
IRIS	Maybe	Worsening symptoms with medication change.
Environmental problems		
ALTITUDE SICKNESS	No	Severe headache, shortness of breath, worse lying.
PLANT POISONING	No	Due to muscarine; much saliva, sweat and urination.
INSECTICIDE POISONING	No	Like muscarine entry above; exposed to insecticide.
SMOKE INHALATION	Maybe	Within 72 hours of inhaling smoke, sudden onset.
Liver likely enlarged, tender or both		
AMEBIASIS	Usual	Pain on right side; holds his side to minimize pain.
LIVER FLUKE[2]	No	Large tender liver, indigestion, general aching.

---

1 *There are two kinds, one in the tropics where dogs live close to people, the other in northern forested areas, where people consume wild food contaminated with animal stool.*

2 *This kind of liver fluke is fascioliasis, present in most areas other than Asia.*

Protocol A.37.B—Cough with green or yellow sputum

▷ SYMPTOMATIC TREATMENT

Have the patient breathe near a cool mist vaporizer or steam. Have him sleep sitting up; a bean bag chair or lazy boy chair is best. A non-drying COUGH SYRUP may be helpful.

Has the patient been ill more than a month and the sputum has a foul, rotten odor?[1]

NO to either	YES to both
|	May be due to a lung abscess which requires surgical care.
See the table below.	

---

1 *Distinguish between the patient's foul breath and foul-smelling sputum. If the problem is sputum, it will still smell foul when in a container that is removed from the patient. This is a major lung problem; it will not likely respond to mouthwash or only antibiotics.*

COUGH WITH GREEN OR YELLOW SPUTUM, NO FOUL ROTTEN ODOR TO THE SPUTUM.

Consider	Fever	Other Characteristics
RESPIRATORY INFECTION	Maybe	Quite short of breath if chronic; otherwise onset after a common cold.
PNEUMONIA	High	Sudden onset, usually after a cold; usually fever.
TUBERCULOSIS	Usual	Gradual onset, weight loss, night sweats.
AMEBIASIS	Usual	Sudden onset after right-sided abdominal or flank pains.
HIV INFECTION	Usual	Diarrhea, loss of appetite, weight loss likely.

Protocol A.37.C—Cough with blood, bloody or brownish sputum

If it's not obvious, distinguish between coughed blood and vomited blood, using your urine dipsticks. With coughed blood the pH of the watery stuff with the blood is 7–8. With vomited blood the pH is 5 or less, maybe 6 if the patient has just eaten. It will never be 7 or more.

Has the patient been ill more than a month and the sputum has a foul, rotten odor?

NO to either	YES to both
|	May be due to a lung abscess: requires surgical care.

Did the patient have bleeding from nose or mouth recently?

NO	YES
|	Do not worry about a small amount; the blood ran down and came up again.
|	If it is part of a general bleeding problem, consult Protocol A.13.E, A.28 or B.7.

Is the patient coughing up clots of pure red blood?

NO	YES
|	RESPIRATORY INFECTION (bronchitis), TUBERCULOSIS, HEART FAILURE or CANCER.
See table, next page.	If it is part of a general bleeding problem, consult Protocol A.13.E, B.7 or B.2.

TOC

SYMPTOMS

DIFFERENTIALS

CONDITIONS

DRUG INDEX

REGIONAL NOTES

INX

ODORLESS BLOODY SPUTUM COUGHED UP FROM THE LUNGS, NOT CLOTS

Consider	Fever	Other Characteristics
Rapid onset, previous good health, mildly to moderately ill.		
ASCARIASIS	Usual	Ate soil-contaminated food in arable tropics.
RESPIRATORY INFECTION	Maybe	Chronic cough, not very sick otherwise.
PNEUMONIA	High, usually	Short of breath, chest pain or both.
PULMONARY EMBOLISM	Low if any	Foamy, pinkish sputum, sudden onset, short of breath.
Rapid onset, probably previous good health, extremely ill.		
PLAGUE[1] (rare)	High	Exposure to plague pus, rapid onset, mental changes.
Sick for a more than a month, maybe more than a year.		
TUBERCULOSIS	Usual	Slow onset, night sweats, weight loss.
AMEBIASIS	Usual	Sudden coughing spell, thick sputum; right side pain.
PARAGONIMIASIS[2]	Unusual	Coughing for a long time, little or no weight loss.

1 *This is usually in an epidemic situation, family members, or healthcare workers. It is contagious and fatal.*

2 *Paragonimiasis; mainly in Asia and Southeast Asia; occasionally India and western Africa; rarely the Americas and Pacific.*

PROTOCOL A.38—BREAST AND OTHER CHEST PROBLEMS

A.38.A—Breast problems   A.38.B—Additional chest problems

Protocol A.38.A—Breast problems

Breast pain: this is normal during adolescence and milk production. Otherwise check MASTITIS, CELLULITIS, ABSCESS, TUBERCULOSIS, FILARIASIS[1] and (rarely) CANCER.

Breast lump: if there is a definite lump so you can feel definite borders, like a marble, and it becomes sore right before menstruation and less sore after, that is probably a cyst. A potentially cancerous lump probably will probably be a non-tender swollen area, irregular in shape, with no definite border. However, only a biopsy can determine for sure if a particular lump is cancerous. Also consider TUBERCULOSIS of the breast. Breast TB is usually painful and tender from the beginning, whereas CANCER is usually initially painless and not tender. Breast TB can be present for years, whereas CANCER usually kills the patient within a year or two.

Breast development: normal with the onset of puberty and with pregnancy. In a newborn, due to mother's hormones; no problem. In an adolescent male, due to hormones during puberty; no problem. This is very common and nothing to worry about; it will go away in 18 months or less. Also may be due to LEPROSY; MUMPS; HEMOCHROMATOSIS;[2] LIVER FAILURE; CIRRHOSIS; KIDNEY DISEASE; THYROID TROUBLE (high-thyroid); MALNUTRITION and some drugs, notably CIMETIDINE, DIGITALIS, GRISEOFULVIN. Premature puberty is potentially serious; send the patient out. You should be aware that breast CANCER does occur in males.

Itchy rash under breast: CANDIDIASIS, CONTACT DERMATITIS

Discharge from the nipple: if the woman has not just given birth to a baby, this is potentially serious. Contact a physician for advice or send out within a week. Send pictures.

Sores on breasts: IMPETIGO is most common; Also consider TREPONARID[3] in the infant, MASTITIS, CANCER. See Protocols A.15 and A.17.

Breast swelling: normal with pregnancy and right before menstruation. May be due to CANCER (in either sex) or TUBERCULOSIS causing large nodes in the arm pit and this may cause swelling of the breast with swollen skin that looks like orange peel. Similar swelling and orange-peel skin may be due to IMPETIGO of the nipple area, MASTITIS, FILARIASIS.[4]

1 *The kind of filariasis affecting the arms and breasts is found only in scattered areas of South Asia, not east of Sulawesi. It is also found in Bangalore, India and west of that location as far as the coast.*

2 *Hemochromatosis; mainly confined to certain ethnic groups who take in excessive iron in the form of blood or beer brewed in iron containers. It may also be hereditary.*

3 *Treponarid: found in arid areas only. The sores are on the breast of the mother who acquires the problem from her breast-feeding, infected infant.*

4 *Asia/Pacific areas only.*

TOC

SYMPTOMS

DIFFERENTIALS

CONDITIONS

DRUG INDEX

REGIONAL NOTES

INX

Protocol A.38 continued | *Village Medical Manual 7th Edition Volume 2* | **A-113**
CHAPTER   PAGE

TOC

SYMPTOMS

DIFFERENTIALS

CONDITIONS

DRUG INDEX

REGIONAL NOTES

INX

Protocol A.38.B—Additional chest problems

Wheezing

Definition: listening through your stethoscope, expiration sounds are the same length or longer than inspiration sounds with a high-pitched whining or squeaking quality to them. The patient will tell you that he has more trouble breathing out than breathing in.

Common causative diseases: ALLERGY, TUBERCULOSIS, MANSONELLOSIS PERSTANS,[1] ASTHMA, ANAPHYLAXIS, HEART FAILURE, ALTITUDE SICKNESS, RESPIRATORY INFECTION, FILARIASIS in expatriates.

Hiccups: see HICCUPS in Protocol A.7.B.

Congestion: ASTHMA, ALLERGY, PNEUMONIA, RESPIRATORY INFECTION, INSECTICIDE POISONING, PLANT POISONING due to muscarine.

Chest pressure: see Protocol A.35.A, chest pain, even if the patient denies that it is really pain.

Skipped beats/palpitations: see Protocol A.3.D.

Vibration felt on the chest wall, synchronous with the pulse, or heart beat: this is equivalent to a heart murmur. Check for signs of HEART FAILURE. If there are none, it can safely be ignored until it is convenient to have it checked out at a major medical center. However you should be careful to treat all infections in this patient. Give antibiotics for all injuries, even minor ones.

Barrel-shaped chest: usually due to RESPIRATORY INFECTION which became chronic; otherwise SICKLE CELL DISEASE,[2] SCURVY.

Bumps on either side of the breastbone: RICKETS, SCURVY, COSTAL CHONDRITIS.

Lump on either side or both sides above collar bone(s) in front: CANCER, TUBERCULOSIS.

Soft swellings on the chest, like abscesses but cool to touch: TUBERCULOSIS.

Sides of lower ribs pulled in: RICKETS.

---

1 *Mansonellosis perstans: found only in Africa (central and west) and in South America (northern Argentina and north of there).*

2 *Sickle cell disease is inherited; it affects those of African genetic origin, mainly in western Africa and the Americas. Some Indians, Greeks and Arabs are also affected.*

VIII—ABDOMINAL PROBLEMS

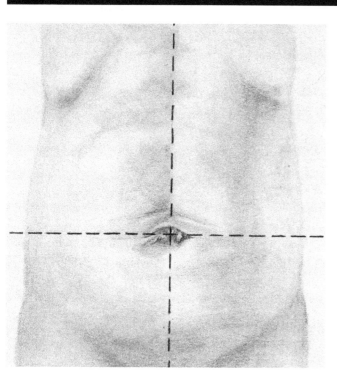

⚠ EMERGENCY

ABDOMINAL PAIN EMERGENCIES

Abdominal pain with *shock* (cool, sweaty skin, rapid pulse, low blood pressure)

Abdominal pain that has lasted *more than 6 hours*, worse with coughing

Abdominal pain that *comes and goes* at regular intervals, 3–25 minutes apart

Abdominal pain with *dehydration* (dry mouth, thirst, rapid pulse, low blood pressure)

Very *sudden onset* of very severe pain

Abdominal pain that goes to the jaw, shoulder or arm

Abdominal pain that goes to the back, thigh, knee, particularly in an older Westerner

Abdominal pain with *loss of consciousness*

Protocol	Subject
A.39	General abdominal complaints
A	Abdominal pain guide
B	Non-localized/middle abdominal pain
C	Acute abdomen: 3 types
A.40	Upper right abdominal problems
A	Upper right abdominal pain
B	Upper right abdominal swelling
A.41	Upper mid- and left-abdominal problems
A	Upper mid- and left-abdominal pain
B	Upper mid-and left-abdominal swelling
A.42	Lower abdominal problems, right or left
A	Lower abdominal pain
B	Lower abdominal swelling
A.43	Flank/waist abdominal problems
A	Flank/waist abdominal pain
B	Flank/waist abdominal swelling
A.44	Lower mid-abdominal problems
A	Lower-mid abdominal pain
B	Lower-mid abdominal swelling

Protocol	Subject
A.45	Groin problems
A	Groin pain
B	Groin swelling
A.46	Abdominal swelling
A	Swelling of entire abdomen
B	Swelling of abdominal organs
A.47	Nausea and vomiting
A.48	Vomiting blood
A.49	Other abdominal problems

Village Medical Manual 7th Edition Volume 2 | **A-115**
CHAPTER PAGE

TOC
SYMPTOMS
DIFFERENTIALS
CONDITIONS
DRUG INDEX
REGIONAL NOTES
INX

PROTOCOL A.39—GENERAL ABDOMINAL COMPLAINTS

A.39.A—Abdominal pains, guide to diagnosis

A.39.B—Non-localized or middle abdominal pain

A.39.C—Acute abdomen - three different types

Protocol A.39.A—Abdominal complaints, guide to diagnosis

▷ SYMPTOMATIC TREATMENT

A warm water bottle is appropriate for abdominal pain. Use no pain medication until the protocol suggests it, a physician orders it or you have at least a tentative diagnosis.

If the patient has a corrected body temperature more than >38.5°/101.3° plus abdominal pain, see Protocol B.9.

Does the patient have definite signs of an ACUTE ABDOMEN (See Protocol A.39.C)?

NO or not sure

YES

Treat as instructed in the Condition Index. Contact a physician.

If the patient has general abdominal swelling see Protocol A.46.

If the pain is in the middle of the abdomen or if it is all over (generalized) or if it seems to be moving around to different locations, go to Protocol A.39.B: non-localized or middle abdominal pain.

If the pain is on the abdominal wall (tender to light touch), not deep inside, then ask the person about an injury; also consider SHINGLES, TRENCH FEVER, SPINAL NEUROPATHY and similar conditions.

If the pain is predominantly localized right, left, upper, lower or to one side, then go to Protocols A.40 to A.45 as indicated on the previous page.

Protocol A.39.B—Non-localized or middle abdominal pain

Definition: the patient points to his navel as the location of the pain or else he tells you that the pain moves around by sweeping his hand over his entire abdomen.

First check for ACUTE ABDOMEN (Protocol A.39.C), if you have not done so already. If there is no ACUTE ABDOMEN and the patient is not very ill and the pain has lasted less than 48 hours, first consider HEAT ILLNESS and IRRITABLE BOWEL. Then pursue another diagnosis if neither of these two diagnoses fit.

Is the patient constipated off and on or continually?

No not constipated

Yes, sometimes constipated

Consider IIRRITABEL BOWEL, IMPACTION, ASCARIASIS, AMEBIASIS, TUBERCULOSIS, OLD AGE, rarely LEAD POISONING.

Has the patient eaten inadequately cooked meat or fish?

NO

YES

Consider TAPEWORM, TRICHINOSIS, INTESTINAL FLUKE.[1]

Has the patient had diarrhea?

NO

YES

Consider GASTROENTERITIS, DYSENTERY, HIV INFECTION, FOOD POISONING,[2] ///
STRONGYLOIDIASIS, TUBERCULOSIS, PIG-BEL,[3] PLANT POISONING, ARSENIC POISONING.

Continued on next page.

Footnotes are at the end of this flow diagram.

Is there blood in the stool: either visible blood or the stool tests positive for blood?

NO	YES
	Nationals and anyone with poor sanitation
	HOOKWORM: areas with sandy soil; ANEMIA is common.
	DYSENTERY: either red blood or black, foul, sticky stools.
	STRONGYLOIDIASIS: itchy rash by rectum off and on.
	TRICHURIASIS: tiny worms, look like whips or coiled springs.
	Anyone, not related to sanitation
	PEPTIC ULCER: burning pain with hunger, relieved by food.
	CANCER: slow-onset symptoms; initially painless.
	Unlikely expatriates
	PIG-BEL:[3] meat meal in a child with prior MALNUTRITION.
	Fresh-water snail exposure
	SCHISTOSOMIASIS MANSONI:[4] bloody diarrhea; liver problems.
See table below	SCHISTOSOMIASIS JAPONICUM:[5] distended abdomen.

1 *Intestinal fluke: not present in Africa south of the Sahara or in the Pacific. In the Americas it is present only in Guyana.*
2 *Eggs, milk and chicken are common causes; pain is severe.*
3 *Pig-bel: developing countries near the equator, ate meat after having a low-protein diet for a long time.*
4 *Schistosomiasis Mansoni: scattered areas throughout Africa, some in the Middle East and the Americas.*
5 *Schistosomiasis Japonicum: in parts of mainland China, the Philippines, parts of the Celebes, the upper Mekong and the Thai-Malaysian border.*

ABDOMINAL PAIN, NO DIARRHEA, NO CONSTIPATION, STOOL NOT BLOODY, NO RARE MEAT

Condition	Fever	Other Characteristics
HERNIA	Unusual	Bulge in groin(s) or by navel, tender to touch.
Patient probably not very ill; he cares for himself.		
STRESS	No	Pain is usually mild and intermittent.
COLIC	No	Otherwise-healthy baby; passing gas relieves pain.
PEPTIC ULCER	No	Burning or aching, aggravated or relieved by food.
INTESTINAL FLUKE[1]	No	Patient may have a swollen face.
Tenderness of the abdominal wall, chest wall or back		
SHINGLES	Maybe	Abdominal wall tender to touch; rash by day three in a band.
COSTAL CHONDRITIS	No	Young adult; tenderness along side(s) of breast bone.
MUSCLE STRAIN	No	After unusual exercise; aching abdominal muscles.
Patient probably very ill, adults mainly		
PANCREATITIS	Maybe	Vomiting; pain goes to the back.
IRIS	Probably	Simultaneous treatment for HIV and (TB or LEPROSY).
Slow-onset or recurrent		
TUBERCULOSIS	Usual	Weight loss, swelling (fluid) or tiny lumps in the belly; adults or children.
TUBERCULOSIS	Usual	Whole abdomen, feels like bread dough or foam rubber inside; adults.
SICKLE CELL DISEASE[2]	Common	Recurrent pains since a young age, family history.
Related to something eaten		
PLANT POISONING	No	Ackee, botulism, coral plant, lolism, manicheel, nicotine.
ARSENIC POISONING	No	Cramping pains, numbness and tingling of limbs, skin changes.
Tenderness present, deep, lower right or left abdomen		
AMEBIASIS	Maybe	History of eating unsanitary food; maybe sticky diarrhea.

1 *Intestinal fluke: not present in Africa south of the Sahara or in the Pacific area. In the Americas, present only in Guyana. It is prevalent in Asia.*
2 *Sickle cell disease: this affects those of African genetic origin, mainly in West Africa and the Americas. Some Indians and Arabs are also affected.*

Protocol A.39.C—Acute abdomen—three different types

Includes appendicitis, intestinal obstruction and perforated ulcer. If the patient has a high fever plus abdominal pain, see Protocol B.9.

> **Before proceeding with this**, inquire about a prior history of severe abdominal pains, sudden onset, maybe with vomiting, lasting for days and then disappearing. These kinds of episodes are classical for tertiary SYPHILIS. You should get a history of either the patient (10+ years ago) or his partner or his parents being exposed. He may have other symptoms of tertiary SYPHILIS. If this is the problem, then treat with PENICILLIN. If this is the first episode, the distinction between this and acute abdomen is impossible. In that case, send him to a surgeon with a note that the problem may be tertiary SYPHILIS. If there were previous episodes that resolved, then treat with benzathine PENICILLIN.

Type 1. Acute abdomen with Shock. The patient has an ashen color, is cool and moist, has a fast pulse, low blood pressure or both. Most often he is lying still, not writhing around. His pain may go to his back, and he may be vomiting. If you lift the patient to a standing or sitting position, he will pass out. He may already be unconscious. If he is a male, usually the pain will have come on suddenly. With females, most often the pain will have come on gradually. Sometimes this kind of acute abdomen is due to injury. Frequently the patient complains of shoulder pain, back pain or both.

Type 2. Acute abdomen with infection (appendicitis type): the patient has had pain for 6 hours or more. It may have started out like ordinary cramps. The patient has lost his appetite. Usually he is vomiting. He frequently is constipated; diarrhea is unusual. Eventually he develops rebound tenderness with at least 2 of the first 3 signs below or (rarely) sign 4 alone being positive. His pain response must be spontaneous. If you must ask him to know if it hurts or not, his response is not spontaneous. (This is assuming your patient is from a Western culture. The criterion of spontaneity may be culturally modified.) Signs are as follows:

a.) *If you ask him to take a deep breath and cough hard twice, he will either refuse or complain of pain the first time; he will definitely not cough hard the second time. He may just clear his throat.*

b.) *If you jar him or the bed on which he is lying, he will wince or verbally complain of pain.*

c.) *If you tap on his abdomen with one finger as if you were hitting a key on a big, old manual typewriter, this also will produce enough pain to make him wince. This pain is not as bad if the patient raises his head up off the bed [using neck muscles, not arms] as it is if his head is down.*

d.) *With the patient lying flat on his back on a table, drop his leg off the side of the table so it hangs down toward the floor from the hip. This markedly aggravates the pain. If you listen to his abdomen with a stethoscope, usually you will hear no bowel sounds.*

In a child with an umbilical hernia (a bulging, soft navel) you can test for type 2 by tapping on the top of the hernia. If the child howls with pain, he has acute abdomen type 2.

Acute abdomen with infection may be caused by injury, appendicitis, perforated ULCER, ASCARIASIS, AMEBIASIS, TUBERCULOSIS or ENTERIC FEVER, as well as other diseases. PELVIC INFECTION, PANCREATITIS and amebic DYSENTERY[1] can be indistinguishable.

Type 3. Acute abdomen with obstruction. The patient has had pain for 6 hours or more and the pain comes in waves, anywhere from 3 minutes to 25 minutes apart. If the pains are quite frequent, the patient is vomiting and may be constipated also. In this case his abdomen might not be distended. If the pains are less frequent, the patient is constipated; he may be vomiting also. In the latter case, the vomit may look and smell like stool. (It is stool.) His abdomen is distended and if you tap it, it sounds hollow. Usually the patient is writhing rather than holding perfectly still. Listening with your stethoscope; as the patient has a pain you will hear silence followed by rushing sounds, possibly followed by tinkles like water dripping into water from a height. The patient may have ASCARIASIS which will cause him to pass roundworms (visible earthworm size), or he may have a hernia that is tender and will not go back inside, or he may have an old surgical scar on his abdomen. This may be caused by ASCARIASIS or TUBERCULOSIS, as well as some other diseases. Occasionally small children have irregular pains and bloody diarrhea with this kind of acute abdomen.

---

1 *Amebic DYSENTERY implies that the person has diarrhea, but frequently there is constipation before the diarrhea. If the intestines perforate (break open into the body cavity), the diarrhea will stop and the person again will be constipated.*

PROTOCOL A.40—UPPER-RIGHT ABDOMINAL PROBLEMS

A.40.A—Upper-right abdominal pain

A.40.B—Upper-right abdominal swelling

Protocol A.40.A—Upper-right abdominal pain

If the patient has a corrected body temperature >38.5°/101.3° plus abdominal pain, see Protocol B.9.

Does the patient have definite signs of ACUTE ABDOMEN (See Protocol A.39 C)?

NO or not sure	**YES**
|	Treat according to directions in the Condition Index.

Try treating with ANTACID and [DICYCLOMINE or CHAMOMILE TEA].
If the treatment fails, go to the next question.

Is the patient 6 months or more pregnant?

NO	**YES**
|	**Consider** TOXEMIA; if it does not fit, follow the 'NO' arm

Does eating change the pain, making it better or worse?

NO	**YES**
|	**Consider** GALLBLADDER DISEASE, PEPTIC ULCER.

UPPER RIGHT ABDOMINAL PAIN, NO ADVANCED PREGNANCY, NO CHANGE WITH EATING

Condition	Fever	Other Characteristics
Most likely, consider these first		
HEPATITIS	Usual	Fatigue, nausea, loss of appetite, maybe JAUNDICE.
AMEBIASIS	Usual	The patient's liver is tender to touch.
PELVIC INFECTION	Maybe	Adult female, pain with intercourse, pus in vagina.
More likely expatriates than nationals		
HEART FAILURE	Unusual	Large, tender liver; exercise intolerance; fatigue, swollen ankles and feet.
CANCER	Seldom	Weight loss and/or lumpy liver edge, initially not tender.
Transmitted by culicoides (no-see-ems that breed in moist locations) see Volume 1, Appendix 10		
MANSONELLOSIS PERSTANS[1]	No	Also joint pains, maybe a rash or short of breath.
Likely nationals and those consuming unsanitary foods		
ASCARIASIS	Maybe	Crampy, episodic pains, especially in children.
LIVER FLUKE[2]	No	Ate raw or rare fish or water plants; liver large and tender.
YELLOW FEVER	Yes	Not immunized, butcher-type body odor, quite sick, only Africa and the Americas.
PLANT POISONING	No	Crotalaria; used to make bush teas; large liver.

1 *Mansonellosis perstans: only in west and central Africa and in South America, northern Argentina and north of there.*
2 *Liver fluke: worldwide, especially in the Far East and Southeast Asia.*

Protocol A.40.B—Upper-right abdominal swelling

See Protocol A.14, Skin Lumps and Bumps if appropriate.

Can you feel an edge of the swelling; and, if so, what is its direction?

No edge felt or rounded. Send the patient out for diagnosis. This may be his gallbladder or a tumor. In any case, there is nothing you can do in a village situation. If there is a lumpy edge, the patient may have CANCER or HYDATID DISEASE.

Horizontal, nearly horizontal or diagonal. The edge runs left to right on the patient; if it is diagonal it is higher (closer to the head) on the left than on the right. The mass in this case is probably the liver. See Protocol A.46, B.2 for the differential diagnosis of an enlarged liver.

Vertical or nearly vertical. The direction is head to foot on the patient—possibly with a notch in the middle of the swelling. The mass is probably a kidney. See Protocol A.46, B.3 for the differential diagnosis of a large kidney.

PROTOCOL A.41—UPPER-MID AND UPPER-LEFT ABDOMINAL PROBLEMS

A.41.A—Upper-mid and upper-left abdominal pain   A.41.B—Upper-mid and upper-left abdominal swelling

Protocol A.41.A—Upper-mid and upper-left abdominal pain

Includes spleen pain. If the patient has a corrected temperature over 38.5°/101.3°, plus abdominal pain, see Protocol B.9.

Does the patient have definite signs of ACUTE ABDOMEN (See Protocol A.39 C)?

NO or not sure

|

Try treating with ANTACID and [DICYCLOMINE or CHAMOMILE TEA].
If the treatment fails, go to next question.

YES

Treat according to directions in the Condition Index.

Is the pain upper-mid abdomen with the right-upper side also hurting?

NO

|
|

YES

Use Protocol A.40.A; the problem is probably with the liver or the gallbladder. The liver extends to the left, a little past the center line.

Has the patient been ill for more than a week, and also have ANEMIA?

NO to either or both

|
|
See table on the next page.

YES to both

Consider MALARIA, TROPICAL SPLENOMEGALY, SPLENIC CRISIS, VISCERAL LEISHMANIASIS,[1] THALLASEMIA, SCHISTOSOMIASIS MANSONI,[2] SICKLE CELL DISEASE.[3]

1 Visceral Leishmaniasis: found in scattered areas of Central and South America, Africa north of the equator, the Mediterranean area, the Indian subcontinent, eastern Europe, central Asia and mainland China.
2 Schistosomiasis Mansoni: scattered areas within Africa, the Arabian peninsula, the Caribbean and parts of eastern South America.
3 Sickle cell disease: this affects those of African genetic origin, mainly in West Africa and the Americas. Some Greeks, Indians and Arabs are also affected.

UPPER-MID AND UPPER-LEFT ABDOMINAL PAIN, NO RIGHT-UPPER PAIN, NO LONG-LASTING ANEMIA

Condition	Fever	Other Characteristics
Likely rapid onset		
SPLENIC CRISIS	Maybe	History of a large spleen which is now tender.
HEART ATTACK	No	Western diet or SYPHILIS; sweaty, nauseous; commonly a sense of doom.
PANCREATITIS	Maybe	Vomiting; severe pain goes to the back.
Only with very poor diets		
BERIBERI	No	Pain worse with food; lower limb weakness.
PELLAGRA	No	Burning pain with swallowing.
Pain likely varies with food intake, gets better or worse		
GASTRITIS	No	Burning pain, upper abdomen, like PEPTIC ULCER.
PEPTIC ULCER	No	Pain aggravated or relieved by food.
GALLBLADDER DISEASE	Maybe	Pain is also felt in right shoulder blade.
Slow onset, weeks to years		
AMEBIASIS	Usual	Center pain, worse with walking; night sweats.
SCHISTOSOMIASIS MANSONI[1]	Unusual	Large liver, large spleen, constipation or diarrhea.
LIVER FLUKE[2]	No	Ate rare or raw fish or water plants; liver large and tender.
CANCER	Seldom	Weight loss and/or lumpy liver edge, initially not tender.

1 *Schistosomiasis Mansoni: scattered areas within Africa, the Arabian peninsula, the Caribbean and parts of eastern South America.*
2 *Liver fluke: present worldwide, especially in the Far East and Southeast Asia.*

Protocol A.41.B—Upper-mid or upper-left abdominal swelling

See Protocol A.14 Skin Lumps and Bumps, if appropriate.

Is there a space between the swelling and the lower rib margins?

> If so, the swelling is probably the kidney, not the liver or spleen.

If you can feel a definite edge to the swelling; start from the groin and carefully feel all the way up:

> upper edge only: kidney, Protocol A.46, B.3.

> lower edge only: spleen Protocol A.46, B.1; left lobe of the liver Protocol A.46, B.2.

> vertical edge only: probably kidney Protocol A.46, B.3; maybe spleen Protocol A.46, B.1.

> U-shaped edge: spleen if it goes up under the ribs on the left side (positive urine urobilinogen); possibly kidney (negative urine urobilinogen and bilirubin, possibly some other urine abnormalities).

No edge felt or a spherical swelling: it may be a tumor or the gallbladder or an enormous liver or spleen. Send the patient out.

If there is a lumpy edge, the patient probably has CANCER or HYDATID DISEASE.[1]

1 *Hydatid disease: there are two kinds, clinically similar. One is prevalent in the arid tropics where dogs live close to people. The other kind is prevalent in temperate and Arctic forests, where people gather plant food and eat it raw or rare.*

PROTOCOL A.42—LOWER ABDOMINAL PROBLEMS, RIGHT OR LEFT

A.42.A—Lower abdominal pain, right or left   A.42.B—Lower abdominal swelling, right or left

Protocol A.42.A—Lower abdominal pain, right or left

If the patient has a corrected temperature, >38.5°/101.3° plus abdominal pain, see Protocol B.9 also.

This protocol is only to be used if the pain is definitely right lower or left lower. If it is not localized to either the right or left, see Protocol A.44. For groin pain (pain in leg crease) see Protocol A.45.

A pregnant woman who has symmetrical pains, both right and left lower, but is not ill, probably has round ligament pain from the enlarging uterus.

Does the patient have symptoms of ACUTE ABDOMEN (See Protocol A.39.C)?

NO or not sure	YES, definitely
	Treat according to directions in the Condition Index.

Is the patient a reproductive woman in severe pain?

NO to either or both	YES to both
	Consider TUBAL PREGNANCY, PELVIC INFECTION. If in doubt, send the patient out to a hospital.

Does the patient have a corrected temperature over 37.5°/99.5°?

NO	YES
	Consider ENTERIC FEVER, KIDNEY INFECTION, DYSENTERY, abdominal TUBERCULOSIS, BRUCELLOSIS, EBOLA VIRUS DISEASE (in West Africa).

LOWER ABDOMINAL PAIN, NOT AN ACUTE ABDOMEN, NOT A FEMALE REPRODUCTIVE CRISIS, NO FEVER

Condition	Fever	Other Characteristics
Most common, consider these first		
Ovulatory pains	No	Female, 2 weeks before her period; use IBUPROFEN.
KIDNEY STONE	Rare	Back or flank pain also; one (either) side only.
SHINGLES	Low if any	Rash in a band after skin pain for 3-4 days; skin tender to touch.
Likely some genital problem		
EPIDIDYMITIS	Maybe	Male with tenderness behind his testicle(s).
SEXUALLY TRANSMITTED DISEASE	Unusual	Also some abnormality of genitals; see Protocol B.1.
Patient has diarrhea		
TURISTA	Unusual	Lower-left crampy pain before episodes of diarrhea.
DYSENTERY	Maybe	Tenderness over the large bowels, right or left.
Likely very slow onset, over weeks, months, or years		
TUBERCULOSIS	Maybe	Slow onset; tender lump in the lower right abdomen.
TUBERCULOSIS	Maybe	Abdomen feels like bread dough or foam rubber inside.
BRUCELLOSIS	Off & On	Slow onset; comes and goes; fatigue, joint pains.
SCHISTOSOMIASIS JAPONICUM[1]	Maybe	Skin exposed to water with infected snails.
CANCER	Seldom	Lump(s) and/or weight loss, initially not tender.

---

1 *Schistosomiasis Japonicum: in areas of mainland China, the Philippines, parts of the Celebes, the upper Mekong and the Thai-Malaysian border.*

TOC

SYMPTOMS

DIFFERENTIALS

CONDITIONS

DRUG INDEX

REGIONAL NOTES

INX

Protocol A.42.B—Lower abdominal swelling, right or left

See Protocol A.45.B, Groin swelling, and/or Protocol A.14 Skin lumps and bumps if appropriate.

Is the swelling also in the central lower abdomen?

NO	YES, definitely
|	See Protocol A.44.B.

Does the mass extend into the upper abdomen?

NO	YES
|	Consult Protocols A.40 and A.41; it is probably kidney or spleen. Otherwise consider CANCER,
|	HYDATID DISEASE,[1] abdominal TUBERCULOSIS.

Is it in the lower right?

NO	YES
|	**Consider** TUBERCULOSIS or send out for diagnosis.

If there is a history of DYSENTERY or constipation, treat as AMEBIASIS. Otherwise send out for diagnosis.

---

1 *Hydatid disease: there are two kinds. One kind is prevalent in tropical areas where dogs live close to people. The other time is prevalent in temperate and Arctic forests where people gather and eat plant products without cooking them first.*

PROTOCOL A.43—FLANK/WAIST/SIDE ABDOMINAL PROBLEMS

A.43.A—Flank/Waist/Side Pain   A.40.B—Flank/Waist/Side Swelling

Protocol A.43.A—Flank/waist/side pain

Pain on either or both sides at the waist, possibly also around to the back or front or both, never down into the legs. See Protocols A.60.B and/or A.63.B if the pain goes to the legs.

Does the patient have bloody or cloudy urine: dipstick-positive for blood, leukocytes or urobilinogen?

NO to all	YES to any
|	**Consider** KIDNEY INFECTION, KIDNEY STONE, TUBERCULOSIS, CANCER, KIDNEY DISEASE,
|	SCHISTOSOMIASIS HEMATOBIUM,[1] PLANT POISONING: djenkol bean;[2] MALARIA.[3]

Does or did the patient have a corrected temperature more than 38.5°/101.3°?

NO to both	YES to either
|	Consider MALARIA,[3] AMEBIASIS,[4] SICKLE CELL DISEASE.[5]

See table on the next page.

---

1 *Schistosomiasis hematobium: present in some areas of Africa and the Middle East.*
2 *Present in Malaysia and Indonesia.*
3 *The pain with MALARIA is either symmetrical or mainly on the left.*
4 *Right side, may be mid-upper also.*
5 *Sickle cell disease: this affects those of African genetic origin, mainly in West Africa and the Americas. Some Greeks, Indians and Arabs are also affected.*

FLANK PAIN, URINE NOT BLOODY OR CLOUDY, NO OR LOW FEVER

Condition	Fever	Other Characteristics
Running pains	No	Crampy pain, onset while running, relieved by rest; no problem.
MUSCLE STRAIN	No	History of unusual exercise or injury; tight, aching pain.
MALARIA	Off & On	Both flanks, also headache, residence in malarious area.
TUBERCULOSIS	Low if any	Dipstick negative for leukocytes, positive for blood, maybe off and on.
AMEBIASIS	Usual	Right side only; patient holds his side with his arm.
KIDNEY DISEASE	Maybe	Urine abnormal in amount or urinalysis; maybe high blood pressure.
CANCER	Seldom	Lump(s) and/or weight loss, initially no tenderness.

Protocol A.43.B—Flank/waist/side swelling

Also see large spleen (left) or liver (right), Protocol A.46.B.

Is the swelling entirely within the abdominal wall, not extending deep inside?

NO, it's deep inside

|
See Protocol A.46 B.3, it is probably kidney.

Also consider A.46 B.2, liver, if it is on the right.

Also consider A.46 B.1, spleen, if it is on the left.

YES, abdominal wall only
See Protocol A.14—Skin Lumps and Bumps

PROTOCOL A.44—LOW MIDDLE ABDOMINAL PROBLEMS

A.44.A—Low middle abdominal pain

A.44.B—Low middle abdominal swelling

Protocol A.44.A—Low middle abdominal pain

If the patient has a corrected temperature more than 38.5°/101.3° plus abdominal pain, see Protocol B.9.

Does the patient have definite signs of an ACUTE ABDOMEN (See Protocol A-39 C)?

NO or not sure   **YES, definitely**

| Treat according to directions in the Condition Index.

Does the patient have a fever or is he/she very ill?

NO to both   **YES to either**

| **Consider** SEPSIS, ENTERIC FEVER, PELVIC INFECTION, a complication of pregnancy or abortion.

Is the patient a male, a new mother or someone with a genital injury?

NO   **YES**

| **Consider** URINARY OBSTRUCTION, URINARY INFECTION, PELVIC INFECTION, PROSTATITIS.

See table on the next page. (In a reproductive female, see Protocol B.1 for a possible sexually transmitted disease.)

LOW MIDDLE ABDOMINAL PAIN, NOT VERY ILL, NO GENITAL INJURY OR URINARY OBSTRUCTION

Condition	Fever	Other Characteristics
Most common, check these first		
Labor	No	Cramping pain at regular intervals.
Menstrual cramps	No	Tight, crampy pain while menstruating.
TUBERCULOSIS	Maybe	Abdomen feels as if there is bread dough or foam rubber inside.
Likely an abnormal urinalysis: including leukocytes, maybe blood also		
URINARY INFECTION	Unusual	Cloudy urine, frequent urination with burning.
PELVIC INFECTION	Maybe	Females; pain with intercourse or tampon insertion.
PROSTATITIS (males)	Maybe	Heavy pain, center pelvis, between penis and rectum.
Likely an abnormal urinalysis, possibly blood alone		
SCHISTOSOMIASIS HEMATOBIUM[1]	Unusual	Most blood at end of urination.
SCHISTOSOMIASIS MANSONI[2]	Unusual	Pain in the bladder and rectal areas.
CANCER	Seldom	Recurrent, increasing frequency and severity.

1 *Schistosomiasis hematobium: present in some areas of Africa and the Middle East.*
2 *Schistosomiasis Mansoni: scattered areas within Africa, the Arabian peninsula, the Caribbean and parts of eastern South America.*

Protocol A.44.B—Low middle abdominal swelling

See Protocol A.14—Skin Lumps and Bumps, if appropriate.

Is the patient an older man, a recently delivered woman or someone with genital injury?

NO	YES
	Consider URINARY OBSTRUCTION.

Is the patient a reproductive female?

NO	YES
	Consider pregnancy; URINARY OBSTRUCTION, otherwise send out for diagnosis. Consider CANCER also.

Send out for diagnosis: **Consider**: CANCER, URINARY OBSTRUCTION, abdominal TUBERCULOSIS

TOC

SYMPTOMS

DIFFERENTIALS

CONDITIONS

DRUG INDEX

REGIONAL NOTES

INX

PROTOCOL A.45—PROBLEMS IN GROIN(S)

A.45.A—Pain in groin(s)   A.45.B—Swelling in groin(s)

Protocol A.45.A—Pain in groin(s)

Are there lumps in the groin—the leg creases or right below them—larger than a pencil eraser? (Smaller are not significant.)

NO	YES or not sure
|	Medium consistency like a ripe peach: see Protocol A.52.B.
|	Very soft like a water balloon: consider ABSCESS, HERNIA.
|	Very hard like a good, fresh apple: consider CANCER.
|	Very tender to touch: consider PLAGUE.

GROIN PAIN, NO LUMPS IN THE GROIN(S)

Condition	Fever	Other Characteristics
MUSCLE STRAIN	No	Had unusual exercise, aching pain, no swelling in groin.
KIDNEY STONES	Rare	Sudden onset, pain shoots down from flank area, urine bloody.
DENGUE FEVER[1]	High	Sudden onset, severe body pains in muscles and bones.
BRUCELLOSIS	Off & on	Gradual onset of feeling generally very wretched.
PROSTATITIS	Maybe	Pain between base of penis and rectum, males only.
EPIDIDYMITIS	Maybe	Swelling and tenderness in back of testicle(s).

1 *Dengue fever: in the Americas only near or north of the equator. In Africa, east coastal, south and west. Prevalent in India, Southeast Asia and the Pacific. Occasionally found in the Mediterranean area. The disease may spread.*

Protocol A.45.B—Swelling in groin, in or above leg creases(s)

See Protocol A.52 if the swelling is below the leg creases also or only.

Is or was previously, the swelling soft like a water balloon?

NO to both	YES to either
|	**Consider**:
|	HERNIA: initially soft, may become hard.
|	SEXUALLY TRANSMITTED DISEASE: hard initially, becomes soft.
|	ABSCESS: hard initially, becomes soft.

Is the swelling firm like a ripe cherry?

NO	YES
|	Swollen lymph nodes which are due to an infection on the legs or feet or due to a
|	genital infection (See SEXUALLY TRANSMITTED DISEASE; see Protocol B.1). If there is
|	a cauliflower-like surface, consider DONOVANOSIS. If this is part of generalized large
|	lymph nodes, see Protocol A.31.B. If extremely tender, consider PLAGUE.

Is the swelling apple-hard and stuck to the skin and surrounding tissue?

NO	YES
|	**Consider** CANCER.

Consider SEXUALLY TRANSMITTED DISEASE Protocol B.1.

TOC

SYMPTOMS

DIFFERENTIALS

CONDITIONS

DRUG INDEX

REGIONAL NOTES

INX

PROTOCOL A.46—ABDOMINAL SWELLING

A.46.A—General or central abdominal swelling

    A1—Abdominal swelling without free fluid

    A2—Abdominal swelling due to free fluid

A.46.B—Swelling of abdominal organs

    B1—Large spleen

    B2—Large liver

    B3—Large kidney

See Protocols A.40.B, A.41.B, A.42.B, A.43.B, A.44.B for guidance in using Protocol A.46.B. If the patient also has severe abdominal pain, first check for ACUTE ABDOMEN (Protocol A.39.C). Use the protocol below only if this is not the problem. Groin swelling: see Protocol A.45.B in or above the leg crease, Protocol A.52 below the leg crease.

Protocol A.46.A—General or central abdominal swelling

Definition: The patient's abdomen sticks out in front more than one would expect from his general physical appearance with reference to the fat (or lack thereof) of his upper arm. Women who have previously given birth, even at a remote time, normally and commonly have protuberant abdomens.

Are the patient's ankles also swollen?

NO	YES
	Consider LIVER DISEASE, LIVER FAILURE, CIRRHOSIS, MALNUTRITION, HEART FAILURE,
	KIDNEY DISEASE, MALABSORPTION, any chronic diarrhea.

Does the patient feel like he has to urinate but cannot?

NO	YES
	Consider URINARY OBSTRUCTION, URETHRAL STRICTURE.

Does the patient complain of a heavy, dragging pain in his upper left abdomen?

NO	YES
	Consider causes of a large spleen: see Protocol A.46.B1.

Does the patient have free fluid in his or her abdomen (see Volume 1, Chapter 1)?

NO	YES
See A.46.A1 (below).	See A.46.A2 (below).

Abdominal swelling without free fluid: table is on the next page.

A.46.A1—Abdominal swelling without free fluid

Most common, check these first

Pregnancy	Lower abdomen, firm mass; Ruler test[1] positive after 6 months.
UMBILICAL HERNIA	Very soft bulge with the naval as a center, no general swelling.
TUBERCULOSIS	Abdomen feels as if it is full of bread dough (adults mostly), slow onset.

Patient probably very ill

ENTERIC FEVER	High fever, abdominal pain, lost appetite or vomiting, lethargic.
SEPSIS	Patient has a high fever (unless infant, elderly or malnourished), not alert mentally.
PANCREATITIS	Severe abdominal pains that go through to the back; vomiting.

Gassy swelling, flicking the abdomen on the side gives a hollow sound.

ASCARIASIS	Passage of "earthworms", crampy pains, constipated.
SPRUE[7]	Severe, foul, watery diarrhea; sore mouth.
PIG-BEL[2]	Poorly nourished children, recent high-protein foods.
TRICHURIASIS	Commonly much gas, abdominal pains, diarrhea and ANEMIA.
LIVER FLUKE[3]	Also constipation, indigestion and nausea.

Probably a solid mass, flicking the abdomen on the side gives a dull, solid sound.

Tumor[4]	Lower abdomen, firm mass, Ruler test[1] positive.
BURKITT LYMPHOMA	Usually children, fast-growing tumor, Ruler test[1] positive.
HYDATID DISEASE[5]	Tropical/arid areas with dogs Ruler test[1] may be positive.

Very slow onset, probably

AFRICAN SLEEPING SICKNESS[6]	Also swollen eyelids, maybe swollen neck or penis; headaches.
TUBERCULOSIS	Night sweats, cough, weight loss or all three, maybe.

1 Ruler test distinguishes the 4 conditions so marked from everything else. Have the patient lie flat on his/her back. Take an ordinary ruler and lay it parallel to the floor crossways on the top of the swollen abdomen. Put it across the navel or a little lower. Hold it down firmly with one finger on each end of the ruler. If the swelling is due to pregnancy, tumor, HYDATID DISEASE, BURKITT LYMPHOMA or URINARY OBSTRUCTION you may feel the patient's pulse in the ruler. This is because there is a solid mass between the large blood vessel by the back bone and the ruler. With any other condition, you will not be able to feel the pulse. Practice with a woman you know to be at least 6 months pregnant to be sure you are doing it correctly.

2 Pig-bel: developing countries near the equator.

3 Liver fluke (Fascioliasis): this is present worldwide except for Southeast Asia. See Regional Notes.

4 This could be due to CANCER or something benign. In any case, you cannot deal with it.

5 Hydatid disease: this may also be found in northern temperate or Arctic areas, in people who eat food that may be contaminated by the stool of wild animals.

6 African sleeping sickness: scattered areas of Africa, south of Bamako, Mali and Lake Chad and north of Lusaka, Zambia.

7 Sprue: in the Americas only near or north of the equator. In Africa only Nigeria and southern Africa. Prevalent in India and Southeast Asia. It is occasionally found in the Mediterranean area.

TOC
SYMPTOMS
DIFFERENTIALS
CONDITIONS
DRUG INDEX
REGIONAL NOTES
INX

A.46.A2—Abdominal swelling due to free fluid

(See also Protocol B.7)

Definition: the patient has a protuberant abdomen; his flanks bulge when he lies on his back, and you can detect free fluid by the procedures outlined in Volume 1, Chapter 1.

Does the patient also have TWO or more of the following?

- A large liver.
- Prominent veins on the front of his abdomen.[1]
- Spots on his skin that resemble little spiders.
- A large spleen.
- Yellow whites of eyes or bilirubin in urine.
- Personality changes.
- Trembling or lethargy.
- Easy bleeding.

One or none of the above symptoms	Two or more of the above symptoms
	Consider CIRRHOSIS, LIVER FAILURE; LIVER DISEASE; determine the cause(s).

Are the patient's feet and ankles also swollen?

NO	YES
	Consider: KIDNEY DISEASE, HEART FAILURE, PERICARDITIS, MALNUTRITION, MALABSORPTION, any chronic diarrhea such as SPRUE,[2] CAPILLARIASIS.[3]

Does or did the patient have severe abdominal pains going through to his back?

NO	YES
	Consider PANCREATITIS.

Consider: abdominal TUBERCULOSIS, CANCER (rarely).

1 *These are wiggly, blue lines, one half to 3 millimeters wide, visible below the skin. They may be hard to see on very dark skin but are easily seen in white or brown skin.*

2 *Sprue: in the Americas only near or north of the equator. In Africa only Nigeria and southern Africa. Prevalent in India and Southeast Asia. It is occasionally found in the Mediterranean area.*

3 *Capillariasis: Philippines mainly; rarely Thailand, found in Egypt with potential of spreading.*

Protocol A.46.B—Swelling of abdominal organs

See also Protocol B.7—Liver and Spleen Problems, if applicable.

Lower abdominal lump: URINARY OBSTRUCTION, pregnancy, TUBERCULOSIS,[1] old, ruptured appendicitis-turned-to-abscess,[2] CANCER, HYDATID DISEASE, a tumor of the ovary (usually benign).

⚠ EMERGENCY

ABDOMINAL LUMP EMERGENCIES

Signs of acute abdomen, any type (See Protocol A.39.B).

Significant weight loss (over 5 kg) in an adult; consider TUBERCULOSIS, CANCER.

Fever: see Protocol B.9.

The patient is not urinating or not able to pass stool.

The lump is quite tender; touching it causes a significant increase in pain.

There has been a recent injury after which the mass appeared or after which the mass became larger or became tender.

Note that lumps in the abdomen are particularly difficult to assess. If there are any symptoms other than a lump, then see other applicable protocols. With rare exceptions you should not trust any diagnosis based on only one protocol.

---

1 *Maybe a lump in the right lower abdomen or a feeling like bread dough within the abdomen.*

2 *In this case the patient will have a history of ACUTE ABDOMEN Type 2 (see Protocol A.39.C.) He must be sent to a hospital.*

TOC

SYMPTOMS

DIFFERENTIALS

CONDITIONS

DRUG INDEX

REGIONAL NOTES

INX

IDENTIFYING AN ENLARGED, SOLID ORGAN IN THE ABDOMEN

Divide the abdomen into four parts by drawing vertical and horizontal lines through the navel, at right angles to each other. Use a marking pen. The vertical line is the same as the midline of the body. The two lines divide the abdomen into four quadrants: right upper quadrant (RUQ); left upper quadrant (LUQ); right lower quadrant (RLQ); and left lower quadrant (LLQ). Now feel the edges of the enlarged organ and draw them on the abdominal surface. How many quadrants are involved?

First see if you can get your hand between the organ and the lower ribs. If you can, then the organ is likely neither spleen nor liver; it may be kidney or tumor. If you tap on a large spleen it sounds solid. If you tap on a large kidney, it is likely to sound hollow, because there is gas-filled bowel between it and the abdominal wall.

One quadrant only: unlikely to be kidney.

Lower, either side: requires higher-level care. Upper: liver on the right, spleen on the left.

Two quadrants vertical: in addition to the conditions listed below, abdominal TUBERCULOSIS can present as a mass.

Either side: kidney if the axis is vertical, or it is not wider on top (toward the chest) and urine bilirubin and urobilinogen are normal. Consider CANCER and HYDATID DISEASE also.

LUQ & LLQ: spleen if it is wider upper (toward the chest) than lower; you might feel a rounded tip or a notch.

RUQ & RLQ: liver (but this is rare) or kidney.

Two quadrants horizontal: in addition to the conditions listed below, abdominal TUBERCULOSIS can present as a mass.
RUQ and LUQ: liver if it is mainly right and spills over to the left. It may be the left lobe of the liver if it is centered and on both sides of the midline in the upper abdomen.

RLQ and LLQ: probably a bladder, pregnancy or tumor.

Three quadrants: determine which quadrant contains most of the mass. In addition to the conditions listed below, abdominal TUBERCULOSIS can present as a mass.

Mainly left upper: spleen mainly LUQ spills over to the lower left and lower right.

Mainly right upper: liver mainly RUQ spills over to the upper left and lower right

Mainly lower: probably a tumor; send the patient out.

▽ LARGE SPLEEN

It may be difficult to tell the difference between a large spleen and a large left kidney. Always check the urine with a dipstick. If the urobilinogen is normal on the dipstick the mass is more likely a kidney than spleen, especially if some of the other tests such as blood, protein or leukocytes are positive. If it is a kidney, see Protocol A-46 B3 below. If most of the mass is toward the middle of the body from the nipple line (a plumb line dropped from the location of a male nipple in a standing patient), then it is likely an enlarged left lobe of the liver.

⚠ EMERGENCY

LARGE SPLEEN EMERGENCIES
- Sudden enlargement after an abdominal blow.
- Spleen tender, maybe with fever.
- A blow to the abdomen, on an enlarged spleen.

Listen to the abdominal mass with your stethoscope: if you hear a humming or scraping noise, then it is spleen. Some, but not all, spleens hum or scrape. Kidneys never make noise.

LARGE LIVER
Upper right abdomen, long axis of the mass is horizontal or diagonal rather than vertical. If it is vertical, then it is probably a kidney: see Protocol A.46.B3, after the tables for an enlarged spleen and an enlarged liver.

DIFFERENTIAL DIAGNOSIS OF A LARGE SPLEEN

Condition	Group[1]	Risk factors	Essential	Maybe	Treatment
Very large spleen, at least down to the navel[5]					
TROPICAL SPLENOMEGALY	Yes	Tropics, malarious areas	Slow-onset; fatigue, anemia, spleen is firm and smooth	Heaviness decreased appetite non-tender[2]	Antimalarials
VISCERAL LEISHMANIASIS[3]	Unlikely or few	Residence in an affected area; bitten by sandflies	Slow-onset; fevers off and on; liver also enlarges	Fatigue, night sweats, poor appetite	Special drugs
Likely prominent fatigue; unable to work for weeks					
BRUCELLOSIS	Maybe, few, area	Contact with cattle or unpasteurized dairy	Slow onset of back or joint pains, feels awful	Fevers come and go	Antibiotics
MONONUCLEOSIS	No	Young age,[4] exposed to the disease	Large tonsils and/or large neck lymph nodes; fever	Extreme fatigue for a week or more	Bedrest only
CANCER	Unlikely	Radiation exposure, old age, hepatitis, other factors	Slow onset, anemia, maybe large lymph nodes	Fevers, frequent infections, bleeding, itching	Difficult
Definite exposure history is likely					
BARTONELLOSIS	Yes, few, area	Peru and adjacent; bitten by sand flies	Bone and joint pains or skin bumps	Fever, fatigue, bleeding ANEMIA	Antibiotics
CAT-SCRATCH DISEASE	Unlikely	A cat scratch or cat flea bite	Swellings between the wound and the trunk	Fevers, rash, fatigue	Antibiotics
SCRUB TYPHUS	Maybe, area	Rural Asia/Pacific; bitten by chigger mites	Fever, constipated, light avoidance, red eyes, fever	Small scab, large lymph nodes, rash	Antibiotics
HYDATID DISEASE	Maybe, few, area	Dogs in tropics or raw forest food, temperate	Slow-onset; not small children; soft lumps	Lumps on liver or spleen	Surgery after medicine
Prominent up and down fevers, maybe erratic at first					
MALARIA	Yes, many, area	Mainly tropics and subtropics; no prophylaxis	Fever and chills, or headaches	Large spleen, fatigue, waist pain, shoulder pain	Antimalarials

1 *"Group" indicates whether the patient is likely to know others who have the same condition; whether these others are few or many; and whether they are from the same family or from the general community (area) where he lives.*

2 *If there is an abscess or a bit of spleen has died, then there will be pain and tenderness See SPLENIC CRISIS.*

3 *Visceral Leishmaniasis is found in scattered areas of Central and South America, Africa north of the equator, the Mediterranean area, the Indian subcontinent, eastern Europe, central Asia and mainland China.*

4 *In the West this is a disease of teenagers; in developing areas it is most often found in younger children.*

5 *For these two conditions the urine dipstick will always show a lot of urobilinogen.*

Table continued on the next page.

DIFFERENTIAL DIAGNOSIS OF A LARGE SPLEEN, CONCLUDED

Condition	Group	Risk factors	Essential	Maybe	Treatment
Sustained fever for most of the first week					
RELAPSING FEVER[1]	Usually	Exposure to lice (crowding) or ticks (camping)	Very sudden onset fever, headache, muscle pains	Joint pains, withdrawn, spleen is tender	Antibiotics
Associated with poor living conditions					
CHAGA'S DISEASE	Maybe a few	C and S America north to the Texas border	Heart trouble, swallowing problems or constipation	History of a swollen eye, lasted more than a day	Dangerous, special meds
TYPHUS	Yes	Mainly tropical, body lice, rodent fleas, poor sanitation	First headache, then fever, back and limb pain, very ill	Musty odor, swollen face, crazy or apathetic, rash	Antibiotics
TRENCH FEVER	Maybe	Poor sanitation, refugee camps, urban homeless, body lice	Fevers and severe joint pains, lasts a long time	Headache, shins painful	Antibiotics
Prominent liver symptoms (liver large, bilirubin in urine)					
CIRRHOSIS	Maybe, few, area	Alcoholics, those with other diseases or toxins	Distended abdomen; bilirubin in the urine	Skin "spiders," easy bleeding	Difficult
SCHISTOSOMIASIS JAPONICUM	Maybe, area	Residence in some parts of Asia; snails in water. Regional notes O, S.	Distended abdomen; exposure in an affected area	History of bloody diarrhea	Praziquantel
SCHISTOSOMIASIS MANSONI	Maybe, area	Tropical Africa, Middle East, Americas, scattered areas: F, M, R.	Present or previous bloody diarrhea	Large liver, free fluid in the abdomen	Praziquantel
SYPHILIS congenital	Maybe family	Prenatal exposure; sibling(s) probably died or miscarried.	Under age 2, also large liver	Peeling hands, runny nose, rash, maybe bone pains	Penicillin
Positive family history					
OVALOCYTOSIS	Yes, family	Asia/Pacific genetic heritage	Anemia and family history of the same	Occasional crises; early deaths in family	Transfusion
SICKLE CELL DISEASE	Yes, family	African, Arab, Greek or Indian heritages; African form is worst	Mostly children, family history of ANEMIA and ill health	Recurrent crises, chest and bone pains	Transfusions, IV fluids, oxygen
THALLASEMIA	Yes, family	Mediterranean, African or Asian heritage	History of ill health in some family members	ANEMIA, fatigue, strange appearance	Transfusions, difficult

1 Relapsing fever: present in tropical and high altitude areas, but not in the islands of SEA and the Pacific.

Table concluded.

TOC

SYMPTOMS

DIFFERENTIALS

CONDITIONS

DRUG INDEX

REGIONAL NOTES

INX

TOC

SYMPTOMS

DIFFERENTIALS

CONDITIONS

DRUG INDEX

REGIONAL NOTES

INX

DIFFERENTIAL DIAGNOSIS OF A LARGE LIVER

Condition	Group[1]	Risk factors	Essential	Maybe	Tender?[2]	Urine[3]	Treatment
Minimal or no liver tenderness							
ALCOHOLISM	Maybe; area	Daily or binge alcohol	Daily or binge drinking	Distended abdomen	N	B(U)	Counseling
Prominent liver tenderness							
AMEBIASIS	Maybe; area	Poor sanitation, dysentery	Pain in right upper abdomen	Hurts to jump, liver is tender to touch	T	B	Metronidazole
LIVER FLUKE	Likely; area	Eating raw fish (Asia) or raw vegetables	Maybe nausea, body pains diarrhea,	No appetite, upper abdominal pains	T	B (U)	Special medicines
Prominent general upper abdominal pain and/or tenderness							
ASCARIASIS	Likely; area	Poor sanitation, raw vegetables, clay soil	Abdominal pain or seeing worms	White "earth-worms" visible in the stool	T	B	Dewormers
Prominent large spleen							
VISCERAL LEISHMANIASIS[4]	Likely; area	Exposed to sandflies in an affected area	Large spleen; slow onset unless HIV+	Night sweats, loss of appetite	N	U(B)	Special meds
Rapid onset; general, whole-body illness with multiple bone and joint pains							
RELAPSING FEVER	Likely: area	Exposure to ticks or lice	Sudden onset of headache, chills	Fatigue, bone, joint muscle pains	T	U(B)	Antibiotics
Slow onset; general, whole-body illness with multiple bone and joint pains							
BRUCELLOSIS	Likely; area	Pastoral areas; raw dairy products, slaughtering	Slow onset joint pains, feeling awful,	Fevers off and on, back and lower limbs	T	B	Antibiotic combinations

1 This specifies if the patient is likely to know others with the same or similar conditions.

2 "Tender?" tells if pushing on it causes increased pain N = not tender; T = tender; T→ N = tender changes to not-tender.

3 "Urine" refers to the dipstick tests for bilirubin and urobilinogen B = bilirubin positive; U = urobilinogen positive;
    letter in parentheses (U) or (B) means maybe positive.

4 Visceral Leishmaniasis is found in scattered areas of Central and South America, Africa north of the equator, the Mediterranean area,
    the Indian subcontinent, eastern Europe, central Asia and mainland China.

Continued on the next page.

DIFFERENTIAL DIAGNOSIS OF A LARGE LIVER, CONTINUED

Condition	Group	Risk factors	Essential	Maybe	Tender?[1]	Urine[2]	Treatment
Likely one or more lumps on or near the liver							
HYDATID DISEASE	Likely, area	Arid rural tropics, temperate forest	Slow onset of a soft tumor	Nothing else	Not initially	B	Dewormers first, then surgery
CANCER	Not likely	Hepatitis, older age	Varies according to kind	Weight loss, lumpy liver edge, jaundice	N→T	Varies	Difficult at best
GALLBLADDER DISEASE	Not likely	Western diet, some worms, malaria	Pain upper central or right abdomen	Light-colored stools, itching	T	B	Usually surgery
Prominent heart symptoms; exercise intolerance							
HEART FAILURE	Not likely	Western diet, prior infection	Short of breath, fatigued or both	Swollen legs and feet, chest pain, tender liver	T→ N	Neither	Special medicines
CHAGA'S DISEASE	Likely; area	Americas; poor housing	Heart failure constipated or trouble swallowing	Had a swollen eye for more than a week	T→ N	Neither	Difficult and dangerous
DIPHTHERIA	Likely	Unimmunized	Sore throat or skin ulcer with swollen edges	Trouble seeing and/or swallowing	T→ N	Normal	Antitoxin— seek higher level care
PERICARDITIS	Not likely	Tuberculosis, other prior infection	Chest pain; fatigue, low pulse pressure	Scraping heart sound or enlarged heart	T→N	Neither	Difficult
Prominent yellow whites of the eyes likely, early in the course of the illness							
HEPATITIS	Maybe area	Poor sanitation, blood exposure	Jaundice or bilirubin in urine	Joint pains, poor appetite	T	B(U)	Supportive, maybe antiviral
INDIAN CHILDHOOD CIRRHOSIS	Likely; ethnic	Indian cultural heritage, bronze drinking vessels	Jaundice and/or fluid in the abdomen	Slow onset	Unknown	B (U)	Very difficult

1 *"Tender?" tells if pushing on it causes increased pain. N = not tender; T = tender; T→ N = tender changes to not-tender.*
2 *"Urine" refers to the dipstick tests for bilirubin and urobilinogen. B = bilirubin positive; U = urobilinogen positive;*
letter in parentheses (U) or (B) means maybe positive.

Continued on the next page.

SYMPTOMS

DIFFERENTIALS

CONDITIONS

DRUG INDEX

REGIONAL NOTES

INX

TOC

TOC

SYMPTOMS

DIFFERENTIALS

CONDITIONS

DRUG INDEX

REGIONAL NOTES

INX

DIFFERENTIAL DIAGNOSIS OF A LARGE LIVER, CONCLUDED

Condition	Group[1]	Risk factors	Essential	Maybe	Tender?[2]	Urine[3]	Treatment
Totally unpredictable symptoms and time course, depending on the kind of poisoning							
PLANT POISONING	Likely; area	Using ethnic remedies or some drugs.	Symptoms vary by kind of poisoning.	Variable	Varies	Probably B(U)	Variable
Geographically very confined to certain areas							
SCHISTOSOMIASIS JAPONCUM[6]	Likely; area	Exposure to water with snails in an affected area; Asia only.	Liver failure, large spleen, weight loss, big abdomen.	Diarrhea, brain damage, cough	N	B(U)	Praziquantel
SCHISTOSOMIASIS MANSONI[4]	Likely; area	Exposure to water with snails in an affected area.	Liver failure or chronic diarrhea, large spleen.	Urinary or reproductive symptoms	N	B(U)	Praziquantel
Likely a positive family history							
SICKLE CELL DISEASE[5]	Likely; family	African, Arab, Indian or Greek genetic heritage.	Anemia; family history.	Recurrent crises with pain	N	U(B)	Transfusions, IV fluids, oxygen
SYPHILIS, congenital	Maybe, family	Parent(s) had syphilis.	Baby under age 2.	Rash, runny nose, ill health	Unknown	??	Penicillin
THALLASEMIA	Likely; family	Genetic heritage African, Asian or Mediterranean.	Family history; recurrent crises, large spleen.	Strange facial appearance	N	U	Transfusions

1 This specifies if the patient is likely to know others with the same or similar conditions.
2 "Tender?" tells if the mass is tender—if pushing on it causes pain. N = not tender; T = tender; T→ N = tender changes to not-tender.
3 "Urine" refers to the dipstick tests for bilirubin and urobilinogen. B = bilirubin positive; U = urobilinogen positive;
   letter in parentheses (U) or (B) means maybe positive.
4 Schistosomiasis Mansoni: scattered areas within Africa, the Arabian Peninsula, the Caribbean and parts of eastern South America.
5 Sickle cell disease: this affects those of African genetic origin, mainly in West Africa and the Americas. Some Indians and Arabs are also affected.
6 Schistosomiasis Japonicum: in areas of mainland China, the Philippines, parts of the Celebes, the upper Mekong and the Thai-Malaysian border.

Table concluded.

LARGE KIDNEY

Is the mass (presumably enlarged kidney) tender to touch?

NO

This may be cyst(s) on the kidney, HYDATID DISEASE or CANCER. Consider BURKITT LYMPHOMA; also consider TUBERCULOSIS of the kidney.

YES

Consider: URINARY OBSTRUCTION; ABSCESS of the kidney; also consider TUBERCULOSIS of the kidney with episodic bloody urine.

PROTOCOL A.47—NAUSEA, VOMITING OR BOTH

This protocol deals only with usual vomiting. See Protocol A.48 if the patient has vomited blood: red liquid, clots or brown stuff that looks like coffee grounds. For regular vomiting that only has streaks of blood, use this protocol; ignore the blood. Since vomiting is very common, it is better to focus on other, less common symptoms.

First check for DEHYDRATION. If your patient is dehydrated, treat him for that while working on the diagnosis. Severe dehydration with loss of consciousness is an emergency; use rectal or intraperitoneal fluids. See Volume 1, Appendix 1

Prompt vomiting of all food right after eating mandates sending the patient for surgery promptly, regardless of age and treating for DEHYDRATION in the meantime using intraperitoneal fluids (Volume 1, Appendix 1).

▷ SYMPTOMATIC TREATMENT	⚠ EMERGENCY
If the problem is not too severe and the patient is not too ill, try the following: give nothing by mouth for 6 hours and have the patient lie as still as possible. At the beginning of this time, pour a bottle or can of Coca Cola into a large-diameter container and let it become warm. After 6 hours, all of the fizz will be gone. Give the patient a teaspoon at a time, every 2-5 minutes. If he keeps this down, advance the amount to a tablespoon at a time. In older children and adults it is acceptable to use PROMETHAZINE or HYDROXYZINE additionally, to settle the stomach.	**VOMITING EMERGENCIES** Projectile vomiting: the vomit shoots out across the room. Vomiting without nausea, in the presence of headache or some brain problem. Severe vomiting with dehydration (thirst, dry mouth). Vomiting in the presence of severe, watery diarrhea. Vomiting in an unconscious patient. Vomiting large amounts of blood.

QUICK AND EASY DIAGNOSES FROM SENSITIVE AND SPECIFIC SYMPTOMS

PERTUSSIS	Severe coughing spells trigger vomiting; young children and elderly mainly.
CHOLERA	Massive watery diarrhea followed by vomiting; rapid onset of dehydration.
MENINGITIS	High fever, severe headache in adults, very ill, maybe stiff neck or seizures.
ASCARIASIS	Whitish, earthworm—sized worms seen in stool or vomit, round in cross-section.

Is the patient an infant, less than 4 months old?

NO

YES

Send him to the hospital if he is losing weight, if he vomits his entire feeding or if the whites of his eyes look yellow. If you cannot send him, consider SEPSIS, KIDNEY INFECTION, ACUTE ABDOMEN type 3. Treat for DEHYDRATION.

Is there a recent-onset, severe whole-body illness with abnormal vital signs, eye symptoms, and/or sweating?

NO to all

YES to any

Consider: DIPHTHERIA, PLANT POISONING due to botulism or water hemlock, TETANUS, RABIES, ENCEPHALITIS, HEART ATTACK. In young children, almost any illness with a fever might cause vomiting.

Does or did the patient have significant abdominal or chest pain, without other significant pain?

NO to both

YES to either

Chest pain

> HEART ATTACK/ANGINA: also sweaty, maybe a sense of doom
> LASSA FEVER[1]: epidemic context in West Africa; fever

No abdominal tenderness

> KIDNEY STONE: sudden onset flank pain; maybe bloody urine
> HEART ATTACK/ANGINA: sweaty; chest pain; Western diet.
> DIABETES: known diabetic or sugar and ketones in urine
> LASSA FEVER[1]: weakness, aching; chest pain common.

Maybe abdominal tenderness

> ASCARIASIS: clay soil, poor sanitation, white "earthworms" in stool
> FOOD POISONING: ingestion within the past week
> INTESTINAL FLUKE[2]: also severe diarrhea.
> ACUTE ABDOMEN: SHOCK, pain over 6 hours or episodic pains.
> PIG-BEL[3]: previously malnourished, had a high-protein meal.

For sure abdominal tenderness

> GASTRITIS or PEPTIC ULCER with burning pains, center front.
> AMEBIASIS; pain and tenderness, upper right or mid abdomen.
> GALLBLADDER DISEASE: upper mid abdominal pain.
> YELLOW FEVER[4]: bilirubin and protein in urine, jaundice.
> PANCREATITIS; pain goes through to the back

Does the patient have a corrected temperature more than 38.5°/101.3° or has he had one recently with this illness?

NO fever

YES, vomiting with fever or history of fever

Extremely ill

> LASSA FEVER[5]: weakness, aching; chest pain common.
> EBOLA VIRUS DISEASE: weakness, aching, diarrhea, Africa epidemic context
> MENINGITIS: severe headache and mental changes.
> HEAT ILLNESS: infant, elderly or exertion in a hot environment.
> IRIS: change in medication in a patient with HIV plus TB.

No rash

> MALARIA: chills, sweats, headaches.
> EAR INFECTION: ear pain, fussiness in small children.
> FAMILIAL MEDITERRANEAN FEVER[12]: recurrent abdominal/joint pains.
> YELLOW FEVER: quite ill, bilirubin and protein in the urine, Africa and Americas.
> INFLUENZA: epidemic context; headache, cough, congestion.

Continued on the next page.

All footnotes are at the end of this flow diagram, next page.

Protocol A.47 continued | *Village Medical Manual 7th Edition Volume 2* | **A-137**
CHAPTER PAGE

TOC

SYMPTOMS

DIFFERENTIALS

CONDITIONS

DRUG INDEX

REGIONAL NOTES

INX

Does the patient have a corrected temperature more than 38.5°/101.3° or has he had one recently with this illness?

NO fever	YES, vomiting with fever or history of fever
	Maybe rash

- RELAPSING FEVER[6]: sudden chills, headache, body pain.
- ENTERIC FEVER: cough or abdominal pain; not alert.
- ROSEOLA: either rash or fever, not both.
- LEPTOSPIROSIS: sudden, red eyes and whole-body pains.
- ARBOVIRAL FEVER: variable symptoms; seek local lore.
- RAT BITE FEVER: inflammed bite wound or red spots.
- TULAREMIA[7]: exposure to small animals and/or ticks.
- HIV INFECTION: positive blood test; weight loss; diarrhea

Prominent rash

- MEASLES: red-spotted or sandpapery rash.
- TYPHUS: whole-body pains; intoxicated-like mental state.
- SPOTTED FEVER[8]: chills, headache, body pains.
- KATAYAMA DISEASE: episodes of fever and hives.

Does the patient also have diarrhea?

NO	YES

Consider CHOLERA if he is like an open faucet. Diarrhea occurs before vomiting.

Identifiable, recent exposure, probably others similarly involved

- ARSENIC POISONING: also skin changes, usually homicidal or industrial
- FOOD POISONING: ate tainted food containing meat
- PLANT POISONING:[9] ate tainted food or took an ethnic medicine
- INSECTICIDE POISONING: also a lot of body fluid: saliva, tears, diarrhea
- RADIATION ILLNESS; history of exposure

No identifiable, recent exposure, stool positive for blood

- DYSENTERY, SCHISTOSOMIASIS MANSONI[10]

No identifiable exposure, probably stool tests negative for blood

- TURISTA, GIARDIASIS, GASTROENTERITIS, INTESTINAL FLUKE[11]

Does the patient also have a severe headache or eye pain?

NO or do not know	YES

Consider ALTITUDE SICKNESS, MIGRAINE, HEAT ILLNESS, CARBON MONOXIDE POISONING, GLAUCOMA, MALARIA.

See the table on the next page.

---

1 Lassa fever: only in the humid, rural areas of Africa.
2 Intestinal fluke: this kind is found only in Asia.
3 Pig-bel: developing countries, near the equator.
4 Yellow fever: found in scattered areas of Africa and the Americas only, thus far.
5 Lassa fever: only in the humid, rural areas of Africa.
6 Relapsing fever: tropical and high altitude, but not in the islands of SEA and the Pacific.
7 Tularemia: North America, central Asia, Europe, Far East, the north coast of Africa; exposure to small animals.

8 Spotted fever: worldwide including the Arctic, but not in the islands of Southeast Asia.
9 Many kinds of plant poisoning cause vomiting.
10 Schistosomiasis Mansoni: scattered areas within Africa, the Arabian Peninsula, the Caribbean and parts of eastern South America.
11 Intestinal fluke: this kind is found only in Asia.
12 Familial Mediterranean fever: this affects persons of Mediterranean genetic heritage such as Jews, Arabs, Turks and Armenians.

VOMITING, NOT AN INFANT, NO HIGH FEVER, NOT A RECENT ONSET ILLNESS, NO ABDOMINAL PAIN, NO DIARRHEA, NO HEADACHE, NO JAUNDICE

Condition	Fever	Other Characteristics
Most common, consider these first		
Pregnancy	No	Missed periods, daily nausea; early pregnancy only
Overfeeding	No	Baby fed too much vomits some; use smaller feedings
PERTUSSIS	Low if any	Vomiting triggered by severe coughing spells, young children and elderly
ASCARIASIS	No	Maybe cramps, constipated, common in children
Abnormal urine dipstick		
KIDNEY DISEASE	Unusual	Eyes swollen in the morning, little or abnormal urine with protein and/or blood
KIDNEY STONE	Unusual	Pain in back, side, groin or genitals, blood in urine
DIABETES	No	Sugar in urine, dehydrated, breathing fast
Related to a recent ingestion		
PLANT POISONING[1]	Unusual	Many types; check history of eating plant
ARSENIC POISONING	No	Numbness, burning in hands; maybe abdominal pains
TRICHINOSIS	Usual	Ate rare pork or game within the last week

1 *Ackee, argemone oil, botulism, claviceps, coral plant, lolism, manicheel, margosa oil, mushrooms, nicotine*

TOC

SYMPTOMS

DIFFERENTIALS

CONDITIONS

DRUG INDEX

REGIONAL NOTES

INX

PROTOCOL A.48—VOMITING BLOOD

Definition: the patient vomits either red blood or else a black substance that resembles coffee grounds
See the list of vomiting emergencies under Protocol A.47.

Distinguish between coughed blood and vomited blood	▷ **SYMPTOMATIC TREATMENT**
With coughed blood the pH of the watery stuff with the blood is 7–8; use your urine dipsticks. With vomited blood the pH is 5 or less, maybe 6 if the patient has just eaten. It will never be 7 or more unless the patient is on medicine for GASTRITIS or PEPTIC ULCER.	Discontinue any alcohol or ASPIRIN the patient may be taking. Encourage the intake of ORS and other liquids. Allow no solid food for several days. CIMETIDINE may be helpful.

If this is part of a general bleeding problem: bloody nose, easy bruising, excessive menstruation, bloody stools, bleeding from minor wounds, then also see Protocols A.13.E, B.2 and B.7.

Is the patient vomiting ordinary vomit with some streaks or small clots of blood in it?

NO	YES
|	Ignore the blood; use the previous protocol.

Is there evidence of SHOCK: cool moist skin, rapid pulse, low blood pressure?

Shock absent	Shock present
|	Treat for SHOCK and send out as soon as possible. **Consider** PEPTIC ULCER if there is a delay.
|	**Consider** CANCER if the patient has had symptoms of increasing frequency and severity.
|	Also follow the other arm for this question.

Check the patient's nose and mouth for bleeding.

Bleeding absent	Bleeding present
|	Patient may have vomited swallowed blood. Consider SCURVY; consider HEMORRHAGIC FEVER
|	(and related diseases) if the patient is very ill.

Does the patient have a corrected temperature of 38.5°/101.3° or more, or a history thereof?

NO	YES
|	**Consider** HEMORRHAGIC FEVER (and related diseases), TYPHUS, YELLOW FEVER, ENTERIC FEVER, MALARIA.

VOMITING SIGNIFICANT AMOUNT OF BLOOD, NO SHOCK, NO MOUTH/NOSE BLEEDING, NO HIGH FEVER.

TROPICAL SPLENOMEGALY	ANEMIA, large spleen, urobilinogen in the urine.
VISCERAL LEISHMANIASIS[1]	Huge spleen, large liver, very slow onset, geography.
LIVER FAILURE	JAUNDICE, distended abdomen, bilirubin in the urine.
LIVER DISEASE	Bilirubin in the urine.
THALLASEMIA	Hereditary ANEMIA; Mediterranean, African or Asian genetic heritage.
INDIAN CHILDHOOD CIRRHOSIS[2]	South Asian children, bronze drinking vessels.
CANCER	Symptoms of increasing frequency and severity; weight loss.

---

1 *Visceral Leishmaniasis: found in scattered areas of Central and South America, Africa north of the equator, the Mediterranean area, the Indian subcontinent, eastern Europe, central Asia and mainland China.*
2 *Indian childhood cirrhosis: affects Indian children in India and elsewhere in the world.*

A good general rule is to send anyone with jaundice or an enlarged spleen to a hospital. Those with normal vital signs and without an enlarged spleen may be given symptomatic treatment, provided that CANCER is unlikely.

Continue to check for SHOCK every few hours. An increase in the pulse rate, even without a drop in blood pressure, should prompt immediate evacuation. Consider a PEPTIC ULCER that has bled.

PROTOCOL A.49—OTHER ABDOMINAL PROBLEMS

Appetite problems: see Protocol A.9.

Abdominal wall stiff and hard like a board: normal in an athletic person. If ill, consider ACUTE ABDOMEN, TETANUS, PLANT POISONING due to strychnine.

Bleeding stump of umbilical cord in a newborn: treat with VITAMIN K by injection; put firm pressure on it meanwhile.

Infected stump of umbilical cord in a newborn: SEPSIS if the baby acts sick, otherwise CELLULITIS which may turn into SEPSIS.

Excessive gas: this is usually due to diet. Otherwise consider GALLBLADDER DISEASE, GIARDIASIS, GASTRITIS, PEPTIC ULCER, DYSENTERY (amebic), CAPILLARIASIS,[1] SPRUE,[2] MILK INTOLERANCE, TRICHURIASIS, MALABSORPTION.

Loud, rumbling bowel sounds: usually due to diet and of absolutely no consequence. Otherwise consider: GIARDIASIS, GASTROENTERITIS, TUBERCULOSIS, CAPILLARIASIS,[1] SPRUE,[2] MALABSORPTION.

Large veins on the abdominal wall: normal in OLD AGE; LIVER FAILURE, CIRRHOSIS, TROPICAL SPLENOMEGALY.

Indigestion: usually this is from a dietary indiscretion. Occasionally it is from PEPTIC ULCER, HEARTBURN, ANGINA or a HEART ATTACK in those who have eaten a Western diet. PELLAGRA, INTESTINAL FLUKE,[3] SCHISTOSOMIASIS MANSONI,[4] CANCER and LIVER FLUKE[5] may also cause chronic indigestion.

Skin ulcer on the abdominal wall: AMEBIC SKIN ULCER, DIPHTHERIA, possibly SEXUALLY TRANSMITTED DISEASE if it is at or near the groin area.

⚠ **EMERGENCY**

AMEBIC SKIN ULCER
An amebic skin ulcer is an emergency; treat it promptly.

---

1 *Capillariasis; mainly in the Philippines; rarely in Thailand; found in Egypt with potential of spreading.*
2 *Sprue: in the Americas only near or north of the equator. In Africa only Nigeria and southern Africa. Prevalent in India and Southeast Asia. Occasionally found in the Mediterranean area. The disease may spread.*
3 *Intestinal fluke: found in Asia and the Middle East.*
4 *Schistosomiasis Mansoni: scattered areas within Africa, the Arabian peninsula, the Caribbean and parts of eastern South America.*
5 *Liver fluke: present worldwide, including temperate climates, but especially common in Southeast Asia.*

TOC

SYMPTOMS

DIFFERENTIALS

CONDITIONS

DRUG INDEX

REGIONAL NOTES

INX

IX—PELVIC AND RECTAL PROBLEMS

PROTOCOL A.50—PELVIC AND RECTAL PAIN

In any sexually active patient, consider also the sexually transmitted diseases which can seldom, if ever, be diagnosed separately without sophisticated lab. See Protocol B.1. The protocols below focus on non-reproductive problems and diseases. Check the lower back. Pelvic and buttock pains can arise from a lower back problem. If pushing on the lower back provokes the same pain, then see the protocols for back problems.

A.50.A—Very ill with a fever
A.50.B—Rectal and/or anal pain
A.50.C—Pain with urination

A.50.D—Genital pain in males
A.50.E—Vaginal and pelvic pain
 in females

A.50.F—Deep bone pain in pelvis,
 both sexes
A.50.G—Muscle pains in pelvis
 and buttocks

Protocol A.50.A—Very ill with a corrected temperature above 99.0°F/37.2°C

Onset likely over two days or less

DENGUE FEVER[1]	Severe bone and muscle pains, sudden onset, eye pain.
PLAGUE	Large, extremely tender lymph nodes with blackened skin on them.
LASSA FEVER[2]	Weakness, chest and general body pains; epidemics.

Onset variable

ACUTE ABDOMEN	SHOCK, increased pain with coughing or both.

Onset likely over more than 2 days

SEPSIS	Recent delivery, ABORTION or miscarriage; infection, injury or both.
ABSCESS	Localized red, swollen, tender area which may feel soft.
SEXUALLY TRANSMITTED DISEASES	Swelling or abnormal holes in the genital area; like an infected injury.
URINARY INFECTION	Burning and pain with urination, possibly with back pains also.

1 *Dengue fever: in the Americas only near or north of the equator. In Africa, east coastal, south and west. It is prevalent in India, Southeast Asia and the Pacific. Occasionally found in the Mediterranean area. The disease may spread.*
2 *Lassa fever occurs in epidemics in west and central Africa.*

Protocol A.50.B—Rectal and/or anal pain

▷ **SYMPTOMATIC TREATMENT**   Sitting in a tub of water may relieve pain.

Conditions	Fever	Other Characteristics
Likely nothing abnormal visible on the outside		
PROCTITIS	Maybe	Pain inside with bowel movements.
PROSTATITIS (males)	Maybe	Heavy, aching pain between the rectum and the penis.
SCHISTOSOMIASIS HEMATOBIUM[1]	Unusual	Like PROCTITIS; maybe bloody urine also.
SCHISTOSOMIASIS MANSONI[2]	Unusual	Like PROCTITIS; maybe bloody urine also.
Likely something abnormal visible on the outside		
HEMORRHOIDS	No	Bluish bulge by rectum or blood on the outside of stool.
SEXUALLY TRANSMITTED DISEASES	Maybe	Large groin nodes, visible sores or both; maybe pus.
ABSCESS	Maybe	Red warm bulge, tender to touch, near the rectum.
FISSURE	No	Split in the skin, severe pain with bowel movements.

1 *Schistosomiasis hematobium: present in some areas of Africa and the Middle East.*
2 *Schistosomiasis Mansoni: scattered areas within Africa, the Arabian Peninsula, the Caribbean and parts of eastern South America.*

Protocol A.50.C—Pain with urination

Definition: the patient has pain either at the beginning of urination, at the end of urination or throughout. Usually there is also urgency (have to go RIGHT NOW) and frequency (frequent urination of small amounts).

First consider SEXUALLY TRANSMITTED DISEASES, Protocol B.1; this and URINARY INFECTION are most common. Any open skin wound can affect the genital area and is likely to cause pain if and when urine touches it. Anytime there is pain with urination you must look at the patient's genital area.

Conditions	Fever	Pain	Other Characteristics
These most common; check these first			
URINARY INFECTION	Rare	Urination	Urine cloudy; probably leukocytes on urine dipstick.
KIDNEY INFECTION	Usual	Back & Urination	Urine cloudy; probably leukocytes on urine dipstick.
URETHRITIS	No	Urination	Genital redness and pus; leukocytes on urine dipstick.
PROSTATITIS	Maybe	Yes, by rectum	Pain between penis and rectum; tender prostate.
METHYLENE BLUE (drug)	Not from drug itself	Urination	This is a malaria drug; the urine turns blue, and there may be pain with urination.
Sudden onset whole-body illness			
HEMORRHAGIC FEVER	High	Yes, place varies	Epidemic setting; consider EBOLA VIRUS DISEASE as one kind.
DENGUE FEVER[1]	High	All bones	Severe bone and muscle pains, sudden onset, headache.
LASSA FEVER[2]	High	Mainly chest	Weakness, chest and body pains, maybe bloody urine.
PLANT POISONING	No	Kidneys	Djenkol bean (Malaysia and Indonesia); bloody urine.
Gradual onset whole-body illness			
TUBERCULOSIS	Usual	With urination	No response to usual antibiotics, blood positive on dipstick intermittently, leukocytes negative on dipsticks.
SCHISTOSOMIASIS HEMATOBIUM[3]	Maybe	Maybe, variable	Urine bloody, especially at the end of urination.
Local genital problem, likely a visible abnormality			
MYIASIS	Maybe	Varies	Maggots (little fat "worms") on genitals or in urine
HERPES	Maybe	Always	Blistery rash, very tender
CHANCROID	No	Varies	Pain with urine touching an ulcer; maybe tender

1   Dengue fever: in the Americas only near or north of the equator. In Africa, east coastal, south and west. Prevalent in India, Southeast Asia and the Pacific. Occasionally found in the Mediterranean area. The disease may spread.

2   Lassa fever occurs in epidemics in west and central Africa.

3   Schistosomiasis hematobium: present in some areas of Africa and the Middle East.

Protocol A.50.D—Genital pain in males

> **▷ SYMPTOMATIC TREATMENT**
>
> Have the patient wear a jock strap or a homemade or cultural equivalent. Have him stay at bedrest and use IBUPROFEN for pain, for an hour or two. Try warmth or cold, whichever feels better.

Visually examine the genital area. The skin of the genital area can be affected just like the skin elsewhere. Check the skin protocols A.14–A.17 in this index if nothing fits from this protocol. Try the symptomatic treatment first.

Two major alternatives to consider:

- ***if there was sudden onset of pain*** in a previously healthy male who has no fever now, and if the pain is not relieved by the symptomatic treatment, then send the patient to a hospital immediately. He may have a twisted testicle which he will lose if he does not have emergency surgery.
- ***if the onset of pain was slow,*** there is a fever or pain was somewhat relieved with the symptomatic treatment, proceed as follows:

Does the patient have a fever or recent history of fever?

NO	YES
|	**Consider**: DENGUE FEVER,[1] FILARIASIS, BRUCELLOSIS, SPOTTED FEVER (in the Americas), MUMPS.

Does the patient have a swollen scrotum?

NO	YES
|	**Onset likely less than 2 weeks:** DONOVANOSIS, LYMPHOGRANULOMA VENEREUM, EPIDIDYMITIS,[2] MUMPS.
|	**Onset likely more than 2 weeks:** HERNIA, BRUCELLOSIS, TUBERCULOSIS, AFRICAN SLEEPING SICKNESS.[3] See also Protocol A.52.A.
See table below.	

1 Dengue fever: in the Americas only near or north of the equator. In Africa, east coastal, south and west. Prevalent in India, Southeast Asia and the Pacific. Occasionally found in the Mediterranean area. It may spread anywhere.

2 If you elevate and support the testicles for an hour, pain is relieved. This distinguishes epididymitis from a twisted testicle; a twisted testicle is an emergency.

3 African sleeping sickness: scattered areas of Africa, south of Bamako, Mali and Lake Chad and north of Lusaka, Zambia.

MALE GENITAL PAIN, NO FEVER, SCROTUM NOT SWOLLEN

Conditions	Fever	Other Characteristics
The abnormal appearance is not exclusively in the foreskin.		
Injury	No	Should see bruising or obtain a history of injury.
SEXUALLY TRANSMITTED DISEASE	Maybe	Blister, ulcer, enlarged groin nodes or swollen penis.
SICKLE CELL DISEASE[1]	Maybe	Painful erection that won't go away.
EPIDIDYMITIS	Maybe	Back side of testicle very tender.
The abnormal appearance is confined to the foreskin and penis tip.		
PARAPHIMOSIS	No	Foreskin pulled back from penis tip and swollen there.
PHIMOSIS	No	Foreskin stuck to the (uncircumcised) tip of the penis.
Genitals not likely visibly abnormal at all.		
PROSTATITIS	Maybe	Heavy aching between the penis and rectum.
SCHISTOSOMIASIS HEMATOBIUM[2]	Rare	Dull aching backside of the scrotum.
SCHISTOSOMIASIS MANSONI[3]	Rare	Dull aching backside of the scrotum.
KIDNEY STONE	Rare	Sharp genital pain, no tenderness;[4] sudden onset.

1 Sickle cell disease: this affects those of African genetic origin, mainly in West Africa and the Americas. Some Indians and Arabs are also affected.

2 Schistosomiasis hematobium: present in some areas of Africa and the Middle East.

3 Schistosomiasis Mansoni: scattered areas within Africa, the Arabian Peninsula, the Caribbean and parts of eastern South America.

4 A lack of tenderness means that gentle pressure on the part does not aggravate the pain.

Protocol A.50.E—Vaginal and pelvic pain in females see also Protocol B.1

If the problem is itching, see VAGINITIS. The skin of the genital area can develop skin problems just like skin anywhere else.

Conditions	Fever	Other Characteristics
Pain with intercourse[1] a likely complaint initially, insertional or deep pain		
SEXUALLY TRANSMITTED DISEASES	Maybe	A visible blister, sore or large groin lymph nodes.
CHANCROID	No	Large, tender groin nodes, maybe without a visible sore.
MENOPAUSE	No	Irritation with intercourse because of dry vagina.
Injury	Rare	Visible or evident from history.
Pain with intercourse a likely complaint initially, likely only deep pain		
PELVIC INFECTION	Usual	Pain with intercourse, tampon insertion or jumping.
TUBERCULOSIS	Usual	Like PELVIC INFECTION; onset over months; maybe cough.
TUBAL PREGNANCY	No	Pain less than a month; more to right or left than center.
Pain with intercourse a likely complaint, likely only insertional pain		
HERPES	Maybe	Blisters, intact or broken, red, raw areas.
CHANCROID	No	A visible ulcer, lips or vaginal wall, red ring on it.
Other symptoms preceded pain with intercourse.		
SCHISTOSOMIASIS HEMATOBIUM[2]	No	Bloody urine, pain with urination, pain with intercourse later.
DYSENTERY, amebic	Maybe	Painful and tender bowels, right, left or both.
KIDNEY STONE	No	Severe pains, one side; usually vomiting, genitals not tender.
MYIASIS	Maybe	Visible maggots (short, fat "worms") in the genital area.
CANCER	Maybe	Abnormal pelvic exam; see Volume 1, Chapter 6.

1 *Distinguish between insertional pain with intercourse (when the penis first touches the vagina) and deep pain (only with vigorous thrusting of the penis). Insertional pain requires examination of the external genitals. Deep pain is likely due to some internal problem. It requires a speculum examination additionally.*

2 *Schistosomiasis hematobium: present in some areas of Africa and the Middle East.*

Protocol A.50.F—Deep bone pain in pelvis, both sexes

Definition: This is an aching pain, worse at night, with high humidity and weight bearing. It is invariably severe.

Check the lower back. Pelvic and buttock pains can arise from a lower back problem. If pushing on the lower back provokes the pain, then see the protocols for back problems also.

Conditions	Fever	Other Characteristics
No fever		
RICKETS	No	Inadequate sun, patient or a nursing baby's mother.
Maybe a fever		
TUBERCULOSIS	Maybe	Slow-onset, one location only, limp; thin thigh muscles.
SICKLE CELL DISEASE[1]	Common	Recurrent abdominal pain, ANEMIA; hereditary.
BRUCELLOSIS	Erratic	Joint pains or shooting pains; slow onset.
BARTONELLOSIS[2]	Yes	General aching, bumps on legs.
YAWS	Maybe	Skin over painful area is inflamed or broken open.
Certainly a fever		
DENGUE FEVER[3]	High	Sudden onset, also limb pains and rash.
OSTEOMYELITIS	High	Increased pain with tapping anywhere on the pelvis.

Footnotes are on the next page.

TOC

SYMPTOMS

DIFFERENTIALS

CONDITIONS

DRUG INDEX

REGIONAL NOTES

INX

Footnotes for the previous table.

1 *Sickle cell disease: this affects those of African genetic origin, mainly in West Africa and the Americas. Some Indians and Arabs are also affected.*

2 *Bartonellosis: scattered areas in Peru and adjacent countries.*

3 *Dengue fever: in the Americas only near or north of the equator. In Africa, east coastal, south and west. Prevalent in India, Southeast Asia and the Pacific. Occasionally found in the Mediterranean area. It may spread.*

Protocol A.50.G—Muscle pains in pelvis and buttocks

Definition: This is an aching pain, worse at night, with high humidity, movement and weight bearing.

Check the lower back. Pelvic and buttock pains can arise from a lower back problem. If pushing on the lower back provokes the pain, then see the protocols for back problems.

Is this part of a general illness with a fever and general whole-body pains?

NO to both	YES to either or both
	See Protocol B.2.

MUSCLE PAINS IN PELVIS AND BUTTOCKS, NEITHER WITH A HIGH TEMPERATURE NOR WITH WHOLE-BODY PAINS.

MUSCLE STRAIN	Patient fell, nearly fell, or did unaccustomed exercise.
PYOMYOSITIS	Warmth and swelling; site of old injection or minor injury; area warm to the touch.
POLIO	Some weakness which is worse in pelvis than in feet and toes.
RICKETS	Inadequate sun, patient or a nursing baby's mother.
CYSTICERCOSIS	History of eating inadequately cooked pork; lumps under the skin.
TRICHINOSIS	Ate rare or raw meat within the past month; muscles swollen, no lumps.

PROTOCOL A.51—RECTAL[1] AND GENITAL ITCHING

1 *The area that is visible on the outside by spreading the buttocks is properly called the anus. However, this vocabulary may not be familiar. Hence the term "rectum" includes both the rectum and anus.*

First consider SEXUALLY TRANSMITTED DISEASES, particularly in females; see Protocol B.1.

▷ SYMPTOMATIC TREATMENT

Wash with cool water and soap. Dry well. Use baby powder. This will frequently relieve itching. If it helps, then it is mucous irritation only, nothing serious. Otherwise consider the following:

Most common, consider these first

VAGINITIS	Itching around or in vagina, maybe discharge or odor. CANDIDIASIS is likely.
Food allergy	Itching 3 or 4 days after eating the offending food; keep a diet diary and eliminate the offending food; most commonly dairy products, fish or peanuts.

Probably a skin rash visible plus scratch marks

CANDIDIASIS	Bright, red rash with some red spots around it.
STRONGYLOIDIASIS	Pricking, itching sensation by rectum and/or buttocks; red raised line or area.
SCABIES	Fine little spots or holes that are extremely itchy.
CONTACT DERMATITIS	History of the patient using some kind of cream or douche; reddened; irregular borders.

Probably something visible other than a rash plus scratch marks

FISSURE	A split in the skin adjacent to the anus; pain with bowel movements.
FISTULA	An abnormal hole between the rectum and the genital area.
HEMORRHOIDS	Red or purple bulge(s) around the anus.
LICE	Moving creatures visible and/or tiny bumps on the genital hairs.

Continued on next page.

SYMPTOMS

DIFFERENTIALS

CONDITIONS

DRUG INDEX

REGIONAL NOTES

INX

TOC

Living creatures visible with hand magnification, maybe without

Beef TAPEWORM	White rectangles visible by anus or in stool
ENTEROBIASIS	Tiny worms visible by the rectum, about 1/2 hour after going to bed
LICE	Very small moving creatures and/or bumps (louse eggs) on pubic hairs

Probably nothing visible except scratch marks

LYMPHOGRANULOMA VENEREUM	History of large, painful lymph nodes in the groin; sexual misbehavior likely, possibly rectal symptoms
Rat TAPEWORM	Try a treatment if rats are common
DIABETES	Known diabetic or sugar in urine, thirst and vomiting

PROTOCOL A.52—ABNORMAL APPEARANCE OF PELVIS AND RECTUM

Note: see Volume 1 Chapter 6 for drawings depicting the normal and abnormal appearances of female genital areas.

A.52.A—Groin and genital swelling   A.52.B—Enlarged groin lymph nodes   A.52.C—Other problems

Protocol A.52.A—Groin and genital swelling

HERNIA is most common. Abdominal swelling can go down into the scrotum in males or the genital lips in females. See Protocol A.46.A if the abdomen is swollen. For skin bumps in the genital area, see the insert at the beginning of Protocol A.14.

Is the patient sexually active (or possibly an abused child)?

NO	YES
|	**Consider** SEXUALLY TRANSMITTED DISEASE, Protocol B.1. Otherwise continue down the "No" arm of
|	this question.

Is the swelling in the scrotum or vaginal area only not extending continuously to the leg creases?

NO	YES	
|	In a dark room, shine a bright flashlight behind the swelling; does the light shine through?	
|	**NO**	**YES**
|	**Consider** EPIDIDYMITIS, FILARIASIS, MUMPS, ABSCESS, LYMPHOGRANULOMA VENEREUM, DONOVANOSIS, TUBERCULOSIS, rarely CANCER (mostly in men under 40 y.o.) In females, consider the conditions pictured in Volume 1, Chapter 6.	**Consider** HYDROCELE (males only)

Is the swelling in the groin only, with the genital area not swollen?

NO	YES
|	**Consider** enlarged groin lymph nodes (see Protocol A.52.B); also consider DONOVANOSIS, HERNIA,
|	ONCHOCERCIASIS,[1] TUBERCULOSIS, ABSCESS. Undescended testicle (empty scrotum on that side).

Is the patient a male with a swollen penis?

NO	YES
|	**Consider**: LYMPHOGRANULOMA VENEREUM, SICKLE CELL DISEASE,[4] DONOVANOSIS,
|	SCHISTOSOMIASIS HEMATOBIUM,[2] AFRICAN SLEEPING SICKNESS,[3] PARAPHIMOSIS, PHIMOSIS,
Go to table below.	CANCER.

1 *Onchocerciasis: scattered areas in Africa, the Middle East, Central America and northern South America.*

2 *Schistosomiasis hematobium: scattered areas of Africa and the Middle East only.*

3 *African sleeping sickness: scattered areas of Africa, south of Bamako, Mali and Lake Chad and north of Lusaka, Zambia.*

4 *Sickle cell disease: this affects those of African genetic origin, mainly in West Africa and the Americas. Some Indians and Arabs are also affected.*

BOTH GROIN AND GENITALS SWOLLEN

By far the most common; either not generally ill or else ACUTE ABDOMEN

HERNIA	Swelling is from the leg creases down into the scrotum or genital lips.

Conditions affecting only below the waist

LYMPHOGRANULOMA VENEREUM	Genital swelling which may be massive, usually with swollen groin lymph nodes.
DONOVANOSIS	Genital swelling which may be massive; groin swelling, if there is any, is not lymph nodes but has a cauliflower surface.
FILARIASIS	Both large nodes in groin and swollen genitals and/or leg(s); it Initially came and went.
CELLULITIS	Skin red and swollen, warm, maybe tender.

Whole-body illnesses, both above and below waist

ONCHOCERCIASIS[1]	Firm bulge or else lumps within "bags" of groin skin; body generally itchy.
BRUCELLOSIS	Gradual onset of back or joint pains, fevers and weakness, feeling awful.
AFRICAN SLEEPING SICKNESS[2]	Gradual onset of fevers, headaches and abnormal sleep-wake cycles.

1 *Onchocerciasis: scattered areas in Africa, the Middle East, Central America and northern South America.*
2 *African sleeping sickness: scattered areas of Africa, south of Bamako, Mali and Lake Chad and north of Lusaka, Zambia.*

Protocol A.52.B—Enlarged groin lymph nodes

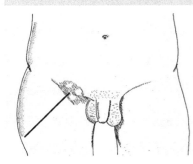

Definition: there are lumps on, right above or right below the crease line, where the upper thigh attaches to the trunk, just to the side of where one can feel the pulse in that area. Enlarged nodes the size of cherries or smaller are normal in anyone who walks barefoot.

First consider SEXUALLY TRANSMITTED DISEASE. If this is not reasonable, then follow the protocol below.

Did the patient have lower limb or genital sore(s) right before the large lymph nodes developed?

NO	YES
	Sores without a whole-body illness
	Injury;[1] history of an injury, scar or infection of legs/groin.
	ABSCESS: there is a warm, swollen area on the legs/feet/genitals.
	CELLULITIS: there is a warm, swollen area on the legs/feet.
	TROPICAL ULCER: crater-like wound on the legs/feet.
	YAWS:[2] some raised areas, some craters, both off-white.
	Sores with a whole-body illness with an elevated corrected temperature (fever)
	SCRUB TYPHUS:[3] fever, headache, muscle pains, small scab.
	SPOTTED FEVER:[4] fever, headache, muscle pains, rash.
	TULAREMIA:[5] fever, chills, headache, muscle pains.
	PLAGUE: blackened skin over tender lymph nodes; maybe scab(s).
	IRIS: patient being treated for both HIV and [TB or LEPROSY]
	RAT BITE FEVER: inflamed wound or a history of a recent bite.

Is the patient a reproductive adult female?

NO	YES
	Question her as to whether she or her partner may have been exposed to an STD. If yes or evasive, then treat her for whatever SEXUALLY TRANSMITTED DISEASE she is likely to have; see Protocol B.1. Many such diseases have no or minor symptoms in females for an extended time. If an STD is unlikely, follow the "No" arm for this question. Consider also HIV INFECTION, seroconversion illness.

Continued on next page, footnotes on the next page.

TOC

SYMPTOMS

DIFFERENTIALS

CONDITIONS

DRUG INDEX

REGIONAL NOTES

INX

TOC

SYMPTOMS

DIFFERENTIALS

CONDITIONS

DRUG INDEX

REGIONAL NOTES

INX

Does the patient have a skin condition affecting below his waist[6]?

NO   **YES**

| **Consider**: LEPROSY reaction,[7] ONCHOCERCIASIS,[8] HIV INFECTION, maybe SPOTTED FEVER,[9]
| MONKEYPOX,[10] FILARIASIS, SYPHILIS.

Does the patient have a very large spleen?

NO   **YES**

| **Consider**: VISCERAL LEISHMANIASIS,[11] AFRICAN SLEEPING SICKNESS,[12] BARTONELLOSIS,[13] SYPHILIS
See table below.   (congenital in an infant), rarely CANCER.

---

1 If the patient walks or works barefoot, it is inevitable that he will have minor injuries which will swell nodes.
2 Yaws: only the humid tropics.
3 Scrub typhus: asia and the Pacific; always fever, eye symptoms, headache, constipation.
4 Spotted fever: worldwide but not in the islands of Southeast Asia.
5 Tularemia: temperate North America, central Asia, Europe, Far East, the north coast of Africa; exposure to small animals.
6 The skin condition may also be above the waist; if it is below at all the answer is, "yes".
7 A leprosy reaction is a sudden change in leprosy, usually in response to drug treatment. It is not an ALLERGY to the medication being used to treat the disease.
8 Onchocerciasis: scattered areas in Africa, the Middle East, Central America and northern South America.
9 Spotted fever: not in the islands of Southeast Asia.
10 Monkeypox: in northern D R Congo and adjacent Central African Republic; rarely in western Africa.
11 Visceral Leishmaniasis: found in scattered areas of Central and South America, Africa north of the equator, the Mediterranean area, the Indian subcontinent, southern Europe, central Asia and mainland China.
12 African sleeping sickness: scattered areas of Africa, south of Bamako, Mali and Lake Chad and north of Lusaka, Zambia.
13 Bartonellosis: scattered areas within Peru and adjacent countries.

LARGE LYMPH NODES, NOT A REPRODUCTIVE FEMALE, NO SORE OR SKIN CONDITION, SPLEEN NOT LARGE

Probable onset within a week

CHANCROID	Groin nodes are tender to touch; genital sore may not be present.
HIV INFECTION seroconversion illness	Flu-type illness, maybe with a measles rash, under 4 weeks post-exposure.
SCRUB TYPHUS[1]	Fevers, very ill, rural areas, bitten by a mite.
PLAGUE	Exquisitely tender, swollen lymph nodes; high fevers; very ill.

Recurrent episodes or slow onset

FILARIASIS	Episodes of pain and swelling of legs/feet/genitals.
HIV INFECTION	Fevers, weight loss, diarrhea, cough; any one or more of these.
SEXUALLY TRANSMITTED DISEASES	Sexually active adult or sexually abused child; See Protocol B.1.
SCURVY	Bleeding gums, easy bruising, eats no fresh fruit or vegetables.
CANCER	A lump or abnormal function; probably loss of appetite, weight loss.
AFRICAN SLEEPING SICKNESS[2]	Erratic fevers, abnormal sleep pattern, maybe uncoordinated.

---

1 Scrub typhus: Asia and the Pacific area; always fever, eye symptoms, headache, constipation.
2 African sleeping sickness: scattered areas of Africa, south of Bamako, Mali and Lake Chad; north of Lusaka, Zambia.

Protocol A.52.C—Other abnormal appearance of pelvis and rectum

Pink, moist bulge hanging out of rectum: RECTAL PROLAPSE.

Pink, moist bulge hanging out of vagina: UTERINE PROLAPSE, Volume 1, Chapter 6.

Cannot tell sex of a newborn: send to a major medical center; **do not guess**.

No testicle in scrotum. Usually with bulge(s) in groin area(s): check again after warming the genital area. If still not there, send out when convenient.

Painless ulcers, cracks or bumps in genital or groin areas: DONOVANOSIS, SYPHILIS, REITER SYNDROME, congenital SYPHILIS, other SEXUALLY TRANSMITTED DISEASES.

Painful ulcers, blisters, cracks or bumps in genital or groin area: AMEBIC SKIN ULCER, CHANCROID, HERPES, FISSURE, FISTULA, MONKEYPOX,[1] SEXUALLY TRANSMITTED DISEASE.

Extra holes in genital area with discharge: FISTULA, GONORRHEA (males), LYMPHOGRANULOMA VENEREUM, DONOVANOSIS, AMEBIC SKIN ULCER, TUBERCULOSIS if the scrotum is swollen.

Large groin lymph nodes that hang down in loose bags of skin: ONCHOCERCIASIS.[2]

Swollen scrotum: see Protocol A.52.A.

Foreskin stuck on end of penis: PHIMOSIS.

Foreskin stuck behind end of penis: PARAPHIMOSIS.

Visible worms: ASCARIASIS (earthworm-size), ENTEROBIASIS (short/skinny), MYIASIS (short/fat), STRONGYLOIDIASIS (under the skin, near rectum), TRICHURIASIS (long, coiled), TAPEWORM (flat, rectangular segments), MYIASIS (under the skin of buttocks).

Scars in groin area: an old injury, prior hernia surgery, maybe SEXUALLY TRANSMITTED DISEASE.

Erection that will not go away: SICKLE CELL DISEASE,[3] RABIES, BRAIN DAMAGE, any spinal cord injury. This is an emergency. It must be dealt with quickly, or it will cause impotence.

Black, discolored dead genital skin: TYPHUS, SPOTTED FEVER,[4] other causes of GANGRENE.

Abnormal genital bumps: MOLLUSCUM CONTAGIOSUM, WARTS, LYMPHOGRANULOMA VENEREUM, DONOVANOSIS, SYPHILIS, FILARIASIS, BARTHOLIN CYST, sebaceous cyst. See Volume 1 Chapter 6.

Tiny pink pearly bumps around the ridge at the base of the pink, moist part of the penis: normal variation in those with dark skin color; without symptoms and without consequences.

---

1 *Monkeypox: northern D.R. Congo and adjacent border area in Central African Republic; rarely West Africa.*

2 *Onchocerciasis: scattered areas in Africa, the Middle East, Central America and northern South America.*

3 *Sickle cell disease: this affects those of African genetic origin, mainly in West Africa and the Americas. Some Indians and Arabs are also affected.*

4 *Spotted fever: worldwide in tropical and temperate climates, also the Arctic, but not in the islands of Southeast Asia.*

TOC
SYMPTOMS
DIFFERENTIALS
CONDITIONS
DRUG INDEX
REGIONAL NOTES
INX

TOC

SYMPTOMS

DIFFERENTIALS

CONDITIONS

DRUG INDEX

REGIONAL NOTES

INX

PROTOCOL A.53—ABNORMAL VAGINAL BLEEDING

A.53.A—Probably not pregnant

A.53.B—First three months of pregnancy

A.53.C—Second three months of pregnancy

A.53.D—Last three months of pregnancy

First check patient's vital signs, check her for SHOCK and treat if necessary.

Protocol A.53.A—Probably not pregnant (as far as the patient can tell)

Definition: vaginal bleeding with no prior missed periods, no sexual activity or used reliable birth control. (Condoms are not reliable birth control.)

If this is part of a general bleeding problem: easy bruising, bloody nose, vomiting blood, bloody stool, etc., see Protocol A.13.E and Protocol B.2 and B.7 additionally.

Is bleeding a heavy menstruation in someone who usually menstruates?

NO	YES
	Try to wait it out, checking frequently for SHOCK and ANEMIA. If either occurs, send her out. You may try BIRTH CONTROL PILLS.
	Consider: THALLASEMIA, SCURVY, TYPHUS, HEMORRHAGIC FEVER, PELVIC INFECTION due to TUBERCULOSIS.

Consider alternatives

- **If the patient just had a baby,** see Chapter 7 of Volume 1.

- **Irregular periods**: ignore for the time being unless they are very heavy and the patient is developing ANEMIA. Consider ENDOMETRIOSIS. Treat ANEMIA if it develops. Have the patient seen by a physician when it is convenient. Otherwise try a few months of BIRTH CONTROL PILLS.

- **Very heavy menses during early menopause, after a miscarriage, or in a girl who is just starting to menstruate**: have her take BIRTH CONTROL PILLS for a few months.

- **Vaginal bleeding in a woman past menopause**: possibly CANCER; needs to be sent out to a medical facility within a few weeks.

- **Bleeding (slight) after intercourse**: usually no problem, but send the patient and her husband to a physician to be checked for SEXUALLY TRANSMITTED DISEASE and CANCER. Use a speculum to distinguish between bleeding in the woman and bloody semen in her husband. Blood in semen is potentially quite serious.

- **Some light bleeding in the middle of the month at the time of ovulation** is common and normal.

- **Vaginal bleeding in a young girl who played in water** is usually caused by sexual assault (bruising and bleach-like smell of semen) or a leech. The leech will exit the vagina if you squirt in clean, strong salt water.

Protocol A.53.B—First three months of pregnancy

(See also Chapter 6 of Volume 1.)

Definition: vaginal bleeding after one or two missed periods in a woman who is sexually active; the upper rim of the uterus is less than half-way between the pubic bone and the navel.

If this is part of a general bleeding problem: easy bruising, bloody nose, vomiting blood, bloody stool, etc., see Protocol A.13.E and Protocol B.2 and B.7 additionally. Consider algid MALARIA, HEMORRHAGIC FEVER or EBOLA VIRUS DISEASE if there is a fever.

If there is a fever or the patient is very ill, see SEPSIS. If the patient is having pain or had pain, consider TUBAL PREGNANCY. Otherwise:

Is bleeding as much as a regular period?

NO, not as much	YES, as much or more.
	Send the patient out or call for advice. Treat SHOCK if it occurs.
Threatened miscarriage: bed rest, no tampons, no intercourse until bleeding stops. If it becomes as much as a regular period, send her out.	

Protocol A.53.C—Second three months of pregnancy

(See also Chapter 6 of Volume 1.)

If this is part of a general bleeding problem: easy bruising, bloody nose, vomiting blood, bloody stool, etc., see Protocol A.13.E and Protocol B.7 additionally. Consider HEMORRHAGIC FEVER.

If bleeding is more than slight, it probably means a spontaneous ABORTION (miscarriage) which may be due to any one of a large number of diseases and/or drugs. Wait it out as these miscarriages usually complete themselves. If there is heavy bleeding (enough to soak 3 pads or more), then send the patient to a hospital right away. If it goes on for more than a day or two, if the patient develops a fever, or she is very sick, see SEPSIS, HEMORRHAGIC FEVER (and related diseases).

Habitual mid or late pregnancy miscarriages are frequently due to SYPHILIS.

Protocol A.53.D—Last three months of pregnancy

(See also Chapter 6 of Volume 1.)

⚠ EMERGENCY CONDITION

Bleeding during the last 3 months of pregnancy, enough to soak more than 1 pad or 2 regular tampons.

If this is part of a general bleeding problem: easy bruising, bloody nose, vomiting blood, bloody stool, etc., see Protocol A.13.E and Protocol B.2 and B.7 additionally.

The patient may be in labor. If so, bleeding enough to soak one pad is normal. If the patient is not (or should not be) in labor or the bleeding is heavier, send her out immediately. If you do not, she and the baby both are likely to die.

PROTOCOL A.54—ABNORMAL VAGINAL DISCHARGE

Definition: the patient has an unusually large amount of watery or creamy liquid flowing out from her vagina, either with or without an odor, either blood-tinged or not, maybe with pain, itching or both.

In the following, "sore" means a visible break in the skin or vaginal surface with raw flesh, something like a skin ulcer, laceration or wound; pain and tenderness vary.

First see SEXUALLY TRANSMITTED DISEASES: Protocol B.1; it is best to treat according to that protocol unless there is some reason not to do so.

If the vaginal discharge looks and smells like stool or urine, the problem is FISTULA; this may be due to childbirth, injury or a SEXUALLY TRANSMITTED DISEASE.

Also see Chapter 7 of Volume 1.

A-152
CHAPTER PAGE

Village Medical Manual 7th Edition Volume 2 | **Protocol A.54 continued. Protocol A.55**

ABNORMAL VAGINAL DISCHARGE

Condition	Sore	Odor	Probable CC[1]	Other Characteristics
Likely painful; corrected temperature over 38.5°/101.3° or abnormally low temperature				
SEPSIS	Maybe	Maybe	Illness	Very ill, severe pain.
Infection after childbirth	Usual	Foul (usually)	Illness	Recent childbirth with tearing; see SEPSIS.
Likely painful, maybe fever				
PELVIC INFECTION	No	Unlikely	Pain	Pus present, usually abdominal pain also.
CHANCROID	Maybe	Maybe foul	Pain	Sore, if there is one, is tender; large nodes.
Likely neither painful nor itching, no fever				
VAGINITIS, bacterial	No	Fishy	Odor	No itching, moderate discharge; bad odor.
Tampon, forgotten	No	Foul, rotten	Odor	Remove tampon, rinse vagina.
MYIASIS[2]	Maybe	Maybe, foul	Varies	Maggots visible (short, fat "worms").
DONOVANOSIS	Yes	Maybe foul	Wound odor	Sore relatively painless; ragged edges.
Likely itching, no fever				
VAGINITIS, trichomonas	No	Little	Discharge Itching	Moderate itching; foamy, yellow-green.
VAGINITIS, candida	No	Little	Itching	Usually much itching; white thick discharge.
ENTEROBIASIS	No	None	Itching	Little worms visible at night.

1 *Chief complaint.*

2 *This only occurs if the patient sometimes lies naked and uncovered in a place where flies can access her genital area. This is generally amongst the poor, disabled and socially disadvantaged.*

PROTOCOL A.55—CONSTIPATION

Definition: the patient has bowel movements much less frequently than his usual pattern, and when he does move his bowels it is difficult to pass the stool. The stool is dry, and it comes out in small pieces. What constitutes constipation varies greatly between cultures and between individuals within a culture. Failure to pass stool after an episode of diarrhea (or severe vomiting) is not constipation; the bowel must fill up from the top before any comes out the bottom.

Note: DEHYDRATION is the most common cause of constipation. Any rectal pain will cause constipation because the patient will try to avoid pain by holding his stool; see Protocol A.50.B if this appears to be so. The most common pain-mediated causes of constipation are HEMORRHOIDS, genital HERPES and FISSUREs. Rectal pain is a common chief complaint in homosexual males.

⚠ EMERGENCY	▷ SYMPTOMATIC TREATMENT
CONSTIPATION EMERGENCY Constipation accompanied by abdominal pains: see ACUTE ABDOMEN, type 3. Also check ACUTE ABDOMEN type 2.	Do not do this if there is a fever or signs of ACUTE ABDOMEN. If there is neither of these and if the bowel sounds are not very active, then you may give the patient prunes. Ex-lax or any culturally equivalent medication obtained from a pharmacy. In tropical areas papaya seeds work well. Enemas may also work.

TOC

SYMPTOMS

DIFFERENTIALS

CONDITIONS

DRUG INDEX

REGIONAL NOTES

INX

Does the patient have definite signs of ACUTE ABDOMEN (see Protocol A.39.C)?

NO or not sure	YES, definitely
|	Send out immediately, treating meanwhile.

Does the patient have alternating diarrhea and constipation?

NO	YES
|	**Consider** IRRITABLE BOWEL, DYSENTERY, IMPACTION, PELLAGRA, SPRUE.[3]

Is the patient taking strong pain medications?

NO	YES
|	Usual side effect; use any laxative to relieve it once you know the patient does not have ACUTE
|	ABDOMEN.

Does the patient have a dry mouth?

NO	YES
|	Drugs that cause a dry mouth also cause constipation. DEHYDRATION also causes both dry
|	mouth and constipation.

Does the patient have a corrected temperature more than 38.5°/101.3°?

No	Yes
|	**Likely recent onset over less than a week.**
|	ENTERIC FEVER, POLIO, /// DENGUE FEVER,[1] TYPHUS, SCRUB TYPHUS,[2] LEPTOSPIROSIS,
|	**Likely remote onset, slow onset or recurrent**
|	BRUCELLOSIS, FAMILIAL MEDITERRANEAN FEVER.[5] See Protocol B.9.

Does the patient have numbness, tingling, weakness or paralysis of his lower limbs or pelvic area?

NO	YES
|	**Consider**: PELLAGRA,[4] SPINAL NEUROPATHY, SYPHILIS, TROPICAL SPASTIC PARAPARESIS, STROKE,
Table below.	ARBOVIRAL FEVER, BRAIN DAMAGE.

1 *Dengue fever: in the Americas only near or north of the equator. In Africa, east coastal, south and west. Prevalent in India, Southeast Asia and the Pacific. Occasionally found in the Mediterranean area. The disease may spread.*

2 *Scrub typhus: Asia and the Pacific. There are always eye symptoms, headache and gradually rising fever.*

3 *Sprue: in the Americas only near or north of the equator. In Africa only Nigeria and southern Africa. Prevalent in India and Southeast Asia. It is occasionally found in the Mediterranean area.*

4 *Pellagra usually causes diarrhea but may on occasion cause constipation.*

5 *Familial Mediterranean fever: this affects persons of Mediterranean genetic heritage such as Jews, Arabs, Turks and Armenians.*

CONSTIPATION, NO FEVER, NO DIARRHEA, NO PAIN MEDS, NO DRY MOUTH, NO LIMB PROBLEM

	May occur in children or adults
ASCARIASIS	Crampy pains also, especially in children; clay soils with poor sanitation.
MALNUTRITION	If adequate food doesn't go down, stool won't come out the bottom.
INTESTINAL FLUKE[1]	Comes from eating raw water plants, e.g. lotus and watercress.
DYSENTERY (amebic)	Crampy pains in lower left abdomen; constipation first, diarrhea will come later.

Footnotes at the end of the table.

Unlikely in children, no localized genital/rectal symptoms

OLD AGE	Most common cause of constipation; use a high-fiber diet.
ENDOMETRIOSIS	Females: constipation along with pain monthly with menstruation.
DIABETES	Definite diagnosis or else excessive thirst and urination.
DEPRESSION	Possibly appetite change; sleep disturbance.

Unlikely in children, local, genital/rectal symptoms

HEMORRHOIDS	Pain with moving bowels, sometimes blood on stool.
HERPES (genital)	Also back pain, history of painful genital blisters.
FISSURE	Extreme rectal pain; small split in skin by the anal opening.
IMPACTION	Commonly with old and disabled persons Frequently DEHYDRATION.

Slow-onset, whole-body illness, almost always adults

HYDATID DISEASE	Tropical/arid areas with dogs or temperate, forested areas.
THYROID TROUBLE	Low-thyroid; always tired, weight gain, slow pulse, brittle hair.
CHAGA'S DISEASE[2]	Also trouble swallowing, maybe HEART FAILURE.
CANCER	Progressive constipation, maybe lumpy liver or weight loss.

Slow-onset illness, maybe fever off and on, may occur in children

INTESTINAL FLUKE[1]	History of eating raw or rare fish or using teeth to peel water plants.
TUBERCULOSIS	Abdominal TB, in children free fluid in the abdomen; in adults abdomen like sponge rubber.
BRUCELLOSIS	Joint pains; sharp, shooting pains; or both; severe fatigue, slow onset.
LEAD POISONING	Also ANEMIA, crampy pains, maybe a metallic taste in the mouth, blue lines on the gums.

1 The kind of intestinal fluke that can cause constipation early in the course of the disease occurs throughout Asia.
2 Chaga's disease: present in scattered areas of the Americas.

PROTOCOL A.56—DIARRHEA

A.56.A—Diarrhea, sudden, recent onset   A.56.C—Persistent diarrhea   A.56.E—Grossly bloody diarrhea
A.56.B—Recurrent diarrhea   A.56.D—Chronic diarrhea

Definition: diarrhea is an increased frequency and volume of stool relative to the patient's usual habits.

Terminology

Kind:
- Watery diarrhea—is 90% or more liquid.
- Mushy diarrhea—is the consistency of runny mashed potatoes.
- Mucous diarrhea contains white, stringy material; it may be mushy or watery.

Amount: (assuming patient is an adult).
- Small—less than a cup at a time.
- Moderate—more than a cup, but less than a liter, at a time.
- Large or huge—a liter at a time or more.

Smell:
- Usual—ordinary stool odor.
- Foul—indicates a particularly offensive and strong odor.

TOC SYMPTOMS DIFFERENTIALS CONDITIONS DRUG INDEX REGIONAL NOTES INX

▷ SYMPTOMATIC TREATMENT	Diarrhea in travelers and returning travelers
Check for DEHYDRATION first and treat for that. If the patient is not vomiting, and does not have DIABETES give him ORS to drink. If he is vomiting, consider rectal fluids if the diarrhea is not so bad. If the patient is having both severe vomiting and severe diarrhea, he is very dehydrated and you cannot send him to a hospital, consider intraperitoneal fluids. See Volume 1, Appendix 1.16. Diarrhea that follows antibiotic usage is best treated with yogurt, brewer's yeast or giving an enema of normal stool dissolved in water. In any case, stop the antibiotic if at all feasible. Yogurt or powdered yogurt culture may be used to treat any kind of diarrhea.	First just put up with the diarrhea for a few days. This will help you develop some immunity and will make subsequent problems less likely. During this time it is good to consume ORS: oral rehydration solution. If ORS does not work, consider a bacterial cause. Amongst bacteria, campylobacter which reportedly responds to DOXYCYCLINE is most likely. Most of the other common bacteria respond to CIPROFLOXACIN except in Asia. Following bacteria, consider various worms. Give a general deworming treatment with MEBENDAZOLE or ALBENDAZOLE. In the SEA/Pacific area, consider CYCLOSPORIASIS. In the Mediterranean/Middle East area and the Indian subcontinent, consider CRYPTOSPORIDIUM.

Protocol A.56.A—Diarrhea, sudden, recent onset, not grossly bloody

Is the patient's mouth very dry, his skin very loose and his eyes sunken?

NO	YES
|	See DEHYDRATION, Volume 1, Appendix 1.16. Rehydrate and arrange transport while you follow the "No" arm.

Is the diarrhea small amounts in a patient who is disabled and otherwise constipated?

NO	YES
|	**Consider** IMPACTION.

Is the diarrhea of recent onset[1] with a history of normal bowel movements for the last 2 months?

YES, recent onset	NO, this has been happening for a while
| | | | |	**Go to one of these protocols:** A.56.B—Recurrent Diarrhea.[2] A.56.C—Persistent Diarrhea.[3] A.56.D—Chronic Diarrhea.[4] See MALABSORPTION.[5]

Is there a very foul odor to the diarrhea?

NO	YES
|	**Consider**: GIARDIASIS,[6] also see Bloody Diarrhea, Protocol A.57.A.

Did the patient eat anything unusual or tainted?

NO	YES
| | |	**Consider**: PLANT POISONING: foods or ethnic remedies of plant origin FOOD POISONING: foods containing animal products.

Does the patient have a corrected temperature of 38.5°/101.3° or more[1]?[3]

NO	YES
| |	**Consider:** MALARIA, MEASLES, ENTERIC FEVER, KATAYAMA DISEASE, SCRUB TYPHUS,[12] VISCERAL LEISHMANIASIS.[7] In children almost any disease with a fever will cause diarrhea, even EAR INFECTION.

Continued on the next page; footnotes at the end of the flow diagram.

SYMPTOMS · DIFFERENTIALS · CONDITIONS · DRUG INDEX · REGIONAL NOTES · INX · TOC

Is the diarrhea watery—it fills a container to the edges with a flat or almost flat surface?

NO, it is mushy	**YES, it is watery**
	For a patient under 2 years old, consider ROTAVIRUS.
	Otherwise consider CHOLERA, GIARDIASIS, CYCLOSPORIASIS or CRYPTOSPORIDIOSIS.
	Try the following treatments, in this order, giving 2 days for each to take effect before moving on:
	1. Give ORS.
	2. Eliminate milk and milk products from the diet.
	3. Treat with DOXYCYCLINE.
	4. Treat with CO-TRIMOXAZOLE.

Is there blood in the stool? Test the stool by shaking it with water and using urine dipsticks.

Stool probably negative for blood	**Stool probably positive for blood**
MALARIA	HOOKWORM
INFLUENZA	SCHISTOSOMIASIS MANSONI[9]
TRICHURIASIS	SCHISTOSOMIASIS JAPONICUM[10]
THALLASEMIA	INTESTINAL FLUKE[11]
ZINC DEFICIENCY	STRONGYLOIDIASIS
LIVER FLUKE[8]	ARSENIC POISONING
DEPRESSION	**Also see Bloody Stool, Protocol A.57.A.**

---

1 *Note that the yes and no arms of this question are reversed. This is not an error!*

2 *Recurrent diarrhea: sudden onset, lasted more than 14 days, more than 2 consecutive days without diarrhea.*

3 *Persistent diarrhea: sudden onset, lasted more than 14 days, less than 2 consecutive days without diarrhea.*

4 *Chronic diarrhea: gradual onset, lasted more than a month.*

5 *Whatever is eaten comes out the bottom quickly.*

6 *In Nepal and Latin America also consider CYCLOSPORIASIS which is indistinguishable but treated differently.*

7 *Visceral Leishmaniasis: found in scattered areas of Central and South America, Africa north of the equator, the Mediterranean area, the Indian subcontinent, eastern Europe, central Asia and mainland China. Not present south of the equator.*

8 *This kind of liver fluke (fascioliasis) is not present in Southeast Asia, eastern Asia or the Pacific.*

9 *Schistosomiasis Mansoni: scattered areas within Africa, the Arabian peninsula, the Caribbean and parts of eastern South America.*

10 *Schistosomiasis Japonicum: in areas of mainland China, the Philippines, parts of the Celebes, the upper Mekong and the Thai-Malaysia border area.*

11 *Intestinal fluke: not present in sub-Saharan Africa or the Pacific. In the Americas it occurs only in Guyana.*

12 *Scrub typhus occurs in northern Australia and throughout the Eastern Hemisphere north of there and east of Afghanistan, as far north as Mongolia*

13 *If the patient is very ill, malnourished, elderly, or an infant, his temperature may be abnormally low rather than abnormally high. In any case, his temperature will not be within normal limits.*

Protocol A.56.B—Recurrent diarrhea

Definition: this is sudden onset, lasted more than 14 days, some diarrhea-free intervals lasting more than 2 days, either watery or mushy, either bloody or not bloody.

Treatment To be treated the same as Protocol A.56.A1, looking for changes in lifestyle that might decrease the numbers of episodes. In particular, look at the availability of clean water, sanitation in food preparation and hand-washing after bathroom duties and before eating. If food sanitation is good, have the patient drink only water that he, or she personally boiled for 30 minutes. Don't trust bottled water; don't trust your maid to boil your water.

Protocol A.56.C—Persistent diarrhea

Definition: this is sudden onset, lasted more than 14 days, less than 2 consecutive days without diarrhea, either watery or mushy, either bloody or not-bloody.

- Frequently associated with another underlying bacterial infection: PNEUMONIA, EAR INFECTION and URINARY INFECTION being the most common. Children with CANDIDIASIS in their mouths, those with MALNUTRITION and those with PNEUMONIA are the most likely to die. It is important to examine children with persistent diarrhea for these other conditions and to treat for them. Treatment for the other conditions may also take care of the diarrhea.
- Tends to occur in malnourished children and increases malnutrition because of wastage of food substances in the stool as well as loss of appetite.
- It is common in children less than 6 months old who are not exclusively breast-fed and who consume water or cow's milk during an episode of acute diarrhea.
- Persistent diarrhea in returning travelers from Nepal or the environs in (Northern Hemisphere) spring or summer is probably due to CYCLOSPORIASIS.
- If there is a group of cases that all start within a few days, consider TRICHINOSIS if there is a history of eating game meat that was insufficiently cooked.

Treatment: try the following treatments in order, leaving 2 days between each to see if it works. If there is one treatment that works in several cases in your area, then elevate that treatment to the #1 position. In any case, provide clean drinking water, preferably as ORS, and nutritious food throughout the episode.

1. Give a general deworming treatment with MEBENDAZOLE, LEVAMISOLE or both in succession.

2. Give METRONIDAZOLE for 5 days to eliminate GIARDIASIS and amebic DYSENTERY.

3. Try at least two different antibiotics in succession: DOXYCYCLINE, CO-TRIMOXAZOLE, CIPROFLOXACIN, AMOXICILLIN, CHLORAMPHENICOL are possibilities.

4. NITAZOXANIDE is a drug that works for some parasites associated with HIV INFECTION.

Protocol A.56.D—Chronic diarrhea

This is diarrhea of gradual onset that has lasted more than 30 days which may or may not be bloody.

This is most often due to coeliac disease, inflammatory bowel disease, hereditary problems, SPRUE,[1] all of which require high-tech diagnosis and/or treatment. Thus these patients must be sent out or they will die. Meanwhile treat DEHYDRATION and provide MULTIVITAMINS, preferably injectable.

---

1 Sprue: in the Americas only near or north of the equator. In Africa only Nigeria and southern Africa. Prevalent in India and Southeast Asia. It is occasionally found in the Mediterranean area.

TOC

SYMPTOMS

DIFFERENTIALS

CONDITIONS

DRUG INDEX

REGIONAL NOTES

INX

Protocol A.56.E. Grossly bloody diarrhea

Definition: the patient passes either bright red blood on or mixed into his stool, or he passes coal-black stool that is mushy and extremely foul-smelling. This is digested blood. He may be vomiting also. If the stool is black but not particularly foul, it is probably due to the patient's consuming iron tablets or black licorice.

Is the patient's skin cool and moist and his pulse rapid, or is he very lethargic or unconscious?

NO	YES
|	Arrange transport immediately. Meanwhile treat SHOCK.
|	

Has the patient recently had symptoms of PEPTIC ULCER and the diarrhea is large amounts?

NO	YES
|	He is bleeding internally. Arrange transport. Treat him meanwhile.
|	

Does he have abdominal pain that is severe enough to prevent his sleeping?

NO	YES
|	**Consider**: ACUTE ABDOMEN, PIG-BEL,[9] DYSENTERY, AMEBIASIS. If none of these fit, then follow
|	the "No" arm.

Is there evidence of a general bleeding problem with bloody urine, heavy menstruation, bloody nose, minor cuts that won't stop bleeding?

NO	YES
|	**Consider**: conditions listed in Protocols A.13.E, B.2 and B.7. Also: THALLASEMIA, SCURVY, TYPHUS.
|	ARBOVIRAL FEVER,[1] HEMORRHAGIC FEVER (and related diseases), ONYALAI.[2]

Does the patient have a corrected temperature more than 38.5°/101.3°?

NO	YES
|	**Individuals or epidemics:** MEASLES, DYSENTERY, ENTERIC FEVER,
|	**Mainly epidemics:** TYPHUS, RELAPSING FEVER,[3] LASSA FEVER,[4] HEMORRHAGIC FEVER (early),
|	YELLOW FEVER.[5]

Was the patient in an area with SCHISTOSOMIASIS?

NO	YES
|	**Consider**: SCHISTOSOMIASIS MANSONI,[6] SCHISTOSOMIASIS JAPONICUM,[7] rarely
Go to table below.	SCHISTOSOMIASIS HEMATOBIUM.[8]

---

1 Arboviral fever can turn into HEMORRHAGIC FEVER; bloody diarrhea might be the first manifestation.

2 Onyalai: this is a hereditary tendency to bleed abnormally, found in southern Africa only.

3 Relapsing fever: tropical and high altitude, but not in the islands of SEA and the Pacific.

4 Lassa fever: found in scattered areas in Africa only, mostly West Africa.

5 Yellow fever: South America north of Sao Paolo, central and western Africa and the Sudan area.

6 Schistosomiasis Mansoni: scattered areas within Africa, the Arabian peninsula, the Caribbean and parts of eastern South America.

7 Schistosomiasis Japonicum: in areas of mainland China, the Philippines, parts of the Celebes, the upper Mekong and the Thai-Malaysian border.

8 Schistosomiasis hematobium: present in some areas of Africa and the Middle East.

9 Pig-bel is found in developing areas near the equator, mostly in New Guinea island.

TOC   SYMPTOMS   DIFFERENTIALS   CONDITIONS   DRUG INDEX   REGIONAL NOTES   INX

BLOODY DIARRHEA, NO BELLY PAINS, NO FEVER, NO SCHISTOSOMIASIS, NO GENERAL BLEEDING.

Commonly children, maybe adults

HOOKWORM	Sandy, moist, shaded areas where people walk barefoot.
DYSENTERY	Blood dark or bright red, with obvious white stringy mucus.
TUBERCULOSIS	Diarrhea off and on with blood and mucus; the blood is mixed with stool.
TRICHURIASIS	Similar to HOOKWORM, similar treatment; ANEMIA uncommon.
PIG-BEL[1]	Malnourished children who suddenly eat a heavy protein meal.

Mostly adults, rarely children

CANCER	Weight loss, probably over 40 years old.
PEPTIC ULCER	Previous history of upper abdominal pains relieved by food.

Adults, localized anal/rectal symptoms

PROCTITIS	Rectal pain, red blood on outside of the stool.

1 *Pig-bel: found in developing countries near the equator, mainly New Guinea.*

PROTOCOL A.57—ABNORMAL STOOL, NOT DIARRHEA

A.57.A—Bloody stool, not diarrhea   A.57.B—Other abnormal stool   A.57.C—Stool incontinence

Protocol A.57.A—Bloody stool, not diarrhea

Definition: either blood-red stool, black tarry stool, or it tests positive for blood.

First check for ACUTE ABDOMEN and for SHOCK. If either is present, immediate evacuation is your only option.

If the patient has neither of these, then proceed with the protocol below.

Did the patient recently consume rare meat or blood?

NO	**YES**
	Ignore the problem for now if not very ill; recheck after four days off rare meat.

Is there bleeding elsewhere: bloody urine, heavy menstruation, minor cuts, bloody nose?

NO	**YES**
	With a fever, recent onset: TYPHUS, YELLOW FEVER,[1] HEMORRHAGIC FEVER (and related diseases), ARBOVIRAL FEVER, EBOLA VIRUS DISEASE.
	No fever, recurrent or slow onset: THALLASEMIA, SCURVY, LIVER DISEASE, LIVER FAILURE, ONYALAI.[2] Also see Protocol B.2 and B.7 and Protocol A.13.E.

Does the patient have a corrected temperature more than 38.5°/101.3°?

NO	**YES**
	Consider: DYSENTERY, ENTERIC FEVER, TYPHUS, MEASLES /// RELAPSING FEVER,[3] LASSA FEVER,[4] ARBOVIRAL FEVER, YELLOW FEVER.[1]

Was the patient in an area with SCHISTOSOMIASIS (see the Regional Notes for your area)?

NO	**YES**
See table below on next page.	**Consider:** SCHISTOSOMIASIS MANSONI,[5] SCHISTOSOMIASIS JAPONICUM,[6] rarely SCHISTOSOMIASIS HEMATOBIUM.[7]

1 *Yellow fever: South America north of Sao Paolo, central and western Africa and the Sudan.*
2 *Onyalai: this is a hereditary tendency to bleed abnormally, found in southern Africa only.*
3 *Relapsing fever: tropical and high altitude, but not in the islands of SEA and the Pacific.*
4 *Lassa fever: found in scattered areas in Africa only.*
5 *Schistosomiasis Mansoni: scattered areas within Africa, the Arabian peninsula, the Caribbean and parts of eastern South America.*
6 *Schistosomiasis Japonicum: in areas of mainland China, the Philippines, parts of the Celebes, the upper Mekong and the Thai-Malaysian border.*
7 *Schistosomiasis hematobium: present in some areas of Africa and the Middle East.*

TOC
SYMPTOMS
DIFFERENTIALS
CONDITIONS
DRUG INDEX
REGIONAL NOTES
INX

BLOODY STOOL, NOT DIARRHEA OR DIETARY, NO HIGH FEVER, NO OTHER BLEEDING

Severe abdominal pain unlikely, at least initially

HOOKWORM	Sandy, moist, shaded areas where people walk barefoot; ANEMIA is common.
TUBERCULOSIS	Diarrhea off and on with blood and mucus; blood mixed with stool.
CANCER	Weight loss, probably over 40 years old.
TRICHURIASIS	Similar to HOOKWORM, similar treatment; ANEMIA uncommon.

Significant abdominal pain likely

DYSENTERY	Blood dark or bright red, with obvious white, stringy mucus.
PIG-BEL[1]	Malnourished children who suddenly eat a heavy protein meal.

Rectal/anal pain likely

PROCTITIS	Rectal pain, red blood on outside of the stool.
HEMORRHOIDS	Blood is on outside of the stool or toilet paper; there may be pain.
FISSURE[2]	Exquisite rectal pain, minimal bright red blood.

1 *Pig-bel: found in developing countries near the equator, mainly New Guinea.*
2 *Fissure may be due to damage to the rectum caused by anal intercourse or by masturbation using sharp objects.*

Protocol A.57.B—Other abnormal stool

White or light stool: HEPATITIS, JAUNDICE from many causes, LIVER FAILURE, GALLBLADDER DISEASE.

Green stool: due to diet (can also be other colors); also common in newborns.

Wormy stool: ASCARIASIS, TRICHURIASIS, STRONGYLOIDIASIS, ENTEROBIASIS, MYIASIS, HOOKWORM, TAPEWORM (flat worm segments, like confetti).

Flat worm segments: TAPEWORM.

Black, sticky stool: see bloody stool, Protocol A.57.A. Black, sticky stool with a foul odor is due to blood in the stool. Without a particularly foul odor, due to iron tablets or black licorice.

Protocol A.57.C—Stool incontinence

Incontinent of stool: diarrhea and OLD AGE are the most common causes. Otherwise consider SEIZURE, SEXUALLY TRANSMITTED DISEASE, STROKE, sometimes after hard childbirth or multiple childbirths, after injury to the neck or back, SYPHILIS (tertiary), SCHISTOSOMIASIS HEMATOBIUM,[1] PLANT POISONING due to lathyrism, TROPICAL SPASTIC PARAPARESIS, SPINAL NEUROPATHY, BRAIN DAMAGE, TYPHUS, CANCER. Disabled people are frequently constipated; liquid stool forms behind the constipated stool, flows around it and comes out. If this is the case, see IMPACTION. This may be due to damage to the rectum caused by anal intercourse or by masturbation with objects that tear the rectal muscles. It may also be caused by a fractured pelvis or RECTAL PROLAPSE; also see Protocol A.59.A.

1 *Schistosomiasis hematobium: found in scattered areas of Africa and the Middle East.*

PROTOCOL A.58—ABNORMAL URINE

A.58.A—Various urinary problems   A.58.B—Bloody urine with a fever   A.58.C—Bloody urine without a fever

Protocol A.58.A—Various urinary problems

Red urine: red urine is not necessarily bloody urine. A urine dipstick (Volume 1, Appendix 2) test for blood is the only way to distinguish blood from other red color. Ask the person if he/she ate red beets or took the drug RIFAMPIN recently. For some people, beets will color the urine. For everyone, RIFAMPIN will color urine orange. CLOFAZAMINE also colors the urine red. Consider vaginal origin of the blood if the dipstick test indicates the red is truly blood. Check the patient's vagina with a speculum or with your gloved fingers; See Volume 1 Chapter 6. If the urine is truly bloody and this is part of a general bleeding problem—nosebleeds and easy bruising—then see Protocols A.13.E, B.2 and B.7.

Full bladder but can't urinate: see Protocol A.59.

Too little urine:[1] DEHYDRATION, TOXEMIA, KIDNEY DISEASE, SHOCK, NECROTIZING FASCIITIS; HYPERTENSION, URETHRAL STRICTURE, CANCER, POLIO.

Too much urine:[2] MALARIA, drinking too much, DIABETES, some kinds of KIDNEY DISEASE, some CANCERs, SICKLE CELL DISEASE, effect of some drugs used to treat HEART FAILURE.

Frequent urination of small amounts: pregnancy, STRESS (bathroom is an escape), possibly KIDNEY INFECTION, TUBERCULOSIS, URINARY INFECTION, SCHISTOSOMIASIS HEMATOBIUM,[3] URETHRITIS, PROSTATITIS, CANCER.

Bed-wetting: usually due to STRESS; also consider ENTEROBIASIS, ATTENTION DEFICIT DISORDER.

Urine is milky or pink milky: FILARIASIS.

Urine is cloudy but not milky: may be normal or URINARY INFECTION, KIDNEY INFECTION.

Pain with urination: see Protocol A.50.C.

Foul-smelling urine: KIDNEY INFECTION, URINARY INFECTION, TYPHUS, sometimes due to drugs or food, possibly VAGINITIS or SEXUALLY TRANSMITTED DISEASE. If there is an abnormal hole between the rectum and the bladder, then stool will pass into the bladder, making the urine foul. The patient will also pass rectal gas out of his penis.

Dark urine but not black or coke colored: DEHYDRATION, HEPATITIS or other LIVER DISEASE, LIVER FAILURE, some medications such as METRONIDAZOLE and TINIDAZOLE.

Other colored urine: usually due to foods or drugs; ignore the problem. METHYLENE BLUE, a drug for MALARIA causes blue urine which burns when passed.

Bloody urine with just a few drops of blood at the end of urination: SEXUALLY TRANSMITTED DISEASE, URINARY INFECTION, SCHISTOSOMIASIS HEMATOBIUM, CANCER of the bladder or urethra, TUBERCULOSIS, BLADDER STONE.

Black or Coke-colored urine: this is likely due to bleeding in the kideys or the tubes connecting kidney with bladder. It may also be due to blackwater fever, a kind of severe MALARIA. The urine dipstick test will be strongly positive for blood. See A.58.B.

---

1 *For normal minimum urine outputs, see the chart under KIDNEY DISEASE.*
2 *Try to distinguish between frequent urination but normal total daily amount vs. frequent urination with increased daily total amount. The maximum daily urine volume for an adult is 3 liters. Local bladder irritation and reduced bladder capacity will make someone urinate more often, but the total amount is normal.*
3 *Schistosomiasis hematobium: present in some areas of Africa and the Middle East.*

Protocol A-58 B. Bloody urine with a fever

If this is part of a general bleeding problem—nosebleeds and easy bruising—then see Protocols A.13.E, B.2 and B.7

Is the urine various colors, some red, some pink, some normal-looking?

NO	YES
|	URINARY INFECTION: similar to KIDNEY INFECTION but the pain
|	is low central abdomen.

BROWNISH URINE, NOT RED, COLOR THE SAME THROUGHOUT, NO CLOTS; FEVER PRESENT:

KIDNEY INFECTION	Severe mid-back pain, one or both sides; burning with urination.
TUBERCULOSIS	Initially the bloody urine is off and on, not continual; maybe weight loss.
MALARIA (severe)	Mostly in patients of Mediterranean ethnic origin; Coke-colored urine; very ill.
TYPHUS	Mental state appears intoxicated; headache, general body pains occur before the fever.
HEMORRHAGIC FEVER	Headache, fever and general body pains first, before bloody urine.
RELAPSING FEVER[1]	Sudden onset of severe fever and chills with headache and general aching.
BARTONELLOSIS[2]	First fatigue, then fever, then general pains, especially chest and back.
YELLOW FEVER[3]	Headache, eye pain, general aching, nausea; patient unimmunized.
SEPSIS	Very sick, unconscious or almost so, usually some other infection or injury.

1 Relapsing fever: tropical and high altitude, but not in the islands of SEA and the Pacific.
2 Bartonellosis: scattered areas within Peru and adjacent countries.
3 Yellow fever: South America north of Sao Paolo, central and western Africa and the Sudan.

Protocol A.58.C—Bloody urine with no or low fever

Consider vaginal origin of the blood in a female if the dipstick test indicates the red is truly blood.

If the urine is truly bloody and this is part of a general bleeding problem, then see Protocols A.13.E, B.2 and B.7.

Bloody urine with a few drops of blood at the end of urination, not all mixed through is from the bladder or the urethra (the tube between the bladder and the genital area): SEXUALLY TRANSMITTED DISEASE, URINARY INFECTION, SCHISTOSOMIASIS HEMATOBIUM,[2] CANCER of the bladder or urethra, TUBERCULOSIS of the bladder, BLADDER STONE.

BLOODY URINE WITHOUT A FEVER OR WITH A LOW FEVER

Brownish urine color the same throughout, no clots

THALLASEMIA	Hereditary ANEMIA; large spleen; maybe a retarded facial appearance.
PLANT POISONING	Djenkol bean;[1] history of eating this bean; also mid-back pain.
KIDNEY DISEASE	Due to nephritis; There is a history of a recent infection; BP is high.

Either brownish or reddish urine

CANCER	Frequently painless initially with no other symptoms.
Injury	History of injury to the middle of the back or to the lower abdomen.
KIDNEY STONES	Sudden onset of severe pain flank(s) and/or groin(s), with nausea and vomiting.
URETHRITIS	Males with a history of pus or another abnormal discharge from the penis tip.
Poisonous snake bite	History of a recent snake bite; see Volume 1, Chapter 9.
SCURVY	Diet devoid of fresh fruits and vegetables; bleeding gums, loose teeth present.
SCHISTOSOMIASIS HEMATOBIUM[2]	From a culture where bloody urine is common in boys.
SCHISTOSOMIASIS MANSONI[3]	Either DYSENTERY, LIVER DISEASE or LIVER FAILURE.
ONYALAI[4]	History of bleeding episodes from other parts of the body.

1 Djenkol bean poisoning occurs in Malaysia and Indonesia.
2 Schistosomiasis hematobium: found in areas of Africa and the Middle East.
3 Schistosomiasis Mansoni: scattered areas within Africa, the Arabian Peninsula, the Caribbean and parts of eastern South America.
4 Onyalai: this is a hereditary tendency to bleed, found in southern Africa only.

PROTOCOL A.59—OTHER PELVIC AND RECTAL PROBLEMS

A.59.A—Bladder and bowel control problems   A.59.B—Sexual dysfunction   A.59.C—Other pelvic and rectal problems

Protocol A.59.A—Bladder and bowel control problems

Definition: the patient has trouble initiating urination or defecation, or he is incontinent—passing urine or stool involuntarily.

BLADDER AND BOWEL INCONTINENCE

Is the problem with ONLY bladder or bowel, or is the problem with both?

One   **Both bowel and bladder**

With mental issues: consider it may be due to this; the patient may be thumbing his nose at the rules of polite society. See Protocol A.6.A. Bizarre behavior.

During a seizure: due to the seizure; see Protocol A.7.A. Does not need to be treated separately.

With lower limb or pelvic numbness, tingling or weakness: the patient has a neurological problem; seek higher level care. Consider POLIO, TROPICAL SPASTIC PARAPARESIS, SPINAL NEUROPATHY., RABIES.

With no lower limb or pelvic numbness, tingling or weakness: the problem is probably a mechanical defect that is interrupting normal waste functions. Consider SCHISTOSOMIASIS (any kind), SEXUALLY TRANSMITTED DISEASEs, CANCER, some injury or childbirth. Consider homosexual activity. This can cause both bowel and bladder problems, but usually not both simultaneously.

The problem is probably some mechanical defect in the pelvis. It is more likely treatable than if bladder and bowel are both involved together, together with (and at the same time as) lower limb and pelvic symptoms. It is usually worth sending the patient out for higher level care. He may need surgery, but send him first to a non-surgeon.

ISOLATED BLADDER PROBLEM, NO BOWEL PROBLEM

Bladder full, cannot urinate or only dribbles: PROSTATITIS, URETHRAL STRICTURE, URINARY OBSTRUCTION, genital HERPES, SCHISTOSOMIASIS (any kind), SYPHILIS, POLIO, any other disease or injury that causes weakness or paralysis of the lower limbs (e.g. SLIPPED DISC), SPINAL NEUROPATHY.

Very small bladder capacity: pregnancy, BLADDER STONE, SCHISTOSOMIASIS HEMATOBIUM,[1] CANCER, previous pelvic radiation, lower abdominal TUBERCULOSIS, any lower abdominal tumor.

Incontinent of urine: SEIZURE, SEXUALLY TRANSMITTED DISEASE,[2] STROKE, URINARY INFECTION, KIDNEY INFECTION, sometimes FISTULA after hard childbirth or multiple childbirths, after injury to the neck or back, SYPHILIS (tertiary), SCHISTOSOMIASIS HEMATOBIUM,[1] PLANT POISONING due to lathyrism, TROPICAL SPASTIC PARAPARESIS, SPINAL NEUROPATHY, BRAIN DAMAGE, TYPHUS, DIPHTHERIA, RABIES, TETANUS. This may be due to overflow: the patient cannot release urine so his bladder fills up to capacity and then the great pressure causes leakage. If this has been present for a long time, a urinary catheter is the best solution.

---

1   *Schistosomiasis hematobium: found in scattered areas of Africa and the Middle East.*

2   *In this case the person is incontinent because there are abnormal holes in the genital areas out of which urine runs. Men may have a watering-can-type area between their legs. Females may have a hole or holes between bladder and vagina. In some cases these problems can be fixed surgically, and in other cases they cannot be fixed.*

ISOLATED STOOL INCONTINENCE, NO BLADDER PROBLEM

Does the patient have severe diarrhea with gas?

NO	YES
|	Most likely the incontinence is because of the diarrhea; address the diarrhea problem and then check again. AMEBIASIS in particular can cause urgency: the need to move bowels **right now**.

Have the patient spread his cheeks as you look at his anus. Do you see an abnormal slit or hole?

NO	YES
|	He has a FISTULA that needs surgery; refer him or tell him to live with it.

Is the patient someone who uses his anus sexually?

NO	YES
|	The problem is most likely due to injury or a sexually transmitted disease; it is beyond your capability to deal with it. Refer him, or tell him to live with it.

Does the patient give a history of pain in his rectal area with some bleeding or visible large veins?

NO	YES
|	**Consider** HEMORRHOIDS, FISTULA.

Does the patient give a history of difficult childbirth, back injury, genital injury or pelvic surgery?

NO	YES
|	**Consider** FISTULA.

Did this just happen when the patient had a SEIZURE?

NO	YES
|	Patients are commonly incontinent during a seizure; deal with the seizure.

Is the incontinence a small amount in a patient who is disabled?

NO	YES
|	Disabled people frequently have IMPACTIONs; liquid stool accumulates behind the impaction and is passed involuntarily. Deal with the IMPACTION.

Does the patient have weakness or a movement disorder in his legs and feet?

NO	YES
|	**Consider**: POLIO, SPINAL NEUROPATHY and its causative diseases; TROPICAL SPASTIC PARAPARESIS. PLANT POISONING due to botulism or lathyrism; DIPHTHERIA, RABIES, TETANUS.

Does the patient have a severe illness with a corrected temperature more than 38.5°/101.3°?

NO	YES
|	**Consider**: TYPHUS, POLIO, ARBOVIRAL FEVER, EBOLA VIRUS DISEASE (Africa).

Stool incontinence can occur with illnesses such as DIPHTHERIA, RABIES, TETANUS without fevers.

Protocol A.59.B—Sexual dysfunction

Impotence *may* be emotional[1] (see STRESS) or else due to OLD AGE, LIVER FAILURE, HOOKWORM, KIDNEY DISEASE, SYPHILIS, SPINAL NEUROPATHY, TROPICAL SPASTIC PARAPARESIS, DIABETES, LEPROSY, ZINC DEFICIENCY, AFRICAN SLEEPING SICKNESS,[2] PLANT POISONING (lathyrism[3]), (previous) MUMPS; could be a side effect of some drugs; and any paralysis could cause it. Regional and rare: HEMOCHROMATOSIS.[4]

Erection that will not go away: see Protocol A-52 C.

Small-sized testicles: LEPROSY, previous MUMPS, LASSA FEVER.[5]

No menstruation in a female: not old enough, pregnant, MALNUTRITION, MENOPAUSE, AFRICAN SLEEPING SICKNESS,[6] SCHISTOSOMIASIS HEMATOBIUM,[7] SCHISTOSOMIASIS MANSONI,[8] sometimes a hormone problem.

Infertility: see Volume 1 Chapter 6.

---

1 One can distinguish emotional from other causes with a simple test. For several consecutive nights, before retiring, place a row of connected small postage stamps snugly around the penis. Moisten the last one to secure the stamps. If there is a night-time erection, in the morning some of the stamps will be separated. This indicates physical ability to achieve an erection and therefore an emotional cause of impotence.
2 African sleeping sickness: scattered areas of Africa, south of Bamako, Mali and Lake Chad and north of Lusaka, Zambia.
3 Lathyrism poisoning occurs in the Indian area, in eastern Africa and in the Mediterranean area where "Khasari" is eaten.
4 Hemochromatosis; mainly confined to certain ethnic groups who take in excessive iron in the form of blood or beer brewed in iron.
5 Lassa fever: found in scattered areas in Africa only, mainly West Africa.
6 African sleeping sickness: scattered areas of Africa, south of Bamako, Mali and Lake Chad and north of Lusaka, Zambia.
7 Schistosomiasis hematobium: found in scattered areas of Africa and the Middle East
8 Schistosomiasis Mansoni: scattered areas within Africa, the Arabian peninsula, the Caribbean and parts of eastern South America.

Protocol A.59.C—Other pelvic and rectal problems

Pus from penis: URETHRITIS, GONORRHEA. See Protocol B.1.

Interrupted urine stream: PROSTATITIS, URETHRITIS, URETHRAL STRICTURE. If he needs to jump up and down to urinate, probably a BLADDER STONE. Send out if possible.

Bloody semen: SCHISTOSOMIASIS HEMATOBIUM, injury, TUBERCULOSIS, CANCER.

Groin scar; any SEXUALLY TRANSMITTED DISEASE; prior surgery.

Redness and itching: VAGINITIS, ENTEROBIASIS, STRONGYLOIDIASIS, SCABIES.

Worm-like creatures: ASCARIASIS, STRONGYLOIDIASIS, ENTEROBIASIS, MYIASIS, TRICHURIASIS, TAPEWORM.

A lump in the scrotum with watery pus dripping out: TUBERCULOSIS

Swelling in pelvic/genital area: see Protocol A.52.

Numbness and tingling in the saddle area between the legs: SPINAL NEUROPATHY

Large amounts of very foul gas: see Protocol A.49.

Foreskin stuck behind the pink part of penis: PARAPHIMOSIS.

Foreskin stuck onto the pink part of the penis: PHIMOSIS.

Passing gas or stool through the penis, vagina or female urinary tract: this indicates a FISTULA which is an abnormal hole between pelvic organs. It requires surgical treatment.

TOC

SYMPTOMS

DIFFERENTIALS

CONDITIONS

DRUG INDEX

REGIONAL NOTES

INX

X—LOWER LIMB PROBLEMS

PROTOCOL A.60—PAIN IN HIPS, LEGS AND FEET

A.60.A—Skin pain, lower limbs

A.60.B—Neuritis, legs and feet

A.60.C—Muscle-type pain, legs

A.60.D—Bone and joint pain

A.60.E—Other pain in lower limbs

⚠ EMERGENCY

LEG PAIN EMERGENCIES

If there is severe pain in (usually) one or (rarely) both legs along with at least two of the following paleness, weakness or paralysis, numbness and tingling, no pulses and the limb(s) feel(s) cold, that is an emergency which requires prompt surgical care or the patient will lose the limb and possibly his life also.

Fast onset and rapid progression of severe pain and tenderness, with a fever, not symmetrical: consider NECROTIZING FASCIITIS.

Protocol A.60.A—Skin pain, lower limbs

Definition: skin pain is any pain that is felt on the surface of the limb, not deep inside.

Also see Protocols A.14–A.18 on skin problems. Conditions which especially affect the legs and feet are listed.

Conditions	Skin	Characteristics
Likely the skin appears abnormal, and this is a recent occurrence		
TINEA	Rash	Cracks between toes with itching and burning, peeling skin.
CELLULITIS	Red or warm	Area red, warm, tender; large groin nodes.
TUNGIASIS[1]	Tiny wounds	Toe or finger tips have black or white spots where sand fleas burrowed in; area touched soil.
TROPICAL ULCER	Wound	Crater in skin of leg; pus or raw flesh in center; definite edges.
GUINEA WORM[2]	Blister	Very painful blister that breaks open.
Likely the skin appears abnormal; it is a long-standing or recurrent problem		
FILARIASIS	Red or warm	Swelling and warmth initially, big groin nodes.
PELLAGRA	Rash, sun-exposed skin	Burning in soles and with swallowing; poor diet, some swallowing or stomach distress.
YAWS	Soles cracked	Skin of soles of feet thick and cracked in adults who had skin sores as children; humid tropics only.
MOSSY FOOT	Thickened	Red clay soil areas, burning foot pain before swelling begins.
Skin likely appears normal		
MALNUTRITION	Normal	Severe pain in feet, unable to tolerate anything touching feet.
HIV INFECTION	Normal	Pain in the area normally covered by stockings.
TROPICAL SPASTIC PARAPARESIS	Normal	Also stiffness of the legs; maybe back pain, incontinence.
VISCERAL LEISHMANIASIS[3]	Normal	Burning foot pain, particularly in Sudan, Africa.
BERIBERI	Normal	Burning in soles; diet of white rice or another carbohydrate mainly or exclusively.

---

1 See Regional Notes for Africa (F), the Americas (M) and South Asia (I).

2 Guinea worm: scattered areas in Africa and the Middle East only.

3 Visceral Leishmaniasis: found in scattered areas of Central and South America, Africa north of the equator, the Mediterranean area, the Indian subcontinent, eastern Europe, central Asia and mainland China. Not present south of the equator.

TOC

SYMPTOMS

DIFFERENTIALS

CONDITIONS

DRUG INDEX

REGIONAL NOTES

INX

Protocol A.60.B—Neuritis, legs and feet

Definition: neuritis is nerve inflammation; it causes pain that is sharp and shooting, though occasionally it is burning or aching. The pain goes up and down the legs, maybe from the back; frequently there is numbness and tingling, muscle cramps or muscle weakness. The big toe side and the little toe side of the lower legs and feet are likely to be affected differently.

Initially examine the patient's lower back. Tap his spine and press next to the spine on both sides. Back problems may present with pain in the legs. If the pain is aggravated by pressure on or movement of the back, then it is probably a back problem, not a leg problem. Consult the appropriate protocol.

Is the patient very ill or disabled, or does he have a corrected temperature over 37.5°/99.5° or both?

NO to all	YES to any
	Rapid onset: DENGUE FEVER,[1] DYSENTERY (bacterial), ARBOVIRAL FEVER.
	Slow onset: BRUCELLOSIS, TUBERCULOSIS, SYPHILIS, tertiary.

Does the patient have severe back pain that shoots down the legs?

NO	YES
	Consider: BRUCELLOSIS, MUSCLE STRAIN, SCIATICA, SLIPPED DISC, TUBERCULOSIS, SPINAL NEUROPATHY, LEPROSY, rarely HYDATID DISEASE.[2]

Does the patient eat a very poor diet?

NO	YES
Table below.	**Consider**: MALNUTRITION, COBALAMIN DEFICIENCY, PELLAGRA, BERIBERI, PLANT POISONING due to cassava.

1 *Dengue fever: in the Americas only near or north of the equator. In Africa, east coastal, south and west. Prevalent in India, Southeast Asia and the Pacific. Occasionally found in the Mediterranean area. The disease may spread*

2 *Hydatid disease: there are two kinds: one is in cattle-raising areas of the tropics where there are dogs that live close to people. The other kind is in temperate, rural areas where there are wild animals and people eat gathered, wild plant life that might be contaminated with the stool of animals.*

NEURITIS, NO FEVER, NOT VERY ILL, NOT CAUSED BY BACK PAIN, DIET IS OKAY

May affect children as well as adults	
ISONIAZID (drug)	Side effect of this TB drug; treatable with vitamins.
DIABETES	Known DIABETES or glucose present in urine.
LOIASIS[1]	Swellings come for a few days and then go.
SYPHILIS (tertiary/congenital)	Lightning pains; patient, partner or parent exposed.
IMMERSION FOOT	Pains on recovery from feet being cold, wet or both; skin changes.
Affects adults almost exclusively	
TROPICAL SPASTIC PARAPARESIS	Also stiffness of the legs; maybe back pain, incontinent of urine.
COBALAMIN DEFICIENCY	Mostly older people of European genetic heritage.
Obvious skin changes, mostly adults	
ARSENIC POISONING	Numbness, tingling and burning in feet, skin changes.
LEPROSY	Skin bumpy or color changes; there may be numbness or lack of pain sense.

1 *Loiasis: present in humid, rural areas of western and central Africa.*

TOC

SYMPTOMS

DIFFERENTIALS

CONDITIONS

DRUG INDEX

REGIONAL NOTES

INX

Protocol A.60.C—Muscle-type pain, legs

Definition: the pain is crampy. The calves, thighs or both are tender when squeezed. Pain is increased when the patient moves his own limbs, but when he relaxes (if he can) and you move his limbs, the pain is not much worse than it is at rest. If this is part of whole-body muscle pains, see also Protocol 10.C.

Initially examine the patient's lower back. Tap his spine and press next to the spine on both sides. Back problems may present with pain in the legs. If the pain is aggravated by pressure or movement of the back, then it is probably a back problem, not a leg problem. Consult the appropriate protocol.

If this is part of a generalized illness with fever, headache and body pains, then see Protocol B.2.

Does or did the pain occur after unusual exercise, heat exposure or standing all day?

NO	YES
|	**Consider**: MUSCLE STRAIN, TENDINITIS, BURSITIS, VARICOSE VEINS, HEAT ILLNESS.
|	

Does the patient have a corrected temperature over 37.5°/99.5°, or does he report a recent fever?

NO to both	YES to either or both	
|	*Was the onset of the illness over 3 days or more?*	
|	|	|
|	**NO, rapid onset**	**YES, over 3 days or more**
|	|	**Consider**: TYPHUS (murine), POLIO, PYOMYOSITIS BRUCELLOSIS, TRICHINOSIS, CYSTICERCOSIS, SPOTTED FEVER,[1] TETANUS.
|	|	
|	|	
|	**Consider**: DENGUE FEVER,[3] INFLUENZA, ARBOVIRAL FEVER, LEPTOSPIROSIS, TYPHUS (louse), SPOTTED FEVER,[1] RELAPSING FEVER,[2] POLIO, RAT BITE FEVER, TRENCH FEVER.	
See table below		

---

1 *Spotted fever: worldwide but not in the islands of Southeast Asia; the pain is mainly in the calves rather than the shins.*

2 *Relapsing fever: tropical and high altitude, but not in the islands of SEA and the Pacific.*

3 *Dengue fever: in the Americas only near or north of the equator. In Africa, east coastal, south and west. Prevalent in India, Southeast Asia and the Pacific. Occasionally found in the Mediterranean area. The disease may spread.*

MUSCLE PAINS, NO UNUSUAL ACTIVITIES, NO CURRENT OR RECENT FEVER

	Most common causes
Night cramps	Older people or pregnant; use QUININE if not pregnant.
OLD AGE	Poor circulation in legs causes a deep, throbbing pain, worse with legs elevated.
ANEMIA	Pale fingernails; leg cramps with walking.
	History of a very poor diet
BERIBERI	Weakness also, broad-based gait; poor diet or alcoholic.
PELLAGRA	Also rash, burning with swallowing, mental changes.
	Distinctive history
CHOLERA	History of severe watery diarrhea before muscle cramps, recent onset.
PLANT POISONING	Claviceps or ergot; aching pain with numbness, feet cool to the touch.
GANGRENE	Similar to claviceps above; skin discolored.

Protocol A.60.D—Bone and joint pain

Definition: a deep, boring, frequently throbbing pain, worse with movement and weight bearing. The pain usually increases as much if someone else moves the limb as if the patient moves it. Firm pressure over the painful areas aggravates the pain.

Initially examine the patient's lower back. Tap his spine and press next to the spine on both sides. Back problems may present with pain in the legs. If the pain is provoked by pressure or movement of the back, then it is probably a back problem, not a leg problem. Consult the appropriate protocol.	**Growing pains in children, treatment not necessary** Not at the start of the day; mainly evenings and night. Child is not ill. He does not limp. He cannot point with one finger to an exact location for the pain.

Does the patient have brittle bones that fracture easily?

NO   **YES**
|
| **Consider**: OLD AGE, paralysis, SYPHILIS,[1] TUBERCULOSIS of the bones, CANCER, THALLASEMIA,
| RICKETS, HYDATID DISEASE.[2]

Is there a visible wound on or near the painful area?

NO   **YES**
|
      Consider: AINHUM, BURULI ULCER, YAWS, CANCER, OSTEOMYELITIS.

Is there only pain without swelling?

NO, there is swelling also   **YES, only pain with no swelling**
|
| **No fever:** MANSONELLOSIS PERSTANS,[4] PELLAGRA, BRUCELLOSIS, ONCHOCERCIASIS.[5]
| **Fever; onset over less than a week, likely previously healthy**
| **No prominent red rash**: HEPATITIS, RELAPSING FEVER,[3] TRENCH FEVER, YELLOW FEVER,[6]
| ARBOVIRAL FEVER, BRUCELLOSIS, TYPHUS.
| **Prominent red rash, now or previously:**
| DENGUE FEVER,[7] RUBELLA, ARBOVIRAL FEVER, TYPHUS.
| **Fever; recurrent problem or slow onset**
| BRUCELLOSIS, FILARIASIS, SICKLE CELL DISEASE,[8] TUBERCULOSIS.
| **A tap on the shin causes severe pain after a delay**
| AFRICAN SLEEPING SICKNESS; scattered sub-Saharan areas.
|

Did the problem start only or mainly over a joint?

NO to both   **YES to either**

See Protocol B.6.B   See Protocol B.6.A.

---

1 *Only in babies less than 2 years old.*
2 *Hydatid disease: there are two kinds: one is in cattle-raising areas of the tropics where there are dogs that live close to people. The other kind is in temperate, rural areas where there are wild animals and people eat gathered, wild plant life that might be contaminated with the stool of animals.*
3 *Relapsing fever: tropical and high altitude, but not in the islands of SEA and the Pacific.*
4 *Mansonellosis perstans: only in west and central Africa and in South America, northern Argentina and north of there.*
5 *Onchocerciasis: present in scattered area in Africa, in the Americas north of the Amazon, in Yemen and Saudi Arabia.*
6 *Yellow fever: South America north of Sao Paolo, central and western Africa and the Sudan.*
7 *Dengue fever: in the Americas only near or north of the equator. In Africa, east coastal, south and west. Prevalent in India, Southeast Asia and the Pacific. Occasionally found in the Mediterranean area. The disease may spread.*
8 *Sickle cell disease is inherited; it affects those of African genetic origin, mainly in western Africa and the Americas. Some Indians, Greeks and Arabs are also affected.*

Protocol A.60.E—Other pain in lower limbs

Condition	Onset	Who	Characteristics
FIBROMYALGIA	Probably days to months	Middle-aged and older	Symmetrical pain with certain tender spots close to joints; fatigue; usually Western ethnicity.
RABIES	Hours to days	Mammal encounter	Either throat spasms with swallowing water or else paralysis.
PLANT POISONING ergot	Minutes to hours	Consumers of the plant	Crampy pain, like a blood pressure cuff left on too long.
FILARIASIS	Months to years	Resident in affected area	Initially recurrent pain and swelling.
VARICOSE VEINS	Slowly, over weeks or months	Adult who stands a lot	Aching legs after standing; big, swollen veins visible on the legs with standing.
ACUTE ABDOMEN	Less than a day	Anyone	Abdominal pains or tenderness along with thigh or knee pain; lower limb is not tender.
CANCER	Weeks to months	Mostly older	Cancer in the lower abdomen may cause thigh or knee pain, similar to acute abdomen.
AFRICAN SLEEPING SICKNESS[1]	Weeks to months	Tropical Africa	Tapping shin causes severe pain after a delay.

1 African sleeping sickness: scattered areas of Africa, south of Bamako, Mali and Lake Chad; north of Lusaka, Zambia.

PROTOCOL A.61—SWELLING OF LEGS AND FEET

A.61.A—Swelling; pitting

A.61.B—Swelling; non-pitting

A.61.C—Join swelling, lower limbs

A.61.D—Swelling of soles of feet

PITTING VS. NON-PITTING LEG AND FOOT SWELLING AND USE OF DIURETICS

Category	Conditions	At first	Later[3]	Diuretics[2]
Obstructed lymph nodes	Some CANCER pregnancy, any mass in the abdomen, MOSSY FOOT, FILARIASIS, local infection such as CELLULITIS.	Non-pitting	Non-pitting[4]	No
Too little protein in the blood	TOXEMIA, nephrotic KIDNEY DISEASE, LIVER DISEASE, LIVER FAILURE, MALNUTRITION, MALABSORPTION.	Pitting	Rapid filling[5]	No[1]
Blood vessels too full	KIDNEY DISEASE, HEART FAILURE, some CANCER.	Pitting	Rapid filling	Yes
Leaky blood vessels	SEPSIS, injuries, EBOLA VIRUS DISEASE, some rare conditions.	Pitting	Rapid filling	No

1 If the patient is truly miserable, small amounts of diuretic may be given or fluid may be drained from his abdomen. He will lose weight and feel better, but his life may be shortened because of it. The watery part of his blood will decrease, so the effect will be the same as his being dehydrated or bled: low blood pressure and rapid pulse.

2 That is, are medications that increase urine output, such as FUROSEAMIDE and HYDROCHLOROTHIAZIDE helpful? When they are not helpful, you should be aware that they are harmful. They decrease the blood volume further in patients who already have a deficient volume because of fluid leaking out of the vessels.

3 The division between first and later is before 1 month and after 3 months.

4 Non-pitting means that one cannot easily make a dent in the swelling that is visible after removing one's thumb.

5 Rapid filling means over less than 40 seconds.

Protocol A.61 continued | *Village Medical Manual 7th Edition Volume 2* | **A-171**
CHAPTER PAGE

TOC

SYMPTOMS

DIFFERENTIALS

CONDITIONS

DRUG INDEX

REGIONAL NOTES

INX

Protocol A.61.A—Swelling; pitting

Definition: press a swollen area to the bone with your thumb and then lift your thumb; there is a dent where you pushed. This dent gradually fills. The most common cause for this is standing or sitting in one place for a prolonged period. If this is not the case, check below. See also Protocol A.61.B.

The protocol below assumes that the swelling is symmetrical or nearly symmetrical left and right. If it is asymmetrical, it is likely to be due to injury (see Volume 1), infection, localized heat or cold injury, ALLERGY, LEPROSY reaction, FILARIASIS, blood clots or CANCER. Infection could be CELLULITIS, ABSCESS, PYOMYOSITIS, OSTEOMYELITIS, GANGRENE, NECROTIZING FASCIITIS. In these cases the swelling is likely to not only be asymmetrical, left vs right leg, but it will also be asymmetrical, involving one part of the limb (inside/outside or top/bottom) more than the other. Occasionally VARICOSE VEINS might be asymmetrical. See also Protocol B.6: limb swelling.

SYMMETRICAL PITTING SWELLING

Is the patient six months or more pregnant?

NO	YES
|	**Consider** TOXEMIA, VARICOSE VEINS.

Does the patient have a skin condition affecting a large part of his body?

NO	YES
| See the table below	**Consider** LEPROSY reaction, KIDNEY DISEASE, MALNUTRITION, FILARIASIS

SYMMETRICAL PITTING SWELLING, NO ADVANCED PREGNANCY, NO PROMINENT SKIN CONDITION

Conditions	Characteristics	Diuretics?
Likely large liver and prominent heart symptoms (exercise intolerance)		
HEART FAILURE	Also fatigued or short of breath on exertion; check out causative diseases.	Yes
CHAGA'S DISEASE[1]	Large liver which may be tender; fatigued or short of breath.	Yes
Prominent liver symptoms likely		
LIVER FAILURE	Yellow eyes, distended abdomen or both.	No
LIVER DISEASE	Yellow eyes, distended abdomen or both; check out causative diseases.	No
Large liver and spleen but without either liver or heart symptoms		
VISCERAL LEISHMANIASIS[2]	Enormous spleen, large liver after the third month, not responsive to anti-malarial medication.	No
Likely liver and spleen not large; there is weight loss, long term		
MALABSORPTION	Severe diarrhea immediately after eating anything.	No
MALNUTRITION	Also brittle hair or hair color change; thin upper arms.	No
Likely a general whole-body illness, weight gain		
KIDNEY DISEASE	Face swollen in the morning; abnormal urine amount or urinalysis.	Yes
Likely a localized or recent-onset illness		
FILARIASIS	Initially swelling is episodic; swollen legs common in the community.	No
VARICOSE VEINS	Soft, bluish bulges on legs; swelling worse at the end of the day.	No
PLANT POISONING	From argemone oil or anything causing KIDNEY DISEASE.	Maybe

1 Chaga's disease: scattered areas in Central and South America.
2 Visceral Leishmaniasis: found in scattered areas of Central and South America, Africa north of the equator, the Mediterranean area, the Indian subcontinent, southern Europe, central Asia and mainland China.

Protocol A.61.B—Swelling; non-pitting

Definition: if you press into the swelling with a finger tip and then let go, the swelling pops right out to where it has been. If you persist and manage to make a dent, it may remain for a long time, gradually filling over much more than 40 seconds. In these cases diuretics are never appropriate.

Does the patient have a corrected temperature over 38.5°/101.3°?

NO   **YES**

| **Consider** PYOMYOSITIS, TRICHINOSIS, CELLULITIS, GANGRENE, OSTEOMYELITIS.

Was the onset of the problem over less than 2 weeks?

NO   **YES**

| **Consider** PYOMYOSITIS, CYSTICERCOSIS, GANGRENE, LOIASIS,[1] IMMERSION FOOT.

Is there a prominent skin condition affecting the swollen limb?

NO   **YES**

| **Consider** LEPROSY, YAWS, FILARIASIS, ONCHOCERCIASIS,[2] GANGRENE, HEMOCHROMATOSIS,[3]
See the table below.   MOSSY FOOT,[4] MYCETOMA, IMMERSION FOOT.

---

1 *Loiasis: humid, rural west and central Africa only.*
2 *Onchocerciasis: scattered areas in Africa, the Middle East, Central America and northern South America.*
3 *Mainly confined to certain ethnic groups who take in excessive iron in the form of blood or beer brewed in iron. There are also some hereditary cases. The skin is generally darkened.*
4 *See Regional Notes F, I, M or S.*

NON-PITTING SWELLING, SLOW ONSET, NO HIGH FEVER, NO PROMINENT SKIN CONDITION.

Most common, check these out first

PYOMYOSITIS	Increasing swelling with tenderness deep in the muscle.
FILARIASIS	Swelling comes and goes by itself early in disease.

Less common than the conditions above

CANCER	Large lymph nodes, groin or upper thigh or abdominal swelling.
TUBERCULOSIS	Most often on or near joints, hip or knee, not symmetrical usually.
Repeated infections	CELLULITIS, ABSCESS or TROPICAL ULCER on the leg, now or previously.
MOSSY FOOT	Red clay soil area; see Regional Notes F, I, M, S, may be locally common.

Protocol A.61.C—Joint swelling, lower limbs

If there is pain with the swelling, see Protocols A.60 and B.6 also.

Are the joints relatively painless even though they are swollen?

NO	YES
|	**Consider**: SYPHILIS (tertiary, congenital), LEPROSY, DIABETES, TUBERCULOSIS.

Are the joints red (or warm) and painful?

NO	YES to both
|	See Protocol B.6.A.

PAINFUL AND SWOLLEN BUT NOT RED OR WARM

SYPHILIS, congenital	5–30 yo; initially painless; symmetrical knee swelling common.
TUBERCULOSIS	Knee or hip swelling before pain; thigh muscles thinner than the other side.
TENDINITIS	Painful motion of the joint, due to repetitive exercise, adults mostly.
RICKETS	Inadequate sunlight exposure; legs bones curved in or out; usually symmetrical.
ONCHOCERCIASIS[1]	Expatriates; also back pains and an itchy rash.
SCURVY	Swollen ankles; also bleeding gums and spontaneous bruising.

1 Onchocerciasis: *scattered areas in Africa, the Middle East, Central America and northern South America.*

Protocol A.61.D—Swelling of soles of feet

YAWS	Skin thick, cracks, very painful; humid tropics only.
LEPROSY	Also parts of fingers or toes missing, poor pain sensation; slow-onset skin condition.
ARSENIC POISONING	Thick skin of palms and soles; belly pains and diarrhea are common.
TUNGIASIS	Black spots near the tips of the toes, with swelling; from sand fleas.
BIG HEEL	Painful swelling of heel along with fever.
REITER SYNDROME	History of a SEXUALLY TRANSMITTED DISEASE or DYSENTERY.

PROTOCOL A.62—OTHER LEG AND FOOT PROBLEMS

Groin pain: see Protocols A.45 and A.52.B.

Groin swelling: see Protocols A.52.A and B.

Appearance: size/shape

Strangely shaped legs: long-standing ARTHRITIS, RICKETS, TUBERCULOSIS, congenital SYPHILIS, YAWS, CRETINISM, any weakness or paralysis such as that caused by POLIO.

Shortening of feet or foot: LEPROSY or MYCETOMA.

One leg shorter than the other: old POLIO, TUBERCULOSIS of the hip, prior injury.

Shins bowed forward: RICKETS; SYPHILIS, congenital; possibly YAWS or TREPONARID.

One toe narrow and then falling off: AINHUM.

SYMPTOMS

DIFFERENTIALS

CONDITIONS

DRUG INDEX

REGIONAL NOTES

INX

Appearance: skin

Abnormal color: GANGRENE, PLANT POISONING: claviceps or ergot; FROSTBITE. See Protocol A.16.

Leg ulcers: THALLASEMIA, SICKLE CELL DISEASE,[1] TROPICAL ULCER, BURULI ULCER, GUINEA WORM,[2] any old, infected wound, rarely TUBERCULOSIS, MYCETOMA, see Protocol A.17.

Slow growth of hard, painless swellings on the feet: TUBERCULOSIS, MOSSY FOOT, MYCETOMA, FILARIASIS, BURULI ULCER, see Protocol A.14.

Big, blue, soft veins on the legs: VARICOSE VEINS.

Function: movement

Painful motion of a joint after exercise or sustained pressure: see Chapter 9 H, Volume 1.

Abnormal gait: see Protocol A.7.C.

Spasms: if cramps, see Protocol A.7.B; if seizures, Protocol A.7.A.

Paralysis or weakness: see Protocol A.8.

Stiff leg muscles: SCURVY, ARTHRITIS, THRITIS, TETANUS, SPINAL NEUROPATHY, TROPICAL SPASTIC PARAPARESIS, PYOMYOSITIS, PLANT POISONING due to lathyrism,[3] also see Protocol A.8.C.

Joints bend abnormally: RICKETS, SYPHILIS, LEPROSY, DIABETES, some hereditary problems.

Function: feeling

Numbness: see Protocol A.10.A.

Cold feet: exposure to cold, IMMERSION FOOT, prior injury, GANGRENE if very ill, OLD AGE.

Itching and peeling skin between toes: TINEA, SCABIES.

Itching soles: ALLERGY; maybe FOOD POISONING due to fish in the Pacific area.

---

1 *Sickle cell disease: this affects those of African genetic origin, mainly in West Africa and the Americas. Some Indians and Arabs are also affected.*

2 *Guinea worm: scattered areas in Africa and the Middle East only.*

3 *Plant poisoning, lathyrism: found in eastern African, Indian area and the Mediterranean area.*

XI—BACK PROBLEMS

PROTOCOL A.63—BACK PAIN

A.63.A—Back pain due to kidney or liver problems

A.63.B—Back pain due to a spine or muscle problem

A.63.C—Back pain due to neuritis (nerve irritation)

> ### ⚠ EMERGENCY
>
> **BACK PAIN EMERGENCIES**
>
> New, severe pain in patient age under 20 or over 55 years.
>
> Sudden onset of severe pain.
>
> Weakness of legs and feet.
>
> Problems with urine or stool.
>
> Pain is worse with rest.
>
> Numbness of legs, feet, groin.
>
> AIDS or CANCER.
>
> Back pain with severe vomiting.
>
> Back pain with loss of consciousness
>
> Back pain radiating to the thighs or knees.
>
> Pain with weight loss.

***If the back pain does not increase with touching or pushing on the back but it does increase with pushing on the abdomen, then the origin of the problem is not the back but is the abdomen. The back pain is referred pain. See Protocol A.39 and the subsequent protocols rather than a protocol below.

See also:

Severe back pain with SHOCK: Protocol A.39.C (ACUTE ABDOMEN).

Pain in the back above the waist: Protocol A.35.

Back pain with abdominal pain: Protocol A.39.

Protocol A.63.A—Back pain due to kidney or liver problems

Definition: the pain is not dead center back but is more to the right, left or both. The pain may travel down to the groin or genitals; it may be felt in the shoulder or shoulder blade. Also see Protocol A.43: Flank Pain or Protocol A.10.C: Aching All Over, if applicable. This kind of pain may be due to enlarged lymph nodes in the back. These nodes drain the pelvic/genital areas as well as the legs. Check for SEXUALLY TRANSMITTED DISEASEs as well as various causes of enlarged lymph nodes in the groin. If the times of onset correlate, any large, tender lymph nodes in the groin may be the cause of back pain as well.

Conditions	Urinalysis	Characteristics
Pain both sides or indeterminate which side is worse		
MALARIA	Urobilinogen?	Fevers, headache, sudden onset; left shoulder pain likely.
SCHISTOSOMIASIS HEMATOBIUM[1]	Blood	Blood in urine, at first just at end of urination.
URINARY OBSTRUCTION or KIDNEY DISEASE	No sample; Varies	The patient is not urinating at all, or he just dribbles. If you get a sample at all it will be abnormal in some way.
PLANT POISONING	Blood	Djenkol bean with bloody urine; Malaysia and Indonesia.
BARTONELLOSIS[2]	Urobilinogen?	Episodic fevers, headaches and ANEMIA.
May occur in children; pain likely one-sided at some point in the illness		
AMEBIASIS	Bilirubin?	Tender liver; pain only right lower chest or upper abdomen.
GALLBLADDER DISEASE	Bilirubin?	Also pain in upper abdomen, center or right; vomiting common.
KIDNEY INFECTION	Leukocytes	Cloudy urine, fever and pain with urination are common; back pain one side.
LIVER FLUKE[3]	Bilirubin	The patient ate raw fish or water plants.

1 *Schistosomiasis hematobium: present in some areas of Africa and the Middle East.*
2 *Bartonellosis: scattered areas in Peru and adjacent countries.*
3 *Liver fluke: worldwide, including temperate climates, especially in Southeast Asia.*

TOC

SYMPTOMS

DIFFERENTIALS

CONDITIONS

DRUG INDEX

REGIONAL NOTES

INX

TOC

SYMPTOMS

DIFFERENTIALS

CONDITIONS

DRUG INDEX

REGIONAL NOTES

INX

Condition	Urinalysis	Other Characteristics
Occurs mostly in adults; pain likely one-sided at some point in the illness		
FILARIASIS	Varies	Swollen limbs common in the community; may have swelling.
HYDATID DISEASE[1]	Varies	Tropical/arid areas with dogs or temperate forested areas.
CANCER	Varies	Swelling, blood in urine, weight loss.
KIDNEY STONE	Blood	Sudden onset of severe pain; urine test positive for blood.

1 *Hydatid disease: there are two kinds: one is in cattle-raising areas of the tropics where there are dogs that live close to people. The other kind is in temperate, rural areas where there are wild animals and people eat gathered, wild plant life that might be contaminated with the stool of animals.*

Protocol A.63.B—Back pain due to a spine or muscle problem

Definition: back pain may be dead center back or slightly off to one side; if it is off to both sides, almost invariably one side will hurt much worse than the other. It may be felt in the thigh, either the front of the thigh (mid-back problem) or the back of the thigh (lower back problem) The pain is aggravated by movement. Urinalysis is normal unless the patient also has a kidney problem. If this is part of general body pains, see Protocol A.10.C. If this problem is part of a general illness with fever, headache and general body pain, see Protocol B.2. If this is part of an illness with prominent fevers, see Protocol B.13.

Condition	Fever	Characteristics
Most common, check these first		
ENDOMETRIOSIS	No	Females; monthly back pains at time of menstruation.
MUSCLE STRAIN	No	Had some unusual exercise; sudden or gradual onset.
No prominent muscle spasms; localized to one part of the back		
BURSITIS and related	No	See Chapter 9H in Volume 1.
TUBERCULOSIS	Maybe	There is a bulge in the spinal column, pain, tenderness or both.
HYDATID DISEASE[1]	No	Relatively soft bulge, very slow onset.
No prominent muscle spasms, but other joint and muscle symptoms likely		
FIBROMYALGIA	No	Pain worst after resting; tender spots; fatigue, sleep disturbance.
ARTHRITIS	Maybe	Painful area of the spine is also warm and tender.
No prominent spasms, whole-body illness likely, slow onset or recurrent		
SICKLE CELL DISEASE[2]	Maybe	Recurrent bone and abdominal pain, problem began before 2 yo.
BRUCELLOSIS	Maybe	Joint pains; fever and illness come and go; fatigue.
ONCHOCERCIASIS[3]	No	In expatriates; also itchy skin, joint pains, large lymph nodes.
Prominent muscle spasms likely		
SLIPPED DISC	No	Very severe pain, onset with some movement; adults; no fever.
RICKETS	No	Also curved leg bones; history of inadequate sun exposure.
POLIO	Usual	Weakness or paralysis after a "cold" or diarrhea; back pains.
TROPICAL SPASTIC PARAPARESIS	Maybe	Also stiffness in legs and some urinary difficulty.
RABIES	Maybe	Also throat spasms with swallowing or a breeze, maybe paralysis.
TETANUS	Maybe	Whole-body spasms; can't open mouth, body arched backward.

1 *Hydatid disease: there are two kinds: one is in cattle-raising areas of the tropics where there are dogs that live close to people. The other kind is in temperate, rural areas where there are wild animals and people eat gathered, wild plant life that might be contaminated with the stool of animals.*

2 *Sickle cell disease: this affects those of African genetic origin, mainly in West Africa and the Americas. Some Indians and Arabs are also affected.*

3 *Onchocerciasis: scattered areas in Africa, the Middle East, Central America and northern South America.*

Protocol A.63.C—Back pain due to neuritis (nerve irritation)

Definition: the back pain is in a band around the back or goes down one or the other leg or both. Urinalysis is normal unless the patient also has a kidney problem. If this is part of General Body Pains, see Protocol A.10.C.

Consider the problems listed above under spine. Also consider SPINAL NEUROPATHY, LEPROSY, SHINGLES, TRENCH FEVER, RADICULOPATHY, SLIPPED DISC, FLUOROSIS.

PROTOCOL A.64—OTHER BACK PROBLEMS

Pain in a band from the back around to the front: SHINGLES, TRENCH FEVER.

Sideways curved backbone with one shoulder blade sticking out: SCOLIOSIS.

Pit or lump along center line in back: old injury; TUBERCULOSIS; birth defect. If it is a birth defect, ignore it if it is on the tailbone. Send out if further up. (Requires a level 4 or 5 facility for treatment.)

Stiff back, arched back: cerebral MALARIA, SEIZURES (see Protocol A.7.A), POLIO, TETANUS, MENINGITIS, TUBERCULOSIS, ENCEPHALITIS, (rarely) HEAT ILLNESS, RABIES.

Lump on back flank area: HYDATID DISEASE,[1] maybe ABSCESS, CANCER.

Hunched back: may be due to weak muscles, OLD AGE, ARTHRITIS, SCOLIOSIS, FLUOROSIS, RICKETS, TUBERCULOSIS, BRUCELLOSIS or an old injury. A very similar condition may be the side effect of the drug PREDNISONE or a similar drug.

Pimples on the back: ACNE.

Back pains with abdominal pains: ACUTE ABDOMEN, PANCREATITIS, PERICARDITIS.

Back pains with chest pains: PERICARDITIS.

Red, warm, swollen area: ABSCESS, CELLULITIS, PYOMYOSITIS, OSTEOMYELITIS, CANCER.

---

1 *Hydatid disease: there are two kinds: one is in cattle-raising areas of the tropics where there are dogs that live close to people. The other kind is in temperate, rural areas where there are wild animals and people eat gathered, wild plant life that might be contaminated with the stool of animals.*

INDEX B: DIFFERENTIAL DIAGNOSIS

INDEX B: INTRODUCTION

- How to use the B protocols
- Assumptions
- Notes on column headings and abbreviations (applies to several protocols)

How to use the B protocols

The objective of these protocols is to enable a health worker to make an educated guess at a probable diagnosis, when working under circumstances where few or no diagnostic facilities are available. If such facilities are available, they should be used. This index is not to be used as a "cookbook"; rather, narrow down the options of possible diagnoses.

In each protocol, a few major presenting symptoms are named in its title. Choose the protocol that covers the prominent symptoms your patient is experiencing. If the patient has symptoms named in more than one protocol, then study each applicable protocol. First go through the list of diseases, eliminating those which are not found in your area. Geographical information is provided. Secondly, check the incubation and onset time, as they may give an indication whether that disease is a possible candidate. Then look at the other columns that give further information on the characteristics of each disease, in order to determine which ones are the most probable. Also pay attention to the column labeled "contagious," included in some of the protocols, In some diseases (e.g., hemorrhagic fever) extreme care must be exercised in dealing with the patient. Look up the most probable diagnoses in the Condition Index to make a final determination.

Assumptions

The following assumptions apply:

1. The reader is in a developing area where the vast majority of medical problems are infectious.

2. There is no Western-type facility available.

3. The reader has a Western education at a minimum through 2 years of college.

4. The reader can both read and understand English fluently.

5. The reader and patient have a common language and good rapport.

6. The reader has mastered the contents of the first volume of this book, and has had supervised practice in using the logic of the second volume.

To the extent that these assumptions are valid the protocols below will be helpful. To the extent that they are not valid, other medical care must be obtained.

Notes on column headings and abbreviations
(applies to several protocols)

Incubation (I): the time from exposure to first symptom. (N/A = not applicable.)

Onset (O): the time from first symptom to the person being sick enough to seek help or sick enough to be bedridden, whatever comes first— Secs = seconds; Mi = minutes; H = hours; D = days; W = weeks; Mo = Months; Y = years.

Group: would one expect to find others in the same community having this disease?

"Yes": definitely expect groups. "No": definitely do not expect groups. Other terms also used: Rare; Maybe; Usual; ?? (indeterminate or unknown); Family (genetically linked diseases); N/A, Not applicable.

For some (not all) diseases which are infectious and for conditions resulting from certain environmental factors, one is likely to find multiple individuals having the same symptoms.

Information about this tendency is useful for diagnostic purposes. If, for example, there is only one person in the community known to have the particular symptoms, it is unlikely to be a disease that is highly contagious. But if there are other similar cases, then one should focus on group diseases. Genetically inherited diseases also tend to occur in family or kinship groups; these are labeled as "Family" in the protocols.

Risk factors: factors in a patient's life that make him likely to get the disease. "Residence" means he lives in an affected geographical area. Absence of risk factors does not eliminate the diagnosis.

Usual symptoms: symptoms in addition to the defining symptoms listed in the title of the chart.

Common symptoms: other symptoms which are frequently also present but may be absent.

Treatment: see the Condition Index for more details on the treatment.

Contagious?: whether the disease can be transmitted directly from one person to another.

PROTOCOL B.1—STDs—SEXUALLY TRANSMITTED DISEASES (and Similar Diseases)

B.1.A—Abstinence or faithfullness counseling

B.1.B—Genital skin ulcers: summary

B.1.A—Abstinence or faithfulness counseling

These protocols are fashioned similarly to those put out by WHO, substituting abstinence outside of marriage and faithfulness within marriage (rather than the use of condoms) as the only feasible way of preventing infection or reinfection with sexually transmitted diseases. Other sexually transmitted diseases promote the transmission of HIV, and the presence of HIV makes the symptoms of some other STD's worse. Condoms fail as contraceptives 10% of the time, which means that sperm pass through or around them. HIV viruses are vastly smaller than sperm. Even when condoms don't break or leak, they do not cover all skin that sheds STD organisms. Recommending condoms is like recommending Russian roulette; the odds are similar.

The problem with abstinence/faithfulness is that the only abstinence/faithfulness one can be sure of is his or her own. A crisis arises within a marriage relationship when one suspects his or her partner of unfaithfulness. In this case it might be feasible to practice abstinence for four months at which time negative HIV and STD tests can again permit a normal marital sexual relationship. This necessarily involves confronting one's partner, which is easier said than done. However, the alternative of continued marital relationships is suicidal. With twice-weekly sexual activity with consistent usage of condoms, within four months one would still have three exposures to STDs including deadly HIV.

Partner treatment

Traditionally this was mere notification—having the patient tell his, or her partner to show up at the clinic and then treating him or her as a separate patient. There are obvious problems with that approach. The current thinking is to give the patient the medicine to take back home for the partner, in addition to urging a separate examination. The partner must be treated at the same time as the patient; otherwise a disease just passes back and forth.

B.1.B—Genital skin ulcers: summary[1]

Disease	Initial	Ulcer	Pain	Big nodes	Long-term
SYPHILIS	Bump	Usually single, oval,[2] swollen.	Rare	Usual; non-tender.	Insanity, ANGINA, blindness, sick babies.
CHANCROID	Bumps	Multiple, ragged edges.	Yes	Big/tender, one side.	Groin scar.
LYMPHOGRANULOMA VENEREUM	Bump or blister Single	Only 50% of patients.	Yes	20% of patients, one side, tender.	Swelling, pain, destruction of genitals causing incontinence.
DONOVANOSIS	Bump	Yes, shape irregular.	Minimal	No	Destruction of genitals causing incontinence.
HERPES	Blister	Shallow if any.	Usual	Maybe	Recurrent.

1 See the lecture entitled "Ulcerative STD's".
2 There commonly are multiple ulcers in the presence of HIV INFECTION.

STD appearance in males

See Chapter 6 in Volume 1 for illustrations of genital ulcers in females.

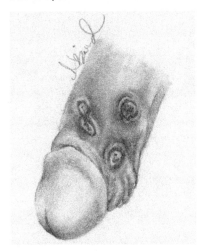

CHANCROID. Note the multiple ulcers with red halos inside the rims. There is not significant swelling below. It is tender to touch. AB

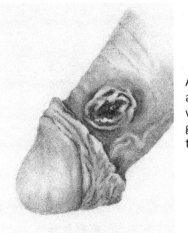

A **SYPHILIS** ulcer. It is single and there is swelling below when it is found on the genitals. It is not tender to touch. AB

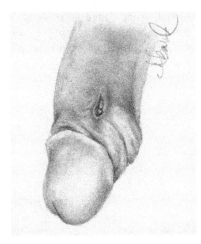

An ulcer of **LYMPHOGRANULOMA VENEREUM** looks just like a little pimple. Most patients skip this stage; they go right on to developing enlarged, tender lymph nodes in their groins, which become abscesses. These abscesses may spread throughout the abdominal wall and internally. AB

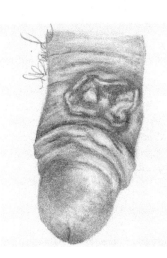

An ulcer of **DONOVANOSIS**. In contrast to the other ulcers which are round, this is irregular in shape. There is some swelling around it. It is not tender to touch. It may smell bad. AB

TOC

SYMPTOMS

DIFFERENTIALS

CONDITIONS

DRUG INDEX

REGIONAL NOTES

INX

B.1.C—Genital ulcer treatment protocol

Is the ulcer

a. *on or very near the abdominal wall?*
b. *discharging some sort of fluid?*
c. *very painful?*

One or none of these apply

Two or three of these apply

Consider AMEBIC SKIN ULCER, and treat it aggressively. Check it daily.

Find out the history and examine him or her: is there a visible genital ulcer (penis in men, vagina in women)?

YES

NO

Find out if there was one that healed. If so have the patient describe it and treat accordingly. If not, counsel abstinence and/or faithfulness.

Are or were there many small blisters, tender to touch?

NO

YES

Treat for HERPES; treat partner(s) also and counsel. Consider REITER SYNDROME in males which may cause sores on the penis indistinguishable from HERPES, but it is not so tender; it is also likely to cause mouth sores.

Treat for SYPHILIS and CHANCROID; also consider DONOVANOSIS and LYMPHOGRANULOMA VENEREUM. Treat partner(s) also and counsel. AZITHROMYCIN treats for all bacterial STD's except for SYPHILIS which requires PENICILLIN additionally. AZITHROMYCIN is expensive, but it is safe in pregnancy. The dosage for MALARIA covers STDs. Beware of counterfeit AZITHROMYCIN.

B.1.D—Male complaining of pain or pus discharge from his penis

Find out the history and examine him. Have him try to push pus out of the tip of the penis. Can you see pus?

NO pus

YES, pus is present

Treat for GONORRHEA and CHLAMYDIA. Also treat his partner(s) and counsel.

Is there a genital ulcer or ulcers?

NO

YES

Use the protocol for genital ulcers.

Recheck in a week.

B.1.E—Male returned with more pus from his penis or burning pain with urinating

Check, as before, if there truly is pus.

YES there is pus

|
|
|
|

NO pus

Check for a genital ulcer. Is there one?

|

YES

Use the genital ulcer protocol.

NO

Counsel.

Did the person fail to take all his medicine, or did he get reinfected?

NO, neither

|

Treat as you would for VAGINITIS due to TRICHOMONAS.
Treat the partner also and counsel. If not improved, refer to a
hospital. Consider counterfeit medicines.

YES, either

Repeat the treatment for CHLAMYDIA and GONORRHEA;
treat partner(s) also; counsel.

B.1.F—Female complaining of vaginal discharge

Do a history and examination. Is there an abnormal discharge?

YES

|
|

NO

Find out if the patient is worried and if so, why; counsel abstinence and/or
faithfulness. (See the genital ulcer protocol B.1.B) if applicable.

*Does the patient have abdominal tenderness and/or pain with pushing a tampon applicator deep into her vagina, and/or
pain with intercourse?*

NO to all

|

YES to any

See the protocol for female lower abdominal pain.

Has she or her husband had illicit sexual contact?

NO

|
|

YES

Treat for GONORRHEA and CHLAMYDIA. Treat the partner also; counsel.

Is there severe itching and a white, cheesy discharge?

NO

|
|
Counsel.

YES

Treat for candida VAGINITIS. Treat her partner(s) at the same time;
counsel. Treat for bacterial VAGINITIS (if there is an odor) and trichomonas
VAGINITIS (frothy with little odor) only. Treat partner at the same time.

TOC

SYMPTOMS

DIFFERENTIALS

CONDITIONS

DRUG INDEX

REGIONAL NOTES

INX

B.1.G—Female complaining of lower abdominal pain

Elicit a history and examine the patient. Does she have any one or more of the following:?

- Missed or late period?
- Recent abortion, miscarriage or delivery?
- Is her pain increased with her coughing or your jarring her bed?
- Does she have bleeding more than an ordinary period?
- Corrected temperature over 38° C/100° F?
- Abnormal mental state?

NO to all	**YES to any or all**
|	Send her to a hospital for treatment immediately.

Is there any one of the following:

- Increased pain with a tampon or fingers being pushed deep inside, to touch the cervix?
- Lower abdomen tender to gentle pushing?
- Vaginal discharge looks like pus?
- Pain with intercourse?

YES to any	**NO to all**
|	Check for genital ulcers; see Protocol B.1.A.
Treat for PELVIC INFECTION; consider SCHISTOSOMIASIS HEMATOBIUM in some areas of Africa and the Middle East. Consider TUBERCULOSIS if the pain is long-lasting but not severe.	

Is the patient improved in a few days?

NO, not improved	**YES, improved**
|	|
Send to a hospital with her partner. **Consider** counterfeit medicines.	|
	|
	Continue the treatment. Treat her partner(s) and counsel.

B.1.H—Male with a swollen scrotum

Is the testis on that side higher than the other or turned around or does the patient give a history of some testicular injury, pain or tenderness?

NO to all

|

Has the patient engaged in risky behavior?

YES or acts guilty

|

|

Treat for LYMPHOGRANULOMA VENEREUM, CHLAMYDIA and GONORRHEA. Keep the patient on bedrest and support his scrotum.

Is he improved in a week?

NO

Send to a hospital.

YES to any

Send to a hospital immediately.

NO

Consider non-contagious causes: HYDROCELE, TUBERCULOSIS, HERNIA, FILARIASIS, CANCER.

YES

|

Continue the treatment. Treat his partner(s) and counsel.

B.1.I—Either sex, swelling in the groin

Elicit a medical history and examine the patient: is there a swollen node or nodes?

YES

|
|
|
|
|
|

Are there skin ulcers present in the genital area?

NO

|

Are there skin ulcers on the legs or feet?

YES

|

|

If the patient has not been involved in risky behavior, then you should treat the leg or feet skin ulcers and see if this clears up the nodes. If he had risky behavior treat for LYMPHOGRANULOMA VENEREUM, SYPHILIS and CHANCROID additionally; treat the partner(s) and counsel.

NO

Is there an abnormal discharge?

YES   **NO**

| Counsel.

Treat according to Protocols B.1.A through B.1.D. Treat the partner(s) also; counsel.

YES

Use the genital ulcer protocol: B.1.C.

NO

Treat for LYMPHOGRANULOMA VENEREUM, SYPHILIS and CHANCROID; Treat the partner(s) also and counsel.

PROTOCOL B.2—FEVER, HEADACHE AND BODY PAINS

B.2.A—Fevers, headache and body pains

B.2.B—Tourniquet test for hemorrhagic fevers

B.2.C—Viral hemorrhagic fevers

B.2.A—Fever (high corrected body temperature), headache and body pains

In a malarious area, first treat MALARIA and then see what, if any, symptoms are left. Be sure to use some form of ARTEMISININ so that the treatment works rapidly. If the patient is not improved within 12 hours, then proceed to use the chart below. If the patient is improved but still quite ill, and has abdominal symptoms, consider ENTERIC FEVER, which frequently coexists with malaria. Also consider the possibility of HEMORRHAGIC FEVER: see Chart B.2.C, below. For the first week, use strict precautions in nursing your patient: gown, gloves, mask, sterilizing eating utensils, care in disposing of waste—until you are sure this is **not** HEMORRHAGIC FEVER. These are also good precautions as regards other contagious conditions.

See introduction to index B: notes on column headings and abbreviations.
Abbreviations for Incubation (I) and Onset (O) times: Secs = seconds; Mi = minutes; H = hours; D = days; W = weeks; Mo = Months; Y = years.

Before beginning this protocol, check out LEPTOSPIROSIS, *bold italic,* on the page following. If this is a possibility, begin treatment on mere suspicion. Treatment must be started within 4 days of the onset of symptoms.

Disease	Incubation Onset	Group	Risk factors[1]	Usual symptoms	Other symptoms	Treatment	Contagious?
Abnormal mental state[2] when the patient is bedridden							
African sleeping sickness[3]	I: varies O: W–Y[4]	Rare	Residence; bitten by a fly that dives.	Swollen bite area or large lymph node(s) at first.	**Heart failure, weight loss, somnolent.**	Difficult, dangerous; fatal if untreated.	No
Enteric fever	I: 1–3 W O: D–W	Maybe	Poor sanitation, food or water.	**Acts "spacy" and belly pain**; fever is high by day 4.	Constipation, diarrhea, vomiting, **body odor.**	Antibiotics; some fatal if untreated.	Yes
Typhus, louse-borne	I: 12 D O: H–D	Usual	Poverty, crowding, body lice.	**Body lice; other symptoms before fever.**	**Mental changes,** musty body odor, **shin pain.**	Antibiotics; may be fatal.	Yes[5]
Typhus, murine	I: 6–14 D O: D–W	Maybe	Rodent contact, fleas or urine.	Muscle pains; **other symptoms before fever.**	Red eyes, rash, musty body odor.	Antibiotics; rarely fatal.	No
Dengue fever	I: 2–15 D O: H	Usual	Tropics, urban, house plants.	**Severe bone pains, eyes red and painful.**	Rash, very ill, **depression.**	Supportive care only.	No
Ebola virus disease	I: 2–21 D O: D	Yes!	Humans, bats, monkeys.	**Vomiting, diarrhea, dizzy, fatigue.**	**Rash, hiccups, maybe bleeding.**	Supportive.	Yes!

1 *Not all patients will have a risk factor.*

2 *An abnormal mental state means that they patient is not as rational as one would expect, given his, or her physical condition.*
   An abnormal mental state might be sleepy; agitated, withdrawn (as in enteric fever and typhus) or depressed (as in dengue fever).
   If the disease is just starting, you might not see the abnormal mental state.

3 *Scattered, small areas throughout Africa, from 15° north to 20° south. The Great Lakes area of East Africa has both kinds; east and south of there it is all Rhodesian; west and north of there it is all Gambian. However, the boundaries move; there may be exceptions.*

4 *West Africa: initial incubation period is a month; mental symptoms start after months to years with slow onset. East Africa: incubation to the first fever is under 3 weeks; mental symptoms start within a month or two, onset over weeks.*

5 *It is not contagious by direct contact, but anyone who touches a person with lice is likely to get a louse bite or two.*

Disease	Incubation; Onset	Group	Risk factors	Usual symptoms	Common symptoms	Treatment	Contagious?
Maybe an abnormal mental state, maybe not							
Arboviral fever	I: varies O: D–W	Some kinds	Residence; insect bite.	Varies with the geography and the kind.	Mental, red eyes, joint pains, bleeding.	Supportive or antivirals	Some kinds
Malaria	I: 3–21 D O: varies[6]	Maybe	Humid tropics and subtropics.	**Shaking chills; headache; sweats.**[7]	Waist and shoulder pains; tired.	Antimalarials; supportive.	No
Normal mental state, variable onset							
Lyme disease	I: 3–32 D O: varies	Rare	**Temperate and sub-tropics;** tick bite, rural.	Rash or history of rash.	**Joints painful, maybe red and swollen.**	Antibiotics; supportive; rarely fatal	No
Serum sickness	I: unknown O Variable	Rare	Coincident with a disease or an injection.	**Fever plus skin rash;** see the next cell.	Headache, body pains, short of breath.	Treat the cause; use anti-histamines and steroids.	No
Q fever	I: 2–4 W O: varies	Rare	Animal exposed.	**Headache**, body pains; **fatigue.**	Like hepatitis or pneumonia.	Antibiotics; supportive.	??
Normal mental state; ordered by onset from most rapid; onset a day or less							
Relapsing fever, louse	I: 2–14 D O: Mi–H	Usual	Refugee camps; head or body lice.	**Fever is high, over 101.3°F/ 38.5°C, sustained for days.**	Short of breath, cough, chest pains, large spleen.	Antibiotics; supportive; may be fatal.	Yes[8]
Relapsing fever, tick	I: 2–14 D O: Mi–H	Maybe	**Caves, abandoned houses, camps**	**Fever sustained** at first, drops in less than 7 days.	Cough, belly pain, quite ill.	Antibiotics, supportive.	No
Leptospirosis	*I: 2–21 D O: H*	*Maybe*	*Exposure to rat urine; flood water; food.*	*Sore eyes or muscle pains or both.*	*Fever goes up and down unpredictably.*	*Antibiotics; must be started soon;[9] may be fatal.*	*No*
Trench fever	I: 4–36 D O: H–D	Usual	**Temperate;** urban, homeless.	Poor hygiene, **body lice.**	**Shin pains,** bone pains.	Antibiotics; supportive.	Yes[10]
Spotted fever, Rocky Mountain	I: 6–10 D O: H–D	Rare	**Americas only;** tick exposure.[11]	Spleen tender, nausea; limb pains.	**Rash begins on wrists and ankles;** black scab.	Antibiotics; supportive; may be fatal.	No

6 Onset is likely to be rapid if the person is not taking prophylactic medicines but slow if he/she was taking them.

7 The shaking chills and sweats are essential if the patient has not taken prophylactic medicines. The medicines might negate these symptoms.

8 Anyone who cares for the patient is likely to acquire a louse or two. It is not otherwise contagious.

9 Antibiotics are totally useless if started after 4 days from onset.

10 It is not contagious by direct contact, but anyone who touches a person with lice is likely to get a louse bite or two.

11 The patient will not necessarily remember the tick, but he will have been exposed to tick-infested flora or fauna.

TOC | SYMPTOMS | DIFFERENTIALS | CONDITIONS | DRUG INDEX | REGIONAL NOTES | INX

Disease	Incubation; Onset	Group	Risk factors	Usual symptoms	Other symptoms	Treatment	Contagious?
Normal mental state; ordered according to onset from most rapid; onset a day or more							
Spotted fever, various	I: < 12 D O: H–D	Maybe	**Tick/ mite exposure**, Eastern Hemisphere.	Rash on limb(s), moderately or very ill.	**Tiny scab(s) from insect bite(s).**	Antibiotics; supportive; may be fatal.	Pox type only
Ebola virus disease	I:2–21 D O: D	Yes	Contact with patient or meat.	Headache, vomiting, diarrhea.	**Chills, muscle pains, rash.**	Supportive; seek recent information.	Yes, very
Syphilis, secondary	I: 2–24 W O: D	Usual	Sexual contact or infant of syphilitic mother.	Spotted skin rash or white mouth patches.	Hair loss, a genital ulcer; **rash on palms and soles.**	Antibiotics prevent tertiary syphilis.	Yes Very
Tularemia	I: 1–14 D O: D	Rare	From small animals or their insects.	**Scab with a red ring around.**	**Red lumps or streaks from the scab to the trunk.**	Antibiotics; supportive.	No
Yellow fever[12]	I: 3–6 D O: D	Usual	Unimmunized; mosquito bitten.	Jaundice or bilirubin in the urine after several days.	Slow pulse relative to fever; **protein in urine; body odor like meat.**	Supportive only; **no drugs**; may be fatal.	No
Rat bite fever 2 kinds	I: 3–30 D O: D	Rare	Rodent bite or urine exposure.	**Open wound, rash or both.**	Wound broke open, nausea, weakness.	Antibiotics to prevent recurrences.	No
Trichinosis	I: < 30 D O: D–W	Usual	**Ate pork or wild game.**	**Muscles swollen and sore.**	**Other eaters also are sick.**	Steroids, no antibiotics.	No
Bartonellosis[13] Oroya	I: 4–16 W O: W–Mo	Maybe	**Peru area; sandfly bite.**	Joint pains, bone pain, chest pain.	Large spleen, large lymph nodes.	Antibiotics; supportive; fatal if untreated.	No

12 *South America north of Sao Paolo, Africa south of the Sahara.*
13 *Only present in Peru and border areas of adjacent countries.*

B.2.B—Tourniquet test for hemorrhagic fever Tourniquet test for hemorrhagic fever

▷B.2.B—TOURNIQUET TEST FOR HEMORRHAGIC FEVER

- *Determine the patient's blood pressure.*
- *Find the number half-way between the higher and lower blood pressure numbers.*
- *Inflate the blood pressure cuff to that number and keep it inflated there for five minutes; the patient will have pain.*
Deflate the blood pressure cuff and look at the arm below the cuff to see if there is a rash. If you can see a rash—little spots like measles or pin-head bruises—then the test is positive. Your patient has a blood clotting problem. The spots may be hard to see in very dark skin; look at the fingernails for black-and-blue marks.

B.2.C—Viral hemorrhagic fevers

Various fevers become hemorrhagic. These are contagious; you can start an epidemic with carelessness. A patient should only be transported in a towed trailer or a medical evacuation vehicle.

(Also consider ONYALAI, LEPTOSPIROSIS, CANCER, SCURVY as possible causes of abnormal hemorrhage, not contagious.)

See Introduction to Index B: notes on Column Headings and Abbreviations.

Abbreviations for Incubation (I) and Onset (O) times: Secs = seconds; Mi = minutes; H = hours; D = days; W = weeks; Mo = Months; Y = years.

Disease	Incubation; Onset	Exposure	Distinctives[1]	Other symptoms[2]	Geography
Lassa fever	I: 5–35 D. O: gradual.	Rodents, humans.	Chest pain, sore throat, swollen face.	Fatigue, red eyes, belly pain, vomiting, diarrhea.	D R Congo, West Africa, south of the Sahara.
Ebola virus disease	I: 2–21 D. O: sudden.	Monkeys, bats, humans, corpses.	Blisters in mouth and throat, very red eyes, bleeding gums, maybe a rash, hiccups.	Belly pain, diarrhea. Bleeding starts from Day 5 to Day 7.	Africa mainly; may spread worldwide.
Marburg fever	I: 3–13 D. O: sudden.	Monkeys, bats, prairie dogs.	Like Ebola.	Like Ebola.	Eastern D R Congo, Uganda, western Kenya.
Crimean-Congo hemorrhagic fever	I: 1–3 D with tick bite; 5–6 D direct. O: sudden.	Farm animals, ticks.	Neck pain, large, tender liver, large lymph nodes, red face.	Bleeding from all over.	Much of Africa, south-eastern Europe, parts of Asia, entire Middle East.
South American VH fevers (3 types)	1. I: 7–16 D. O: gradual onset. 2. I: 5–19 D; O: ? 3. O: gradual onset.	Rodents, farm animals, humans.	1. Low back pain; brain damage, bleeding. 2. Maybe brain damage. 3. Sore throat.	1. Red eyes. 2. Fatigue. 3. Red eyes.	1. Argentine pampas. 2. Beni area of Bolivia. 3. Plains of Venezuela.
Rift Valley fever[3]	I: 2–7 D. O: sudden.	Sick or aborting farm animals.	Back pains, eye symptoms.	Jaundice, rash, may cause blindness.	Kenya and across sub-Saharan Africa and the Middle East.

1 *Distinctives are symptoms that are not present with most of these diseases but ones that should alert you to the fact that this patient may be contagious. It is important, if you note a distinctive symptom, to do the tourniquet test which will tell you if this person is likely to have a hemorrhagic fever.*

2 *This lists symptoms in addition to fever, headache, general body pains and distinctives.*

3 *It is unknown if this is transmissible from patient to patient. It is treated as if it is, because it can be transmitted from animal blood to humans.*

PROTOCOL B.3—FEVER, FATIGUE AND ANEMIA (Large Spleen, Jaundice)

Be sure to use the corrected body temperature. Use this protocol if the patient does not have a fever at the moment, but she has a history of fevers. See Introduction to Index B: notes on Column Headings and Abbreviations.

Abbreviations for Incubation (I) and Onset (O) times: Secs = seconds; Mi = minutes; H = hours; D = days; W = weeks; Mo = Months; Y = years.

Disease	Incubation; Onset	Group	Risk factors[1]	Usual Symptoms	Common Symptoms	Treatment	Contagious?
Onset more than a week; geographically confined areas only							
African sleeping sickness[2]	I: varies O: W–Y[3]	Rare	Residence; bitten by a fly that dive-bombs.	**Headache,** body pains, swollen bite area, big nodes.	**Mental symptoms,** loss of weight, sleepiness, large spleen.	Special drugs, supportive; dangerous, may be fatal.	No
Bartonellosis[4] Oroya	I: 4–16 W O: W–Mo	??	**Peru area;** bitten by sandflies.	Joint pain, anemia came on rapidly.	Chest pain; lymph nodes and liver are big.	Antibiotics, supportive; may be fatal.	No
Tropical splenomegaly	I: Y O: Mo–Y	Usual	Malarious area; humid tropics.	Heaviness, left upper abdomen; **big spleen.**	**Urobilinogen in the urine;** dry cough; liver normal.	Antimalarials, long-term.	No
Visceral Leishmaniasis[5]	I: 10 D–3 Y O: Mo–Y	??	Residence; bitten by sandflies.	Large liver, weight loss, big spleen.	**Urobilinogen in the urine.**	Special drugs Difficult.	No
Onset more than a week; geographically widespread							
Cancer	I: N/A O: Mo–Y	No	Many; old age; radiation, hepatitis.	Pale tongue and fingernails.	Lump(s) somewhere, weight loss, bleeding.	Difficult and expensive; supportive.	No
Tuberculosis any kind	I: W–M O: Mo–Y	Usual	Contact with a coughing adult; unimmunized.	Varies with the organs infected with the TB.	Cough, large neck lymph nodes, weight loss.	Special antibiotics; supportive.	Yes if > 10 y.o.

1 Not all patients will have risk factors.

2 This is present in Africa between 15° north and 20° south. Both kinds are present in the Great Lakes area of East Africa; west and north of there it is all Gambian whereas east and south of there it is all Rhodesian. The boundaries might move, and there may be exceptions.

3 The West African form comes on slowly over years after an initial incubation of a month, followed by a brief illness. The East African form comes on rapidly over weeks after an incubation of less than 3 weeks.

4 This occurs only in Peru and the border areas of adjacent countries.

5 This is present in scattered areas of Africa, the tropical Americas, the Mediterranean and Asia; may be locally common.

Fever, fatigue and anemia, continued.

Disease	Incubation; Onset	Group	Risk factors	Usual symptoms	Common symptoms	Treatment	Contagious?
Onset indeterminate, geographically widespread							
Dysentery	I: 2–14 D O: H–D	Usual	Poor sanitation, water or food	Bloody diarrhea, maybe mucus	Pain, lower abdomen	Antibiotics Metronidazole	Yes
Hemorrhagic fever	I: varies O: varies	Usual	Residence; bitten by insects	Fever, body pains, headache, bleeding	Varies by the kind; bleeding	None or difficult	Some kinds yes
Malaria	I: 3–21 D O: H–W[6]	Usual	Humid tropics and sub-tropics mostly	Chills, headache, sweating	Waist, shoulder, joint pains	Antimalarials, (antibiotics[8])	No
Family history or recurrent problem; urobilinogen in the urine							
Ovalocytosis	I: N/A O: Mo-Y	Family	Family affected; Malaysia and Papua	Large spleen; urobilinogen in urine	Sometimes recurrent crises	Transfusion	No
Sickle cell disease	I: N/A O: Mo–Y	Family	Family affected; early deaths[9]	Child—big spleen, but not adult(s)	Bone pain, chest pain, jaundice	IV's, oxygen, transfusion	No
Thallasemia	I: N/A O: Mo–Y	Family	Genetic heritage	Family history of ill health	Bone pain, growth problems, strange facial appearance	Transfusion	No

6 *The onset is likely to be rapid if the person was not taking preventive medication; it is likely to be gradual otherwise.*

8 *Some ordinary antibiotics also are active against malaria, but they are weak antimalarials.*

9 *This affects mainly those with an African genetic heritage; some Arabs, Indians and Greeks are affected but rarely and not severely.*

▷ **SUPPORTIVE TREATMENT if you can't begin to get a medical history.**

- Bedrest sitting up.
- Give antimalarials in malarious areas.
- Give a high-protein diet.
- Give CHLOROQUINE if on the island of Borneo.
- Give VITAMIN B_{12} and FOLIC ACID.

PROTOCOL B.4—SHORTNESS OF BREATH (Fever, Chest Pain, Cough)

Be aware that respiratory distress with noisy inhalations is an emergency: send out!

See Introduction to *Index B*: notes on Column Headings and Abbreviations. Abbreviations for Incubation (I) and Onset (O) times: Secs = seconds; Mi = minutes; H = hours; D = days; W = weeks; Mo = Months; Y = years.

Condition	Incubation; Onset	Group	Risks[1]	Usual Symptoms	Common Symptoms	Treatment	Contagious?
Most common, check these first							
Anemia from any cause	I: varies O: varies	??	Blood loss, poor diet, hereditary.	**Pale tongue or fingernails if anemia is severe; fatigue.**	Dizzy, jaundice, can't exercise.	Various, transfusion.	Some kinds
Respiratory infection	I: recurs O: varies	??	Smoke, heredity.	**Congestion, breathing labored.**	Chest pain, cough, fever.	Steam; antibiotics.	Maybe
Instantaneous onset likely							
Pneumothorax	I: Sec–H[2] O: Sec–Mi	No	Maybe chest wound.	**No breath sounds one side.**	Chest pain one side.	Emergency surgery.	No
Related to an environmental exposure							
Altitude sickness	I: N/A O: Mi-H	Maybe	**Recent ascent to 2000+ meters.**	Rapid respiration, rales in lungs, cough.	Headache, confused, no fever.	Descent, oxygen, sitting position.	No
Carbon monoxide poisoning	I: Mi–D O: Mi–D	Maybe	**Fire or engine exhaust exposure.**	Nausea, headache.	Red inside the mouth, no fever.	Oxygen.	No
Smoke inhalation	I: Sec–3 D O: Mi–3 D	Maybe	**Exposure to a smoky fire.**	Smoke exposure, cough.	**Sputum has black flecks.**	Oxygen, high-tech.	No
Some swelling is evident somewhere on the body							
Anthrax	I: <7d O: H–D	Likely	Animal meat or hides.	**Massive swelling.**	Fever; sore not painful.	Antibiotics.	Pus is infective
Filariasis[3]	I: 4–18 Mo O: D–W	Usual	Rainy season, tropics, expatriates.	**Wheezing, fever, chills, swelling.**	Swollen limbs are common in the area.	Special drugs.	No
Diphtheria	I: 1–6 D O: varies	Maybe	Exposure to diphtheria; unimmunized.	**Swollen neck or painful wound; low fever if any.**	**Muscles weak;** sweet odor.	Anti-toxin; antibiotics.	Yes, very
Sepsis	I: H–W O: varies	Rare	Previous infection, stress.	**Fever unless elderly, infant.**	Abnormal vital signs.	IV antibiotics.	Maybe

1 Not all patients will have risk factors.

2 This is the time, when caused by trauma, from the causative event until the lung collapses.

3 This occurs in coastal South America, the Caribbean and scattered areas through out the tropics of the Eastern Hemisphere, especially the Pacific. Only diagnose this if you commonly see swollen limbs in the neighborhood.

SHORTNESS OF BREATH, CONTINUED

Condition	Incubation; Onset	Group	Risks[1]	Usual Symptoms	Common Symptoms	Treatment	Contagious?
Related to a chronic or recurrent condition							
Asthma	I: N/A O: Mi–H	No	Expatriates; Western culture, rare in nationals.	**Wheezing or struggling to breathe.**	**Recurrent,** no fever, breathing fast or slow.	Special drugs.	No
Familial Mediterranean fever	I: N/A O: varies	Family	**Mediterranean genetic heritage; family history.**	Skin or mental or abdominal symptoms.	Varies, fever; recurrent problems.	Diet, special drugs.	No
Sickle cell disease	I: recurs O: Mi–Y	Family	African, Arab, Indian or Greek heritage.	**Chest pain, anemia, growth delay.**	Bone pain, kidney trouble, leg ulcers.	High-tech, oxygen, IV's.	No
Heart failure	I: varies O: D–Mo	Rare	Western diet; prior infection(s).	**Exercise intolerant.**	Heart murmur or chest pain.	Special drugs.	No
Tuberculosis	I: Mo–Y O: Mo–Y	Usual	Exposed to a coughing adult; not immunized.	**Slow onset, productive cough, night sweats.**	Chest pain, **weight loss,** pale skin, phlegm.	Special drugs, antibiotics.	Yes
Cancer	I: N/A O: H–Y	No	Old age, Western culture, some toxins, smoking, tumor.	Cough or abnormal breath sounds.	**Weight loss,** chest pain, fever, coughing blood.	Difficult and high-tech.	No
Related to a new illness in a previously healthy patient							
Pneumonia	I: varies O: H–D	??	Previous cold or another illness.	**Fever, cough, fast breathing.**	Chest pain worse with breathing.	Antibiotics.	Yes
Q fever	I: 2–4 W O: varies	??	Newborn animal contact, esp. the Middle East.	**Fever, head-ache, chills, fatigue.**	Jaundice, joint pains; large tender liver.	Antibiotics.	Unknown
Pertussis	I: 1–2 W O: D–W	??	Unimmunized; infants and elderly mostly.	**Violent coughing followed by noisy breathing in.**	Vomiting from coughing hard; bloody eyes.	Supportive, oxygen, maybe antibiotics.	Yes

---

▷ SUPPORTIVE TREATMENT for when obtaining a history is impossible.

- Elevate the head of the bed.
- Take the patient to a lower altitude.
- Use AMINOPHYLLIN for wheezing.
- Provide a nourishing liquid diet.

- Treat fever if necessary.
- Check for ANEMIA; use Protocol B.3.
- Give CHLOROQUINE if on the island of Borneo.

TOC   SYMPTOMS   DIFFERENTIALS   CONDITIONS   DRUG INDEX   REGIONAL NOTES   INX

PROTOCOL B.5—FEVER, JAUNDICE (Large Liver, Tender Liver)

Be sure to use the corrected body temperature. See Page A-5.
See Introduction to *Index B*: notes on column headings and abbreviations.
Abbreviations for Incubation (I) and Onset (O) times: Secs = seconds; Mi = minutes; H = hours; D = days; W = weeks;
Mo = Months; Y = years.

Condition	Incubation; Onset	Group	Risk factors	Usual elements	Likely elements	Urine[1]	Treatment	Contagious?
Peru and adjacent countries only								
Bartonellosis Oroyo	I: 2–16 W O: D–W	??	Peru area; bitten by sand flies.	**Fatigue, headache, joint pains.**	Big spleen & liver; craziness.	?U ?B	Antibiotics.	No
Illness is recent, within the last few weeks, in someone previously healthy								
Malaria	I: 3–21 D O: varies	Maybe	Tropics, rainy season.	**Fever, chills, headache.**	Fatigue, waist pain.	?U	Antimalarial meds.	No
Hepatitis	I: varies	Maybe	Unsanitary water, food; blood contact.	**Joint pains, no appetite, liver pain.**	Yellow eyes, fatigue.	B	Supportive.	Usually
Related to a long-lasting, chronic or recurrent condition								
Brucellosis	I: 2–4 W O: Mo	Rare	Pastoral areas; hides, meat, milk, cheese.	**Back pain,** joint pains, no swelling.	**Feels awful;** fevers episodic.	??	Three antibiotics for 6 weeks.	No
Hepatitis	I: varies O: H–D	??	Poor sanitation, blood exposure.	**Jaundice or urine bilirubin.**	Joint pains, vomiting, weight loss.	B ?U	Supportive; high-tech medicines.	Some kinds
Cancer	I: unknown O: Mo–Y	Rare	Old age; smoking; refined diet; hepatitis; toxins.	Symptoms vary; initially painless.	**Weight loss;** lumpy liver; light-colored stool.	?B; ?U	Surgery; difficult.	No
Sickle cell disease	I: recurs O: varies	Family	**African genetic heritage; stress.**	**Episodic bone pain, fatigue, anemia.**	Chest, bone pain, poor growth.	U	Complex; high-tech, transfusions.	No
Visceral leishmaniasis[2]	I: 3D–3Y O: W–Mo	Rare	Residence; sandflies.	**Large spleen,** weight loss.	**Large liver;** fever episodes.	U	Special medicines.	No
Thallasemia	I: N/A O: sudden	Family	Mediterranean or Asian genetic heritage.	**Sudden onset after food or medication.**	Profound fatigue, short of breath.	U	Transfusion.	No

1 *Urine: whether bilirubin (B) or urobilinogen (U) is found in the urine. A question mark (?) before the letter means "maybe." Any time there is bilirubin, there may also be excess urobilinogen. If only U appears, it implies that bilirubin is absent. These are general rules; there are exceptions.*

2 *Present in scattered areas of Africa, the tropical Americas, the Mediterranean and Asia. May be locally common.*

TOC   SYMPTOMS   DIFFERENTIALS   CONDITIONS   DRUG INDEX   REGIONAL NOTES   INX

PROTOCOL B.6—LIMB SWELLING, PAIN OR BOTH (FEVER, STIFFNESS)

B.6.A—Limb swelling and pain, initially and only or mainly over joints

B.6.B—Limb swelling and pain, **not** initially and only or mainly over joints

B.6.A—Limb swelling and pain, initially and mainly or only over joints

If the pain and swelling started out somewhere on the limb other than right in or on a joint, then it moved to a joint, see Protocol B.6.B below. **See Introduction to** Index B: **notes on Column Headings and Abbreviations.**

Abbreviations for Incubation (I) and Onset (O) times: Secs = seconds; Mi = minutes; H = hours; D = days; W = weeks; Mo = Months; Y = years.

Condition	Incubation; Onset	Group	Risk factors	Usual elements	Common elements	Treatment
Likely no hot, red, swollen joint(s)						
Arthritis, osteoarthritis	I: N/A O: Y, comes and stays	No	Rough sports or excessive stress on the joint(s).	Slow onset; **adult patient or prior injury; no fever.**	Not red, minimally swollen.	Anti-inflammatory medicines.
Tendinitis, bursitis	I: N/A O: H–D	No	**Unaccustomed exercise or pressure on the part.**	Pain worse with active than passive motion.	Tenderness at a point or small area.	Anti-inflammatory medicines. See Chapter 9.H.
Brucellosis	I: 2–4 W O: Mo	Maybe	Pastoral areas; hides, meat, milk, mostly arid.	**Complaining bitterly, back pain,** fevers.	Joints not red; tender; minimal swelling.	3 antibiotics for six weeks.
Rickets	I: varies O: W–Mo	Usual	**Little or no sun exposure for weeks.**	History; deformity of bones.	Not red/hot; chest deformity in children.	Vitamin D, surgery.
Scurvy	I: Mo O: W–Mo	Usual	**No fresh produce in the diet.**	History; swelling, bleeding, stiffness.	Loose teeth, putrid-sweet body odor.	Vitamin C.
Arthritis, tuberculous	I: Mo–Y O: W–Y	Rare	Much TB in the community.	**Slow onset,** pain, stiff, swollen, abnormal shape.	Joint not tender; thin muscles, **abnormal gait.**	Anti-TB medicines, surgery.
Patient likely has a skin condition: a rash, bumps or scars						
Syphilis tertiary	I: Yrs adult I: ? child O: W–M	Family	Middle aged or born to syphilitic mother.	**Swelling worse than pain,** very movable joints, gait problems.	Skin bumps or ulcers, curved bones.	Antibiotics to prevent worsening.
Syphilis congenital	I: N/A O: < 2 yrs	Family	Mother has syphilis.	Baby refuses to move limbs because of pain.	Spontaneous fractures.	Penicillin.
Leprosy	I: 2–10 Y O: Mo–Y	Maybe	Residence in an area with much leprosy.	**Skin condition or history of same;** limb numbness.	Painless deformed joints with abnormal motion.	Special medicines Antibiotics.
Likely hot, red, swollen joints, at least some symmetry some of the time						
Arthritis, rheumatoid	I: N/A O: H–D	No	**Western culture;** family history, rare in poor nationals.	**Multiple joints, symmetry, migrates; stiff mornings.**	Joints red and swollen; fever, hands affected.	Anti-inflammatory medicines.

Table continues on next page.

Condition	Incubation; Onset	Group	Risk factors	Usual elements	Common elements	Treatment
Likely hot, red swollen joints, indeterminate symmetry						
Rheumatic fever[1]	I: Weeks O: H–2 D	Rare	Strep infection, poorly treated.	**Arthritis usually symmetrical, may not be.**	**Red/hot joints; migrates**, heart murmur.	Anti-inflammatory; antibiotics.
HIV infection	I: Y; recurs O: H–D	Usual	Sexual or blood exposure; **Africa** mostly.	**Large joints**; not small joints, **high fever.**	Red/hot, comes and goes.	Special medicines.
Reiter syndrome	I: 1–3 W O: unknown	??	Sexual exposure or dysentery.	**Single large joint or one digit; fever.**	**Skin, mouth, penis sores, little or no pain.**	Antibiotics, special medicines.
Likely hot, red swollen joints, symmetry unlikely						
Arthritis, septic	I: varies O: H–D	No	Injury; infection, poor immunity.	**Single joint**, rarely two.	**Red/hot joint; swollen, fever.**	Surgery, antibiotics.
Gonorrhea	I: 2 W–Mo[2] O: H–D	Usual	Sexual exposure; body secretions.	Sudden onset, **single joint** or two.	**Red/hot joint; swollen, fever.**	Antibiotics.
Gout	I: N/A O: H	No	**Affluent**; from some medicines; rich diet.	**One big toe or ankle**; severe pain and tenderness.	**Red/hot joint; very swollen.**	Special medicines.
Osteomyelitis	I: varies O: slow usually	Rare	Prior injury or infection.	Severe pain, fever, **skin on top abnormal.**	Red/hot joint,[3] maybe **pus drainage through skin.**	Antibiotics for 6 weeks.
Indeterminate whether there are hot, red swollen joints						
Lyme disease[4]	I: 3–32 D Recurs O: varies	Rare	**Temperate rural areas; exposure to ticks.**	Initial rash; one or few joint pains recur; swelling.	History of fever and fatigue; knees most common.	Antibiotics for 2–6 weeks.
Bartonellosis[5] Verugga	I: 4–16 W O: D–W?	??	Residence; sandfly bitten.	**Fever drops** with bumpy swellings appearing.	**Skin bumps**; face affected also.	Antibiotics.
Chikungunya fever	I: 2–4 D O: 2–4 D	Always	Bitten by mosquitoes, day-biters.	**Fever**, headache, **joint pains.**	Rash, vomiting, severe pains.	Pain medication only.
Arboviral fever	I: D–W usual O: H–D	Usual	Bitten by insects or ticks; maybe contagious.	Headache, **fever**, joint pain, **general body pains.**	Bleeding, red eyes, muscle pains.	Supportive only.
Rat bite fever	I: 3–30 D O: 3 D	No	Bitten by a rodent.	Fever, chills, headache; **wound breaks open or else there is a rash.**	Fever sustained, then drops and relapses.	Antibiotics, supportive.

1 Although this is usually symmetrical, it is put here since it must be treated on mere suspicion.

2 The incubation is on the order of 2 weeks for males but months for females.

3 Osteomyelitis is a bone infection. If it happens to be near a joint, it is indistinguishable from septic arthritis.

4 It occurs in the temperate Northern Hemisphere plus subtropical areas such as the north coast of Africa and coastal Australia.

5 This occurs only in Peru and adjacent countries.

> ▷ **SUPPORTIVE TREATMENT** if getting a history is impossible.
>
> - Bedrest, elevate and rest the affected joint(s).
> - Provide a high-protein diet and multivitamins.
> - Use ASPIRIN or IBUPROFEN as needed for pain.
> - Treat for RHEUMATIC FEVER with PENICILLIN if there is any symmetry.
> - Provide supportive care: Volume 1 Appendix 8.

B.6.B—Limb swelling and pain, *not* initially and only or mainly over joints

See Introduction to *Index B*: notes on column headings and abbreviations. Abbreviations for Incubation (I) and Onset (O) times: Secs = seconds; Mi = minutes; H = hours; D = days; W = weeks; Mo = Months; Y = years.

Condition	Incubation; Onset	Groups?	Risk factors	Usual Elements	Common Elements	Varies?[1]	Treatment
History of ingestion of rare pork or game meat within the past month							
Trichinosis	I: < 30 D O: unknown	Usual	**Ate poorly cooked pork or wild game.**	**All limbs swollen**, trunk swollen also; then fever.	General whole-body pains, **symmetrical.**	No	Difficult or impossible.
Recurrent condition and/or family history							
Sickle cell disease	I: N/A O: H–D	Family	**African** genetic heritage.	Child, both hands swollen or recurrent crises.	**Anemia**; delayed growth, pain episodes.	Maybe	Oxygen, IV's, complicated.
Likely a prominent skin condition over more than one area, not only one limb							
Arsenic poisoning	I: varies O: varies	??	Ethnic meds, occupational, homicidal.	**Numbness, tingling, weakness, burning.**	Skin is rough, dry, flaky, face swells.	??	High-tech.
Leprosy reaction	I: < 6 Mo[2] O: H–D	No	**Leprous patients on medication.**	Symmetrical bumpy skin rash before starting meds.	Missing toes and fingers; skin ulcers.	Maybe	Special medicines.
Likely localized swelling, not the entire limb circumference, not pitting							
Tendinitis or bursitis[3]	I: N/A O: H–D	No	Exercise or pressure on the part.	Pain worse with active than passive motion.	**Tenderness at a point or small area.**	No	See Chapter 9.H.
Abscess	I: varies O: D–W	No	Prior injury, even slight.	**Single, swollen, warm area, initially firm.**	Center spot; becomes soft; tender, large lymph nodes.	No	Surgery.
Cellulitis	I: H–D O: D	Rare	Prior injury, even slight.	**Swelling, warmth in a confined area of the skin.**	Red streaks from the area to the trunk.	No	Antibiotics, maybe surgery.
Loiasis	I: 1 Y O: H–D; recurs	Rare	**Humid central or western Africa.**	**Bumps** that arise here and there, then disappear, size of small eggs.	Patient reports a worm in his eye.	Only at random times	Dewormers.

1 *Varies: this is whether the swelling gets better and worse with the limb up and down or if it stays the same all the time, regardless of limb position.*

2 *This is the time from starting the leprosy medication until the reaction occurs. It is not the incubation period for the leprosy itself.*

3 *This may be either over joints or adjacent to joints. It is usually not on a limb remote from a joint.*

Condition	Incubation; Onset	Group	Risk factors	Usual Symptoms	Common Symptoms	Varies[1]	Treatment
Likely a prominent skin condition, a large area swollen, swelling is not pitting							
Mossy foot	I: Y O:Years	Yes	**Barefoot on red clay soil in childhood.**	**1st burning & itching feet; then skin thickens, clumsy gait.**	Some symmetry; moves from feet to trunk.	Slightly at first	Shoes, soaking, maybe surgery.
Filariasis[2]	I: < 18 Mo O: < 2 Y	Usual	Tropical, humid, crowded.	**Comes and goes at first; skin rough.**	Maybe symmetry moves upper to lower.	At first only	Medicines early; surgery later.
Anthrax	I: D O: H-D	??	**Exposed to ill animals, meat, hides.**	Skin bump or ulcer, then fever and swelling.	**Severe swelling,** little pain, maybe itching.	No	Antibiotics.
Likely bumps and lumps, not tender, not symmetrical, swelling not pitting							
Cancer	I: N/A O: W–Y	No	HIV-positive, toxins, radiation, old age.	**Weight loss,** big lymph nodes, **not symmetrical.**	Painless at first.	No	Difficult and high-tech.
Cysticercosis	I: unknown O: ??	Rare	From pork tapeworm.	Muscles swollen and sore.	**"Split peas" under the skin.**	No	Not much.
Swelling is likely pitting; non-tender, symmetrical, whole circumference							
Heart failure	I: N/A O: varies	No	Western diet, rheumatic fever, infection.	**Fatigued or short of breath or both, symmetrical.**	Chest pain, heart murmur, fast respiration.	Yes	Special medicines, surgery.
Kidney disease	I: varies O: varies	No	Some illnesses and poisonings.	**High BP or abnormal urinalysis.**	Little urine or much protein in urine.	Yes	High-tech, and/ or difficult.
Liver failure	I: varies O: W–Y	No	Alcoholics, drugs and toxins.	**Jaundice or swollen abdomen.**	Skin spiders, fatigued, waddling gait.	Yes	Diet, maybe high-tech.
Malabsorption	I: varies O: varies	??	Any one of a large number of conditions.	**Severe diarrhea, weight loss.**	Swollen legs, worse the end of the day.	Yes	Variable.
Malnutrition	I: varies O: varies	Usual	Famine, poverty; cancer.	**Poor diet,** symmetrical swelling.	Swollen legs, worse the end of the day.	Yes	Good food.
Swelling non-symmetrical and tender; patient feverish & won't let you try to push on it							
Osteomyelitis	I: varies O: varies	No	Prior injury or illness.	**Severe bone pain, keeps awake at night,** fever.	Swelling feels hot, may see pus, one place.	No	Antibiotics, maybe surgery.
Pyomyositis	I: varies O: D-W	No	Prior injury or injection.	**Muscle pain,** one place.	Fever, swelling feels hot.	No	Drain pus and give antibiotics.

1 *Varies: this is whether the swelling gets better and worse with the limb up and down or if it stays the same all the time, regardless of limb position.*

2 *Coastal South America, the Caribbean and scattered areas throughout the tropics of the Eastern Hemisphere, especially in the Pacific. Only diagnose this if you see a lot of swollen limbs in the area.*

PROTOCOL B.7—LIVER [AND SPLEEN] ENLARGED (SWOLLEN ABDOMEN, JAUNDICE)

How to use this protocol

Outline of Symptoms and Conditions

Guide to Causative Diseases

B.7.A—Cirrhosis = slow-onset liver failure

B.7.B—Fulminant = rapid-onset liver failure

B.7.C—Common drugs and plants causing liver failure

B.7.D—Causes of ascites (free fluid in the abdomen)

B.7.E—Causes of a large spleen, no visible veins

B.7.F—Causes of KIDNEY DISEASE

B.7.G—Causes of JAUNDICE

B.7.H—Causes of easy bleeding

B.7.I—Causes of BRAIN DAMAGE

How to Use this Protocol

This protocol is for sorting out problems involving the liver and spleen. The first table and the following diagram with the rectangles and lines, serve as guides to the tables in the remainder of this protocol. The first column in the table lists various conditions; some of these conditions are syndromes (groups of symptoms) and some are disease clusters. The second and third columns define what you and the patient will observe, if he has the stated condition—what he is likely to complain of and what you will see when examining him.

If the symptoms and results of the physical exam fit **only one** of the conditions listed in Column 1, then go to the subsections of this protocol listed in Column 4. See also the other references given in Column 5.

If the patient shows symptoms and physical exam results that correspond to **more than one** of the conditions in Column 1, then he probably has liver failure.

There are two kinds of liver failure:

Cirrhosis or slow-onset develops over 6 months or more.

Fulminant or rapid-onset develops over less than 3 months.

If the problem has been going on for well over 6 months, then it is slow-onset, but if it has been developing for less than 3 months, then it may be either type. You can only wait and see.

You need to decide:

Does your patient have liver failure?

Which kind of liver failure does your patient have?

Which disease(s) is/are the likely cause(s)?

Might your patient have a treatable disease that mimics ordinary liver disease?

Might your patient be exposed to toxins that should be eliminated?

To do that, consult the diagram with the rectangles on the following page. Not all patients will have all conditions. Most will lack at least one. The causative disease(s) must also be treated. The urgency of referral is greater with rapid-onset than with slow-onset liver failure. Aside from high-tech facilities in the West, treatment of liver failure entails only supportive care. A patient is not likely to do better in a city hospital than in his or her own rural community.

Outline of Symptoms and Conditions

Conditions	Symptoms	Physical exam	Causative disease lists	Reference for diagnosis and diseases
Ascites: free fluid in abdomen.	Clothes fit tight, maybe ankle swelling.	Abdomen distended but not lumpy.	B.7.D, 1 for only ascites, no other conditions.	Volume 1, Chapter 1 Symptom Protocol A.46.
Large spleen without big veins on the abdominal wall.	Heavy, dragging feeling in the left upper abdomen.	Abdomen distended, you can feel a left upper abdominal mass.	B.7.A; B.7.D, 2 for only a large spleen, no big veins, no other conditions.	Volume 1, Chapter 1 Symptom Protocol A.46 Condition Index: TROPICAL SPLENOMEGALY.
Large spleen with big veins on the abdominal wall.	Heavy, dragging feeling in the left upper abdomen.	As above and the abdominal wall has bluish, wiggly veins.	B.7.A	Volume 1, Chapter 1 Symptom Protocol A.46 Condition Index: TROPICAL SPLENOMEGALY.
Kidney disease	Fatigue, little urine or abnormal urine.	High blood pressure, maybe nosebleeds, urinary body odor.	B.7.A; B.7.D, 3 for only kidney disease, no other conditions.	Volume 1, Chapter 1 Condition Index: KIDNEY FAILURE.
Jaundice	Yellow eyes, loss of appetite, dark urine, fatigue.	Yellow whites of the eyes; yellow below the tongue, bilirubin in urine.	B.7.A; B.7.B; B.7.D 4 for only jaundice, no other conditions.	Volume 1, Chapter 1 and Appendix 2;. Condition Index: JAUNDICE.
Bleeding	Nosebleeds, heavy periods, bloody urine, stool, vomits blood.	Urine tests positive for blood; there is spontaneous bruising.	B.7.A; B.7.B; B.7.D, 5 for only bleeding, no other conditions.	Volume 1, Appendix 2.
Brain damage	Difficulty understanding; moving uncoordinated.	Abnormal mental state, bizarre behavior or lethargy; trembling; uncoordinated.	B.7.A; B.7.B; B.7.D, 6 for only brain damage, no other conditions.	Condition Index: BRAIN DAMAGE.

Guide to Causative Diseases

The dark gray boxes state which disease lists apply to each of the conditions associated with liver and spleen problems below in the light gray boxes.

The white boxes below the conditions show the two types of liver failure caused by those conditions: cirrhosis and fulminant. Not all patients will have all of these conditions. Most will lack at least one.

B.7.A and B.7.B list the most common conditions which cause liver failure.

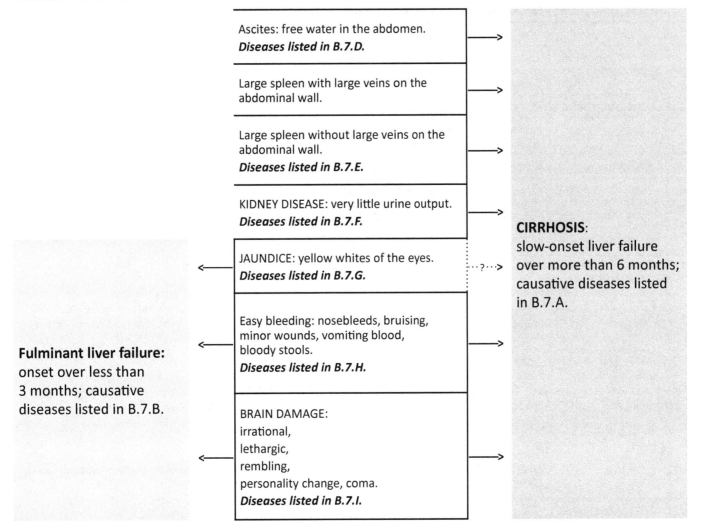

Ascites: free water in the abdomen.
Diseases listed in B.7.D.

Large spleen with large veins on the abdominal wall.

Large spleen without large veins on the abdominal wall.
Diseases listed in B.7.E.

KIDNEY DISEASE: very little urine output.
Diseases listed in B.7.F.

JAUNDICE: yellow whites of the eyes.
Diseases listed in B.7.G.

Easy bleeding: nosebleeds, bruising, minor wounds, vomiting blood, bloody stools.
Diseases listed in B.7.H.

BRAIN DAMAGE:
irrational,
lethargic,
rembling,
personality change, coma.
Diseases listed in B.7.I.

CIRRHOSIS:
slow-onset liver failure over more than 6 months; causative diseases listed in B.7.A.

Fulminant liver failure: onset over less than 3 months; causative diseases listed in B.7.B.

TOC · SYMPTOMS · DIFFERENTIALS · CONDITIONS · DRUG INDEX · REGIONAL NOTES · INX

B.7.A—Cirrhosis: slow-onset liver failure

Slow-onset, over more than 6 months. This is frequently due to ALCOHOLISM but may also be due to various drugs and poisonings as listed under B.7.C.

Condition	Usual Characteristics
Alcohol consumption[1]	Not a teetotaler; daily drinker or binge drinker.
Arsenic poisoning	Slow-onset; due to occupational exposure, ethnic remedies or homicidal intent.
Brucellosis	Pastoral area; exposed to cattle, hides, meat or unpasteurized milk.
Cancer	Varied; usually weight loss; liver may feel lumpy without being tender.
Drugs and herbs[2]	Ingests a liver-toxic substance.
Gallbladder disease	Pain or lump in upper central abdomen; may be tender; shoulder pain is common; may be associated with liver flukes.
Hemochromatosis	History of blood transfusion, high iron diet or heredity.
Hepatitis	Large, tender liver; frequently joint pains, nausea, jaundice.
Hydatid disease	1. Arid tropics with dogs or 2. Food gathered from temperate forests; mostly adults.
Schistosomiasis	Exposure to fresh-water snails in an area with S. Mansoni or S. Japonicum.

1 *Don't discount this diagnosis if the patient drinks but does not drink excessively. Some people have very sensitive livers which will fail with only a nightly glass of wine.*

2 *Of the drugs listed in this manual, it is likely one in which liver failure is listed as a side effect or a consequence of an overdose. Seek information on other drugs. Many natural herbs and ethnic remedies are toxic to the liver and might cause cirrhosis. See the drugs and herbs listed under B.7.B. Ingesting small amounts over a long period of time rather than a one-time overdose might result in cirrhosis rather than fulminant liver failure.*

B.7.B—Fulminant (rapid-onset) liver failure

Onset over less than 3 months: this is mostly due to drugs and poisons; PLANT POISONING from crotalaria and other bush teas; overdose of ACETAMINOPHEN; sometime from ISONIAZID and other medicines for TUBERCULOSIS.

Does or did the patient have a fever or severe abdominal pain and/or a general body illness?

YES	NO
|	The problem is probably due to drugs, or herbs. See the chart B.7.C (below) for the most common
|	offending substances.

Consider:	
Hepatitis	Obvious yellow whites of the eyes; poor sanitation or blood exposure.
Pancreatitis	Severe pains go to the back.
Leptospirosis	Exposure to flood waters or rat urine; erratic fevers; muscle pains, red eyes or both.
Malaria	Chills, headaches, cyclical or sustained fevers.
Toxemia	Related to pregnancy or delivery.
Yellow fever	Prominent headache, nausea, only Americas and Africa.

B.7.C—Common drugs and plants causing liver failure

Substance	Characteristics
Acetaminophen	Usually suicidal overdose.
Isoniazid	Tuberculosis drug, usually patients over 40 years old.
Chlorpromazine	Jaundice, light stool, dark urine, severe itching, rapid onset.
Gallbladder of raw fish	Chinese traditional medicine for poor eyesight.
Mushrooms	Those picked in the wild—usually more than 6 hours delay before symptoms occur.
Other drugs[1]	Usually only when used in excess, but may be quickly problematic in sensitive patients. See the list of drugs in the footnote.
Plant poisoning[2]	Most of these are used as "natural" herbal remedies. Some are used in herbal teas. Most people need to take large amounts before they get liver failure, but some people are very sensitive. See the list of plants in the footnote.

1 *Drugs known to cause liver failure: acetaminophen, acetazolamide, acyclovir, albendazole, atovaquone, cephalosporin (some kinds), chlorpromazine, cloxacillin, codeine, co-trimoxazole, dapsone, dicyclomine, diphenhydramine, doxycycline, furosemide, gentamycin, griseofulvin, halofantrine, hydralazine, hydrocortisone, ibuprofen, isoniazid, ketoconazole, levamisole, metronidazole, pyrazinamide, quinidine, quinine, rifampin, suramin, thiacetazone.*

2 *Plants known to cause liver failure: camphor. cascara sagrada. *castor beans. chaparral. *comfrey. *crotalaria. *ephedra. *heliotropium. *jequarity beans. *kavakava. kombucha. ma-huang. *margosa oil, pennyroyal oil, ricin, sassafras, *senecio, *valerian.*
Those herbs with * next to them have a more extensive description under PLANT POISONING in the Condition Index. For the others, you need to find independent information.

B.7.D—Causes of ascites (free fluid in the abdomen)

Condition	Characteristics
Cirrhosis[1]	Usually due to alcohol, HEPATITIS or SCHISTOSOMIASIS.
Abdominal tuberculosis	Children and others with only ascites, no other symptoms of liver failure; maybe numerous, pea-sized lumps in the abdomen. There is no swelling of the ankles and feet, no bilirubin in the urine.
Kidney disease (nephrotic)	Also urine contains much protein, swollen eyes in the morning, swollen ankles.
Heart failure	Difficulty breathing lying down or fatigued; heart murmur, infection or Western diet in an adult, swollen ankles the end of the day.
Malnutrition	Also swollen legs but no other symptoms of heart failure or kidney disease.
Malabsorption	Same as malnutrition; this is malnutrition due to losing foodstuff in the diarrhea.
Pericarditis	Swollen ankles, large liver, maybe abnormal heart sounds are very quiet or raspy.
Cancer (Rare)	May resemble abdominal TB.

1 *Initially there may not be big, easily visible veins on the abdominal wall, but eventually these will develop.*

TOC

SYMPTOMS

DIFFERENTIALS

CONDITIONS

DRUG INDEX

REGIONAL NOTES

INX

B.7.E—Causes of a large spleen, no visible veins (See also Protocols A.46, B.1)

Condition	Characteristics	Onset	Spleen huge?
Geographically very confined;			
African sleeping sickness	Sub-Saharan Africa only; changed mental state, fevers, whole-body illness.	Slow in west; over weeks in the east	Unknown
Bartonellosis	Peru area; ANEMIA also, maybe JAUNDICE.	Slow	
Chaga's disease	Americas only; HEART FAILURE also.	Slow	
Associated with an illness with a fever; onset less than a week			
Relapsing fever	Body lice associated with poor sanitation, rapid onset with severe prostration.	Over hours	No
Enteric fever	Unimmunized patient,[2] onset of abdominal symptoms over days, high fever.	Over days	No
Malaria	Humid tropics; chills, fevers, headaches, general body aching.	Rapid or slow	No
Mononucleosis	Tonsils look bad, extreme fatigue, child or adolescent.	Over days	No
Hereditary; family history			
Ovalocytosis	Hereditary ANEMIA, mostly Malaysian and Pacific islanders, some Europeans (spherocytosis).	Unknown	Unknown
Sickle cell disease	Hereditary, mostly West African genetic heritage, some Greeks, Arabs, Indians.	Rapid or slow	Yes
Thallasemia	Hereditary ANEMIA, Mediterranean, African or Asian genetic heritage.	Slow	Yes
Associated with a slow-onset illness			
Malaria	See TROPICAL SPLENOMEGALY.	Slow	Yes
Brucellosis	Joint pains, feels awful, pastoral area or patient consumed unpasteurized milk products. Especially common in the Middle East and Mediterranean areas.	Slow	No
Cancer	Frequently ANEMIA, maybe easy bleeding.	Slow	Maybe
Cirrhosis	See the page above with the diagrams.	—	—
Tuberculosis	Children, weight loss, loss of appetite, history of exposure to tuberculosis.	Slow	Unknown
Hydatid disease	Arid rural areas with dogs or temperate, forested areas, from gathering plants.	Slow	Yes
Visceral Leishmaniasis	Geographically confined--see the maps for your region; fevers, weight loss, night sweats, slow-onset illness.	Slow	Yes

1 Onset is rapid if it is over a week or less and the spleen is tender; it is slow if it is over more than three weeks. These designations are not absolute. Also, they refer to the spleen enlargement, not the disease onset. Generally rapidly enlarging spleens are tender to touch and slowly enlarging spleens are not.

2 That is, patients not immunized against typhoid fever.

B.7.F—Causes of KIDNEY DISEASE

See the listing under this title in the *Condition Index*. When kidney disease occurs as a result of liver failure, it presents as very little urine.

B.7.G—Causes of JAUNDICE

See the listing under this title in the *Condition Index*. If there is a fever, see Protocol B.5.

B.7.H—Causes of easy bleeding

There are five major categories of causes:
1. Liver problems, preventing the liver from making the chemicals necessary for normal clotting. In this case there will be other signs of liver failure: a large or tender liver, jaundice, ascites. The most common causes are alcoholism, certain drugs in sensitive people, various ethnic remedies, hepatitis and malnutrition.
2. Bone marrow or blood problems, preventing the proper number and/or function of platelets which are the blood cell fragments necessary to initiate clotting. Aspirin and ibuprofen are the most common drugs causing this.
3. Even with a healthy bone marrow, a large spleen is apt to destroy the platelets, leaving a dearth of functional platelets.
4. An overwhelming infection that causes abnormal clotting within the body, thus using up the clotting elements in the blood so that there is easy bleeding. Sepsis and Ebola virus disease are some examples.
5. Excessively fragile small blood vessels that burst at the slightest provocation. This is the least common cause.

B.7.I—Causes of BRAIN DAMAGE

See the listing under this title in the *Condition Index*.

▷ **SUPPORTIVE CARE if a history and physical exam are not possible.**

- Bedrest
- Low-fat diet; some authorities recommend low-protein also.
- Avoid any and all drugs, especially those that cause liver failure in overdose.
- Give multivitamins.
- Give supportive care (see Appendix 8.)

PROTOCOL B.8—EYES BOTH RED AND PAINFUL

See Introduction to Index B: notes on column headings and abbreviations.

Condition	Group	Risk factors	Ill?[1]	Usual elements	Common elements	Treatment
Symptoms predominantly eye rather than whole-body, no skin rash						
Old age	No	Age.	No	Slow onset.	Eyes dry and irritated.	Artificial tears.
Eye infection	Usual	Poor sanitation; flies.	No	More irritation than pain.	Eyes stick shut, maybe pus.	Antibiotics and antibiotic ointment.
Glaucoma (acute)	Maybe	Genetic heritage, old age.	Yes	Hard eyeballs.	Sudden nausea with the pain.	Ophthalmologist.
Iritis	Rare	Some illnesses, eye injury.	??	Pupil(s) not round.	Some other illness.	Ophthalmologist.
Loiasis[3]	Usual	Humid Africa only, fly bitten.	Maybe	Worm in the eye, comes and goes, no fever.	Worms cause swellings under the skin.	Deworming medicines, ophthalmologist.
Trachoma	Usually	Poor hygiene, flies.	No	Bumps under the upper lid; lashes scratch cornea.	Cloudy cornea starts on top.	Antibiotics, surgery.
Keratitis	Rare	Prior injury or infection.	Maybe	Cloudy corneas, severe pain, tearing.	White spot(s) on cornea(s).	Ophthalmologist.
Likely a prominent fever and generalized body pains, maybe a rash						
Arboviral fever	Usual	Residence; insect bitten.	Yes, severe	Fever, headache, aching all over.	Varies with the type.	Supportive, maybe high-tech.
Hemorrhagic fever[2]	Maybe	Residence; insect-bitten.	Yes, severe	Fever, headache, general body pain.	Bleeding.	High-tech, problematic.
Leptospirosis	**Usual**	**Exposed to flood water or rat urine.**	**Yes**	**Sudden onset, erratic fever, headache.**	**Sore muscles, calves, back.**	**Antibiotics, start within 4 days.**
Dengue fever	Usual	Child, urban, tropical Asia, Pacific; house plants.	Yes, severe	Sudden onset, high fever, headache, severe bone pain.	Rash, depression.	Supportive only.

1 Ill?—Is the patient generally ill with a whole-body illness (yes) or are only the eyes affected (no)?
2 Hemorrhagic fever—present in some scattered areas of Africa, southern Asia and the Americas. See Protocol B.2.
3. This is only found in humid western and central Africa.

SUPPORTIVE CARE

- Put in antibiotic eye drops every 2 hours.
- Use no antibiotic by mouth if the skin is blistering.
- Use DOXYCYCLINE with a whole-body illness, onset less than 4 days ago (LEPTOSPOROSIS).
- Use PENICILLIN if there is a skin condition without blistering.
- Use CHLORAMPHENICOL if there is visible pus or the eyeball is swollen

PROTOCOL B.9—ABDOMINAL PAIN WITH FEVER

Be sure to use the corrected body temperature. See Page A-5. See Introduction to **Index B**. Abbreviations for Incubation: (I) and Onset (O) times: Secs = seconds; Mi = minutes; H = hours; D = days; W = weeks; Mo = Months; Y = years.

Condition	Incubation; Onset	Group	Risk Factors[1]	Other symptoms[2]	Treatment
Prominent family history and recurrent					
Sickle cell disease	I: N/A O: H–D	Family	Genetic heritage.[3]	Anemia, recurrent painful crises of bone, abdomen, chest pain.	IV fluids, Special meds.
Familial Mediterranean fever	I: N/A O: H	Family	Genetic heritage.[4]	Family history of recurrent pains, and/or mental illness and/or rash.	Special meds.
Prominent headache and limb pains					
Arboviral fever	I: varies O: H–D	Usual	Residence, insect bitten.	Varies; maybe rash or mental changes.	Supportive[5] high-tech.
Enteric fever	I: 1–3 W O: D	??	Poor sanitation, not immunized.	Mentally 'out of it'; constipation early, diarrhea later; fever is sustained.	Antibiotics, supportive.
Relapsing fever louse or tick-borne	I: 2–14 D O: Mi–H	Usual	Crowding—lice Camp-ticks.	Onset over minutes; whole-body aching, headache; rash.	Antibiotics, supportive.
Scrub typhus	I: 4–11 D O: H–D	??	Asia-Pacific; chigger mites.	Red eyes, constipation, rash; eye pain, general body pain.	Antibiotics, supportive.
Ebola virus disease	I: 2–21 D O: H–D	Yes	Humans, bats, monkeys.	Vomiting, diarrhea, fatigue, maybe a rash, hiccups.	Supportive; maybe other.
Typhus, louse or murine	I: 6–14 D O: H-louse D-murine	??	Tropics, crowding, poor sanitation, rodents.	Other symptoms for days before the fever started; musty body odor; mental changes; headache; body pains; rash.	Antibiotics, supportive.
Dengue fever	I: 2–15 D O: H	Usual	Residence.	Severe bone pains, rash; headache; fever may drop and recur; depression.	Supportive only.
Pain all over the abdomen; headache and limb pains, if any, are not prominent.					
Kidney infection	I: varies O: H–W	Rare	Female, sexually active, poor.	Cloudy urine, usually mid-back pain also; prior bladder infection.	Antibiotics, ? surgery.
Strep infection	I: 1–4 D O: H-D	??	Exposed to strep infection.	Sore throat or skin infection.	Antibiotics.
Enteric fever	I: 1-3 W O: D	??	Poor sanitation, not immunized.	Mentally 'out of it'; constipation early, diarrhea later; fever is sustained.	Antibiotics, supportive.

1 *Not all patients will necessarily have a risk factor.*

2 *These are symptoms in addition to fever and abdominal pain and symptoms listed in subheadings. Not all patients will have all of these symptoms.*

3 *Usually African genetic heritage; some Arabs, Indians and Greeks are affected but usually not as severely as Africans*

4 *Heritage of one of the Mediterranean countries, particularly Greece, Turkey, Spain, Israel, Italy or North Africa.*

5 *This means simply making the patient comfortable. See Appendix 8.*

Condition	Incubation; Onset	Group	Risk factors	Other symptoms[6]	Treatment
Pain predominantly localized in the abdomen, below the navel					
Urinary infection	I: varies O: varies	No	Female, child or sexually active, poor hygiene.	Cloudy urine, painful urinating or incontinent; pain is lower abdomen.	Antibiotics, drink a lot of water, supportive.
Pelvic infection	I: D–Mo O: H–D	Usual	Sexually active female.	Pus from vagina or pain with intercourse; pain is lower abdomen.	Antibiotics, surgery.
Dysentery	I: D O: H–D	Usual	Poor sanitation, food and water.	Bloody diarrhea, small amounts frequently; pain is lower abdomen, either side or both sides.	Antibiotics, supportive.
Pain predominantly localized in the abdomen, at or above the navel					
Yellow fever[7]	I: 3–6 D O: 1–2 D	??	Residence, mosquitoes, unimmunized.	Headache, general aching, eye pain, maybe JAUNDICE, protein in urine; pain is upper right.	Supportive only.
Kidney infection	I: varies O: H–W	Rare	Female, sexually active, poor.	Cloudy urine, usually mid-back pain also, either side or both; prior bladder infection.	Antibiotics, maybe surgery.
Gallbladder disease	I: varies O: varies	??	Western diet, malaria, some worms.	Focus of pain upper central abdomen, maybe to shoulder; vomiting is common.	Higher-level care; surgical.
Malaria	I: varies O: H–D	Usual	Tropics, mosquito bitten.	Headache, waist pain, chills and sweats; pain left, shoulder pain, vomiting, diarrhea.	Antimalarials.
Mononucleosis	I: 1–2 M O: D	??	Age < 25 y.o.	Fatigue, large, tender spleen; large lymph nodes; sore throat.	Supportive only.
Pneumonia	I: varies O: H–1 D	Rare	Prior "cold".	Rapid respirations, cough with sputum, short of breath, pain is upper, either side.	Antibiotics, supportive.

6 *These are symptoms in addition to fever and abdominal pain; not all patients will have all of those listed.*

7 *This is present in scattered areas throughout Africa and in the Americas from 22° North to 28° South latitude.*

> ▷ **SUPPORTIVE CARE when obtaining a history and doing a physical exam are impossible.**
>
> - Bedrest
> - Gram-negative antibiotics
> - Bland, liquid diet
> - Antimalarial medications

TOC SYMPTOMS DIFFERENTIALS CONDITIONS DRUG INDEX REGIONAL NOTES INX

PROTOCOL B.10—LETHARGY OR CONFUSION

B.10.A—Lethargy or confusion plus a high fever
B.10.B—Lethargy or confusion, no fever or low fever

B.10.A—Lethargy or confusion plus a high fever

The fever does not have to be present currently; a history of a fever during this illness suffices. See Protocol B-10B for low or no fever. Be sure you use the corrected temperature. A high fever is a corrected temperature over 38.5°C/100.3°F.

Lethargy or confusion plus a fever is most likely due to a physical cause, though mentally disturbed patients can also get fevers for other reasons. In this case the mental symptoms predate the fever. See Protocol A.5. In elderly people, any simple infection such as urinary tract infection or pneumonia will cause confusion, possibly without a fever.

See Introduction to Index B: notes on column headings and abbreviations.
Abbreviations for Incubation (I) and Onset (O) times: Secs = seconds; Mi = minutes; H = hours; D = days; W = weeks; Mo = Months; Y = years.

Condition	Delay;[1] Onset	Group	Epidemics?	Risk factors	Other symptoms[2]	Treatment
Symptoms uncertain or variable						
Bartonellosis[3]	D: 2–16 W O:D–W	??	Maybe	**Residence in Peru and adjacent;** sand fly bites.	Fatigue, headache, joint pains, up and down fevers, short of breath.	Antibiotics.
HIV infection[4]	D: Years O: varies	Usual	Yes	Sexual or blood exposure; born to an infected mother.	**Recurrent infections; weight loss; diarrhea.**	Complicated Expensive.
Prominent headache plus significant whole-body pain						
Arboviral fever	D: varies O: H–D	??	Maybe	Residence, insect bites.	Varies with the type; see the Condition Index.	Supportive only.
Brucellosis	D: 2–4 W O: H–D	Unusual	Unlikely	Mediterranean and Middle East, cattle, unpasteurized milk.	**Headache, vomiting,** maybe seizures.	Multiple antibiotics for 6 weeks.
Leptospirosis	D: 3D–3W O: H	??	Maybe	Flood water; rat urine contact.	**Red eyes, muscle pains,** jaundice, liver pain.	Nothing helps.[5]
Spotted fever	D: 6–10 D O: H–D	??	Rare	Tick exposure; rural.	Rash starts on limbs..	Antibiotics.
Measles	D: 9–14 D O: D	Usual	Yes	Childhood, unimmunized, black skin, malnourished.	Initial 'cold'; **rash starts on the forehead; peeling skin late;** vomiting, diarrhea.	Supportive and antibiotics.

1 "Delay" is the time from first symptom to being lethargic or confused.
2 Symptoms in addition to fever and lethargy or confusion; not all patients will have all of those listed.
3 Found only in Peru and adjacent countries.
4 This usually manifests as follows: trouble concentrating, mood changes, disorientation, withdrawal, lethargy, talking nonsense, being "hyper", having totally irrational ideas.
5 Antibiotics are helpful for leptospirosis if they are begun within 4 days of first symptoms. By the time the patient is lethargic or confused, it will have been more than 4 days. Hence, antibiotics at this time are useless.

TOC

SYMPTOMS

DIFFERENTIALS

CONDITIONS

DRUG INDEX

REGIONAL NOTES

INX

Condition	Delay;[5] Onset	Groups?	Epidemics	Risk factors	Other symptoms[6]	Treatment
Prominent headache; not much other pain						
Encephalitis	D: varies O: H–D	??	Maybe	Viral illnesses and/or insect bites.	**Headache, numbness, weakness, clumsy, mental changes.**	Supportive.
Malaria, cerebral	D: N/A O: H–W	Rare	N/A	**Prior malaria,** tropical area.	Vomiting, seizures, headache, jaundice.	Antimalarials Antibiotics.
Meningitis	D: H–D O: H–D	Some kinds	Yes	Crowding, Africa, residence, not immunized.	Vomiting, **severe headache,** maybe stiff neck, peeling skin.	Antibiotics.
Heat illness	D: varies O: varies	Usual	Maybe	**Elderly, infants, exercising, hot environment.**	Sweaty or hot and dry; fever very high.	Cooling and high-tech.
Relapsing fever, tick or louse-borne	D: 2–14 D O: H	Usual	Yes	**Body lice, crowding; or tick exposure rural area.**	Headache, rapid onset, chills and sweats.	Antibiotics.
Toxoplasmosis	D: 1–3 W O: W-Mo	Rare	Rare	Exposure to lamb meat or cat stool; may be HIV+.	Big lymph nodes and/or spleen; weight loss, **prominent fatigue.**	Special meds.
African sleeping sickness[7]	D: D–Mo O: W–Y	Rare	Unusual	Residence, fly bite.	Increasing **sleepiness;** weight loss.	Difficult and dangerous.
Prominent headache plus significant other pain that likely is localized						
Enteric fever	D: 1–3 W O: D–W	??	Maybe	Poor sanitation; bad food or water.	**Abdominal symptoms; body odor like bread.**	Antibiotics.
Necrotizing fasciitis	D: unknown O: sudden	No	No	Prior wound; poor health.	**Very severe pain in a body part, with a prominent skin manifestation.**	Surgery.
Plague	D: 2–15 D O: H	Usual	Yes	Exposure to dead or dying rodents or to animal fleas.	**Extreme pain, rapid onset; blackened, painful lymph nodes.**	Antibiotics.
Brucellosis	D: 2–4 W O: W–Mo	Rare	Unusual	Pastoral area; meat, milk, cheese, hides.	**Complaining, joint pains and/or back pain; weight loss.**	3 antibiotics for 6 weeks.
Typhus; louse or murine (fleas)	D: 6–14 D O: D—W	Usual	Maybe	Exposure to lice or to rodent fleas.	**Ill for days before the fever starts; musty body odor; maybe rash, limb and back pains.**	Antibiotics.
Sepsis	D: varies O: varies	No	Yes	**Previous illness;** ill health; injury, childbirth, newborns.	Maybe heart murmur, short of breath, cloudy urine.	Antibiotics.

5 *"Delay" is the time from first symptom to being lethargic or confused.*

6 *These are symptoms in addition to fever and lethargy or confusion; not all patients will have all of those listed.*

7 *This is present in scattered areas of Africa from 15° north to 20° south. Both kinds are present in the Great Lakes area of eastern Africa. North and west of there it is mostly Gambian; south and east of there it is Rhodesian.*

B.10.B—Lethargy or confusion, no fever or low fever

Be sure you use the corrected temperature. See Page A-5. This protocol deals with decreased mental functioning—confusion or new-onset stupidity in the absence of a fever or in the presence of a low fever (under 38.5° C or 101.3° F).

—In newborns, the elderly, diabetics and those malnourished, see also B.10.A. These patients may not manifest a fever with diseases that ordinarily have high fevers.

—In elderly people, any simple infection such as a urinary tract infection or pneumonia will cause confusion.

—If a person cannot talk, he will appear to be confused; check his ability to speak by telling him what to say, having him repeat after you. If he cannot speak, ask him to look up or look down and see if he follows your command. There is a rare condition in which a patient cannot respond in any way except to look up or down, yet he is totally alert and needs to be treated as such—talked to, entertained, included in conversation, comforted. Confusion may also arise from Alzheimer disease, which is decreased mental functioning without another reason.

See Introduction to Index B: notes on column headings and abbreviations.
Incubation (I) and Onset (O) times: secs = seconds; Mi = minutes; H = hours; D = days; W = weeks; Mo = Months; Y = years.

Condition	Delay;[1] Onset	Group	Risk factors[2]	Other symptoms[3]	Treatment
Prominent emotional component likely; related to a bad diet					
Beriberi	D: W–Mo O: W–Mo	Usual	Poor diet; alcohol consumption; white rice.	Unaware; wide-based gait, heart failure, weight loss, weak.	Thiamine, diet.
Pellagra	D: varies O: D–Mo	Usual	Poor diet; only one kind of grain, usually corn.	Diarrhea; rough rash; may be unaware.	Vitamins, diet.
Prominent emotional component likely, not related to diet					
Addiction	D: N/A O: W–Y	N/A	Recreational drug usage.	Varies with the type of addiction; denial is common.	Difficult.
Attention deficit disorder (crisis)	D: N/A O: H	N/A	Western culture, male, heredity.	Adjustment problems since childhood.	Counseling, special meds.
Demonization	D: N/A O: varies	??	Occult activity or cursed.	Symptoms don't make medical sense; religious context.[4]	Prayer and exorcism; godly national pastors may be helpful.
Stress	D: N/A O: varies	N/A	Emotional problems; personal disaster.	Trembling, crying, insomnia; patient is aware of the problem.	Emotional support and counseling.
Alcoholism	D: N/A O: W–Mo	N/A	Daily or binge drinking.	Denial is common; distended abdomen, red nose.	Counseling.

1 *"Delay" is the time from the first symptom to being lethargic or confused.*

2 *Patients do not necessarily have risk factors; these are relatively sensitive, but not completely.*

3 *These are symptoms in addition to the confusion or lethargy. Not all patients will have all the other symptoms.*

4 *"Context" refers to problems arising during religious experience: either Christian worship, in which case it may be disruptive activity or participation in some occult ritual.*

Confusion or lethargy, no fever or low fever, concluded.

Condition	Delay;[5] Onset	Groups?	Risks Factors	Other symptoms[6]	Treatment
Likely related to a short-term event or illness, rapid onset likely					
Distinctive history					
Dehydration[7]	D: N/A O: varies	N/A	Vomiting, diarrhea, not drinking, diabetes.	**Very dry mouth, sunken eyes, loose skin, thirsty if conscious.**	Fluids; treat the causative condition(s).
Hypothermia	D: N/A O: H	Maybe	Cold exposure, very young and very old.	**Low body temperature, below 36.4°/97.6°.**	Warming.
Malaria (PMNS)	1W-2M after malaria Rx	No	**Successfully treated severe malaria.**	Incoordination, maybe seizures.	Prednisone.
Head injury	D: N/A O: Mi-D	N/A	Epilepsy, adventurous sorts, young males.	Headache, vomiting, seizures, abnormal movements.	Hospitalization, surgery.
History may or may not be distinctive					
Drug side effect	D: N/A O: varies	No	Taking a new drug, especially elderly.	Varies with the type.	Stop the drug if possible.
Lyme disease[8]	D: 3-32 D O: Mo	Rare	Temperate, rural; tick bitten.	Prior rash, arthritis and ill health.	Antibiotics.
Seizure[9]	D: N/A O: secs	Rare	Epilepsy, head injury; in a child sudden onset of fever.	Rhythmic jerking of limbs, eyes or facial muscles.	Special medicines.
Stroke	D: N/A O: < 1 Mi	No	High blood pressure; elderly; sickle cell anemia.	Sudden onset of weakness or paralysis, speech problem.	Special medicines and/or procedures.
Plant poisoning	D: varies O: varies	??	Ethnic remedies.	Varies according to type.	Varied.
Meningitis[10]	D: varies O: H-Mo	Rare	Newborns, elderly, previous tuberculosis, crowding.	Headache, stiff neck, vomiting, cough, abnormal eye movements	Antibiotics.

5 *"Delay" is the time from the first symptom to being lethargic or confused.*

6 *These are symptoms in addition to the confusion or lethargy. Not all patients will have all the other symptoms.*

7 *This is a condition but not a diagnosis. You still must find out what caused the dehydration.*

8 *This may be acquired in subtropical and temperate regions, not the tropics.*

9 *"Seizure" is a condition but not a diagnosis. You still must find out why the patient has seizures. It is important to check for subtle seizure activity; blinking, twitching, lip-smacking or any apparently automatic, repetitive movement (status epilepticus). If you find such repetitive motions, stopping them is an emergency. Seek higher-level care immediately.*

10 *Meningitis usually causes a fever. However, in newborns (less than 4 weeks old), in the elderly and in anyone who is malnourished, there may be little or no fever.*

▷ **SUPPORTIVE CARE**
• PENICILLIN for tertiary SYPHILIS if the patient is unaware of his mental state • Nutritional, low-salt diet • Treat dehydration with fluids • Stop any new drugs if possible • Use PREDNISONE if there is a history of recent malaria

PROTOCOL B.11—SKIN ULCER AND WHOLE-BODY ILLNESS

The conditions marked with * do not by themselves cause a general illness, but they may have a secondary infection. Bold faced items are relatively sensitive.

See Introduction to *Index B*: notes on column headings and abbreviations. Bold-face characteristics are sensitive.

Abbreviations for Incubation (I) and Onset (O) times: Secs = seconds; Mi = minutes; H = hours; D = days; W = weeks; Mo = Months; Y = years.

Condition	Incubation;[1] Onset	Group	Risk factors	Usual location	Other characteristics	Treatment
Probably not round or oval; likely an irregular broken-open area						
Cancrum oris	I: ?? O: H–D	No	Malnourished child.	Face or a sucked finger.	**Dead-looking flesh; foul odor to the pus.**	Surgery, diet, antibiotics.
Gangrene	I: ?? O: varies	No	Severe injury or ill health, poor nutrition.	Injured part or fingers or toes.	**Dead-looking flesh;** pain, numbness.	Surgery and antibiotics.
Tuberculosis	I: ?? O: W–Mo	Usual	**Patient or family member has/had tuberculosis.**	Head and neck; may be elsewhere.	Varies very much.	TB medicines.
Syphilis, tertiary	I: years O: Mo	No	**Patient, partner or parent exposed.**	Anywhere.	**Scalloped edges,** large ulcer from merging small ulcers.	Penicillin.
Necrotizing fasciitis	I: D O: H–D	No	**Some minor wound.**	Anywhere.	**Very rapid progression, very severe pain.**	Antibiotics, surgery.
Likely a discreet, round or oval skin sore, probably more than 2 cm in diameter						
Amebic skin ulcer	I: ?? O: D–Mo	No	Poor sanitation, prior dysentery.	**Trunk or genitals only.**	**Painful; discharges pus or another liquid.**	Metronidazole, maybe surgery.
Bedsores	I: ?? O: D	No	Bedridden patient, not moving about.	**Body surface with constant pressure.**	First red and swollen; patient either very ill or paralyzed.	Wound care; see Tropical ulcer.
Buruli ulcer	I: ?? O: W	??	Tropics, swamps.	Limbs.	Ragged, **overhanging edges.**	Surgery.
Diphtheria	I: D O: D	Maybe	**Unimmunized;** urban areas.	Anywhere.	**Doughnut rim; painful,** moist.	Antitoxin; antibiotics.
Rat bite fever	I: 3–30 D O: D–W	??	Rodent bite or urine exposure; mostly Asia.	Limbs but it can be anywhere.	**Healed and then broke open or a generalized rash.**	Antibiotics.
Tropical ulcer	I: ?? O: W	??	Tropics; poor hygiene, malnutrition.	Usually legs, feet.	Gradual onset, **first swollen then breaks open and enlarges.**	Antibiotics, supportive.

1 *Incubation: many of these diseases are late complications so that the incubation cannot be known.*

Skin ulcer plus whole-body illness, concluded.

Condition	Incubation;[2] Onset	Group	Risk factors	Usual location	Other characteristics	Treatment
Likely a discreet, round or oval skin sore, size quite variable						
Anthrax	I: 1–3 D O: D	??	Contact with sick animals, hides, meats, bioterrorism.	Above the waist.	Not painful but may itch; **much swelling; black scab.**	Antibiotics, supportive.
Tularemia	I: 1–14 D O: H–D	Maybe	Small animal exposure, 'temperate climates.	Anywhere.	General flu-like illness, bedridden early.	Special antibiotics.
Sexually transmitted disease[3]	I: varies O: D–W	Usual	Sexual, or health care exposure.	**Exposed to secretions: genitals, hands, face.**	Varies by the type of disease; see protocol B.1.	Antibiotics, surgery.
Likely discreet, round or oval scab(s) less than 1 cm in diameter						
Plague	I: 2–15 D O: H–D	Usual	Contact with other cases or with rodents or their fleas.	Limbs but it can be anywhere.	**Big lymph nodes with blackened skin over top**; tiny scab.	Antibiotics, supportive.
Scrub typhus	I: D–W O: D–W	??	**Rural tropical Asia Pacific,** chigger mite bite.	Commonly genital or lower limbs.	Headache, **red eyes**, large spleen, **constipation.**	Antibiotics, supportive.
Spotted fever (Eastern Hemisphere}	I: < 12 D O: D	??	Mostly Africa and the Mediterranean; tick bites; **rural areas.**	Anywhere.	Headache, stiff neck, red eyes, rash heaviest on the wrists and the ankles.	Antibiotics, supportive.
Spotted fever (Rocky Mountain)[5]	I: 6–10 D O: D	??	North, Central and South America; tick bites; **rural areas.**	Anywhere.	Headache, fatigue, joint and muscle pains, rash heaviest on the wrists and the ankles.	Antibiotics,[4] supportive.
Tularemia[6]	I: 1–14 D O: H–D	Rare	Residence; child or hunter; rural.	Upper or lower limbs; anywhere.	**Exposure to a small animal or insect.**	Antibiotics, supportive.

3 *This includes chancroid, Donovanosis, herpes, lymphogranuloma venereum, syphilis.*
4 *These must be started on the mere suspicion of the disease. The blood tests don't turn positive until the patient is beyond hope of survival.*
5 *This occurs throughout the United States, Central America and northern South America, not just near the Rocky Mountains.*
6 *This occurs in the Northern Hemisphere, temperate and sub-tropical, as far south as the northern coast of Africa.*

▷ SUPPORTIVE CARE if you can't begin to get a history.

- Provide local treatment, keeping the ulcer clean, dry and covered.
- Provide a high-protein diet.
- Use METRONIDAZOLE for ulcers between the waist and upper thighs or if there is a rotten odor.
- Use DOXYCYCLINE if the patient has a fever.
- Treat for a genital ulcer (Protocol B.1) if the patient is sexually active or abused.

PROTOCOL B.12—LARGE LYMPH NODES WITH FEVER

The corrected body temperature is over 37.1°/99°

Incubation (I) and Onset (O) times: Secs = seconds; Mi = minutes; H = hours; D = days; W = weeks; Mo = Months;

Reliable elements of the diagnosis are **bold-face**.

Condition	Incubation; Onset	Group	Related wound[1]	Risk factors	Specific characteristics	Treatment
Prominent rash likely						
Strep infection	I: 1–4 D O: H–D	??	No	Child, young adult, poor hygiene, crowding.	**Sore throat; rapid onset; no cold symptoms; red tonsils.**	Antibiotics.
Measles	I: 9–14 D O: D	Usual	No	**Unimmunized**; crowding.	**Red eyes**, cough, fever, vomiting, diarrhea.	Vitamin A, supportive.
Drug eruption	I: N/A O: H–D	No	No	Western culture; drug usage.[2]	**Related in time to taking the drug.**	Stop drug.
Prominent swelling likely						
Anthrax	I: <7 D O: H–D	??	Yes	**Cattle, meat, hides, bioterrorism.**	**Marked swelling**; sore with black scab, not painful.	Antibiotics.
Chaga's disease[3]	I: varies O: D–W	??	No	**Residence**; poor housing.	**History of swollen eye;** constipation, or heart failure.	Difficult.
Skin condition in relationship to the nodes with no or only a trivial injury history						
African sleeping sickness[4]	I: varies O: D–Mo[5]	Rare	No	**Residence**; fly bite.	Headache, fevers off & on; swelling of bite site.	Difficult and dangerous.
Cellulitis	I: varies O: H–D	Rare	Maybe	Minor wound, poor hygiene.	**Area of redness and swelling;** maybe fever; **tender.**	Antibiotics.
Plague	I: 2–15 D O: H–D	??	Yes	Rodent flea or patient contact.	Little scab(s), pain; skin blackened; fevers, **mental changes.**	Antibiotics.
Scrub typhus	I: 3–10 D O: H–D	??	Yes	**Rural Asia Pacific;** bitten by mite.	Moderately very ill; fevers, rash, **constipation, eye problems.**	Antibiotics.
Tularemia	I: 1–14 D O: H–D	Rare	Yes	**Contact-small mammal or insects, rural.**	Fever, general whole-body illness, **red bumps by wound.**	Antibiotics.

1 *Related wound indicates whether one is likely to see an open wound nearby or on a limb beyond the location of the large lymph nodes.*

2 *These drugs are common causes: allopurinol; cephalosporins; hydralazine; penicillin; phenytoin; pyrimethamine; quinidine; sulfa.*

3 *Chaga's occurs in scattered areas in the Americas between the 41° south and the northern border of Mexico. The Caribbean and the Amazon basin are largely spared.*

4 *This is present in scattered areas of Africa, from 15° north to 20° south. See Regional Notes F.*

5 *In western Africa the large nodes develop within weeks to months; in eastern Africa they may develop rapidly, within days to weeks.*

Large lymph nodes with fever, concluded.

Condition	Incubation; Onset	Group	Related wound[6]	Risk factors	Specific characteristics	Treatment
Skin near the large nodes has a history of sexual contact						
Sexually transmitted disease	I: varies O: varies	Usual	Yes	**Sexual contact or contact with secretions.**	Usually genital symptoms or history thereof; not very ill.	Antibiotics.
Skin near the nodes or beyond them suffered a significant wound.						
Wound infection	I: varies O: H–D	No	Yes	Poor sanitation, **dirty wound, poor nutrition.**	Maybe fever, visible pus, bad odor.	Surgery, antibiotics.
Cat-scratch disease	I: 3–30 D O: H–D	Rare	Yes	**Cat contact, scratch or licking open wound.**	Lumps in a line between wound and trunk.	Antibiotics, supportive.
Tularemia	I: 1–14 D O: H–D	Maybe	Yes or tonsillitis	**Northern Hemisphere, temperate.**	Skin wound; large, red tonsil; or an eye infection.	Special antibiotics.
Prominent joint pains or history thereof, onset over hours to days						
Serum sickness Katayama disease	I: ? D–W O: H–D	No	No	Western culture; drug usage,[7] some illnesses.	**Fever plus allergy symptoms**; hives, joint pains.	Special.
Prominent joint pains or history thereof, onset over weeks or more						
Arthritis rheumatoid	I: N/A O: W	No	No	Western culture; old age, females, affluent.	**Symmetrical joint pains migrate; morning stiffness.**	Anti-inflammatory.
Brucellosis	I: 2–4 W O: W–Mo	Rare	No	Pastoral areas or raw milk, cheese, meat, hides.	Pains in back and/or lower limbs; **complaints of feeling awful.**	3-antibiotic combination.
Lyme disease[8]	I: 3–32 D O: W	Rare	No	Residence; **rural; tick bite.**	**Fevers and rash or history of such, joint pains.**	Antibiotics, supportive.
Likely very slow onset or recurrent symptoms						
Cancer	I: N/A O: W–Mo	No	Maybe	Old age; HIV infection, toxins.	Weight loss; fatigue; easy bleeding; **nodes hard or matted.**	High-tech.
Tuberculosis	I: M–Y O: W–Mo	Usual	No	Young person, contact with a coughing adult.	Beer-like odor; **neck nodes not tender,** may be matted.	Special medications.
HIV infection	I: Y O: W–Mo	Usual	Maybe	Sexual or blood exposure.	**Repeated infections; weight loss, diarrhea,** mental changes.	Difficult expensive.
Prominent severe fatigue likely, onset over hours to days						
Mononucleosis	I: 1–2 Mo O: H–D	??	No	**Child (national), teenager (expatriate).**	**Extremely tired;** large tonsils with scum; fever, sore throat.	Supportive.

6 *Related wound indicates whether one is likely to see an open wound nearby or on a limb beyond the location of the large lymph nodes.*

7 *These drugs are commonly involved: allopurinol; cephalosporins; hydralazine; penicillin; phenytoin; pyrimethamine; quinidine; sulfa.*

8 *Lyme disease is found, at present, in temperate and subtropical areas of the Northern Hemisphere plus along the north coast of Australia.*

TOC SYMPTOMS DIFFERENTIALS CONDITIONS DRUG INDEX REGIONAL NOTES INX

PROTOCOL B.13—BACK PAIN WITH FEVER

Be sure to use the corrected body temperature. See Page A-5.

See Introduction to Index B: notes on column headings and abbreviations.

Abbreviations for Incubation (I) and Onset (O) times: Secs = seconds; Mi = minutes; H = hours; D = days; W = weeks; Mo = Months; Y = years.

Abbreviations for Midline?: is the pain in the midline (center line) of the back or is it off to one or both sides? M = midline; S = sides; B = both; ?? = unknown or variable.

Condition	Incubation; Onset	Group	Risk factors[1]	Type of pain	Midline?	Other characteristics[2]	Treatment
Prominent mental symptoms							
Typhus	I: 6–14 D O: D	??	Lice or rodent flea exposure.	Part of body pains; rash.	B	Lethargic; **musty body odor, mental changes.**	Antibiotics.
Meningitis	I: varies O: H–W	??	Residence; epidemics; tuberculosis.	Neck pain; lies arched back.	M	**Headache,** vomiting; mental changes.	Antibiotics.
Pain probably not symmetrical right and left							
Pneumonia	I: varies O: H–D	Rare	Poor immunity; children; prior cold.	**Chest area; worse with breathing.**	S	Cough, rapid or slow breathing.	Antibiotics.
Polio	I: ?? O: D	??	Unimmunized; child.	**Muscle spasms.**	S	Some weakness, **not totally symmetrical.**	Supportive.
Kidney infection	I: ?? O: H–W	No	Female; sexually active; previous urine infections.	One or both sides, just above waist.	S	**Tenderness** to gentle punch; cloudy urine, leukocytes on urine dipstick.	Antibiotics.
Very slow onset or recurrent, maybe with a family history							
Brucellosis	I: 2-4 W O: W–Mo	Rare	Hides, meat, milk, especially Mediterranean and Middle East areas.	Lower back, slow onset.	M, S[4]	**Feels generally awful,** leg weakness, maybe numbness.	3 antibiotic combination.
Sickle cell disease[3]	I: N/A O: H–D	Family	**Genetic heritage;** any stress.	Variable.	??	**Anemia;** bone pains, stress.	Varies, mostly high-tech.
Tuberculosis	I: W–Y O: Mo–Y	Usual	Exposed to a coughing adult or coughs.	**One part** of spine painful and tender.	M	Maybe cough, weight loss, night sweats, maybe a midline bump.	Special drugs.

1 *A patient will not necessarily have one of the risk factors, but if he does, the diagnosis is more likely.*

2 *These are symptoms in addition to the back pain and fever. Not all patients will have all of these symptoms.*

3 *This affects persons of African, Arab, Indian and Greek genetic heritage.*

4 *In the upper back it is apt to be midline; in the lower back it is apt to be on either one or both sides.*

Part of general, whole-body pain, including headache and symmetrical limb pains.							
Condition	Incubation; Onset	Groups	Risk factors	Type of pain	Midline?	Other characteristics[5]	Treatment
Distinctive history likely							
Tetanus	I: 4–20 D O: H–D	No	**Prior burn or wound; not immunized.**	General muscle spasms; stiff neck.	B	**Can't open mouth**, grimacing.	Mostly high-tech.
Trench fever	I: 4–36 D O: H–W	Usual	**Refugee, urban, body lice.**	Part of general body pains.	M	**Shin pains**, headache.	Antibiotics, supportive.
Trichinosis	I: <30 D O: D–W	Usual	**Ate rare pork or game within the past month.**	Muscles swollen and very sore.	S	Patient looks muscular, weight loss.	Varies.
Rabies	I: 4D–Y O: H–D	Rare	**Bitten by mammal;** not immunized; bat exposure.	Muscle spasms; stiff neck.	M	**Can't swallow water**, headache, maybe paralysis.	Supportive until death.
Distinctive history less likely, still possible							
Leptospirosis	**I: 3D–3W O: H–D**	??	**Exposure to flood waters, rodents, urine.**	**General joint pains.**	U	Red eyes, jaundice, muscle pains, rash.	**Antibiotic started within 4 days.**
Malaria	I: 3D–3W O: H–W	Usual	Tropics; mosquito bitten, pregnant, no prophylaxis.	Shoulder area, waist, other joints.	B	**Headache, chills, sweats**; spleen pain.	Antimalarials.
Dengue fever	I: 2–15 D O: H	Usual	Tropical especially Asia-Pacific; urban; house plants.	**Severe general bone pains.**	B	Rash, depression, red eyes, fever may relapse.	Pain meds only.
Relapsing fever	I: 2–14 D O: H	Usual	Lice or tick exposure; poor sanitation.	Part of body pains, **calf pain.**	B	Chills/sweats the same day.	Antibiotics, supportive.
Spotted fever	I: <14 D O: varies	??	Residence; tick exposure.	Part of general body pains.	??	**Red spotted or blistery rash.**	Antibiotics, supportive.
Arboviral fever	I: varies O: H–D	Usual	Residence, insect bitten.	Part of general whole-body pains.	??	Headache, rash, red eyes, sore muscles.	Supportive, maybe higher level care.

5 *Symptoms in addition to the back pain and fever. Not all patients will have all of these symptoms.*

PROTOCOL B.14—MALABSORPTION (Severe Diarrhea)

Malabsorption is the prompt fecal elimination of anything eaten, severe enough to cause weight loss.
See Introduction to Index B: notes on column headings and abbreviations.

Abbreviations for Incubation (I) and Onset (O) times: Secs = seconds; Mi = minutes; H = hours; D = days; W = weeks;
Mo = Months; Y = years.

Condition	Incubation; Onset	Group	Risk factors	Sensitive characteristics	Specific characteristics	Treatment
Related to a poor or strange diet; onset slow, over weeks or months						
Capillariasis[1]	I: ?? O: W	??	Residence, **ate raw fish.**	Loud bowel sounds, loss of appetite.	Same.	Dewormers.
Pellagra	I: N/A O: D–W	Usual	**Corn diet,** malnutrition.	Rash on sun-exposed skin.	Mental symptoms, burning foot pain.	Vitamins, Niacin.
Intestinal fluke[2]	I: 2–3 Mo O: W–Mo	??	**Raw fish or water plants; poor sanitation.**	Abdominal pain, body swelling, abdominal fluid.	Same.	Special meds.
Related to something eaten or drunk immediately before; onset less than a week						
Milk intolerance	I: N/A O: Mi–H	No	Genetic heritage; child; recently sick.	Vomiting, gas.	Only with milk products.	Diet or lactase.
Pig-bel	I: 1–7 D O: H–D	Usual	Near equator; meat meal after malnutrition.	Severe abdominal pain.	Bloody stool, diarrhea.	Antibiotics Surgery.
Plant poisoning	I: varies O: Mi–H	Rare	Herbal remedies.	Varies; maybe severe pain; vomiting.	History of ingestion or homicidal attempt.	Various.
Vomiting likely; onset less than a week						
Cryptosporidiosis	I: 1–14 D O: Mi–H	Usual	Children; HIV+; poor sanitation.	Cramping, vomiting, gas.	Diarrhea is explosive.	Antibiotics, supportive.
Cyclosporiasis[3]	I: 1–11 D O: Mi–H	Usual	Residence; spring and summer; poor sanitation.	Vomiting, much gas, fatigue, maybe fever.	Geography.	Antibiotic, supportive.
Giardiasis[4]	I: 1–45 D O: Mi–H	Usual	Water; poor sanitation.	Vomiting, much gas, no fever.	Loss of appetite, explosive diarrhea, loud bowel sounds.	Metronidazole, Tinidazole, supportive.
Pancreatitis	I: N/A O: H–D	No	Adults; alcohol, injury, gallstones.	**Severe pain goes to back**; vomiting.	Same; maybe symptoms of DIABETES.	Hospitalization.

1 *Capillariasis: currently known to be in parts of the Philippines, Thailand, Java and Egypt. There is potential for its spreading to other areas.*

2 *Most kinds of intestinal flukes don't cause malabsorption. The kind that does, fasciolopsiasis, is found only in Asia.*

3 *Cyclosporiasis may be locally common in scattered areas worldwide. At present it is mostly found in Nepal and Latin America.*

4 *Giardiasis: very common worldwide in Arctic, temperate and tropical areas. It is by far the most common cause of malabsorption in most areas.*

Malabsorption concluded.

Condition	Incubation; Onset	Group	Risk factors	Sensitive characteristics	Specific characteristics	Treatment
Large liver, bloody stool or free fluid in the abdomen likely; slow onset						
Schistosomiasis Japonicum[5]	I: Y O: D–W	??	Residence; fresh water with snails.	Exposure to fresh water in an endemic area.	Bloody stool; fluid in abdomen; liver disease.	Praziquantel.
Schistosomiasis Mansoni[6]	I: Y O: D–W	??	Residence; fresh water with snails; adult.	Exposure to fresh water in an endemic area.	Maybe bloody stool; fluid in abdomen; liver disease.	Praziquantel Artemisinin.
Sore mouth and mental changes						
Sprue[7]	I: < 6 Mo O: varies	Rare	Residence; adult; expatriates.	Residence, gradual onset.	Much gas, mental symptoms, mouth pain, red tongue.	Antibiotics Vitamins.
Visible abnormality by the rectum						
Strongyloidiasis	I: ?? O: varies	??	Residence; poor sanitation, sandy soil.	Residence in a community where this is known to occur.	Itching by rectum, visible worms, maybe bloody stool.	Dewormers.
Trichuriasis	I: ?? O: D–W	??	Poor sanitation, clay soil, humid areas.	Residence in a community where this is known to occur.	Visible coiled worms; maybe bloody stool; cravings.	Dewormers.
History of exposure to a tuberculous adult or unpasteurized milk products						
Tuberculosis	I: Mo–Y O: W–Mo	Rare	Poverty; crowding; raw milk or cheese.	Residence in a community where TB is common.	Possibly right lower abdominal pain, swelling, and/or tenderness.	Special meds Antibiotics.

5 *Schistosomiasis Japonicum: some scattered areas within Asia, including the SEA islands.*
6 *Schistosomiasis Mansoni: some scattered areas within Africa and the Americas.*
7 *Sprue: present mainly in Asia and the Caribbean.*

PROTOCOL B.15—WHOLE-BODY SWELLING

Detecting swelling by physical examination: in trichinosis, muscles are swollen, so gravity does not affect the swelling. In other kinds of swelling gravity tends to pull the swelling down. Hence, in standing patients, it is the legs, ankles and feet that are swollen. In bedridden patients, it is the small of the back that is swollen, sometimes the buttocks also. Press your thumb firmly.

Condition	Onset	Fever[1]	Groups?	History	Sensitive	Specific	Treatment
Arms also swollen; patient looks muscular, upper and lower body similarly swollen							
Trichinosis	Hours to days	Usual	Usual	Ate poorly cooked game or pork.	Muscle pains, weight loss.	**Muscle pains, muscles swollen, looks muscular.**	Deworming maybe prednisone.
Related to poor diet							
Beriberi	Weeks to months	No	Usual	Diet of white rice or any one grain.	**Weak muscles, can't exercise well.**	Rapid response to treatment.	Thiamine, no diuretics
Malnutrition	Weeks to months, usually	Unusual	Usual	Poverty, **famine conditions.**	Thin upper arms, low BMI.	Hair color changes, flaky skin.	Food, initially low-protein, warmth.
Likely a fever							
Sepsis Ebola virus disease	Variable	Usual	No	**Prior infection, Exposure to a prior patient.**	Fever or abnormally low temperature.	Mental changes, low blood pressure.	No diuretics! Give IV fluids.
Tuberculosis[2]	Weeks to months	Usual	Maybe	Cough or TB exposure.	**Poor appetite.**	Cough, bloody sputum, weight loss.	TB meds plus diet.
Likely normal urinalysis and no fever							
Heart failure[3]	Variable	Maybe	No	Sore throat, Western lifestyle.	Excessive fatigue or **can't exercise well.**	Short of breath lying down; tender large liver or both.	Diuretics, sit up to sleep; referral.
Thyroid trouble	Months	Low body temperature	Unusual	Recent child-birth, swelling lower front neck.	Very tired all the time, sleeps a lot.	**Low body temperature,** slow pulse, hair and skin changes.	Thyroid hormone.
Likely an abnormal urinalysis and no fever							
Kidney disease	Variable	Maybe	No	Malaria, urinary complaints.	BP high, abnormal urine dipstick result.	**Face swollen in the morning,** body odor of urine, white flakes on skin.	Referral, diuretics, blood pressure meds.
Liver failure	Weeks to months, usually	Unusual	No	Hepatitis, consumption of alcohol or ethnic medicines.	**Bilirubin in urine.**	Yellow whites of eyes.	Diet and multivitamins; referral usually not helpful.

1 *Be sure you are using the corrected body temperature. See Page A-5.*
2 *With tuberculosis, the decrease in appetite is the cause of malnutrition which causes swelling.*
3 *Consider that beri-beri might be a cause of heart failure. It partakes of the characteristics of both heart failure and malnutrition.*

INDEX C: CONDITION INDEX

CONDITION CLASSIFICATION

Class 1: you can treat safely, assuming a correct diagnosis.

Class 2: you will have an occasional death or disability that a medical profession would not.

Class 3: you will mistreat 20%–80% of patients.

Class 4: you will mistreat 80% or more of patients whom a doctor could adequately treat.

TERMINOLOGY

Who = what habits, foods and other factors tend to provoke the condition

y.o. = years old

Send out = arrange transportation to a hospital

Levels of care:

1 = village clinic with a health worker

2 = hospital in a developing area with some local physician staff

3 = hospital in a developing area, specialty or expatriate staff, surgical, lab, imaging facilities

4 = major referral hospital in a developing country or a community hospital in a Western country

5 = referral hospital in a Western country

Results = time after initiating treatment when you should see some improvement

Entry category:

disease = a single ailment with a single cause

disease cluster = a group of ailments with common elements so they are lumped together

syndrome = symptoms which occur together but may be caused by different diseases

Words in UPPER CASE refer to entries in the Condition Index or Drug Index

REGIONAL NOTES CODE LETTERS

E = Eastern Europe and western Asia

F = Sub-Saharan Africa

I = Indian subcontinent

K = Central Asia; the former USSR

M = Central and South America

N = Arctic region

O = Eastern Asia

R = Mediterranean area and the Middle East

S = Southeast Asia

U = South Pacific and Oceania

CONDITION ROSTER

ABORTION
ABSCESS
ACNE
ACROMEGALY
ACTINOMYCOSIS
ACUTE ABDOMEN
ADDICTION
African sleeping sickness.
AFRICAN tick typhus
AIDS
AINHUM
ALBINISM
ALCOHOLISM
ALLERGY
ALTITUDE SICKNESS
ALZHEIMER DISEASE
AMEBIASIS
AMEBIC SKIN ULCER
ANAPHYLAXIS
ANEMIA
ANGINA
ANTHRAX
APHTHOUS STOMATITIS
ARBOVIRAL FEVER
ARSENIC POISONING
ARTHRITIS
ASCARIASIS
ASTHMA
ATTENTION DEFICIT DISORDER (ADD)
BARTHOLIN CYST / ABSCESS
BARTONELLOSIS
BEDSORE
BELL'S PALSY
BERIBERI
BIG HEEL
BLADDER STONE
Boutonneuse fever
BRAIN DAMAGE
BRAIN TUMOR
BRUCELLOSIS
BURKITT LYMPHOMA
BURSITIS
BURULI ULCER
CANCER
CANCRUM ORIS
CANDIDIASIS

CAPILLARIASIS
CARBON MONOXIDE POISONING
CARPAL TUNNEL SYNDROME
CATARACT
CAT-SCRATCH DISEASE
CELLULITIS
CEREBRAL PALSY
Chaga's disease
CHANCROID
CHICKEN POX
CHIKUNGUNYA [FEVER]
CHLAMYDIA
CHOLERA
CIRRHOSIS
COBALAMIN DEFICIENCY
Coccidiomycosis
COLIC
CONCUSSION
Congo-Crimean hemorrhagic fever (CCHF)
CONTACT DERMATITIS
COSTAL CHONDRITIS
CRETINISM
CRIMEAN-CONGO HEMORRHAGIC FEVER (CCHF)
CRYPTOSPORIDIOSIS
CUTANEOUS LEISHMANIASIS (CL)
CYCLOSPORIASIS
CYSTICERCOSIS
DEHYDRATION
DELIRIUM TREMENS
DEMONIZATION
DENGUE FEVER
DEPRESSION
Dermatitis
DIABETES
Diarrhea
DIPHTHERIA
DONOVANOSIS
DOWN SYNDROME
DRUG ERUPTION
DYSENTERY
EAR INFECTION, EXTERNAL
EAR INFECTION, MIDDLE
Ebola virus disease

ECZEMA
ELEPHANTIASIS
ELLIPTOSYTOSIS
ENCEPHALITIS
ENDOMETRIOSIS
ENTERIC FEVER
ENTEROBIASIS
EPIDIDYMITIS
EPILEPSY
Erythema infectiosum
ERYTHEMA MULTIFORME
ERYTHEMA NODOSUM
EXFOLIATIVE DERMATITIS
EYE INFECTION
FAMILIAL MEDITERRANEAN FEVER (FMF)
Favus
FEBRILE SEIZURE
FELON
FIBROMYALGIA
FIBROSITIS
FIFTH DISEASE
FILARIASIS
FISSURE
FISTULA
FLEAS
FLUOROSIS
FOOD POISONING
FROSTBITE
Fungal Infection
G6PD DEFICIENCY
GALLBLADDER DISEASE
Gallbladder of raw fish
GANGRENE
GASTRITIS
GASTROENTERITIS
GIARDIASIS
Gingivitis
Glandular fever
GLAUCOMA
GOITER
Gondou
GONORRHEA
GOUT
GUINEA WORM
Hand-foot-mouth disease
HANGOVER

HAVERHILL FEVER
HEART ATTACK
HEARTBURN
HEART FAILURE
HEAT ILLNESS
HEMOCHROMATOSIS
HEMORRHAGIC FEVER
HEMORRHOIDS
HEPATITIS
HERNIA
HERPES
HIVES
HIV INFECTION
HOOKWORM
HYDATID DISEASE
HYDROCELE
Hyperimmune malarial splenomegaly
HYPERTENSION
HYPERVENTILATION
HYPOGLYCEMIA
HYPOTHERMIA
IMMERSION FOOT / TRENCH FOOT
IMPACTION
IMPETIGO
INDIAN CHILDHOOD CIRRHOSIS (ICC)
INFLUENZA
INSECTICIDE POISONING
INTESTINAL FLUKE
IRIS
IRITIS
IRRITABLE BOWEL
JAUNDICE
JET LAG
KATAYAMA DISEASE
KELOID
KERATITIS
Keshan Disease
KIDNEY DISEASE
KIDNEY INFECTION
KIDNEY STONE
Kyasanur Forest disease
Lactose intolerance
LARVA MIGRANS (LM)
Lassa fever

LEAD POISONING
LEISHMANIASIS
LEPROSY
LEPTOSPIROSIS
LICE
LIPOMA
LIVER DISEASE
LIVER FAILURE
LIVER FLUKE
Loiasis
LYME DISEASE
LYMPHOGRANULOMA
   VENEREUM (LGV)
MALABSORPTION
MALARIA
MALNUTRITION
Mansonellosis perstans
MASTITIS
MASTOIDITIS
MEASLES
Mediterranean tick typhus
MELIOIDOSIS
MENINGITIS
MENOPAUSE
MENSTRUAL CRAMPS
MENTAL ILLNESS
MIGRAINE HEADACHE
MILK INTOLERANCE
Miscarriage
MOLLUSCUM CONTAGIOSUM
MONGOLIAN SPOT
Mongolism
Monkey fever
Monkeypox
MONONUCLEOSIS
MOSSY FOOT
MUSCLE STRAIN
MYCETOMA
MYIASIS
Nairobi eye
NECROTIZING FASCIITIS
NEURALGIA, NEURITIS,
   NEUROPATHY
OLD AGE
ONCHOCERCIASIS
Onyalai
OSTEOMYELITIS
OVALOCYTOSIS /
   ELLIPTOCYTOSIS

Overdose
Palpitations
PANCREATITIS
PARAGONIMIASIS
PARAPHIMOSIS
PARKINSON'S DISEASE
PARONYCHIA
Parovirus
PELLAGRA
PELVIC INFECTION (PID)
PEPTIC ULCER
PERICARDITIS
PERTUSSIS / WHOOPING
   COUGH
PHIMOSIS
PIG-BEL
PINGUECULA
Pinta
PLAGUE
PLANT POISONING
PLEURISY
PNEUMONIA
PNEUMOTHORAX
Poisoning
POLIO
PORPHYRIA
POST-MEASLES CACHEXIA
POSTPARTUM SEPSIS
PREMENSTRUAL TENSION
PROCTITIS
PROSTATITIS
PTERYGIUM
PULMONARY EMBOLISM (PE)
PYOMYOSITIS
Q FEVER (QF)
RABIES
RADIATION ILLNESS
RADICULOPATHY
RAT BITE FEVER
RECTAL PROLAPSE
REITER SYNDROME / REACTIVE
   ARTHRITIS
RELAPSING FEVER (RF)
RESPIRATORY FAILURE
RESPIRATORY INFECTION
RHEUMATIC FEVER (RF)
RHEUMATOID ARTHRITIS (RA)
RHINITIS
RICKETS

Rickettsial pox
Rickettsiosis
ROSEOLA
ROTAVIRUS INFECTION
RUBELLA
SAND FLY FEVER
SCABIES
Scarlet fever
Schistosomiasis
SCHISTOSOMIASIS MANSONI
   (SM)
SCIATICA
SCOLIOSIS
SCRUB TYPHUS
SCURVY
SEABATHER'S ERUPTION
SEIZURES
SEPSIS
Septic abortion
SERUM SICKNESS
SEXUALLY TRANSMITTED
   DISEASE: (STD)
SHINGLES
SHOCK
SIBERIAN TICK TYPHUS
SICKLE CELL DISEASE (SCD)
SLIPPED DISC
SMALLPOX
SMOKE INHALATION
SPINAL NEUROPATHY
SPLENIC CRISIS
SPOTTED FEVER
SPRUE
STD
STREP INFECTION; STREP
   THROAT
STRESS
STROKE
STRONGYLOIDIASIS
SWIMMER'S ITCH
SYPHILIS (venereal)
TAPEWORM
TB
TENDINITIS
TETANUS
THALLASEMIA
THYROID TROUBLE
TICK PARALYSIS
Tick typhus

TINEA
TORTICOLIS (spontaneous)
TOXEMIA
TOXOPLASMOSIS
TRACHOMA
TRENCH FEVER
TRENCH FOOT
TREPONARID
TRICHINOSIS
TRICHURIASIS
TROPICAL SPASTIC
   PARAPARESIS (TSP)
TROPICAL SPLENOMEGALY
   (TSS)
TROPICAL ULCER
TUBAL PREGNANCY
TUBERCULOSIS (TB)
TULAREMIA
TUNGIASIS
TURISTA, TRAVELER'S
   DIARRHEA
TYPHUS
ULCERATIVE COLITIS
ULCERS
UMBILICAL HERNIA
URETHRAL STRICTURE
URETHRITIS, MALES
URINARY INFECTION (UTI)
URINARY OBSTRUCTION
UTERINE PROLAPSE
VAGINITIS and VAGINOSIS
VARICOSE VEINS
VINCENT STOMATITIS
VISCERAL LEISHMANIASIS (VL)
Vitamin A deficiency
VITILIGO
WARTS
WEST NILE VIRUS
Worms
XEROPHTHALMIA
Yanonga
YAWS
Yellow fever
ZINC DEFICIENCY

ABORTION

Regional Notes: F.

Definition: abortion refers to either the spontaneous process (in which case this is synonymous with miscarriage) or else to the deliberate act of interrupting a pregnancy.

Clinical

The initial symptoms are usually cramping pains, like labor, and vaginal bleeding. See Volume 1, Chapter 6 for a complete description.

Complications: SEPSIS, ANEMIA, subsequent infertility.

Treatment

Prevention: good nutrition, malaria prophylaxis, boil the drinking water of pregnant women.

Referrals: if it is after the third month, send the patient to a hospital, preferably level 3 or 4, but level 2 is better than nothing. She should be seen, ideally, by an obstetrician/ gynecologist or at least by a surgeon or midwife.

Patient care: none in the village situation unless there is SEPSIS or ANEMIA.

ABSCESS

Includes: perirectal abscess, boil.

Definition: an abscess is a localized infection that causes the accumulation of a pocket of pus.

Cause: bacteria.

Mildly to moderately ill; class 1–2, class 3 in the presence of a pulse,[1] venereal disease, PLAGUE, severe ANEMIA, OSTEOMYELITIS; an abscess of the eyeball, chest wall or kidneys. Worldwide, common in developing areas.

Age: any. **Who:** anyone, especially diabetics, weakened, malnourished, old injuries, nursing mothers (breast abscesses). **Onset:** 1–7 days.

Clinical

Necessary: if it is near the surface, it is a warm or red, painful, tender, swollen area on the body, like a pimple or a water balloon. If it is deep and not yet ready to drain, it may be firm, warm or red and tender. In the mouth an abscess may cause swelling of the gums or the outside of the face. In the breast it causes local pain and swelling as well as a fever. If it is deep in the muscle, it appears to be a generally swollen muscle, usually the thigh, the buttock or anywhere the skin was broken. Rectal abscesses are usually to the right or left of the anus, and the onset of pain is gradual. Near the rectum it causes severe pain with bowel movements and walking.

Probably: at first the skin over the abscess will look normal. If the abscess is near the surface; as it ripens (becomes ready to drain) the surface skin first becomes shiny and then thin and scaly. When its texture changes from hard to soft the abscess is ready to drain. Probably the lymph nodes adjacent to the abscess will be swollen.

Maybe: fever, pus draining out of the swollen area, a center spot or hole in the swelling.

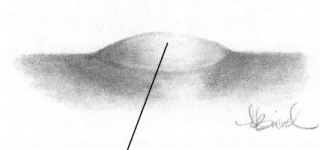

This abscess is ready to drain. It is soft to the touch with very thin skin on top. At an earlier stage the abscess was simply a red, swollen, tender area on the skin; at that stage it was not ready to drain. AB

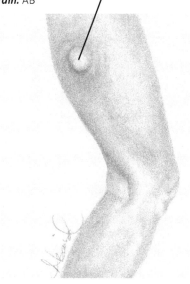

This is the appearance of an abscess on a thigh. AB

Complications: if the abscess is not cared for properly, it will come back, and the patient may develop SEPSIS and die.

Similar conditions: see Protocol B.6.

Cold abscess: likely due to TUBERCULOSIS. *Black scab on the swelling*: ANTHRAX, TUBERCULOSIS. *Abscess in the genital area:* SEXUALLY TRANSMITTED DISEASE, PELVIC INFECTION (females). *No center spot:* CELLULITIS (near surface), PYOMYOSITIS, OSTEOMYELITIS (deep in). *Jaw:* ACTINOMYCOSIS *Hands and feet swollen in a child:* SICKLE CELL DISEASE

Treatment

Prevention: cleanliness in caring for injuries. Use only sterile needles for injections.

---

1 *That is, you can feel the patient's heartbeat by resting your fingers lightly on the top of the abscess.*

Referrals: send out if possible. Laboratory: possibly helpful if level 2 or 3. Practitioner: general practitioner or surgeon, level 2 or more; some nurses might do this.

Patient care: don't do anything to an abscess with a pulse in it! Otherwise, to check if an abscess is ready to drain, (or to drain it in the case of the diseases listed above), pierce it with a sterile 18 gauge needle attached to a disposable syringe (since it is very hard to clean pus out of a glass or nylon syringe); if you can withdraw pus, it is ready. See Appendix 1.

If it is not ready, lay warm wet towels on it, renewing them as they cool. Cover them with thin plastic. Do this until it is ready, checking it daily. Then drain the abscess according to Appendix 1 in Volume 1 after giving a single dose of antibiotic. Rinse the abscess cavity daily after draining; squirt clean water into it with a syringe. PHENYTOIN powder sprinkled into the cavity daily will hasten healing.

Antibiotics are not helpful unless the patient has a fever. In any case, they are no substitute for draining the pus. If there is fever treat with ERYTHROMYCIN plus SULFADIAZINE. CIPROFLOXACIN and RIFAMPIN (one or the other) are also good choices but expensive. RIFAMPIN is particularly good if there is a foreign body (e.g. bullet or splinter) in the abscess cavity. Switch to CHLORAMPHENICOL or CO-TRIMOXAZOLE if the fever does not drop in 48 hours. Some more expensive antibiotics that work more reliably are AUGMENTIN, CLOXACILLIN or one of the CEPHALOSPORIN antibiotics. Be sure the patient eats a diet adequate in protein; otherwise he will not heal. If the pus smells very foul, then use PENICILLIN plus METRONIDAZOLE. In patients or cultures that have had prior medical care, substitute CLINDAMYCIN for PENICILLIN.

Results: improved in 3 days, healed in 3 weeks. If the patient still has pain or is not healed, continue antibiotics, supplement his diet with protein, and send him out for further medical care.

ACNE

Definition: small, localized infections of the hair follicles, mainly in teenagers.

Cause: bacteria or mites.

Not ill; class 1; worldwide, worse in humid, tropical climates.

Age: teenagers, sometimes middle aged. **Who:** those with oily skin. **Onset:** over days.

Clinical

Pimples on the face or back.

Similar conditions: with a fever: ENTERIC FEVER, SPOTTED FEVER (Rickettsial pox), CHICKEN POX (in the early phase).

Treatment

Have the patient wash with soap and warm water four times a day. Some surface washing agents like BENZOYL PEROXIDE may be helpful. Use oral ERYTHROMYCIN. DOXYCYCLINE works but it may be dangerous to use; it masks the signs of appendicitis in those who still have an appendix.

ACROMEGALY

Entry category: syndrome, worldwide, rare.

Definition: acromegaly is an excess of growth hormone, causing a child to grow to excessive height or causing growth of only the face, hands and feet in adults. In either case the facial features are heavy and coarse. Send the patient to a major medical center.

Cause: tumor or hormone problem.

Referrals: level 4 or 5, endocrinologist.

ACTINOMYCOSIS

This is an infection with bacteria that behave like fungi. It affects males more than females, middle-aged more than young or old and especially those with poor dental hygiene. It causes a slow-growing tumor in the mouth which breaks open on the cheek and discharges a thick fluid with yellow granules in it. It is treatable with high doses of MINOCYCLINE, PENICILLIN or AMOXICILLIN for 2–6 weeks, followed by lower doses for 6 to 12 months. The problem might resolve on its own. When this affects the deeper tissues of the body, it is indistinguishable from other diseases which are much more common. Diagnosing this in a Third-World setting is hopeless.

ACUTE ABDOMEN

Regional Notes: F, I, S

Entry category: disease cluster.

Synonyms: surgical abdomen.

Includes: PANCREATITIS, perforated ulcer, TUBAL PREGNANCY, appendicitis, volvulus, obstructed bowel and other problems too numerous to mention.

Definition: an acute abdomen is a diseased abdomen which requires the services of a surgeon.

Cause: variable.

Moderately to very ill; class 4; worldwide, type is regional, generally not common, not rare.

Age: any. **Who:** anyone. **Onset:** sudden to 4 days or more.

Clinical

Necessary: the patient has abdominal pain. He is sick enough not to be walking around and doing his usual work or play. The pain is either of sudden onset, or else it has lasted for 6 hours or more. The symptoms match one of the types listed below.

Maybe: The pain may extend down the inner thigh to the knee.

TOC SYMPTOMS DIFFERENTIALS CONDITIONS DRUG INDEX REGIONAL NOTES INX

TYPE 1: WITH SHOCK

The patient has an ashen color, his skin is cool and moist, he has a rapid pulse rate and possibly a low blood pressure. Generally he is lying still, not writhing about. He is unconscious, or he becomes unconscious if you lift him to an upright position. Usually the onset is sudden in males and slow in females. This kind of acute abdomen may be due to injury to the abdomen or a complication of TUBAL PREGNANCY, amebic DYSENTERY, SPLENIC CRISIS or PEPTIC ULCER. Sometimes the patient has shoulder or back pain. In this case his shoulder or back is not tender. Pushing on the abdomen, however, increases the shoulder or back pain.

> Very sudden onset of severe pain may be a catastrophe. Proceed with the diagnosis; simultaneously make arrangements to transport the patient to higher level care.

TYPE 2: DUE TO INFECTION

Appendicitis is the most common form. The patient has pain for six hours or more. There is a loss of appetite and frequently vomiting or constipation. (But the pain usually comes before the other symptoms.) Pushing on the abdomen makes the pain worse; with simple abdominal cramps, pushing relieves the pain. There is rebound tenderness—the patient will not cough hard twice, because it hurts too much after coughing the first time. Jarring the bed or tapping on the abdomen firmly with one finger causes pain. Frequently bowel sounds are absent. The pain is constant. If there is fever, it probably is not high. Usually, the abdominal wall is stiff so that the patient is unable to relax it. There may be hiccups or DEHYDRATION. The pain may be felt in the pelvis or rectum. Acute abdomen due to infection may be caused by appendicitis, injury, ENTERIC FEVER, abdominal TUBERCULOSIS and quite a number of other conditions. (Also see Protocol A.39, Abdominal Pain, in the Symptom Index; it is more complete than the preceding description.)

> **USUAL CHRONOLOGY OF APPENDICITIS:**
> 1. Upper abdominal pain
> 2. Nausea and vomiting
> 3. Pain shifts to lower right (rarely left).

TYPE 3: DUE TO BOWEL OBSTRUCTION

The patient has had pain for six hours or more, coming in waves, anywhere from 3 to 25 minutes apart. If the pains are closer together, the patient is vomiting and may be constipated also. If they are further apart, he will be constipated, may vomit also, and the vomit may look and smell like stool. (It is stool.) Usually the patient is writhing about.

Bowel sounds may be absent, or they may be rushing, followed by tinkles like dripping water. The most frequent causes are ASCARIASIS, previous surgery, a HERNIA that will not go back, intestinal TUBERCULOSIS and HYDATID DISEASE. Small children sometimes have lethargy, irregular pains, a soft lump in the abdomen and bloody diarrhea. There is a more complete description in Symptom Protocol A.39.C.

Similar conditions:

Type 1: SEPSIS may be indistinguishable; both require hospitalization.

Type 2: if the respiratory rate is twice normal or more, the patient may have PNEUMONIA, which can closely mimic this. If there is a history of this pain happening monthly in a female, consider ENDOMETRIOSIS. Consider PELVIC INFECTION, abdominal TB and TUBAL PREGNANCY. ENTERIC FEVER involves a sustained, high fever which acute abdomen seldom has. Consider FAMILIAL MEDITERRANEAN FEVER for patients with a Mediterranean genetic heritage; there may be a family history of recurrent abdominal pain. AMEBIASIS and GALLBLADDER DISEASE cause local tenderness in the mid or right upper abdomen. Some patients with SYPHILIS (tertiary) have this kind of pain that lasts for days and then spontaneously disappears before happening again. If the patient has a history of this, he may not need to be sent out.

Type 3: check for IMPACTION before transporting a patient for this. If you cannot send the patient out, then consider abdominal TUBERCULOSIS.

Bush laboratory: check hemoglobin and urinalysis. (See Appendix 2.) These are usually normal in acute abdomen. Hospital labs can do blood counts and imaging to determine diagnosis. If you have the kind of thermometer that is a strip of plastic, check the temperature of the right lower abdomen if you suspect Type 2. If it is higher than the skin temperature of the rest of the abdomen, appendicitis is likely. You can try to relieve the pain with DICYCLOMINE or CHAMOMILE TEA. This will relieve many other abdominal pains but not the pain of an acute abdomen.

Treatment

Referrals: speedy evacuation is essential; see Volume 1, Appendix 13 for referral guidelines. Laboratory: possibly helpful if level 3 or more. Essential capability is doing blood counts, urinalysis, blood chemistries. Facilities: on occasion x-ray, ultrasound or CT scan may be helpful. A surgical theatre is essential. Practitioner: level 3–4, surgeon and anesthesiologist. Some general practitioners can cope.

If it is Type 3 in a disabled patient, first check for IMPACTION; pulling stool out with your fingers might be curative. Otherwise send the patient to a surgeon as soon as possible.

Patient care:

- Give the patient nothing to eat or drink, only a wet cloth to moisten his mouth. The patient will become dehydrated, but this is unavoidable if you do not have IV fluids. If you do have IV fluids, start an IV and give the usual maintenance fluid. Do not use intraperitoneal fluids, especially not for type 2.

- Put a stomach tube in, preferably large diameter, but small diameter is better than nothing. (See Appendix 1 of Volume 1.)

- Empty the patient's stomach frequently with a syringe.

- During a delay in transport for Type 2, give the following antibiotics: (TINIDAZOLE or METRONIDAZOLE), plus AMPICILLIN plus GENTAMYCIN. CHLORAMPHENICOL can substitute for GENTAMYCIN. CIPROFLOXACIN is also a good choice.

- For all types, in malarious areas, also treat for MALARIA.

- Consult a medical doctor; he may have additional advice.

- Do not give pain medication unless either the receiving physician orders it or you are sure it will be worn off before reaching the hospital. (Medication is worn off if it is an hour or more past the time for the next dose.)

ADDICTION

Regional Notes: F, O, R, S, U.

Entry category: syndromes

Synonyms: drug abuse, drug dependency.

Definition: the continued use of a drug in spite of its having an adverse effect on social and economic functioning. The routine use of a drug per se does not constitute addiction or abuse.

Class 1–3; worldwide: which drug or drugs are used or abused varies with place and ethnic group. Some areas and cultures have major problems, others have minor or no problems.

Age: any, but mostly preteen to adult. Infants of addicted mothers will be addicted at birth and have withdrawal problems. **Who:** anyone, with individual variations. Some people become addicted readily while others do not. **Onset:** variable. Addiction seldom occurs with less than a week of drug use, and it usually requires several weeks to several months.

Clinical

Necessary: the patient takes a drug regularly and seeks it in spite of its having a negative effect on his social and economic status. There are three main types of abused drugs. If a patient takes a drug, it will give a drug effect. If he has taken a drug regularly for over a week and then suddenly stops, he may have withdrawal effects.

Sometimes: people with ATTENTION DEFICIT DISORDER may have reverse effects with uppers and downers; they will become calm with uppers and stimulated with downers. Some of them lack a brain hormone; they use "uppers" to be calm enough to function socially.

UPPERS

Uppers speed up bodily and mental processes.

Drug effect: loss of appetite, trembling, rapid pulse and respiration, fast speech, hyperactivity, confusion, nervousness. Some uppers can cause fevers and high blood pressure. There may be weight loss with a good appetite. Betel nut causes a red/black discoloration of the tongue and mouth.

Withdrawal effect: excessive sleep, depression, incoordination, low blood pressure, drug-seeking behavior.

Examples: caffeine, amphetamines, cocaine, khat, betel nut.

DOWNERS

Downers slow down bodily and mental processes.

Drug effect: slurred speech, sleep, slow pulse and respiration, incoordination, lowered blood pressure.

Withdrawal effect: nervousness, rapid pulse, anxiety, seizures. Withdrawal from narcotics causes excessive saliva.

Examples: ALCOHOL, tranquilizers, barbiturates, KETAMINE and NARCOTICS; sometimes cannabis (marijuana).

OUTERS

Outers cause crazy behavior.

Drug effect: dangerous, violent or bizarre behavior; nonsense speech; hallucinations.

Withdrawal effect: none, but flashbacks are common.

Examples: LSD, KETAMINE, some mushrooms, sometimes cannabis (marijuana). Drugs taken in connection with animistic rituals are frequently in this class.

Similar conditions:

Uppers addiction or downers withdrawal: ATTENTION DEFICIT DISORDER may appear similar but has been present since childhood. THYROID TROUBLE with high-thyroid or MALARIA (cerebral) involves a fever also. Consider DEMONIZATION. Withdrawal of downers may cause trembling similar to PARKINSON'S DISEASE or HYPOGLYCEMIA or LIVER FAILURE. DELIRIUM TREMENS due to alcohol withdrawal is a type of downers withdrawal.

Downers addiction or uppers withdrawal: consider HYPOGLYCEMIA (also sweaty); THYROID TROUBLE, low-thyroid (also low body temperature). In Africa consider AFRICAN SLEEPING SICKNESS. See Protocol B.10.

Outers effect: if there is a fever, consider MALARIA, (cerebral) and similar conditions. DEMONIZATION does not cause a fever. LIVER FAILURE may also cause bizarre behavior. Consider TOXEMIA in a pregnant woman, BERIBERI or PELLAGRA in a malnourished patient, SYPHILIS (tertiary), HIV INFECTION which has progressed to full-blown AIDS.

Treatment

Referrals: laboratory: level 4 only, capability of blood and/or urine tests to determine the kind of drug and amount. Practitioner: level 3–4; general practitioner or internal medicine. Competent nursing is essential. a psychiatrist, counselor or clergy might be helpful.

Patient care:

Uppers: excessive drug effect may be treated with downers if there is no history of ATTENTION DEFICIT DISORDER. Withdrawal from uppers must be done slowly.

Downers: excessive drug effect must be treated with assisting the patient's breathing until the drug wears off. Withdrawal from downers must be done slowly.

Outers: excessive drug effect should be treated with a quiet, semi-dark, calm environment with someone to talk quietly to the patient and reassure him. It frequently takes two or three days for these effects to wear off. Withdrawal is not a problem. Flashbacks should be treated like excessive effects.

African sleeping sickness

See Regional Notes F.

AFRICAN tick typhus

See SPOTTED FEVER. African tick typhus is one form of Boutonneuse fever, listed under SPOTTED FEVER. It is frequently fatal. The other form of Boutonneuse fever is Mediterranean tick typhus, a similar disease but not so severe.

AIDS

See HIV INFECTION. AIDS refers to HIV INFECTION that has progressed enough to cause severe symptoms: repeated infections; weight loss; diarrhea; failure to thrive in children.

AINHUM

Cause: unknown.
Regional: present in South Africa, African Americans, Pacific Islanders and South Asians.

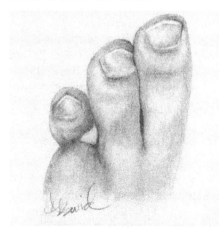

Ainhum of the little toe; note the narrowing. It may be at the base of the toe or farther up. AB

Clinical

A narrowing develops around the little toe and gradually tightens until the toe falls off. It may or may not be painful. This may subsequently happen to adjacent toes.

Treatment

Referrals: practitioner: level 2–4, general practitioner or surgeon. If the little toe is amputated when this starts, the process will not spread to the other toes.

ALBINISM

Cause: birth defect.

This is a condition characterized by a complete lack of brown skin pigment. The skin is very fair, the hair is a very light blond, and there are eye problems connected with it. You can do nothing about it except to advise avoiding sunburn. Albino skin is very vulnerable to skin CANCERs. It is important to assure the family that the condition was not caused by marital unfaithfulness.

ALCOHOLISM

Definition: the continued use of alcohol, either as regular drinking or as occasional binges, in spite of its causing adverse physical and/or social consequences.

Cause: ADDICTION.

Not ill to very ill; class 1–4; worldwide, common.

Age: adults. **Who:** anyone, but especially those who are impulsive or who have a family history of alcoholism. **Onset:** over weeks to years.

Clinical for condition

Necessary: the person cannot control his drinking, and it interferes with his social functioning at least some of the time.

Usually: he has been drinking excessively for months to years. He usually denies that his drinking is a problem.

Occasionally: he has a sore tongue. A chronic alcoholic may have a red face with a red, bumpy nose. He may have swollen cheeks, especially right in front of his ears. DEPRESSION is a common cause as well as a common effect of alcoholism.

Clinical for withdrawal

Usually: symptoms include sweating, nervousness and desperate alcohol-seeking behavior.

Commonly: patients have SEIZURES.

Sometimes: withdrawal involves DELIRIUM TREMENS (DT's). It begins 2–4 days after the last drink and lasts 3–10 days. The patient is not aware of his surroundings; he is hyperactive. Without professional care (IV fluids), many people die, but sedative medication may be helpful.

Complications: BERIBERI, HEART FAILURE and CIRRHOSIS.

Similar conditions: see Protocol B.10 for confusion and lethargy. See Protocol B.7 for liver disease which is a consequence of alcoholism. *Indistinguishable from alcohol withdrawal:* ADDICTION, HYPOGLYCEMIA. *Mental symptoms:* ATTENTION DEFICIT DISORDER, LIVER FAILURE, DEMONIZATION. *Swollen cheeks:* MUMPS, MALNUTRITION, HIV INFECTION.

Treatment

Referrals: send out for treatment if possible, having a responsible adult watch the patient during withdrawal. Laboratory: level 2 or more, basic capabilities. Practitioner: general practitioner or internal medicine; psychiatrist, counselor or clergy might be helpful.

Patient care: usually alcoholics are malnourished; treat them with MULTIVITAMINS. Minor tranquilizers such as DIAZEPAM may be useful for withdrawal. Seizures should be treated with DIAZEPAM, not with PHENYTOIN. Large hospitals with psychiatric units have treatment programs which may be successful. For nationals in remote areas, pastoral counseling is most appropriate once the initial withdrawal stage is past.

ALLERGY

Entry category: syndromes, worldwide, common.

Synonym: mango fever

Includes: hives, hay fever, ASTHMA, vernal conjunctivitis.

Definition: allergy is an illness caused by the body's reaction against some substance inhaled, eaten or encountered through skin contact.

Mildly to moderately ill; class 1–4; worldwide, common in developed areas.

Age: any. **Who:** anyone, but especially those with prior episodes of allergy or a family history of allergy. PENICILLIN, IRON shots and bee stings frequently cause severe reactions. **Onset:** seconds to one day; onsets tend to be rapid with lung symptoms.

Clinical

This commonly occurs in three forms: lungs, head and skin. Any one, two or all three may be present in any patient. In severe cases the patient may faint or develop ANAPHYLAXIS. Other forms of allergy are SERUM SICKNESS and DRUG ERUPTION.

Hives are very itchy, raised, flat-topped bumps on the skin.

Complications: allergy that affects the lungs may make a person susceptible to RESPIRATORY INFECTION. Sometimes patients die from severe allergic reactions.

THREE FORMS OF ALLERGY

HEAD	Eyes	Red, tearing, swollen, itchy.
	Nose	Stuffy, runny, sneezing.
	Throat	Swollen, itchy.
	Face	Swollen, itchy, bluish.
	Ears	Itchy.
LUNGS		Short of breath.
		Long expiration.
		Noisy inspiration.
		Congestion.
SKIN		Itchiness, swelling.
		HIVES.
		ECZEMA.
		CONTACT DERMATITIS.

VERNAL CONJUNCTIVITIS

A common form of allergy that affects the eyes in dry climates.

Not ill; class 1–2; regional, in hot areas.

Age: any but especially 3–16 y.o. Who: anyone. Onset: usually gradual.

Clinical: the patient has itching of the eyes, with a white, mucous discharge. With time there is thickening of the clear membrane that covers the white part of the eye, with a dark ring forming around the cornea. The lining of the eyelids may also thicken.

Similar Conditions: TRACHOMA, EYE INFECTION, XEROPHTHALMIA, ONCHOCERCIASIS. See Protocol B.8: red, painful eyes.

Higher-level care: send out if possible.

Laboratory: Level 3–4, culture capabilities

Practitioner: general practitioner or ophthalmologist

Treatment: send out if possible for a firm, definitive diagnosis. PREDNISOLONE EYE DROPS are very helpful; they clear the condition in a few days. However, they are dangerous. They must not be used for more than 2 weeks at a time. Once the condition is cleared, CROMOGLYCATE eye drops will keep the eyes clear.

Causative diseases: allergy plus fever or ASTHMA plus fever may indicate TUBERCULOSIS (mainly adults), SWIMMER'S ITCH, KATAYAMA DISEASE or possibly KIDNEY INFECTION. See also SERUM SICKNESS and DRUG ERUPTION. HYDATID DISEASE, GUINEA WORM and MANSONELLOSIS PERSTANS and some other infections may also cause allergic symptoms.

Similar conditions: ANAPHYLAXIS is a form of severe allergy with a sudden onset. ANTHRAX swelling may look similar, but there is always a scab.

Bush laboratory: check the urine dipstick. Occasionally liver problems (bilirubin in the urine) or URINARY INFECTION (leukocytes or nitrites in the urine) may cause hives. Blood tests are not helpful.

Treatment

Prevention: clean the person's environment. One of the common causes of allergy is the presence of insects. When insects die their parts contaminate dust, causing allergy.

Referrals: send out if possible. Laboratory: generally not helpful. Practitioner: level 2–4, general practitioner or internal medicine.

Patient care: for a bee sting or an injection, see ANAPHYLAXIS. If the patient is short of breath, but this is not due to bee sting or an injection, see ASTHMA. IPRATROPIUM may be helpful.

Treat SERUM SICKNESS, DRUG ERUPTION, ECZEMA and CONTACT DERMATITIS according to their own descriptions.

Allergy without trouble breathing: treat with DIPHENHYDRAMINE, CHLORPHENIRAMINE or DEXCHLORPHENIRAMINE. If you have some HYDROCORTISONE or PREDNISONE, and the problem is either severe or recurrent, use it for up to 5 days, but not longer unless a physician so orders. There are better drugs than those listed here, available in Western facilities.

Allergy with trouble breathing: see ANAPHYLAXIS.

ALTITUDE SICKNESS

Entry category: disease.

Synonym: acute mountain sickness; mountain sickness, high altitude illness.

Includes: high altitude cerebral edema (HACE), and high altitude pulmonary edema (HAPE).

Definition: altitude sickness is an illness caused by problems in the body's adaptation to high altitudes.

Moderately to very ill; class 4; high altitudes only.

Age: any. **Who:** those at an altitude of 2000 meters (6000 feet) or more for mild illness. It is more likely if the patient has previously been at high altitudes and/or previously had altitude sickness. It affects a few percent of climbers. **Onset:** usually 12–24 hours after arriving at high altitude; sooner with rapid ascent and exertion.

Clinical

Necessary: there are three types; the second and third types are life-threatening. Usually it begins with the first type and then progresses to the second or third type. Altitude sickness does not cause fever.

MILD ALTITUDE SICKNESS

This consists of fatigue and mild shortness of breath and/or headache, worse with exertion. The headache is similar to a hangover.

HACE (BRAIN SWELLING)

The patient has a severe headache and mental changes, with slurred speech or crazy behavior. He may be uncoordinated. This starts within 48 hours of ascent.

HAPE (LUNG SWELLING)

The patient is very short of breath, and he has abnormal lung sounds. He may faint. The shortness of breath is worse lying than sitting. His respiration is rapid, irregular or both, and he may turn blue. You may hear fine crackles or wheezing in his chest with your stethoscope. The patient may have a pressure-type chest pain or a cough which is either dry or productive of white or foamy sputum. This starts 2–4 days after ascent; it is worse at night.

Complications: HEART FAILURE, RESPIRATORY FAILURE, STROKE.

Similar conditions: HYPERVENTILATION is similar, but the patient's hands are cramped; they are never cramped with altitude sickness. ASTHMA may be indistinguishable. CARBON MONOXIDE POISONING involves exposure to a fire or an engine. See Protocol B.4 for other causes of shortness of breath. See Protocol B.10 for other causes of confusion and lethargy.

Treatment

Prevention: ascend gradually, spending a day or two at intermediate altitudes. Altitude gain above 9000 feet should be only 1000 feet per day for those prone to altitude sickness. Consider using ACETAZOLAMIDE before ascent.

Referrals: laboratory: generally not helpful. Practitioner: level 2–4; general practitioner or internal medicine; a nurse might be adequate.

Patient care: **Mild illness** and to hasten acclimatization, give ACETAZOLAMIDE daily for 3 days. **Do not use FUROSEAMIDE for treatment!**

Moderate to severe illness

- Have someone arrange to take the patient to a lower altitude. This is essential.
- Keep the patient on bedrest, sitting up.
- Give DEXAMETHASONE but only with HAPE.
- Keep track of vital signs and make repeated efforts to get the patient to a lower altitude.
- Give the patient oxygen.
- No diuretic other than ACETAZOLAMIDE.

ALZHEIMER DISEASE

This is a loss of mental functioning in adults, generally elderly, presenting as inability to care for oneself plus some difficulty in coordination. It is always slow-onset. There is no proven effective treatment. There is some anecdotal evidence that adding substantial quantities of coconut oil to the diet may be helpful.

AMEBIASIS

Regional Notes: E, F, I, K, M, O, R, S, U.

Entry category: disease.

Synonym: amoebiasis (British spelling).

Includes: amebic liver abscess, amebic dysentery, ameboma; (amoeboma in UK)

Excludes: amebic skin ulcer, listed separately.

Definition: amebiasis is an inflammation of the liver or the bowel, either a formed tumor or abscess or one in the process of forming, caused by the protozoa *Entameba histolytica.*

Cause: protozoa.

Moderately to very ill; class 3–4; worldwide, mostly in areas where there is poor sanitation. The disease is frequently carried by cockroaches and flies which contaminate food and water.

Age: rare in children. **Who:** *dysentery:* anyone, especially those who are malnourished. Males are much more susceptible than females. Homosexuals transmit the disease sexually. *Liver disease:* more Europeans than nationals. This usually starts within the first month after the bowel infection. The use of alcohol predisposes to it. **Onset:** slowly usually; if it appears abruptly the patient will admit to having had prior symptoms if he is asked. Incubation is 1–2 weeks if the exposure is minor; it is days for major exposures.

There are three forms of initial presentation: amebic dysentery, amebic liver disease and ameboma (rare).

Clinical

AMEBIC DYSENTERY

Most common in adults and in malnourished children, it has a gradual onset; patients usually have the disease more than a week before seeking help.

Usually: bowel movements are not excessively frequent (1–4 daily). They are large and incredibly foul, their odor resembling that of very rotten meat. There may be alternating constipation and diarrhea. There is frequently bloody mucus smeared on the outside of otherwise-normal soft stool. The cramping abdominal pains are usually localized to the right or left lower abdomen, or they may be felt in the back. If the onset is rapid, they may be felt in the central abdomen. In that case there may also be headache, vomiting and fever.

Sometimes: there is fever. The pattern of bowel movements may vary greatly. Women may have vaginal or pelvic pain. With time the patient will lose weight and develop ANEMIA. If the disease is mild, there may be only fatigue, abdominal discomfort and either diarrhea or constipation. After the disease has lasted a long time the patient may be incontinent of stool. Hiccups indicate a bad prognosis.

Complications: amebic liver disease (see below) is most common. Other complications are ACUTE ABDOMEN and AMEBIC SKIN ULCERS. In homosexuals, the disease tends to be very aggressive.

AMEBIC LIVER DISEASE

Usually: fevers, chills or night sweats; loss of appetite or nausea; pain or burning in the upper abdomen or (usually) the right shoulder, side or back which is worse with walking, with a gentle punch or with pushing between the ribs in the painful area.

Sometimes: the patient may have only weight loss without pains or fever.

Maybe: vomiting; tender, soft lump in upper right abdomen; large, tender liver; mild JAUNDICE; cough (5–7%); pain with breathing; diarrhea; insomnia; general lethargy and fatigue. If it is advanced, then jumping up and down causes severe pain in the liver.

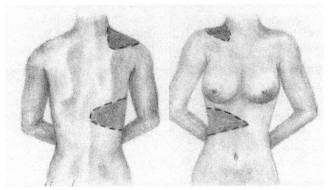

The pain of amebic liver disease is most often felt in the shaded areas. The shoulder pain is worse if the patient bends her head forward, chin on chest. The abdomen is tender, but the shoulder is not. Pressing on the liver is apt to increase the shoulder pain. AB

AMEBOMA

On occasion amebae may form a mass or tumor in the abdomen. It is indistinguishable from another tumor.

Complications: ANEMIA, HICCUPS, spread to the brain causing STROKE or SEIZURES. In Africans and Asians especially, the amebae may eat through the diaphragm, and the pus in the liver pour into the chest. (PREDNISONE and related drugs may provoke this.) The patient then suddenly develops a cough with lavender or brown (occasionally yellow or green) sputum, severe PLEURISY-type chest pains and sometimes a scraping sound that can be heard through a stethoscope with each breath. If the pus breaks out into the abdomen, he will develop an ACUTE ABDOMEN. In both cases the patient must be sent to a hospital quickly.

Similar conditions: ENDOMETRIOSIS causes pain synchronous with monthly menstrual cycles. PEPTIC ULCER also involves burning pain, but the pain varies with hunger or a full stomach. HEART FAILURE is a cause of a tender, enlarged liver. KIDNEY INFECTION on the right may look similar, but the urine is cloudy and tests positive for leukocytes. PNEUMONIA, HEPATITIS and GALLBLADDER DISEASE are of more sudden onset. With HEPATITIS the JAUNDICE is apt to be intense, not slight. CANCER may look similar, but the lower border of the liver is lumpy. MALARIA and SEPSIS can have a similar fever pattern, but the liver is not so tender. HYDATID DISEASE shows an enlarged liver; check the geography for your area. See Protocol B.5 for other causes of fever and jaundice.

Bush laboratory: the urine may contain bilirubin and possibly urobilinogen and protein. You may find positive ketones also. Blood, leukocytes or nitrites in the urine indicate a kidney problem.

Treatment

Prevention: filter or boil drinking water; do not eat cold or lukewarm food from street vendors.

Referrals: send out if possible. See Volume 1, Appendix 13. Laboratory: level 3–4, capable of blood chemistries. Hospital labs may check stool for amebae. The test is not at all sensitive (there are many false negatives), but it is specific (rare false positives). The stool test must be done and found to be negative seven times on seven different, very fresh specimens before you can be sure the patient does not have the disease. It is easier to just treat on the basis of history. Facilities: x-ray, ultrasound, CT scan: level 3–4. Practitioner: general practitioner, may need a surgeon.

Patient care: severe cases frequently need surgery. However, you can try METRONIDAZOLE or TINIDAZOLE. The patient will improve within 72 hours if the treatment will ultimately be successful. If he is not improved within this time, he must be sent to a hospital for surgery. ORNIDAZOLE and SECNIDAZOLE are new, related drugs. PROMETHAZINE might be helpful for nausea.

Results: some improvement before one week.

AMEBIC SKIN ULCER

Entry category: disease, regional, tropical.

Definition: a skin ulcer, found on the genitals or on the trunk, due to the protozoa *Entameba histolytica*.

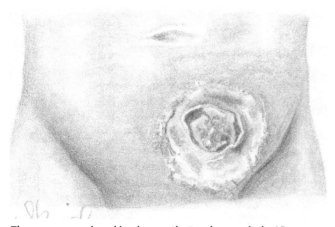

The appearance is a skin ulcer on the trunk or genitals. AB

It is sometimes due to amebae which have infected the bowel and now are eating a hole through the abdominal wall. It might be due to a direct skin infection with amebae. The ulcer is very painful, and there is usually a lot of discharge from the wound. It is essential to start treatment soon since these ulcers can progress rapidly, and the bowel contents can spill out through them. They can destroy the genitals within a few days to a week.

Similar conditions: see Sexually Transmitted Diseases, Protocol B.1, which may be indistinguishable from this although other STDs do not usually have a discharge from the ulcer. See Protocol B.11 for skin ulcer plus general illness.

Treatment

Referrals: send out if possible; see Volume 1, Appendix 13. Laboratory: level 3–4, capable of culturing bacteria, doing stained smears for amebae. Practitioners: level 3–4, internist, possibly a surgeon.

Patient care: the treatment is the same as for AMEBIASIS above. The ulcers usually respond rapidly to treatment.

ANAPHYLAXIS ⚠ Life-threatening, treat immediately!

Regional Notes: M.

Synonyms: anaphylactic shock.

Definition: an overwhelming allergic reaction to some substance, usually inhaled or injected.

Cause: allergy.

Very ill; class 1–4; worldwide but relatively rare.

Age: any. **Who:** anyone, especially after an injection of PENICILLIN or IRON or an insect sting. This may occasionally come from food, particularly nuts, milk and eggs. **Onset:** sudden, over seconds to minutes.

Clinical

Necessary: the patient has one or more of the following: sudden swelling of the face or throat, shortness of breath, blue skin color, wheezing, loss of consciousness, sudden death. The blood pressure may drop. The patient may vomit or develop hives. He may have abdominal pain. After a severe episode, he may develop KIDNEY DISEASE or SHOCK (which must be treated).

Causative diseases: HYDATID DISEASE as well as PLANT POISONING due to claviceps or cassava can cause anaphylaxis.

Similar conditions: anaphylaxis is a severe form of ALLERGY.

With cramped hands: HYPERVENTILATION. *With a sore and fever:* ANTHRAX

TOC SYMPTOMS DIFFERENTIALS CONDITIONS DRUG INDEX REGIONAL NOTES INX

Treatment

EPINEPHRINE 1:1000 injection. Repeat this every 5–10 minutes as long as the patient is either unconscious or blue, and then every 30 minutes as long as he is having severe symptoms but conscious and not blue.

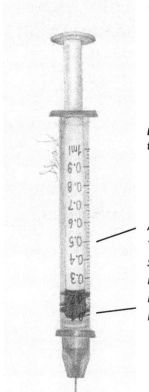

Epinephrine dosage in ml according to the size of the patient. AB

Adult 0.5 ml
Teenager 0.4 ml
School age 0.3 ml
Kindergartener 0.2 ml
Preschooler 0.1 ml
Infant 0.05 ml

Referrals: sending out is not possible since the problem progresses rapidly over minutes. The exception is if you live across the street from a level 3–4 hospital, in which case you should not be using this manual.

Start CIMETIDINE, DIPHENHYDRAMINE and PREDNISONE as soon as the patient can swallow. Continue the DIPHENHYDRAMINE and CIMETIDINE for 2–3 days but give only 1–2 doses of PREDNISONE.

Result: a few minutes after the epinephrine injection.

ANEMIA[1]

Regional Notes: F, I, M, N, O, S, U.

Entry category: syndrome.

Definition: anemia is not enough hemoglobin in the blood. Hemoglobin is the red stuff in the blood. It combines with oxygen in the lungs and releases oxygen in the organs of the body. Anemia is defined as a hemoglobin of less than 10 (11–18 is normal at sea-level; normals are higher at high altitude). Anemia puts a stress on all the organs of the body.

Cause: variable.

Not ill to very ill; class 3–4 in a pregnant woman with paleness. Class 2–3 in non-pregnant people who are pale or have a hemoglobin of 7 or less; class 1 in non-pregnant people who are not pale. Worldwide, extremely common.

Age: any. **Who:** anyone, especially children, pregnant women, those with a poor diet or suffering from various diseases. In agricultural areas it is frequently due to HOOKWORM. A diet of goat's milk causes folic acid deficiency anemia. A diet deficient in animal products causes vitamin B_{12} anemia. In women, anemia increases with the number of children, the use of IUD's and an early age of first pregnancy. In most cultures, more than 50% of pregnant women have anemia. **Onset:** usually over weeks to months unless there is obvious blood loss, then over hours to days.

Clinical

Necessary: the patient feels tired, dizzy or both.

Usually: if the hemoglobin is less than 8, he will have pale skin, fingernails, inner lower eyelids and tongue or inner mouth; the fingernails usually turn pale before the inner eyelids or mouth. He will have a rapid pulse and respiration and a high pulse pressure if the anemia is severe. He may feel short of breath.

Maybe: he will be dizzy and faint easily. Some patients have scooped-out fingernails or bluish whites of the eyes. The tongue may be sore. There may be leg cramps with climbing stairs. The skin may turn a darker color if the problem is a lack of vitamin B_{12}.

With anemia due to lack of iron, there may be difficulty swallowing, splits at the angles of the mouth, long ridges on the fingernails and intolerance of cold. There may also be numbness and tingling. His heart size may be large (see Volume 1, Chapter 1), and he may develop HEART FAILURE.

At high altitudes other symptoms (such as shortness of breath) occur before paleness. The table below shows the kinds of symptoms one is likely to find with various levels of hemoglobin at various altitudes.

The normal hemoglobin range is 11–17 mg/dl or 110–170 mg/liter. A hemoglobin of 6 mg/dl is considered severe anemia at low altitude, while 8 mg/dl is severe at high altitude or in pregnant women. Papers to measure anemia are sometimes indexed as % of the normal, the normal being 15 or 16. See Volume 1, Appendix 2, Procedure 10.

Instructions in using an inexpensive laboratory system for determining hemoglogin are in Volume 1, Appendix 2, Procedure 9.

---

1 See the anemia *Powerpoint lecture on www.villagemedicalmanual.org.*

TOC SYMPTOMS DIFFERENTIALS CONDITIONS DRUG INDEX REGIONAL NOTES INX

Table of hemoglobin levels vs. symptoms at low and high altitudes.

Hemoglobin mg/dl[1]	Hemoglobin mg/liter	%	Low altitude symptoms	High altitude symptoms
12	120	80%	None	Fatigue
10	100	70%	Fatigue	Can't exercise
8	80	52%	Can't exercise	Short of breath at rest
6	60	38%	Short of breath at rest	Maybe heart failure
4	40	25%	Maybe heart failure	Heart failure, may die
2	20	13%	Heart failure, may die	Survival unlikely

1 dl = deciliter, i.e., one tenth of a liter.

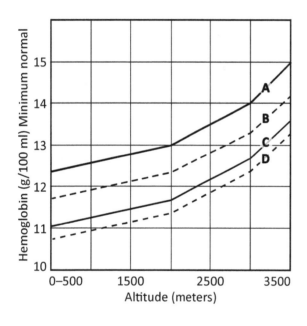

Graph of minimum normal hemoglobins for various people at different altitudes.

A: males >11 y.o. & pregnant females

B: females >11 y.o. and not pregnant

C: children 5–12 years old

D: children < 5 years old

OUTLINE OF CAUSES OF ANEMIA		
1. Blood lost outside the body	Hemorrhage	Visible bleeding
		Invisible, in urine or stool
	Pregnancy	Blood to make a baby
2. Blood destroyed within	Malaria	Destroyed by parasites
	Large spleen	Destroyed by spleen
	Hereditary conditions	Fragile red cells
3. Deficient blood manufacture	Lack of raw materials	Vitamin deficiency
		Iron deficiency
	Bone marrow problems	Chronic illness
		RADIATION
		Drugs
		CANCER

ANEMIA DUE TO BLOOD LOSS

This may be visible or invisible. If it is visible, sudden and large amounts, then at first the hemoglobin does not drop. As the body detects a drop in blood volume, it replenishes the loss with water and thus dilutes the hemoglobin, revealing the anemia. A patient may lose a lot of blood in stool without the stool looking bloody. The most common cause of blood loss in stool is HOOKWORM. The patient should be able to tell you of any visible blood loss. If he has not had any visible loss, ask about black and tar-like stools, and check his stools for blood. There are special tests to check for blood in stool, or you can put some stool in a tin can, add a little water, shake it and then use a urine dipstick to check for blood in the water.

ANEMIA DUE TO RED CELL DESTRUCTION

This occurs in THALLASEMIA, MALARIA, SICKLE CELL DISEASE, OVALOCYTOSIS, BARTONELLOSIS and any spleen enlargement. It may also occur as a complication of bacterial DYSENTERY. There is usually urobilinogen in the urine. The patient may have JAUNDICE. Usually his spleen is enlarged. See Protocol B.7.

ANEMIA DUE TO DEFICIENT RAW MATERIALS: LACK OF VITAMINS

This occurs with fish TAPEWORM, PELLAGRA, any MALNUTRITION, MALABSORPTION or THALLASEMIA. It occurs after 3 years on a strict vegan diet. In those on vegan diets, the problem is lack of VITAMIN B_{12}. In those who eat no vegetables, the problem is lack of FOLATE.

In those of northern European or African genetic heritage, a condition called pernicious anemia occurs which requires VITAMIN B_{12} injections. See COBALAMIN DEFICIENCY if the patient has the symptoms without evident paleness.

Clinical, lack of vitamins

Frequently the patient has darkening of the creases on the palm side of his hands and dark discoloration of his tongue. His skin may darken. Numbness and tingling of the hands and feet develop first. Thereafter he may have trouble walking. The gait is stiff, or it might be just uncoordinated without weakness. These symptoms are symmetrical (or nearly so), right and left. He may lose bladder and bowel control. There may be easy bruising, excessive bleeding, premature graying, burning of the tongue and susceptibility to infection. Sometimes there are mental changes—emotional upset—and this may predate the obvious anemia.

Treatment

You should treat with both VITAMIN B_{12} and FOLATE. **Don't treat with folate if the person eats no animal products and you have no B_{12}.**

ANEMIA DUE TO DEFICIENT RAW MATERIALS: IRON

In addition to the symptoms of all anemias, with anemia due to lack of iron, there may be difficulty swallowing, splits at the angles of the mouth, long ridges on the fingernails and intolerance of cold. There may be crampy pains in the legs when walking up stairs.

Iron deficiency anemia is usually due to MALNUTRITION (not eating enough iron), blood loss or pregnancy (using iron to make the baby). It may be due to rapid growth with a poor diet. Ask about diet to see if she takes in enough IRON in the form of red meats, blood, sorghum or IRON-containing medicines.

ANEMIA DUE TO BONE MARROW PROBLEMS
Chronic disease harms bone marrow.
This may be indistinguishable from that due to IRON deficiency. Check the patient for TB and other chronic diseases. Chronic diseases are those that last a long time; usually their onsets are slow.

TOXINS HARM BONE MARROW
This comes from RADIATION ILLNESS or from a side effect of CHLORAMPHENICOL or some other drug. This type of anemia is not treatable in a remote setting.

CHILDHOOD ANEMIA
You can guess from the age in many cases.

> **0–3 months:** some hereditary problems, congenital SYPHILIS, bacterial infection, (RESPIRATORY INFECTION, KIDNEY INFECTION, SEPSIS most common).
> **3–24 months:** bacterial infections as above, MALARIA, THALLASEMIA, nutritional anemia from a malnourished mother; SICKLE CELL DISEASE.
> **2–5 years:** anemia from IRON deficiency; vitamin deficiency (responds to FOLATE) occurs occasionally. In vegan families, this responds to VITAMIN B_{12}.
> **5–15 years:** almost all anemia is due to iron deficiency, usually from HOOKWORM, beginning menstruation in females or rapid growth.

Complications: HEART FAILURE, RESPIRATORY FAILURE, other complications depending on the cause.

Similar conditions: also see Protocol B.4 if the patient is *short of breath,* Protocol B.10 for other causes of *lethargy Pale skin:* TUBERCULOSIS, MALNUTRITION

Bush laboratory: the patient's hemoglobin must be 8 or less before you will notice paleness inside the lower lids. The Copack paper test will give you a rough idea; do not trust other tests that compare the color of a drop of blood to a standard. See Appendix 2, Procedure 10, and the lecture on anemia. Most hospital labs can determine hemoglobin. If the anemia is due to red blood cell destruction, there will be excess urobilinogen in the urine, as seen on a urine dipstick. (Note: 1+ urobilinogen is normal; 2+ or more is excess.)

Treatment

Prevention: all pregnant women should take IRON and folate. Those in malarious areas should also take MALARIA-preventive medication throughout pregnancy. They should eat some animal products in order to get VITAMIN B_{12}. Educate people on the best diet to eat, using local foods.

Treat all HOOKWORM and other worms.

Referrals: send out if possible, see Volume 1, Appendix 13. Laboratory: level 3–4. Capability of blood smears, a microscope and sometimes blood chemistries. Most labs will be able to do stool tests for various kinds of worms. With severe anemia a blood bank might be helpful. Large labs can also do specific tests for the various kinds of anemia. A good technician or physician can guess the cause from examining the blood smear. It is important that hospitals check transfused blood for HIV, and don't use blood that tests positive. If there is a delay in finding blood and/or transfusing it and if the patient is somewhat improved in the meantime, then refuse transfusion. Patients who truly need blood need it quickly. Even blood that tested negative can transmit HIV INFECTION in the developing world. Facilities: blood bank, IV fluids and associated equipment. Practitioner: level 3–4: pathologist is ideal; internist or general practitioner might suffice.

Patient care: hemoglobin 25% or less at low altitude, 45% or less at high altitude: send to a hospital for transfusion. In patients who are elderly or have prior heart problems, HEART FAILURE is common; these patients need transfusion. Anyone with severe anemia plus pregnancy or any major illness is likely to die without transfusion.

Patient care: hemoglobin above 25% at low altitude, above 45% at high altitude: treat both the anemia and the cause.

If you are not sure of the cause of the anemia, treat the patient with IRON, FOLATE and MULTIVITAMINS. Also treat for HOOKWORM, and treat for MALARIA if you are in a malarious area. If the patient has evidence of HEART FAILURE or PNEUMONIA, treat that also. A boiled egg weekly will supply enough VITAMIN B$_{12}$.

If you are fairly certain of the cause of the anemia:

- anemia **due to red cell destruction** is treated with FOLATE alone if the patient eats meat, with FOLATE plus IRON if he eats no meat.

- anemia **due to vitamin deficiency** is treated with FOLATE and either injected VITAMIN B$_{12}$ or ground raw beef liver[1]. Usually these patients require IRON also.

- anemia **due to iron deficiency or chronic disease** is treated with both IRON and FOLATE. Add VITAMIN B$_{12}$ if the diet does not include animal products. Anemia due to chronic disease usually does not respond unless the underlying disease is treated.

Results: some improvement in 2 weeks. Recheck the patient every 4 weeks for 3 months.

ANGINA

Entry category: syndrome.

Definition: angina is chest pain caused by a heart problem. **Age:** usually middle-aged or older. **Who:** usually Westerners or affluent. **Onset:** usually rapid, over seconds; sometimes gradually, over hours.

Clinical

It is heavy, aching or burning; center front, going to the neck, left shoulder, left jaw or left arm. Frequently there is nausea and/or vomiting, shortness of breath, severe sweating, poor (possibly bluish) skin color and an irregular pulse. It goes away in less than 20 minutes. A longer duration may indicate a HEART ATTACK.

Similar conditions: muscle spasm of the chest wall might appear similar. In that case there is chest wall tenderness which angina does not cause. The pain of angina usually has a delayed onset after the beginning of exercise and a delayed relief with rest. Also, leg as well as arm exercise triggers the pain.

Treatment

Referrals: send out if possible. Laboratory: level 3–4: EKG machine, blood chemistries. Facilities: oxygen, heart monitors. Practitioners: level 3–4: a cardiologist is ideal; internist or general practitioner might suffice.

Patient care: have the patient rest quietly in a sitting position and give him his usual angina medication if he has any. Oxygen may be helpful.

ANTHRAX

Regional Notes: E, F, I, K, M, R, U.

Entry category: disease, mainly tropical, worldwide, maybe terrorist-related.

Synonyms: charbon, malignant edema, malignant pustule, ragpickers' disease, woolsorters' disease.

Definition: anthrax is a bacterial infection causing a localized infection where it enters the body, as well as consequent surrounding swelling.

Cause: bacteria (*Bacillus anthracus*).

Moderately to very ill; class 2–4; the material from a skin sore is infectious, but the respiratory form is not contagious. Most prevalent in the early and late rainy seasons, in areas with animals, where the soil is neutral or alkaline.

Age: any. **Who:** anyone who has not already had the disease, especially those who process skins and bone meal, handle sick animals, eat their meat or drink their milk. Lab technicians who handle material from a patient are also vulnerable. **Onset:** incubation less than a week.

---

1 *This should be an act of desperation; raw liver is dangerous; it transmits some nasty diseases.*

TOC   SYMPTOMS   DIFFERENTIALS   CONDITIONS   DRUG INDEX   REGIONAL NOTES   INX

The initial bump or blister becomes a big sore in 3–4 days; a black scab forms within a week. The respiratory incubation is 1–3 days.

Clinical

SKIN

90% of all infections are the skin form, usually on exposed part(s) and above the waist. A tiny pimple or blister appears, which then enlarges over one day to become a sore with a black scab. It is painless, but it may prick or itch initially. There is no pus. It is regular and round, with raised edges, and there may be blistery satellite sores. It may be red or black and blue. The patient develops a fever, fatigue, headache and severe pitting swelling which may involve half his body; the swelling fills rapidly when it is pressed to make a dent. The swelling always involves the lymph nodes; the nodes may be painful. This may disappear very slowly or the patient may develop SEPSIS and die. It takes 6 weeks to heal; the delayed healing does not necessarily imply antibiotic failure. It scars as it heals. Antibiotic treatment does not hasten the healing, but it does prevent serious complications.

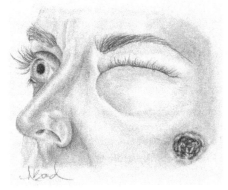

An early anthrax sore on the face with swelling only around the eye. The swelling may become much more severe than this, involving half of the head and neck. AB

RESPIRATORY

The respiratory form is the same, except that the pimple and swelling are within the throat and windpipe; death is almost inevitable since the swelling cuts off air flow. The disease might dominate on left or right. The patient may have pain with swallowing and shortness of breath. It is caused by inhaling contaminated body fluids or dust. This can, at times, progress to MENINGITIS.

INTESTINAL

This form is indistinguishable from bacterial DYSENTERY. It can also be similar to ENTERIC FEVER. SEPSIS and death are common. It is found almost exclusively in Africa and comes from eating contaminated, poorly cooked meat.

Similar conditions: see Protocol B.4 for *shortness of breath,* B.6 for *limb swelling,* B.11 for a *skin ulcer* plus general illness, B.12 for *large lymph nodes. Sore(s) with black scab(s):* PLAGUE, SPOTTED FEVER, SCRUB TYPHUS, TULAREMIA, CANCRUM ORIS, TUBERCULOSIS. *Severe swelling:* DIPHTHERIA, MUMPS, ABSCESS, CELLULITIS.

Treatment

Prevention: human immunization is available. There are two kinds; both give partial but not complete protection. Immunize animals against the disease. Be extremely careful when handling body fluids from the patient. If you inadvertently inhale some of the material from the anthrax wound, immediately seek immunization plus take DOXYCYCLINE for 60 days.

Referrals: send out of possible. See Volume 1, Appendix 13. Laboratory: level 4; capable of Gram stain with very high-tech laboratory safety precautions. An excellent hospital lab can do cultures and Gram stain, but handling the material is dangerous. There is a skin test for this that is better and safer than bacterial culture for diagnosis. Practitioner: level 3–4; infectious disease specialist is ideal; internist or general practitioner might suffice.

Patient care: use (CIPROFLOXACIN or LEVOFLOXACIN or DOXYCYLINE) plus (CLINDAMYCIN or RIFAMPIN). Otherwise use PENICILLIN or AMPICILLIN. Don't use any CEPHALOSPORIN except for Cefoperazone.

If the patient is very ill, initially give antibiotics intravenously until he is improved, then change to oral. It is essential to treat for the entire 60 days.

In case of swelling involving the head or neck, use high doses of PREDNISONE by mouth or intravenous HYDROCORTISONE, as for severe ENTERIC FEVER, just until the swelling subsides. IV works faster than oral or IM medication. It might also be helpful to use cold compresses on the swelling and to give DIPHENHYDRAMINE or another antihistamine.

APHTHOUS STOMATITIS

Definition: aphthous stomatitis is a viral infection of the inner surface of the mouth.

Cause: virus.

Not ill to mildly ill; class 1; worldwide.

Age: any. **Who:** anyone. **Onset:** variable.

Clinical

The patient has grayish ulcers in his mouth, anywhere. They are 1–1.5 cm in diameter. The normally pink surface is red around the ulcers, and the ulcers are painful. They may be associated with REITER SYNDROME which is an after-effect of some infectious diseases.

Similar conditions: HERPES occurs mainly at the junction of the pink and the skin, and where the pink moist surface is right over bone.

Treatment

None. These go away by themselves.

ARBOVIRAL FEVER

Regional Notes: E, F, I, K, O, R, S, U.

Entry category: disease cluster.

Includes: numerous diseases; most contain the name of a location. See Regional Notes as follows: Rift Valley fever (F); Ross River fever (S, U); West Nile virus (F); Igbo Ora virus (F); Crimean-Congo hemorrhagic fever (E, F, R); Sand Fly fever (E, F, I, R). Some of these are also discussed under HEMORRHAGIC FEVER. In some cases there is uncertainty about how a disease is transmitted, by insect or otherwise.

Definition: arboviral fever is a large class of viral diseases that are transmitted to humans by various insects. Some are contagious.

Mildly to very ill; class 1–4; some contagious; worldwide; caused by many different viruses.

Age: any. **Who:** anyone, especially mosquito-bitten anywhere. It may be transmitted by hard ticks. Sometimes it comes from direct contact with a sick patient or from milk. **Onset:** sudden, usually.

Clinical

Symptoms are quite variable depending on the local virus. Seek local lore. Many times local place names followed by the word "fever" are used to identify the various forms of this.

There are seven groups of symptoms in arboviral diseases; any one disease may have more than one group of symptoms. See the table below to determine what disease you are dealing with.

There generally are not good treatments for any of them in remote areas, but it is important to know if you are dealing with something highly contagious and life-threatening.

UNDIFFERENTIATED

This form causes a general flu-like illness with fever, headache and aching all over. All arboviral fevers start out with this symptom group.

ENCEPHALITIC OR MENINGITIC

This form causes, in addition to the undifferentiated symptoms, a very severe headache with a stiff neck and possibly seizures, mental symptoms (personality changes lasting over 24 hours) or lethargy or coma. There may also be asymmetrical limb weakness and problems with bladder and bowel function. See ENCEPHALITIS for a specific description. West Nile virus is occasionally in this category, particularly in the elderly. It occurs worldwide.

ARTHRITIC OR ARTHRALGIC

This form, in addition to the undifferentiated symptoms, causes pains and possibly swelling and redness of the joints. See ARTHRITIS.

The pattern of the joint problems varies. Clues include its happening in an outbreak; a sudden onset of a fever, possibly with a rash. There can be any pattern of joint pains: small or large joints, with or without symmetry, with or without relapse and migration.

The description of the manifestations of arboviral fever is continued on page 20.

TABLE OF ARBOVIRAL FEVERS

- Determine the characteristics of your patient's illness, referring to the heading row on the chart. What are the most distressing symptoms? If you are not sure, for example *eyes just slightly red*, then don't list it.

- Find which diseases have the "yes" answers that match your patient. Disregard the discrepancy if your patient does NOT have something marked "yes". However, if he definitely has something marked "no", that eliminates the diagnosis.

- Now from the list of possible diagnoses, eliminate those diseases that do not occur in your geographic area. Consider where the patient traveled recently.

- From the possibilities, determine if any is/are contagious. If so, notify the local health authorities. Be very careful about hand-washing, gowns, gloves, masks and the like. Keep children away from the patient and his family. Be sure your will is up to date. Don't send the patient out on public transport.

NOTES ON THE TABLE FOLLOWING

1 This refers to unusual lethargy or crazy behavior, inability to move body parts or abnormal, involuntary movements, along with a severe headache and possibly changes in sensation: numbness and tingling are most common. See the entry ENCEPHALITIS in the Disease Index.

2 This refers to abnormal blood clotting. It may manifest as nosebleed, bleeding gums, vomiting blood, bloody or black stools, excessive menstruation, bleeding from minor wounds, spontaneous black and blue marks from little or no injury.

3 This refers to a prominent cough or shortness of breath.

4 This means you can get it directly from a patient without an intervening bug bite.

5 There may be severe depression.

6 An alternative name is monkey fever. Do not confuse this with monkeypox.

7 This refers to the kind of sand fly fever of the Eastern Hemisphere. The fever of the Western Hemisphere called sand fly fever is entirely different.

Table of arboviral fevers, their geographies and symptoms

Disease	Index	Region	Flu-like	Encephalitis[1]	Arthritis	Skin rash	Eyes	Bleeding[2]	Lungs[3]	Contagious[4]
Chikungunya	C	E,F,I,M, O,R,S,U	Y	Rare	Y, severe	Y	Red	Rare	Rare	N
Crimean-Congo hemorrhagic fever	C	F,R,I	Y	Y	N	N	Red	Y	Y	Y
Dengue fever	C	Tropics	Y	N[5]	Y	Y	Pain	Rarely	N	N
Japanese encephalitis	C	I,S,O	Y	Y	N	N	N	N	N	N
Kyasanur Forest diease[6]	I	I,R	Y	Y	N	Y	Red	Y	Y	Maybe
Murray Valley encephalitis	C	S Pacific	Y	Y	N	N	Red	N	N	N
Rift Valley fever	F	Africa	Y	Y	N	N	Red	Y	N	Maybe
Ross River fever	U	S Pacific	Y	N	Y	Y	N	N	N	N
Sand fly fever[7]	C	F,R	Y	N	N	N	Red	N	N	Maybe
Tick-borne encephalitis	C	Europe/Asia	Y	Y	N	N	N	N	N	N
West Nile virus	C	Worldwide	Y	Y	Y	Y	Red	N	N	N
Yellow fever	F,M	F,M	Y	N	N	N	Red	Y	N	N

SKIN

There are prominent rashes in addition to the undifferentiated symptoms.

EYES

Eyes are red and possibly sore also.

HEMORRHAGIC

This causes abnormal bleeding, usually after several days of the undifferentiated symptoms. See HEMORRHAGIC FEVER.

RESPIRATORY

There are prominent respiratory complaints in addition to the undifferentiated symptoms: cough, chest pain, shortness of breath.

Complications: long-term consequences of the encephalitic form are common: weakness of the limbs, depression, chronic fatigue, personality changes, blindness, deafness, trembling. This may be permanent or last for a long time, and it may occur with mild as well as severe disease.

Similar conditions: see Protocol B.2 for fever/headache/body pains; B.6 for limb swelling; B.8 for red painful eyes; B.9 for fever plus abdominal pains; B.10.A for fever plus lethargy, B.13 for fever plus back pain. The most common similar condition is INFLUENZA; pursue one of the diagnoses listed on the chart only if the condition is obviously more serious than simple flu: temperature over 101.3° F (38.5° C), and the patient is totally bedridden. Also, if it is a malarious area treat MALARIA. *With a rash and fever:* RAT BITE FEVER, SCRUB TYPHUS. *With prominent joint pains:* HEPATITIS, FIFTH DISEASE, RUBELLA. *With prominent mental symptoms:* cerebral MALARIA; AFRICAN SLEEPING SICKNESS, MONKEYPOX and LASSA FEVER in Africa only. EBOLA VIRUS DISEASE may be indistinguishable, particularly if there is no bleeding.

Bush laboratory: none and it's best not to handle blood, urine or stool.

Treatment

Prevention: keep patients under mosquito nets to avoid infecting local mosquitoes and thus transmitting the disease. It is essential to consider one of the contagious hemorrhagic fevers, especially if you are in Africa! Your own health is at risk, and you can cause a major, worldwide epidemic by indiscreetly transporting a contagious patient on public transportation. See Protocol B.2

Referrals: see Volume 1, Appendix 13. Send out if possible unless the patient might be contagious. See the chart in Protocol B.2. Also consult the Regional Notes for your area. Laboratory: level 4–5 only; a level 3–4 lab might be helpful to exclude alternatives. The definite diagnosis of the various arboviral fevers requires a large lab in a Western university. The other possibilities can be excluded by small to middle-sized hospital labs. Practitioner: level 4–5; an infectious disease specialist is ideal; a hematologist might be helpful; an internist or general practitioner is adequate in some cases. Hospitals may be able to use RIBAVIRIN or serum from patients who have recovered.

Patient care: treat the patient with ACETAMINOPHEN. Have him stay in bed. Sore joints may linger for months. Deaths are not common unless HEMORRHAGIC FEVER develops. However, disabilities are common with ENCEPHALITIS.

ARSENIC POISONING

Entry category: disease, toxic.

Definition: arsenic poisoning is a type of poisoning due to the heavy metal, arsenic.

Cause: pesticides, herbicides, ethnic herbs and medicines, some old medicines. Some of these products are: crocodile bile, crude red pills, crude tan pills.

Age: any. **Who:** suicide or homicide victims; work-related exposures, those using some herbal products. This is especially common in Taiwan, Mexico, Chile, India and Bangladesh. It can come from drinking water, from mines, glass work, metal work, burning plywood or the manufacture of semiconductor computer chips. Arsenic is found in wine, glues and pigments. It can be absorbed through the skin from pressure-treated wood. **Onset:** variable. With frequent small amounts, there is a latency period (like the incubation for infections) between exposure and symptoms. Large amounts cause immediate symptoms.

Clinical

TAKEN IN A LARGE DOSE

There is a garlic odor to the patient's breath. Arsenic causes nausea, vomiting, bloody diarrhea, a burning pain in the hands, feet, mouth and throat, bleeding gums and abdominal pains with diarrhea. It causes death by KIDNEY DISEASE, LIVER FAILURE or bleeding into the bowel.

TAKEN IN SMALL AMOUNTS OVER A LONG PERIOD

The patient develops numbness, tingling, burning and a weakness of the hands and feet which then moves toward the trunk. His eyes, throat and windpipe become red and irritated. His skin becomes dry, scaly and flaky, his face and limbs swell, and a horizontal white line forms on his fingernails. The skin changes are an essential element of the diagnosis.

Similar conditions: see Protocols B.7: Liver/Spleen problems and B.6: Limb Swelling. Check other causes of KIDNEY DISEASE and LIVER FAILURE. *Skin changes and burning, tingling:* PELLAGRA, BERIBERI, other nutritional diseases, tertiary YAWS. *Diarrhea:* CHOLERA, DYSENTERY or FOOD POISONING.

Treatment

Referrals: requires a level 4 or 5 laboratory and sophisticated drugs and monitoring. A large laboratory can analyse hair and fingernails for arsenic. See Volume 1, Appendix 13.

Aside from stopping exposure, treatment involves a physician and hospital facilities at level 4–5.

ARTHRITIS

Outline of this entry

I Introduction

II Clinical elements   General

Approach to diagnosis

Charts for differential diagnosis

Arthritis-only conditions

Logic of diagnosis

Trial treatments

III Treatment   Treatments

I. Introduction

Regional Notes: F, I, M, O, U.

Entry category: syndrome.

Includes: arthralgia, rheumatoid arthritis, osteoarthritis; septic arthritis, which includes that caused by GONORRHEA.

Definition: arthritis is a syndrome consisting of pain, redness or warmth and swelling of a joint or joints. Arthralgia is pain without the redness, warmth or swelling. Usually these conditions start out as arthralgia and progress to arthritis.

Cause: variable.

Well to moderately ill; class 2–4; worldwide, prevalence varies, no predictable pattern.

Age: any, even children. **Who:** anyone; see causative diseases below. **Onset:** over months, usually; occasionally rapid.

II. Clinical

Since arthritis is a syndrome, once you have diagnosed this far, you need to determine the cause. In the West most arthritis is autoimmune; the management thereof is complex and risky. In developing areas most arthritis is due to infectious causes and injuries. With autoimmune conditions there usually is a family history. With some infectious causes there may be, since families that live together are prone to developing similar infectious diseases.

Necessary: the patient has swollen, red, warm, and/or painful joints.

Approach to diagnosis:

1. Determine the context of this illness in this patient, if there are others with the same illness at this time. Determine if family members have had similar illnesses.

2. Determine if this is part of a general body illness involving a fever and skin abnormalities.

3. Key to the diagnosis is which joints[1] are involved and how. Large joints are the joints of the arms (shoulders through wrists) and of the legs (hips through ankles). Joints of the backbone and pelvis are considered large joints also. Small joints are the joints of the hands and feet.

4. Symmetry is whether the same joints are involved right and left. Symmetry does not have to be absolute. The number of joints refers to how many are painful at the present time. If there is only one joint involved or if the joints are in the back midline, then there is no symmetry.

5. A joint is inflamed if the pain does not decrease or disappear with rest. Starting a movement causes maximal pain. An inflamed joint will be abnormally warm.

6. The timing of the joint pains is likewise a key to diagnosis. The onset may be fast (over hours to days) or slow (over weeks to months). Pain relapses if it comes and goes. Relapsing refers to days, weeks or months, not to minutes or hours. Of course, if this is a first episode, you cannot know if it will disappear and relapse. Also, pain may migrate; that is, it travels from joint to joint during one episode. With ordinary migration the first joints improve as others become painful; with additive migration the pain moves to other joints without the first ones improving.

---

1 *It is not always obvious which joint is problematic. Sometimes a problem in one joint manifests with pain in another. This is particularly common with hips. Hip problems may manifest with knee pains. Push on the painful joint. If this aggravates the pain, then that joint is problematic. If it does not aggravate the pain, then push on adjacent joints. It is the joint that is tender (that is, pressure on that joint annoys the patient) that is the joint affected by the arthritis.*

BASIC ELEMENTS OF THE ILLNESS   L = likely; Y = yes; M = maybe; R = rarely; O = occasionally

CONDITION[1]	CONTEXT[2]			FEVER		SKIN PROBLEM[3]		RISK FACTORS
	Family	Many	Sporadic	Yes	None	Present	Absent	
Arboviral fever	Note 5 below	L		L		M	M	Tropics, creatures.
Brucellosis			L	M	M	R	L	Animals, milk, hides.
Chikungunya		Y		L		M	M	Mosquitoes.
Dengue		L		L		L		Mosquitoes.
FMF[6]	L		R	L, early		M	M	Ethnicity.
Gonorrhea[8]			L	M	M	M	M	Sexual.
Gout	M		L	Y, early	M	Red	L	> 30 y.o.
Hepatitis	M	M	M	M	M		L	Water, blood.
HIV infection	M	M	M	M	M	M	M	Sexual, blood.
Lyme disease			L	M		M	M	Temperate, woods.
Osteoarthritis			L		Y		L	Over 30.
Rat-bite fever			L	L		M	M	Asia, rat exposure.
Reiter syndrome			L	L		L	M	Expatriate.
Rheumatic fever			L	L		M	M	Children > Adults.
Rheumatoid arthritis			L	M	M		L	Adults > Children, expatriate.
Septic arthritis			L	M	M		L	Prior infection.
Sickle cell	L			M	M	M	M	Ethnicity.
Syphilis, infant			L		Y	M	M	Under 2 yr.
Syphilis, congenital			L		Y		L	2–30 y.o., mother infected.
Syphilis, acquired			L	M	M	M	M	Sexually active.
Tuberculosis			L		Y		L	TB exposure.
Viral arthritis[7]		L		L		L		Children/teens > adults.

1 These conditions are all in the Condition Index, but they are not upper case here for formatting reasons.

2 That is, in the community there are many patients with this disease at the same time. Sporadic means there are never many at the same time.

3 This may be a rash, but it may also be something like an ulcer or hole. It is prominent. The L under absent means there is likely no skin abnormality.

4 L = likely; Y = yes; M = maybe; R = rarely; O = occasionally

5 A blank cell in the table means that the author was unable to find information regarding that element.

6 Familial Mediterranean fever (FMF); the fever and pain are maximum at or before 48 hours. The rate of disappearance varies widely.

7 Viral arthritis is rubella, fifth disease and other childhood diseases with rashes, which commonly cause arthritis, particularly in older children and adults.

8 There are two kinds of gonorrhea arthritis: one is the same as septic arthritis; the other is the same as Reiter syndrome.

IDENTIFYING THE JOINTS[1] L = likely; Y = yes; M = maybe; R = rarely; O = occasionally

CONDITION[2]	JOINT SIZE[3]		SYMMETRY[4]		NUMBER OF PAINFUL JOINTS			INFLAMMED[5]
	Small	Large	Symmetry	Asymmetry	One	2–4	>4	
Arboviral	L	L		M				Varies.
Brucellosis	No	Y		M	M	L		Unlikely.
Chikungunya[7]	M	Y	L				L	L
Dengue	M	M						
FMF[8]	No	Y		Y	L	M		M, minimal warmth.
Gonorrhea	O	Y if one	R		M	M	M	Y, extreme pain.
Gout	M late	Early	M late	Early	L	M	R	Y, extreme pain.
Hepatitis	M	M	L			M	M	Unlikely.
HIV		L		M		M		Y
Lyme		L		M	M	M		Y
Osteoarthritis	M	L		M	M	M		No
Rat-bite fever	Y	Y				M	L	M
Reiter syndrome	M	Y		Y	M	M		Y
Rheumatic fever		Y	L	M	R	M	M	Y
Rheumatoid arthritis	M	M	L	M		M	M	Y
Septic arthritis	M	M		Y	L			Y, extreme pain.
Sickle cell	Y	Y		Y	L			Y
Syphilis, infant[9]		Y	L	M		M	M	M
Syphilis, congenital[10]	No	Knees	Y			2		No
Syphilis, acquired	M	Y	M		L	M		No
Tuberculosis		Y		Y	L			Unlikely.
Viral arthritis	Y	M	L				L	Unlikely.

1 Be sure the pain is in the joints, not only in the bones adjacent to the joints. Have the patient use one finger to show you where the pain is the worst. If that is not a joint, then consult the protocols for bone pain in the Symptom Index. The problem is not arthritis. If the pains are both in the joints and in the long bones, the diagnosis is probably dengue fever, sickle cell disease or syphilis.

2 The conditions are all in the Condition Index, but they are not upper case here for formatting reasons.

3 Small joints are the joints of the hands and fingers mainly, sometimes of the feet also. They are joints smaller than the wrist. The joints of the midline skeleton are considered large joints.

4 Symmetry is whether the right and left sides are similarly affected. Symmetry does not have to be absolute in order to qualify as symmetrical.

5 Inflammed, that is, rest does not much relieve the pain, but motion aggravates it.

6 A blank cell in the table means that the author was unable to find information regarding that element.

7 Chikungunya commonly involves the joints of the backbone.

8 FMF = Familial Mediterranean fever. The joint involved is apt to be one that previously was stressed or injured, maybe minor.

9 That is, onset before age 2 years, usually during the first 4 weeks.

10 That is, onset after age 2; the onset may be up to age 30.

TIME-COURSE OF THE ILLNESS L = likely; Y = yes; M = maybe; R = rarely; O = occasionally

CONDITION	ONSET[1]		RELAPSE[2]		MIGRATION[3]	RELATIVELY SENSITIVE
	fast	slow	relapse	continual		
Arboviral	L				Vaaries	Fever and general body pains.
Brucellosis		L	M	M	M early None late	Slow onset, back or lower limbs, present in the community.
Chikungunya	L			Y	M	Pain is incapacitating.
Dengue	L		L		None	Non-joint bone pain also, eye pain.
FMF	L		Y		None[6]	Healthy between attacks.
Gonorrhea	L			M	M, additive[4]	Sexually active or abused.
Gout	L		Y		Late	Extreme pain; affluent.
Hepatitis	M	M			None	Jaundice when joints improve.
HIV	Varies		M	M		Weight loss, other infections.
Lyme disease			L		Maybe	Temperate climate with ticks.
Osteoarthritis		L			None	Joints with injury or wear and tear.
Rat-bite fever			L		L	Rats common; large & small joints, away from the trunk.
Reiter syndrome	Y			M	M, additive[4]	Prior dysentery or genital symptoms.
Rheumatic fever	L		U		L	Sore throat history common; spectacular relief with aspirin.
Rheumatoid arthritis		L	L		L	Morning stiffness, in developing areas mostly expatriates.
Septic arthritis				L	None	History of prior infection common.
Sickle cell disease		L		L	M	Family history is usual; a variety of episodic pains beginning <5y.o.
Syphilis, infant	M	M		L	None	Ill newborn, mother maybe had prior miscarriages, stillbirths, infant deaths.
Syphilis, congenital		L		Y	None	Symmetrical knee swelling, not very painful.
Syphilis, acquired		L		Y	None	Worse with warmth and at night.
Tuberculosis		L		Y	None	Swelling more than pain, slow onset.
Viral arthritis	L			Y	Maybe	Epidemic context with rashes.

1 *A fast onset is within hours to days. A slow onset takes weeks, months or years.*

2 *Relapse means that the problem went away on its own and then came back. Continual means that the problem has not gone away. If it started recently, then it might appear to be continual now because it is too soon for it to disappear and then relapse. Arthritis is considered relapsing even if subsequent episodes involve different joints, as long as the kind of pain is the same.*

3 *Unqualified migration means that the pain in the present joints gets better as new joints become involved.*

4 *Additive migration means the first joints don't get better as the pain migrates to other joints.*

5 *During one episode the pain stays in one joint, but with other episodes it may involve another joint.*

6 *The pain does not migrate during any one episode, but different episodes may involve different joints.*

COMPARISON BETWEEN THE MOST COMMON TYPES OF ARTHRITIS-ONLY DIAGNOSES

GOUT

Age: adult, usually middle-aged or older. **Who**: affluent, men, eating a Western diet. **Onset**: rapid for the particular episode.

Clinical: pain, redness, warmth, swelling of a single joint, usually the base of a large toe or an ankle for the initial episode. Subsequent episodes may involve the upper limbs, some symmetry and small joints. The pain is extreme.

Similar diseases: when advanced, RHEUMATOID ARTHRITIS, but the history is different. Septic ARTHRITIS and GONORRHEA may be indistinguishable, particularly for the initial episode in an ankle.

Treatment: there are special drugs. See the separate entry, GOUT.

Rheumatoid arthritis

Age: any, but middle-age is more common than younger. **Who**: especially affluent, Western culture, family history. **Onset**: usually rapid for each episode.

Clinical: pain, redness, warmth, swelling of (usually) multiple joints, symmetrical, comes and goes by itself, with morning stiffness that improves during the day.

Similar diseases: RHEUMATIC FEVER, BRUCELLOSIS, REITER SYNDROME.

Treatment: high-dose ASPIRIN is best, another anti-inflammatory drug may be helpful if aspirin is not available.

Septic arthritis

Age: any. **Who**: anyone, especially those with a prior infection or a wound. **Onset**: varies; usually rapid.

Clinical: pain, redness, warmth, swelling of a single joint or two, not symmetrical, maybe with a fever and general illness. The pain is extreme.

Similar diseases: GONORRHEA, FILARIASIS, LYME DISEASE, REITER SYNDROME.

Treatment: send to higher level care to drain the pus from the joint and rinse it out. The patient needs antibiotics, but this is no substitute for drainage. Use a third-generation CEPHALOSPORIN or a combination of Gram-positive and Gram-negative antibiotics.

Osteoarthritis

Age: adults, older unless this is due to a specific, known injury. **Who**: history of injury to the joint(s) involved; history of stressing the joints repeatedly as in rough sports. **Onset**: gradual, usually.

Clinical: joint pains with little or no redness, warmth or swelling. The severity of the pain varies, but it is not extreme. There is symmetry if the prior injury or stress was symmetrical, such as hips in football players. This does not cause fever.

Similar diseases: BRUCELLOSIS, LYME DISEASE, SYPHILIS.

Treatment: pain medications and anti-inflammatory medications. Higher level care is only appropriate if there is the option of implanting an artificial joint. This requires a level 4 or 5 hospital.

Viral arthritis

Age: any. **Who**: anyone, particularly those coming down with HEPATITIS, CHIKUNGUNYA, RUBELLA or ARBOVIRAL FEVER. **Onset**: usually rapid; may be slow.

Clinical: in the process of developing a viral illness, the patient also develops painful, swollen, tender, red or warm joints. The knuckle joints of the middle of the hand are frequently involved; there may be large-joint involvement also. The arthritis is usually symmetrical. There may be morning stiffness.

Similar diseases: rheumatoid arthritis, REITER SYNDROME, LYME DISEASE.

Treatment: pain medication and anti-inflammatory medicines such as ASPIRIN or IBUPROFEN.

Condition	Context	Fever	Skin	Risk	Joint size	Symmetry	Number	Inflammed	Onset	Relapse	Migrate	Sens
Arboviral												
Brucellosis												
Chikungunya												
Dengue												
FMF												
Gonorrhea												
Gout												
Hepatitis												
HIV												
Lyme disease												
Osteoarthritis												
Rat-bite fever												
Reiter syndrome												
Rheumatic fever												
Rheumatoid arthritis												
Septic arthritis												
Sickle cell disease												
Syphilis, infant												
Syphilis, congenital												
Syphilis, acquired												
Tuberculosis												
Viral arthritis												

LOGIC OF DIAGNOSIS:

In each cell on the chart above, put a symbol, perhaps a colored dot, as to whether that characteristic is a vote for the diagnosis, a vote against it or neutral. Then a simple glance at the chart will indicate which condition descriptions you need to read in detail, in order to make a best-guess diagnosis.

TRIAL TREATMENT

If there is any history of injury, treat the patient with pain medication: ASPIRIN or IBUPROFEN is best. If the arthritis is non-inflammatory, this is all you can do for him. It is also the only treatment for some types of inflammatory arthritis. It is appropriate in all cases, with the exception of some medications which should not be used for GOUT. Even with a history of injury, do pursue further diagnosis. Sometimes diseases settle in joints that have previously been injured. Also keep contact with the patient for the next week. Sometimes joint pains are the first symptom of viral diseases such as HEPATITIS, RUBELLA and some ARBOVIRAL FEVERs.

Consider a trial treatment for infectious arthritis. Symptoms indicating an infection-related cause are as follows: sudden onset; the condition migrates from joints to joints; whole-body symptoms like fever; redness (or warmth) is more prominent than swelling; at least one hip is involved.

CONDITIONS SIMILAR TO ARTHRITIS:

MANSONELLOSIS PERSTANS and ONCHOCERCIASIS are parasitic diseases, confined to certain parts of Africa and the Americas, that can cause a condition of chronic joint pains. They are not included in the list above. They affect mostly expatriates.

III. Treatment of arthritis

Prevention: treat all DYSENTERY, GONORRHEA and STREP THROAT. Treating arthritis earlier rather than later prevents permanent damage to the joints.

Referrals: laboratory: level 3 might be helpful; generally level 4 or 5 is necessary. Facilities: x-ray may be helpful. Surgical theatre might be helpful; also there are some sophisticated drugs available at level 4. Practitioner: initially internal medicine at a level 3 or higher facility. A surgeon with level 4 or higher capabilities might be necessary at some point.

Patient care: in all cases except GOUT, use anti-inflammatory drugs: ASPIRIN, IBUPROFEN or DICLOFENAC. If you suspect GOUT, then use COLCHICINE but avoid ASPIRIN. If it is a single joint, send the patient out for surgery. Without surgery antibiotics do no good. Do use a CEPHALOSPORIN while awaiting surgery.

Treat RHEUMATIC FEVER on mere suspicion. In someone sexually active, cover GONORRHEA , SYPHILIS and REITER SYNDROME. If you try an antibiotic MINOCYCLINE is best; some forms of arthritis respond to it.

Results: 48–72 hours improvement.

ASCARIASIS

Regional Notes: F, I, K, O, R, S, U.

Entry category: disease.

Synonyms: ascaridiasis, roundworm.

Definition: ascariasis is a disease caused by the infestation of the bowels with the worm *Ascaris lumbricoides.*

Not ill to very ill; class 1–3; worldwide, tropical mainly, most common where soil is clay or loam and humidity is high. It is not likely to be a big health problem in areas with less than 1200 mm rainfall per year. If it is a problem in your area, people will report occasionally passing light-colored "earthworms" by rectum or by mouth.

Age: any, but especially children. **Who:** those eating raw foods which have not been peeled or soaked in bleach- or iodine-water. (Washing does not eliminate the worm eggs.) **Onset:** usually gradual, but may be without symptoms and then have sudden onset. The initial cough, if it occurs, comes 4–16 days after eating the contaminated food.

Clinical

Necessary: cramping abdominal pains, or the patient reports seeing worms in his stool or in his mouth or nose. Ascaris worms are the size and shape of earthworms or larger; they are the only worms that are in this size range.

Maybe: there is an initial cough and fever for 2–3 months after eating the offending food. The sputum coughed up may be bloody. If the case is severe there will be vomiting. The abdomen may be distended, and the patient may be constipated. There may be pain in the right upper abdomen. Diarrhea is unusual. MALNUTRITION occurs even with mild cases; there may be refusal to eat or a good appetite, but in both cases there is weight loss. (Children will have a growth spurt after deworming.) Strange cravings may occur. With heavy infections or with fasting, worms migrate into the mouth and nose; they may be vomited.

Complications: ACUTE ABDOMEN, MALNUTRITION, RESPIRATORY INFECTION, HEART FAILURE. It may occasionally cause liver problems similar to AMEBIASIS. The worms may cause GALLBLADDER DISEASE; children have pains every 15–30 minutes, lasting 5–10 minutes and their upper-right abdomens are tender. The gallbladder is enlarged so it is possible to feel it; there is greenish-yellow discoloration of the whites of the eyes; the patient has general, whole-body itching without a skin rash; the patient's stool is light-colored.

Similar conditions: IMPACTION is likely in disabled or bed-ridden patients. TUBERCULOSIS of the abdomen may be indistinguishable; treat for ascariasis first and see what happens. In areas where TUBERCULOSIS is common, treat for that if two treatments for ASCARIASIS don't help. HYDATID DISEASE is found in very few areas. The early stage of ascariasis (cough and fever) is indistinguishable from ordinary PNEUMONIA and RESPIRATORY INFECTION.

Treatment

Prevention: encourage the use of outhouses. Wash hands well, and clean fingernails. Peel foods or soak food in bleach or iodine water between market and use; see Chapter 2. Simple washing does no good. If you treat everyone in a village, the treatment should be repeated every 6 months.

Referrals: laboratory: stool examination for worms, level 2 or higher. Almost any hospital lab with a microscope can find the ascaris eggs in one stool specimen. The test is both sensitive and specific, so both a positive test and a negative test are significant. During the initial 2–3 months' migration through the lungs, the blood count will show many eosinophils, but the stool will be negative for eggs. Once the eggs appear in the stool, then the eosinophils disappear from the blood. Practitioner: general practitioner, pediatrician or internist for diagnosis; for complications, a surgeon.

Patient care

- With ACUTE ABDOMEN or GALLBLADDER DISEASE, do not kill the worms! If there is GALLBLADDER DISEASE, initially use LOPERAMIDE rather than one of the worm medicines. Kill the worms only after the symptoms have abated.

- Without complications, to kill the worms, ALBENDAZOLE, LEVAMISOLE, MEBENDAZOLE, IVEERMECTIN or PYRANTEL PAMOATE are the best drugs. FLUBENDAZOLE, THIABENDAZOLE, BEPHENIUM HYDROXYNAPHTHOATE NITAZOXANIDE and PIPERAZINE may be effective. If symptoms are severe, give repeated small doses before giving full doses.

ASTHMA

Regional Notes: F, M, O, U.

Entry category: disease.

Synonyms: asthmatic bronchitis, bronchospasm.

Definition: asthma is an allergic reaction to some substance, causing narrowing of the airways and shortness of breath.

Cause: allergy.

Mildly to very ill; class 2–4; worldwide, common in developed countries.

Age: 1–10 y.o. usually, for first attack. **Who:** anyone, especially those affluent with allergies or family allergies. **Onset:** minutes to hours for each attack. Asthma tends to recur.

TOC SYMPTOMS DIFFERENTIALS CONDITIONS DRUG INDEX REGIONAL NOTES INX

Clinical

Necessary: the patient is short of breath; it is always harder for him to breathe out than in. He is either wheezing, or he has a tight, dry cough without wheezing[1].

Sometimes: he is blue around the lips. He may have other symptoms of ALLERGY. He is probably congested. The patient usually has a fast respiratory rate and a fast pulse. In severe cases, his respiratory rate may be normal or slow, but then he is obviously struggling to breathe. In long-lasting cases the patient may have an irregular pulse.

Complications: asthma may result in RESPIRATORY FAILURE, HEART FAILURE, RESPIRATORY INFECTION.

Causative diseases: adult-onset asthma is frequently due to TUBERCULOSIS or ALLERGY to ASPIRIN. MANSONELLOSIS PERSTANS is possible in Africa or South America. STRONGYLOIDIASIS is a common cause in the tropics and subtropics. HYDATID DISEASE and SMOKE INHALATION may cause asthma. If there is a fever, consider SERUM SICKNESS and the underlying infections that cause it. In areas where FILARIASIS is common, asthma may be due to that; try treating for FILARIASIS.

Similar conditions: see Protocol B.4: in allergic people, any kind of RESPIRATORY FAILURE may present as if it were asthma. *Shortness of breath.* HEART FAILURE may be indistinguishable; treat with THEOPHYLLINE only if this is likely. GOITER can also cause wheezing. ALTITUDE SICKNESS should be obvious if you know your location.

Treatment

Prevention: discourage people from smoking within the patient's home, whether the patient is there at the time or not. Dust, sweep or otherwise raise dust only when the patient will be absent for several hours. Sometimes asthma is caused by a tiny insect, in which case regular spraying of the house with an insecticide may be very helpful.

Referrals: see Volume 1, Appendix 13. Laboratory: level 3 or higher; a respiratory care team, ability to determine blood gases. Facilities: chest x-ray, level 3; occasionally more sophisticated tests at level 4 or 5. Monitored bed, anesthesia equipment, ventilator, oxygen if there is severe distress. Practitioner: general practitioner, internist or pediatrician. *Patient care:* at level 3 or above referral hospitals, there are likely to be excellent inhaled medications for asthma that work much better than the medications listed below. These older medicines are listed because they are more commonly available and much less expensive. In areas with FILARIASIS or STRONGYLOIDIASIS, treat for it or them, since these are common causes of "asthma"

Mild attack: THEOPHYLLINE or ALBUTEROL.

Severe attack: THEOPHYLLINE and EPINEPHRINE. You may also add either HYDROCORTISONE or PREDNISONE for severe or recurrent asthma. IPRATROPIUM or METAPROTERENOL may be helpful.

Results: 15 minutes improvement with EPINEPHRINE, 60 minutes with the other drugs except for PREDNISONE which takes 6 hours. Entirely well in 7–10 days, unless the patient has a second attack or is a chronic asthmatic.

ATTENTION DEFICIT DISORDER (ADD)

Synonyms: ADD, ADHD, hyperactivity.

Definition: attention deficit disorder is a hereditary condition causing a "sticky valve" effect as regards attention.

Cause: heredity; lack of a brain hormone.

Not ill; class 1–3, depending on severity.

Age: any, but the problem is more common and obvious in children than adults. **Who:** members of affected families; boys more than girls; common in adopted children. Some ethnic groups are more affected than others. **Onset:** chronic and recurrent problems dating from birth or early childhood; adult onset is rare.

Clinical

Necessary: the person either has trouble paying attention or trouble switching attention in a calm, controlled manner. Some people are physically hyperactive; others not.

Common consequences of this are as follows, but not every patient has every symptom: nervousness; impulsive behavior; inner rage; addictions; learning disabilities,[2] sleep disorders,[3] inconsistent performance in school,[4] lack of depth perception,[5] incoordination,[6] lack of social skills and conscience; emotional immaturity; irritability (for example, from labels in clothing); reverse response to sedative or stimulant medications.[7]

Similar conditions: if there is a crisis, consider the conditions in Protocol B.10. Consider various forms of malnutrition, e.g. PELLAGRA and BERIBERI, which can cause mental symptoms. ADDICTION may be indistinguishable except for age of onset. Also consider DEMONIZATION. If the patient has a fever, consider MALARIA, TYPHUS and similar conditions.

Treatment

Referrals: laboratory, facilities: nothing is helpful. Practitioner: pediatrician, psychiatrist, counselors, level 4 or above.

---

2 *Reading disability, left/right and north/south/east/west disorientation are common manifestations of this.*

3 *This may take the form of insomnia, abnormally deep sleep or bed-wetting.*

4 *The student will get an A without trying in one subject and struggle for a D in a closely related subject.*

5 *This will manifest as inability to judge speed and distance with consequent incoordination and poor judgment when driving.*

6 *This may be either fine (handwriting) or gross (sports) or both.*

7 *The person may be calmed by stimulants such as caffeine, theophyllin and Ritalin, but become agitated with sedatives.*

---

1 *Wheezing is high-pitched, squeaky sounds, usually during a long expiration. If wheezing is severe, you can hear it without a stethoscope.*

Patient care: avoid large-group situations. Avoid fluorescent lights. Since conscience development is deficient, parents should stress consequences of actions. Medication may be helpful. Reportedly the anti-seizure drug CARBAMAZEPINE works for this. THEOPHYLLIN may help. Adults should seek counseling with someone who is familiar with the phenomenon.

BARTHOLIN CYST / ABSCESS

In both cases, this is a lump next to the vagina in a female. If it is warm, red and tender, it is an abscess. If it is not, it is a cyst. An abscess should be drained. A cyst can be removed by a physician or nurse practitioner. See Volume 1, Chapter 6 for a picture.

BARTONELLOSIS

See Regional Notes M. The term also recently refers to CAT-SCRATCH DISEASE and sometimes TRENCH FEVER. In this work, the term only refers to the disease found in Peru and adjacent countries. Others may use the term with a broader definition.

BEDSORE

Definition: this is an open sore that spontaneously arises due to the person's putting pressure on the same part of his body for an extended period of time. It is indistinguishable from TROPICAL ULCER and is treated the same, whether or not the patient is in the tropics. See Protocol B.11 for similar conditions.

Treatment

Prevention is easier than treatment; turn any patient who does not turn himself, at least every two hours during the day and every four hours at night to avoid constant pressure on one part of his body.

Referrals: laboratory and facilities: level 3 or above are helpful in stubborn cases. Practitioner: physicians or nurses with experience in long-term care facilities might be most helpful. The treatment is labor-intensive and takes a long time, but is not difficult. Even an email contact—send close-up pictures of the wound and get advice—can be very helpful.

You might be able to train a national to do the hands-on work. Detailed instructions are beyond the scope of this book.

Patient care: see TROPICAL ULCER. Tend the patient's nutrition.

Results: slow improvement over weeks and months.

BELL'S PALSY

Regional Notes: E, F, I, R.

Entry category: syndrome.

Synonym: seventh cranial nerve paralysis.

Definition: this is a paralysis of the muscles on one side of the face.

Cause: variable.

Not ill to mildly ill; class 2–3; worldwide, not common, not rare.

Age: any, especially adults. **Who:** anyone. **Onset:** suddenly.

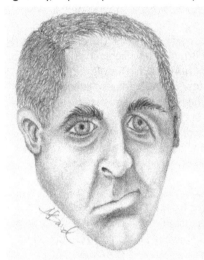

Bell's palsy on the right side. The left side is normal, even though the eye has a peculiar shape. The patient cannot completely close the eye on the right side. When he smiles the right side of his mouth does not move. AB

Clinical

Sudden drooping of the face (usually only one side) with inability to close the eye on that side, usually with no pain, no warning and no other symptoms. This is easily confused with STROKE. The problem may occur for no known reason or may be due to RELAPSING FEVER (never with the first fever, always with a relapse), POLIO, LEPROSY, LYME DISEASE (may be on both sides with this), DIPHTHERIA or EAR INFECTION, MIDDLE (which may be due to ordinary bacteria or TUBERCULOSIS). A child with a draining ear plus Bell's palsy most likely has TUBERCULOSIS.

Treatment

Referrals: practitioner: general practitioner, internist, pediatrician. A neurologist is most helpful.

Patient care: it usually goes away by itself in a matter of weeks or months and is treated only by keeping the eye moist. ARTIFICIAL TEARS are best. Sterile saline will do. See Volume 1, Appendix 1, Procedure 1. Put drops or ointment in the eye and patch the eye.

BERIBERI

Regional Notes: F, I, O, R, S.

Synonyms: thiamine deficiency.

Includes: dry and wet beriberi, Wernike-Korsakoff syndrome.

Definition: beriberi is an illness caused by a deficiency of the vitamin thiamine. Thiamine is vitamin B_1.

Cause: poor nutrition (thiamine deficiency).

Mildly to severely ill; class 1; worldwide, areas with white rice or any starch-only diet.

Age: any, including infants of mothers with marginal thiamine intake. **Who:** those eating a diet deficient in THIAMINE, especially those who also consume ALCOHOL. (See ALCOHOLISM.) It is most common in cultures consuming polished white rice that is milled by machinery. (Rice milled by hand retains enough THIAMINE.) THIAMINE is found in yeast, brown rice, peanuts, wheat, barley, millet, pork, liver and to a small extent in legumes. Beriberi may be associated with any physical stress such as hard work, fevers, alcohol consumption, pregnancy or nursing. **Onset:** usually slow, maybe rapid, may come and go repeatedly. It requires a few weeks on a deficient diet to develop the condition.

Clinical

Necessary: the patient (or his mother) eats a diet without whole grains or meats. Initially he has whole-body itching or a sensation of bugs crawling on his skin. Additionally, he has symptoms of one or more of the 4 types: infant, paraplegic, wet or mental. The various types may blend into each other. There is no fever due to this.

INFANT BERIBERI

These are the breastfed babies of malnourished women. They have a hoarse or silent cry or SEIZURES, abnormal eye movements and vomiting. They might have large livers.

PARAPLEGIC (DRY) BERIBERI

Limbs: this causes general weakness of the limbs, with numbness, tingling, burning pains and loss of muscle. The pains are increased with warmth. Squeezing the calves causes pain. The muscles may twitch. There is ascending weakness, from the feet up towards the trunk. The skin is shiny. Because of the weakness, the patient is uncoordinated. He walks with his feet wide apart and may lift his legs high with each step, letting them flop down, since it is hard for him to raise his toes. The legs are affected first and mainly; he may also have arm symptoms later if the problem is severe.

Eyes: the pupils gravitate inward, toward the nose. There may be pain in the eyes, flashing lights or a mist in the center of his vision.

WET BERIBERI

This causes HEART FAILURE in addition to the symptoms of dry beriberi, usually with a sudden onset. The patient, however, has little or no protein in his urine. His urine specific gravity will be high. He may have abnormal heart sounds. His blood pressure will have a very low second number, so his pulse pressure will be high. His ankles are always swollen. His liver and face may swell also. He may have a heart murmur. He may have abdominal pains made worse with food.

MENTAL BERIBERI

This usually involves one of the other types also. The patient has severe and persistent loss of appetite. In addition, the patient is confused and makes up fantastic stories. This is especially common in alcoholics. It may be precipitated by diarrhea, SEPSIS or MALARIA.

Similar conditions: most similar conditions also cause fever, which beriberi does not. See Protocol A.10.B and the conditions outlined below. *Infant:* congenital SYPHILIS. *Paraplegic and mental:* tertiary SYPHILIS is different in that it causes sharp, shooting, rather than burning pains. Mental symptoms can be similar. Also consider DEMONIZATION. STROKE usually involves weakness on one side only; beriberi weakness is roughly symmetrical. PLANT POISONING onset is rapid. ARSENIC POISON may be similar; look for the rough rash. DIPHTHERIA may cause paralysis, but this always follows problems with the mouth and eyes. *Wet beriberi:* HOOKWORM can also cause HEART FAILURE, but burning pains and specific leg weakness are not present. Consider other causes of HEART FAILURE.

Diagnosis is by trying the treatment. The symptoms improve spectacularly over a couple of hours or less with injected THIAMINE. Complete recovery takes a couple weeks.

Treatment

Referrals: laboratory, facilities are generally not helpful. Send out for wet or mental beriberi, treating in the meantime. Practitioner: general practitioner, internist, pediatrician. A dietician might also be helpful.

Patient care: give THIAMINE, preferably by injection, but by mouth is acceptable. If you don't have the vitamin, give thiamine-containing foods. See Volume 1, Chapter 5. It is good to add multivitamins, since multiple deficiencies are common.

Results: some symptoms resolve rapidly, some slowly. If the diagnosis is correct, you should see some improvement within a day. Severe HEART FAILURE, however, may not improve.

BIG HEEL

This is an unusual condition that occurs in Ghana, Taiwan and possibly elsewhere. There is a sudden onset of fever. The patient develops pain and tenderness with swelling of one or both heels. Neither cause nor cure is known.

BLADDER STONE

Regional Notes: F, I, O, R.

Clinical

A stone forms in the bladder, usually in school-aged boys. They pull on their penises to begin urinating and their stream may be interrupted at times as the stone blocks the urine. If it is not taken care of, when they get older they may have to jump up and down or lie down to urinate. If the stone becomes large, it can decrease the capacity of the bladder.

Treatment

Surgery which is simple and effective; at a level 3 or above, possibly some level 2 facilities.

Boutonneuse fever

African tick typhus or Mediterranean tick typhus, both listed under SPOTTED FEVER.

BRAIN DAMAGE

Regional Notes: F, I, O, R, S, U.

Entry category: syndrome.

Synonym: encephalopathy.

Definition: brain damage is a malfunction of the brain due to some injury or illness.

Cause: variable.

Clinical

Necessary: symptoms of brain damage are any combination of the following: lack of muscle control with abnormal gait; trembling, jerking or seizures; weakness or paralysis (stiff after a few weeks); retention or incontinence of urine or stool; inability to concentrate; confusion or mental retardation; dizziness, blindness, deafness, loss of smell; difficulty understanding or speaking; trouble swallowing; abnormal pupil size and/or eye movements; irregular respirations; drooping of one side of the face.

Causative diseases: HIV INFECTION, LIVER FAILURE (see Protocol B.7), PELLAGRA, BERIBERI, ADDICTION, TRICHINOSIS, SICKLE CELL DISEASE, CYSTICERCOSIS, ENCEPHALITIS, EPILEPSY, head injury, HEAT ILLNESS, MALARIA (cerebral), MEASLES, MENINGITIS, RADIATION ILLNESS, SCHISTOSOMIASIS JAPONICUM, SCHISTOSOMIASIS MANSONI, STROKE, SYPHILIS. See CEREBRAL PALSY also. Any symptoms that have been present over six months probably will be permanent. LIVER FAILURE might cause this—mild involves just confusion, more severe a tremor in addition and very severe, SEIZURES or coma. In this case the damage may be reversible with treatment. *Similar conditions:* SPINAL NEUROPATHY and the conditions listed in Protocol B.10.

Treatment

Referrals: there is no sense in sending the patient out to a facility with less than level 4 capabilities.

Patient care: until sending out, attend to SEIZURES, DEHYDRATION, MALNUTRITION and be sure that the patient is breathing adequately, and does not choke on his secretions. See Volume 1 Appendix 8.

BRAIN TUMOR

This refers to any abnormal lump in the brain. It may be an ordinary tumor (benign or malignant) or else something like HYDATID DISEASE or CYSTICERCOSIS. There may be no symptoms at all, or it may cause symptoms of BRAIN DAMAGE listed above. It may also cause headache, the most common pattern being an intermittent, localized headache, with increasing frequency and severity of pain. Sending the patient to a level 4 or above facility is mandatory.

BRUCELLOSIS[1]

Regional Notes: E, F, I, K, M, N, O, R, S, U

Entry category: disease.

Synonyms: Bang's disease, Malta fever, Mediterranean fever, undulant fever, Gibraltar fever, Danube fever.

Definition: Brucellosis is a slow-onset bacterial infection of animals and secondarily of humans, caused by the bacteria *Brucella abortus* or *Brucella melitensis.*

Cause: bacteria, Gram-negative.

Mildly to very ill; class 2–4: contagious, any direct contact; worldwide, mainly tropical, pastoral, mainly in the Mediterranean and Middle East, the northern part of Mexico, Mongolia, the Sahel and Central Asia.

Age: any, but mostly adults. **Who:** anyone handling meats or domestic animals and those consuming unpasteurized milk products. It can come from breathing dust in pastoral areas. It is transmitted by human breast milk. It may be sexually transmitted. **Onset:** varies, usually slow.

Clinical

The chief complaint is always one of the following: fatigue, joint pains, fevers, episodes of sweating.

Necessary: the patient should have all of the characteristics, a–c, and at least one of the conditions listed under d.

a. a setting of exposure to animals or their products in an environment without adequate veterinary public health: animal husbandry, slaughter, meat packing, working with wool or hides, consumption of rare or raw meat, or consumption of unpasteurized milk.

b. a slow-onset, recurrent whole-body illness with episodic fevers, fatigue and accelerating misery that has lasted 10 days or more.

c. symptomatic dysfunction of at least one organ systems:

  • abdomen—loss of appetite, vomiting, constipation, weight loss;

  • brain--weakness, incoordination, difficulty with seeing and hearing, headache, stiff neck, abnormal emotions and behavior;

  • skeletal system—sore joints in the lower body, with pains that migrate before settling down to one or a few joints.

---

1 See the Powerpoint lecture entitled *Brucellosis.*

d. additional symptoms:

- *common*: swollen painful scrotum, a single swollen joint in a child, no shaking chills with fevers, large liver, large spleen, family or personal history of Brucellosis.

- *uncommon* but specific: pain in eyes with looking sideways; pain in cheeks with chewing; fever without feeling feverish; rash; bizarre behavior, incoordination; weakness of lower limbs; headache; stiff neck; constipation, thirst.

Sometimes: There are symptoms not listed here. Additional symptoms should not negate the diagnosis.

If in doubt about the diagnosis, try the treatment. Sometimes the first dose of medicine makes the patient sicker. **Do not stop treatment for this. It is evidence that the diagnosis is correct**. If the patient does not get either better or worse within 4 or 5 days, the diagnosis probably is not correct. If the patient has a relapse, give a full second treatment.

Complications: HEART FAILURE, STROKE, BRAIN DAMAGE. ABORTION in pregnancy. LIVER DISEASE, destruction of testicles and infection in bones resembling TUBERCULOSIS. The disease persists at low levels throughout life, and it will reactivate when the immunity is down.

Similar conditions: see Protocols B.10 and B.12. With Brucellosis there is a slow onset; fever, sweats or both; and large joints only. Take the patient's temperature several times a day for a week. If he never has a fever, he probably does not have Brucellosis. Also see Protocol A.12: Large Lymph Nodes if applicable. *Bone and joint pains:* various kinds of ARTHRITIS; ARBOVIRAL FEVER. RHEUMATIC FEVER joints are always red or warm as well as painful and swollen; the joints of Brucellosis are not usually red or warm, though they might be. In areas where MANSONELLOSIS PERSTANS occurs, try a treatment for that first. It may be indistinguishable. The normal changes of OLD AGE may be very similar.

Bone TB pain never migrates like Brucellosis pain initially does. In the spine the two conditions may be indistinguishable. See Protocol B.6: Limb Swelling or Protocol B.13: Fever plus Back Pain.

Inflammation of the testicles may resemble MUMPS, TYPHUS, FILARIASIS, EPIDIDYMITIS or TB. *JAUNDICE:* see Protocols B.5 and B.7. *Flu-like symptoms:* Brucellosis is distinguishable from ENTERIC FEVER and SEPSIS in that the highest daily fever occurs at noon or early afternoon. In these other conditions, the peak fever occurs near sunset. *Mental symptoms:* see Protocol B.10.

Bush laboratory: sedimentation rate is elevated in 50%, so it is not helpful. There may be protein in the urine, but this also occurs in some other diseases.

Treatment

Prevention: destroy affected animals, pasteurize milk.

Referrals: sending out to a level 4 facility is very desirable. See Volume 1, Appendix 13. Laboratory: blood cultures can be done in level 3 or above hospitals. They must be held for 6 weeks before they are thrown out as being negative. A negative result does not exclude the diagnosis, particularly in longstanding (>1 year) cases. An antibody test is available. Level 2 and some level 3 laboratories are probably useless. Facilities: level 4 or above, x-ray might be helpful. Practitioner: infectious disease specialist with tropical/travel expertise is essential. The diagnosis is elusive and the treatment is complex. Since the problem is no longer of public health concern in the West, medical text books don't write much about it. Therefore physicians (both national and Western) are frequently not familiar with it. If you send the patient to a hospital be sure the hospital personnel are experienced in diagnosing and treating this. Otherwise just try treating.

Patient care: treatment is with at least 3 drugs, for 6 weeks if the symptoms have been present for less than a month, for 3 months if the symptoms have been present for more than a month. After a year the treatment should be extended to 6 months. One or two drugs are inadequate. It is better to not treat at all than to treat inadequately. Choose three of the following for the entire time. (STREPTOMYCIN or GENTAMYCIN), DOXYCYCLINE, CO-TRIMOXAZOLE, CIPROFLOXACIN (or a related medication), RIFAMPIN, CEPHALOSPORIN (ceftriaxone), CHLORAMPHENICOL. Evidence indicates that adding LEVAMISOLE to the antibiotics hastens recovery. In pregnancy avoid STREPTOMYCIN, DOXYCYCLINE and CIPROFLOXACIN. The patient may feel much worse the first few days that he takes the medicine; this confirms the diagnosis, and it will pass. Warn him not to discontinue the meds.

Results: gradual, over weeks and months.

BURKITT LYMPHOMA

Regional Notes: F, M, R, U.

Entry category: disease, a type of CANCER.

Definition: a childhood cancer of the lymph nodes.

Cause: variable.

Moderately to very ill; class 4; regional, occurring in highly malarious areas, mostly in Africa and New Guinea, but also elsewhere in the tropics. It exists only with rainfall over 500 mm (20 inches) per year, a mean temperature over 16°C (60°F) and only between 10° north and 10° south of the equator.

Age: children, mainly 5–7 years old. **Who:** those with chronic MALARIA, possibly interacting with some viruses. **Onset:** over hours to days.

Clinical

This is a CANCER which begins with swelling of the face (usually the middle of the face) or abdomen; it progresses very rapidly. It is surprisingly painless, which distinguishes this from tooth ABSCESS.

Complications: damage to the spinal cord with paralysis or tumor in the brain with BRAIN DAMAGE.

Similar conditions: MUMPS, DIPHTHERIA, ANTHRAX, TUBERCULOSIS (abdominal).

Treatment

Referrals: it is treatable and frequently curable if it is treated early. Do not give any immunizations to patients who have this disease. See Volume 1, Appendix 13. Laboratory: a level 3 or above hospital can do a biopsy which is both sensitive and specific. Practitioner: hematologist/oncologist is ideal. A pediatrician or internist with tropical/travel medicine expertise may be adequate.

BURSITIS

Definition: pain and swelling of a bursa, which is a small slippery water balloon-type structure that helps muscle slide smoothly over bone.

Cause: unknown.

Age: mainly those over 40 years old. **Who:** history of sustained pressure on the affected part. **Onset:** variable.

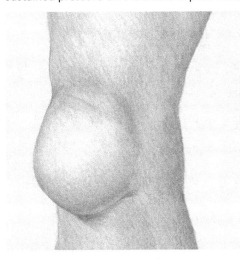

This is bursitis of the knee. It comes from excessive kneeling. Deep bursitis may not be visible. OW

Treatment:
Patient care: treat bursitis like ARTHRITIS without a fever. For an abscess, see Volume 1, Appendix 1, Procedure 19.

Referrals: facilities: x-ray might be helpful to exclude alternative diagnoses. Practitioner: general practitioner, internist, pediatrician. If the bursitis becomes an abscess, it may require surgical drainage.

BURULI ULCER

Regional Notes: F, M, U; this does not occur in Europe or the Middle East. It is found mostly in east and west Africa and in the Pacific region.

Entry category: disease.

Synonym: Bairnsdale ulcer (in Australia).

Definition: Buruli ulcer is a skin ulcer caused by Mycobacterium ulcerans.

Cause: bacteria, acid-fast, related to TB and LEPROSY.

Mildly to moderately ill; class 3 if advanced; worldwide, tropical, south of 10° north of the equator in swampy areas of West Africa, Southeast Asia and Australia.

Age: any, but most common in older children. **Who:** those with minor skin injuries, especially near swamps or flooding; the water might be stagnant or slow-flowing. **Onset:** slowly, over weeks, not hours and not days.

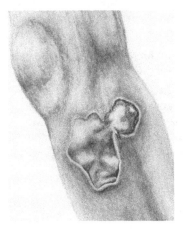

This is a close-up of a Buruli ulcer. The edges overhang the wound proper. AB

Clinical

Necessary: a skin ulcer which occurs on areas of the body not covered by clothing, the arms and the legs. There is no preference for right or left, for upper or lower limbs.

Occasionally: it might occur on the trunk, head or neck. About half the time it is over joints. It commonly occurs near old, healed Buruli ulcers.

At first: this starts out with a firm, spontaneous lump under the skin, more than 1 cm in diameter. The bump is attached to the skin, so one cannot move the skin back and forth over top of the bump. It may look like a piece of cardboard, more than 2 cm in diameter, sitting on the skin. There will be swelling. It may or may not itch, but it is not painful. The swelling may be severe but the area is not hot or red. The patient has no fever.

Later: the bump breaks open to form a round, oval or star-shaped, open skin ulcer. The edges of the ulcer are somewhat raised, slightly ragged, discolored, firm rather than soft and swollen. There may be surrounding dark discoloration. There is a large overhang of skin over the ulcer base; one can put half a toothpick under the skin edge. Joints near the ulcer might be painful. The ulcer itself is not painful unless there is secondary infection with other bacteria.

Still later: usually it enlarges slowly over months but may enlarge rapidly over weeks. Satellite ulcers may form around the main ulcer. The ulcer is likely to last for 3 years or so and then spontaneously heal. It commonly recurs or relapses.

Complications: this may become secondarily infected, resulting in SEPSIS. The patient may develop TETANUS. The infection may enter the bones and become OSTEOMYELITIS. In the presence of HIV infection, the ulcer may be very aggressive.

Similar conditions: see Protocol B.11: Skin Ulcer plus "Flu" if applicable.

Treatment

Prevention: BCG vaccine for TUBERCULOSIS gives only short-term protection.

Referrals: laboratory; a level 3 or above, possible a level 2 hospital can do a smear and stain of a scraping from the base of the ulcer. Practitioner: tropical/travel medicine expertise for diagnosis, surgeon for treatment.

Patient care: if possible, send out for a surgical consult; drugs do no good if the disease is advanced. Otherwise:

- Daily cleaning and dressings. A healthy, healing wound will be reddish only; this just needs cleaning with sterile saline-bleach. If there is dead tissue (off-white, yellow or dark), that should be removed. Put absorbent cotton on the wound after removal and keep the wound moist with bleach-saline.

- Sprinkle PHENYTOIN in the ulcer.

- If diagnosed early, treat with STREPTOMYCIN plus RIFAMPIN as they are used for TUBERCULOSIS for 8 weeks.

- CLARITHROMYCIN.

- Support the patient nutritionally.

CANCER

Regional Notes: E, F, I, K, M, O, R, S, U.

Entry category: disease cluster.

Synonyms: neoplasia, neoplasm, neoplastic disease, carcinoma, sarcoma.

Definition: abnormal growth of some cells of the body, some of which then break off and go to other parts of the body and grow abnormally there.

Cause: variable.

Not ill to very ill; class 4; Worldwide with widely varying manifestations. Leukemia (blood cancer) is rare in nationals in developing areas.

The following is only a brief summary, as these problems cannot be treated by non-medical people in remote areas. Any medical problem that does not respond to ordinary medicines in a reasonable length of time needs to be sent to a medical facility, whether it is cancer or something else.

Clinical

Symptoms of cancers anywhere in the body:

- An abnormal lump or swelling, usually initially painless, usually slow-growing. If it is on the right or the left, that side is different from the opposite side. (Cancers do not grow symmetrically right and left.) If it is in the midline, it will usually not be exactly symmetrical, i.e. the same right and left. These are general rules, but any lump needs to be biopsied to determine if it is cancer.

- An abnormally colored spot or an open sore or lump on the skin or the moist, pink parts of the body. It does not heal, and it changes color or shape slowly. It does not respond to repeated washing and dressing changes.

- Any persistent evidence of obstruction or inflammation of one of the tubes or hollow parts of the body: constipation, indigestion, stuffy nose, hoarseness or trouble breathing, trouble swallowing, cough, difficulty urinating, a lump in the vagina or by the rectum. Suspect cancer when these symptoms do not respond to treatment for infection.

- Any persistent enlargement of an organ, particularly when the organ in question feels lumpy (rather than just large but normal shape) and, at least initially, is not tender to touch.

- General whole-body itching without a corresponding skin rash.

- Cancer may cause fevers.

- Loss of appetite with weight loss.

- Enlarged lymph nodes which are typically painless and apple-hard to the touch. There may be multiple nodes matted together.

In the tropics, lung, colon and rectal cancer are common only amongst the affluent. Cancer of the cervix in women is common throughout the tropics, especially with poor hygiene, early marriage, promiscuity and uncircumcised male partner(s). For other cancers that are common in your area, see your Regional Notes.

CANCER SYMPTOMS

Body part	Usual first symptom(s)	Associated factors (sometimes)
Esophagus	Trouble swallowing	Unknown
Head	Lump or ear pain[1]	Tobacco
Nose	Swelling or obstruction	Family origin southern China
Liver	Weight loss, yellow eyes, itching all over	HEPATITIS B, moldy peanuts or grains
Abdomen	Increased girth	Pain, free fluid in abdomen
Penis	Sore or bump	Poverty, poor hygiene, uncircumcised
Thyroid	Lump in neck	Radiation
Blood	Bleeding, large lymph nodes, itching	Virus, radiation
Breast	Lump	Westerner; women from areas with GOITER
Skin melanoma[2]	Bump on the skin; asymmetrical; irregular border, black or multicolored, larger than a pencil eraser	Fair skin; sun exposure, hands and feet of those with dark skin.

1 *In particular, constant or worsening, dull ear pain on one side only.*

2 *This is a particularly dangerous kind of skin cancer.*

Similar conditions: too many to list. See applicable protocols. Any patient that does not respond to treatment needs hospitalization for evaluation. A particular problem is distinguishing TB of the breast from breast cancer. TB of the breast tends to cause an aching pain initially whereas breast cancer is usually initially painless. If the lump is removed and cut in two, the inside of the lump will be like cheese if it is due to TB and most likely not if it is cancer. TB of the gastrointestinal tract is another common mimic of cancer. HYDATID DISEASE can look similar; if exposed, seek laboratory tests for hydatid disease before consenting to surgery for cancer. Surgery can be disastrous if the diagnosis is in error.

Treatment

This must be done in a hospital. In remote areas, you might be obliged to provide terminal care for very ill patients.

See Appendix 8 in Volume 1. It is important to provide pain relief, even if this shortens the patient's life. CHLORPROMAZINE does not relieve pain, but it relieves suffering by making the patient not care if he has pain. DIPYRONE is an excellent non-narcotic pain reliever that is frequently available in developing areas. TRAMADOL is a good narcotic-type pain reliever.

Referrals: see Volume 1, Appendix 13. Laboratory; a level 3 or above hospital can do a biopsy for diagnosis. Practitioner: at a minimum a general practitioner or internist or pediatrician. An oncologist and a surgeon will probably be necessary, as well as the facilities of at least a level 3 hospital. If HYDATID DISEASE is a possibility, seek tropical/travel medical advice.

CANCRUM ORIS

Regional Notes: I, O

Synonyms: noma, gangrenous stomatitis.

Definition: an infection of the lower face in malnourished children, causing extensive destruction.

Cause: spirochete.

Very ill; class 3–4; requires surgery. Worldwide, tropical, found mainly in Africa, the Indian subcontinent and South America south of the equator.

Age: mostly children. **Who:** malnourished only, mostly with a recent illness such as MALARIA or MEASLES. **Onset:** over days, mostly during the dry season.

Clinical

Necessary: there is a spontaneous facial wound which eats a big hole in the child's cheek. It develops from first symptoms to a hole within 2 weeks. It may also destroy an eyelid or a thumb or finger that is sucked. The wound will have a foul/rotten odor.

Similar conditions: see Protocol B.11. In the Americas consider CUTANEOUS LEISHMANIASIS that has become mucocutaneous. Also consider TUBERCULOSIS of the skin and GANGRENE; cancrum oris is a kind of GANGRENE. Tertiary YAWS can look similar; it affects the nose, and the patients are older.

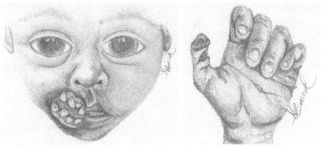

Cancrum oris creates a hole into the mouth. The black discoloration is usually more extensive than that shown. A sucked thumb or finger may also be affected. AB

Treatment

Referrals: speedy referral to a level 3 or above hospital is mandatory if the child is to live.

Patient care:

- Use PENICILLIN and METRONIDAZOLE to stop the infectious process. DOXYCYCLINE[1] might be helpful if you lack PENICILLIN.
- Treat other diseases the child may have (WORMS, MALARIA, etc.).
- Treat the wound(s) like a TROPICAL ULCER.
- Treat for MALNUTRITION.

Results: these children generally do poorly and frequently die in spite of best efforts.

CANDIDIASIS

Synonyms: Candidosis, Monilia.

Entry category: disease

Includes: thrush, crotch itch, diaper rash

Definition: an infection with a fungus. In people with good immunity, it is usually annoying but not serious; in those with poor immunity it can be life-threatening.

Cause: fungus.

Mildly ill; class 1–4; worldwide, especially humid tropics.

Age: any. **Who:** anyone, especially those with white skin, HIV patients, those who have taken antibiotics and the poorly nourished. **Onset:** over days.

Clinical

Necessary: the patient has a very itchy, very red rash. It is either entirely spotted or else solid red in the center with satellite red spots around. It develops first and possibly only on the warmer parts of the skin: the groins, the armpits, under large breasts, between rolls of fat, sometimes in the ear canals.

Commonly: includes the scrotum and the rectal area. In patients with good immunity, when it involves the skin only, it does not cause fever.

---

1 *Don't worry about discolored teeth.*

Sometimes: in the mouth it is painful, and it looks like white scum on the pink surface. If the patient also has pain with swallowing, the candida has invaded his esophagus. It may cause cracks at the sides of the lips. In some areas, when this problem recurs or will not respond to treatment, it is likely that the patient has HIV. In these patients it may cause diarrhea and fevers. For vaginal candidiasis, see VAGINITIS.

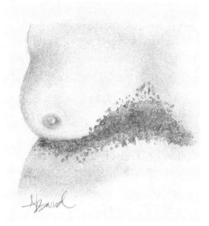

Candidiasis :
1. *There is a red, roughened center to the area.*
2. *There are satellite spots around the area, rather small.*
3. *The location is a warm, moist area of the body.* AB

Similar conditions: ECZEMA occurs in people with a family history of allergies; in the developing world, this is usually the more affluent. CONTACT DERMATITIS is found in an area of contact with a particular substance. In the rectal area, ENTEROBIASIS may seem similar; check for the worms.

Treatment

Prevention is by frequent showering.

Referrals: laboratory: level 3, possibly level 2 can do a skin scraping. HIV testing might be helpful in severe cases. Practitioner: general practitioner, internist, pediatrician.

Patient care: send the patient out if he is ill. Otherwise:

- Treat with NYSTATIN, CLOTRIMAZOLE, MICONAZOLE or KETOCONAZOLE.
- Frequent washing, drying and use of baby powder is also helpful. GENTIAN VIOLET or tincture of IODINE may help.
- Exposing the affected area to direct sunlight (not filtered through glass) for a half-hour daily usually will clear it promptly.
- In the mouth, GENTIAN VIOLET or NYSTATIN are best.

CAPILLARIASIS

Regional notes: R.

Entry category: disease.

Synonym: intestinal capillariasis.

Cause: worm.

Regional: it is found in tropical coastal regions of northern Luzon, the Philippines; occasionally in south and northeast Thailand; in northern Java; in Egypt. A related parasite is found in Iran, but it is rare and causes entirely different symptoms. The disease is listed here rather than in the Regional Notes because of its potential for spreading to other areas.

Mildly to severely ill; class 2.

Age: usually adults. **Who:** those eating raw fish. **Onset:** slowly.

Clinical

The patient has diarrhea with loud, rumbling bowel sounds and much gas for a long time. He loses his appetite, gradually loses weight and develops various vitamin deficiencies and swelling of the ankles and feet. He will die of MALNUTRITION eventually if he is not treated.

Similar conditions: MALABSORPTION and the causes thereof are indistinguishable from this. See Protocol B.14.

Treatment

Prevention: discourage the consumption of raw or poorly cooked fresh-water fish.

Referrals: laboratory: stool specimen for diagnosis of this and other worms.

Patient care: MEBENDAZOLE, ALBENDAZOLE, THIABENDAZOLE. ALBENDAZOLE is best. It must be treated for 30 days.

CARBON MONOXIDE POISONING

Cause: toxic gas.

Definition: poisoning by this toxic gas that is generated by internal combustion engines and fires.

Class 3–4.

Clinical

Exposure to fumes from an internal combustion engine, furnace or a fire in an enclosed space leads to carbon monoxide poisoning. Symptoms are nausea, vomiting, shortness of breath and headache initially; lethargy progressing to loss of consciousness if severe. The face (in Whites), and the inside of the mouth will be redder than normal. There is no fever due to this.

Similar conditions: see Protocol B.4 if the patient is short of breath. ALTITUDE SICKNESS looks similar, but the inside of the mouth is never bright red. SMOKE INHALATION is similar and may be present along with this.

Treatment

Patient care: remove the patient to fresh air. Giving oxygen hastens the clearing of the carbon monoxide from the body. There can be delayed symptoms.

Referrals: laboratory: at least level 3: blood gases, respiratory care team. Facilities: oxygen is essential. At level 4 a hyperbaric oxygen chamber helps. Practitioner: pulmonologist is ideal; internist or pediatrician or general practitioner might be helpful.

CARPAL TUNNEL SYNDROME

Cause: pressure on one of the nerves that travels from the spine to the hand as it goes through the wrist area.

Entry category: syndrome.

Age: middle-aged **Who***:* females more than males, short more than tall, fat more than thin, mostly those doing work requiring repetitive hand motion such as factory workers. It may be the result of a one-time injury. It is very uncommon in rural, developing areas. **Onset:** days to months.

Clinical

Necessary: there is pain, numbness and tingling, maybe weakness on the palm-thumb side of the hand, the thumb, index and middle fingers. It may involve both hands.

Usually: it starts in the dominant hand and is worse at night. It is initially relieved with awakening and shaking the hand or hanging the hand down over the side of the bed.

Treatment

There are both surgical and non-surgical treatments. Medication such as IBUPROFEN may be helpful. Splinting the wrist in a neutral position might help. Sometimes local steroid injections are helpful, but usually surgery is required eventually.

CAT-SCRATCH DISEASE

Entry category: disease

Synonym: subacute regional lymphadenitis. The bacterium is related to the causative organism of BARTONELLOSIS but the disease is entirely different. It should not be called Bartonellosis and is not called so in this book.

Definition: cat-scratch disease is an infection with the Gram-negative bacillus *Bartonella henselae*.

Not ill to mildly ill in patients with good immunity; moderately to very ill with poor immunity. Class 2: probably worldwide.

Age: any, especially children; adults may experience more serious symptoms. **Who:** those who have been scratched by a cat or bitten by cat fleas. Infected cats are not ill. **Onset:** incubation 3–30 days.

Clinical

Necessary: the patient has large, tender lymph nodes closer to the trunk than where the cat scratched or the flea bit.

Probably: initially the wound might look like a small bump or blister, reddish brown in color. The large lymph nodes persist for 3 weeks and then go away. They may be soft and resemble ABSCESSes. There may be fever, weight loss, large spleen, a (non-itchy) rash or fatigue connected with this.

Complications: sometimes this causes SEPSIS, ENCEPHALITIS, ERYTHEMA NODOSUM, PNEUMONIA and abnormal bleeding.

Similar conditions: see Protocol B.12 for other causes of large, tender lymph nodes. TULAREMIA may be indistinguishable.

Treatment

RIFAMPIN, CIPROFLOXACIN, AZITHROMYCIN, ERYTHROMYCIN, DOXYCYCLINE or GENTAMYCIN work fine for treatment, given for 10 days. Choose one of these. CO-TRIMOXAZOLE works about half of the time. Other antibiotics are not usually helpful.

CATARACT

Regional Notes: F.

Entry category: symptom.

Definition: opacities in the lens of the eye.

Cause: variable.

Not ill; class 2–4, depending on hospital facilities; worldwide, more common in arid and high altitude tropics, especially in the Indian subcontinent.

Age: any, common in older people but occurs in babies. **Who:** anyone; MALNUTRITION, DEHYDRATION, RADIATION ILLNESS and bright sunlight contribute to it. When it is present from birth it may be hereditary or else due to prenatal infection, such as RUBELLA, HERPES or SHINGLES. **Onset:** slowly in older children and adults.

Clinical

Necessary: the pupil of the eye looks cloudy (white or gray rather than the normal black) and the patient gradually loses vision with blurring being worse in bright than in dim light. He may see halos around lights. Early cataract is hard to diagnose; there are streaks of gray or white on the pupil.

Treatment

Prevention: bright sunlight as well as DEHYDRATION seems to increase the rate of development of cataract. Issue plain sun glasses to those with early cataract.

Referrals: surgical referral is mandatory; An ophthalmologist is ideal. Be sure the eye you are referring has light perception. Cataract surgery is useless if the eye will be blind anyway, afterward.[1]

Patient care: there is some evidence that daily, small doses of ASPIRIN might slow the development of cataract. Some hospitals can do surgery for cataract but the person usually must wear glasses thereafter. If he refuses to wear glasses or is likely to break or lose them, the surgery will do no good. An alternative is having a lens implant put into the eye; in that case glasses are necessary just for reading. Babies born with cataract must have surgery within 6 months.

---

1 Cover the other eye. The patient should be able to tell when you shine a non-LED flashlight directly into the eye with cataract. If he can, then surgery may be helpful.

CELLULITIS

Regional Notes: F

Entry category: disease cluster.

Includes: erysipelas.

Definition: an infection of the skin usually caused by Gram-positive bacteria.

Cause: bacteria.

Mildly ill; class 1–2 if previously healthy; class 3–4 if previously ill; probably not contagious in most cases, but use good hygiene; worldwide, erysipelas is common.

Age: any. **Who:** anyone, especially those with poor hygiene, chronic illness or both. **Onset:** few days to a week or two; faster with bites, embedded foreign bodies and in hot, humid climates.

Clinical

Necessary: an area of skin is reddened or warm. It matches one of the clinical conditions described in the table on the following page. It is never itchy, although it might arise on skin that had been itchy; it is seldom symmetrical; the redness and swelling do not go away with raising the body part above the level of the heart.

Frequently: it is painful and tender to the touch. There may be swelling. The lymph nodes closer to the trunk may be enlarged and tender. If the area is on an arm or a leg, there may be red streaks from the reddened area going towards the trunk.

Commonly: this involves the breast. If it involves the stump of the umbilical cord in a newborn, check for SEPSIS.

Occasionally: there is fever.

⚠ WARNING

Ordinary cellulitis involves obvious redness and/or warmth and some (but not extreme) pain and tenderness. There is a type of cellulitis called **NECROTIZING FASCIITIS** which can look similar. Early on the area is red, warm, swollen, tender; over hours to days it darkens and is bluish, maybe with large blisters forming. Pain is extreme; swelling is not pitting; the patient is generally ill, usually with a history of some injury or infection. Over time there may be thin, foul-smelling, watery pus resembling dishwater. First underlying fat and structures rot with gangrene; then the skin becomes gangrenous and rots off. The pain is extreme, all out of proportion to the redness and warmth. Ordinary cellulitis looks worse than it feels. NECROTIZING FASCIITIS feels much worse than it looks. Treatment is IV broad-spectrum antibiotics as well as emergency surgery; seek outside advice. **The patient must get to a hospital, at least level 3, before 3 days from onset, or evacuation is hopeless. He will die.**

Similar conditions: see Protocol B.6 for limb swelling and/or B.11 for skin ulcer plus illness. B.12 for large lymph nodes; B.8 if the problem involves the eye(s), B.13 if it involves the back. If the area involved is the genital area, then see Protocol B.1. If there is a *raised area with a center spot*, see ABSCESS. *Redness and swelling over a joint,* see ARTHRITIS. *With deep bone pain, see* OSTEOMYELITIS. *Mediterranean genetic heritage, see* FAMILIAL MEDITERRANEAN FEVER.

FILARIASIS can look similar, but with this the red streak moves away from the heart; with cellulitis it moves toward the heart. (You can decide which way it is moving by marking the end of the streak with a pen and then checking it again the next day.)

Treatment

Prevention: frequent use of soap and water, care of wounds.

Referrals: laboratory: at level 3 or more, culture and blood count might be helpful. There may be other appropriate tests. Practitioner: general practitioner, internist, pediatrician, maybe a nurse; infectious disease expertise is helpful. A surgeon is essential if there is necrotizing fasciitis.

Patient care: if the cellulitis is in the leg or groin, check the genitals and foot for an infected wound. Likewise, check the hand for a wound or wounds if the cellulitis is between the wrist and the shoulder. See Chapter 10 in Volume 1 for treatment of an infected wound. Send the patient out to a hospital if at all possible. Treat ordinary cellulitis as follows:

- Bedrest with elevation of the body part is helpful for severe cases.

- Treat with an appropriate antibiotic for 10 days, according to the table on the next page.

- If there was an animal bite then use both Gram-positive and Gram-negative antibiotics. See the table on the next page.

- If it is due to exposure to contaminated water, then use Gram-negative antibiotics: DOXYCYCLINE, CHLORAMPHENICOL or GENTAMYCIN. See the table following.

- Other drugs that might help (but are expensive) are AZITHROMYCIN, CLARITHROMYCIN, OFLOXACIN.

- If there is a relapse after a partial treatment, give a full treatment. If there is a relapse after a full treatment, then use CEPHALOSPORIN or CLOXACILLIN. Use these in the first place in a child with multiple sites, visible pus and a fever.

Results: 4 days.

BACTERIA CAUSING CELLULITIS

Type of Bacteria	History	Appearance	Symptoms	Treatment
Erysipelas (most common)	Various.	Red or warm swollen skin.	Usually on the face or by a wound.	Gram-positive antibiotic(s).[1]
Aeronomas	Exposed to fresh or salt water.	Watery pus, gas bubbles.	Pain excessive, fever, more swelling than redness, rapidly progressing, foul smell.	Emergency surgery and IV antibiotics.
Clostridium	Major wound or fracture; dead tissue.	Watery pus, gas bubbles	Pain excessive, fever, more swelling than redness, rapidly progressing, foul smell.	Emergency surgery, IV antibiotics.
NECROTIZING FASCIITIS	Various.	Large area, large blisters.	Pain excessive, fever, more swelling than redness, rapidly progressing, foul smell.	Emergency surgery and IV antibiotics.
Staph	Maybe Western context.	Usually redness and swelling, pus, maybe blisters also.	Variable, maybe fever, maybe mild or serious.	Anti-staph Gram-positive antibiotics.
Pasteurella	Dog or cat bite or contaminated wound.	Ordinary wound infection—swollen and red.	Few, if any.	Various[3]
Vibrio vulnificus	Sickly patient and salt water exposure.	Red rash becomes big blisters become ulcers, dead centers.	Low blood pressure Many deaths.	Doxycycline plus a third-generation CEPHALOSPORIN.

1 *You must treat both staph and strep: [AMOXICILLIN plus CLAVULANIC ACID] or else [CLOXACILLIN] for staph, plus [first generation CEPHALOSPORIN, ERYTHROMYCIN or PENICILLIN V.] for strep.*

2 *Clindamycin is particularly good since it prevents some complications.*

3 *Amoxicillin with calvulanate, doxycycline, ciprofloxacin, a second or third generation CEPHALOSPORIN.*

⚠ CELLULITIS EMERGENCIES

REASONS TO EVACUATE THE PATIENT FOR SURGERY
- Blisters along with very ill or severe pain
- Low blood pressure
- Watery pus with gas bubbles
- Rapid progression of symptoms
- Purplish discoloration of the skin
- Agitation, confusion or new-onset crazy behavior
- Pain out of proportion to the appearance of the cellulitis

CEREBRAL PALSY

Regional Notes: F, I, S.

Entry category: syndrome.

Definition: this is a type of BRAIN DAMAGE, a permanent problem of movement and coordination, possibly due to lack of oxygen at birth, being born prematurely, ENCEPHALITIS, cerebral MALARIA, poisoning, head injury, untreated JAUNDICE after birth and sometimes other diseases.

Clinical

The patient has uncoordinated movements and garbled speech. Most often these people are mentally normal, though their inability to speak clearly and their incoordination gives the impression of retardation.

Treatment

Obtain professional advice from a physical therapist or another appropriate professional.

Chaga's disease

At present this is confined to Central and South America. The insects that carry it are present in the Pacific area, so it might spread. See Regional Notes M, U.

CHANCROID

Regional Notes: O, S, U

Synonyms: soft chancre, soft sore, ulcus molle

Definition: a sexually transmitted (venereal) disease caused by the bacterium *Hemophilis ducreyi.*

Cause: bacteria.

Not ill to mildly ill; class 1–2; contagious; worldwide, more in tropical areas, especially sub-Saharan Africa and South Asia.

Age: sexually mature or sexually abused. **Who:** sexually active; symptoms are more common in males than females, more common in uncircumcised than in circumcised males. Females are likely to have no symptoms whatsoever if the genital ulcers are inside the vagina. **Onset:** incubation from exposure to a bump is 1–3 days; exposure to an ulcer is 3–60 days. Large lymph nodes develop within a week.

Clinical

This disease varies greatly in its manifestations.

Necessary: the patient has or had small red pimple(s) which became ulcer(s) with irregular (not smooth) edges on the genitals. When there are more than one, they tend to form on surfaces that normally touch each other. They bleed easily if they are disturbed.

Usually: they are painful and may be tender to touch, but there is no swelling around them. There is a red halo around the inside rim of the ulcer(s). The center has a yellowish appearance. The groin lymph nodes on one side are large and tender, possibly rupturing and spilling pus. They subsequently heal with scarring.

In females, the pimples and ulcers may be inside the vagina so only the enlarged lymph nodes are visible. The internal ulcers may be painless and non-tender.

Maybe: the ulcer may have a foul odor. Females may have pain with intercourse, pain with urination or a visible ulcer on the outside genitals. The ulcers may simply disappear.

Occasionally

- Ulcers coalesce.

- The initial bump stays as a bump, and does not develop into a full ulcer.

- The ulcer, rather than being depressed below the skin surface, may be raised up above the skin surface. There may just be pain with urination and/or pus coming from the hole in the penis rather than a visible ulcer. The large, swollen lymph nodes in the groin may develop without there being a visible ulcer or pus in the genital area.

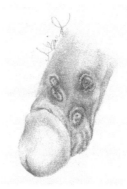

Chancroid: 1. Swelling is minimal. 2. Ulcers are not deep. 3. They are usually multiple. 4. Red halos are common. 5. They are tender. See Chapter 6, Volume 1 for the appearance in females. AB

Complications: if there is secondary infection, there may be a foul discharge from the ulcer, and there may be rapid destruction of the genitals. Chancroid can cause PHIMOSIS.

Similar conditions: see Protocol B.1. Common diseases that cause genital ulcers like this are impossible to distinguish from each other except for HERPES which is usually distinctive. However, chancroid ulcers may, at times, resemble HERPES. Chancroid is more common than herpes in developing countries. You should treat for all genital ulcers unless you are certain of the diagnosis[1]. The *swollen nodes in the groin* might be due to any lower limb infection. LYMPHOGRANULOMA VENEREUM is commonly confused with this. If you consider either, treat for both.

Bush laboratory—is useless.

Treatment

Prevention: discourage promiscuity. Prostitutes spread the disease. In some large tropical cities, the majority of the prostitutes are infected.

Referrals: laboratory: only a level 4 or level 5 hospital lab is worthwhile. *Practitioner;* a sexually transmitted disease clinic is ideal. A general practitioner or internist can provide decent care. A surgeon can drain the pus from the groin nodes.

---

1 *An example would be if the patient's sexual partner had a laboratory diagnosis of chancroid.*

TOC   SYMPTOMS   DIFFERENTIALS   CONDITIONS   DRUG INDEX   REGIONAL NOTES   INX

Patient care: patients should be treated according to Protocol B.1: SEXUALLY TRANSMITTED DISEASES. The following drugs work for chancroid: AZITHROMYCIN (single oral dose), ceftriaxone (CEPHALOSPORIN), CIPROFLOXACIN, ERYTHROMYCIN, RIFAMPIN. Withdraw the pus from the lymph node with a syringe: **do not cut it to drain it**. It is important to treat all sexual partners.

Results: few days. Uncircumcised males do not respond as well as circumcised.

CHICKEN POX

Regional Notes: F, I, O, S.

Definition: a viral infection that usually causes a mild disease in children.

Cause: virus.

Synonym: varicella.

Mildly to moderately ill; class 1–4; contagious; worldwide, common, usually in small epidemics.

Age: any, especially young children. **Who:** anyone not immunized who has not yet had the disease. **Onset:** over days; 10–23 days incubation.

Clinical

Necessary: a fever and a rash which consists of red spots initially. The spots become tiny, soft blisters on red bases, appearing in crops, first here and then there. Spots become blisters over hours. They start drying very quickly after forming. They are on the trunk first and heaviest, then the head, neck, upper arms and legs. The blisters break, crust over and heal.

Maybe: there are blisters on the white of the eye and inside the mouth.

Sometimes: in older children there is a low fever and fatigue first; the rash comes later. In young children the fever and rash occur together. The disease may be fatal with MALNUTRITION.

Complications: HYPOGLYCEMIA, IMPETIGO. Adults— ENCEPHALITIS. Reye's Syndrome is a rare complication characterized by severe vomiting. It is a major emergency requiring immediate evacuation.

Similar conditions: see Protocol B.8 for other causes of red, painful eyes. *If blisters break out at one time, progress from spots to blisters all at once,* consider MONKEYPOX, SMALLPOX.[2] *Skin bumps firm like warts with center holes*: MOLLUSCUM CONTAGIOSUM. *Blisters in one area of skin or a band*: SHINGLES. *Few, countable blisters*: SPOTTED FEVER (Rickettsial pox), GONORRHEA. Resolving chicken pox and resolving SCABIES may appear similar, but SCABIES never involves the face with blisters *if only the hairy back of the hand is involved, not the face or trunk*: HAND-FOOT-MOUTH DISEASE.

Treatment

Prevention: isolate the patient until the skin spots are dry. There is a vaccine.

Referrals: laboratory: there is nothing helpful. *Practitioner:* expert nursing care, a pediatrician or an internist may be helpful.

Patient care: sending out is desirable for adults. Send out immediately for vomiting in this context.

- Treat the fever but use no ASPIRIN.
- Use DIPHENHYDRAMINE for itching.
- Feed malnourished children.

CHIKUNGUNYA [FEVER]

Regional Notes: M, U.

Entry category: disease—a type of ARBOVIRAL FEVER.

Definition: this is an arboviral infection. It is very common in Reunion Island and in India. It occurs in the Caribbean.

Age: any, but children are not likely to develop serious forms of the disease. **Who:** those bitten by mosquitoes; they are day biters and generally not susceptible to DDT. The disease is maintained in monkeys and possibly rodents. People do not get it twice. It occurs in outbreaks, not isolated cases. **Onset:** Very sudden after an incubation of 2–4 days.

Clinical

Necessary: fever, chills, headache, joint pains (always more than one joint). The pain is disabling.

Usually: pains may precede or follow the fever by up to 2 days. They are usually symmetrical and involve the large joints and spine, sometimes the small joints. They also involve joints that were previously injured. The joint pains are worse on getting up from resting; patients resist moving. There may or may not be joint swelling.

Maybe: the fever may disappear and recur. Descriptions don't mention the pain migrating from joint to joint, but they do mention the similarity to RHEUMATOID ARTHRITIS, which does migrate. There may be morning stiffness. A rash is common. It is red spotted in fair skin, sandpapery or blistery in dark skin; it may itch, peel or both. Older people have more joint pains and less fever; younger, more fever and less joint pains.

Complications: HEART FAILURE, HEPATITIS, ENCEPHALITIS, HEMORRHAGIC FEVER (rare and usually mild). There may be floppy paralysis similar to POLIO. In the young, joint pains may persist for up to five years; in older and previously ill patients, they may persist indefinitely.

---

2 *Smallpox blisters are present for several days before they start to dry; chickenpox blisters start to dry within a day after they arise.*

Similar conditions: RHEUMATIC FEVER is similar, but the joint pains migrate, and there is no headache connected with it. LEPPTOSPIROSIS may be similar. Other ARBOVIRAL FEVERS, EBOLA VIRUS DISEASE and DENGUE FEVER are indistinguishable. The treatments are similar.

Treatment

Prevention: care for patients under mosquito nets.

Patient care: RIBAVIRIN, an antiviral medication, may be helpful. Other than that, just give pain and fever medications. Patients need to have absolute bedrest during the initial symptoms in order to minimize long-term problems.

Prognosis: severe initial symptoms, prior chronic illness, old age and involvement of fingers and toes indicate a bad prognosis.

CHLAMYDIA

Synonym: non-gonococcal urethritis.

Definition: this is infection with the bacterium *Chlamydia trachomatis.*

Mildly to moderately ill; class 2; contagious, sexually; worldwide, common everywhere.

Age and Who: sexually active adults; sexually abused children; babies of infected mothers. **Onset:** unknown incubation, unknown onset.

Clinical

There are three forms to this infection

- TRACHOMA when it affects the eyes, listed separately.

- LYMPHOGRANULOMA VENEREUM, (LGV), a form of genital infection listed separately.

- Genital chlamydia infection, described here.

Genital chlamydia

In many cases there are no symptoms at all. Nevertheless, the disease is present. It is passed on through sexual relations and late complications can develop. When there are symptoms, they are as follows

Males: burning pain with urinating, possibly with pus discharge from the hole at the end of the penis. It may cause EPIDIDYMITIS with painful swelling of the scrotum.

Females: a white or yellowish, opaque vaginal discharge, possibly with some blood; it may cause vaginal pain, pain with urination, pain with intercourse or symptoms of PELVIC INFECTION. It may also cause perihepatitis, the sudden onset of pain in the right upper abdomen with infection and inflammation of the surface of the liver.

Either sex: it can cause genital ulcers—usually just small bumps—and large lymph nodes in the groin. The nodes are painful and may extend down into the upper leg. Initially these are separate but then stick together and develop ABSCESSes in and around them. Where there has been rectal intercourse, the ulcers and associated large lymph nodes might be in or near the rectum. This can cause itching and a pus discharge. It may cause PROCTITIS.

It can cause REITER SYNDROME which consists of pain with urinating, pain with intercourse in women, eye infection and a painful, swollen large joint or tendon—usually on the lower body, on one side only. It may also cause mouth sores: see APHTHOUS STOMATITIS. In the eyes, it can cause burning, itching or red eyes or all of these.

Complications in adults: genital ELEPHANTIASIS; persistent genital sores; rectal cancer; healing with scarring, making the anus narrow; massive genital swelling; formation of fistulas: abnormal holes between bladder, rectum, vagina or penis and the outside of the body. *Babies* of infected females: EYE INFECTION or PNEUMONIA.[1]

Similar conditions: it is impossible for you to distinguish between this and other SEXUALLY TRANSMITTED DISEASEs. Thus it is best to treat by symptoms: Protocol B.1. REITER SYNDROME might resemble other forms of ARTHRITIS. An infection of the rectum might resemble DYSENTERY, but other dysentery usually does not cause rectal pain. Females with perihepatitis might be misdiagnosed as having AMEBIASIS, or HEPATITIS. Chlamydia does not cause bilirubin in the urine dipstick; HEPATITIS does.

Treatment

Referrals: laboratory: this is not helpful unless it is level 4 or 5. *Practitioner;* a sexually transmitted disease clinic is ideal. A general practitioner or internist might be helpful.

Patient care: treat according to Protocol B.1.

- In milder cases you may use AZITHROMYCIN, AMOXICILLIN, ERYTHROMYCIN, OFLOXACIN or DOXYCYCLINE. Treatment should continue for 7 days.

- *Pneumonia in babies* of infected females should be treated with ERYTHROMYCIN for 14 days.

---

1 *This type of pneumonia occurs before 6 months of age. The symptoms are listlessness; cough; a rapid respiratory rate; and bluishness of the lips, fingers and toes.*

CHOLERA

Regional Notes: E, F, I, M, O, R, S, U.

Definition: an epidemic bacterial infection that causes sudden, severe dehydrating diarrhea, due to the bacterium *Vibrio cholerae*

Cause: bacteria, Gram-negative.

Moderately to very ill; class 3; contagious, very; worldwide, tropical, it occurs mainly in epidemics in times of drought or flood. Areas where the problem is common are those with stagnant or sluggish water, frequent flooding and less than 100 meters (300 feet) elevation, i.e., near the coast. The organism can live in salt water.

Age: any. **Who:** anyone, especially children and those with prior stomach surgery or who are on ulcer medicines. Half of family members will develop the disease within 2 days of the first case. **Onset:** sudden, incubation time a few hours to 5 days.

Clinical

Necessary: the patient has huge amounts of watery diarrhea, then vomiting also. Sometimes vomiting comes first.

Sometimes there is a fever, usually in children. After a half-hour or more, the patient experiences weakness, SHOCK, low temperature, fast pulse rate, fast respiratory rate, low blood pressure and painful muscle cramps in his arms and legs. Vomiting and diarrhea are both forceful. They both resemble rice water after the first few bouts. The diarrhea may have a mild fish or egg odor; if you test it with your urine paper, the pH is more than 7 in true cholera. It may be different with other massive diarrhea. A peculiar characteristic of cholera is that there may be a difference of more than 3°F (1.5°C) between the armpit and the rectal temperatures. Hiccup is common.

Sensitive	Specific
Sudden onset of severe, dehydrating diarrhea	Diarrhea like rice water with a mild odor

Complications: death if not treated, HYPOGLYCEMIA and SEIZURES in children, possibly KIDNEY DISEASE.

Similar conditions: see MALARIA, choleraic form, as this may be easily confused with cholera, with disastrous results. If in doubt, treat for both. The hand and foot cramps associated with this look like the cramps of HYPERVENTILATION. There is no need to distinguish this from severe, ordinary diarrhea, since the same treatments apply.

Bush laboratory: if you draw blood, it is an abnormally dark color. There is commonly protein in the urine.

Treatment

Prevention: avoid sewage contamination of water supply. Wash your hands after cleaning up diarrhea or vomit. Protect both the diarrhea and vomit, as well as food and water, from flies. Use DOXYCYCLINE for family members; 5 days is ideal, but even one dose helps. There are live and killed oral vaccines available for cholera that are both safe and effective, available in Europe. They should only be used when one anticipates exposure to contaminated water with the inability to secure clean reliable water supplies.

Referrals: speedy referral is essential unless you can start an IV or give intraperitoneal fluids. *Laboratory:* hospitals can stain or culture stool, but this does not affect treatment. *Facilities:* IV fluids, level 2 or more. *Practitioner:* nurse or any physician, level 2 or more.

Patient care: send the patient out. Meanwhile treat as follows: this treatment is good for any severe diarrhea.

- *In mild cases* if the patient is vomiting, give IM PROMETHAZINE and wait a half-hour before giving fluids by mouth or stomach tube.

- *In severe cases* give the PROMETHAZINE but immediately give IV or intraperitoneal fluids.

- As soon as possible, give this cholera rehydration fluid by mouth: to 1 liter of water add 1/2 tsp. (2.5 ml) salt, 1/2 tsp. baking soda and 8 tsp. (40 ml) of sugar. Also add 1/4 tsp. (1.25 ml) salt substitute (KCl) if available. Regular ORS diluted 50:50 with plain water is acceptable also. Give as much of this fluid as the patient will take; continually give small amounts at a time. Use a stomach tube if necessary. See Volume 1, Appendix 1, Procedures 4 and 13. With very severe diarrhea, adults get 1 liter an hour, children get 250–500 ml/hour until their vital signs are reasonably normal and their mouths are moist.

- Collect the diarrhea, measure its volume and give this volume of rehydration fluid by mouth in addition to the amount specified above.

- Do not give LoMotil, loperamide or other anti-diarrhea drugs! METOCLOPRAMIDE might be helpful.

- Use antibiotics: if the diarrhea seems to be the result of other antibiotic usage, treat with METRONIDAZOLE or TINIDAZOLE. Otherwise CO-TRIMOXAZOLE, CHLORAMPHENICOL, CIPROFLOXACIN or SULFA medications are helpful. DOXYCYCLINE works fine for adults. **An antibiotic is no substitute for giving fluids.**

- If the patient vomits the rehydration fluids consider intraperitoneal fluids: Volume 1, Appendix 1, Procedure 17.

- Low dose CHLORPROMAZINE will decrease vomiting.

- CALCIUM GLUCONATE is useful for spasms.

Results: usually in 24–48 hours. Recovered or dead within 7 days.

CIRRHOSIS

Regional Notes: F, I, O, R, S.

Definition: this is scarring of the liver which occurs over months. It may be due to ALCOHOLISM, certain drugs and herbs, HEPATITIS, SCHISTOSOMIASIS, LIVER FLUKE and various other diseases that affect the liver. Eventually it causes LIVER FAILURE with the following symptoms:

Clinical

- Change in size of the liver, at first large, later shrunken.

- JAUNDICE : the whites of the eyes are yellow and/or there is bilirubin in the urine.

- Bleeding problems because the blood won't clot normally: nosebleeds, easy bruising, excessive menstruation, excessive bleeding from minor wounds, vomiting blood, bloody stool or urine.

- Free fluid in abdomen, with prominent veins on the abdominal wall in front, usually painless unless it is caused by CANCER or PANCREATITIS or the patient develops a secondary bacterial infection in the fluid. One manifestation of the prominent veins are small, spider-like, red or blue spots on the skin; see the illustration below.

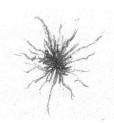

This is a skin spider, about ten-times actual size. AB

- A large spleen, but this may be difficult to feel if there is much fluid.

- Breast development in males because of a lack of male hormone.

- Whole-body itching, on occasion. When this happens, the jaundice will be intense, there will be light-colored stools and dark urine. There will be much bilirubin in the urine.

- BRAIN DAMAGE which at first responds to treatment and later does not:

  o personality changes;

  o poor mental functioning;

  o abnormal involuntary body movements;

  o seizures (only some cases);

  o lethargy with loss of consciousness.

Similar conditions: these symptoms may also develop with rapid-onset LIVER FAILURE. See Protocol B.7 also.

It is sometimes desirable to remove fluid in order to help the patient breathe better. However, that should not be done in remote areas, because it is easy to introduce bacteria with disastrous consequences.

Treatment

Referrals: it may be useful to send a patient out to a higher-level facility, both for diagnosis (some types of cirrhosis can be treated successfully) and relief of symptoms. It may be futile by the time full-blown CIRRHOSIS has developed. See LIVER DISEASE.

Patient care

- Low-sodium diet; no salt or baking powder.

- Give no DIURETICS (a physician might).

- Good nutrition; some authorities recommend low-protein and others recommend high-protein.

- Multiple vitamins and minerals, including ZINC.

- Medications for itching: DIPHENHYDRAMINE or CHOLESTYRAMINE.

- Avoid the following drugs which may harm the patient: IBUPROFEN and related medications; AMOXICILLIN/ CLAVULANIC ACID; KETOCONAZOLE, ISONIAZID, GENTAMYCIN and related antibiotics; ERYTHROMYCIN and related drugs; CHLORPROMAZINE and similar drugs; all herbal teas and ethnic medicines.

COBALAMIN DEFICIENCY

This is a deficiency of vitamin B_{12}, a vitamin found in animal products. Strict vegans (eating no animal products at all) may develop this and also some persons who don't absorb vitamin B_{12} adequately. The latter are usually of European genetic heritage. There are two syndromes; usually the patient will have one or the other, not both:

1. ANEMIA

2. nerve problems: pains, numbness, tingling and incoordination of the legs and feet.

The condition can be cured by cobalamin injections. An alternative is eating raw, ground beef liver. However, in developing areas, there are some nasty infections that can be acquired from the liver.

Coccidiomycosis

See Regional Notes M.

COLIC

Entry category: syndrome.

Definition: abdominal pains caused by excessive gas, usually in babies from 2 weeks to 4 months old. It may be due to dietary indiscretion in adults.

Cause: unknown.

Clinical

Crampy abdominal pain that comes and goes, causing a baby to draw his legs up to his trunk. In adults, the pain varies greatly as to time and location. It is at least partly relieved by pushing on the abdomen. If pushing on the abdomen aggravates the pain, this diagnosis is incorrect.

Similar conditions: see Protocol A.39.

Treatment

Referrals: laboratory, facilities: only helpful to exclude other possible diagnoses. *Practitioner:* pediatrician, general practitioner, internist.

Patient care: for colic in babies, try peppermint or CHAMOMILE TEA. Do not use DICYCLOMINE or similar drugs. You should burp the baby more frequently or turn him bottom up and spread his buttocks to help gas come out of his rectum. This problem normally goes away by three months of age. *Adults*: use DICYCLOMINE or CHAMOMILE TEA.

CONCUSSION

See Head Injury in Chapter 9 of Volume 1.

Definition: concussion refers to head injury with loss of consciousness and temporary confusion, but no permanent BRAIN DAMAGE.

Congo-Crimean Hemorrhagic Fever (CCHF)

See CRIMEAN-CONGO HEMORRHAGIC FEVER.

CONTACT DERMATITIS

Definition: an allergic skin reaction caused by and confined to the area of skin that touched a particular substance.
Cause: allergy.
Aggravated, not ill; class 1; worldwide.

Age: any. **Who:** anyone, especially those with other allergies or allergies in the family. **Onset:** usually suddenly, over hours.

Clinical

There are two different types: irritant, in which case most people exposed will have the effect; and allergic, in which case only a minority of people, those who are sensitive, will have the effect.

Necessary: the patient has a rash where some substance, such as leather or metal, touched his skin. This may take any one of a number of forms. There may be a red spotted rash. This may be coarse like MEASLES or fine like SCARLET FEVER. With a poison ivy-type rash, there are tiny blisters with fluid.

Almost always: the rash will itch. In the case of an allergy to laundry soap or detergent, the rash will be widespread on the body, especially on those areas where cloth and skin touch.

Usually: the offending agent is not something new; an allergy develops to something that has been used before without causing problems.

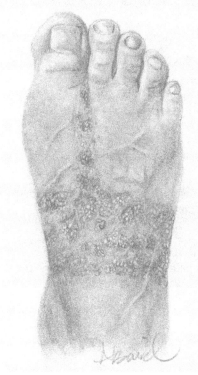

Contact dermatitis: this rash came from an allergy to the leather on sandals; note the pattern on the foot. The pattern of something touching the skin is the clue to the diagnosis. AB

Similar conditions: SCABIES can look very similar, but if you smear some ink over the area and then wash it off, you will see little lines where the ink entered the burrows of the scabies mites. ECZEMA is also an allergic skin rash, but without a defined area of contact. TINEA is similar. Treat for an allergic skin problem first if the patient is from a family with allergic tendencies. Treat for TINEA if many other people in the area have a similar problem. PELLAGRA may appear very similar in those who eat a poor diet with much corn. It starts on sun-exposed parts of the body, and does not itch.

Treatment

Referrals: this is not helpful except to exclude alternative diagnoses.

Patient care:

- For contact dermatitis other than diaper rash, use CORTISONE CREAM locally.

- For diaper rash, a cream with zinc oxide is best or else plain petroleum jelly (Vaseline). If the rash does not clear promptly, then treat it like CANDIDIASIS, because that is probably what it is.

- Do detective work to discover what is causing the problem and advise the patient to change his lifestyle to eliminate contact. With ALLERY-caused problems, HYDROCORTISONE or PREDNISONE may be helpful.

- Ice packs might help, but be careful to avoid FROSTBITE.

COSTAL CHONDRITIS

Synonym: Tietze's Syndrome.

Definition: inflammation of cartilage at the joints where the ribs attach to the breast bone.

Cause: probably virus.

Not ill; class 1; worldwide, common.

Age: older children, young adults. **Who:** anyone. **Onset:** sudden.

Clinical

Necessary: the joints on one or both sides of the breast bone, where the ribs attach, become inflamed. They are tender if pushed.

Maybe: the muscles of the abdomen attaching to the lower joints go into spasm, causing abdominal pain also.

Treatment

Patient care: send out to confirm the diagnosis. Use IBUPROFEN or any mild pain medication. Whether treated or not, the problem will go away, though it may recur. There are no serious consequences.

CRETINISM

Regional Notes: F, I, M, O, S, U

Synonym: congenital hypothyroidism.

Definition: birth defect caused by a thyroid problem in the mother during pregnancy.

Cause: birth defect.

Disabled, not ill; class 1–2; worldwide, present where GOITER is common.

Age: any; always present from birth. **Who:** those living in areas where GOITER is common, mostly inland and mountainous. **Onset:** before birth.

Clinical

There are two kinds of cretinism.

FIRST KIND

With the first kind, the main symptoms are hearing and speech defects and deformed, uncoordinated, stiff limbs; the patient cannot walk normally. Stature is normal.

SECOND KIND

The second kind of cretinism causes short stature, badly formed teeth and symptoms of THYROID TROUBLE of the low-thyroid type.

BOTH KINDS

There is severe mental retardation, mongoloid appearance and possibly crossed eyes. An infant is likely to have decreased activity with poor feeding and weight gain, floppy muscles and a hoarse cry. He may have a large tongue, a large soft spot that stays open and cool, dry skin.

Similar conditions: DOWN SYNDROME, THALLASEMIA.

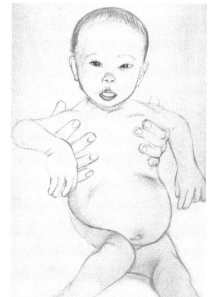

This is a cretin baby of African genetic heritage. In infancy it is impossible to distinguish the two kinds. OW

Treatment

Prevention: if there are any cretins in your area or more than one or two cases of GOITER, treat all young women with low doses of IODINE.

Referrals: laboratory; a level 3 or above lab might be helpful. *Practitioner:* pediatrician, internist, physical therapist.

Patient care: symptoms of THYROID TROUBLE can be treated with medicines. Mental retardation and deafness will not change.

CRIMEAN-CONGO HEMORRHAGIC FEVER (CCHF)

Regional Notes: E, F

Also see HEMORRHAGIC FEVER and Protocol B.2.

This disease likely is a contagious hemorrhagic fever! This is found in the Middle East; the western portion of the Indian subcontinent; Asia west of China; the Crimean, Caspian and Ural Sea areas; eastern, central and southern Africa; Nigeria and Mali. It is common in NE Turkey and in SE Iran. It is most common during the spring and summer, in males and at time of civil unrest, when there is less agriculture and more wild animals. The virus does not make the animals sick, but almost all human cases have had contact with animals or else they are healthcare workers. It is frequently associated with domestic animals being moved in herds and/or slaughtered.

Age: most patients are teens or older. **Who:** the disease is directly infective from handling infected animal products, but it may be transmitted by the bite of a tick—*Hyalomma*—or from crushing a tick. **Onset:** sudden. Incubation is 1–7 days, longer in patients exposed to infected blood rather than a tick bite.

Clinical

Necessary: there is a severe headache first, with dizziness; a painful, stiff neck; eyes that are sore, red and sensitive to light; fever, chills, vomiting, diarrhea and general body pains.

Usually: the fever tends to come and go. The patient's emotional state may be sleepy, confused, depressed or aggressive.

Maybe: the pulse may be slow relative to the fever. There may be a sore throat, red eyes or hair loss. The liver, spleen and lymph nodes may be enlarged. Most cases develop hemorrhage about day 4 or 5. A rash of tiny black-and-blue marks may appear, which may become large bruises. There may be abnormal bleeding from nose, mouth, genital or rectal areas. Patients typically seek care about the fourth day. 40–60% of patients die, usually between the fifth and fourteenth day of illness. Recovery takes months.

Bush laboratory: the sedimentation rate will be elevated; the test is sensitive but not specific.

Treatment

Prevention: Use gowns and masks when caring for a patient. Avoid tick bites. Only transport a patient in a towed trailer.

Patient care: the drug RIBAVIRIN may be helpful. Avoid using ASPIRIN, IBUPROFEN or similar drugs. ACETAMINOPHEN is acceptable. Avoid injections.

CRYPTOSPORIDIOSIS

Regional Notes: I, K, M, N.

Entry category: disease.

Definition: cryptosporidiosis is a bowel infection with *Cryptosporidium parvum*

Cause: protozoa.

Mildly to very ill; class 1–3; contagious; worldwide, especially in developing areas, generally common.

Age: any, especially 1–5 years old; also in adults, especially those with poor immunity, as in HIV infection. **Who**: those drinking contaminated water, eating contaminated food, those in contact with manure from domestic animals. **Onset**: sudden; incubation 1–14 days.

Clinical

Necessary: watery diarrhea, resembling GIARDIASIS, it may be severe. The disease tends to hang on unless treated.

Maybe: cramping and vomiting. With normal immunity the diarrhea persists from 2–26 days.

Complications: DEHYDRATION is common. The patient may develop REITER SYNDROME.

Similar conditions: see Protocol B.14.

Treatment

Prevention: the protozoa are resistant to chlorine so soaking vegetables in bleach-water does not help. They can be killed by heating water to 140° F or 65° C for 30 minutes; this may be accomplished with a hot water heater set on high.

Referrals: laboratory: level 3 or above, stool for parasites; not detected in normal tests; a test for this must be specifically ordered. The test is not very sensitive so you should submit at least 2 specimens before believing a negative report. The parasites are small, but they stain well with the stains usually used for TUBERCULOSIS. *Facilities:* IV's and fluids. Some of the drugs may only be available at level 4 or above facilities. *Practitioner:* level 3 or above, pediatrician, internist, general practitioner.

Patient care: treat DEHYDRATION. No drugs work reliably everywhere. Try PAROMOMYCIN, AZITHROMYCIN, CLARITHROMYCIN or NITAZOXANIDE.

CUTANEOUS LEISHMANIASIS (CL)

Regional Notes: E, F, I, K, M, R.

Entry category: disease, tropical.

Synonyms: Aleppo boil, Baghdad boil, Delhi boil, Oriental sore.

Definition: a skin infection caused by protozoa transmitted by the bites of sand flies.

Cause: protozoa.

Includes: localized cutaneous Leishmaniasis (LCL); mucocutaneous Leishmaniasis (MCL); diffuse cutaneous Leishmaniasis (DCL).

Excludes: VISCERAL LEISHMANIASIS (VL) and a complication of it called post-kala-azar dermal Leishmaniasis (PKDL).

Not ill to mildly ill; class 2–3; regional, does not occur in the Pacific area.

Age: any, but mostly children and teenagers. **Who:** bitten by sand flies, males more than females, rainy season more than dry season. These sand flies (see Volume 1, Appendix 10) bite especially at dusk but they feed throughout the night. **Onset:** variable according to geography and different types of organisms; see the chart on page 49 and the *Regional Notes*.

A **leishmania complex** is a group of leishmania species that ordinarily cannot be distinguished. You should first determine the species or complex to which your patient might have been exposed. The Web site, www.who.int/Leishmaniasis, shows distribution maps. Local lore usually is more reliable than published maps.

Present in Europe, Africa, the Middle East and Asia

Leishmania Donovani and *Leishmania infantum* which usually manifest as VISCERAL LEISHMANIASIS

Leishmania Major.

Leishmania Tropica.

Leishmania Aethiopica (Ethiopia only).

Present in the Americas: there are two main complexes

Leishmania Mexicana

(Mexicana, Amazonensis, Venezuelensis).

Leishmania Viannia

(Braziliensis, Guyanensis, Panamensis, Peruviana).

(There is also a third Leishmaniasis complex, which causes VISCERAL LEISHMANIASIS)

CUTANEOUS LEISHMANIASIS and VISCERAL LEISHMANIASIS (VL) are caused by similar organisms but the diseases are entirely different. Two unusual manifestations of CUTANEOUS LEISHMANIASIS are listed below: mucocutaneous (MCL) and diffuse cutaneous (DCL). Unusual manifestations occur in people with decreased immunity due to HIV INFECTION, MALNUTRITION, CANCER or OLD AGE.

Clinical, general picture

Necessary: the patient has been in an area where CUTANEOUS LEISHMANIASIS occurs, and the skin problem develops slowly, and it does not hurt much, and it has one or more of the following characteristics:

- it starts as tiny, painless, maybe-itching pimples which enlarge to ulcers with raised edges, or rough raised bumps.

- one can feel that part of the sore lies underneath the skin; it does not have the appearance or feel of being right on the surface. It may be saucer-shape, with raised edges and a depressed center or the center may be raised.

- it occurs on parts of the body not ordinarily protected with clothes. The face is common.

Clinical, specific forms

LOCALIZED CUTANEOUS LEISHMANIASIS: LCL

LCL is the most common form of cutaneous Leishmaniasis. It causes spontaneous lumps or sores which may become ulcers, shaped like craters or flattened volcanoes with raised edges. The color is reddish or purplish on white skin but dark-colored on dark skin. Sometimes they are nodules, lumps under the skin or bumps on top of the skin; pain or itchiness is not severe unless there is secondary infection from bacteria. There may or may not be satellite sores—tiny sores that form around the outside of the main sore.

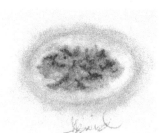

This is a close-up of a typical sore; the appearance may vary greatly. AB

Healing is always with scarring: usually pink or white scars on light skin and dark scars on dark skin though the scars may be normal skin color but have a wrinkled appearance (especially with Aetheopica).

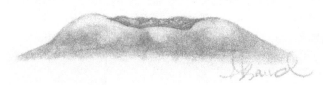

This is a side-ways view of a leishmania sore. AB

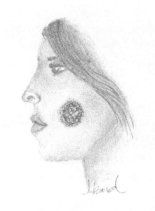

This is the appearance of this sore on the face of a woman. Note the satellite spots around the central ulcer. AB

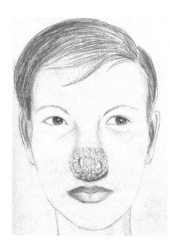

On the nose, the sores are raised up, dry and scaly. OW

Similar diseases: TUBERCULOSIS of the skin; skin CANCER, DOOVANOSIS.

Mucocutaneous Leishmaniasis: MCL

MCL is found mainly in the Americas though it may appear elsewhere. It is a highly destructive disease which affects the pink moist parts of the body—in the mouth, the nose and possibly the genital area, in addition to the skin. The most common cause is *Leishmania Viannia Braziliensis;* the second most common cause is *Leishmania Mexicana.* It causes big, disfiguring holes and wounds that ulcerate, may become secondarily infected and cause difficulty in breathing and eating. It can be fatal. It usually occurs after the skin is infected. The history of the previous skin sore and progression over a week or more distinguishes it from CANCRUM ORIS, which it otherwise resembles.

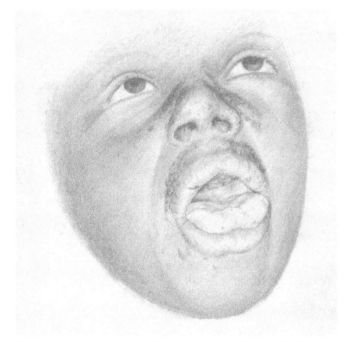

This is a typical appearance of mucocutaneous Leishmaniasis, MCL.

Diffuse cutaneous Leishmaniasis: DCL

DCL is a form of the disease where the skin sores spread over a wide area of skin, rather than staying as few well-defined bumps or ulcers. The color is reddish or purplish on white skin; either purplish, lighter or darker on dark skin. There usually are not ulcers. They spread slowly over months to years and never heal spontaneously. The scarring causes deformity of the body part. The appearance of DCL can be like cobblestones on the face, very similar to lepromatous LEPROSY. It also may resemble post-kala-azar dermal Leishmaniasis, PKDL, a complication of VISCERAL LEISHMANIASIS. DCL is a rare complication of cutaneous Leishmaniasis, due to a decreased immunity.

Treatment for all forms

Prevention: the sand flies that cause this are weak fliers; they have trouble biting in a breeze. A fan is protective. Use insecticide on dogs and in rodent burrows. Use insect repellent on exposed skin. A fine-mesh mosquito net is helpful, especially if it is treated with insecticide or insect repellent.

Referrals: see Volume 1, Appendix 13; this requires tropical/travel expertise. *Laboratory:* the following may be done in a clinic or hospital, probably level 4 or above.

Leishmanin Skin Test: Montenegro test: This is positive in any kind of cutaneous Leishmaniasis except for diffuse cutaneous Leishmaniasis, in which case it is negative. It does not show that the current problem is due to CL but merely shows that the patient has been exposed to Leishmania.

Obtaining materials for microscopic examination: several areas should have samples taken; the edges of open sores are best, but with intact bumps samples should be taken from the center. The material can be taken by scraping with the edge of a knife blade, by pulling material into a syringe with a needle or by cutting out a chunk of tissue, i.e. a biopsy. The parasites are very small and difficult to find. They can only be seen with a 100x lens, using immersion oil.

Serological tests: these are blood tests that show whether there are proteins in a person's body to fight the disease. These tests are very sensitive for VL and reasonably sensitive for MCL (you can usually believe a negative result), but they are generally negative in simple, localized CL. Positives may persist after the disease has been treated and cured. *Facilities:* IV's and fluids; some of the drugs are hard to obtain and require technology to administer. *Practitioner:* experience with this disease is most desirable. An infectious disease specialist is ideal. Otherwise an internist or general practitioner might be helpful. A surgeon can get tissue for microscopic examination.

Patient care: (if sending out is not possible):

Injectable drugs: alternatives are: STILBOGLUCONATE; PENTAMIDINE; AMPHOTERICIN B given daily or every other day, for 20 – 40 days. Injectable medicine is essential in cases where mucocutaneous disease might develop. Additional forms which require injectable drugs are cases which involve lymph nodes, body joints, the outer ear or extensive areas of skin. In addition to whole-body medicines, you can try the following topical treatments. Some work in some geographical areas and others in other areas; none works really well. Local lore is particularly valuable.

VARIETIES OF CUTANEOUS LEISHMANIASIS, ACCORDING TO GEOGRAPHICAL AREAS

Area	Species or Complex	Appearance of skin	Incubation	Healing	Usual Form	Unusual Forms
Europe Americas NW Africa	*Donovani* and *Infantum*	Face, many small bumps, ulcers unusual	Days to years	1–3 years	VL	LCL, DCL
Africa Mideast India Asia	*Major*	Moist sores, no satellites, 2–6 cm round, oval or irregular; inflamed, maybe multiple, lymphatic spread[1]	1–10 weeks	2–8 months	LCL	DCL MCL
Africa Mideast India	*Tropica*	Dry; reddish satellites; ulcers are crusted; 1–4 cm, usually single, usually on face, may be chronic	2–4 months	2 years	LCL	VL
Ethiopia only	*Aethiopica*	Bumpy, usually single, satellites common, wet or dry; no crusting or ulceration	??	2–5 years	LCL	DCL
Americas	*Mexicana*	Single, bump or ulcer, face and ears commonly	Less than 6 months	6–8 months	LCL	DCL VL
Americas	*Viannia*[2]	Various; may spread by lymph nodes	??	??	LCL,	MCL, DCL, VL

1 *In this case one will feel rows of lumps underneath the skin in a line, usually along the long axis of a limb.*

2 *In this case one will feel rows of lumps underneath the skin in a line near the sore. See the chart in Regional Notes M.*

Oral drugs: KETOCONAZOLE, ITRACONAZOLE, ALLOPURINOL work slowly. MILTEFOSINE might work. Reportedly FLUCONAZOLE works for CL Major; it is quite expensive. SITAMAQUINE is newer than the other drugs. An article from Baghdad states that oral zinc sulfate, 5–10 mg/kg daily, cures the problem. If it works, that would be great because the stuff can be purchased by the kilogram from chemical companies.

Topical (surface) drugs: for Major and Tropica-type CL in the Old World and for New World CL in Mexico, injecting STIBOGLUCONATE-type drugs into and under the sore may work well, about 1 ml of the undiluted drug every other day or twice a week for 2–3 weeks. This avoids the toxicity of whole-body drug injections.

AMINOSIDINE in 15% methylbenzethonium chloride can be used as a skin cream.

PAROMOMYCIN ointment; apply locally twice a day for 10–20 days.

Results: the sore first becomes flat and then heals. It may only heal partially during the treatment but the healing will likely be completed after treatment. It will heal as much as it is going to heal by 6 weeks after treatment, so if it is still open then, it needs retreatment. If and when the problem relapses, it usually does so around the outer edges of the scar. DCL, Leishmaniasis on the nose or ear and chronic Leishmaniasis are particularly difficult to treat.

CYCLOSPORIASIS

Cause: protozoa.

Not ill to moderately ill; class 2; nearly worldwide in pockets; especially in Nepal and Latin America.

Age: any; more common in children than adults. **Who:** those who travel and those who consume contaminated food or water or have contact with contaminated soil; it is not transmitted person to person. Chlorination does not kill the cysts. It is seasonal. **Onset:** sudden after an incubation of 1–11 days.

Clinical

Necessary: there is a sudden onset of diarrhea, which may be explosive and fatigue, loss of appetite, nausea, much gas and abdominal cramps. There may be a low fever. The problem lasts for weeks to months. In patients with normal immunity, it cures itself; in people with poor immunity, it may be fatal.

Similar Condition: this is indistinguishable from GIARDIASIS which is much more common and from CRYPTOSPORIDIOSIS. See Protocol B.14.

Treatment

CO-TRIMOXAZOLE is the only thing that works consistently. CIPROFLOXACIN is an alternative that works sometimes. NITAZOXANIDE might also work. Use standard doses for 7 days in the absence of HIV INFECTION; for 10 days in the presence of HIV INFECTION.

CYSTICERCOSIS

Regional Notes: F, I, M, O, R, S, U.

Definition: an infection of the larval form of pork tapeworm.

Cause: worm larva.

Not ill to very ill; class 3; regional.

Age: generally only older children and adults. **Who:** those who live in areas where pigs are raised in such a way that they can come into contact with human waste. It is caused by swallowing any substance contaminated by human stool with pork tapeworm eggs. It may occur in Muslim families who employ foreign house workers. **Onset:** unknown.

Clinical

This is a form of pork TAPEWORM that forms lumps the size of dry green peas. The lumps go to the skin, the muscles and the brain. In the skin, they are underneath the surface. One can feel them easily; the skin will move back and forth over them, and they are not tender. There usually are many. In the muscles they cause soreness and frequently tremendous swelling. In the brain they usually cause no symptoms at all for 3–5 years. Then they cause headache, SEIZURES and BRAIN DAMAGE. SEIZURES most often involve only one part of the body; they are not generalized.

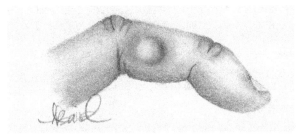

This is a typical cysticercal nodule on a finger. Rheumatic fever may cause similar nodules. AB

Similar conditions: check the causes of SEIZURES and BRAIN DAMAGE if the patient has either. The skin lumps along with muscle pains are distinctive. In some geographic areas consider HYDATID DISEASE.

Treatment

Prevention: don't consume pork that was raised in areas without sanitation. Overcook all pork before eating it. Wash your hands carefully after using a toilet.

Referrals: laboratory; a skin or muscle biopsy is needed to confirm the diagnosis. *Facilities:* if the patient has any evidence of seizures or BRAIN DAMAGE, then a CT scanner is essential. *Practitioner;* a surgeon and a pathologist. A general practitioner, pediatrician or internist is helpful for treatment.

If there are signs of BRAIN DAMAGE, a neurologist or neurosurgeon is desirable.

Patient care: send the patient to a hospital. Otherwise:

- in the absence of SEIZURES, use (PRAZIQUANTEL and ALBENDAZOLE both) plus DEXCHLORPHENIRAMINE. It is good to treat with PREDNISONE or DEXAMETHASONE from 2 days before the deworming drugs until 2 days after.

- FLUBENDAZOLE is a veterinary drug which may work without significant side effects.

- treat SEIZURES with ordinary seizure medicines. Hospitals use high doses of PRAZIQUANTEL + ALBENDAZOLE, plus (PREDNISONE or DEXAMETHASONE) plus CIMETIDINE. It is safer for you to use the lower dose unless you are sure your patient does not have STRONGYLOIDIASIS or AMEBIASIS.

DEHYDRATION

Entry category: syndrome

Definition: lack of an adequate amount of body water.

Cause: body fluid loss.

Not ill to very ill; class 1–3; worldwide, very common everywhere. **Not a diagnosis!** Look for the cause of dehydration. Frequently the patient, if a child, also suffers from MALNUTRITION.

Age: any, especially children. **Who:** those with vomiting, diarrhea, not drinking or DIABETES. **Onset:** 1/2 hour to 2 days.

Clinical severity of dehydration

MILD DEHYDRATION

The patient is thirsty. The top of his tongue is dry but it is moist beneath his tongue[1]. He may have a rapid pulse and respiration.

MODERATE DEHYDRATION

The patient is thirsty. It is dry both on top of and beneath his tongue. His eyes are somewhat sunken and his skin a bit loose on his upper, inner thighs[2]. He is not unconscious from the dehydration. He has a rapid pulse and respiration. His blood pressure is lower than usual, and he faints easily.

SEVERE DEHYDRATION

The patient is unconscious or lethargic. He may have a fever from dehydration alone. His skin is very loose, his eyes are sunken and his entire mouth is dry. His pulse is fast and his breathing is both fast and deep.

Complications: KIDNEY DISEASE, CATARACT.

---

1 *If the patient is mouth-breathing, his tongue will normally be dry. In this case, check the inside of his lower lip; if that is dry, he is dehydrated.*

2 *In elderly people whose skin is naturally loose, check the skin on the forehead. That remains tight longer than other skin.*

Bush laboratory: the patient's urine will be an intense yellow color unless the cause of dehydration is DIABETES. In that case the urine will be a light color, but it will test positive for sugar with a urine dipstick.

Treatment

Referrals: level 2 or above. Laboratory; a hospital blood test will show an elevated blood urea nitrogen. Facilities: IV's and fluids. Practitioner: general practitioner, internist, pediatrician, senior nurse.
Patient care: see Appendix 1 for detailed instructions.

- If he is vomiting, try to settle his stomach with PROMETHAZINE.

- A severely dehydrated vomiting patient who does not have diarrhea may be given plain, half-strength non-sterile saline by enema. He should be sent to a hospital, but this will help him meanwhile.

- In case of vomiting plus diarrhea in a severely dehydrated patient, use intraperitoneal fluid. See Procedure 17 in Appendix 1, Volume 1. Intraperitoneal fluids are acceptable to use with DIABETES.

- Protect the eyes. With severe dehydration, the eyes are sunken so the lids do not properly cover them. The cornea is exposed, resulting in damage to the eyes and consequent blindness. You can prevent this by putting ANTIBIOTIC EYE OINTMENT in the eyes and then covering them. The patient will pull the eye covers off when he wakes up.

- Consider your patient's nutrition. If the patient is unable to eat or drink over more than a few days, he should be given calories, protein and vitamins as well. Give the refeeding mixture used for malnourished children as described in Chapter 5. Use a stomach tube if necessary. For an adult, give about 1/4 to 1/3 of his daily fluid requirement as refeeding mixture. Once a day crush a multivitamin tablet and give this also.

DELIRIUM TREMENS

This is a complication of alcohol withdrawal. See ALCOHOLISM. The patient is disoriented, agitated, trembling and sweating; he may have an increased pulse, rapid breathing and fever. See the withdrawal paragraph under ALCOHOLISM.

DEMONIZATION

Entry category: syndrome.
Definition: this refers to abnormal physical or mental conditions, usually not following recognized disease patterns, brought on by occult powers.

Age: usually older children or adults. **Who**: it can affect anyone, and those most susceptible are those who believe that it does not exist or that it cannot happen to them. Some drugs, both recreational and prescription, can make one vulnerable. **Onset**: highly variable; if it is sudden, it is commonly after an occult or emotionally traumatic experience.

Clinical

Usually: violent emotional upset, speaking in other voices, lethargy, weakness, seizures, jerking, day-night reversal, fatigue, paralysis, panic attacks and unusual susceptibility to disease are common patterns. There may be depression, decreased appetite and difficulty walking.

Commonly: the symptoms vary widely both qualitatively and in severity over hours and days; they are not constant. The following are common characteristics:

- an illness that does not make sense medically.

- a medical crisis right before a critical ministry obligation.

- an irrational hatred of a godly person.

- a seizure, panic attack or other disruptive behavior in the context of worship.

Similar conditions: see Protocol B.10.B. Demonization does not generally cause fevers; if there is a fever or history of fevers, consider cerebral MALARIA, BRUCELLOSIS and similar conditions. Other similar problems are ADDICTION, ALCOHOLISM, ATTENTION DEFICIT DISORDER, BERIBERI, PELLAGRA, RADIATION ILLNESS. PLANT POISONING due to mushrooms can both mimic and be a causative factor in this. Demonization can coexist with any of these.

Treatment

Referrals: this is essential only to rule out medical causes of the problem. Referral should be to level 3 or 4 at least. If the problem is due to demons, a Western-trained practitioner will probably tell you that it is psychiatric or psychogenic.
Patient care: this is problematic since anyone with a Western education is likely to think you are crazy for suggesting the diagnosis. It is important also to avoid psychotropic medications, in particular CHLORPROMAZINE and related medications. The effects are sometimes reversed by audible prayer in the name of Jesus. National clergy with allegiance to Jesus are frequently helpful with treatment. It is essential to avoid treatment by traditional healers who may use occult means which will make the final problem worse.

DENGUE FEVER

Regional Notes: F, I, M, O, R, S, U.

Synonym: breakbone fever.

Definition: a general whole-body viral infection, a type of ARBOVIRAL FEVER, caused by a virus transmitted by *Aedes* mosquitoes, mainly tropical. The mosquito that transmits the disease in urban and semi-urban areas of the Eastern Hemisphere is black with white spots on the joints of its limbs and white spots along the sides of its body.

Includes: dengue hemorrhagic fever (DHF), dengue shock syndrome (DSS).

Cause: virus.

The geography of this disease is continually changing. It potentially may manifest anywhere that *Aedes* mosquitoes live. This is from 40° north to 40° south in the Western Hemisphere; the northern limit may be up to 50° north in Europe and western Asia.

Mildly to severely ill; class 1–3; not directly contagious; it requires mosquito transmission.

Age: mostly children in Asia and the Pacific; both children and adults in the Americas. **Who**: mosquito-bitten, especially urban dwellers, some rural people, mostly during the rainy season. There are major epidemics every 3–5 years in Asia and the Americas. The epidemics are every 5–6 years in the Pacific area. In the Americas there are additional small outbreaks every year. Dengue hemorrhagic fever is most likely to arise in areas that normally have many dengue cases. There are 4 kinds of dengue fever; 1, 2, 3, 4; each person can get each kind only once. Their clinical pictures are identical. **Onset:** suddenly, 2–15 days after the bite.

Clinical

Necessary: sudden onset of high fever and severe general body pain. The length of time from the first symptom to when the patient is in bed is less than 12 hours.

Usually: the patient has a fever which drops to normal about day 4 and then rises again after 1/2 to 3 days. With this second fever rise, the pains and depression are worse than before. He has aching or shooting pains all over, especially in the front of his head, in his back and his eyes; the pains are particularly severe in his muscles, joints and bones. His eyes hurt worse when he moves them to look sideways.

Commonly: patients believe they will die. There is insomnia, nightmares and depression. Constipation is usual. The patient may have a slow pulse relative to the fever with the second rise in temperature. Local lore is helpful as the disease varies from place to place. The symptoms in any one epidemic are consistent, but they vary from one epidemic to another.

Frequently: an intensely itchy rash that fades with pressure develops with the first fever. It is more common in children than in adults. It looks like a sunburn, measles or scarlet fever on fair skin. It may be invisible or sandpapery on dark skin. It starts on the chest and the trunk and moves from there to the limbs and the face. It does not last long. There are two subsequent rashes which may or may not occur.

During early recovery a peculiar rash develops; in fair people, the skin is red with white dots. It starts on the hairy surfaces of the hands and feet, moving up the limbs, possibly to include the whole body. It itches and may peel.

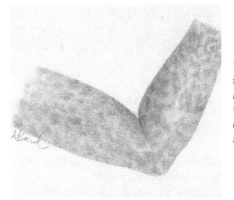

This drawing is of the second rash; it resembles HIVES with red, raised areas of irregular shapes. AB

Lymph nodes may be large and the abdomen tender, causing confusion with ACUTE ABDOMEN. Watch for the rash and bone pain which are not present with ACUTE ABDOMEN.

Sometimes: he has chills, loss of appetite, fatigue, stiffness and possibly a strange sense of taste. The liver may be large.

Occasionally: symptoms include weakness, dizziness, light avoidance, red eyes, drenching sweats, sore throat, cough, nosebleed, pain with urination, pain in the groin and testicles and crazy behavior. There may be neurological signs with dengue: lethargy, irritability, drowsiness, coma, seizures, a stiff neck, sharp shooting pains down limbs or paralysis. This might occur in either dengue fever or dengue hemorrhagic fever (DHF) and in both adults and children. It may result in paralysis or recurring seizures (EPILEPSY). About 10% of patients with neurological symptoms die from the disease. Occasionally the illness looks just like ENTERIC FEVER in adults. Strange symptoms also might occur with this; do not discount the diagnosis just because your patient has some other symptom not listed here.

Complications of dengue fever: DEPRESSION may last for years. In some cases Reye syndrome, a type of LIVER FAILURE, develops during recovery. Its manifestation is severe vomiting. It requires immediate evacuation. When a pregnant woman gets dengue fever near term, the infant may die.

Similar conditions: see Protocols B.2, B.8, B.9, B.13. Dengue is different from ARTHRITIS in that the pains are not exclusively in the joints. Also its onset is very rapid.

Bush laboratory: check hemoglobin, urine and stool. Lab should show only ketones in urine unless HEMORRHAGIC FEVER has developed. In that cases there will also be blood in the urine. Do a tourniquet test. The tourniquet test is not sensitive, but it is specific for some bleeding problem:

Tourniquet test

Inflate a blood pressure cuff on an upper arm and leave it inflated for 5 minutes at a pressure half-way between the lower number and the higher number; then deflate it.

The test is positive if there are more than 3 red spots per square centimeter on the skin below where the cuff had been. These might not be visible on very black skin. However, you will see the spots on the fingernails in that case.

Referrals: see Volume 1, Appendix 13. *Laboratory;* a very sophisticated lab, level 4 or above, can definitely diagnose the disease. In a level 2 or above laboratory, there will be an increased hematocrit with DHF. Rapid diagnostic tests do not become positive until late. *Facilities:* at level 3 or above, IV equipment and fluids; a blood bank; monitoring equipment is desirable. *Practitioner:* an infectious disease specialist is ideal. A general practitioner, internist or pediatrician is acceptable.

DENGUE HEMORRHAGIC FEVER (DHF)

Entry category: disease complication

This is a major problem in Asia, the Pacific region and Latin America. There have been major epidemics since WW2 in Thailand, the Philippines, Indonesia, the South Pacific, Cuba, Nicaragua and Brazil. It can occur almost anywhere in the tropics and subtropics.

Age: any in the Americas; usually children and teens only in other areas. Who: those for whom this is a second dengue infection. Risk factors are older age, malnutrition, female. Onset: sudden, usually after 3–4 days of ordinary dengue fever.

Clinical: there may or may not be the ordinary signs and symptoms of dengue. With DHF the pulse will become rapid, and the blood pressure will drop because the watery part of the blood leaks from the small veins. There may be abnormal bleeding.

Treatment: you can do nothing for patient care; either send the patient out or tell the family he will die.

Treatment of dengue fever

Prevention: mosquito control: don't keep house plants. Nurse your patient under a mosquito net. Prevent mosquito contact with patients for 5 days after the onset of the illness. Dengue mosquitoes bite during the day. In rural areas discourage monkeys from being around your house, since they are a reservoir for the disease, keeping the local mosquitoes infected. Keep fish in containers that collect water; they eat mosquito larvae. Lids or screens on water collection surfaces help. Clean water collection containers often. Temphos is a chemical that kills the mosquito larvae.

Patient care: prevent DEHYDRATION and keep the patient in bed. **Antibiotics are not helpful.** However, you may give ACETAMINOPHEN for fever, MILK OF MAGNESIA for constipation, pain medicines, etc. Do not use ASPIRIN since it may trigger bleeding or Reye's syndrome (a form of rapid-onset LIVER FAILURE). Use MULTIVITAMINS.

Results: varies. Case fatality rate is 1–15%.

DEPRESSION

Regional Notes: F, O.

Entry category: syndrome.

Definition: either a feeling of sadness or a group of physical symptoms commonly associated with emotional sadness.

Cause: variable.

Mildly to very ill; class 1–4; worldwide.

Age: mid-childhood and older. **Who:** those dealing with guilt or anger, especially if they find it hard to express the anger; religious people who are angry with God; anyone who has experienced a significant loss. (The loss is not always obvious. A job promotion may involve the loss of significant relationships.) **Onset:** may be sudden or gradual.

Clinical

If the person cries or acts sad, depression is obvious. Many times, however, the patient is not consciously sad. Loss of appetite or eating binges (depending on whether the person is genetically slim or overweight) and change in bowel habits (either constipation or diarrhea) are usual.

The patient may have a pressure-type chest pain. He may sigh or breathe irregularly. The most frequent symptom is alteration of the sleep cycle; the person has no trouble falling asleep, but wakes up very early and cannot get back to sleep. He may complain only of chronic fatigue. Also see STRESS as this is invariably associated.

Causative diseases: DEMONIZATION may be causative. Depression may also be physiological. Childbirth, DENGUE FEVER, BRUCELLOSIS, DIABETES, TUBERCULOSIS, HEAT ILLNESS and chronic pain from any cause are some of the possible causes. Some families are prone to depression, so any stress will provoke it. Some women become depressed each month during the menstrual cycle.

Similar conditions: malnourished patients: BERIBERI, PELLAGRA, ALCOHOLISM. *History of occult activity:* DEMONIZATION. *History of drug abuse:* ADDICTION. *Patient has an enemy:* ARSENIC POISONING, DEMONIZATION, RADIATION ILLNESS. *History of a recent illness with a fever:* DENGUE FEVER, ENTERIC FEVER, ARBOVIRAL FEVER.

Treatment

Referrals: laboratory, facilities: useful to exclude alternative diagnoses. Practitioner: general practitioner or internist is adequate; a psychiatrist is ideal. Send the patient out if at all possible.

Patient care:

- Do not try to cheer the person up by telling him how good his life is! This only adds guilt to his depression.

- Teach him to mistrust his feelings; feelings do not reflect reality.

- Point out some aspect of his work that was helpful to you or someone else.

- Listen to him, encourage him to talk and do not be critical of what he says.

- Urge him to exercise in spite of his depression; go for walks or go swimming together.

- Ask him about suicidal thoughts and if he admits having them, ask if he has thought of how he would do it. Someone who has a specific suicide plan requires more help than you can give. Suicidal people are relieved to have someone ask; others do not take offense at this question. Take away the gun, rope, medication or whatever he intended to use to kill himself.

- Beware of the person who was depressed and now is cheerful. One can attain peace by deciding on a suicide plan.

- If a depressed person gives away valuable possessions he intends suicide even if he denies it. His gifts are a cry for help. In these cases, keep the person in view of a responsible adult until he can be sent out for professional care.

- Be aware that antidepressant medicines (with few exceptions) are potent suicide agents. Giving a bottle of these to a depressed patient is asking for trouble.

Dermatitis

See CONTACT DERMATITIS, TINEA and CANDIDIASIS.

DIABETES

Regional Notes: F, I, S, U.

Definition: lack of the hormone insulin which enables sugars to enter into the cells of the body. This results in the starvation of the cells for lack of sugar and excess sugar in the blood.

Cause: hormone deficiency (Insulin).

Mildly to very ill; mild is class 2 and severe is class 4; worldwide, variably common.

Age: any. **Who:** anyone, especially older folks and relatives of diabetics; this may be a consequence of severe MALNUTRITION, PANCREATITIS or PLANT POISONING: cassava. **Onset:** usually over weeks.

Clinical

In mild diabetes, the patient has thirst, excessive urination, increased appetite and weight loss.

With severe diabetes he will additionally have rapid respiration, rapid pulse, low blood pressure, vomiting, DEHYDRATION, SHOCK and loss of consciousness. His breath may smell like glue (acetone). He may lose his sense of smell. He is apt to be lethargic before he becomes unconscious.

Complications: blindness, heart problems and bad circulation which may result in STROKE, KIDNEY DISEASE or GANGRENE. There may be impotence or sharp shooting pains in the legs and feet. Females who are diabetic during pregnancy may have very large babies. Diabetics are prone to CANDIDIASIS.

Similar conditions: if the patient is lethargic, see Protocol B.10. TAPEWORM can cause the increased appetite with weight loss. The subsequent abdominal pain, vomiting, etc. can look like INFLUENZA. There is no fever with diabetes. The leg pains might resemble BERIBERI, SYPHILIS or rarely ARSENIC POISONING. The symptoms of low blood sugar with treatment may resemble alcohol intoxication.

Bush laboratory: urine has sugar and possibly ketones in it. Sugar plus ketones is more serious than sugar alone. Glucose is another name for sugar.

Treatment

Prevention: prevent MALNUTRITION or treat it early. Urge people to properly process cassava. Avoid a high-sugar diet and obesity.

Referrals: see Volume 1, Appendix 13. *Laboratory*; a level 2 or above laboratory blood test shows a high blood sugar, positive serum ketones and possibly abnormal blood electrolytes. *Facilities*: IVs and fluids, monitoring equipment if the patient is very ill. Practitioner: an internist is ideal, a general practitioner or pediatrician might be helpful. A Western-educated diabetic who is managing his own diabetes might be helpful if other care is unavailable. *Patient care:* varies according to the severity of the disease. Check the urine and then seek advice. Send out if at all possible; there is not much you can do otherwise.

Complications of treatment: an Indian and Chinese vegetable, karela, lowers the blood sugar and can cause problems with diabetes control. Too much insulin, too much exercise, insufficient food or another illness may drop the blood sugar too far; the patient becomes sweaty, shaky and hungry. He may have SEIZURES, lose consciousness and have permanent BRAIN DAMAGE. He needs sugar by mouth, stomach tube or rectum.

Results: 2 hours to 1 day.

Diarrhea

This is a symptom, not a condition. See Protocol A.56 in the Symptom Index. The PowerPoint lecture might also be helpful.

DIPHTHERIA

Regional Notes: E, F, I, K, M, O, S, U.

Includes: veld sore (skin diphtheria).

Definition: this is an infection causing a severe illness in unimmunized people, usually children.

Cause: virus-infected bacteria.

Usually very ill; class 2–4; contagious, very; worldwide, related to crowding and lack of immunization, more common in cooler areas. Frequently occurs in epidemics. The skin ulcer form is most common in hot dry environments and during conditions of war.

Age: mostly children over 6 months old and older adults. Deaths occur mostly in those under 5 y.o. or over 40. **Who:** not immunized or insufficiently immunized; the D of DPT stands for diphtheria, as does the D in DT and Tdap. Occasionally an immunized person may get it. **Onset:** during the cooler months; incubation 1–10 days, variable onset; patients seek help within several days.

Clinical

Necessary: fever, if any, is not high. There is fatigue and headache; throat or nose pain; and a white, black or gray leathery scum on the normally moist pink tonsils. It extends from a small spot to a large area in hours. Nasal diphtheria starts out as a simple head cold with congestion and a slightly bloody runny nose. Other symptoms vary according to the site of the infection.

Commonly: if it affects the throat, the patient may be very ill, have foul breath, hoarseness and a swollen neck. The presence or absence of fever varies. There may be HEART FAILURE after one or more weeks. The pulse is rapid relative to the fever. Weakness is more prominent than numbness.

Maybe: with nasal diphtheria there may be significant blood loss from the nose. He may not be able to open his mouth wide enough for you to see his throat. He may not be able to swallow, talk or move his eyes normally. If it affects the throat, he may be short of breath or unable to speak at all.

Sometimes: the liver and spleen may be large and soft. If it infects just the nose, it is a mild disease with no heart problems, but it makes a rash on the upper lip resembling IMPETIGO.

Occasionally: diphtheria also infects the eyes, the ears, wounds and the genital area, causing pain. It may also cause incontinence, sweating, light avoidance, dizziness, dry mouth, sexual dysfunction and wild swings in vital signs.

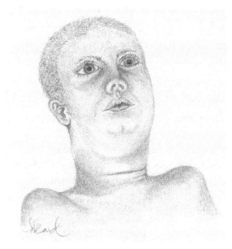

Note the swelling on both sides of the upper neck. The boy is staring into space; he looks sick. One may have diphtheria without this swelling or the swelling might be much worse than this. AB

Usual order of weakness

1–2 weeks: throat problems with trouble swallowing, regurgitating through the nose, change in voice.

2–5 weeks: double vision, crossed eyes.

3–4 weeks: face asymmetrical with smiling or frowning; difficulty chewing.

Complications: sudden death is possible up to eight weeks after the original illness. HEART FAILURE may start early in the disease or during convalescence. PNEUMONIA is common.

Prognosis: hoarseness, shortness of breath and cough are bad signs. Paralysis may last for months, but usually recovery is complete.

Similar conditions: if the patient is short of breath, see Protocol B.4. *Nasal diphtheria early on:* consider RESPIRATORY INFECTION, a common cold, croup. *Neck swelling:* both diphtheria and ANTHRAX can cause massive swelling of the face and neck. Other causes are VINCENT STOMATITIS and ALLERGY. *Skin diphtheria:* if the sore is on the genitals, hands or face, see Protocol B.1: Sexually Transmitted Diseases. IMPETIGO may look similar but it does not make the person ill.

Bush laboratory: there is almost always protein in the urine.

Treatment

Prevention: immunize. The D of DPT stands for diphtheria. Do not allow unimmunized people near the patient until after 7 days of antibiotic. If you have been exposed, take ERYTHROMYCIN or benzathine PENICILLIN as for STREP INFECTION.

Referrals: see Volume 1, Appendix 13. Laboratory: hospitals, level 3 or above, can do a culture and a stain. Facilities:

there is a wide variety of equipment, level 4 or above, that might be helpful. Antitoxin is extremely important; that is unlikely to be available below a level 4 facility. Practitioner: anesthesiologist for airway management; infectious disease specialist, neurologist, general practitioner, pediatrician, internist, surgeon.

Patient care: send the patient out if the receiving facility has antitoxin. He will probably die otherwise. If this is out of the question, treat as follows

If the skin is infected, treat it with ANTIBIOTIC OINTMENT. PENICILLIN, ERYTHROMYCIN or CLINDAMYCIN must also be used; it must be injectable. The patient must stay in bed for 3 weeks to decrease the chances of HEART FAILURE. Immunize him (even while he is ill) since having the disease does not confer immunity.

DONOVANOSIS

Regional Notes: F, I, M, O, S, U.

Synonyms: granuloma inguinale, granuloma venereum.

Definition: a sexually transmitted disease caused by a bacterium, *Klebsiella granulomatis*.

Cause: bacteria, Gram-negative.

Not ill to very ill; class 1–3; contagious by direct contact between warm moist body parts; worldwide, mainly large urban areas and/or ports, particularly in South Africa, Brazil, India (southeast coast), New Guinea, New Britain and aboriginal Australia. It is also found in Vietnam, the Caribbean, Zambia and Zimbabwe. It is associated with poverty, prostitution and poor personal hygiene.

Who: sexually mature and sexually abused. Males more than females, nationals more than expatriates; poverty and poor hygiene promote transmission. **Onset:** incubation 3 days to 3 months, occasionally up to 1 year.

Clinical

Everybody who has the disease has symptoms, in contrast to other venereal diseases which may be without symptoms. However, in females where the sore is deep inside the vagina, the disease might not be obvious on the outside, and there may be a delay before she knows she has it. There is no fever or fatigue unless there are complications with secondary infection. When this happens the prognosis is poor. The disease affects the genitals in 90% of the patients and the groin in the other 10%. There are 4 kinds of presentations.

- Red ulcers which bleed.
- Ulcers with rotting flesh that smell bad.
- Swellings with cauliflower-type surfaces.
- Areas with scarring.

Necessary: the disease begins with a little painless pimple or crust on the skin; it may be dry or wet. It may resemble genital warts, a SYPHILIS ulcer or have a raised, cauliflower-like surface. The surface rubs off, and it exudes a discharge. It bleeds readily. The disease spreads from the penis to the groins in males, from the genital lips or vagina to the groins in females.

Maybe: ulcers may may develop on adjacent skin. There are no enlarged lymph nodes unless another infection starts on top of this, but there may be a raw, pink or red, cauliflower-type bump(s) in the groin(s) that may be mistaken for large lymph nodes. The disease extends slowly on skin surfaces which then heal with scarring. It extends rapidly on the moist pink areas which then do not heal. Pregnancy makes the disease more aggressive.

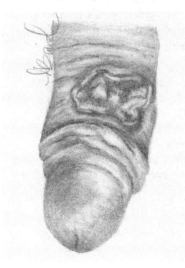

The shape is irregular. The center bleeds readily. The edges are swollen. AB

Commonly: there is shiny, deep tissue showing in the middle of the ulcer. The ulcer looks more painful than it is. Pain, if any, is minimal. If there is secondary infection in addition to the Donovanosis, there may be a foul-smelling discharge.

Sometimes: instead of an ulcer there may be a round area without any skin, with a raised-up, beefy-red, cauliflower-like raw surface. Sometimes this raised-up area has a split down the middle. The appearance of these raised areas are like the meat of a half-walnut lying flat-side down, but red instead of tan. If the sores develop internally, in women especially, they may become rapidly fatal due to severe tissue destruction.

Uncommonly: there may be some spontaneous healing in which case there is bumpy scar tissue, similar to KELOIDS. The disease may infect the inside of the mouth, causing swelling, bleeding and loose teeth. A primary sore might be on the skin other than the genital area, usually the head or neck.

Complications in females and homosexual males: in the vagina or rectum, the ulcer may cause widespread destruction, forming holes into the bladder, rectum or both. Urine or stool then passes through these holes, causing incontinence and bacterial infection. These holes need surgery. After antibiotics the scarring may interfere with urination, bowel movements, sexual activity and childbirth. Untreated women may have massive fatal bleeding at the time of childbirth.

Complications in uncircumcised males are PHIMOSIS or PARAPHIMOSIS.

Complications in either sex: the genitals may be swollen and eventually roughened like ELEPHANTIASIS. This may cause the person to retain urine or stool, unable to pass it normally. There may be bony lesions—a kind of OSTEOMYELITIS—associated with weight loss, fevers, night sweats and fatigue. It can affect the leg, spine or pelvis with dastardly consequences. See SPINAL NEUROPATHY.

Similar conditions: *on the face*: CUTANEOUS LEISHMANIASIS, CHANCROID, SYPHILIS, TUBERCULOSIS. *In the mouth*: like on the face and also SCURVY. *Wart/cauliflower surface:* secondary SYPHILIS, WARTS. With SYPHILIS the wart-like lesions are white or pale; with Donovanosis they are red. SYPHILIS clears within 1 week of PENICILLIN treatment; Donovanosis lesions do not clear at all with penicillin. With appropriate treatment Donovanosis heals over 2 weeks or more.

Treatment

Referrals: laboratory; a stained smear can be done by a hospital lab, level 3 or above. The name of the stain is Giemsa (GEEMsuh); if you have opportunity, ask before sending the patient. Practitioner; a sexually transmitted disease clinic is ideal. Previous experience in dealing with this is essential A surgeon is necessary in advanced cases.

Patient care: follow Protocol B.1 if you are not sure of the diagnosis. If you are sure of the diagnosis, then treat as follows.

• Clean the area four times a day.

• Treat with an antibiotic: AZITHROMYCIN, DOXYCYCLINE, ERYTHROMYCIN, CO-TRIMOXAZOLE, CHLORAMPHENICOL, STREPTOMYCIN, CIPROFLOXACIN or CEFTRIAXONE. If there is no response at all in a few days, add a second antibiotic; patients who are HIV infected should get two drugs in the first place. If the patient has intolerable side effects from the antibiotic or if there is no improvement in a week, then the antibiotic needs to be changed. Generally a minimum of 14–21 days of antibiotic is recommended. Treat the patient until he or she is totally healed and then for another week thereafter.

• Be sure to treat the sexual partner or partners for the disease.

• If you are not totally sure of the diagnosis or if the disease is not known to be common in your area, also treat for other genital ulcers according to the Protocol B.1.

• Childbirth should be in a hospital; it is important to treat the newborn.

Results: there is usually severe scarring. Healing is slow, over 2 weeks or more.

DOWN SYNDROME

Synonyms: trisomy 21, mongolism.

Definition: Down syndrome is a birth defect, caused by an extra chromosome.

Cause: birth defect.

Age: the problem is evident from birth, though the parents might not initially recognize or admit it. **Who:** anyone can give birth to a Down syndrome child; nothing can prevent it aside from prenatal diagnosis and abortion. **Onset:** from conception, evident from birth.

Clinical

This is a common kind of mental retardation; the degree of retardation varies greatly. The child's eyes are widely set and slant downward from the temples to the nose. The bridge of his nose is low. The tops of the outer ears may be folded down. His mouth usually hangs open, showing a large tongue. The crease on his palm, closest to his fingers, may go across his hand without interruption. His fingers are shorter than normal. Heart problems are common. CRETINISM and THALLASEMIA may look similar. There is no good treatment.

Complications: HEART FAILURE, CANCER of the blood (leukemia), frequent infections, ALZHEIMER DISEASE, premature graying of the hair.

DRUG ERUPTION

⚠ EMERGENCIES WITH DRUG ERUPTIONS

If the patient has large blisters and/or large areas of peeling skin, he should be treated as if he has a burn. See Chapter 9 in Volume 1. If this covers over 30% of his body surface area, he probably will die. Any referral should be to a level 3 hospital or above.

Clinical

This is a reaction to a drug which can be seen with PENICILLIN therapy for SYPHILIS, GRISEOFULVIN or KETOCONAZOLE for TINEA or DIETHYLCARBAMAZINE for ONCHOCERCIASIS. It involves older more than younger patients and frequently causes swelling of lymph nodes. There are two types:

IMMEDIATE REACTION

This is from the **first dose**, due to bacterial debris liberated by the death of micro-organisms. The reaction is characterized by fever; large tender lymph nodes; sore joints; transient bumps or HIVES on the skin; and worsening of the skin rash of the original disease. You should not stop treatment, because symptoms resolve with continued therapy.

DELAYED REACTION:

This occurs **7 to 20 days after starting** a new drug or within hours after restarting a drug that was used previously. Serious reactions are of five types and **for these the drug must be stopped:**

- Blistering and/or peeling skin (EXFOLIATIVE DERMATITIS.)
- Red/raised/target-like round skin swellings.
- Significant swelling, abnormal bruising and areas of skin or flesh that appear to be dead.
- A reaction that affects the moist, pink parts of the body.
- Anything that looks like a sunburn but is not sunburn by history.

Similar conditions: see Protocol B.12 if the patient has large lymph nodes. Also see SERUM SICKNESS and KATAYAMA DISEASE. These diagnoses may overlap.

Treatment

Immediately stop the offending drug or drugs, but only for a delayed reaction.

Referrals: any facility that has IV capabilities is likely to be helpful, though a level 4 facility would be ideal.

Patient care: give IV fluids to keep the patient hydrated; use PREDNISONE or a related drug; check vital signs frequently; email to request further advice, sending pictures and a detailed history.

DYSENTERY

Entry category: disease cluster.

Regional Notes: E, F, I, M, O, R, S, U; largely but not exclusively tropical.

Includes: bacterial and amebic dysentery

Definition: an infection with bacteria or amebae which affects the lining of the bowel, causing diarrhea with blood, mucus or both; plus fever, abdominal pain or both, lasting over 48 hrs.

Cause: variable.

Mildly to very ill; class 1–4 depending on severity; contagious; worldwide, relatively common, causes vary by region.

Age: any. **Who:** anyone, especially where sanitation is poor. For amebae the disease tends to be worse in children under 1 year old, in the malnourished, in pregnant women and in persons taking PREDNISONE or related drugs. **Onset:** variable. Sometimes there is a long history (weeks) of vague abdominal discomfort. Shigella (a type of bacterial dysentery) has an abrupt onset after a 2–4 day incubation. For amebae, the incubation is 1–2 weeks for small exposures but only days for major exposures.

Clinical

Necessary: the patient has either constipation with lower abdominal pain (right or left) or else he has diarrhea with mucus, blood and sometimes pus.

Sometimes: he may have cramps, headache, nausea and vomiting or fever. His abdomen may be tender. DEHYDRATION will develop if the diarrhea is severe. Listed below are some of the characteristics of the two kinds.

BACTERIAL DYSENTERY

Most common in children; the incubation is less than a week. It has a sudden onset, usually with more than one patient. The diarrhea stools are small in amount, frequent (perhaps 100 times a day), gelatinous and almost odorless or with a slight odor resembling rancid fat. The patient becomes ill rapidly; he usually **seeks help within 5 days**; the stool blood is bright red rather than reddish brown or black.

Severe cramping pains are common. If the abdomen is tender, it is tender all over. The patient may have a high fever. The pulse is rapid relative to the fever. The blood pressure may be low. *Complications:* REITER SYNDROME; red lumps under the skin; sharp shooting pains in limbs; SEPSIS; and death. There may be new ANEMIA and KIDNEY DISEASE.

AMEBIC DYSENTERY

See also AMEBIASIS. Bowel movements are infrequent (1–4 daily), large and sometimes incredibly foul, their odor resembling that of very rotten meat. With time the patient will lose weight and develop ANEMIA. There may or may not be fever. *Complications:* dysentery due to amebae may result in ACUTE ABDOMEN and in AMEBIC SKIN ULCERS.

Similar conditions: see Protocols B.1, B.3, B.9, B.11, B.14. *In a female during menstruation* consider ENDOMETRIOSIS. *With anal pain:* consider CHLAMYDIA, LYMPHOGRANULOMA VENEREUM. *With heavy blood loss:* if the bloody stool is part of a general bleeding problem (also with easy bruising and nosebleeds), see Protocols B.2 and B.7. HOOKWORM is a common condition that can be nearly indistinguishable. Hookworm tends to occur in areas with sandy or loam soil, not clay.

Fever and/or very sick: ACUTE ABDOMEN—watch carefully for this; falciparum MALARIA, ENTERIC FEVER, MEASLES, abdominal TUBERCULOSIS, KIDNEY DISEASE, SEPSIS. *No fever, not real sick:* TRICHURIASIS, STRONGYLOIDIASIS, HOOKWORM or ARSENIC POISONING may also look similar. Consider SCHISTOSOMIASIS in some regions.

Bush laboratory: shake up the stool with some water and use your urine dipsticks. Stool tests positive for blood in both kinds and also positive for leukocytes with bacterial dysentery. Urine is normal except possibly for ketones.

Treatment

Prevention: eliminate flies, roaches, contamination of water supply. Avoid food from street vendors. Boil, filter or treat all water. Soak food in iodine water or cook it. Bleach water does not kill amebic cysts. Wash hands after moving bowels; teach people to use leaves or toilet paper rather than rags to wipe themselves.

Referrals: see Volume 1, Appendix 13. *Laboratory:* hospital laboratories, level 3 or more, can examine stools for white cells which indicate bacteria as a cause; they can culture the stool and can examine it for amebae. A lab report for bacteria in stool means nothing; all stool **is** 50% bacteria. The microscope test for amebae is specific but not sensitive. You need to have 7 negative tests done by experienced technicians on very fresh stool before you can conclude that there are no amebae. Usually it is easier to just treat.
Practitioner: level 3 or more, internist, general practitioner, pediatrician; tropical/travel expertise is helpful.
Patient care: if there is severe abdominal pain plus fever or if the diarrhea is associated with ground beef ingestion, then he may develop new ANEMIA and KIDNEY DISEASE. It is best not to use CO-TRIMOXAZOLE as this may increase the likelihood of this complication.

- Rehydrate just as you would for plain diarrhea. (See TURISTA.)

- Use antibiotics for bacterial dysentery; treat with DOXYCYCLINE, CO-TRIMOXAZOLE, AMPICILLIN or CIPROFLOXACIN, assuming that it is bacterial. Also ceftriaxone or another 2nd or 3rd generation CEPHALOSPORIN is ideal. If it appears that the problem is due to Shigella[1,] avoid using AMPICILLIN. AZITHROMYCIN works in a single dose, but it is very expensive. With a very sick patient, use CIPROFLOXACIN first; treat until a week after the diarrhea stops. NORFLOXACIN is a new, expensive, unproven drug that might work where others fail.

- If the patient is both very sick and a child, pregnant or taking PREDNISONE (or a related medication), then treat for dysentery due to amebae also.

- For amebic dysentery, treat with METRONIDAZOLE, SECNIDAZOLE, TINIDAZOLE or with [DOXYCYCLINE plus CHLOROQUINE]. ERYTHROMYCIN may be used if the symptoms are not severe. The patient should respond within 2 days. If he does not, he may need surgery. After the treatment, clear the remaining amebic cysts from the bowel with DILOXANIDE FUROATE, IODOQUINOL or PAROMOMYCIN. NIRIDAZOLE is an old, dangerous drug that might be available in some areas. Do not use it.

- PAROMOMYCIN is a drug that works for both bacterial and amebic dysentery.

- If the dysentery responds to neither treatment for amebic nor for bacterial dysentery, treat for HOOKWORM, STRONGYLOIDIASIS or TRICHURIASIS. Since the cause of dysentery varies so much from one area to the other, seek local lore.

- Give half-strength ORS.

- If the patient is a baby, encourage continued breast feeding.

Results: 2–3 days.

EAR INFECTION, EXTERNAL

Regional Note: N

Synonyms: otitis externa, swimmer's ear.

Definition: infection of the ear canal.

Cause: variable.

Mildly to moderately ill; class 1; worldwide; common everywhere.

Age: any. **Who:** anyone, especially swimmers and those who have cleaned wax out of ears. **Onset:** usually over minutes to hours.

Clinical

Necessary: the patient has ear pain, maybe severe, made worse with moving the external ear.

Usually: he has no fever. If you have an otoscope, you will see red, possibly swollen, ear canals. The eardrums will be normal, but you probably will not be able to see that far in.

Complications: pus in the ear canal. In this case try to suck out the pus with a syringe. Do not squirt anything in.

Treatment

Referrals: laboratory: level 3 or more: if there is visible pus, a hospital can do a smear or culture. Practitioner: ear-nose-throat specialist, general practitioner, internist, pediatrician.

Patient care: if there is a fever treat for CELLULITIS. Otherwise mix CORTISONE CREAM or OINTMENT and ANTIBIOTIC CREAM or OINTMENT, 50:50. Use the kinds labeled "ophthalmic" rather than the kinds intended for outer skin. Thin creams with water; thin ointments with oil. Put a few drops of this into the canal(s) four times a day until it is better plus two more days; you may use it more often.

---

1 *Very frequent stool passage; the stool consists of small amounts of almost pure blood and pus.*

You may also use otic medication, drops intended for this problem. Injectable CIPROFLOXACIN, made up to a 0.2 to 0.5% solution in normal saline is appropriate. Put a cotton wick in the ear canal to absorb the drops and keep them against the inflamed walls. Use pain medicines. See Volume 1, Appendix 1 for directions for the ear wick. *Results:* one day.

EAR INFECTION, MIDDLE

Regional Notes: N, U.

Synonym: otitis media.

Definition: infection of the middle ear, the part between the ear drum and the brain.

Cause: variable.

Mildly to moderately ill; class 1;. worldwide, generally common where colds are common.

Age: any. **Who:** anyone, especially children after a cold. **Onset:** hours to a day or two.

Clinical

Necessary: moderate or severe ear pain. A young child pulls on his ear or is fussy.

Maybe: he may have a fever and vomiting. Moving the external ear does not worsen the pain. The patient may feel dizzy, off-balance, tilting, spinning or being in a spinning room. Through the otoscope you will see red or opaque-white eardrums. There may be visible pus in the ear canal or enlarged lymph nodes in the neck.

Complications: MENINGITIS, MASTOIDITIS, hearing loss if not properly treated, FEBRILE SEIZURE.

Similar conditions: a chronic, painless, draining ear that does not get better with antibiotics is probably due to TUBERCULOSIS. In children too young to localize pain, ear infection may resemble GASTROENTERITIS, MALARIA, URINARY INFECTION or RESPIRATORY INFECTION. In all these conditions, there may be fever, vomiting and diarrhea.

Treatment

Prevention: HIB immunization prevents some kinds.

Referrals: laboratory: level 3 or above: if there is visible pus, a hospital can do a smear or culture. Practitioner: most physicians unless the problem is recurrent.

Patient care:

- Treat with PENICILLIN in adults, in children over 7 y.o. and in those under 7 y.o. who have had HIB vaccine.

- Use AMOXICILLIN in children under 7 y.o. who have not had the vaccine.

- In PENICILLIN-allergic patients, use either ERYTHROMYCIN with SULFADIAZINE or else CO-TRIMOXAZOLE alone as a substitute for AMOXICILLIN. Use ERYTHROMYCIN alone as a substitute for PENICILLIN.

- CHLORAMPHENICOL can be used if other drugs are not available. AZITHROMYCIN and CLARITHROMYCIN are helpful but expensive.

Results: 3–5 days for ordinary infection.

Ebola virus disease

See Regional Notes F.

ECZEMA

Definition: an allergic skin disease causing roughness and peeling of the skin.

Cause: autoimmune.

Not ill to mildly ill; class 1–2; worldwide amongst affluent.

Age: any. **Who:** anyone, family history of ALLERGY, affluent more than poor. **Onset:** begins over a day or two; changes over that period.

Clinical

Necessary: the patient's skin has a roughened rash, in circular patches or large areas. The skin may peel.

Commonly: it affects hands frequently immersed in soapy water. It may be itchy; may be on any part of the body.

Similar conditions: CANDIDIASIS may be indistinguishable. Treat for ECZEMA first if the patient is from an allergic family; treat for CANDIDIASIS first if the area is hot and humid. CUTANEOUS LEISHMANIASIS is never symmetrical. Also consider SCABIES (much more itchy), TINEA (may be indistinguishable), PELLAGRA (malnourished patient), ARSENIC POISONING.

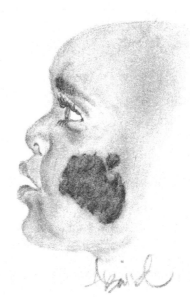

Eczema is commonly on the face and symmetrical The shape is irregular with indistinct margins. The center is rough but it is not raised up much. Usually the contrast between normal skin and eczema is not as marked as is pictured here; the appearance is more subtle. AB

Treatment

Referrals: practitioner: dermatologist

Patient care: find the cause and remove it. Use local ice packs 15 minutes three times a day. HYDROCORTISONE OINTMENT may be helpful. Some stronger steroid ointments may be available. In severe cases, PREDNISONE for a few days may help.

ELEPHANTIASIS

Definition: elephantiasis is massive swelling of a body part. The skin is rough like an elephant's. It is a tropical condition.

Leg elephantiasis causes: (1) non-endemic, caused by FILARISIS infection (see FILARASIS) and (2) endemic, also known as MOSSY FOOT.

Genital elephantiasis causes: FILARIASIS, LYMPHOGRANULOMA VENEREUM, DONOVANOSIS.

Arm or breast: only FILARIASIS causes this.

ELLIPTOSYTOSIS

See OVALOCYTOSIS. The difference is merely academic, the conditions indistinguishable.

ENCEPHALITIS

Regional Notes: E, F, I, K, M, N, O, R, S, U.

Entry category: disease cluster or syndrome.

Definition: an inflammation of the brain, usually due to a viral infection.

Cause: usually virus.

Very ill; class 1–4, depending on type; worldwide, but not real common anywhere.

Includes: many specific types carry geographic names, e.g., Japanese encephalitis (for which see ENCEPHALITIS, Regional Notes S). Many are listed under ARBOVIRAL FEVER. HERPES and HIV INFECTION can also cause encephalitis.

Very ill; class 3; usually not contagious; worldwide, not common except during epidemics.

Age: any. **Who:** usually those insect-bitten or tick-bitten; see Volume 1, Appendix 10. Sometimes a complication of childhood diseases. **Onset:** sudden; incubation about a week.

Clinical

See the following chart.

ENCEPHALITIS CLINICAL DIAGNOSIS entails at least one symptom from each set, lasting over 24 hours.
Set 1
Lethargy, unawareness, coma
New-onset personality aberration
New-onset impaired judgment
New-onset emotional changes
Set 2
Fever
Seizure, new-onset
Headache, eye pain, stiff neck
Changes in sensation[1]
Changes in body motion[2]
Difficulty hearing, seeing or swallowing

Complications: BRAIN DAMAGE, death.

Causative diseases: this may be caused by HERPES, MUMPS, MEASLES, CYSTICERCOSIS, TOXOPLASMOSIS, LARVA MIGRANS, ARBOVIRAL FEVERs, AFRICAN SLEEPING SICKNESS, MONKEYPOX or LOIASIS. HERPES encephalitis presents with a 1–7 day history of a "cold" and then headache, fever and bizarre psychiatric symptoms. If you see this pattern, sending for further care is very worthwhile, because there are good medications to treat this, whereas most of the other causes are not very treatable.

Similar conditions: see Protocol B.10 and/or Protocol B.13. FEBRILE SEIZURE may look similar, but the patient is totally normal once the fever is treated. It may be indistinguishable from TYPHUS,[3] cerebral MALARIA, PMNS, HEAT STROKE or MENINGITIS. If in doubt, treat these also. RELAPSING FEVER may also be indistinguishable. The brain damage effects of LIVER FAILURE might be similar to encephalitis; sometimes a simple change of diet can make a big difference.

Treatment

Prevention: keep an ill patient under a mosquito net to avoid infecting local mosquitoes and transmitting the disease. There is an immunization available for Japanese encephalitis and for tick-borne encephalitis (Asia). These should be used in those considering long-term residency or a trip to a rural area.

---

1 *Sensation changes: new-onset numbness, tingling, unaware of body position, hot/cold insensitivity, loss of pain sensation.*

2 *Motion abnormality: new-onset, weakness or paralysis, trembling, incoordination.*

3 *With TYPHUS there are other symptoms for a matter of days before the onset of the fever.*

Referrals: speedy referral is necessary. See Volume 1, Appendix 13. Laboratory; a very sophisticated laboratory, level 4 or above, can test the blood to determine the cause of the encephalitis. This can provide a prognosis. Facilities; a well-equipped level 4 or above intensive care unit. Practitioner: infectious disease specialist, internist, pediatrician, neurologist, anesthesiologist, expert nursing care.

Patient care: the patient will probably not survive in your care. Treat for SEIZURES if they occur.

In malarious areas treat for MALARIA. For some types of encephalitis some viral drugs work well. If you cannot send out, place a stomach tube to provide food and water through the tube. See Volume 1, Appendices 1 and 8

ENDOMETRIOSIS

Entry category: disease.

Cause: some uterus lining escapes into the abdomen and pelvis, causing monthly symptoms.

Not ill to moderately ill; class 1–3; not contagious; common.

Age & Who: reproductive females. **Onset:** symptoms develop before menstruation, are worst during menstruation and subside gradually thereafter.

Clinical

Usually: the patient has pain that comes and goes with her menstrual cycle. It may be generalized abdominal or pelvic pain, or it may be localized to one part of the lower trunk or back.

Sometimes: there may be constipation or diarrhea, menstrual irregularity or bloody urine.

Complications: infertility.

Similar conditions: the most common is PELVIC INFECTION. With endometriosis there is usually a history of cyclical pain in the past, whereas with pelvic infection this history is usually lacking. Also consider ACUTE ABDOMEN and SEXUALLY TRANSMITTED DISEASES (Protocol B.1).

Treatment

Referrals: gynecologist, nurse practitioner, surgery at times may be helpful.

Patient care: BIRTH CONTROL PILLS, the kind that contains both estrogen and progesterone; give these for at least 3 months.

ENTERIC FEVER

Regional Notes: E, F, I, M, O, R, S, U.

Entry category: two similar diseases.

Synonyms: salmonellosis typhi, typhus abdominalis.

Includes: typhoid fever, paratyphoid fever.

Definition: an infection, primarily of the bowel, but extending to the body as a whole, caused by the bacterium *Salmonella typhi, Salmonella paratyphi* or related organisms.

Cause: bacteria, Gram-negative.

Moderately to severely ill; class 1–3; contagious through body secretions; typhoid is present worldwide and common in areas of unsanitary food and water supply; paratyphoid is mainly from unsanitary food. Both are most common in the Indian subcontinent, in Southeast Asia and in the Caribbean.

Age: in nationals it is most common in children and young adults; in travelers there is no age selection. **Who:** anyone not immunized, particularly those eating foods from street vendors or prepared in an unsanitary environment; those eating shellfish taken from water with sewage pollution; those who are taking treatment for GASTRITIS or PEPTIC ULCER. Those who have SCHISTOSOMIASIS are prone to relapse, because the bacteria can hide in the parasites, away from the body's defenses. **Onset:** usually incubation 1–3 weeks and onset over 3–4 days in typhoid which is more severe; may be sudden with a short incubation period in paratyphoid, which is milder. A longer incubation time implies a more serious illness.

Clinical

CLASSICAL TYPHOID FEVER
The diagnosis is difficult because of many symptoms in common with other diseases.

Necessary: the patient has a fever (unless he is malnourished, an infant or elderly). Either the fever is sustained (it goes up and down but is never less than 99.5°F [37.5°C]), and/or the patient has at least one of the following symptoms: headache, apathetic or crazy behavior, abdominal pain with constipation (early in the disease) or diarrhea (more common later in the disease), a cough, congestion, aching all over.

Usually: other symptoms are extremely variable by region and by patient. Children over 2 y.o. are likely to have abdominal pain and a large, soft spleen, possibly also a large liver; those under 2 y.o. are more likely to have vomiting and diarrhea. The pulse is slow relative to the fever, a specific phenomenon that develops during the second or third week in those over 2 years old. Bowel sounds are decreased or absent, and the abdomen is swollen. The patient will not eat normally; he has loss of appetite and weight loss. His tongue has a gray-yellow coating.

Commonly: the patient is bedridden by the third day with typhoid, each day sicker than the previous day. Diarrhea, when it occurs, is usually in the third week, sometimes earlier; it looks like pea soup and smells foul. Late in the disease there are nervous changes: SEIZURES, mania or extreme apathy, depression, confusion, dizziness, crazy behavior, trembling, incoherent speech, incoordination (see ENCEPHALITIS). The spleen or liver is sometimes enlarged and tender. When the spleen is enlarged it is not greatly enlarged. Lymph nodes may also be enlarged.

Sometimes: there may be a red, sore throat or nosebleed. There are symptoms of PNEUMONIA (cough, chest pain), KIDNEY INFECTION (pain with urination, back pain) or MENINGITIS (severe headache, stiff neck). There may be a peculiar body odor similar to that of freshly baked bread. If there is a rash, it is mainly or completely on the abdomen, occurs in fair skin only and looks like very slightly raised, rose-colored freckles, 2–4 mm in diameter. If you push on them, they disappear but quickly reappear when the pressure is released. They first occur on the seventh to the tenth day of illness. As each disappears it leaves a brown stain in the skin.

Complications: deafness, ANEMIA, PNEUMONIA, ACUTE ABDOMEN Type 2, BRAIN DAMAGE, MENINGITIS, HEART FAILURE, HEPATITIS, SEPSIS, BRONCHITIS. The disease may become chronic and relapsing, especially with SCHISTOSOMIASIS. The patient may bleed into his bowel and have bloody bowel movements, particularly after the first week of illness; he may be incontinent of urine and stool. This signifies a bad prognosis.

Similar conditions: see the chart in Protocol B.2 for general fever, headache and aching; see Protocol B.4 if the patient is short of breath, B.7 for liver/spleen involvement, B.9 for abdominal pain, B.10 for lethargy and B.12 for large lymph nodes. BRUCELLOSIS and typhoid are frequently confused. The onset of BRUCELLOSIS is slower, and the joint pains tend to be worse than the abdominal symptoms. Patients with Brucellosis are loud complainers; those with enteric fever are withdrawn. *Diarrhea:* DYSENTERY and similar conditions. *With mental symptoms* consider MENINGITIS, ENCEPHALITIS, MALARIA, HEAT STROKE and similar conditions. TYPHUS may be indistinguishable; treat for both. *Mediterranean genetic origin,* consider FAMILIAL MEDITERRANEAN FEVER.

Bush laboratory: there may be protein in the urine. Stool may be positive for blood. The sedimentation rate will be high. Enteric fever does not cause urobilinogen in the urine, but MALARIA does cause this.

MALARIA PLUS TYPHOID:
This is rare but vastly overdiagnosed. When it occurs, invariably there is a sustained fever, abdominal pain and persistence of fever for more than 24 hours after initiation of malaria drugs.

MILD PARATYPHOID:
This is just like ordinary INFLUENZA or GASTROENTERITIS; it resolves without treatment.

Treatment for all enteric fever:

Prevention: immunize. Both oral and injectable immunizations are available. Neither of these gives absolute protection; one must still be careful of sanitation in water, food and personal hygiene. The immunizations only protect against typhoid, not paratyphoid.

- From Merieux (company), a single injection with minimal side effects, only for those over 18 months old; immunity lasts for 3 years.

- Oral vaccine, Ty21a, one capsule every other day for 3 or 4 doses, also gives protection for 3 years. The oral immunization capsules must be swallowed whole and they must be kept cold until they are taken. The patient must not take PROGUANIL at the same time as the oral immunization; if he does, the immunization is likely to not work.

Referrals: see Volume 1, Appendix 13; speedy referral is necessary. Laboratory: the Widal test is totally useless. Latex agglutination is not reliable until after 9 days of illness. Culture of blood, stool and urine is difficult; many must be done for one to be positive and the test takes 48 hours. There are some new, better tests available: Typhidot, Typhidot-M, Tubex typhoid fever, ELISA. Typhidot is positive in about half of the cases; it is insensitive. A malaria smear will be negative and a white count will be normal. Facilities: at level 3 or above, IV fluids and IV antibiotics. Practitioner: infectious disease, internist, general practitioner; a surgeon is helpful for complications.

Patient care

- Antibiotics of choice: for mild to moderate illness only, use AZITHROMYCIN. For severe disease Ceftriaxone (see CEPHALOSPORIN) is best if it has not recently been abused.

- Alternatives: CHLORAMPHENICOL, CO-TRIMOXAZOLE, AMPICILLIN or AMOXICILLIN in areas where there has not been much prior medical care. In areas where there has been prior care (especially India), one must use a CEPHALOSPORIN, CIPROFLOXACIN[1], OFLOXACIN or GENTAMYCIN. CHLORAMPHENICOL might work in areas where it has not been used for the last decade.

- Supplementary treatment: in very sick patients, use additionally (METRONIDAZOLE or TINIDAZOLE) plus (DEXAMETHASONE, PREDNISONE or HYDROCORTISONE) for the first 3 days. This considerably reduces the death rate. Do not use ASPIRIN for fever.

---

1 *CIPROFLOXACIN is useless in many areas of the world, so if the patient is very ill, it is best to start with another antibiotic. Another –oxacin antibiotic might work.*

ENTEROBIASIS

Regional Notes: E, F, K, U.

Synonyms: oxyuriasis, Pinworm (American[2] term).

Definition: a bowel infestation caused by the worm *Enterobius vermicularis.*

Cause: worm.

Not ill; class 1; contagious; common worldwide, especially crowded areas.

Age: any, but especially children. **Who:** anyone. **Onset:** over a day or two.

Clinical

Necessary: the patient has no symptoms at all or else rectal and genital itching, mainly at night; small children may just be restless and fussy at night.

Commonly: the child loses his appetite or starts to wet his bed after being dry for some time. Vaginal discharge is common in little girls. If you look at the rectal area with a flashlight a half-hour after bedtime, you will see little, white, wiggly worms that look like pieces of thread. They are mainly around the rectal opening and are less than a half centimeter long. They may be seen in the stool. They may cause vaginal itching.

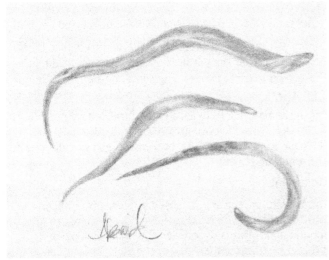

The pictures of the worms are greatly magnified; the actual size is just a few millimeters long, like a tiny snip of white thread. AB

Similar conditions: TAPEWORM, dwarf TAPEWORM, CANDIDIASIS and food ALLERGY may produce similar rectal itching. There are no other kinds of worms that look the same.

Treatment

Prevention: treat all family members at the same time, as well as children's friends. Recommend daily washing of bedding and pajamas for 2 weeks, very meticulous hand-washing after toilet or diaper change, frequent cleaning of fingernails. Reinfection is common.

Referrals: laboratory: the eggs, deposited by the rectum, can be picked up on a piece of scotch tape which is then checked with a microscope. This procedure is not sensitive; you need 7 negative results before excluding the diagnosis.

Patient care: it is usually necessary to treat the whole family and to repeat the treatment weekly for 4 weeks. Use MEBENDAZOLE, ALBENDAZOLE, PYRANTEL PAMOATE or THIABENDAZOLE. IVERMECTIN is 85% effective. PIPERAZINE works but must be given for 6 days.

EPIDIDYMITIS

Definition: epididymitis is an infection of the collecting tubules of the testes, found on the back side of the testes within the scrotum.

Mildly ill; class 1; worldwide, common.

Age: teens and older. **Who:** males only; especially sexually active, physically strained. **Onset:** minutes to hours, sometimes a day or two.

Clinical

ORDINARY EPIDIDYMITIS
Necessary: the patient has pain, swelling or both in his scrotum. His testicle is tender, swollen or both on its back side.

Maybe: fever may be present. The patient is tender into his groin and lower abdomen.

Occasionally: both testicles are involved.

Complications: rarely ABSCESS formation—check for a localized, tender red area of skin.

Causative diseases: this may be due to a SEXUALLY TRANSMITTED DISEASE. If you suspect this, then you should treat the patient's sexual partner(s) as well.

TUBERCULOUS EPIDIDYMITIS:
There is slow, painless and non-tender swelling of the testicle. There may be holes through to the outside of the scrotum. The epididymitis (the back side of the testicle) will be hard and large, with an irregular surface. It may be misdiagnosed as CANCER.

Similar conditions: *indistinguishable*: MUMPS, FILARIASIS (early). *Pain but no tenderness,* consider KIDNEY STONE.
Generalized illness: BRUCELLOSIS, TUBERCULOSIS, CANCER.
Mediterranean genetic origin: consider FAMILIAL MEDITERRANEAN FEVER.

---

2 In the UK, "pinworm" refers to STRONGYLOIDIASIS.

TOC | SYMPTOMS | DIFFERENTIALS | CONDITIONS | DRUG INDEX | REGIONAL NOTES | INX

Treatment

Referrals: laboratory: evaluation for various SEXUALLY TRANSMITTED DISEASEs, level 3 or above. Practitioner: urologist is ideal; an internist or general practitioner is okay.

Patient care: if elevation and support of the testicle does not relieve the pain within an hour, the patient may have torsion (twisting) of his testicle, which needs surgery within 6 hours of the onset of pain.

- *Ordinary epididymitis*: keep the patient in bed, support his scrotum with towels between his legs, apply warmth to his scrotum and use AMOXICILLIN, SULFADIAZINE or CO-TRIMOXAZOLE. Follow Protocol B.1: Sexually Transmitted Diseases, if there was an exposure.

- *Tuberculous epididymitis:* treat for TUBERCULOSIS.

Consider FILARIASIS or CANCER if the problem does not respond to treatment.

Results: 2–3 days usually; 3–4 weeks for TUBERCULOSIS.

EPILEPSY

Regional Notes: F, R.

Entry category: syndrome.

(See also SEIZURES.)

Definition: recurrent seizures.

Age: any. **Who:** those with prior head injuries, with reactions to various drugs or with hereditary seizures. Some children who have had a FEBRILE SEIZURE develop epilepsy. It may be a consequence of various illnesses; see ENCEPHALITIS and similar conditions. Those who begin to have SEIZURES as adults without any prior illness, or head injury probably have CYSTICERCOSIS if they eat pork. MEFLOQUINE, CHLOROQUINE and CIPROFLOXACIN are drugs that occasionally cause this. LARVA MIGRANS may also cause this. **Onset:** each seizure onset is sudden, but the pattern of frequent seizures develops slowly over days to weeks.

Clinical

See the description of seizures under FEBRILE SEIZURE. Not all seizures are like that; they vary greatly. Seek further information from other sources. Petit mal epilepsy manifests as staring, fluttering eyelids, lasting only a few seconds. Sometimes this occurs on awakening in infants and in teens.

Similar conditions: see Protocol B.10. DEMONIZATION can cause seizure-like activity which usually happens in the context of Christian worship or prayer. People can fake seizures, but they usually have pelvic thrusting, which real seizures never cause.

Treatment

Referrals: see Volume 1, Appendix 13. Laboratory: level 4 and above—EEG, many different blood tests. Facilities: level 4 and above. Practitioner: neurologist is ideal; a neurosurgeon, internist or pediatrician may be appropriate.

Patient care: send out if at all possible. The greater the frequency of seizures, the more urgent this is. Patients should be started on medicine to control the seizures. This should be done under a physician's supervision, but lacking that, see PHENYTOIN or PHENOBARBITAL in the Drug Index. Those who have been on medication and have either gained weight or had a period of STRESS may again have seizures. They need to have their seizure medication dosage increased. In areas with ONCHOCERCIASIS, treat for that also.

Erythema Infectiosum

See FIFTH DISEASE.

ERYTHEMA MULTIFORME

Clinical

Necessary: this is a skin condition characterized by red (warm in those with dark skin), irregular areas on or under the skin, shaped like circles, targets or doughnuts.

Maybe: these are symmetrical on knees, elbows, palms, soles, sometimes all over, sometimes on moist pink surfaces. With time the skin may become crusted.

Commonly: there is a lighter red ring around a darker, inner reddened area. The problem usually starts on the limbs, usually the hairy surfaces. The center of the targets might be pale or purple. The individual areas last at least 7 days.

Causative diseases: HERPES, a type of PNEUMONIA, AFRICAN SLEEPING SICKNESS, LYME DISEASE, TUBERCULOSIS, LEPROSY, RHEUMATIC FEVER or some drugs[1], vaccinations or environmental toxins.

Treatment

This is symptomatic. If it is caused by a drug (see DRUG ERUPTION), then you must stop the drug. If there are spontaneous blisters or sores on the moist pink parts, or if this involves more than 10% of the body surface, this is very serious, and the patient must be sent out. Do not use STEROIDs for treatment.

---

1 *Commonly antibiotics (especially sulfa-type), IBUPROFEN and related pain medications and medicines for SEIZURES.*

ERYTHEMA NODOSUM

Definition: a skin condition characterized by red (warm in those with dark skin) lumps under the skin.

Age: mostly children age 5–15; it usually does not affect the elderly. **Who:** mostly young females are affected. It is related to an initial infection. **Onset:** unknown.

Clinical

Necessary: the patient has lumps on the front of her lower legs or arms, larger than a normal pimple, about 0.4 to 4 cm in diameter, with ill-defined edges. They are symmetrical and appear to be under or in the skin rather than on the skin. They vary in size. There are a countable number. They become purplish and very tender. They change from hard to soft, change color and possibly cause the skin to peel. They last less than 4 weeks.

Sometimes there are also sore joints, fever and fatigue. The joint pains last longer than the skin problem, but eventually they disappear. The skin redness might look like targets at some points. There may be a similar lump on a warm moist surface of the body.

Causative diseases: STREP INFECTION, FUNGAL INFECTION, COCCIDIOMYCOSIS, CHLAMYDIA, DYSENTERY (bacterial), LEPTOSPIROSIS, TUBERCULOSIS, RESPIRATORY INFECTION, TULAREMIA, TYPHUS, CAT-SCRATCH DISEASE, LEPROSY (being treated) or drugs such as PENICILLIN, BIRTH CONTROL PILLS, SULFA DRUGS; sometimes pregnancy or no discernible cause.

Treatment

This is symptomatic with pain medication and anti-inflammatory drugs. The lumps do not become ulcers; they heal in weeks without scarring.

EXFOLIATIVE DERMATITIS

Entry category: syndrome.

Includes: toxic epidermal necrolysis, scalded skin syndrome, Stevens-Johnson syndrome.

Definition: exfoliative dermatitis is a skin condition in which the outer layer of skin peels off.

Cause: variable.

Moderately to very ill; class 2–4; worldwide, quite rare.

Age: any, but especially children and the elderly. **Who:** malnourished, poor immunity, taking antibiotics. **Onset:** usually sudden, over hours to a day.

Clinical

Necessary: the skin blisters and then peels off in sheets, leaving a raw red surface beneath. There may also be spontaneous inflammation of the pink moist parts of the body.

Maybe: there is a high pulse pressure. (See Symptom Protocol A.2.C.)

Similar conditions: burns, which you can distinguish by history. Also with certain kinds of MENINGITIS, some MALNUTRITION and SEPSIS, a similar condition may occur. ONYALAI in South Africa may appear similar, but the blisters are bloody.

Treatment

Referrals: see Volume 1, Appendix 13; speedy referral is necessary. Laboratory: level 3 or above, blood chemistries to monitor the patient's fluid balance; possibly blood counts and cultures. Facilities: if severe, a level 4 monitored bed and intensive care unit; in a hot dry climate this is essential for all cases. Practitioner: dermatologist, infectious disease specialist, internist, pediatrician.

Patient care: if the patient is a malnourished child who is not taking medicine, treat him with AUGMENTIN, one of the CEPHALOSPORINs or CLOXACILLIN.

- If this developed in a patient who was taking an antibiotic, stop the antibiotic. Treat him with HYDROCORTISONE intravenously if you have it or PREDNISONE, using high doses initially.

- In either case, treat the patient with large amounts of fluid as if he had a 50% burn. (See Volume 1, Chapter 9.)

- Furnish a high-protein diet.

Results: some improvement within 48 hours.

EYE INFECTION

Regional Note: M.

Entry category: disease cluster.

Synonyms: conjunctivitis, pink eye. See also TRACHOMA. *Includes:* sty.

Definition: eye infection (in this context) is an infection, usually bacterial, of the surface structures of the eye.

Cause: bacteria, virus.

Mildly ill; class 1–3; contagious, very; worldwide, common.

Age: any. **Who:** anyone, especially those with poor hygiene. **Onset:** hours to 1–2 days.

Clinical

Necessary: any one of the following: an irritated eye with pus; a red, painful bump on the upper or lower lid or the inside corner of the eye; a red, (burning) painful eye with tears; an eye that is swollen, with red lids and red around the eye or with visible pus within the eye.

Maybe: the clear membrane over the white of the eye may be swollen. The patient may have an enlarged lymph node on his cheek in front of his ear.

Occasionally: an infection caused by a virus causes a burning pain in the eye with a watery discharge. This continues for several days and then the white of the eye may turn partly or completely blood red. This cures itself. ANTIBIOTIC EYE OINTMENT prevents additional bacterial infection, but it does not cure the viral eye infection.

Sometimes: patients with this problem develop an illness resembling POLIO: they are paralyzed for a period of time, but the paralysis eventually disappears.

Causative diseases: GONORRHEA, TULAREMIA, (in Europe, Asia and the north coast of Africa), CHLAMYDIA.

Similar conditions: REITER SYNDROME, ARSENIC POISONING, TRACHOMA, KERATITIS. See Protocol B.8 if the eyes are both red and painful. XEROPHTHALMIA can mimic and also may be associated with eye infection. Xerophthalmia causes foamy white stuff in the corner of the eye, sometimes with wrinkles in the thin membrane next to the cornea. Check carefully! It is an important preventable cause of blindness, and it can be subtle.

If eye infection occurs in a sexual context, right after birth or if it is due to GONORRHEA or CHLAMYDIA, it may cause loss of vision very quickly. Treat for GONORRHEA and CHLAMYDIA both.

ALLERGY (vernal conjunctivitis) causes discharge that is thick, white and sticky.

See Protocol B.1 if this may be due to a SEXUALLY TRANSMITTED DISEASE.

Treatment

Prevention: keep flies away from the patient's eyes. Wash the faces of children who come near the patient. Wash your hands after touching his face. If the patient is a newborn who developed the infection at less than a week of age, you should also treat both parents for GONORRHEA and CHLAMYDIA, whether or not they appear to have it. See Protocol B.1: Sexually Transmitted Diseases.

Referrals: laboratory; a level 3 or above hospital lab can do a smear or culture or both. This will help to predict which antibiotic will work best. Practitioner: ophthalmologist is ideal; internist or pediatrician might be helpful.

Patient care: never patch an infected eye.

- A discharge of pus indicates a bacterial infection which requires ANTIBIOTIC EYE OINTMENT plus (oral or injectable antibiotics). In newborns, treat for both CHLAMYDIA and GONORRHEA since it is hard to tell the difference without laboratory support. It is important, in all cases, to use antibiotic by mouth or injection in addition to ointment.

- In all cases, treat both eyes even if only one is infected. Be sure to use drops or ointment intended for eyes; the product must be labeled "ophthalmic".

- Use ANTIBIOTIC EYE DROPS every hour while awake, every 2 hours during the night until the problem improves. Then decrease the frequency to half that until it is entirely better, plus 2 more days. Once the problem is improved ANTIBIOTIC EYE OINTMENT may be used every 4–6 hours instead. Ointment will blur vision for about 10 minutes.

- If there is a fever, swollen red eyelids or a bulging eyeball, send the patient to a hospital. If you cannot, treat with PENICILLIN plus CHLORAMPHENICOL; this is potentially very serious.

- Infection with a small, localized bump on the eye requires only drops or ointment. Gently massaging the bump may be helpful. Never patch an infected eye.

Results: should be evident in 2 days.

FAMILIAL MEDITERRANEAN FEVER (FMF)

Synonym: recurrent hereditary polyserositis.

Cause: heredity.

Mildly to moderately ill; class 2; Mediterranean genetic heritage wherever they are located. The ethnic groups mainly affected are Jews (Sephardic, not Ashkanazi), Arabs, Armenians and Turks. The carrier state affects between 1/3 and 1/5 of the population. It is autosomal recessive.

Age: onset is <age 20. **Who:** males more than females. **Onset:** sudden; the pain and fever peak at 12–24 hours and then gradually gets better over days to weeks. The problem recurs from weekly to a couple times a year.

Clinical

Episodic fevers plus some of the following symptoms; a diagnosis requires one major element or two minor elements. Attacks occur irregularly and unpredictably. Each patient usually has only one kind of attack, but sometimes more than one. The attacks subside by themselves over days to weeks, and the patient is healthy between attacks.

Major criteria: abdominal pain mimicking ACUTE ABDOMEN; chest pain worse with breathing; chest pain relieved by bending over forward; pain and swelling in a single large joint, occasionally more than one. This may involve the spine. It tends to affect joints that have been previously injured or stressed.

Minor criteria: family members have had episodic fevers and pains; first episode was at age less than 20, Mediterranean genetic heritage; the pain is severe, requiring bedrest; the pain spontaneously goes away.

Other associated symptoms: headaches; sore throat; eye problems; swollen, painful testes; failure to grow in children.

Complications: PERICARDITIS, ARTHRITIS.

Similar conditions: many, including those listed above. If the patient is short of breath, see Protocol B.4; see B.9 for fever and abdominal pain. The recurrent nature of the disease and the family history should help distinguish this. The pattern of ARTHRITIS is similar to that in HIV INFECTION in Africa.

Treatment

Referrals: laboratory: none. This diagnosis is entirely clinical. Practitioner: someone with experience in dealing with this.

Patient care; a diet low in fat and avoiding chocolate, aged cheeses and wine might be helpful. COLCHICINE taken daily will prevent attacks.

Favus

See Regional Notes R.

FEBRILE SEIZURE

Entry category: syndrome.

Definition: whole-body shaking due to the rapid onset of a fever in a child less than 6 years old.

Cause: fever (in children).

Moderately ill; class 1; worldwide, common.

Age: 3 months to 6 y.o. only, never older; patients younger than 3 months probably have MENINGITIS. **Who:** any child who has a fever of sudden onset and rapid rate of rise, especially with MALARIA and EAR INFECTION. **Onset:** sudden.

Clinical

Necessary: a whole-body seizure, which is a rhythmic jerking of the muscles of the body, usually including all 4 limbs plus the face, in a patient who is unconscious. A febrile seizure lasts less than 15 minutes and is always associated with a fever over 101.3° F or 38° C. After the seizure stops, the child may sleep for up to an hour. He is alert an hour after the seizure. Physical exam is normal except for evidence of whatever illness originally caused the fever.

Caution: if the seizure involves just a part of the body; if it lasts more than 15 minutes or if there is more than one seizure, then there is something else wrong with the child, and he should be sent out for further care.

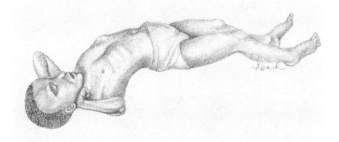

The drawing shows a seizure. A still picture cannot capture the violent shaking that occurs. AB

Complications: rare if the seizure lasted less than 15 minutes. Occasionally EPILEPSY complicates febrile seizures for children who seize at age less than 1 year old.

Similar conditions: watch carefully for MENINGITIS and cerebral MALARIA. If the fever responds to cooling and ASPIRIN or ACETAMINOPHEN, and the child is alert an hour after the seizure stopped, it is unlikely that he has cerebral MALARIA or MENINGITIS. If he is still lethargic or has a second seizure in spite of being cooled, consider these options as well as HEAT ILLNESS and ENCEPHALITIS.

Treatment

Prevention: train mothers to cool children with fevers.

Referrals: this might be helpful, but usually there is no time to get the patient there. If the seizure recurs, then it is not an ordinary febrile seizure. It is cerebral MALARIA, MENINGITIS, ENCEPHALITIS or some other problem. These problems all require at least a level 3 hospital.

Patient care: institute immediate cooling. Use ACETAMINOPHEN or IBUPROFEN. Diagnose and treat whatever illness prompted the fever.

FELON

Cause: bacteria.

This is a painful, tightly swollen, red or warm tip of a finger. See Chapter 10 in Volume 1 whether or not there is a history of a wound.

FIBROMYALGIA

This is a condition that occurs worldwide, affects women more than men, older more than younger. It involves symmetrical pain in the muscles, both above and below the waist and in the backbone area. There may be stiffness. Even minimal exertion seems to trigger pain. Sleep disorders and chronic fatigue are also common. There are specific points that are tender to touch. No one knows from whence this arises. The condition should be treated by a medical professional, but beginning the treatment is not urgent. Usually antidepressants help more than anything else. The trigger points can be injected with LIDOCAINE to provide relief.

FIBROSITIS

This is inflammation of the tissues around joints, not within joints. It may be a side-effect of a medication, or it may occur as a result of some disease, particularly a sexually transmitted disease. The pain is always worse first thing after resting; with movement it improves. Treat it with IBUPROFEN.

FIFTH DISEASE

Synonyms: parovirus B.19 infection, erythema Infectiosum. *Cause:* virus; parovirus B.19.

Not ill to moderately ill; class 1; contagious; probably worldwide.

Age: mostly children. **Who:** those who have not yet had the disease. **Onset:** sudden after an incubation period of about one week.

Clinical

In children, initially there is a fever which responds poorly to fever medications, but there are no other symptoms. Then the fever suddenly drops as the patient develops a rash, first on the cheeks and then mainly on the trunk. The rash lasts for about 3 weeks. It has a lacy appearance. There is an area around the mouth without rash, but the rash may involve the palms and the soles.

In adults, there may additionally be sore joints, possibly with redness and swelling. It usually involves the large joints and is symmetrical. It resolves, usually, in 3 weeks but may last longer.

Complications: in patients with any kind of ANEMIA, their anemia may suddenly worsen. Occasionally there may be long-term BRAIN DAMAGE. This may cause ABORTION in pregnant women.

Similar diseases: SYPHILIS, secondary.

Treatment

Referrals: this is usually not helpful unless it is necessary for ANEMIA or BRAIN DAMAGE.

Patient care: none, since the disease will run its course and cure itself. Transport to a hospital for transfusion might be necessary for patients with ANEMIA.

FILARIASIS

Regional Notes: F, I, M, O, R, S, U.

Synonym: elephantiasis, non-endemic.

Includes: Bancroftian filariasis (Wuchereriasis) and Brugian filariasis. Excludes: MANSONELLOSIS PERSTANS (see F and M Regional Notes).

Definition: an infection of the body with either *Wuchereria bancrofti* or *Brugia malayi;* these are worms. It is a tropical disease. Bancroftian filariasis is the common kind and is most widespread. It is largely urban, prevalent in areas with poor sanitation. Brugian filariasis occurs in Asia. It is largely rural, in areas with clean unpolluted waters.

Not ill to very ill; class 2; regional; mostly below 1200 meters (4000 feet), mostly rainy season, mostly heavily populated areas.

Age: usually adults, both sexes. **Who:** mosquito-bitten. See Volume 1, Appendix 10. In infected areas, almost everyone has the parasites. However, only expatriates and those with large numbers of parasites are apt to have symptoms. **Onset:** variable; incubation is usually 8–12 months, never less than 4 or more than 18 months. In expatriates, symptoms may first occur after the person has left the tropics.

Full-blown filariasis occurs within 1–2 years of the initial symptoms, except in children under 5 years old in whom it may take longer.

Clinical INITIAL SYMPTOMS

Usually: the patient has or had episodes of sudden onset of fever with headache, chills and sweats, resembling MALARIA. Expatriates tend to have a more sudden onset and a more rapid progression of the disease than nationals. Initially they may have just cough and wheezing, resembling ASTHMA.

Sometimes: there are no obvious symptoms like those listed above, but the patient has enlarged lymph nodes.

Clinical full-blown filariasis thereafter

The patient has one or more of the following symptoms. With the first four symptom groups listed, there are frequently multiple attacks which come and go until the problem finally persists. In Bancroftian filariasis, the upper and lower legs and genitals may all be affected; in Brugian filariasis, the genitals are rarely affected, and the legs are affected only below the knees. However, the arms and breasts are commonly affected.

- A body part is painful, red, swollen and stiff, with large, tender lymph nodes in the armpit, groin, neck or elbow areas, maybe with a mild fever and a general flu-like illness. The inflammation starts in the lymph nodes and progresses away from the trunk.

- The patient's scrotum, arm, leg or breast is painful and swollen, maybe of sudden onset with a high fever.

- The lymph nodes in the patient's groin are swollen; they may or may not be painful. Sometimes these are so large, they look and feel as if there were a pile of cooked macaroni underneath the skin.

- The patient's urine is milky, and it may be pinkish also. He had flank or belly pain before his urine turned milky. He may have a fever.

- In advanced filariasis, the patient may have ELEPHANTIASIS: darkened, thickened skin and a huge limb, breast, arm or scrotum. The swelling usually progresses from the trunk to the feet. In the illustration below, note that the foot is swollen, but not as much as the leg.

- The patient may have a painful, swollen joint, usually a knee or ankle, which promptly gets better with DIETHYLCARBAMAZINE (DEC).

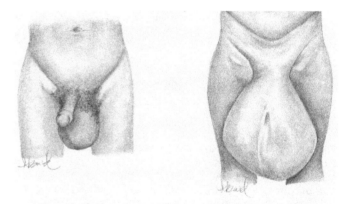

On the left, the patient's left testicle is mildly swollen. On the right the genitals are moderately swollen.[1] His penis is up in the fold of skin that has been pulled down from his lower abdominal wall. The swelling does not extend up into the groins. The wide skin at the top of the genitals is lower abdominal skin that has been pulled down. AB

---

1 *A massively swollen scrotum may need to be transported in a wheelbarrow.*

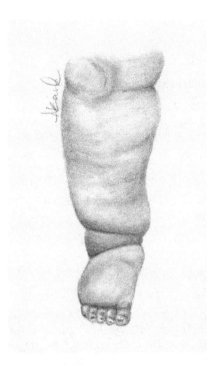

With filariasis, the leg swells first and most. The foot swells second and less. When far advanced, the leg and foot may be swollen comparably. AB

Complications: ARTHRITIS, KERATITIS, GLAUCOMA Another complication is tropical pulmonary eosinophilia (TPE). Patients have a severe, dry cough and wheezing that is worse at night, and many eosinophils (a kind of white blood cell) in their blood. It responds to DEC. TPE is neither common nor rare. It is more common in Westerners than in nationals.

Similar conditions: *limb swelling:* Protocol B.6.B. *Breast swollen:* MASTITIS is indistinguishable and far more common in most areas. *Scrotum swollen or painful:* HYDROCELE, EPIDIDYMITIS, KIDNEY INFECTION, HERNIA (skin thin or normal, not thick), FAMILIAL MEDITERRANEAN FEVER. *Swollen legs with roughened skin:* MOSSY FOOT looks just like this. The difference is that with MOSSY FOOT the swelling starts on the feet and moves up to the legs. The feet are always as swollen or more swollen than the legs. With filariasis, the legs are more swollen than the feet, at least at first. When far advanced the two may be indistinguishable.

Bush laboratory: urine may test positive for blood. Urine may be milky. Milky urine due to filariasis, if it is left to settle in a glass jar, will divide into three layers: creamy on top; milky in the middle; and red, muddy urine on the bottom.

Treatment

Prevention: eliminate mosquitoes and treat infected persons. The mosquitoes that cause this in most places are night-biters. Mosquito nets are helpful in disease prevention. To prevent the disease, use DIETHYLCARBAMAZINE (DEC) once a month.

An alternative is DEC-medicated salt, using 4 parts DEC to 1000 parts salt and keeping the community on it for at least 6 months out of the year. If you put a whole community on preventive medicine, the problem in the mosquitoes will disappear; then even those who do not take DEC will not become infected. Check the precautions in the Drug Index. IVERMECTIN may also be used for mass treatment or mass prevention.

Referrals: laboratory: hospitals can do a blood test for the disease, but usually the test will be negative until the disease has been present for a very long time. They either draw blood at night or give a dose of medicine before drawing. If a hospital lab accidentally finds the parasites in someone who does not have any symptoms, this does not need to be treated. Usually an ordinary blood count shows many eosinophils. Practitioner: tropical/travel expertise is helpful.

Patient care: first give DOXYCYCLINE daily for 4–6 weeks. This kills the bacteria which are essential to the worms' survival. In areas with ONCHOCERCIASIS do no more. In other areas follow this by one of the regimens below.

- Medications to kill worms: any two of these three: IVERMECTIN, ALBENDAZOLE, DIETHYLCARBAMAZINE.
- Some patients who have multiple episodes of redness and swelling respond well to PENICILLIN. Benzathine penicillin, one injection every 2–3 weeks, can prevent these episodes.
- Patients with milky urine should stay in bed with the foot of the bed raised up on cinder blocks.
- For swollen legs, wrap the entire foot and leg in an elastic bandage, from the foot up, not too tightly.
- DIPHENHYDRAMINE is helpful for both red streaks on the legs and reactions to DIETHYLCARBAMAZINE; HYDROCORTISONE or PREDNISONE may be used in severe cases. Reactions can be severe. You must have DIPHENHYDRAMINE and EPINEPHRINE available. Keep the patient near you for about an hour after the first dose.

Results: advanced elephantiasis of the lower limbs usually does not improve much with drug therapy; swelling of the upper body will decrease over 2–4 years with treatment.

FISSURE

Synonyms: rectal fissure.
Definition: an abnormal crack in the perimeter of the anus.
Cause: unknown.
Mildly ill; class 1; worldwide, neither rare nor common.
Age: any, infants and children as well as adults. **Who:** anybody. **Onset:** days to weeks.

Clinical

Necessary: severe pain with bowel movements.

Maybe: pain between bowel movements, small amounts of blood on the stool or on the toilet paper, a visible crack by the rectum. There is so much pain that the patient holds his bowel movements and thus becomes constipated.

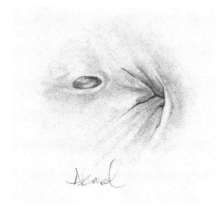

*This fissure is obvious; the condition may be subtle.
It may be difficult to see, being hidden in the normal folds of the anus.* AB

Similar conditions: the pain of HEMORRHOIDS and some SEXUALLY TRANSMITTED DISEASEs are similar, but the appearance of the rectum is different. Also consider Protocol B.1: Sexually Transmitted Diseases.

Treatment

Referrals: laboratory, level 3 or above can eliminate alternative diagnoses. Practitioner; a surgeon is most appropriate; a general practitioner might be helpful.

Patient care: use warm sitz baths for 10–15 minutes after each bowel movement. See the directions in Appendix 1 of Volume 1. Use laxatives or enemas if needed and suppositories with LIDOCAINE OINTMENT smeared on the outside. The suppositories must be held half-way in with the fingers; if they go all the way in, they do no good. *Results:* slow healing over 1–2 weeks.

FISTULA

This is an abnormal hole that forms between the rectum and the vagina or the outside of the body. It may also occur between the bladder and the vagina or the outside of the body between the legs. It may be due to AMEBIASIS, DONOVANOSIS, CANCER, TUBERCULOSIS or some other infection, or it may be due to injury from sexual activity or childbirth. The end result is that gas and stool from the rectum passes out through the vagina (in females) or through the penis (in males) or to the outside of the body in either. This might be corrected surgically. When referring the patient, it is important that you ascertain the probable cause, whether that is disease or trauma, so the receiving physician knows.

FLEAS

Entry category: infestation.

Cause: insect. (See Appendix 10 in Volume 1.)

Aggravated but not ill; class 1; contagious; worldwide.

Age: any, but especially children. **Who:** those near animals or other humans who have fleas. **Onset:** almost immediately after exposure.

Clinical

Necessary: there are visible fleas (little jumping creatures, usually black, the size of a period in print.)

Sometimes: little, itchy, red spots are visible where the fleas bit the patient.

Complications: rodent fleas[1] can transmit some TAPEWORMS, PLAGUE, SPOTTED FEVER, TULAREMIA and TYPHUS.

Similar conditions: lice, ticks, MYIASIS, very tiny flies. Bedbug bites look similar, but the creatures are nocturnal. They do not jump and they are very seldom seen. The red bite marks appear each morning, frequently in straight lines.

Bush laboratory; a strong magnifying glass will help to identify these as fleas. See Volume 1, Appendix 10.

Treatment

Prevention: it is unwise to kill rats and other rodents without first treating their holes with insecticide; fleas leave dying animals to bite humans. Use flea collars on pets. Wash floors weekly with 5–10 ml of 50% MALATHION in a bucket of water.

Patient care: bathe. Remove and wash all clothing, towels and sheets. 0.5% MALATHION[2] and pyrethrin flea powder work well for humans.

FLU

See *Influenza* on page C-95 of this volume.

FLUOROSIS

Cause: excessive fluoride.

Regional Notes: F.

Definition: fluorosis is toxicity from excess fluoride, usually in water.

Not ill to very ill; class 1–4; regional in very few places.

Age: mostly children. **Who:** anyone drinking from a particular contaminated water source; nursing infants of affected mothers. There will generally be multiple cases. **Onset:** variable.

---

1 There are many kinds of fleas. Each kind prefers one kind of host. Hence there are rodent fleas, human fleas, chicken fleas, cat fleas and dog fleas. If the preferred host is not available, fleas will bite whatever warm-blooded creature they can find. Hence humans might be bitten by rodent fleas.

2 This is 10 ml of malathion concentrate (50%) in a liter of water.

Clinical

Necessary: the patient has dark, irregular discoloration of the teeth and bone deterioration in the neck.

Sometimes: the neck bones may put pressure on the spinal cord, causing symptoms resembling SLIPPED DISC: sharp shooting pains in the shoulders, arm and hands, a heavy feeling in the arms, plus floppy weakness of some part(s) of the upper limb(s). See SPINAL NEUROPATHY. The bones of the back may curve, causing the patient to bend forward.

Similar conditions: bone TUBERCULOSIS or BRUCELLOSIS, in which case there is likely a fever, at least off and on. Otherwise SLIPPED DISC which may occur because of some injury or for no good reason at all. The dark teeth discoloration can resemble a side effect of TETRACYCLINE taken during childhood.

Treatment

Prevention: the fluoride cannot be removed by boiling or filtering. An entirely different water source must be found.

Referrals: probably only level 5; a toxicologist should manage the patient.

Patient care: none in the village situation and possibly none in regional hospitals. The advice of a toxicologist by email or telephone might be helpful. A toxicologist can be contacted through the internet.

FOOD POISONING

Regional Notes: N, O, S, U.

Entry category: disease cluster.

Definition: this description refers mainly to meats and cooked foods with meat in them. Poisoning from plants, traditional medicines and oils is listed under PLANT POISONING. ARSENIC POISONING is listed separately, as is LEAD POISONING. For botulism, see PLANT POISONING for a description, although sausage is a common offender.

Cause: bacteria, toxins.

Mildly to very ill; class 2–4, depending on severity; worldwide, generally common.

Age: any except exclusively nursing infants. **Who:** anyone eating tainted food. **Onset:** sudden; from a few hours to 2 days after the meal.

Clinical—four kinds:

ORDINARY FOOD POISONING
Necessary: the patient has severe abdominal cramps with vomiting, diarrhea or both.

Usually: pain is extreme, but tenderness to touch is minimal. Pushing on the abdomen does not greatly aggravate the pain. Everyone eating together becomes ill within a few hours of each other.

BOTULISM
This is caused by homemade sausages mostly; it can be from beans. At first there is vomiting and diarrhea followed by weakness, (especially as regards the head and neck), double or blurred vision, difficulty swallowing, dry mouth, then followed by weakness of the rest of the body, possibly with urine and stool retention. See also the entry under PLANT POISONING.

AFLATOXIN
This is a poison that comes from a kind of mold. It causes liver CANCER, with a slow onset. It is mostly in animal products (dairy, seafood and poultry), but it may also occur in plant products such as peanuts and grains.

MARINE TOXINS
- **Shellfish toxins** are found worldwide. Onset is 30 minutes. The toxin is destroyed by thorough cooking. Symptoms are neurological[3]. Mortality is 10%. There is only symptomatic treatment.

- **Shark liver poisoning** onset is less than 30 minutes. The toxin is not destroyed by heat. After nausea, vomiting, abdominal pains, diarrhea, it becomes neurological; see the footnote on the entry above.

- **Ciguatera poisoning** occurs on tropical shore areas, mainly the Caribbean and South Pacific. Onset is 1–6 hours. It is not destroyed by heat. Symptoms are abdominal pains and neurological[4].

- **Tetrodon/Puffer fish** poisoning occurs in Asia. Onset is rapid. The toxin is not destroyed by heat. Symptoms are respiratory failure and low blood pressure. It is 60% fatal within a day. Treatment is only symptomatic.

- **Scrombotoxin** is due to badly preserved fish of the tuna family. Its onset is in minutes. It is not destroyed by heat. Symptoms are nausea, vomiting, abdominal pains, diarrhea and symptoms of ALLERGY. There are rare deaths. Treatment is with antihistamines.

Treatment

Referrals: laboratory and practitioner: level 3 or more might be helpful. If the patient has botulism, higher-level care is critical. There is an antitoxin which is most useful. Antibiotics don't help.

---

3 There are changes in sensation such as numbness, tingling and burning; this starts on the head and goes down the body. Then there may be incoordination, inability to speak and various spasms, pains and weaknesses.

4 There is profound weakness and changes in sensation so hot feels cold and cold feels hot. There is twitching, seizures and incoordination, any one or more of these symptoms. There may be an abnormal heart beat and low blood pressure. Relapses and chronic fatigue are common.

Patient care: if you cannot send the patient, then do as follows:

- Use PROMETHAZINE for vomiting. Give ORS for diarrhea. Use pain medications. DICYCLOMINE and CHAMOMILE TEA often help with abdominal cramping. It will not eliminate the pains, but may make them tolerable.

- If the incubation period was less than 6 hours, do not use antibiotics. If the incubation period was more than 6 hours plus there is fever, use DOXYCYCLINE if the abdominal pain is mild to moderate. Use ERYTHROMYCIN if the abdominal pain is severe or if the doxycycline does not work. Check for DEHYDRATION and treat it.

FROSTBITE

Definition: cold injury of the skin.

Clinical

The skin surface is white, and it may be frozen hard. Depending on the severity, the patient may or may not have pain.

Treatment

Referrals: this is mandatory for severe cases. *Patient care:* initially, gently warm the body part. Then treat it like a burn. See Chapter 9 in Volume 1.

Fungal Infection

Fungal infection of the skin: see TINEA and CANDIDIASIS. Fungal infection of the vagina: see VAGINITIS.

G6PD DEFICIENCY

Regional Notes: E, F, I, M, O, R, U.

This is a genetic variant, mainly in persons of Mediterranean heritage: Jews, Arabs, Turks, Spaniards, Greeks, Slavs, Italians; also some ethnic groups in Southeast Asia. It also occurs in the Irish and in Hispanics in the Americas, because of migrations. It is more common in males than females since it is inherited recessively on the x chromosome. Generally there are no symptoms unless the person takes certain medications. The most common problematic medication is PRIMAQUINE.

GALLBLADDER DISEASE

Regional Notes: F, I, O, S, U.

Entry category: disease cluster.

Synonyms: gallstones, biliary colic.

Includes: cholecystitis, cholangitis.

Definition: gallbladder disease is a malfunction of the gallbladder. This inhibits the bile made by the liver from being properly stored and released.

Cause: variable.

Moderately to very ill; class 2, class 3 with fever; worldwide.

Age: 20's to 50's, occasionally younger; children with ASCARIASIS. **Who:** anyone, especially females who have had children, those overweight and those who have THALLASEMIA or ASCARIASIS. High-fat diets contribute to risk. **Onset:** suddenly for a given attack, usually within a few hours of eating. Recurs unpredictably.

Clinical

Necessary: the patient has severe upper-right or upper-middle abdominal pain which goes to the right shoulder, shoulder blade.

Usually: the pain lasts 2–5 hours and goes away by itself. The patient passes excessive gas.

Sometimes: the patient vomits. Pressing on the abdomen, just to the right of center and below the ribs, as you have him inhale deeply, reproduces or aggravates the pain.

Occasionally: patients may have fever or JAUNDICE. Children with ASCARIASIS causing this have pains every 15–30 minutes, lasting 5–10 minutes, and they vomit.

Complications: PANCREATITIS and ACUTE ABDOMEN.

Causative diseases: LIVER FLUKE in regions E, N, S and O only. It also occurs in those eating a high-fat diet.

Similar conditions: see Protocol B.7 since liver and spleen problems are frequently indistinguishable. Also see Protocol B.9 for fever plus abdominal pain. *With JAUNDICE:* see Protocol B.5. *With a fever:* consider ENTERIC FEVER, HEPATITIS, AMEBIASIS, PNEUMONIA involving the right lower front of the lung. *With no fever:* consider HYDATID DISEASE (check geography), ACUTE ABDOMEN, GASTROENTERITIS (pain all over, not so localized). MANSONELLOSIS PERSTANS may be similar, but it causes joint pains also.

Treatment

Referrals: see Volume 1, Appendix 13. Laboratory facilities; a level 4 hospital can do blood tests, x-ray and ultrasound. Practitioners: see an internist first; a surgeon might be necessary.

Patient care:

- Try DICYCLOMINE and a low-fat diet. Send out for surgery when it is convenient if there is no fever; send immediately if there is a fever, meanwhile treating with GENTAMYCIN or an injectable CEPHALOSPORIN.

- With ASCARIASIS, give pain medication and LOPERAMIDE and wait for worms to emerge, up to 6 weeks if there is no ACUTE ABDOMEN. Do not give any medication to kill the worms until after the symptoms are gone; then kill them.

- If the patient has a complication, send out quickly, treating for ACUTE ABDOMEN in the meantime. There are occasional deaths.

Gallbladder of Raw Fish

See Regional Notes O, S. This is used as an ethnic remedy.

GANGRENE

Definition: gangrene is the death of tissue.
Age: mostly older. **Who:** mostly poor health, obese or both.
Onset: variable.

Clinical

The problem is usually in a limb, with the first symptoms being pain and a feeling of heaviness. Then there is coldness, color change, swelling, maybe a fever and lethargy and frequently a watery discharge or pus with a bad smell. There may be dark blisters that break and peel or the limb may become pale. The skin might be chalk white or coal black and crusty. The patient may have a fast pulse out of proportion to the fever and pain out of proportion to the appearance. There may be gas bubbles coming out of the skin.

Causative conditions: this can be caused by poisonous snake bite, injury, TROPICAL ULCER, DIABETES, PLANT POISONING with claviceps or ergot and occasionally SPOTTED FEVER, TYPHUS, BARTONELLOSIS or FROSTBITE. It may be caused by the plant toxin, ricin (see PLANT POISONING ricin), CANCRUM ORIS and tertiary YAWS (affecting the nose).

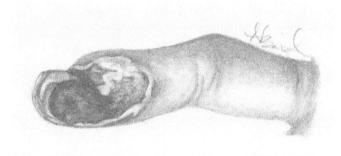

The gangrene has eaten away this fingertip. Earlier the tip would have been present. Some of the dead flesh has fallen off. AB

Similar Condition: see Protocol B.11. CANCRUM ORIS is a type of gangrene.

Treatment

Referrals: this is mandatory; a surgeon at a level 4 or above facility. See Volume 1, Appendix 13. Speedy referral is necessary.

Patient care: sending the patient out or amputating the limb (see Chapter 11 in Volume 1) is the only way to save his life. There is no sense in wasting antibiotic if surgery is out of the question. Awaiting surgery, antibiotics should treat all possible germs: use CEPHALOSPORIN, plus CIPROFLOXACIN, plus METRONIDAZOLE.

GASTRITIS

Definition: gastritis is an inflammation of the stomach.

Cause: bacteria, sometimes drug side effects, dietary indiscretion, pregnancy.

Clinical

See PEPTIC ULCER. Gastritis is similar except it is not an ulcer. The person is likely to have burning upper abdominal pain that is worse with hunger and partially relieved by food. At times the pain may be aggravated by food, especially by hot-spicy foods and by coffee. The patient may also have nausea, vomiting and a lot of gas passed by rectum.

Treatment

Referrals: laboratory and a gastroenterologist might be helpful to exclude alternative diagnoses.

Patient care: this is the same as PEPTIC ULCER. Usually diet change and ANTACIDS suffice. Sometimes antibiotics are necessary. CIMETIDINE may be helpful.

GASTROENTERITIS

Regional Notes: F, R, S.

Entry category: syndrome.

Synonyms: gastroenteropathy, stomach flu.

Definition: gastroenteritis is (usually) a viral infection of the stomach and intestines causing nausea, vomiting, diarrhea, abdominal pain; any combination of these.

Cause: virus, dietary indiscretion, other.

Mildly to moderately ill; class 1; worldwide, very common.

Age: any, especially infants. **Who:** anyone, especially travelers and recently weaned children. **Onset:** variable.

Clinical

The patient does not have a significant fever with this (not over 99.5°F or 37.5°C).

Necessary: the patient has any one or more of the following: abdominal pain, nausea, vomiting, diarrhea. The diarrhea contains no blood or mucus.

Frequently: he has very active bowel sounds and some abdominal tenderness.

Similar conditions: with a fever: if the patient has a significant fever, he probably has something other than simple gastroenteritis. Most childhood diseases present this way. *With no fever:* consider ACUTE ABDOMEN; HEAT ILLNESS; GIARDIASIS; GALLBLADDER DISEASE; FOOD POISONING; KIDNEY DISEASE; PLANT POISONING: castor beans, mushrooms; RADIATION ILLNESS.

Treatment

Referrals: this excludes other diagnoses.

Patient care:

- Treat diarrhea with ORS.

- Treat vomiting according to Protocol A.47.

- Use DICYCLOMINE or CHAMOMILE TEA for abdominal cramps.

- Check for DEHYDRATION, sending the patient out if it develops and you cannot keep up with fluids.

- If the problem is persistent, severe or both, try ERYTHROMYCIN, as this helps for one particular type of gastroenteritis; stop the drug if it makes the problem worse.

- In infants it is essential to give high-calorie food supplements for at least 1–2 weeks after the problem resolves. See MALNUTRITION.

GIARDIASIS

Regional Notes: E, F, I, N, O, R, S, U.

Synonyms: beaver fever, giardia enteritis, lambliasis.

Definition: giardiasis is an infection by *giardia lamblia*. It is not only in the tropics.

Not ill to very ill; class 1; contagious (fecal-oral transmission). worldwide; it occurs in dry as well as humid areas and cold as well as warm. It is common throughout the United States and Canada.

Age: any except exclusively breast-fed infants. **Who:** those drinking contaminated water, children more than adults, expatriates more than nationals, particularly those who had no prior exposure to the disease. It spreads by person-to-person contact, both sexual and otherwise or through contaminated food. Animals get the disease and pass it on to humans via their droppings into water supplies. People can develop immunity to giardiasis, but only after multiple exposures. **Onset:** incubation 1–45 days, usually 1–2 weeks; onset is then sudden.

Clinical

Note: giardiasis does not cause fever! Also, it is no worse in HIV-infected persons than in others.

Necessary: in nationals the disease is without symptoms or else causes a mild, chronic diarrhea. Babies have a persistent, odorless, watery diarrhea, possibly with nausea, vomiting or both. Expatriate adults have watery diarrhea, frequently explosive, with much gas. It may come so fast that the patient is incontinent. It is foamy, floating and very foul-smelling. In mild cases foul gas alone may be present.

Usually: there are loud, rumbling bowel sounds.

Maybe: there is mild to moderate abdominal pain. Nausea and vomiting are common.

Occasionally: children fail to thrive and gain weight, but they have neither diarrhea nor vomiting. MALNUTRITION from giardiasis can be severe and sometimes fatal.

Complications: in severe cases, there may also be loss of appetite and vomiting with consequent DEHYDRATION and weight loss from both the diarrhea and vomiting. Patients may develop MILK INTOLERANCE from having giardiasis. The problem may cure itself or become MALABSORPTION. See Protocol B.14. It may result in IRRITABLE BOWEL or chronic fatigue.

Similar conditions: GASTROENTERITIS, TURISTA, FOOD POISONING, KIDNEY DISEASE, CHOLERA (spectacular diarrhea and painful muscle spasms), MALABSORPTION from any other cause, MANSONELLOSIS PERSTANS (fatigue), MILK INTOLERANCE.

Treatment

Prevention: filter or boil all drinking water or treat it with IODINE in an emergency. Bleach does not work for giardia; heating water to almost boiling works for giardia but not for ENTERIC FEVER. Use outhouses and keep animals away from wells.

Referrals: level 2 or above. Laboratory: stool or fluid withdrawn from the duodenum may be checked with a microscope. Many specimens may be required before one is positive; the test is not sensitive, but it is specific. It will almost always be negative early in the disease. ELISA is a test to detect giardia in stool—both sensitive and specific but unlikely to be available in developing areas. Blood tests are not helpful since they remain positive for a long time after the infection is gone. Facilities: IV fluids and associated equipment. Practitioner: general practitioner, pediatrician or internist.

Patient care:

- TINIDAZOLE single dose is best. Otherwise: METRONIDAZOLE. MEBENDAZOLE and SECNIDAZOLE are alternatives. NITAZOXANIDE or ALBENDAZOLE may work.

- YOGURT is helpful if the patient has MILK INTOLERANCE (a common complication).

- Treat DEHYDRATION; IP fluids may be necessary.

- If the patient has ANEMIA, VITAMIN B_{12} might be helpful.

- Oral PAROMOMYCIN may work in pregnant women; it is not absorbed into the blood stream and therefore does not affect the baby. Use the same dose as for amebic DYSENTERY.

Gingivitis

This refers to infected gums; treat like CELLULITIS.

Glandular fever

This is a British term for MONONUCLEOSIS.

GLAUCOMA

Regional Notes: F.

Definition: glaucoma is an abnormally increased pressure of the fluid within the eyeball.

Cause: unknown.

Not ill to very ill; class 3–4 depending on type and drugs you have; worldwide, not common.

Age: usually adults. **Who:** anyone; susceptibility varies with race. **Onset:** suddenly for acute, slowly for chronic.

Clinical

In both kinds, if the patient closes his eyes and you gently push on his eyeball through the lid, the eyeball feels hard in comparison to a normal eyeball. In acute glaucoma pushing makes the pain worse.

ACUTE GLAUCOMA

This causes a sudden onset of sharp, aching eye pain, frequently with nausea. The patient is almost always over age 60. The eye is red, the cornea is hazy and vision is poor. The patient may see rainbows or halos around lights. This may happen and then go away and then happen again several times before one final severe attack. It is usually on one side only and usually happens when the patient is in dim light. The white of the eye may have a bluish cast. The pupil may be irregular or oval rather than round, with a vertical long axis.

CHRONIC GLAUCOMA

This causes gradually decreased vision with peripheral vision decreasing first and most. The patient develops very narrow tunnel vision. This may occur on both sides. The patient may see halos around lights. It is painless.

Similar conditions: see Protocol B.8.

Treatment

Referrals: facilities: hospitals may have a special instrument to measure eye pressure. Practitioner: optometrist, ophthalmologist, some general practitioners, internists.

Patient care: send the patient out if possible. Speed is of utmost importance in acute glaucoma. Put drops in the eye to make the pupil small. (This is the opposite of the kind used for a scratched cornea.) PILOCARPINE is most frequently used. ACETAZOLAMIDE, a water pill used to hasten acclimatization to high altitude, is useful also. PILOCARPINE drops alone are used in chronic glaucoma. They must be used for the rest of the patient's life.

GOITER

Regional Notes: F, I, O, R, S, U.

Entry category: symptom.

Definition: goiter is a swelling of the thyroid gland on the lower front of the neck.

Cause: iodine deficiency or excess, tumor.

Usually not very ill; class 2; regional, especially inland and high altitude areas.

Age: any. **Who:** those living in affected areas; those eating a diet high in cassava, cabbage, soy beans, bamboo shoots or food originating in the salt water seas. **Onset:** months to years, usually during childhood and adolescence.

Clinical

Necessary: swelling of the center-front of the lower neck, just above the breastbone, maybe extending to the sides. It is generally not tender. The patient may complain of difficulty swallowing and a choking sensation. The patient may wheeze or be short of breath when lying down or raising his arms.

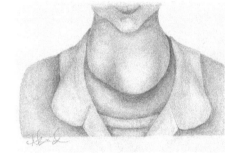

This goiter is very large and lumpy. More commonly a goiter is smaller and smoother. AB

Occasionally: there may be a vibration felt over the goiter, or it may be possible to hear sounds synchronous with the pulse. There may be symptoms of THYROID TROUBLE, usually low-thyroid but occasionally high-thyroid. Babies born to mothers with goiter may have CRETINISM. Iodine deficiency may cause frequent spontaneous ABORTIONs.

Similar conditions: none.

Treatment

Prevention: in areas where most of the diet is derived from the sea, the problem is too much iodine. In these areas, supplement the diet with food grown inland. In areas remote from the sea or where people do not eat sea foods, use iodized salt, treat drinking water with iodine occasionally, or use any kind of sea food in moderate amounts. If the cause is cassava, the water in which the cassava is boiled should not be used and the cassava should be properly processed before being eaten. In some areas public health officials inject young teens with iodinated oil.

Referrals: laboratory: blood tests may be helpful to determine what medication, if any, is most useful. This will require a level 4 or 5 facility. Practitioner: internist for initial evaluation; a surgical referral might be necessary. The surgery is one that can easily go wrong, so it is important to get a surgeon who has extensive experience with this.

Patient care: if it is not possible to send the patient out don't treat patients who have lumpy goiters with iodine. It will not reduce the size of the goiter, and it may cause major problems.

- If there is no CRETINISM in the area or if there is only one patient with goiter, do not use the following treatment! Send the patient to a level 4 or more hospital; he may have CANCER.

- Give IODINE made up as straight LUGOL'S SOLUTION or else tincture of IODINE diluted 1:3 with water; use this in the same dose as LUGOL'S SOLUTION. (See the Drug Index for details.) You can put small amounts of iodine solution in a plastic bag and have the patient put her finger in once a week and lick it. This will be sufficient iodine to make the goiter become smaller over a long period of time. Caution the patient against becoming impatient and overdosing.

Complication of treatment: THYROID TROUBLE of the high-thyroid type. Watch for this and discontinue iodine treatment at the first sign.

Gondou

See YAWS. This is a late complication in which the bones of the middle face swell symmetrically.

GONORRHEA

Regional Notes: F, U.

Synonyms: clap, dose, gleet, strain, drip.

Definition: gonorrhea is a sexually transmitted bacterial infection of the genital tract, caused by the bacterium *Neisseria gonorrhea.*

Cause: bacteria

Not ill to very ill; class 1–3; contagious; worldwide and very common everywhere.

Age: usually adults or newborns, sometimes children. **Who:** sexually active, sexually abused and infants born to infected mothers. **Onset:** symptoms begin in males within two weeks of exposure; in infants within the first 10 days of life; in women usually only many months after exposure.

Clinical

There are almost always symptoms in men, but most women have no symptoms at first. However, even without symptoms they have the disease, pass it on and develop complications.

ORDINARY GONORRHEA:

Necessary: pain with urination (either sex) or a discharge (at first scant mucus, later much pus) coming from the urinary tract, eyes or vagina. A woman might mistake the pus for normal vaginal discharge. There may be a history of these symptoms without their being present when the patient is seen.

Sometimes: the affected part may be red. Eyes always are. Shortly after exposure, the disease may cause mild URINARY INFECTION symptoms in females, similar to URETHRITIS in males. Female patients commonly have a vaginal discharge and abdominal pain. Pain with intercourse develops late. There may be a tender, red, swollen gland on the genital lips. See Volume 1, Chapter 6.

RECTAL GONORRHEA

This may occur in females with contamination from the vagina. In men it is most often from homosexual acts. Many times there are no symptoms. There may be a pus discharge, rectal pain or itching, burning with passing stool, bleeding or constipation.

WIDESPREAD GONORRHEA

There may be inflamed tendons over the hairy surfaces of the wrist, hand, knees or ankles. Along with this there may be (in either sex) a rash consisting of small bumps or blisters with red halos around them, mostly near the joints of the hands and feet, usually less than 40 of them. These are painless but tender to touch. They start out as little bumps which then become pimples with gray centers. Fever, if any, is low. Then ARTHRITIS develops.

THROAT GONORRHEA

This is most often from oral sex. Many times there are no symptoms. If there are symptoms they are likely to be fever, sore throat, visible redness or sores in the throat and large lymph nodes in the neck.

GONORRHEA ARTHRITIS

This usually occurs 1–3 weeks after the urinary symptoms. Initially there are pains in joints on both sides of the body, usually less than 4 joints, without obvious redness and swelling. Then intense swelling develops, affecting one or more joints. It is usually the large joints or the knuckle joints of the hand. The pain is severe, even at rest; it is out of proportion to other symptoms.

Complications: gonorrhea may cause KIDNEY DISEASE, septic ARTHRITIS, HEART FAILURE, PELVIC INFECTION and MENINGITIS. Males may have holes through the skin in the crotch through which urine leaks out. The hole at the end of the penis may swell shut, then heal and scar so urine does not pass easily. There may be swollen lymph nodes in the groin (either sex); a warm, tender swollen testicle; and infection of the prostate (PROSTATITIS), bladder or both. It may cause male infertility, but that is rare. It is the most frequent cause of female infertility.

Similar conditions: penis: URINARY TRACT INFECTION, URETHRITIS of other causes, CHLAMYDIA. *Female genitals:* CHLAMYDIA. *Eyes:* EYE INFECTION. *Throat:* STREP THROAT, MONONUCLEOSIS, DIPHTHERIA, TULAREMIA. *Skin:* CHICKEN POX, insect bites, pimples, SHINGLES, SPOTTED FEVER (Rickettsial pox).*Joint swelling:* Protocol B.6.

Treatment

Prevention; anyone who is exposed to a known case of gonorrhea must be treated. After the treatment, the person is still contagious for 48 hours; he should abstain from sexual activity during that time.

Referrals: laboratory; a smear of pus is stained or a culture may be done. Practitioners: initially a general practitioner, internist or pediatrician; a referral to a surgeon might be necessary.

Patient care: see Protocol B.1 for Sexually Transmitted Diseases. It may be resistant to PENICILLIN and DOXYCYCLINE.

- Gonorrhea in homosexuals or acquired in urban areas: do not use CIPROFLOXACIN, OFLOXACIN or similar drugs. One of the CEPHALOSPORINs is best in this case.

- Gonorrhea acquired in rural areas: AZITHROMYCIN or DOXYCYLINE are best because they also treat CHLAMYDIA. DOXYCYLINE given for 2 weeks (but not AZITHROMYCIN) also works for SYPHILIS which frequently coexists. CIPROFLOXACIN; ceftriaxone or cefixime (see CEPHALOSPORIN); and SPECTINOMYCIN all work for gonorrhea. CIPROFLOXACIN and OFLOXACIN work fine for this, but they do not treat SYPHILIS which frequently coexists.

- Throat infections: use ceftriaxone or CIPROFLOXACIN; SPECTINOMYCIN does not work well.

- Widespread infections: use ceftriaxone or SPECTINOMYCIN at increased dosages; see the Drug Index. CIPROFLOXACIN is no longer appropriate in the western USA or in infections that originated in Asia or the Pacific regions. Give antibiotics for at least 1 week.

- Eye infections: treat eye infections with oral antibiotic as well as ANTIBIOTIC EYE OINTMENT.

GOUT

Definition: gout is a form of ARTHRITIS that usually affects the big toe, sometimes the ankles or wrists.

Cause: heredity, diet, some drugs.

Age: usually adults; in men over age 30, in women almost all post-menopausal. **Who:** more men than women; usually affluent Europeans; it is rare in Africans; it is especially common amongst the Maori of New Zealand. **Onset:** usually sudden; maximally painful in 8–12 hours.

Clinical

Necessary: an ARTHRITIS causing such extreme pain that the patient will scream at the vibration caused by someone's walking by. The joint returns to normal between attacks.

Usually: it initially affects a single joint, particularly the base of the big toe or ankle, possibly the knee. There may be a fever. Pain is maximum within hours, subsides gradually over days to weeks. Attacks occur mostly in the spring and fall. They may recur with increasing frequency and increasing duration of each attack, involving increasing numbers of joints. After 10 years or more the disease might become continual. After it has been present for a long time it can involve upper limbs and finger joints, resembling rheumatoid ARTHRITIS. Frequently there are hard lumps under the skin of the outer ear.

Sometimes: the character of the pain may vary from minute to minute. The patient is restless due to pain.

Complications: gout may cause KIDNEY STONES, especially during DEHYDRATION.

Similar conditions: see Protocol B.6. GONORRHEA and septic ARTHRITIS are two important considerations. Characteristics of gout are that pain is excessive and initially the joint returns to normal between attacks. Skin bumps on the ear may resemble LEPROSY or CUTANEOUS LEISHMANIASIS.

Bush laboratory: the sedimentation rate is always high; a normal rate eliminates this as a diagnosis.

Treatment

Referrals: level 3 or above hospital laboratories can do blood tests for this. Some advanced drugs may be useful. Fluid may be taken from the joint and tested. *Patient care:* weight reduction, low-fat diet, no alcohol, no organ meats, minimal other meats, no shellfish. There are some special medicines that are more helpful than the usual ARTHRITIS medicines, but these should be obtained from and supervised by a physician. ASPIRIN should not be used. ALLOPURINOL is useful to prevent attacks, but it will increase the pain when used during an attack. COLCHICINE works well for treating an acute attack. PROBENECID is sometimes used.

GUINEA WORM

Regional Notes: F, I, R.

Synonyms: dracontiasis, dracunculiasis

Cause: worm

Mildly to moderately ill; class 1; regional, in rural agricultural areas where water is obtained from wells into which people step. There has been a big WHO effort to eliminate the disease. Therefore the maps are no longer reliable. The WHO states that this is only present in Sudan, Ghana, Mali, Niger and Nigeria; they state that it has been eliminated from the Indian subcontinent and from the Middle East.

Age: any. **Who:** those who drink water contaminated with microscopic larvae. **Onset:** variable; usually about 1 year after drinking infected water.

Clinical

Necessary: a small bump forms on the skin, usually on the leg but it may be any part of the body that is frequently cold and moist. This bump enlarges to become a blister. It is itchy and frequently burning; the pain is relieved by cold. When the blister breaks, one can see the end of the worm. There is only one worm per bump and each worm is 30–70 cm (12–28 in.) long. A very painful sore forms in place of the blister. The worm discharges a milky fluid which contains embryos.

Complications: severe infections may develop. When parents are infected their children tend to suffer from MALNUTRITION because of lack of care.

Bush laboratory: none; no lab is required.

Similar conditions: MYIASIS is a skin ulcer with many short, fat "worms". The disease may initially cause KATAYAMA DISEASE. The very painful bump which becomes an ulcer may resemble skin DIPHTHERIA.

Treatment

Prevention: encourage well design which eliminates the possibility of stepping into the water. A simple sand filter works well to eliminate parasites from contaminated water or you can use Temphos (Abate) to treat affected water.

Patient care before the blister forms: the best treatment is for the worm to be surgically removed. This is a relatively easy procedure; it can be done at a level 2 or 3 facility. It reduces the period of disability from weeks to two days. It is feasible for you to learn how to do the procedure.

Patient care: once the blister forms: immerse the blister or sore in cold water. The worm cannot be removed until all the milky fluid with embryos are discharged from the worm's uterus. After the embryos are all discharged, the worm becomes limp, and it sticks out of the skin far enough so one can tie a thread on its end. IBUPROFEN helps to hasten this process. Wind the worm on a small clean stick, a few centimeters a day, not so tightly that the worm breaks. (If it breaks give the patient one of the drugs listed below.) This will gradually draw the worm out. If the patient is bedridden anyway, keeping the area continually wet will draw the worm out faster (in 2 weeks rather than 8–12 weeks). Otherwise keep the area clean and dressed with ANTIBIOTIC OINTMENT to prevent secondary infection. A number of different drugs are also useful, such as METRONIDAZOLE, TINIDAZOLE, MEBENDAZOLE and THIABENDAZOLE. NIRIDAZOLE is a dangerous old drug that should no longer be used.

HAND-FOOT-MOUTH DISEASE

Cause: virus

Mildly to moderately ill; class 1–3; contagious; worldwide, in small epidemics

Age: children usually; **Who**: those exposed to others with the disease; **Onset**: unknown; incubation 4–6 days

Clinical

Necessary: at first a fever and general fatigue, then a blistery rash on the hairy sides of the hands (not the palms).

Sometimes the problem goes away by itself; sometimes there are complications with RESPIRATORY FAILURE or ENCEPHALITIS, requiring higher-level care. The complications are more likely in younger children.

Similar diseases: CHICKEN POX, SMALLPOX, MONKEYPOX, SPOTTED FEVER (Rickettsial pox).

Treatment

Referrals: it is particularly important to send out children less than 5 years old to a level 3 or above hospital.

Patient care: antibiotics do no good. Keep the blisters clean and dry; apply antiseptic. If there are no complications, then the problem usually resolves within a week.

HANGOVER

Entry category: syndrome.

This is a headache and general aching without a fever the morning after ALCOHOL excess. It should not be treated.

HAVERHILL FEVER

See RAT BITE FEVER for a complete description. Haverhill fever is one type of rat bite fever which can also be caused by drinking contaminated milk. It causes a migrating large joint ARTHRITIS that relapses over about 2 weeks. It is a bacterial infection, Gram-negative.

HEART ATTACK

Regional Notes: O.

Synonyms: myocardial infarction, coronary occlusion.

Definition: a heart attack is the death of a portion of heart muscle, usually from blockage of one of the heart's arteries.

Cause: heredity; Western diet; SYPHILIS.

Mildly to severely ill; class 3–4; regional; consider this diagnosis only in those who have eaten Western diets or had SYPHILIS.

Age: generally over 40 y.o. **Who:** affluent nationals and Westerners; achiever types, smokers, those with HYPERTENSION, DIABETES, obesity or SYPHILIS. **Onset:** usually sudden.

Clinical

Necessary: the patient has one or more of the following.

- Chest pain, usually pressure-like, which lasts 20 minutes or more and is not aggravated by deep breathing; the painful area is not tender to touch. The left arm or jaw may also be painful; it is not tender.

- Pale, ashen, sweaty skin.

- A feeling of weakness along with an abnormal pulse rate and a drop in blood pressure.

- Shortness of breath which is worse lying down than sitting up; the patient might turn blue with this.

- An overwhelming sense of doom.

Sometimes: nausea, vomiting, indigestion, coughing up frothy sputum, loss of consciousness, HEART FAILURE. This may be painless in some, especially with DIABETES.

Similar conditions: ANGINA is the pain of a threatened heart attack that doesn't progress to actual heart damage; the pain lasts less than 20 minutes. If it lasts more than 20 minutes, then damage is likely, and the patient should be sent to a hospital. If the frequency and severity of the pain increases, this likewise warrants evacuation to a hospital.

HEARTBURN is likely more of a burning than a pressure pain.

PERICARDITIS pain is relieved somewhat by leaning forward; it is aggravated by lying on one's back. PLEURISY is aggravated by deep breathing. DEPRESSION can cause a general chest heaviness that does not vary much with time. GALLBLADDER DISEASE can cause pain identical with heart attack, but the pain is more on the right, whereas the pain of a heart attack is likely on the left.

Treatment

Referrals: laboratory; a level 3 or more hospital can do an electrocardiogram and some blood tests. A level 4 or 5 hospital may have lifesaving surgical facilities. Facilities: oxygen, intensive care unit, monitored bed, specialized imaging and facilities to dissolve clots in the heart. Practitioners; a cardiologist is ideal; a general practitioner or internist can manage fine. A referral to a level 4 or 5 hospital in a Western nation might be appropriate.

Patient care: send out immediately, having the patient sit up meanwhile. Oxygen is helpful. Relieve pain if you can.

HEART FAILURE

Regional Notes: F, I, M, O, S, U.

Entry category: syndrome cluster.

Synonyms: congestive heart failure, CHF.

Includes: right and left heart failure.

Definition: heart failure is the inability of the heart to perform up to the body's demands.

Cause: variable.

Moderately to very ill; class 2–4 depending on severity; worldwide, highly variable frequency. Dilated (floppy) heart failure in the context of childbirth occurs in tropical Latin America, Africa south of the Sahara, India, China and Korea.

Age: any, including children. **Who:** anyone. It may occur with no obvious cause; in infants it is commonly due to a birth defect. **Onset:** gradual over weeks to months unless the patient is quite sick with a fever or has a HEART ATTACK. It can also be sudden in an infant with a heart murmur (see Volume 1, Chapter 1).

Clinical

Necessary: the patient is short of breath, worse lying than sitting; he becomes lethargic; he has a swollen back or ankles; or a combination of these symptoms. He always has diminished exercise tolerance.

Maybe: his skin color may be bluish. In severe cases the patient may have loss of appetite, dizziness and swelling of the abdomen with a large, tender liver and spleen. His pulse may be slow, fast or irregular. His blood pressure may be high or low. His respiration may be fast, irregular or labored. He may have a low body temperature. He may have a cough or wheezing. Children might have delayed sexual development.

There are 4 types of HEART FAILURE

- dilated (floppy.)
- restrictive (tight.)
- hypertrophic (muscular.)
- valvular (bad valves.)

In any particular geographic area, one or another type of heart failure will be most common. At times an individual might have a combination of two types of heart failure.

DILATED HEART FAILURE

The heart is large and floppy. The patient is usually very short of breath while lying down; he sits up to rest. The blood pressure is not high. Frequently the pulse is irregular and heart sounds are soft. The beat is not easily felt or heard on the chest wall. The liver may be large and the ankles swollen. This occurs in BERIBERI, DIPHTHERIA, many viral diseases and sometimes in connection with childbirth. When it is due to childbirth, it occurs 2–20 weeks after delivery. Sometimes the patient dies and sometimes she recovers. This problem is frequently caused by severe ANEMIA.

RESTRICTIVE HEART FAILURE

In restrictive heart disease, the heart size is usually small or normal. The veins in the neck are distended, and the heart beat can be seen in them. Fatigue with exercise bothers the patient more than shortness of breath with lying down. The two numbers of the blood pressure are not far apart, and the pressure is never high, e.g., 110/96. The liver may be enlarged and tender. This occurs with PERICARDITIS, with TUBERCULOSIS and sometimes for unknown reasons.

HYPERTROPHIC HEART FAILURE

The heart is large and muscular. The patient may be short of breath with lying down. He will have either HYPERTENSION or chest pain. The heartbeat is easily felt on the chest wall unless the patient is fat. The veins in the neck may be swollen, and the pulse easily seen there.

VALVULAR HEART FAILURE

There is a murmur. It might be possible to feel the murmur as a vibration on the chest wall. In addition, there are signs of hypertrophic disease, dilated disease or a mixture of these. There may be an abnormally large or small difference between the two blood pressure numbers (e.g., 130/20 or 120/110), or the patient may faint immediately after exercise or at unpredictable times. It may cause clubbing of the fingernails (see below). The patient may have blue lips.

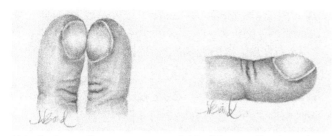

Valvular heart disease may cause clubbed fingernails. The nails are wide and shaped like inverted bowls. AB

This type is most common in developing countries; it is seen in SYPHILIS, RHEUMATIC FEVER, in children with birth defects and sometimes SPOTTED FEVER.

Causative diseases: in a patient with a high fever and sudden heart failure, who was perfectly healthy previously, consider SEPSIS and RHEUMATIC FEVER. RHEUMATIC FEVER may also cause slow-onset heart failure. Heart failure may be associated with AFRICAN SLEEPING SICKNESS, ALCOHOLISM, ALTITUDE SICKNESS, ANEMIA, BERIBERI, BRUCELLOSIS, CHAGA'S DISEASE, childbirth, DIPHTHERIA, DOWN SYNDROME, HEART ATTACK, HOOKWORM, HYPERTENSION, LASSA FEVER, LOIASIS, MALARIA, PERICARDITIS, Q FEVER, RELAPSING FEVER, SCHISTOSOMIASIS JAPONICUM, SCURVY, SEPSIS, SICKLE CELL DISEASE, SYPHILIS, TOXEMIA, TRENCH FEVER, TRICHINOSIS, TUBERCULOSIS, TYPHUS and viral infections.

Similar conditions: body swelling: see Protocols B.6 and B.7. LIVER FAILURE also causes body swelling, but the patient is not short of breath with lying down, and the veins on the surface of his abdomen may be very visible. KIDNEY DISEASE also can cause swelling. Either the blood pressure will be high or the urine dipstick will be abnormal or both. *Shortness of breath* See Protocol B.4; this can be similar to RESPIRATORY INFECTION and diseases similar to that; both are worse lying down and better sitting up. Finger clubbing: TRICHURIASIS can also cause finger clubbing and growth retardation. *Confusion/lethargy:* see Protocol B.10.

Treatment

Referrals: see Volume 1, Appendix 13. Laboratory; a level 3 or above hospital may offer blood tests, electrocardiogram. Facilities; a level 3 or above intensive care unit, monitoring equipment, oxygen and imaging technology might be helpful. Practitioners; a cardiologist is ideal; a general practitioner or internist might be helpful. Consider that the cause may be a tropical/travel disease. A surgical referral might be appropriate, but this must be to a Western level 4 or above.

Patient care:

- Keep the patient in bed, sitting up. Use THEOPHYLLINE if he is wheezing.

- Treat for MALARIA if it is prevalent in your area.

- Consider what diseases in your area might cause heart failure, question the patient as to other present or prior symptoms and treat whatever you think might have caused it.

- Treat patients who have severe ANEMIA with DIGOXIN, HYDROCHLOROTHIAZIDE, IRON, VITAMIN B$_{12}$ and FOLIC ACID.

- In areas with a lot of BRUCELLOSIS, if the patient has consistent symptoms, consider treating for that. It is a frequent cause of heart failure.

HEART MEDICATIONS

In *dilated disease*, use DIGOXIN and HYDROCHLORTHIAZIDE. Give the patient the patient an ASPIRIN each day if his pulse is irregular.

In *restrictive disease,* use HYDROCHLOROTHIAZIDE and HYDROCORTISONE.

In *hypertrophic disease,* HYDROCHLOROTHIAZIDE is helpful, as well as PROPRANOLOL. DIGOXIN might be helpful. Treat HYPERTENSION until the blood pressure is near-normal. Reduce the blood pressure gradually.

In *valvular disease,* HYDROCHLOROTHIAZIDE is safe if the patient is short of breath. DIGOXIN may be used additionally, if necessary, but PROPRANOLOL must not be used unless a physician directs you to do so. Use AMPICILLIN for one day when the patient requires any surgical or dental procedure or delivers a baby. FUROSEAMIDE may substitute for HYDROCHLOROTHIAZIDE.

Results: 1–24 hours with drugs.

HEARTBURN

Entry category: syndrome.

Definition: heartburn refers to a burning chest pain caused by stomach acid.

The symptoms are similar to HEART ATTACK. The patient has a burning sensation underneath his breastbone and an acid taste in his mouth. He may also have indigestion. Treat with ANTACID, and have the patient sit upright for 2 hours after eating. CIMETIDINE might be helpful.

HEAT ILLNESS

Includes: heat exhaustion, heat stroke. The difference between these is the severity.

Definition: heat illness is a failure of the body to adapt to a hot environment.

Cause: hot environment.

Mildly to very ill; class 1–3; worldwide in hot climates, especially humid; mild is common; heat stroke is uncommon.

Age: any, especially very young and very old. **Who:** there are two classes of people who are particularly susceptible to heat illness: (1) Those who are very old or very young or in poor health; and (2) Those in good health, especially expatriates, doing physical work in a hot climate or having a sleep deficit. Drugs for diarrhea and/or nausea tend to aggravate or precipitate the problem. **Onset:** minutes to hours.

Clinical

Necessary: the patient is exposed to a very hot environment. If it is dry heat, he is thirsty; if it is humid heat he is or was sweating profusely and may also be thirsty.

HEAT EXHAUSTION (MILD HEAT ILLNESS)

This causes fatigue; headache; nausea; vomiting; muscle cramps in the arms, legs and abdomen. The skin is warm and moist. There is sometimes a rash with tiny bumps. The blood pressure may drop, causing fainting. Initially there is no or a low fever. Sometimes there are mental changes; the person may be irritable and irrational. He may lose his appetite and complain of dizziness. If he is not treated, it may progress to heat stroke.

HEAT STROKE (SEVERE HEAT ILLNESS)

Initially there are symptoms of heat exhaustion, as given above. Thereafter

- In babies and the elderly, there is little sweating but very rapid respiration.

- Previously healthy patients who are exercising tend to be very sweaty and may have HYPOGLYCEMIA.

- In all cases there is likely to be loss of consciousness; wild combative behavior or SEIZURES. Body temperature will be high, at least 40°C (104°F) and possibly up to 44°C (111°F). If the patient is not cooled immediately he will die.

Complications: BRAIN DAMAGE, death.

Similar conditions: heat exhaustion may coexist with and be similar to ZINC DEFICIENCY; treat both. It is also similar to GASTROENTERITIS, INFLUENZA and early HEPATITIS. Heat stroke is indistinguishable from cerebral MALARIA, ENCEPHALITIS and sometimes MENINGITIS. If you suspect any of these, you should treat for all of them. Also see Protocol B.10.A.

Bush laboratory: with heat stroke, the patient's urine might look like machine oil and test strongly positive for both protein and blood.

Treatment

Prevention: use salt in the diet and drinking water on hot days. Patients who are taking diuretic medicines should decrease the dose. Low-salt diets should be abandoned when much salt is being lost in the sweat, but monitor the blood pressure. Frequent cooling is helpful. Restrict exercise and avoid sleep deficits.

Referrals: see Volume 1, Appendix 13. Speedy referral is essential with heat stroke. Laboratory: A level 3 or above hospital will probably have a variety of blood tests which will help manage the complications of heat stroke. Facilities: in countries that are usually very hot, there might be special cooling units at level 2 or above. In areas with a moderate climate, such cooling units are only found at level 4 and above. Practitioners: an internist is ideal; a general practitioner can manage.

Patient care:

- Heat exhaustion: have a conscious patient drink 1–2 liters of ORS. If this diagnosis is at all possible, try the treatment. Check for DEHYDRATION and treat that also. If the patient is not acclimatized to the hot environment, ZINC might also be helpful. *Results:* 1–2 hours.

- Heat stroke: cool the patient as rapidly as you can. Packing him in ice is best, but immediate care is more important than ideal care. CHLORPROMAZINE will lessen shivering. If he has SEIZURES, keep him from hurting himself. Try to give sugar water if he is able to swallow, or put down a stomach tube. Be aware that patients are usually combative when they awaken. Send him to a hospital even after he has regained consciousness.

- If there is falciparum MALARIA in your area, treat that; it is indistinguishable. DIAZEPAM is best for SEIZURES, and it may also prevent combative behavior.

Complications are numerous and unpredictable. If evacuation is impossible, give the patient plenty of fluids. Give him baking soda in sufficient quantity to keep his urine pH between 8 and 9. (Measure pH with urine dipsticks.)

HEMOCHROMATOSIS

Definition: too much iron which causes failure of multiple organs. The common causes thereof are blood transfusions, some hereditary problems and an abnormally high dietary iron intake.

Cause: iron overload.

Clinical

LIVER DISEASE, LIVER FAILURE, DIABETES, reproductive dysfunction, ARTHRITIS, JAUNDICE, free fluid in the abdomen (increased abdominal girth), HEART FAILURE, increased skin pigmentation.

Treatment

Send to a hospital, level 2 or above.

HEMORRHAGIC FEVER

Regional Notes: E, F, I, M, O, R, S, U.

Entry category: disease cluster.

Includes: Kyasanur Forest disease, CRIMEAN-CONGO HEMORRHAGIC FEVER and many others, most of which contain names of places. There are separate entries for EBOLA VIRUS DISEASE, MARBURG FEVER, LASSA FEVER and DENGUE HEMORRHAGIC FEVER.

Definition: hemorrhagic fever is a group of viral illnesses which cause the blood to fail to clot properly. Because of this there is abnormal bleeding.

Cause: virus.

Very ill; class 3–4; some kinds contagious; regional, mostly tropical, Africa, Middle East and southern Asia.

Age: any. **Who:** anyone, but especially bug-bitten.
Onset: variable; incubation period varies by type.

Clinical

The patient has a fever and general illness. He then begins to bleed: nosebleed; bleeding gums; bloody urine, vomit and stool; very heavy menstruation; and heavy wound bleeding are common. The patient may have bleeding into the whites of his eyes (does not need treatment) or into his skin, causing a bruised appearance. If the bleeding is severe the patient becomes dizzy with a rapid pulse and low blood pressure. He develops SHOCK and dies.

Similar conditions: LIVER FAILURE, MALARIA, TYPHUS, LEPTOSPIROSIS, SEPSIS and any disease that causes a very large spleen (see Symptom Protocol A.46.B) can cause abnormal bleeding.

Bush laboratory: do a tourniquet test:

> *Determine the patient's blood pressure. Choose a number about half-way between the two numbers of the blood pressure.*
>
> *Inflate the blood pressure cuff on the arm to that half-way number and leave it inflated for 5 minutes. (This will cause some pain.)*
>
> *Look at the arm below the cuff. If there are multiple bruise marks, then the patient may have hemorrhagic fever.*
>
> *Check the fingernails if the patient has very dark skin.*

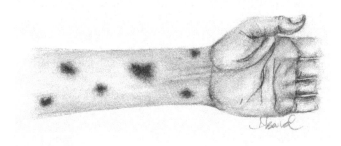

This is a severe case of hemorrhagic fever. The spots may be subtle. They may be provoked with a blood pressure cuff. 1. They are various sizes. 2. They are flat, not raised up. 3. The color is initially purple, then changes over days, like an ordinary bruise. AB

Treatment

Prevention: transport a patient only in a towed trailer. Talk to local or government medical personnel to find the source of the problem locally. Then institute public health measures to prevent the underlying disease. See Protocol B.2.

Referrals: see Volume 1, Appendix 13 and prevention above. Laboratory: hospitals at level 3 or above can do blood tests and may be able to transfuse blood. Facilities: blood bank, IV fluids and means to give them, an intensive care unit with isolation; a monitored bed. Level 4 or above is desirable.

Practitioners; a hematologist and an infectious disease specialist with tropical/travel expertise. An internist or general practitioner might be helpful.

Patient care: VITAMIN K injections may help if there is JAUNDICE. Treat SHOCK with fluids until you can get the patient to a hospital. Transfusions are frequently necessary. RIBAVIRIN may be available at a hospital. Reportedly it works for all kinds of viral hemorrhagic fevers except EBOLA VIRUS DISEASE. Do not use ASPIRIN or IBUPROFEN. ACETAMINOPHEN is okay. Use TRAMADOL for pain.

HEMORRHOIDS

Synonym: piles.

Definition: hemorrhoids are veins by the anus or rectum that become abnormally large and bulge out, causing pain, bleeding or both.

Cause: variable.

Mildly ill; class 1–2 depending on severity; worldwide, variable frequency.

Age: adult, usually middle-aged and older. **Who:** anyone, related to constipation, eating low fiber diets, sitting on a toilet reading, pregnancy, LIVER DISEASE, CIRRHOSIS, LIVER FAILURE and OLD AGE. **Onset:** days to weeks.

Clinical

Necessary: the patient passes bright red blood by rectum, coating the outside of his stool. Pain is worse with bowel movements.

Sometimes: the pain may be so severe that the patient becomes very constipated. You may see big, blue veins protrude from the rectum; sometimes you can feel veins with rectal exam, but frequently examination is normal.

Maybe: there is rectal itching, soiling of underwear, passage of mucus. If external hemorrhoids clot, they become suddenly painful. The pain lasts 1–2 weeks and then disappears.

Bush laboratory: check for ANEMIA.

Similar conditions: TUBERCULOSIS of the rectum or anus may cause rectal bleeding, as may various SEXUALLY TRANSMITTED DISEASEs.

Treatment

Referrals: a surgeon may be helpful.

Patient care: use sitz baths; see Appendix 1 in Volume 1 for directions. Recommend a high-fiber diet. Correct constipation with MILK OF MAGNESIA or another laxative. Hemorrhoids are not serious unless the patient has a large blood loss. However, they usually require the services of a hospital and a surgeon.

HEPATITIS   .

Regional Notes: E, F, I, K, M, N, O, R, S, U

Entry category: disease cluster.

Includes: hepatitis A, B, C, D (Delta), E, G[1]. It also includes toxic hepatitis from industrial or waste substances, drugs and many ethnic medicines.

Definition: hepatitis is an inflammation of the liver, caused by a virus or toxin.

Mildly to very ill; class 1–3, depending on severity; viral hepatitis is worldwide, generally common.

Age: any. **Who:** anyone, usually from unsanitary water, food, personal contact or blood exposure; may be due to drugs, chemicals, excessive ALCOHOL or poisonous fumes. Expatriates are vulnerable to viral hepatitis, especially the unimmunized. Some common liver-toxic herbs are listed under PLANT POISONING. Many drugs are liver-toxic, especially those used to treat TUBERCULOSIS. Hepatitis E is associated with consumption of pork liver. **Onset:** this varies with toxic exposures, depending on the amount of poison and the duration of exposure. For viral hepatitis the onset is over a few days to a week or two. Incubation is 2–8 weeks for water-borne and 2–6 months for blood-borne.

Clinical

For all kinds of hepatitis, the general symptoms are similar. The length of the illnesses and the prognoses vary according to the type of hepatitis.

Necessary: nausea, loss of appetite and fatigue occur first. A large, painful tender liver and either JAUNDICE, bilirubin in the urine or both are present after the first week or two.

---

1 *Hepatitis A is water-borne. It is the mildest type of hepatitis, seldom fatal. There are no severe long-lasting consequences. An immunization is available.*

Hepatitis B is blood-borne and sexually transmitted. There is some evidence that it is also transmitted within families in areas of poor hygiene. It is long-lasting. Sometimes patients recover and sometimes they develop a very severe form and die. Hepatitis B is also a cause of liver cancer. There is an immunization for hepatitis B.

Hepatitis C is also blood-borne, but it is rarely or never sexually transmitted. It is usually mild initially, but many patients develop severe, chronic hepatitis over the longer term. No immunization is available but some anti-viral drugs may work.

Hepatitis D is a blood-borne virus which does not infect people by itself, but is associated with hepatitis B. It causes severe illness. The hepatitis B immunization also protects against hepatitis D.

Hepatitis E is a water-borne hepatitis, which occurs in southern Asia, the Middle East, Latin America and Africa. It causes mild illness in most people. Immunization has been developed; seek recent information on availability. It is becoming common in industrialized countries. Hepatitis E acquired in the west is generally not as serious as that acquired in the developing world.

Hepatitis G is a blood-borne virus and most common in the India area. It is sexually transmitted as well as mother to baby. It is a cause of chronic hepatitis.

Commonly: the patient will walk with his hand over his upper, right abdomen. He will likely feel the pain in his right shoulder.

Maybe: fever less than 101.3°F (38.5°C), very dark urine, light-colored stool, itching all over. Usually there are joint pains along with general itching, nausea and fatigue for 2 days to 6 weeks before the jaundice starts. When the patient develops jaundice, the other symptoms improve. The joint pains are mostly in the hands, sometimes the knees and ankles.

Warning concerning a hepatitis diagnosis.

With a continuous high fever after the onset of jaundice, the diagnosis is more likely MALARIA than hepatitis.

Drowsiness or mental aberrations make death likely.

A rapid pulse and low blood pressure may indicate internal bleeding.

Hepatitis is the most common erroneous diagnosis in fatal MALARIA.

Complications: abnormal bleeding, liver CANCER, LIVER FAILURE (cirrhosis type), ABORTION, death. A common terminal event is a condition resembling ENCEPHALITIS. If mild, there is confusion, hallucinations or apathy; if severe, seizures and coma.

Similar conditions: the initial illness with joint pains can easily be confused with RUBELLA in adults, with ARTHRITIS and with early BRUCELLOSIS. KIDNEY DISEASE might also appear similar. If the patient had shaking chills at the beginning, the diagnosis is probably not hepatitis; check out LEPTOSPIROSIS (especially in males) and MALARIA.

Once JAUNDICE develops: see Protocols B.5 and B.7. Falciparum MALARIA may easily be confused with hepatitis with disastrous results. If in doubt, treat MALARIA. LEPTOSPIROSIS causes severe muscle aching, red eyes or both; the fever is higher than in hepatitis. It requires prompt treatment.

Also consider GALLBLADDER DISEASE (usually episodic localized pains), AMEBIASIS (also localized pains), HEART FAILURE (swollen ankles), THALLASEMIA (anemia), RELAPSING FEVER (higher fever), SPOTTED FEVER (higher fever), SYPHILIS (secondary with a rash), LIVER FLUKE (check geography), MONONUCLEOSIS (also large, tender spleen), SEPSIS in a newborn. PELVIC INFECTION in females can cause liver tenderness mimicking hepatitis. If the patient had contact with newborn animals, the hepatitis might be due to Q FEVER, in which case it might respond to DOXYCYCLINE or RIFAMPIN. Seek local professional medical advice.

Bush laboratory: urine shows bilirubin, maybe ketones and urobilinogen. If you put the urine in a closed glass container and shake it, there will be foam on top similar to soapy water, and the foam will be yellowish. Compare this to a sample of normal urine, the same amount of urine in the same kind of container. Stool may test positive for blood.

Treatment

Prevention: boil all drinking water during an epidemic. This will eliminate all but hepatitis B. Filtering and chemical treatment are not adequate. Dispose of sewage away from water supply. Wash hands and foods before eating. Avoid illicit sexual contacts.

Pressure cooker treatment of needles and syringes is mandatory. **No amount of boiling will kill hepatitis B.** Use gloves when handling wounds. Take extreme care to avoid any blood or sewage contamination.

Injection with GAMMA GLOBULIN gives short-term protection against hepatitis. This is not the same as immunization. The American product prevents hepatitis A only; the French product prevents both hepatitis A and hepatitis E. It must be refrigerated.

Immunizations are available for hepatitis A and hepatitis B. Hepatitis B immunization also prevents hepatitis D. Infants of mothers who carry hepatitis B should be immunized right after birth. Note that the hepatitis B immunization must not be given in the buttock. The intradermal hepatitis B immunization does not give as good long-term immunity as the intramuscular does.

Referrals: see Volume 1, Appendix 13. Laboratory: level 4 and above can do specific blood tests to determine the type of hepatitis and how severe it is. Facilities: level 4 and above may have drugs that are helpful. Practitioners: an infectious disease specialist is ideal; an internist or general practitioner may be adequate.

Patient care: send the patient to a hospital for treatment. There are now good drugs (although they are high-tech) to treat hepatitis B and C.

- If the disease was caused by drugs, chemicals or fumes, remove the offending substance.

- Advise bed rest and good food, avoiding ALCOHOL, chocolate and fatty food.

- Watch vital signs carefully, checking for DEHYDRATION and weight loss. Send out if vital signs become very abnormal.

- VITAMIN K injections may help for bleeding.

- RIBAVIRIN, a new anti-viral drug, may work for some kinds of hepatitis and may be tried in severe cases.

- ARTEMISININ (in particular the dry leaf powder of *Artemisia annua*) may work for HEPATITIS B.

Results: gradual recovery over 1–12 months for water-borne hepatitis (A and E). Hepatitis B and C can cause LIVER FAILURE and result in death. Hepatitis A might be fatal in patients over 50 years old. Hepatitis E might be fatal to pregnant women or their newborn infants.

HERNIA

Regional Notes: F, M.

Synonym: rupture.

Definition: a hernia is a weak spot on the abdominal wall, where a piece of bowel can (and usually does) pass through the deeper layers of the wall until it lies right underneath the skin.

Not ill to very ill; class 1–4; worldwide, common.

Age: any. **Who:** anyone, especially males. **Onset:** sudden or may be there since birth.

Clinical

Necessary: the patient has a soft bulge in his groin, in his groin or on his abdominal wall. A groin hernia may extend part or all the way into the scrotum on that side, causing the scrotum to hang down as far as the knees. The swelling is soft like a water balloon, unless it has become painful and tender. Then it may become hard.

Maybe: if it is not tender and no one has pushed on it within the last 20 minutes, you can hear bowel sounds in it with your stethoscope.

Complications: navel hernias that have been present since birth and scar hernias seldom cause problems. Groin hernias and acquired navel hernias can cause ACUTE ABDOMEN. In this case there is general abdominal pain as well as pain and tenderness in the hernia.

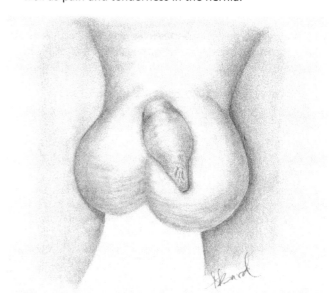

These are fairly large hernias, both right and left; note that the swelling extends up to the leg creases. A small hernia may be just a little bulge on the leg crease. See Volume 1, Chapter 1. AB

Similar conditions: an ordinary hernia is not tender.

Non-painful, non-tender scrotal swelling: HYDROCELE (light shines through); with HYDATID DISEASE (check geography), TUBERCULOSIS and CANCER, light doesn't shine through.

Painful, tender scrotal swelling: FILARIASIS (probably common in the community), ABSCESS, EPIDIDYMITIS. *Groin swelling only; scrotum appears normal:* swollen lymph nodes or an abscess from any infection on the legs or feet or from SEXUALLY TRANSMITTED DISEASE. If the swelling is black and tender, in a very sick patient consider PLAGUE.

Treatment

Referrals: a level 2 or above hospital with anesthesia, a surgical theatre and a surgeon are most helpful.

Patient care: a patient with a tender hernia or signs of ACUTE ABDOMEN must be sent to a hospital immediately; otherwise send him when convenient if a physician agrees to repair the hernia. A hernia that can be ignored goes back into the abdomen easily. Most large ones do so with gentle pushing. To encourage a stubborn groin hernia to go back into place, put the foot end of the patient's bed on concrete blocks and give him a sedative. If it still will not go back in, send him out for repair within 48 hours. If stool drains out of a spontaneous hole in the groin skin, put a diaper on it. Do not try to close the hole.

HERPES

Regional Notes: I.

Synonyms: herpes simplex, cold sore, fever blister

Includes: genital herpes.

Definition: herpes is a viral infection of the skin or of moist pink surfaces, e.g., in the mouth or genital areas.

Cause: virus.

Mildly to very ill; class 1–3; contagious; worldwide; it is the most common genital ulcer disease in both developed and developing countries.

Age: any. **Who:** anyone, especially those who have had the problem before. Patients with HIV are especially prone to this. **Onset:** over a day or two. In the tropics the incubation is 2–14 days if the problem is in the genital area.

Clinical

ORDINARY HERPES

Necessary: first there is a reddened area of skin. Then that red area becomes swollen. Then painful blisters form on a red halo in or near the mouth or the genital areas, occasionally on the skin or in the eyes. They are multiple, small, close together and tender to touch. The blisters may break and then blend into each other to make shallow ulcers. Episodes of blisters and ulcers come and go multiple times. The first episode is the worst, with a large area involved, and it is most likely to be symmetrical, i.e. the same or nearly the same right and left. See the drawing, Volume 1 Chapter 6.

The symptoms are at their worst about a week after the infection started.

Maybe: in young people the pain subsides between attacks; in old people the pain may persist. The skin or blisters might itch, burn or tingle. There may be pain with urination. The patient might have fever and chills or enlarged lymph nodes. The enlarged nodes are tender to touch. He may have fatigue and loss of appetite. His neck might be stiff. The surfaces might peel. The disease can cause blindness if the eye is affected. With an eye infection, light will hurt the eye(s). Herpes may cause pain so severe that a child refuses to eat or drink. He may require a stomach tube for nourishment and fluids. Babies born to mothers with herpes may have CATARACT at birth.

Complications of genital herpes: secondary infection, MENINGITIS, constipation, urinary retention (can't release urine); pains down legs.

HERPES AND HIV

Herpes increases the likelihood of acquiring HIV INFECTION. HIV INFECTION makes the symptoms of herpes worse. With HIV INFECTION, herpes is frequently resistant to ACYCLOVIR.

INFANTS OF WOMEN WITH HERPES

These babies have multiple problems that you will not be able to handle. They should be sent out for care. ACYCLOVIR is not an approved drug during pregnancy, but a physician might justify its use to prevent a disastrous outcome for the newborn.

Similar conditions: see Protocols B.1 (genital) and B.8 (eyes). In the mouth, consider APHTHOUS STOMATITIS, REITER SYNDROME. For herpes that affects the eye, see KERATITIS. SHINGLES is a closely related disease that also causes painful blisters. Burns may appear similar.

Treatment

Referrals: large hospital laboratories and those with special kits can do tests for this.

Patient care:

- Pain medication may be helpful.

- Cool wet-to-dry compresses and sitz baths may be helpful. See Appendix 1 in Volume 1.

- ACYCLOVIR is available in both cream and pill form. Famciclovir is a similar, related drug. Since the disease is recurrent, you should try to give your patient medication to start taking as soon as he feels another episode starting. When started early, even just one day of medication can prevent a full-blown episode.

- You can try using a paste made of crushed BISMUTH SUBSALICYLATE tablets to treat sores on the mouth.

- Eye doctors can treat infected eyes; the patient must be sent out promptly.

Results: herpes in the absence of HIV INFECTION will usually go away in two weeks without treatment. However, it is likely to recur, and the patient may still be contagious during the time when he has no symptoms.

HIV[1] INFECTION

Regional Notes: E, F, I, K, M, O, R, S, U.

Synonyms: retroviral Infection, AIDS.

Includes: ARC (AIDS-Related Complex) and full-blown AIDS.

Definition: infection with the human immunodeficiency virus, type 1 or type 2, also called retrovirus.

Cause: virus.

Not ill to very ill; class 1–4; contagious; those infected with both HIV and TUBERCULOSIS are particularly contagious; HIV is present worldwide.

Age: any, including the 5–16-year age range. **Who:** babies born of infected mothers; sexually active and sexually abused; those who receive contaminated blood transfusions or needle sticks. **Onset:** incubation between the infecting event and the development of a positive antibody blood test (seroconversion illness) is 2–12 weeks. After that the disease is dormant for 5–15 years before it manifests as AIDS. The incubation to AIDS is shorter in older people, in those with severe or long-lasting symptoms of the seroconversion illness and in those whose infection was caused by blood transfusion.

Clinical

The disease occurs in three stages.

SEROCONVERSION ILLNESS

This is a mild, flu-like illness 2–4 weeks after infection, lasting 1–2 weeks but occasionally longer. At times this may cause ENCEPHALITIS. The symptoms are as follows: fever; fatigue; a sore throat; a measles-like rash, not painful or itchy; general aching; night sweats; enlarged lymph nodes. Occasionally there is general body itching, hair loss and sores in the mouth. During this time there is an abnormally high sedimentation rate: [see Volume 1, Appendix 2]. This becomes normal again during the second incubation period of years. The infection is highly contagious during seroconversion.

EARLY AIDS[2]

This occurs 5–15 years after the seroconversion illness. The symptoms are as follows: weight loss; diarrhea; fever; symmetrical, non-tender enlarged lymph nodes at two or more sites, especially on the face near the ears (chipmunk look); tiredness; night sweats; sores in the mouth; reddish face; rash; SHINGLES; increased symptoms from some SEXUALLY TRANSMITTED DISEASES.

ADVANCED, FULL-BLOWN AIDS

This develops gradually from early AIDS and causes more and more infections which become increasingly difficult to treat. In about 20% of patients the virus affects the brain causing poor concentration and memory, poor coordination, abnormal emotions and behavior, pains in the hands and feet in the areas normally covered by stockings and gloves, weakness in the hips and shoulders with muscle pains and stiff weakness of the limbs. The spleen may be enlarged.

There are two kinds of arthritis associated with HIV: one is from the virus itself; the other is a form of REITER SYNDROME. The presence of full-blown AIDS encourages the development of some malignancies, the most common being Kaposi's sarcoma, which is a skin CANCER appearing as black bumps on the skin surfaces, with some surrounding red halos. It is most often on the lower limbs, initially painless and symmetrical.

WOMEN WITH AIDS

Kaposi's sarcoma (a kind of CANCER) is less common than in men. With female circumcision, there is an increase in HIV transmission. The following genital conditions are worse in women with AIDS than those without: CANCER, HERPES, PELVIC INFECTION. Babies born to these women are more likely to die before or shortly after birth; they are more likely to have low birth weight. Malaria during pregnancy is both more common and worse in HIV-positive women.

NEWBORNS WITH HIV

Those born by C-section are less likely to acquire HIV than those born vaginally. Some HIV is acquired through breast milk, but survival is still better in most developing areas by having the children exclusively breast fed than by using bottle feeds.

CHILDREN WITH HIV

There is slower growth, and development is delayed; there may be a stiff weakness and a very small head. PNEUMONIA is common. There may be swelling of the glands in front of the ears, giving a chipmunk-type appearance. There may be swelling of the finger tips associated with breathing difficulties. There will be a poor response to immunizations, so you might see clinical diseases against which the child has been immunized. Also there will be delayed closure of the soft spot on the head of an infant and delayed teething, even if the child is not otherwise ill.

Similar conditions: see Protocols B.6 (limb swelling); B.12 (large lymph nodes); B.10.A (fever and lethargy). TUBERCULOSIS may be indistinguishable. VISCERAL LEISHMANIASIS may also appear similar, as may the weight loss that follows MEASLES. RADIATION ILLNESS may also appear similar. MALNUTRITION as well as MUMPS and ALCOHOLISM can cause similar swellings by the ears. RICKETS causes similar developmental delays, as does congenital SYPHILIS.

Diseases interacting with HIV infection: most diseases make HIV infections worse and the presence of HIV infection makes other diseases worse.
Diseases not interacting with HIV infection: LEPROSY, AFRICAN SLEEPING SICKNESS, CHAGA'S DISEASE, SCHISTOSOMIASIS, FILARIASIS.

Treatment

Prevention: dispose of used syringes and needles and/or pressure cook them or use bleach water to wash and then boil them. Use gloves when suturing and handling blood or other body fluids. Wash your hands. Avoid promiscuity. Avoid injections of any sort. Avoid dental care in heavily infected areas. Even if your dentist is conscientious, it's likely that he hires a low-paid employee to do his cleaning and sterilizing.

---

1 HIV stands for human immunodeficiency virus.
2 Acquired immunodeficiency syndrome

TOC   SYMPTOMS   DIFFERENTIALS   CONDITIONS   DRUG INDEX   REGIONAL NOTES   INX

In case of an inadvertent exposure (blood or rape), there are preventive medications that might be helpful. An appropriate protocol and a reserve supply of medicines should be kept by each family residing in a remote area. The best protocol changes from time to time, and there are coexisting conditions that contraindicate the use of these medicines.

Referrals: see Volume 1, Appendix 13. Laboratory: there are varying tests of varying accuracy. Almost all the tests in developing countries are antibody tests, which means that they measure the proteins in the body that fight the virus rather than the virus itself. So if the person got infected recently, his test will be falsely negative. It might also be falsely negative if he has such advanced disease that his body ceases to fight the infection anymore. Two simple rapid tests especially for developing countries are the particle agglutination assay and the dot immunobinding assay.

Hospital tests:

p24 becomes positive at less than one month.

IgM becomes positive at less than 6 months.

IgG becomes positive at less than 1 year. The standard diagnostic test is ELISA which, however, may fail to detect some infections, and it may be falsely positive. The Western Blot test can differentiate the two kinds of HIV (1 and 2), and it is needed to confirm a positive ELISA. Beware of a positive test that does not make sense; it might be due to laboratory glassware not having been washed well. Have the test repeated at a different, more elite facility.

Following the course of the disease: in Western laboratories CD4 lymphocyte counts are determined. CD4 lymphocytes are a kind of white blood cell. If the CD4 count is 500 or more, then the patient still has decent immunity. If the CD4 count falls below 200, then immunity is poor, and the patient is at risk of infection. A substitute for CD4 count is the total lymphocyte count. If the total lymphocyte count falls below 1000, this indicates a probable CD4 count of less than 200, since CD4 lymphocytes constitute 20% or less of the total lymphocytes.

If a person has a CBC (complete blood count) that includes a total white cell count and also gives the percent of the different types of white cells, one can guess at the CD4 count. Multiply the total white cell count by the percent of lymphocytes (converted to a decimal); this gives the total lymphocyte count. For example, if the total white count is 8,000 and the percent of lymphocytes is 25%, then the lymphocyte count is 8,000 x 0.25 = 2,000. Then the CD4 count may be estimated to be not greater than 20% of this number (2000 x 0.20 = 400, indicating a borderline immunity). But if the total white cell count is 2,000 and the percent of lymphocytes is 40%, then the lymphocyte count is 800, and the CD4 count is probably below 200. Facilities: IVs and advanced drugs at level 3, 4 or 5 might be helpful. Practitioners: an infectious disease specialist is ideal; a general practitioner, internist or pediatrician might be helpful.

Patient care: CO-TRIMOXAZOLE for all HIV-positive patients. It may be useful to give prophylactic CO-TRIMOXAZOLE to infants of HIV-positive mothers. Some retroviral drugs are: ABACAVIR, INDINAVIR, LAMIVUDINE, LOPINAVIR, NEVIRAPINE, RITONAVIR, ZIDOVUDINE. The treatment of HIV infection is beyond the scope of this book, and thus only those drugs used in prevention after an HIV exposure are listed. You should not be using these drugs for infected people. See Volume 1 Chapter 2 for body fluid exposures; Volume 1 Appendix 14 for evaluation post sexual assault.

- The program of anti-retroviral drugs is called HAART. HAART must be used under professional medical supervision. Do not give HAART drugs at the same time as RIFAMPIN[3] because RIFAMPIN will make them ineffective. Either delay the HAART until after the patient has finished RIFAMPIN or else choose drug(s) other than RIFAMPIN (and related drugs). When using HAART avoid St John's wort, garlic and vitamin C. Fish oil is good to take with HAART drugs.

- There are some reports that deworming HIV+ patients may delay the disease progression.

- If the patient has persistent diarrhea that is not responsive to the usual treatments, it may respond well to ALBENDAZOLE or else a change in diet. Avoid wheat and rye, substituting corn and rice for other grains.

- PNEUMONIA might respond to PENTAMIDINE if other antibiotics fail.

- Keep the patient on CO-TRIMOXAZOLE permanently. It prevents certain kinds of infections as well as covering MALARIA prevention.

- There are some unsubstantiated reports that the antimalarial herb, Artemisia annua (see ARTEMISININ) will reverse some of the symptoms of advanced AIDS when it is given together with Moringa olifiera plus a high-protein diet, multivitamins and minerals. Lemon grass tea is helpful to improve the appetite. ALOE VERA might also improve the patient's health.

- A high-protein diet with vitamins and minerals helps.

- ZINC supplements of 12–15 mg of elemental zinc per day may delay immune failure and help with diarrhea.

---

3 *RIFAMPIN is a mainstay drug for TUBERCULOSIS.*

HIVES

See ALLERGY and/or DRUG ERUPTION. Hives are very itchy, raised, flat-topped bumps on the skin. These may arise from exposure to something injected, eaten or inhaled. Hives from ALLERGY start within 10 minutes of the exposure, and they last less than 24 hours once the substance is removed. Hives that last more than a day arise from some underlying disease. Treatment is complex; the underlying disease must be diagnosed and treated.

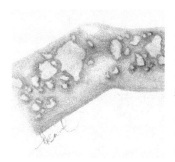

Hives are very itchy. They are raised up above the skin surface, like a bas relief map. Sizes and shapes are variable and irregular. Larger ones are relatively flat-topped, not peaked. They start out pale with red rings around them; then they change to being red without rings; see the next illustration. AB

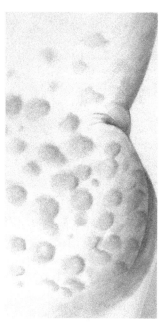

These are also hives. In this case the bumps are a reddish color, darker than the surrounding skin. They may be very difficult to see on very black skin. OW

HOOKWORM

Regional Notes: F, I, M, O, S, U.

Includes: ancylostomiasis, necatoriasis, uncinariasis.

Definition: hookworm is a bowel infestation with either one of two similar species of worms: *Necator americanus* or *Ancylostoma duodenale*. The worms are barely visible to the naked eye.

Not ill to very ill; class 1–2; worldwide, mostly with sandy, moist, shaded soil. Unusual with clay soil. Occurs almost exclusively in tropical areas below 2000 meters (6000 feet) in areas with loam or sandy soil.

Age: any. **Who:** those whose skin touches contaminated soil; those eating contaminated food. **Onset:** rash develops rapidly; other symptoms develop over weeks.

Clinical

May be without symptoms but diagnosed by a medical laboratory; without lab, one should suspect it in a patient with ANEMIA in the arable tropics.

Initially: a rash might appear on skin exposed to soil, usually on soft skin (e.g., between toes).

Days to weeks later: symptoms of PNEUMONIA or ASTHMA occur as the worms travel through the lungs.

Then: upper abdominal pain (which may be relieved by food) and ANEMIA develop. With severe infections the patient may have black, tarry, obviously bloody or mucous diarrhea stool like DYSENTERY.

Later still: he may have shortness of breath, leg swelling, loss of appetite, leg cramps with walking. Men may become impotent.

Occasionally: in severe cases there may be general body swelling and HEART FAILURE. Children may have strong food cravings.

Similar conditions: *The initial rash* might resemble SCABIES. *The lung migration phase* is indistinguishable from PNEUMONIA or ASTHMA.

In the bowel phase, the disease resembles other types of WORMS, DYSENTERY or other causes of ANEMIA.

Severe ANEMIA from hookworm may cause HEART FAILURE. In this case it may be difficult to distinguish from wet BERIBERI

Bush laboratory: check stool for blood three times; it should be positive at least once. Check for ANEMIA.

Treatment

Prevention: wear shoes; encourage use of outhouses.

Referrals: laboratory: those that have microscopes, possibly level 2, certainly level 3, can check stool for hookworm eggs; it is an easy and reliable test. It is moderately sensitive but very specific; three negative samples from 3 days, collected and processed fast, would eliminate the diagnosis. There are commonly false-negatives if any time elapses—as little as 3 hours—between the patient passing the stool and the lab examining it. Before the stool is positive for the eggs (for a couple weeks to a couple months), there will be an increase in the number of eosinophils in the blood. However, other diseases can also cause this. Facilities: with severe ANEMIA, a blood bank for transfusion might be helpful. Practitioner: general practitioner, internist, pediatrician.

Patient care: treat ANEMIA using IRON and MULTIVITAMINS. Use MEBENDAZOLE, PYRANTEL PAMOATE, TETRACHLOROETHYLENE[1] or ALBENDAZOLE. FLUBENDAZOLE, BEPHENIUM HYDROXYNAPHTHOATE, NITAZOXANIDE or LEVAMISOLE may work also. Treat a second time a week later if possible, but one treatment is better than none.

---

1 *This drug does not work against ASCARIASIS. Therefore, if you use it, you should treat for ASCARIASIS first if it occurs in your area. You will know that ASCARIASIS occurs if anyone says he has passed worms by rectum or by mouth. ASCARIASIS worms are the size of earthworms or larger.*

HYDATID DISEASE

Regional Notes: E, F, I, K, M, N, O, R, S, U

Entry category: two indistinguishable diseases.

Synonyms: echinococcosis, unilocular echinococcosis, multilocular echinococcosis.

Definition: hydatid disease is an infestation with a larval form of animal hookworm, causing tumor(s) or cyst(s) that grow slowly, over decades. There are two kinds: granulosus and multilocularis. Granulosis affects any organ, but mostly the lungs. Multilocularis affects the liver almost exclusively.

Cause: tumor, caused by animal hookworm.

Not ill to very ill; class 2–4; regional: Greece, Argentina, Xinjiang China, Australia and Kenya's Turkana region. It is also common in the rural, semi-rural and suburban areas of western Europe, related there to the fox population. Multilocularis is rampant in the Arctic.

Age: symptoms in any above 5 y.o. **Who:** common in ethnic groups that keep dogs, where the dogs live close to the people; it also occurs in temperate, forested areas, where people gather and eat foods contaminated with the stool of wild animals. **Onset:** slowly; the incubation period is measured in years.

Clinical

This depends on the organ(s) affected. The following are from the most to the least common.

LIVER

The liver enlarges. There may be a lump on the liver's edge. The lump may burst causing sudden ANAPHYLAXIS, ACUTE ABDOMEN or both.

LUNG

Cough, shortness of breath, fever and PLEURISY. He may have symptoms of ALLERGY. If the cyst ruptures, the patient will cough up a mouthful of salty fluid.

BOWEL

Abdominal swelling leading to ACUTE ABDOMEN, Type 3.

SKIN

A lump is under the skin; it feels like a water balloon.

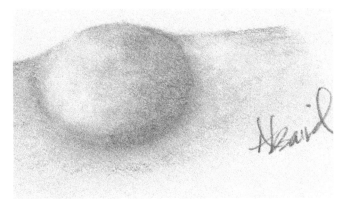

This is a lump under the skin due to hydatid; it is soft and non-tender. Similar conditions are ABSCESS, LOIASIS and LIPOMA. AB

BREAST

A lump which feels like a water balloon.

BONE

Pain, possibly with spontaneous fracture.

SPLEEN

Similar to liver, but on the left side.

BRAIN

STROKE, BRAIN TUMOR.

KIDNEY

A big bulge develops in the back waist area, possibly with pain. KIDNEY DISEASE may occur after a time.

Complications: ANAPHYLAXIS, ALLERGY, ASTHMA, all common with dog-transmitted disease. Also consider LIVER FAILURE, RESPIRATORY FAILURE, ACUTE ABDOMEN, KIDNEY DISEASE, STROKE, BRAIN DAMAGE.

Similar conditions: see Protocol B.7 for other causes of a large liver and/or spleen.

Liver: AMEBIASIS, GALLBLADDER DISEASE, liver CANCER. *Lung*: PNEUMONIA, TUBERCULOSIS. *Bowel*: ASCARIASIS, abdominal TUBERCULOSIS. *Skin*: SYPHILIS (tertiary), CYSTICERCOSIS. *Breast*: MASTITIS, CANCER, TUBERCULOSIS. *Bone*: TUBERCULOSIS, CANCER. *Spleen*: TROPICAL SPLENOMEGALY. *Brain*: CYSTICERCOSIS and similar diseases. *Kidney*: CANCER.

Treatment

Referrals: see Volume 1, Appendix 13. Laboratory: hospitals can do blood tests, x-rays or ultrasound. The blood tests are more reliable in the wild animal-transmitted than in the dog-transmitted forms of the disease. Facilities: ultrasound is most helpful; in some cases a surgical theatre is necessary. Practitioners: infectious disease specialist with tropical/travel expertise is ideal; a general practitioner or internist might be helpful. A surgeon may be necessary.

Patient care: traditionally this has always been surgical, only after the patient has taken a full course of deworming medication. ALBENDAZOLE is the drug of choice. FLUBENDAZOLE may work well. Reportedly PRAZIQUANTEL might be helpful. The combination of ALBENDAZOLE and PRAZIQUANTEL may be helpful.

HYDROCELE

Cause: unknown.

Clinical

Hydrocele is a swelling next to one or both testicles in males of any age, due to a pocket of watery fluid. Both sides are affected. The swelling does not go all the way up into the groin. There is an illustration in Volume 1 Chapter 1.

Similar conditions: it differs from a hernia in that the swelling is confined to the scrotum, not extending up to the groin. It differs from tumor in that a small light placed behind the swelling in a dark room shows it to be translucent; only the testicle is opaque. It generally is not at all painful or tender. The testicle is totally surrounded by water so it cannot be felt within the scrotum.

Treatment

Hydrocele can be corrected with surgery whenever it is convenient to do so. Send the patient to a hospital.

Hyperimmune malarial splenomegaly

See TROPICAL SPLENOMEGALY.

HYPERTENSION

Regional Notes: E, F, U.

Entry category: syndrome.

Synonym: high blood pressure.

Definition: adult resting BP over 140/90 for Westerners and 130/80 for nationals, both at rest.

Cause: variable.

Not ill to moderately ill; class 1–4, depending on severity; it is somewhat related to salt consumption.

Age: any, but mainly adults. **Who:** anyone, but especially Westerners and those with KIDNEY DISEASE. Many of the medicines used for ASTHMA can cause this, as well as licorice (a kind of black or red candy). **Onset:** over months; more rapidly in pregnancy and KIDNEY DISEASE.

Clinical

Necessary: blood pressure is higher than normal, even at rest and this has been found at least 3 times.[1]

Maybe: the patient may have no symptoms, or he may have headaches.

Complications: if the pressure goes very high, he will have HEART FAILURE, KIDNEY DISEASE or STROKE. He may become blind. Hypertension can both cause KIDNEY DISEASE and be caused by it. It may cause nosebleed which can be severe and will not stop until the blood pressure is lowered.

Similar conditions: TOXEMIA, STROKE, KIDNEY DISEASE and HEART FAILURE are associated with hypertension. Check for these, but do not fail to treat the hypertension in the meantime.

Bush laboratory: urinalysis might show protein.

Treatment

Prevention: frequent blood pressure checks; avoid eating salt.

Referrals: see Volume 1, Appendix 13. Laboratory: level 3 and above hospital labs can do blood tests and electrocardiograms to check for possible causes and for complications. Facilities; a monitored bed is desirable in critical cases. Practitioner: internist, obstetrician/gynecologist, possibly other specialists if there is a specific cause.

Patient care: higher-level care is very desirable as you are incapable of determining the specific cause. In every case, tell the patient to avoid salt and baking powder in his diet; to lose weight if he is overweight and to exercise regularly.

(Subtract 10 points off the following blood pressures for non-Westerners in developing areas.)

140/90 to 160/100: HYDROCHLOROTHIAZIDE, 50 mg by mouth daily and a low-salt diet. If KIDNEY DISEASE is not a problem, then (and only then) also increase dietary potassium intake (e.g., eat apricots, avocados, bananas, coconut water, dates, papaya, potatoes, pumpkin, spinach, tomatoes or citrus fruits).

160/100 to 190/110: drug and diet as above plus LISINOPRIL or NIFEDIPINE. Those with African genetic heritage might not respond to LISINOPRIL. Anyone with blood pressure over this must be sent out, treating as above in the meantime.

HYDRALAZINE may substitute for NIFEDIPINE. PROPRANOLOL or VERAPAMIL may be added.

FUROSEAMIDE may substitute for HYDROCHLOROTHIAZIDE. If you substitute another drug, use the dose for that drug rather than for the original drug. In the presence of KIDNEY DISEASE, use that diet rather than the one listed above.

Do not stop or reduce treatment when the pressure comes down to normal levels, but do reduce doses if the pressure goes below the normal range. Seek other advice.

Results: 2 weeks for HYDROCHLOROTHIAZIDE alone; 6 hours for both drugs.

---

1 *Do not treat high blood pressure on the basis of only one or two readings. Be sure the cuff is large enough in a patient who is obese.*

HYPERVENTILATION

Regional Notes: O.

Entry category: syndrome.

Definition: hyperventilation is the state in which a patient is breathing deeper and faster than necessary for the amount of air exchange he requires.

Cause: anxiety.

Very ill during an episode; class 1; worldwide, related to culture.

Age: usually only adults. **Who:** more females than males, more emotional than stoical. **Onset:** suddenly over minutes.

Clinical

Necessary: the patient breathes rapidly, feeling very short of breath. He is dizzy and very anxious or panicked. He is not blue and his breathing is not noisy.

Maybe: he might feel numb around the lips, have numbness, tingling and cramping of the hands, lose consciousness and have a SEIZURE.

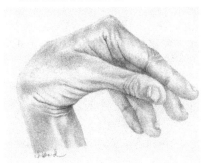

This hand is cramped because of hyperventilation. The wrist is flexed. The fingers are stiff. The thumb is close to the other fingers, not spread out. The knuckles may be flexed as they are here or they might be extended. AB

Similar conditions: with ANAPHYLAXIS the patient's hands are never cramped. Persistent vomiting, CHOLERA, RICKETS and some hormonal problems can cause similar hand cramping without shortness of breath.

Treatment

Put your cupped hands or a paper bag over the mouth and nose of the patient so he re-breathes some of the air he breathes out. (Never use a plastic bag.) This should solve the problem within 5 to 10 minutes. Deal with emotional causes if necessary.

HYPOGLYCEMIA

Regional Notes: F, M.

Entry category: syndrome.

Synonyms: low blood sugar, insulin reaction.

Definition: hypoglycemia is the state of too little sugar in the blood.

Mildly to very ill; class 1–3; worldwide with varying causes.

Age: any. **Who:** anyone, especially those with MALARIA or MALNUTRITION. **Onset:** slow onset and recurrent usually. Rapid onset when caused by various diseases, drugs or poisons.

Clinical

Necessary: the patient is either weak, sweaty and shaky, or he is sweaty and unconscious[2]. Sugar abolishes the symptoms.

Maybe: the patient may be quite emotional, laughing or crying with the slightest provocation. He may appear to be drunk. He may have SEIZURES. His pulse will be rapid, and he is likely to be lethargic or fatigued.

Causative diseases: MALARIA and/or the QUININE used to treat it; MALNUTRITION; PLANT POISONING due to akee; poisoning with drugs used to treat DIABETES (especially INSULIN).

Similar conditions: alcohol withdrawal, see ALCOHOLISM; RELAPSING FEVER treatment; SHOCK from any cause.

Bush laboratory: there are blood dipsticks, similar to urine dipsticks, that can indicate if the blood sugar is low, normal or high.

Treatment

Referrals: laboratory: level 2 or above. Facilities: in severe cases, IV's with fluids are helpful. Practitioners: general practitioner, internist, pediatrician.

Patient care: if the patient is not alert, prompt treatment is essential. Use IV fluids with sugar or use a stomach tube with sugar water.

For the spontaneous type in an alert patient, recommend six small, sugar-free meals a day. Sugar helps the problem immediately but tends to provoke more episodes. Provide nourishment in MALNUTRITION.

HYPOTHERMIA

Regional Notes: F.

Entry category: syndrome, environmental.

Synonyms: exposure.

Definition: hypothermia is an abnormally low body temperature.

Cause: cold exposure.

Moderately to very ill; class 1–3 depending on how cold the patient is.

Age: any. **Who:** inadequately clothed and exposed to cold, especially infants, old people and those wet or hungry. **Onset:** variable.

---

2 *Some people who are on heart drugs such as PROPRANOLOL may fail to be sweaty or shaky and will just be unconscious or lethargic. This kind of drug is generally only available in developed areas; it is usually prescribed for people who have HYPERTENSION, who have had ANGINA or a HEART ATTACK.*

Clinical

Necessary: the patient has been exposed to cold, maybe lost and wet and cold overnight. He has a low body temperature, 35.5°C (96°F) or less.

Maybe: he is either very lethargic or unconscious and may have a low or no blood pressure and a slow or no pulse.

Complication: GANGRENE.

Similar conditions: see Protocol B.10.B.

Treatment

Even if you do not find a blood pressure or pulse, the patient may be alive. The patient is not certainly dead until he is warm and dead, unless he is frozen solid!

- Remove cold wet clothing. Warm him gently with heated blankets. As soon as one blanket cools, replace it with another warm dry one. If he is conscious, give him hot tea to drink.

- Breathe for the patient if he is unconscious, and does not appear to be breathing adequately.

- Watch closely for signs of life. Give up after a few hours or after the body is warm and dead.

- If you are successful (and he was unconscious), send him out. This is not necessary if he never lost consciousness.

- Check for FROSTBITE and treat this if it occurs.

IMMERSION FOOT / TRENCH FOOT

This is tissue damage caused by exposure to cold, water or both. Initially the feet are cold, swollen and white, possibly with a bluish tinge. They are numb. With warming, they become red, hot and dry. They are also weak. About 10 days later there are sharp, shooting pains in the feet. It may take weeks to recover from the numbness and weakness. Once this happens, the patient is prone to its happening again. The symptoms may vary somewhat, depending on if the problem is wet cold or dry cold. GANGRENE is a possible complication.

IMPACTION

Definition: an impaction is hard-packed stool in the rectum, which the patient is unable to pass.

Cause: constipation in bedridden people.

Mildly to moderately ill; class 1 usually; worldwide.

Age: any. **Who:** chronically ill, old, paralyzed. **Onset:** days.

Clinical

Necessary: the patient is constipated. If you put a gloved finger in the rectum, you will feel it packed with hard stool.

Sometimes: he has small amounts of watery diarrhea that flows past the hard stool. Abdominal pain is frequent.

Similar conditions: ACUTE ABDOMEN, Type 3; always check first for impaction and remove the stool before sending the patient out. It may make the hospital trip unnecessary. ASCARIASIS, abdominal TUBERCULOSIS, CANCER and HYDATID DISEASE can cause bowel obstruction, but in these cases there is no hard stool in the rectum.

Treatment

Referrals: for severe or recurrent problems, a level 3 or above hospital with a surgeon might be helpful.

Patient care: remove hard stool by pulling it out with your gloved fingers. Then try an oil enema. Do not use laxatives or large volume enemas until some stool is out.

Results: within a day.

IMPETIGO

Regional Notes: U.

Synonym: pyoderma.

Definition: impetigo is a bacterial infection of the outer layers of the skin, almost always Gram-positive.

Cause: bacteria.

Not ill; class 1; contagious; worldwide and very common everywhere.

Age: any, especially babies and children. **Who:** anyone; usually a history of some minor injury or scabies. **Onset:** hours to a day or two.

Clinical

Necessary: an area of skin is rough, with irregular bumps like pimples or blisters which are broken open and weeping. These form an off-white to dark brown to honey-colored crust with a rough, variously colored surface. In some cases the skin resembles sandpaper. The area might be painful or itch, but not intensely.

Maybe: fever occurs if the problem is severe. There may be visible pus.

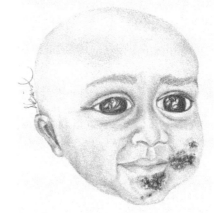

Impetigo on the face usually has a mixture of dark-colored and gold crusts. It is common in children. AB

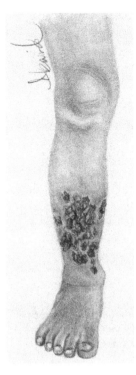

Impetigo on the legs usually has dark-colored crusts; it is also called pyoderma. AB

Complications: KIDNEY DISEASE, nephritic type; TETANUS, other bacterial infections.

Similar conditions: DIPHTHERIA which affects the nose, causing a similar skin condition on the upper lip. YAWS has discreet circles, both bumps and ulcers on the same patient, whereas impetigo is over irregularly shaped areas. CUTANEOUS LEISHMANIASIS is also discreet, with either bumps or ulcers but not both. SEXUALLY TRANSMITTED DISEASE causes spontaneous wounds on the genital area or near the mouth. Lupus vulgaris, a form of skin TUBERCULOSIS, may be indistinguishable.

Treatment

Prevention: cleanliness; encourage the use of soap.

Patient care: washing with warm water and soap and drying well 4 times a day will usually suffice if there is no fever. Cover the area with IODINE ointment or ANTIBIOTIC CREAM or ANTIBIOTIC OINTMENT between washings. Use an oral antibiotic such as PENICILLIN, ERYTHROMYCIN, CEPHALOSPORIN or AZITHROMYCIN if the problem is severe.

Results: it should improve within a week.

INDIAN CHILDHOOD CIRRHOSIS (ICC)

Entry category: disease, probably toxic.

Definition: ICC is a severe, progressive type of LIVER FAILURE which affects Indian children both in India and elsewhere.

Cause: it is thought to be caused by feeding milk from bronze drinking vessels. It occurs less often where bronze drinking vessels are not used.

Age: children. **Who:** it affects boys more than girls, middle class more than upper class or poor and Hindus more than non-Hindus. It tends to run in families, mostly in families originating in southern India, Calcutta and Punjab. **Onset:** the disease begins gradually, but once it begins death is almost inevitable.

Clinical

There may be a low-grade fever. The child is irritable, and has a tender, swollen abdomen full of fluid (See Volume 1, Chapter 1). The liver is first enlarged and then it shrinks. The spleen is enlarged and hard. There is JAUNDICE. There may be abnormal bleeding: nosebleeds; bloody urine, stool or vomit; bleeding gums; excessive bleeding from minor wounds. Sometimes HYPERTENSION develops.

Treatment

It is difficult, but there are some newer treatments that permit survival.

Referrals: a level 3 or above hospital is essential to confirm the diagnosis and eliminate more treatable causes of liver failure. Find someone familiar with this disease. Most physicians don't know about it.

INFLUENZA

(New definition, epidemic influenza)

During the past decade 'influenza' has come to mean very specific virus infections with designations such as H1N1, or H3N2. Each year immunizations are developed that address that year's particular virus. Some of these viruses are very serious, with substantial mortality even amongst previously healthy patients. Whereas by the previous definition one could only offer supportive care, with the epidemic influenzas there are now blood tests for diagnosis and effective drugs for treatment.

The usual symptoms are fever, cough, sore throat, nasal congestion, headache in adults, vomiting and diarrhea additionally in children. General muscle aches may or may not be present. In other words, it presents like a severe cold (RESPIRATORY INFECTION in this manual), with a fever higher than one would usually find with an ordinary cold. Thus the essentials for diagnosis are:

    a. an epidemic setting; and

    b. a 'cold' with an unusually high fever.

It is nearly indistinguishable from an ordinary cold and from the initial symptoms of measles.

Treatment involves supportive care first of all. Evacuation to a level 4 or 5 hospital is entirely warranted, especially for the very young and very old who are most at risk of dying from the condition. Level 4 and 5 hospitals can offer better supportive care, plus definitive diagnosis and curative medications.

Cross-references: B-2, measles, respiratory infection, nasal congestion.

Regional Notes: E.

Synonym: flu.

Definition: influenza is a viral infection of the body, causing muscle aching amongst other symptoms.

Mildly to moderately ill; class 1; usually contagious; worldwide and common everywhere.

Age: any. **Who:** anyone. **Onset:** over a day or two.

Clinical

Necessary: the patient feels tired and his muscles ache all over.

Usually: he has nausea, vomiting, abdominal pain, diarrhea, fever under 38.5°C (101.3°F) and headache.

Rarely: complication in children, Reye's Syndrome, causes mental changes and severe persistent vomiting. This requires hospital treatment; give sugar in the meantime.

Similar conditions: see Protocol B.2. In malarious areas treat for MALARIA if there is a fever.

Treatment

Patient care: keep the patient in bed and treat fever, but do not use ASPIRIN or antibiotics.

INSECTICIDE POISONING

Cause: toxin.

Clinical

Insecticides vary one from another, but generally they cause an outpouring of body fluids and activate involuntary muscles. As a result the patient has tearing, much saliva, sweating, coughing due to secretions in the respiratory tract, much urine and diarrhea. See PLANT POISONING, muscarine; the effects are similar. Those exposed to small amounts over a long time may develop PARKINSON'S DISEASE.

Treatment

ATROPINE, giving repeated doses frequently, as much as necessary to counteract the symptoms. This may involve giving much more than the usual dose.

INTESTINAL FLUKE

Regional Notes: E, I, M, O, R, S. This is not known to occur in Africa.

Includes: fasciolopsiasis, heterophyiasis, metagonimiasis, echinostomiasis, gastrodisciasis.

Definition: intestinal fluke is a bowel infestation of any one of the flukes (flat worms) named above.

Cause: worm.

Not ill to very ill; class 1.

The problem occurs in all major regions of the world except Africa south of the Sahara, the Arctic, and the Pacific area. It is a tropical disease. The different varieties of intestinal flukes are found in different areas:

- Fasciolopsiasis is found throughout Asia (Regions I, O, S); it is the most serious.

- Heterophysiasis is found throughout Asia also (Regions I, O, S), plus throughout the R region. It is second in seriousness.

- The other kinds, metagonimiasis, echinostomiasis, gastrodisciasis, are found in Regions E, I, O, S and in Guyana.

Age: any except nursing infants. **Who:** those eating raw or rare fish. Fasciolopsiasis may also be acquired by eating raw water plants or by peeling them with the teeth. **Onset:** incubation 2–3 months; slow insidious onset.

Clinical

This varies by type and geographic area:

FASCIOLOPSIASIS

Most patients have no symptoms at all. In heavy infections, they may have diarrhea alternating with constipation and abdominal pain when hungry, relieved by food. With very severe disease, the patient will have loss of appetite, nausea, vomiting, continuous abdominal pain and swelling of the face and body. He may develop MALABSORPTION, a severe, watery diarrhea causing weight loss. He may accumulate fluid in his abdomen, making him look pregnant.

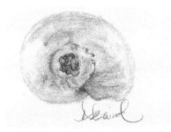

This is the appearance of the snail that carries fasciolopsiasis. AB

HETEROPHYSIASIS

This causes indigestion, abdominal pain, diarrhea like dysentery and occasionally HEART FAILURE or sudden death.

ECHINOSTOMIASIS, GASTRODISCIASIS, METAGONIMIASIS:

These each cause only diarrhea with no long-term consequences.

Similar conditions: *abdominal pain relieved by food:* PEPTIC ULCER. *Alternating constipation and diarrhea:* IRRITABLE BOWEL. *Severe diarrhea:* MALABSORPTION. See Protocol B.14.

Treatment

Prevention: cook fish and water plants well before eating. Do not use teeth to peel raw plants.

Referrals: laboratory: level 3 or above. When the disease is fully developed worm eggs might be found in the stool. Earlier there will be a large number of eosinophils in a blood smear. However, other diseases can also cause that.

Patient care: PRAZIQUANTEL is the drug of choice for most kinds; seek local lore. TETRACHLOROETHYLENE might be more available and/or cheaper. Give a low-fat meal in the evening. Give PROMETHAZINE in the morning, then give TETRACHLOROETHYLENE; 4–5 hours later give MILK OF MAGNESIA or something else to cause diarrhea.[1] NICLOSAMIDE also works but it is not safe.

---

1 *The diarrhea flushes the worms out of the bowel.*

IRIS

This acronym stands for Immune Reconstitution Inflammatory Syndrome. It is a phenomenon in which a patient has increasing symptoms as his immune system recovers its function. The most common scenario is for symptoms of TUBERCULOSIS to begin, recur or worsen within a couple days to a couple months after starting treatment for HIV INFECTION. This may also happen at the beginning of treatment for TUBERCULOSIS without involvement of HIV drugs; LEPROSY treatment can also cause IRIS in the presence of HIV treatment.

Clinical

Fever, large lymph nodes (neck, armpit and groin) and worsening respiratory symptoms. The patient may develop ABSCESSes. There may be mental changes and symptoms of BRAIN DAMAGE.

Treatment

Extremely difficult. The management of the condition should be left to physicians; frequently PREDNISONE is used and IBUPROFEN for symptomatic relief.

IRITIS

Regional Notes: F, R.

Synonyms: uveitis.

Definition: iritis is inflammation of the iris and the surrounding structures of the eye, behind the cornea but in front of the eye's lens.

Cause: variable.

Mildly ill; class 2–3; worldwide.

Age: any. **Who:** anyone, especially those with LEPROSY, TUBERCULOSIS, SYPHILIS, LARVA MIGRANS, REITER SYNDROME, BRUCELLOSIS LEPTOSPIROSIS (during the recovery phase) or eye injury. **Onset:** usually sudden, may be gradual.

Clinical

Necessary: the patient has pain in the eye(s) and his vision is blurred. His pupil is small and irregular, not round; the shape is like a key-hole, oval or scalloped. This is more obvious if you use drops to dilate the eye (HOMATROPINE OPHTHALMIC).

Usually: the white of the eye is red, but the redness is more around the cornea than further out (in contrast to other problems in which the redness is either worse further out or the same all over). The patient avoids light since it aggravates the pain; he has increased tears. The pain may be aggravated when a light is shone into the opposite (good) eye or when the patient shifts between near and far vision. If the problem has been for a long time, he may have little or no pain but only blurry vision.

Occasionally: the patient has a fever.

If you have an ophthalmoscope, move the magnification to +20–30. If you look at the eye, you will see black dots on the shiny red pupil.

Similar conditions: see Protocol B.8. SYPHILIS (tertiary) might cause iritis. Also consider TB of the eye and XEROPHTHALMIA (poor vision in dim light).

Treatment

Referrals: a level 3 or above facility with an ophthalmologist (an optometrist at a minimum) is most helpful. *Patient care:* do not treat for this unless you are sure of the diagnosis! If the pupil has an irregular shape and this is not the way it was before, and there is no facial rash, then treatment might be safe. But you should still seek outside advice. Use steroid eye drops, such as PREDNISOLONE EYE DROPS (labeled ophthalmic), using one or two drops every hour until the inflammation has subsided; then use them 4 times a day for 4 days, no longer.

IRRITABLE BOWEL

Regional Notes: F, I, M.

Synonyms: spastic bowel, spastic colitis.

Definition: irritable bowel is a bowel prone to cramping, constipation or diarrhea. It may occur for no good reason, or it may be caused by stress, unfamiliar foods or dietary indiscretion.

Mildly ill; class 1; worldwide, related to culture.

Age: any. **Who:** anyone, especially those who have had this before. **Onset:** variable. Some people have this on occasion, some their whole lives.

Clinical

Necessary: the patient has crampy abdominal pain with either diarrhea, constipation or both alternating. The location of the pain is around the navel or all over, or the location moves. (However, if it just moves from upper or center abdomen to the lower-right and then stays there, it may be ACUTE ABDOMEN.) There is no fever. The patient does not howl if you jar the bed. The diarrhea does not awaken him at night.

Maybe: the abdomen may be tender all over.

Causative diseases: GIARDIASIS, MANSONELLOSIS PERSTANS, TOXOPLASMOSIS, MONONUCLEOSIS, other infections.

Similar conditions: STRONGYLOIDIASIS may be similar but it causes an itchy rectum. Check for a blue line on the gums; if you find it, the patient may have LEAD POISONING. ENDOMETRIOSIS, GASTROENTERITIS and FOOD POISONING (if the patient eats alone) might be indistinguishable. Early DYSENTERY due to amebae might be similar. Various WORMS might cause similar symptoms.

Treatment

Referrals: laboratory: level 3 or above might be useful to eliminate other possible diagnoses. Practitioner: general practitioner, internist, pediatrician.

Patient care: use DICYCLOMINE or CHAMOMILE TEA to relieve the pain. Address stresses in the patient's life.

JAUNDICE

Cause: variable.

Regional Notes: F, M, O, S, U.

Entry category: syndrome cluster; See Protocol B.7 to arrive at a diagnosis.

Definition: jaundice means yellow skin, yellow whites of the eyes or both.

Clinical

ORDINARY JAUNDICE, NOT NEWBORN
When mild, the yellow color is first visible underneath the tongue, in the tab of tissue that holds the tongue to the floor of the mouth in the center line. It is easiest to see in sunlight and hardest to see under fluorescent lights. With true jaundice, the whites of the eyes are yellow. The urine will test positive for bilirubin, urobilinogen or both.

JAUNDICE IN NEWBORNS
Normally jaundice in newborns becomes visible the first or second day. If it is after the second day, then it is probably due to some illness, not the normal transient jaundice that many babies have. It is seen first on the face and forehead. Firm pressure on the skin makes it more visible. After that it is seen on the trunk and limbs. The infant is apt to be drowsy. If there are stiff or floppy muscles, SEIZURES or a change in voice, this mandates immediate transfer to a hospital. This jaundice occurs more in east Asians and at high altitudes, less in African babies.

THERE ARE 3 CAUSES OF JAUNDICE:

DUE TO DESTRUCTION OF RED BLOOD CELLS
In this case the jaundice is a pure yellow. There is urobilinogen in the urine but no bilirubin. (It is normal to have 1+ urobilinogen in the urine. Only 2+ and more are abnormal.) This is the usual kind that newborns have, not due to disease.

Diseases that cause jaundice by destroying red cells (resulting in more urobilinogen than bilirubin in the urine): MALARIA, SICKLE CELL DISEASE, TROPICAL SPLENOMEGALY, THALLASEMIA, BARTONELLOSIS, OVALOCYTOSIS, VISCERAL LEISHMANIASIS.

DUE TO LIVER DAMAGE
In this case the jaundice is orangish-yellow, and there is bilirubin in the urine. There is more bilirubin than urobilinogen. If you don't have the urine dipsticks to check for bilirubin, put some of the patient's urine in a clear glass container. Put some normal urine in a similar container. Shake them both. If there is bilirubin in the patient's urine, it will get a larger head of foam on the top than normal urine, and the foam will be yellowish.

Diseases that cause jaundice by liver damage (resulting in more bilirubin than urobilinogen in the urine): MALARIA, HEPATITIS, PNEUMONIA, SCHISTOSOMIASIS JAPONICUM, SCHISTOSOMIASIS MANSONI, YELLOW FEVER, INDIAN CHILDHOOD CIRRHOSIS, LIVER FLUKE.

DUE TO BILE BLOCKAGE
The bile cannot pass from the liver to the intestines. In this case the jaundice is greenish-yellow. There is bilirubin in the urine. Frequently jaundice from this cause will result in severe, whole-body itching. The patient will say that he itches deep inside his body, where he can't scratch. If the jaundice is intense, the stool is likely to be white or very light-colored.

Diseases that cause jaundice by blocking bile flow (give light-colored stools): ASCARIASIS, GALLBLADDER DISEASE, LIVER FLUKE, CANCER.

Similar conditions: *s*ee Protocols B.5 (Fever + Jaundice) and B.7 (Liver/Spleen Problems). *With excess consumption of yellow/orange foods* such as carrots, the skin will turn yellow, but the whites of the eyes are still white. This is not true jaundice; it will pass with a dietary change.

Help with diagnosis and treatment:

- Jaundice with fever: Protocol B.5.
- Jaundice without fever; painless in middle age: check CANCER. Also consider MALARIA if the patient is seen when the temperature happens to be down.
- Newborn: see Volume 1, Chapter 6.
- Infant: see MALARIA, HEPATITIS, TUBERCULOSIS; SYPHILIS, SEPSIS; check similar diseases listed under these.

Treatment

Referrals: laboratory; a level 3 hospital can do a blood test to determine the seriousness of the jaundice and sometimes the cause. Facilities: many imaging and other facilities at a level 3, 4 or 5 might be helpful. Practitioner; a gastroenterologist is ideal. A general practitioner or internist is appropriate initially.

Patient care, newborns: put the infant under a special intense light, no more than 50 cm (20 inches) away. Sunlight also works but not as well as the specially made artificial lights. Newborns who have jaundice may have green teeth later in life.

Patient care, not newborns: one can only treat symptoms. For itching due to jaundice: try CHOLESTYRAMINE; RIFAMPIN; sun exposure 1–2 hours daily.

JET LAG

Definition: jet lag is a problem of a change in day and night cycles, frequently with profound emotional changes (irritability, DEPRESSION) which lasts for up to 2 weeks after travel over 6 or more time zones. It is worse with traveling east than traveling west. It is treatable with MELATONIN (see Drug Index.)

KATAYAMA DISEASE

Regional Notes: F, I, O, R.

Cause: allergy

Definition: Katayama disease is an allergic reaction to a germ or worm infestation. It is the initial stage of a number of diseases, especially KIDNEY INFECTION, HYDATID DISEASE, GUINEA WORM and SCHISTOSOMIASIS (any kind but especially JAPONICUM). How common it is and which diseases it is related to in a particular area, varies greatly. It is one particular type of SERUM SICKNESS. Also see SERUM SICKNESS.

Mildly to severely ill; class 2–3; worldwide.

Entry category: syndrome.

Age: any **Who:** those exposed to these diseases, usually expatriates. **Onset:** usually rapid, 3–8 weeks after exposure.

Clinical

Katayama disease causes fever, HIVES, nausea, diarrhea, headache, fatigue, loss of appetite or any combination of these symptoms. About half the patients have respiratory symptoms. It may resemble ASTHMA. It may be severe and life-threatening. At least initially, the symptoms tend to come and go.

Usually the respiratory complaints are first, and the abdominal complaints follow thereafter. The patient may give a history of having had SWIMMER'S ITCH 3–6 weeks before.

Similar conditions: consider ASTHMA and ALLERGY though in these cases there usually is no fever. TRICHINOSIS can be similar, but it is rare except in outbreaks with a number of patients.

Bush laboratory: when the cause is SCHISTOSOMIASIS, the stool might (or might not) have eggs in it. Eventually it will have eggs, in a matter of days or weeks. You might be able to check this yourself with the lab procedure for hatching the eggs. See Appendix 2. The sedimentation rate will be elevated.

Treatment

Prevention: reportedly, ARTEMISININ, taken shortly after exposure, prevents Katayama disease. It is uncertain if it prevents the infection or only the symptoms.

Referrals: laboratory; a blood count may show an abnormally large percentage of eosinophils (over 5%). However, there are a number of other diseases that will also cause this. Facilities: it is safest to treat this in a level 3 or higher facility with IV's and a monitored bed. Practitioners: general practitioner, internist, pediatrician, tropical/travel expertise.

Patient care: ASPIRIN and, if absolutely necessary, HYDROCORTISONE or PREDNISONE. Also treat for whatever seems to be the most likely cause. Be sure to use PREDNISONE together with PRAZIQUANTEL.

KELOID

Cause: hereditary.

Clinical

Keloid is a skin condition, found mostly in Africans, causing huge scars in response to any injury, however minor. Something as trivial as a pimple or an insect bite can result in a bumpy lumpy scar which may be small or huge. Once formed, the scars remain.

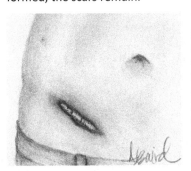

This keloid is on the scar from an appendectomy; it is relatively small. Keloids may become as large as a dinner plate. They have rough surfaces, are very firm, non-tender. The appearance does not change rapidly. Frequently their coloration is darker than normal skin. AB

Treatment

You can do nothing about it, nor can most physicians. Some plastic surgeons can remove the scars.

KERATITIS

Cause: variable.

Includes: corneal abrasion, corneal burn, corneal ulcer, herpes keratitis. Interstitial keratitis.

Definition: keratitis is an inflamed (painful) cornea caused by some irritation of the corneal surface.

Entry category: syndrome.

Age: more often adults than children. **Who:** those who have a scratched cornea, a foreign body in the eye, exposure to UV light (such as in welding) or a variety of diseases such as TRACHOMA, HERPES, SYPHILIS, ONCHOCERCIASIS or LEPROSY. It may occur because of the eyes being dry. In hot humid areas corneal ulcers due to fungi form around corneal foreign bodies of vegetable origin. At high altitudes or sea shores keratitis may be caused by sunlight which reflects off white rocks, snow or sand. This causes burned corneas, similar to those of welders who do not wear special glasses. **Onset:** sometimes immediately after the injury, but many times after a delay of 2–12 hours. With diseases the onset is unknown.

Clinical

Necessary: unless the eye is numb, there is severe pain and watering.

Usually the whites of the eyes are somewhat red. The patient complains that light hurts his eyes. With SYPHILIS, ONCHOCERCIASIS and LEPROSY, the patient may see halos or rainbows around lights. His vision is distorted.

Keratitis due to congenital SYPHILIS starts in the middle of the cornea; that due to TRACHOMA starts in a ring around the outside of the cornea. If the problem is due to HERPES and you stain the cornea(s) with fluorescein, you will see a stained branching or a puddle-of-water shape.

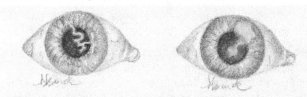

Keratitis is a whitening and opacification of the normally clear cornea. These are two common appearances when due to HERPES. The one on the left has a curvy line. The one on the right is irregular, like a mud puddle. AB

Complications: IRITIS, blindness.

Similar conditions: see Protocol B.8. TB of the eye causes a little white blister right at the border between the cornea and the white of the eye. Also check for XEROPHTHALMIA.

Treatment

Referrals: facilities; a level 3 or above hospital with a slit lamp. If the problem is due to HERPES there are expensive, antiviral eye drops available in major medical centers. Practitioner: an optometrist or ophthalmologist is most helpful.

Patient care:

- Check for GLAUCOMA before treating for keratitis.

- Treat the causative disease(s).

- If the problem is due to ONCHOCERCIASIS, LEPROSY or SYPHILIS, PREDNISOLONE EYE DROPS may be helpful but their use requires accurate diagnosis which is best done in a hospital.

- If the problem is due to a fungus, try ANTIBIOTIC EYE OINTMENT made with sulfadiazine or else oral THIABENDAZOLE.

- See Chapter 9 in Volume 1 for removing any foreign body; this must be done before the keratitis will heal. Thereafter, use ATROPINE, HOMATROPINE or TROPICAMIDE EYE DROPS to make the pupil big; then put in some ANTIBIOTIC EYE OINTMENT and patch the eyes for 72 hours. Renew the ointment every 6 hours. If you use ANTIBIOTIC EYE DROPS the drops must be renewed every 2–4 hours. The patient may require oral pain medication, repeated HOMATROPINE or both.

Keshan disease

See Regional Notes O.

KIDNEY DISEASE

Regional Notes: F, I, M, O, R, S, U.

Entry category: syndrome cluster.

Synonyms: renal disease, renal failure. Kidney failure is kidney disease that has progressed.

Includes: glomerulonephritis, nephrotic syndrome, hydronephrosis.

Definition: kidney disease is the inability of the kidney to adequately eliminate body waste.

Cause: variable.

Moderately to very ill; class 3–4; worldwide, related to MALARIA, crowding and level of medical care. It is commonly due to tropical disease.

Age: any. **Who:** anyone, mainly children and elderly; mostly a complication of other diseases but it may happen for no obvious reason. In the developing world, untreated KIDNEY INFECTION is the most common cause. LIVER FAILURE may cause kidney disease also. **Onset:** days, usually; maybe weeks or months.

Clinical

There are six types of kidney disease, according to causation, with some symptoms peculiar to each. These are listed in the table below: Types of Kidney Disease.

The following symptoms are common to all but nephrotic:

Necessary: fatigue, ANEMIA, dry and flaky skin, urine which is abnormal either in amount[1] or in dipstick test. Except for nephrotic type, there is rapid or irregular respiration. There is always some urine output. If the urine flow is

---

1 *See the table for minimum urine output below.*

absolute zero, then the problem is obstruction of the flow out of the bladder or an extensive cancer (inevitably fatal in a Third-World context). See URINARY OBSTRUCTION, Condition Index.

If the bladder is distended, then it is an outflow problem. If the bladder is not distended, then it is more likely CANCER.

Commonly: high blood pressure. There is nausea, vomiting and a decrease in appetite. The patient's eyes are swollen in the morning; his ankles and feet are swollen later in the day. He may have itchy skin. In severe cases his whole body, including his abdomen, may swell. He may have pain over his kidneys. There may be an abnormal skin color—a yellow/bronze. He may have abnormal taste or a loss of taste.

Occasionally: he has a headache, insomnia or mental changes. He may have a body odor resembling ammonia or urine. In some cases he has involuntary twitching or trembling, similar to LIVER FAILURE. He may have SEIZURES. He is likely to have muscle cramps. He may have abnormal bruising of the skin or bloody diarrhea. Males may develop breast tissue like females. Sexual dysfunction occurs. In advanced cases the patient cannot lie flat to sleep, because he becomes short of breath.

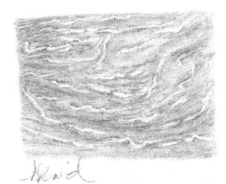

This is a highly magnified view of the white flakes found on the skin.
AB

Nephrotic syndrome causes the kidneys to put a lot of protein in the urine. This causes total body swelling.

Similar diseases

See Protocols B.6, B.7, B.10 and B.13. All types or most types: GASTROENTERITIS, HEPATITIS, GIARDIASIS, PARKINSON'S DISEASE, DYSENTERY, SCURVY, HEART FAILURE, LIVER DISEASE, LIVER FAILURE, CIRRHOSIS, abdominal TUBERCULOSIS, HEMORRHAGIC FEVER.

Bush laboratory: blood tests can demonstrate kidney disease, the extent and sometimes the cause. Urinalysis might be helpful.

Treatment

Seek higher level care within a few days; See Volume 1, Appendix 13. Only treat if sending out is impossible. Treat any causative disease. CHOLESTYRAMINE helps for itching.

TOC | SYMPTOMS | DIFFERENTIALS | CONDITIONS | DRUG INDEX | REGIONAL NOTES | INX

Table of minimum urine output: kidney disease

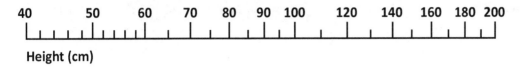

Height (cm)

On this chart find your patient's minimum urine output by putting a straight edge between his height on the top line and his weight on the bottom line. Read his minimum urine output off the middle line.

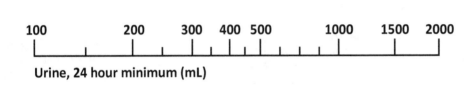

Urine, 24 hour minimum (mL)

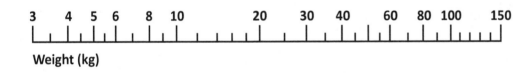

Weight (kg)

The following diagram shows the time course of kidney disease that has progressed to failure. The order of development of the symptoms is reasonably accurate; the total length of time from beginning to death or recovery is quite variable. This may be from 3 to 30 days; the chronology is on the assumption that it lasts for about 10–14 days. If it is more severe and lasts for a shorter period of time, then the symptoms are compressed into a shorter interval; if it has a slower onset and thus lasts a longer time, then the symptom development is also prolonged. After this period of poor urine output, sometimes there is a sudden burst of excessive urine output. Otherwise the patient dies at about 14–21 days.

Lab: urine specific gravity is
near 1.010

    Urine is positive for protein and blood.

							Body swelling			Muscle weakness				
Lethargy						High blood pressure	Diarrhea			Abnormal heart rhythms				
Nausea							Vomiting	Excessive sleep		Muscle twitching, maybe asymmetrical				
1	**2**	**3**	**4**	**5**	**6**	**7**	**8**	**9**	**10**	**11**	**12**	**13**	**14**	**15**

Days of inadequate urine production

Treatment: restrict salt and water intake.
        diet only carbohydrates; no fats or protein.
        no high-potassium foods (see POTASIUM in the Drug Index).

Types of kidney disease and treatments thereof

Type	Most Common Causes	Usual Symptoms	Urinalysis	Treatment
Nephrotic (leaky)	Variable.[1]	Swollen eyes mornings; swollen legs and feet evenings; urine may be frothy.	Always much protein. [2]	Diet,[3] Bedrest. PREDNISONE or HYDROCORTISONE. Give no DIURETICS!
Nephritic (inflamed)	Any skin infection, other.[4]	High blood pressure.[5] Sudden onset of making very little urine; rapid weight gain, whole-body swelling over a matter of days, eyes swollen in the morning.	Positive for blood, maybe positive for protein. SG about 1.020; acid pH, < 7.	Diet,[6] bedrest, sitting. HYDROCHLORTHIAZIDE, PREDNISONE, HYDROCORTISONE.[7]
Obstructive (blocked)	FILARIASIS, KIDNEY STONE, HYDATID DISEASE, PROSTATITIS, TUBERCULOSIS, URINARY OBSTRUCTION, CANCER.	Side pain or low abdominal pain, but may be painless, especially early in the disease.	Maybe no urine, urinalysis variable.	Treat cause. Surgical removal of a single diseased kidney may help.
Infective or toxic (poisoned)	MALARIA, SEPSIS, TRICHINOSIS, LEPTOSPIROSIS, drugs and poisons, ARSENIC POISONING, ENTERIC FEVER, PLANT POISONING.	Decreasing quantity of urine, otherwise like nephritic type.	Varies, always abnormal, commonly bloody.	Treat cause. Send out. Diet,[6] bedrest, sitting. HYDROCHLOROTHIAZIDE.[7] Surgical removal of a single diseased kidney may help.
Prerenal (dehydrated)	SEPSIS, burns, injuries, DEHYDRATION.	Decreasing quantity of urine, followed by huge quantities, see the chronology.	Urinalysis probably is normal.	Fluid balance.[8] Treat cause.
Hemolytic (bloody)	MALARIA, THALLASEMIA, DYSENTERY, SICKLE CELL DISEASE, some drugs.	Similar to prerenal; see the chronology	Urobilinogen probable, maybe bilirubin, maybe blood.	Give a lot of fluids. Give baking soda to raise urine pH to 8–9.

1   The most common cause of nephrotic kidney disease is MALARIA. Other causes are TUBERCULOSIS, STREP THROAT, SYPHILIS, HEPATITIS, SICKLE CELL DISEASE, HIV INFECTION, CANCER, ALLERGY, SCHISTOSOMIASIS MANSONI and ENTERIC FEVER. Some drugs may also cause this. It has a poor prognosis.

2   See laboratory procedures, Volume 1, Appendix 2.

3   Diet: high-protein, high-carbohydrate, low-salt, low-potassium. (There is much potassium in avocados, bananas, coconut, citrus fruits, dates, papayas, potatoes, pumpkin, spinach.)

4   Other causes of nephritic kidney disease are STREP THROAT, FILARIASIS, some WORMS, LEPROSY, HYPERTENSION, SICKLE CELL DISEASE and DIABETES.

5   Use HYDRALAZINE to bring the pressure down to near normal.

6   Diet: low-protein, low-carbohydrate, low-salt, low-potassium, high-fat and high-calorie. (There is much potassium in avocados, bananas, coconut, citrus fruits, dates, papayas, potatoes, pumpkin, spinach.)

7   FUROSEAMIDE may substitute.

8   Fluid balance: treat DEHYDRATION. If he has signs of HEART FAILURE, give him FUROSEAMIDE and restrict his fluid intake to just the amount of urine that he puts out. If he shows signs of neither HEART FAILURE or DEHYDRATION his total daily fluid intake is restricted to his urine output plus 600 ml per day for adults or plus 12 ml per kg per day for children. Do this whether the urine produced is too much or too little. This might require very small or enormous amounts of fluid!
In arid areas the patient will lose a lot of water through evaporation. In this case these directions must be modified; seek professional advice. Results: if the patient does not start urinating in a week, he will probably die. None of these problems is properly treated in the village; send the patient to a hospital.

KIDNEY INFECTION

Regional Notes: F.

Synonym: pyelonephritis.

Definition: kidney infection is a bacterial infection (usually Gram-negative or tuberculous) of the upper urinary tract.

Cause: bacteria.

Mildly to moderately ill; class 1 first episode; class 2 subsequently; worldwide, common.

Age: any. **Who:** anyone, especially females and babies; may be caused by ENTERIC FEVER. **Onset:** hours to days or weeks; weeks to months for TUBERCULOSIS.

Clinical

Usually: the patient has pain in his back, at the level of his waist, on one or both sides of the spine. These areas are tender. His urine looks cloudy.

Maybe: the patient may feel pain in his abdomen, in any portion or in his entire abdomen. The urine may have a foul odor. He may be quite sick with fevers, have pain with urination, nausea and vomiting. He may be incontinent of urine. Children may have only abdominal pain. Newborns, especially low-birth-weight males, may have fever, jaundice and failure to gain weight.

Occasionally: fever plus ALLERGY symptoms which may come and go.

Complications of repeated infections: SEPSIS, KIDNEY DISEASE. Sometimes there is a kidney ABSCESS in which case the patient will not respond to antibiotics. He will have tender kidneys and possibly swelling in the flank area.

Similar conditions: see Protocols B.9 and B.13.

Bush laboratory: urine will test positive for leukocytes and/or nitrites if the cause is ordinary bacteria. These will not be positive if the cause is TB. Sometimes there is just a very high pH, but these other tests are negative. The urine might test positive for blood additionally with either TB or ordinary bacteria. With infection due to TB, the urine tests positive for blood off and on or continually. The urine dipstick is negative for leukocytes, but white cells are evident under a microscope.

Treatment

Referrals: laboratory; a hospital laboratory can do a complete urinalysis and possibly a culture. Facilities: IV fluids with special antibiotics might be helpful. Practitioners: most general practitioners, internists and pediatricians.

Patient care: use SULFADIAZINE or CO-TRIMOXAZOLE. AMPICILLIN also usually works. CHLORAMPHENICOL might work. PENICILLIN will not work. CIPROFLOXACIN and OFLOXACIN are good for adults. Some CEPHALOSPORINS may work. If treatment with two different drugs fail, then consider TUBERCULOSIS or fake drugs as a cause of the problem.

Results: 1–2 days. Continue treatment for 3–5 days for a first episode, for 10 days for subsequent episodes, for 6–8 months for TUBERCULOSIS.

KIDNEY STONE

Regional Notes: F.

Synonym: ureteral colic.

Definition: a kidney stone is a small piece of hard crystal formed by the salts in urine.

Cause: variable.

Moderately ill, usually severe pain; class 2–3; worldwide.

Age: any, but not usually children. **Who:** anyone, but especially males; those with DEHYDRATION; sometimes it runs in families. Common in arid locations, and in Muslims during Ramadan. **Onset:** sudden, recurrent.

Clinical

Necessary: the patient has pain in the side, back, groin(s), testicle(s) or vagina.

Sometimes: the pain shoots from the back (the right or left flank) or side to the lower abdomen, groin or vagina.

Frequently: the patient sweats and vomits. If there is an infection also the patient may have fever or chills.

Complications: KIDNEY DISEASE, obstructive type. KIDNEY INFECTION with a stone can be exceedingly serious.

Similar conditions: ACUTE ABDOMEN is tender; kidney stones cause no tenderness unless there is a tear in the urinary tract. KIDNEY INFECTION and FILARIASIS onsets are slower.

Bush laboratory: blood in the urine. It is usually too little to be seen; it should be detected with a urine dipstick or a microscope.

Treatment

Referrals: facilities: there is some special equipment that can locate, snag and remove kidney stones; hospital level 3 or above. Practitioners; a urologist is ideal; a surgeon might be helpful.

Patient care: have the patient drink large amounts of water, using PROMETHAZINE to keep him from vomiting. Treat KIDNEY INFECTION, if present. Use strong pain medications if you have them. Strain all urine through a cloth; save the stone if one passes, and send it to a hospital. (A stone looks like a grain of sand.)

Results: the patient will feel better when the stone passes into the bladder. When this happens is totally unpredictable; it can happen in 10 minutes, or the problem can last weeks.

Kyasanur Forest disease

See Regional Notes I.

Lactose intolerance

See MILK INTOLERANCE.

TOC

SYMPTOMS

DIFFERENTIALS

CONDITIONS

DRUG INDEX

REGIONAL NOTES

INX

LARVA MIGRANS (LM)

Regional Notes: E, F, I, K, O, R, S, U.

Synonym: creeping eruption (skin type).

Includes: cutaneous larva migrans (skin), gnathostomiasis, toxocariasis, visceral larva migrans (deep).

Definition: larva migrans is a human infestation of the larvae of worms which ordinarily affect animals.

Not ill to severely ill; class 1–4; worldwide, type varies, mostly tropical.

Age: any, frequently children. **Who:** skin type: skin-soil contact, like HOOKWORM. The deep type may be caused by eating something contaminated with dog or cat stool. In Asia a deep type (gnathostomiasis) is acquired by handling raw meat with one's bare hands. **Onset:** usually rapid.

Clinical

SKIN LARVA MIGRANS
There is a red outline of a worm visible, moving beneath the skin. Sometimes the patient can only feel the movement and there is swelling in the area. It is extremely itchy.

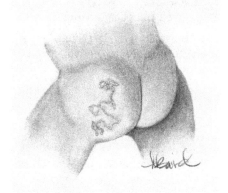

This is a fairly obvious case of skin LM; the condition might be subtle. The line is wiggly, raised and red. The end of the line moves over a matter of hours; mark its location with a pen. AB

DEEP LARVA MIGRANS
Symptoms vary with the organ of the body that is affected. In the eye there may be itching, pain or loss of vision. In the liver it may mimic HEPATITIS, LIVER DISEASE or LIVER FAILURE. In the brain it will cause ENCEPHALITIS, SEIZURES, STROKE and frequently death.

Complications: deep LM can damage any organ, depending on where it is. In Southeast Asia, a kind of deep LM can cause SERUM SICKNESS.

Similar conditions: skin LM is similar to STRONGYLOIDIASIS and MYIASIS. In larva migrans the lines are more definite, and they last for weeks rather than for hours. With STRONGYLOIDIASIS there is more red, and a definite track is hard to see. *Deep LM* may mimic almost any other disease as the worm, in migrating, might damage any internal organ. In Africa, consider LOIASIS.

Treatment

Prevention: treat pets for worms; keep them indoors. Don't use sandals or sit on the ground without something thick under you. In Southeast Asia, use rubber gloves to handle raw meat and fish to prevent gnathostomiasis. Cook meat well before eating it.

Referrals: for deep larva migrans speedy referral is essential; see Volume 1 Appendix 13. Laboratory; a white blood count shows a large number of eosinophils; however, this is also found in some other diseases. Facilities: level 4 or above imaging might be helpful. Practitioners: at times an infectious disease specialist or a surgeon is appropriate.

Patient care: skin LM near the buttocks should be treated as STRONGYLOIDIASIS. Other skin LM can be treated with ALBENDAZOLE or IVERMECTIN. Reportedly 10% THIABENDAZOLE in hand cream is effective when rubbed on the surface of the skin.

Deep LM patients should be sent to a hospital for care. IVERMECTIN or ALBENDAZOLE might be helpful.

Results: the symptoms resolve in weeks to months after the larvae die. The patient will have itching until then.

Lassa fever

See Regional Notes F.

LEAD POISONING

Cause: lead ingestion.

Slightly ill to very ill; class 3–4; worldwide, more urban than rural, related to cottage industries involving batteries, ceramics, fishing weights, paints. There is frequently lead in illegal alcoholic drinks. Lead poisoning may result from a retained bullet or shrapnel fragments. Occupations associated with poisoning include lead mining, scrap metal work, glass-making, printing and welding.

Age: any. **Who:** lead poisoning occurs when people, especially children, breathe fumes or ingest chemicals containing lead. It is seen in gold and silver workers who extract precious metals by heating them to high temperatures with lead. Some native eye ointments (e.g. kohl) contain lead. Children get the ointment on their hands which then enter their mouths. Paints and fuels may contain lead. Those who drink water that has drained from lead-painted roofs may be poisoned. Many herbal supplements contain lead, including the following: alarcon, alkohl, ayurvedic tonic, azarcon, bali goli, clamshell powder, coral calcium, crocodile bile, crude pills, deshi dewa, gilasard, greta, liga, paylooah, rueda, and surma. **Onset:** usually slow.

Clinical

The symptoms of lead poisoning are ANEMIA that does not respond to treatment and sometimes symptoms of a slow-onset MENINGITIS. Adults get crampy abdominal pains, a sweet metallic taste in the mouth, constipation and loss of appetite. A blue line may be seen on the gums above the teeth. The gums in the mouth may bleed. There may be a fever, but it is usually low.

Similar conditions: TB MENINGITIS, BRUCELLOSIS affecting the nervous system, IRRITABLE BOWEL. The blue line on the gums is diagnostic.

Treatment

Prevention: have parents shower and change their clothes at work. Keep children away from dangerous cottage industry work.

Referrals: see Volume 1 Appendix 13. Laboratory: large hospital laboratories can sometimes test for lead poisoning. Lead causes a peculiar appearance on an ordinary blood smear which some technicians can detect. Facilities: there are some special medications to bind and remove lead from the body at level 4 and 5 Western hospitals. Practitioners; a toxicologist is ideal.

Patient care: not feasible in the bush.

LEISHMANIASIS

See CUTANEOUS LEISHMANIASIS if the condition involves mainly skin; see VISCERAL LEISHMANIASIS if the condition mainly involves the abdomen.

LEPROSY

Regional Notes: E, F, I, M, O, R, S, U.

Synonym: Hansen's disease.

Definition: leprosy is a slow-onset bacterial disease of the nerves which secondarily affects the skin and other structures of the body. It is not tropical.

Cause: bacteria—*Mycobacterium leprae*.

Not ill to moderately ill; class 2–3; contagious, mildly;[1] worldwide with variable frequency; most common in India, Brazil, Congo, Nepal, Mozambique, Tanzania.

Age: any, but rare under 2 y.o. School-aged and older children tend to get tuberculoid leprosy. **Who:** living or having lived in a community where the disease is common. Africans tend to get tuberculoid. Europeans and Chinese tend to get lepromatous. The presence of HIV in a patient does not seem to have any effect on the development of leprosy. **Onset:** slowly over weeks to months. The incubation period averages 5 years; minimum incubation is 6 months.

Clinical, all leprosy

There are areas of skin that have changed appearance. The affected nerves are at first swollen, painful and tender; later they become non-tender. Infected nerves feel like strings of irregular diameter right underneath the skin. Hairs fall out on the affected areas.

---

1 *The only contagious leprosy patients are those with lepromatous (bumpy) leprosy. These are contagious through their respiratory secretions, mainly sneezing and coughing. No leprosy is contagious by touching intact skin. Some lepromatous leprosy might be transmitted by inoculation, e.g. sitting with a bare bottom on a rough surface that a leprous patient with buttock involvement had just vacated.*

TYPES OF LEPROSY: NEW SYSTEM

There used to be four kinds as described in the table below, but these are now considered under two headings, because the treatment varies according to two classes, not four. Which kind a person gets depends on his body's resistance; it does not depend on the kind he was exposed to. All kinds of leprosy are more common and worse on the cooler parts of the body, head and limbs rather than groin and armpits.

PAUCIBACILLARY

The kinds of leprosy previously called indeterminate and tuberculoid are now called paucibacillary. Only one or few nerves are affected; each nerve involves only one side, right or left, on the face or trunk. If it is a limb, only the thumb/big toe side or only the little finger/little toe side is affected. There is an area of the skin where the patient cannot tell the difference between hot and cold. There may be fine, dry scales so it looks like TINEA. **There are fewer than 5 abnormal areas on the skin.**

MULTIBACILLARY

The old classification of borderline and lepromatous is now called multibacillary leprosy. Multiple nerves are involved so there are multiple areas of skin affected, generally more than five. There are symptoms on more than one limb or on a limb and the face and/or more than one side of a limb, and/or both right and left sides of a limb or face.

It is important to test the patient for nerve function.

- Check for temperature sense by asking the patient to tell the difference between hot and cold.

- Check for light touch by having the patient close his eyes and tell you when you touch him with a wisp of cotton. Don't use your finger.

- Check for pain by having the patient distinguish the sharp and dull ends of a new hypodermic needle.

OTHER MANIFESTATIONS

Limbs: the muscles of the thumb side of the palm are wasted, so there is no bulge on the palm below the thumb. Compare the two hands and feet. There may be painless wounds, shortening and abnormal shapes. The patient may not be able to move the hand or foot normally. A hand may look like a claw. Fingers and toes may be missing. The foot may hang down and turn inward so the patient must lift his leg high at the hip and knee to avoid injuring his foot.

Head: there is likely to be a lack of eyebrows or eyelashes. One side of the face or both may droop. There may be bumps on the face, especially the earlobes. The eyes may not close all the way. The corneas may be scarred or even totally opaque. The eyes may be excessively wet or dry. Vision is apt to be poorest in bright light. There may be pus coming from the nose. Most patients have sores in their noses, but they may not notice them; you have to look. There may be hoarseness or decreased smell and taste. Mental apathy is very common.

Eye leprosy may cause inability to close the eye, eyelids rolled in or out, KERATITIS or IRITIS; blindness is common.

Genital: female reproductive capacity is not diminished. Testicular involvement causes shrinking of the testicles, impotence and breast development. Teens have delayed sexual development.

OLD SYSTEM OF CLASSIFICATION

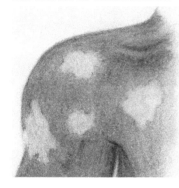

Indeterminate/ paucibacillary: AB

Appearance: light or reddish coloration.[1] Flat. Margins indistinct.

Distribution: it involves one or few areas only, not symmetrical.

Disability: the patient cannot feel hot or cold in the discolored areas. There are no pains, hair loss or paralysis.

Tuberculoid/ paucibacillary: AB

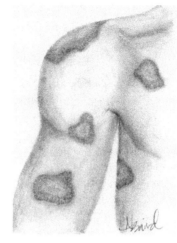

Appearance: color like indeterminate, but the areas may be dry and roughened, flat or only slightly raised.

Distribution: fewer than 6 spots; may have some symmetry, but usually none.

Disability: there is decreased light touch[2] Pain, hair loss and weakness are common.[3]

Borderline/multibacillary: AB Appearance mostly red. The areas are raised or rings with depressed centers. The areas are not shiny.

Distribution: there are over 5 spots; there is some symmetry.

Disability: there is poor pain sense. There may be shooting pains, weakness, hair loss or paralysis.[4]

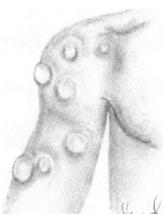

Lepromatous/multibacillary: AB

Appearance: red, shiny, smooth cobblestones of many sizes, many to innumerable.

Distribution: always the ear lobes, generally on the cooler parts of the body. Much symmetry.

Disability: the eyes, hands, feet and testes may be affected.

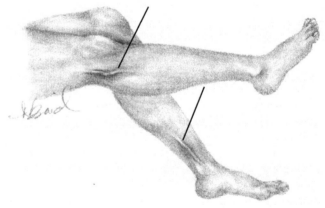

Swollen nerves are subtle; you have to look for them. They may be in many places. When and where the nerves are swollen, most likely the patient will have sharp, shooting pains. The nerve is swollen on the outside of the right knee (upper pointer). The nerve is swollen on the inside of the left leg, just above the ankle (lower pointer). AB

---

1 *Light means resembling the normal skin of a fairer ethnic group. The skin will appear reddish in fair skin. The transition between the colors is indistinct, not at a sharply defined line.*
2 *That is, the patient cannot discern when you are stroking his skin with a wisp of cotton. Don't use your finger to test.*
3 *The patient cannot consistently say "now" whenever he is touched by a wisp of cotton. The pains are sharp and shooting along the course of a nerve. Head hair loss occurs only in Europeans and Japanese. Anyone may have loss of eyebrows.*

---

4 *Poor pain sense means that the patient cannot distinguish the sharp and dull ends of a needle on the affected skin. See the previous footnote for hair loss.*

TOC   SYMPTOMS   DIFFERENTIALS   CONDITIONS   DRUG INDEX   REGIONAL NOTES   INX

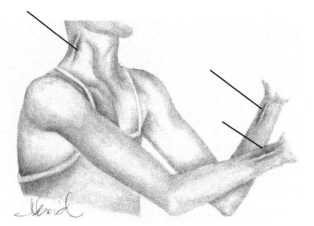

In this case you can see swollen nerves in the neck, on the inside of the left wrist and on the outside of the right wrist. AB

Clinical leprosy reactions to treatment

These reactions are most common in patients who are more than 20 years old.

TYPE 1 REACTION TO TREATMENT

This reaction occurs in borderline leprosy only. It occurs within the first 6 months of multi-drug therapy and in women near the time of childbirth. This reaction causes sudden fever, possibly lasting for months, redness and swelling of the skin, rash and possibly the formation of skin ulcers. The hands and feet may be swollen. There are severe pains along nerves, perhaps with weakness or paralysis.

TYPE 2 REACTION TO TREATMENT

This reaction occurs in lepromatous leprosy during treatment. It can be associated with pregnancy, birth, breast feeding, trauma or some other infection. It causes fever, red bumps that last just a few days, sometimes swollen areas with sores forming, large lymph nodes, large liver and spleen, swollen and tender nerves, swollen testicles and IRITIS. It is a kind of ERYTHEMA NODOSUM. It is most common in young females during pregnancy.

Other Complications: loss of limbs, blindness, vulnerability to injury, decreased immunity to other diseases, IRIS.

Similar conditions: *paucibacillary (tuberculoid) type:* the most common in those with dark skin is scarring from an old skin condition such as diaper rash. Also check VITILIGO (always flat and roughly symmetrical, except on the face), TINEA (itchy). *Multibacillary (lepromatous) type:* tertiary SYPHILIS and tertiary YAWS may cause bumps under the skin, but never any numbness. VISCERAL LEISHMANIASIS PKDL may be very similar. MYCETOMA may look similar but one can see dry grains, and it is almost never symmetrical. Consider also CUTANEOUS LEISHMANIASIS, BARTONELLOSIS. *Nerve damage:* PARKINSON'S DISEASE or BELL'S PALSY can also cause a droopy face, as can STROKE. SCHISTOSOMIASIS and deep LARVA MIGRANS can cause nerve damage.

If there is ulceration: TUBERCULOSIS of the skin (lupus vulgaris) and CUTANEOUS LEISHMANIASIS can cause ulceration (spontaneous, open skin wounds), but there is never nerve damage. *Leprosy reaction:* see Protocol B.6 for limb swelling and B.8 for eye symptoms.

Treatment of leprosy disease

Prevention: BCG immunization (used for TB) also gives partial protection against leprosy.

Referrals: see Volume 1 Appendix 13. Laboratory: most hospitals can make skin scrapings on lepromatous leprosy; the bacteria show up under the microscope, but the test is difficult to do correctly; there are many false negatives and some false positives. Level 3 and above hospitals can biopsy any leprosy to diagnose it. Blood tests for SYPHILIS may be false-positive in leprosy patients. Facilities; a specialty hospital that treats large numbers of leprosy patients is most helpful. Practitioners: nurses, general practitioners and surgeons with experience in treating this disease.

Surgery can be helpful for leprosy patients. Make contact with your closest receiving hospital to find out what sorts of patients they can care for and which surgeries are done. In general, surgeons can care for eyes that will not close and for feet that hang down so that they easily become injured. They can also care for injuries and fit patients with orthopedic appliances to help them manage their lives better.

Patient care: the most important part of treatment is the education of the patient in how to care for his body. It is entirely beyond the scope of this book to outline this, let alone describe it in detail. If there is an established leprosy program in your country, see if you can visit it and learn. Spend at least two weeks. Books and other learning materials may be obtained from Health Books International in the UK. It is possible to visit their location which is accessible by British Rail from London. There is very much to learn about the management of this disease with all its social and psychological implications.

Drug therapy is not difficult, but it is time-consuming; it requires that you be with the patient for 6 months to 2 years. Do not begin a treatment that you cannot complete! Check the Drug Index before beginning treatment.

- *Single skin spot only:* give a single dose of RIFAMPIN plus OFLOXACIN plus MINOCYCLINE.

- *Paucibacillary:* indeterminate, tuberculoid and mild borderline leprosy: RIFAMPIN once a month, plus DAPSONE daily for 6 months. An alternative is daily RIFAMPIN plus OFLOXACIN, both supervised, both for one month.

- *Multibacillary*: definite borderline and lepromatous types: RIFAMPIN once a month plus DAPSONE daily, plus CLOFAZAMINE daily with a monthly larger dose. This is continued for at least 2 years.

- Treat skin ulcers due to leprosy like a TROPICAL ULCER. PHENYTOIN powder (ground tablets), sprinkled into the ulcers, hastens healing. Give the patient ZINC also to hasten healing.

- At night use ARTIFICIAL TEARS to keep eyes that don't close adequately from drying out. Patch the eyes.

- Pregnancy: RIFAMPIN, DAPSONE and CLOFAZIMINE are considered to be reasonably safe.

There are four antibiotics that seem to work for leprosy. They are expensive unless you can get free samples: MINOCYCLINE, CLARITHROMYCIN, OFLOXACIN and PEFLOXACIN. Only change from the old schedule on good authority; don't use hearsay drugs or dosages.

Treatment of leprosy reactions

ASPIRIN alone for ordinary Type 1 that is not too severe. Add PREDNISONE (for 3–4 days only) if it is severe. For Type 2, use CHLOROQUINE and either HYDROCORTISONE or PREDNISONE. In both cases do not stop the usual leprosy drugs! They must be continued. PREDNISOLONE EYE DROPS might be helpful for IRITIS.

LEPTOSPIROSIS[1]

Regional Notes: E, F, I, M, O, R, S, U. It is not common in Europe, the Mediterranean and the Central Asian Republics.

Synonyms: canicola fever, hemorrhagic jaundice, mud fever, swineherd's disease Weil's disease.

Definition: leptospirosis is a whole body infection caused by one of the spirochetes, a type of bacterium.

Moderately ill; class 2; contagious; worldwide temperate as well as tropical areas, especially common in China, Brazil and Southeast Asia. In temperate climates, it is most common in summer and fall; in tropical climates it's most common during the rainy season. It occurs in epidemics at times.

Age: any; children are less sick than adults. **Who:** mainly males; water, plant, soil, animal or patient contact. Usually from wading through flood or stagnant waters contaminated by rodent urine. The disease can be acquired by blood transfusion. **Onset:** sudden; incubation from a few days to 3 weeks.

Clinical

Necessary: fever and either sore red eyes (without pus), severe muscle pains or both. Muscle pains are especially in the calves, back and abdomen.

Maybe: other symptoms are variable. Sometimes a patient will have the germ without being sick at all. Usually a high fever rises and falls unpredictably, and there is headache. There is frequently a rash on the back part of the roof of the mouth.

Sometimes: the patient loses his appetite and vomits. He is usually constipated. He may have JAUNDICE beginning the second or third day. He might have red lumps on his shins. He may have a swollen abdomen and a tender liver.

If there is no JAUNDICE, the initial symptoms last 4–7 days and then go away by themselves, even without treatment. Then the fever starts again after 1–3 days. This second stage lasts 4–30 days. During this time symptoms of MENINGITIS are common, as are eye symptoms[2] (IRITIS as well as visual loss). Mental symptoms indicate a bad prognosis. The fever disappears either suddenly or gradually.

If there is JAUNDICE, the symptoms are more constant, without the relapsing quality.

Complications: PNEUMONIA, RESPIRATORY FAILURE, LIVER FAILURE, KIDNEY DISEASE, MENINGITIS, HEART FAILURE, STROKE, HEMORRHAGIC FEVER, ANEMIA due to destruction of red cells, SHOCK and death. Older patients are more likely to die than younger ones. Relapses are common.

Convalescence is long, 8–10 weeks in severe cases. The patient may be lethargic during this time, and he may develop IRITIS. Chronic fatigue is common after recovery.

Similar conditions: see Protocols B.2, B.5, B.7, B.8, B.10, B.13. In MALARIA jaundice occurs the first week; with leptospirosis it occurs the second week. Be particularly wary of PLAGUE, which may present with red eyes and severe muscle pains. Look for a blackened area of skin.

Bush laboratory: protein may be in the urine with the second temperature rise and bilirubin, blood or urobilinogen at any time.

Prognosis: if the patient coughs up blood, his prognosis is poor; a rapid pulse, rapid respiration or low oxygen content in the blood is worrisome. Cigarette smokers fare badly.

Treatment

Prevention: wear a gown, mask and gloves while caring for the patient. Be very careful to dispose of body secretions properly in an area free of rodents.

Referrals: see Volume 1 Appendix 13. Laboratory: hospitals can do darkfield examination of the blood for leptospires. Tests that measure antibodies will be negative until the patient has been ill for 5 days, at which time treatment is useless. You should initiate treatment on mere suspicion. Facilities: IV fluids and antibiotics might be helpful, but only before 5 days. Practitioner: an infectious disease specialist with tropical/travel medicine expertise is ideal.

---

1   See the Powerpoint lecture: Intermediate Organisms *on the website www.villagemedicalmanual.org.*

2   *There is a specific but not sensitive appearance of the eyes: the bloodshot appearance of the eyes is more intense toward the outsides of the whites and less intense around the cornea. Seeing this clinches the diagnosis; its absence does not eliminate the diagnosis.*

Patient care: antibiotics do no good whatsoever if started after 4 or more days. Therefore, **if you think of this diagnosis, treat it.** PENICILLIN, DOXYCYCLINE, CHLORAMPHENICOL, ERYTHROMYCIN, AMPICILLIN and AMOXICILLIN all work. A third-generation CEPHALOSPORIN may also work. The patient may become sicker with his first dose (higher fever, low blood pressure, short of breath), but do not stop the antibiotic. Since it is difficult or impossible to distinguish leptospirosis and other intermediate organisms (spirochetes and Rickettsiae), it is safest to use DOXYCYCLINE. If he has mental symptoms, consider sending him to a facility that can give him IV or IM MAGNESIUM SULFATE.

LICE

Regional Notes: I.

Entry category: infestation.

Synonyms: pediculosis.

Includes: body lice, head lice, pubic lice.

Cause: insect.

Not ill to mildly ill; class 1; contagious; worldwide, related to crowding, common all over.

Age: any, especially children. **Who:** anyone, especially poor hygiene. Lice like some people and not others. **Onset:** soon after exposure.

Clinical

Necessary: there are little moving creatures on hairy areas of the body: head, genitals, eyebrows. Louse eggs appear as little bumps on hairs or the seams of clothing. With head lice the heaviest infestation is behind the ears. After a person has had body lice he may feel ill for several days with general fatigue and aching all over, the origin of the term "feeling lousy".

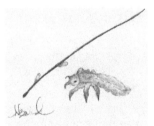

The bumps on the hair are louse eggs glued on. This is a body louse, greatly magnified. In real life it is barely visible. Head lice are similar. Pubic lice are more rounded than long. AB

Similar conditions: fleas also live on humans and bite, but they are bigger, black, and they jump, which body lice do not. (Some lice change color to blend with the color of the skin or hair, which makes them very hard to see.) Bedbugs don't live on skin; they just bite at night and then leave. They are rarely seen.

Treatment

- MALATHION, 0.5% kills only the lice, not the eggs. The eggs can be washed off the body with showering, but they do not wash out of hair. The eggs must be eliminated from cloth by immersing the cloth in boiling water or by ironing it.

- Repeatedly comb the hair with a fine comb to get the eggs off. MALATHION must be repeated weekly until the eggs are all hatched or combed out. The nightly use of mosquito nets impregnated with insecticide discourages head lice.

- Kill lice and eggs by sealing clothing/stuffed toys/bedding in a plastic bag for 12 days. IVERMECTIN cures both scabies and lice.

- Alternatives are BENZYL BENZOATE, PERMETHRIN or 1% LINDANE. Phenothrin and carbaryl are available in England.

- Total shaving works for head lice. Reportedly shampooing with kerosene also works for head lice, but it must be repeated to kill the louse eggs.

- Custard apple (Annoa squamosa) seeds, ground and soaked in coconut oil, kills head lice in less than an hour.

LIPOMA

This is a kind of benign fatty tumor that does not need treatment. It forms right under the skin. Its texture is similar to that of gelatin that has set. It is not as soft as a water balloon, but not as hard as a ripe peach. It is painless and non-tender. It does not cause whole body illness.

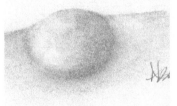

There is a lump under the skin, soft like gelatin refrigerated in a balloon. Similar conditions: ABSCESS (warm and tender), LOIASIS (comes and goes), HYDATID DISEASE (very slow-growing). AB

LIVER DISEASE

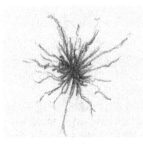

Skin spiders associated with liver disease are flat and smooth red spots. They have reddish or bluish wiggly lines radiating out. There are a countable number, usually on the trunk. This illustration is magnified about 20 times. AB

See LIVER FAILURE. This is a milder form. It is a disease cluster, not a diagnosis. There is bilirubin in the urine. There may be yellowing of the whites of the eyes. In dark-skinned people, liver disease may make the facial skin darker. Over time, liver disease will cause scarring of the liver, described under CIRRHOSIS, or else it may quickly deteriorate into LIVER FAILURE—see the next entry.

The urine test for bilirubin is both sensitive and specific for liver disease. If the bilirubin is positive the liver is diseased. If it is negative, the liver is not diseased.

TOC   SYMPTOMS   DIFFERENTIALS   CONDITIONS   DRUG INDEX   REGIONAL NOTES   INX

Effects of liver disease

This chart reflects general rules but the symptoms may vary with the nature of the liver disease. Symptoms also vary from person to person.

	Mild	**Moderate**	**Severe**
Liver	? large ? tender	Large, usually	Small, usually
Kidneys	—	—	Decreased urine
Blood	—	Anemia	Won't clot
Food	Poor appetite	same	same
Mental	—	Personality change, trembling	Unconscious, seizures
Lung	—	—	Short of breath
Yellow eyes	None	Some	Severe
Sexual dysfunction	Maybe	Probably	Yes

LIVER FAILURE

Regional Notes: F, M, O, S, U.

Entry category: syndrome or disease cluster.

Synonym: hepatic failure.

Definition: liver failure is the diminution or cessation of liver function.

Causes: various infections and toxins. TOXEMIA of pregnancy might also cause this. The most common causes are LEPTOSPIROSIS, PLANT POISONING, BRUCELLOSIS, SCHISTOSOMIASIS, HEPATITIS, HEMOCHROMATOSIS, GALLBLADDER DISEASE, TOXOPLASMOSIS, ARSENIC poisoning, BIRTH CONTROL PILLS and occasionally other drugs.

Moderately to severely ill; class 3–4; maybe a contagious cause; worldwide, many causative diseases are tropical.

Age: any, adults more often than children. **Who:** those who have underlying disease or who take certain drugs, or herbal supplements.[1] **Onset:** variable—over months to years for CIRRHOSIS, over days to weeks for acute (sudden) LIVER FAILURE.

Clinical

For a diagrammatic picture see Protocol B.7. There are two types: both involve free fluid in the abdomen and a large spleen.

CIRRHOSIS

This is scarring of the liver which develops over months to years, causing gradual symptoms, though some event may worsen the problem rapidly. See the separate entry for this.

ACUTE (FULMINANT) LIVER FAILURE

This develops over days to weeks. It is most often due to drugs, HEPATITIS B, herbal toxins (in anyone), or HEPATITIS E in pregnant women.

- The liver is either tender, large or both if the disease just started. Later on the liver might shrink and no longer be tender.

- JAUNDICE: the whites of the eyes are yellow. A urine dipstick tests positive for bilirubin and perhaps urobilinogen.

- Bleeding problems because the blood won't clot normally: nosebleeds, easy bruising, excessive menstruation, excessive bleeding from minor wounds, vomiting blood, bloody stool or urine. Sometimes, with some causes, there may be intolerable whole body itching.

- BRAIN DAMAGE which at first responds to treatment and later does not:

  o Stage 1: apathy, restlessness, confusion, poor handwriting, day/night reversal.

  o Stage 2: drowsiness, disorientation, trembling, mood and behavior changes.

  o Stage 3: sleeps all the time but can be awakened, very active reflexes, episodes of craziness.

  o Stage 4: seizures and coma.

Complications: SHOCK, KIDNEY DISEASE, SEIZURES, coma and death.

Similar conditions: for other causes of free fluid in the abdomen, see Symptom Protocol A.46.A. For other causes of a large spleen, see Symptom Protocol A.46.B. Also see Protocols B.6, B.7 and B.10.

Bush laboratory: normally there is some urobilinogen in the urine. With most causes of liver failure there will be more than normal urobilinogen and excessive bilirubin.

---

1 *herbal supplements associated with liver failure are as follows: camphor, cascara sagrada, chaparral, comfrey, ephedra, germander, jin bu huan, kava kava, kombucha, margosa oil, pennyroyal oil, heliotropium, crotalaria, sassafras, valerian.*

With some causes of liver failure that may respond to surgery (i.e. it is worthwhile to send the patient out), the urobilinogen in the urine will be zero, the bilirubin in the urine will be very high, the stools will have a light color and the patient will have intolerable itching.

Treatment

Referrals: it is useful to send a patient out to a higher-level facility, both for diagnosis (some types of cirrhosis can be treated successfully) and relief of symptoms. It is sometimes desirable to remove fluid from the abdomen in order to help the patient breathe better. However that should not be done in remote areas because it is easy to introduce bacteria with disastrous consequences. Facilities that can transfuse the patient can also deal with bleeding tendencies. A gastroenterologist is the most appropriate specialist; also consider tropical/travel expertise for treating causative diseases.

Patient care: it may be futile by the time full-blown liver failure has developed, but try the following:

- low-sodium diet; no salt or baking powder.

- a nutritious diet; some authorities recommend low-protein and others recommend high-protein. Try low-protein first.

- multiple vitamins and minerals, including ZINC.

- medications for itching: DIPHENHYDRAMINE or CHOLESTYRAMINE.

- avoid the following drugs which may harm the patient: IBUPROFEN and related medications; AMOXICILLIN/CLAVULANIC ACID; KETOCONAZOLE, ISONIAZID, GENTAMYCIN and related antibiotics; ERYTHROMYCIN and related drugs; CHLORPROMAZINE and similar drugs; all herbal teas and ethnic medicines.

- if liver failure develops as a result of medications for treating TB, then stop ISONIAZID, RIFAMPICIN and PYRAZINAMIDE. Treat the person with only ETHAMBUTOL, STREPTOMYCIN and CIPROFLOXACIN until the jaundice is entirely gone. Then introduce the other drugs again, one by one. Usually the liver problems do not recur.

LIVER FLUKE

Regional Notes: E, F, I, K, M, N, O, R, S, U

Entry category: disease cluster.

Includes: fascioliasis, chlonorchiasis, opisthorciasis.

Definition: liver fluke is the infestation of the human body with one of the following creatures: *fasciola hepatica, opisthorcis viverni, opisthorcis felineus* or *chlonorchis sinensis.*

Cause: worm.

Mildly to moderately ill; class 2.

Regional

- Fascioliasis occurs worldwide wherever there are sheep-raising areas with low, wet pastureland harboring snails. It occurs in Siberia and Tibet as well as the tropics. It is very common in the Altiplano region of Bolivia, the Andes, Cuba, Iran, western Europe, Egypt and Wisconsin.

- Opisthorciasis occurs in central and eastern Europe and throughout Southeast Asia and the Far East. It is decreasing in Thailand, but is common in Laos and China. A variant of this occurs in Poland, Kazakhstan, Russia, Ukraine, Siberia: Tyumen and Khanty regions.

- Chlonorchiasis occurs throughout Southeast Asia and the Far East; it is similar to opisthorciasis.

Age: any except nursing infants. **Who:** *fascioliasis*: those who eat raw watercress or drink contaminated water. Larvae of the worm develop in the snails, *Galba trunculata. Opisthorciasis and chlonorchiasis:* those who eat raw or pickled fish. **Onset:** slow for fascioliasis, 1–3 months incubation; may be sudden for opisthorciasis and chlonorchiasis.

Clinical

FASCIOLIASIS
The disease may be entirely without symptoms. If there are symptoms they will be indigestion, a large tender liver, nausea, diarrhea, general aching all over, loss of appetite, cough, itchiness, HIVES, JAUNDICE or any combination of these. There may be a high fever and chills. Usually the problem resolves itself, but it may become chronic.

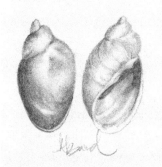

This is the appearance of the snails that carry the liver fluke, fasciola hepatica. AB

OPISTHORCIASIS AND CHLONORCHIASIS
Most patients are without symptoms, but there may be fever, muscle aches, diarrhea, loss of appetite, upper abdominal pains and sometimes a large tender liver. It may lead to serious GALLBLADDER DISEASE. Chlonorchiasis may cause SERUM SICKNESS in the initial stages.

Similar conditions: HEPATITIS and AMEBIASIS may be indistinguishable. For SCHISTOSOMIASIS MANSONI and SCHISTOSOMIASIS JAPONICUM, check the geography.

Treatment

Referrals: laboratory: early in the disease, a blood count will probably show increased eosinophils. Later on a laboratory with a microscope can check stool for the eggs of these flukes. Sometimes it takes many specimens before an egg is found. The eggs do not appear until the patient has been ill about 4 months in fascioliasis. Antibody tests remain positive long after the infection is gone. Stool antigen tests should be helpful. Practitioner: tropical/travel expertise is most helpful.

Patient care: for fascioliasis; a veterinary drug, TRICLABENDAZOLE (brand name Fasinex), is recommended by the WHO. There is resistance to this in disease acquired in developed countries (because of vet usage). ARTEMISININ given additionally may help. TRIBENDIMIDINE does not work. NITAZOXANIDE or METRONIDAZOLE may work.

Opisthorciasis/chlonorchiasis: ARTEMISININ is said to work for these, same dose as MALARIA. PRAZIQUANTEL (which may not work), BITHIONOL, EMETINE (very toxic), possibly ALBENDAZOLE given at twice the usual dosage. Hexachloroparaxylol is used for opisthorciasis, but it is not as good as PRAZIQUANTEL. TRIBENDIMIDINE reportedly works well and is not toxic. Use it for 3 days. Adding KETOCONAZOLE increases the cure rate.

Loiasis

See Regional Notes F.

LYME DISEASE[1]

Regional Notes: E, K, N, O, R, U.

Note that Eurasian Lyme disease looks quite different than North American. See the E and K notes for a description.

Synonym: Lyme borreliosis.

Definition: Lyme disease is an infection with a spirochete.

Cause: spirochete.

Moderately to severely ill; class 3; not contagious; regional; found in Europe and Asia west of the Ural mountains, along the north coast of Africa, some locations in east Asia, in coastal Australia and in North America, particularly east of the Mississippi and along the west coast.

Age: any. **Who:** bitten by a tick. **Onset:** variable, probably gradual in most cases. Incubation to first symptoms is 3–32 days.

Clinical

STAGE 1

There is a fever, fatigue and aching all over, along with a rash consisting of red circles, doughnuts, targets or ovals with clearing centers. The circles on the skin are 5 cm or more in diameter.

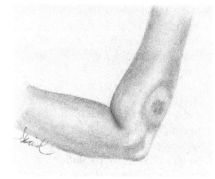

This is a target spot, typical of Lyme disease. A similar pattern might be caused by, AFRICAN SLEEPING SICKNESS or a number of other illnesses. AB

STAGE 2

This may cause BELL'S PALSY, perhaps on both sides. The patient may have abnormal eye movements. He may have difficulty in thinking and remembering. There may be transverse myelitis, a condition that affects the spinal cord with loss of sensation, weakness, paralysis in limbs, and/or disturbances in bowel and bladder function, depending on where the spinal cord is affected. There may be ARTHRITIS.

STAGE 3

This is the same as stage 2, but it becomes chronic.

Similar conditions: see Protocols B.2: Fever/Headache/General pains; B.6: Limb Swelling; B.10: Confusion/Lethargy; B.12: Large Lymph Nodes. *Initial stage:* similar to diseases listed under ARBOVIRAL FEVER, but the rash is distinctive. *Subsequent stages* are similar to MENINGITIS, BELL'S PALSY, ARTHRITIS, or HEART FAILURE of other causes. RELAPSING FEVER can appear quite similar, but it is of more rapid onset.

Treatment

Prevention: avoid tick bites by using DEET repellent. After a tick bite, give antibiotics only if the tick is engorged with a lot of blood or if the patient gets any kind of rash at the site of the bite. Look for a rash daily for 30 days after a bite[2]. A tick is engorged if the dark-colored head part is less than 1/3 of the whole body area, looking down at the tick from above.

Referrals: see Volume 1 Appendix 13. Laboratory; a level 4 or above laboratory will probably show a positive blood test result after 2 weeks of illness. Practitioner: an infectious disease specialist.

Patient care: DOXYCYCLINE (first stage only), PENICILLIN, AMOXICILLIN, CHLORAMPHENICOL, CEPHALOSPORIN. The patient may become sicker with the first dose. Duration of treatment: Stage 1: 14 days; stage 2: initially 30 days oral; change to 30 days IV if there is no cure. Treatment during stage 3 must be continued for 6 weeks. CEPHALOSPORIN (ceftriaxone) given intravenously is usually used in advanced stages. Use injected antibiotics if the patient has a severe headache and/or symptoms of HEART FAILURE.

---

1 See the Powerpoint lecture entitled Intermediate Organisms *on the website www.villagemedicalmanual.org.*

2 *This is a reddening of the skin in an irregular oval area around the site of the bite, with some measles-like spots around the red area, possibly a small black ulcer in the middle of the red. There may be a target-like appearance.*

LYMPHOGRANULOMA VENEREUM (LGV)

Regional Notes: R, U.

Synonyms: climatic bubo, esthiomene, lymphogranuloma inguinale, tropical bubo.

Definition: lymphogranuloma venereum is a sexually transmitted bacterial infection caused by *Chlamydia trachomatis*.

Not ill to mildly ill; class 1–4; contagious; worldwide, especially ports and urban areas. It is particularly common in sub-Saharan Africa, India, South America, the Caribbean and Southeast Asia.

Age: any; usually sexually mature, but sexually abused children may get it. **Who:** promiscuous partner or more than one partner, especially sailors and prostitutes in port cities. Accounts for about 3% of all SEXUALLY TRANSMITTED DISEASES in these areas. **Onset:** incubation period 4–21 days from exposure to primary; 3–16 weeks to secondary.

Clinical

This usually affects the genitals but may affect other areas of the body which have had sexual contact: hands, mouth and breasts.

PRIMARY

A minority of cases have this. A small bump forms on the skin, less than 6 mm in diameter. This becomes an ulcer or a little blister. It is painless, but urine touching it causes burning pain. It disappears in 2–5 days. It is more common in women than men.

SECONDARY

There is a fever. The lymph nodes on one side of the groin enlarge, both above and below the leg crease, creating a firm bulge with a groove down the middle. They may extend down into the thigh. They are painful. Females have lower abdominal and back pain. The patient may have headaches, loss of appetite, nausea and vomiting. The large nodes may become an ABSCESS which will rupture, releasing pus; it heals with scarring.

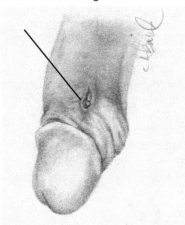

This is a primary skin ulcer. Most patients skip this stage. It is small, subtle, easily missed. Most directly develop a groin abscess. AB

TERTIARY

The genital area becomes swollen, possibly with anal itching and PROCTITIS. Ulcers, ABSCESSes and abnormal holes form between rectum, bladder and vagina or penis to the outside of the body. See FISTULA. Urine, stool, menstrual blood and semen come out of abnormal places. In females it can cause PELVIC INFECTION and infertility. In either sex (but more often women), it may cause gross swelling of the genitals. It may cause narrowing of the rectum and rectal CANCER. The swelling and scarring may cause retention of urine and stool.

Similar conditions:

Primary: see Protocol B.1.

Secondary: CELLULITIS or OSTEOMYELITIS of the legs can cause large nodes, fevers and pains. Generally the leg problem is obvious. CHANCROID may be indistinguishable. TYPHUS is similar but has a peculiar musty body odor. PLAGUE lymph nodes are extremely tender whereas LGV nodes are mildly tender. ENDOMETRIOSIS may be similar, but there are no tender large groin nodes in this case.

Tertiary is similar to advanced DONOVANOSIS which may coexist or be indistinguishable. Treat both.

Treatment

Referrals: laboratory: large hospitals may be able to do a culture or a blood test. Facilities and practitioners; a specialty clinic for sexually transmitted diseases is most helpful.
Patient care: use Protocol B.1 for treatment in most cases.

- *Primary:* DOXYCYCLINE is the drug of choice; use ERYTHROMYCIN or AZITHROMYCIN in pregnancy. CIPROFLOXACIN might work. The minimum duration is for 3 weeks but longer is good, especially in the presence of HIV INFECTION. AZITHROMYCIN does not work as well as DOXYCYCLINE.

- *Secondary:* same drugs plus pierce the swelling with a syringe and large needle to draw off the pus. Do not drain the pus by cutting with a knife.

- *Tertiary:* can be managed only by surgery.

MALABSORPTION

Regional Notes: F, I, O, S, U.

Entry category: syndrome.

Definition: malabsorption is the failure of the bowel to absorb food and water taken in by mouth; the result is that they pass directly from mouth to anus.

Cause: variable. See Protocol B.14.

Moderately to severely ill; class 2; worldwide, but the cause varies from one region to another.

Age: any. **Who:** anyone, but especially expatriates and those with MALNUTRITION. **Onset:** usually slow, over weeks; may be sudden.

TOC   SYMPTOMS   DIFFERENTIALS   CONDITIONS   DRUG INDEX   REGIONAL NOTES   INX

Clinical

The patient has a large quantity of diarrhea, sometimes with abdominal pain. Whenever the patient eats he loses it promptly with foul-smelling diarrhea which has fat in it, floats on top of the toilet water, is hard to flush and leaves residual oil droplets on the water. There is usually much rectal gas. Usually he has loss of appetite, weakness, lethargy, weight loss (or failure to gain weight in children), general abdominal swelling and possibly a sore tongue and mouth. The problem lasts a week or more.

Complications: these are associated with MALNUTRITION: fluid in the abdomen and symptoms of ANEMIA, PELLAGRA, BERIBERI, XEROPHTHALMIA, SCURVY. There may be abnormal bleeding because of lack of vitamin K. The patient may have SEIZURES.

Similar conditions: for diarrhea that is somewhat milder than that described above, see the Symptom Index.

Treatment

Referrals: see Volume 1, Appendix 13. Laboratory: large hospital labs, level 4 or above, may be able to determine stool fat content to diagnose this; other tests on stool or blood may be done to diagnose the cause. Practitioner: tropical/travel disease expertise is important since many of the causes are tropical; otherwise a gastroenterologist.

Patient care: since this is a syndrome, not a disease, the treatment depends on the cause which should be discovered by working through Protocol B.14. Treat the possible causes for your patient, one at a time; try first whatever is common in your area. Give ORS also. FOLATE and other vitamins should be given whatever the cause is. Other helpful medications might be DOXYCYCLINE, PYRANTEL PAMOATE or TINIDAZOLE.

MALARIA[1]

I. Introduction

II. Clinical

   A brief history

   Kinds of malaria

   Ordinary malaria (mostly non-falciparum)

   Knowlesi malaria

   Severe malaria (mostly falciparum)

   Subcategories of severe malaria

   Malaria and pregnancy

   Malaria in children

   Table: diagnosing malaria in children

   Complications for both adults and children

   Similar conditions

   Bush laboratory

III. Prevention

   Table: methods of malaria prevention

IV. Treatment of malaria: principles

   A. Treatment of ordinary malaria, not severe

   B. Treatment of severe malaria

   C. Treatment of complications

V. Higher-level care in developing countries

VI. Higher level care in Western countries

I. INTRODUCTION

Regional Notes: E, F, I, K, M, O, R, S, U.

Includes: blackwater fever; bilious remittent malaria, algid malaria, cerebral malaria, Knowlesi malaria.

Definition: malaria is an infection with one of the plasmodia protozoa. "Falciparum malaria" is caused by *Plasmodia falciparum* and is the most serious kind; "non-falciparum malaria" is caused by any other Plasmodia (*P. vivax, P. malariae, P Knowlesi* or *P. ovale*).

Cause: protozoa.

Not ill at all to very ill; mild is Class 1; severe falciparum malaria is Class 3. Widespread in the tropics, more common at low altitudes. In large tropical cities with substantial air pollution, the adult anopheles mosquito cannot survive and thus there is no malaria transmission. Falciparum malaria is common between latitudes 15° north and 15° south. Vivax malaria is present throughout the tropics and as far north as the North Korea-China border in Asia. Knowlesi malaria was originally only found in Borneo; it is now spreading throughout Southeast Asia.

Age: usually over 6 weeks old, more common in well-nourished children and expatriate adults. **Who:** bitten by anopheles mosquitoes. In many areas of the world these mosquitoes bite without being noticed. See Volume 1, Appendix 10. Expatriates, pregnant women and HIV patients are especially vulnerable. HIV infection makes malaria worse, and malaria makes HIV infection worse, but the effects both ways are not spectacular. Malaria is more severe in patients who have had their spleens removed. **Onset:** variable; it might be sudden or gradual. If the fever and chill cycle is of sudden onset, and has typical every-other-day timing, the malaria is likely to be sensitive to CHLOROQUINE. **Incubation:** usually about 2 weeks; it may be as short as 3 days. If the patient is a national from a malarious area or if he has taken any malaria medication, then the incubation can be much longer. Sometimes the incubation period of non-falciparum malaria from temperate climates is very long—measured in months.

---

1 *See the Powerpoint lecture entitled* Malaria *on the website* www.villagemedicalmanual.org.

II. CLINICAL

A BRIEF HISTORY

The following clinical descriptions of malaria differ from most medical texts. Starting in 1917, tertiary syphilis patients were treated with transfusions of malarious blood. The descriptions of malaria in Western texts were based on these cases. Donors and (consequently) recipients both had regular cycles of chills and fevers; the textbook writers assumed that all malaria presents like that. This is not true; naturally acquired malaria fevers are erratic at first; they only become regular after a considerable time.

Another problem is that blood smears of transfusion-induced malaria were positive for all donors and recipients. But when the disease becomes severe, particularly with falciparum malaria, smears may be negative even though the infection is overwhelming. This is also at odds with medical orthodoxy, but it has been well substantiated.

The end result of these misunderstandings has been that in the USA malaria patients commonly die. Since the disease is rare, physicians don't consider the diagnosis. Those who do expect periodic fevers and insist on seeing a positive malaria smear before treating. Hence, treatment is frequently delayed, sometimes with disastrous results.

KINDS OF MALARIA

There are five kinds of human malaria; for convenience we will consider them under three categories: falciparum, non-falciparum and Knowlesi.

Usually a patient will be infected by only one of the three categories; if an expatriate has falciparum malaria, he will be much sicker than with non-falciparum. However, if there is infection with both forms, he will not be as ill; his risk of dying will be less than infection with falciparum alone.

Non-falciparum tends to last long and relapse, but it does not kill quickly. Non-falciparum causes ordinary malaria in most patients and occasionally severe malaria. Two kinds (vivax and ovale) have forms that hide in the liver and erupt at unpredictable times, perhaps years after the last exposure.

Knowlesi malaria progresses rapidly; it kills through RESPIRATORY FAILURE.

Falciparum kills quickly, but it is also totally curable. Most falciparum causes severe malaria in expatriates; it initially causes ordinary malaria in nationals.

ORDINARY MALARIA (MOSTLY NON-FALCIPARUM)

Non-falciparum malaria in expatriates (and national children) may cause erratic fever or regular up and down fevers, every day, every other day or every third day. The longer the illness has lasted, the more likely it is that the fevers and sweats have regular timing. Shaking chills alternate with episodes of sweating; the patient's temperature goes up when he feels cold and comes down when he feels feverish, the opposite of what one would expect. There are usually at least 12 hours between chills and sweats. He may have previously felt somewhat ill.

Other symptoms are general aching, shoulder pain, dizziness, lethargy, headache, eye pain, left upper abdominal or waist pain, appetite loss. There is likely to be a large urine production, nausea and vomiting. The spleen may be large and tender. Children commonly have rapid respiration, cough and SEIZURES with simple malaria, but these symptoms are uncommon in adults.

- Pregnancy: malaria is more severe in pregnant than in non-pregnant women. It may be fatal, especially around the time of delivery.

- Newborns: occasionally babies are born with malaria. They have ANEMIA, JAUNDICE and a large spleen.

- Ethnic considerations: occasionally non-falciparum malaria may become severe malaria in persons of Mediterranean genetic heritage. See severe malaria below.

- Relapses of ordinary, non-falciparum malaria that has been acquired in tropical areas tend to occur 3–6 weeks after the first illness; those acquired in subtropical or temperate areas tend to relapse after much longer intervals—months or years. In both cases taking preventive medication will make those intervals longer. In either case, the relapse is more likely than the original illness to have a sudden onset and regular cycles of fever and chills.

KNOWLESI MALARIA

Knowlesi malaria has 24 hour cycles (rather than 48 or 72). It causes prominent respiratory symptoms, so it looks like a severe form. However it does not respond to most medications for falciparum. It needs to be treated with CHLOROQUINE.

SEVERE MALARIA (MOSTLY FALCIPARUM)

Definition: severe malaria is malaria with one or more of the following *complications:*

Shortness of breath that is worse lying than sitting	
Coma	Rapid respirations
KIDNEY DISEASE	Spontaneous bleeding
HYPOGLYCEMIA	Unable to sit up
Severe ANEMIA	JAUNDICE
Low blood pressure	Bloody urine

It is usually caused by falciparum malaria. In persons with G6PD DEFICIENCY, it may be caused by non-falciparum. The onset is frequently gradual in adults and sudden in children. Malnourished patients seldom develop severe malaria; it is almost always those who were healthy beforehand.

Fever may be continuous or may go up and down, cycling every 24 or 48 hours. As in non-falciparum malaria, there are at least 12 hours between chills and sweats. Expatriates usually have continuous fevers. In mild cases this may look like non-falciparum malaria. JAUNDICE and ANEMIA are common when the patient has been ill for some time.

Adults may develop KIDNEY DISEASE with little or no urine output; the urine appears bloody. This may happen initially, or it may happen as the patient is recovering. Severe shortness of breath likewise may happen initially or during recovery. Restlessness is worrisome.

SUBCATEGORIES OF SEVERE MALARIA

Cerebral malaria causes a severe headache and fever. The patient may appear drunk or crazy, may be unconscious and may have SEIZURES. His respiration may be irregular or rapid. Malaria, MENINGITIS, ENCEPHALITIS and HEAT STROKE might be indistinguishable. The eyes may become crossed. There may be abnormal lip movements. The legs are likely to be stretched out straight and stiff with the arms also stiff or else flexed at the elbows with the hands on the chest. **Patients with cerebral malaria are never completely alert and able to identify the date.** About 1/3 have JAUNDICE. Negative blood tests are common because all the infected red cells are stuck onto the walls of the blood vessels. **Anyone who has been exposed to malaria, and has both a fever and mental symptoms must be treated for falciparum malaria. Awaiting laboratory confirmation is likely to prove fatal.**

Blackwater fever always occurs in patients who have been resident in malarious areas for a long time and have had prior malaria. There are fever, chills, back pain and vomiting. The patient's urine is dark red or black. He probably has JAUNDICE. Hiccup indicates a bad prognosis. He is very sick and may be unconscious; death is likely. Blackwater fever occurs under three conditions.

1. Severe falciparum malaria under-treated with QUININE.

2. Any malaria treated with QUININE if the patient has a Mediterranean genetic heritage with G6PD deficiency (this can be tested in Western countries).

3. Patients with G6PD DEFICIENCY who take PRIMAQUINE, FANSIDAR or related drugs.

Algid malaria causes vomiting, diarrhea, SHOCK, low temperature, JAUNDICE and severe ANEMIA. The blood pressure is low, and the pulse is rapid. It is difficult to distinguish from CHOLERA and DYSENTERY, so it is good to use DOXYCYCLINE for treatment. It is rare.

Bilious remittent malaria causes LIVER FAILURE, KIDNEY DISEASE, hiccups, vomiting (possibly bloody), diarrhea and possibly JAUNDICE.

Choleraic malaria causes a watery diarrhea, very similar to CHOLERA.

Pulmonary malaria causes lung damage and death through shortness of breath. It begins 2–3 days into treatment. Symptoms are rapid respiration, sitting up to breathe and a cough. There is a 50% mortality rate even with treatment. Lung damage and RESPIRATORY FAILURE might occur even after all the malaria parasites have been cleared out of the blood. This complication is particularly common in Southeast Asia, caused there by Knowlesi malaria. Knowlesi malaria is sensitive to CHLOROQUINE.

Malaria plus typhoid is vastly overdiagnosed. When it occurs, invariably there is a sustained fever, abdominal pain, an apathetic mood and persistence of fever for more than 24 hours after initiation of malaria drugs.

MALARIA AND PREGNANCY

In areas with much malaria (most symptomatic patients are children), pregnant women are more anemic and babies weigh less when they are born. In areas with less malaria (most symptomatic patients being adults), women tend to give birth early if they become ill late in pregnancy. Pregnant women are also at increased risk of developing severe malaria, and when they do the maternal (and fetal) death rate is high. Postpartum maternal death from malaria is also common and commonly fatal.

MALARIA IN CHILDREN

The clinical summary on the next page may be helpful:

Newborns who are born with malaria have fevers and large livers and spleens. They are anemic. There is always a history of maternal malaria within the 2–3 weeks prior to delivery. In areas with very much malaria (most symptomatic patients are children), babies under 2 years old do not commonly get severe falciparum malaria, but they do commonly develop ANEMIA. Older children, however, do get severe malaria which tends to progress rapidly; there is a high mortality rate, and death may occur in less than 24 hours. KIDNEY DISEASE is not a common complication in children. Common symptoms right before death are rapid respiration and deep coma: (the patient does not respond to pain such as rubbing one's knuckles on his breastbone).

DIAGNOSING MALARIA IN CHILDREN

Votes FOR malaria in an ill child
History of shaking chills
Skin hot to the touch
Examiner is able to feel the spleen
Urobilinogen in urine
Acts sleepy

Votes AGAINST malaria in an ill child
Prominent rash
Productive cough
Curious or playful
Leukocytes in urine
Good appetite

COMPLICATIONS, ADULTS AND CHILDREN

- *Bacterial infection:* PNEUMONIA, URINARY TRACT INFECTION, ENTERIC FEVER are common, especially in children.

- *SEPSIS* will cause a sudden drop in blood pressure with loss of consciousness during recovery.

- *KIDNEY DISEASE* is a common complication in adults but not in children.

- *HYPOGLYCEMIA* may develop either as a result of the malaria or as a result of QUININE treatment, especially in young children and pregnant women.

- *BRAIN DAMAGE* and *STROKE*.

- Malarial *SHOCK* may develop the second or third day of treatment, especially in pregnant women and those recently delivered.

- *Cough* and *HEART FAILURE*.

- *ANEMIA* due to destruction of red blood cells and, over the longer term, lack of FOLATE and VITAMIN B_{12}.

- *SPLENIC CRISIS* is the death of a portion of the spleen, causing spleen pain, treated with pain control as long as vital signs are good.

PMNS: post-malaria neurological syndrome
This happens within 2 months after successfully treated severe malaria. It seems to be associated with MEFLO-QUINE usage. There are two kinds.
1. *Simple incoordination without any change in mental functioning. This resolves by itself over months.*
2. *Changes in consciousness, possibly with seizures also.*
It can be treated with PREDNISONE or related drugs.

Similar conditions

See Protocols B.2, B.3, B.5, B.7, B.9, B.10, B.13, B.14.

Similar to both kinds of malaria: all the diseases listed in B.2.

Similar to chronic malaria: HEPATITIS is the most common misdiagnosis. Also consider MALNUTRITION, EAR INFECTION, TUBERCULOSIS, KIDNEY INFECTION, MONONUCLEOSIS, VISCERAL LEISHMANIASIS. See Index B.

With yellow eyes, see Protocol B.5.

Cerebral: may be indistinguishable from MENINGITIS, ENCEPHALITIS and HEAT STROKE. Treat for all of the above. Consider HYPOGLYCEMIA which may coexist or be caused by MALARIA or the treatment thereof.

Algid: may be indistinguishable from bacterial DYSENTERY. Use DOXYCYCLINE for treatment.

Blackwater fever: very similar to HEPATITIS. Also see Protocol B.5 and B.7.

Bilious remittent: see Protocol B.7. Consider also other causes of LIVER FAILURE. Bilious remittent malaria may be indistinguishable from HEMORRHAGIC FEVER.

Choleraic: similar to CHOLERA and may be indistinguishable. Treat for both.

Bush laboratory: urinalysis may show positive urobilinogen when the patient has fever. Ketones are positive if the patient is not eating. Blood and protein are positive in blackwater fever; protein alone may be positive in chronic malaria. The patient may have ANEMIA. Some of the antibody blood tests listed below under higher level care are appropriate; they are expensive.

III. PREVENTION

- Learn the breeding habits of anopheles mosquitoes in your area, and eliminate breeding sites.

- Malaria mosquitoes bite between dusk and dawn. Use repellents, mosquito netting or both at night. (Mosquito nets impregnated with insecticide also help to eliminate LICE and bedbugs.)

- Put screens on houses.

- Drugs for prevention are useful in some areas, especially for pregnant women and young children. See the following table. Unfortunately, no option is a sure guarantee against getting malaria. Which option is best depends on drug resistance patterns and the drug side effects for the individuals.

- HIV-positive pregnant women and their babies are particularly susceptible to malaria, and preventive treatment is essential. In locations where small shopkeepers stock and dispense chloroquine for "headache plus fever", the incidence of malaria will decrease. Immunization for malaria is on the horizon, but that has been so for 20 years or more.

OPTIONS FOR MALARIA PROPHYLAXIS

Method	Malaria type	Adult dose	Advantages	Disadvantages
Avoid bites	All	N/A	No drugs	Hassle
Chloroquine	Non-falciparum	300 mg base weekly	Old/safe	Falciparum resistant, bitter taste, vision damage after years
Chloroquine + chlorpheniramine	All	150/4 mg twice weekly	Old/safe drugs, new usage	Dry mouth, sleepiness, bitter taste, vision damage after years. May not work in the Western Hemisphere.
Mefloquine	Mainly falciparum	250 mg weekly	Weekly	Seizures, expensive, nightmares
Proguanil	Mainly falciparum	200 mg daily	Old/safe okay in pregnancy	Daily dose, must use with chloroquine
Chlorproguanil	Mainly falciparum	20 mg twice weekly	Weekly	Twice weekly dose, must use with chloroquine
Fansidar	All	1 tablet weekly	Weekly	Sulfa drug, some fatalities, not recommended, much resistance
Pyrimethamine	Falciparum	50 mg weekly	Weekly	Also take chloroquine, unreliable, dangerous used alone
Maloprim (pyrimethamine + dapsone)	Falciparum	12.5/100 mg weekly	Weekly	Must take chloroquine; dangerous with G6PD DEFICIENCY
Primaquine	Non-falciparum	30 mg daily for 14 days	Old/safe	Only prevents relapse, dangerous with G6PD DEFICIENCY
Doxycycline	Mainly falciparum	100 mg daily	Safe	Sun sensitivity, belly pain, expensive
Malarone (atovaquone + proguanil)	Mainly falciparum	1 tablet daily	No resistance	Expensive, daily dose
Co-trimoxazole	All	2 SS tablets daily	Oral, cheap, useful in HIV INFECTION	Occasional bad reactions with peeling skin.

Avoid bites by using screens on houses, sleeping under mosquito nets and using insect repellent just before sunrise and just before sunset.

The safe upper limit for chloroquine is an average of 2.5 mg/kg/day of base.

Chlorpheniramine is an antihistamine, an ingredient of cold tablets, a very old drug. It has been found to reverse the resistance of falciparum malaria to chloroquine in the Eastern Hemisphere.

Mefloquine sometimes causes seizures in Europeans. The stigma of having had a seizure will haunt a person when he applies for a driver's license.

There have been reports of deaths in children who use pyrimethamine alone for prophylaxis. It is thought to delay diagnosis until it is too late.

In theory, doxycycline works for all kinds of malaria. However in my experience it works very poorly for non-falciparum. It also makes some fair skin sensitive to sunburn.

IV Treatment

Consult the Worldwide Antimalarial Resistance Network for current information on drug resistance.

A. Ordinary malaria, that is—

- The patient can be awakened and is able to speak as rationally as usual. (A baby should do some things appropriate to his age.)

- His mouth is moist underneath his tongue. Vomiting is not excessive.

- His urine is not brown or black, and the amounts are reasonable.

- The whites of his eyes are not yellow.

- He is not short of breath at rest.

- His body is not swollen.

Give a multivitamin tablet to all malaria patients. It is good to add a single dose of PRIMAQUINE at the end of each treatment. This prevents transmission of the disease to mosquitoes. ARTEMISININ-type drugs also prevent transmission of the disease to mosquitoes.

Option #1: CHLOROQUINE, if this has worked in your area in the past.[1] This should be followed by a course of PRIMAQUINE.

Option #2: CHLOROQUINE plus CHLORPHENIRAMINE. CHLORPHENIRAMINE appears to reverse resistance of falciparum malaria to CHLOROQUINE in Africa, maybe elsewhere.

Option #3: day 1: oral medication of the ARTEMISININ variety. Days 2 and 3: MEFLOQUINE plus ARTEMISININ-type medication. This is particularly good in patients who are from Southeast Asia where there is much malaria resistant to QUININE. Do not use this option for chloroquine-resistant vivax malaria (mostly in the Pacific area).

Option #4: in non-pregnant females and in children over seven years old, use QUININE for three to five days along with DOXYCYCLINE for at least seven days. The patient must have sugar with quinine.

Option #5: QUININE alone which must be used for seven days since it is eliminated rapidly from the body. The patient must have sugar with quinine.

Option #6: ARTEMISININ-type medication for 7 days.

Option #7: ATOVAQUONE-PROGUANIL which is very expensive.

Option #8: PIPERAQUINE or PYRONARIDINE or MEFLOQUINE in a fixed combination with one of the ARTEMISININ-type drugs.

Option #9: ARTEMISININ for 3 days followed by a curative dose of MEFLOQUINE.

Option #10: new combinations. Independent information is necessary.

- ARTEMISININ (as Artesunate) 4 mg/kg plus DAPSONE 2.5 mg/kg plus PROGUANIL 8 mg/kg, all daily for 3 days.

- ARTEMISININ plus LUMEFANTRINE in fixed combination. The brand name is Co-artem, and it is safe to use in children and pregnancy. It is commonly counterfeit.

- Artesunate ½ mg/kg plus fosmidomycin 30 mg/kg, both every 12 hours for 3 days.

- Tafenoquine 200 mg base per day for 3 days, then 200 mg base weekly for 8 weeks.

- Fosmidomycin 30 mg/kg plus CLINDAMYCIN 10 mg/kg, both every 12 hours for 3 days.

- METHYLENE BLUE, combined with CHLOROQUINE and ACT's.

- AZITHROMYCIN, an expensive antibiotic, reportedly works.

B. Treatment of severe malaria

- Keep the patient in bed. Check vital signs every two hours. MULTIVITAMINS and FOLATE are helpful for nutritional support.

- Give malaria medication, using PROMETHAZINE or HYDROXYZINE to prevent vomiting. Choose an option from the malaria medications listed above, but not option # 1.

- Use option #2 if the patient is short of breath and you are in Southeast Asia.

- Use sugar for all patients (caution with diabetics) and DIAZEPAM additionally if the patient has SEIZURES.

- Cool the patient with damp cloths and use ACETAMINOPHEN. Do not use DEXAMETHASONE, HYDROCORTISONE, PREDNISONE or any other similar drug.

- If the patient is not drinking, manage his fluids to prevent DEHYDRATION; see DEHYDRATION in Volume 1, Appendix 1. Also, in adults watch for KIDNEY DISEASE and treat that appropriately. If the patient is a nursing baby, empty his mother's breasts and put the milk down a stomach tube if you can do it without making him vomit.

- Monitor breathing: if breathing is deep and rapid, give fluids with sugar as long as there is no KIDNEY DISEASE. Raise the patient to a sitting position. If the respiration is slow with some foaming at the mouth and abnormal eye movements, the problem is probably SEIZURES; treat him accordingly. If respiration is grossly irregular, most likely the patient is dying.

- Transfer the patient to a hospital as soon as possible. There are many more options at a hospital than what you have in a village situation. For severe malaria transfusion might be helpful provided the hospital uses only HIV-negative blood. If there is a delay in finding blood and/or transfusing it and if the patient is somewhat improved in the meantime, then it is good to refuse transfusion. Even blood that is tested can transmit HIV. General transfusion guidelines are as follows.

---

1 In some areas of the world, vivax malaria is becoming resistant to chloroquine. As of 2011, this has been reported from Southeast Asia, the Pacific area, central Madagascar, Ethiopia, Syria, northern India, northern Pakistan and South America north of Uruguay.

o If the patient is pregnant, near delivery and her hemoglobin is 7 or below,[1] she should be transfused.

o For a non-pregnant patient, a hemoglobin of 4–5 or less should be treated with transfusion if and only if the patient is very short of breath. A hemoglobin of over 5 should receive no transfusion. At high altitudes all patients with anemia symptoms should be either transfused or quickly transported to a lower altitude.

C. TREATMENT OF COMPLICATIONS

o KIDNEY DISEASE: sending the patient for kidney dialysis is worthwhile, because usually kidney function will resume in a week or two; you are not committing to life-long dialysis.

o HEART FAILURE: must be treated like ordinary HEART FAILURE as well as continuing the malaria treatment. If the patient is short of breath due to HEART FAILURE, you can try using HYDROCHLOROTHIAZIDE or a related diuretic. However, if he is also has KIDNEY DISEASE, this won't work.

o ANEMIA: if ANEMIA is severe enough to cause shortness of breath, then transfer to a hospital for blood transfusions is essential.

o SEIZURES: use appropriate medication for seizures.

V. HIGHER-LEVEL CARE IN DEVELOPING COUNTRIES

If the patient is too sick to carry on a conversation, then speedy referral is necessary. See Volume 1, Appendix 13.

Laboratory

Blood smears are commonly available. Usually, if the technician is experienced, the thick smears will read positive by the time of the first fever. However, with severe falciparum malaria, even when properly and repeatedly done, smears may be negative. They will usually be negative in blackwater fever and in any expatriate. On the other hand, an adult national might not be ill at all and yet have a positive blood smear, because he has developed immunity. Expatriates often have to be extremely ill before a malaria blood smear will turn positive; false negatives are very common.

There are two kinds of blood smears: thick and thin. A thick smear examines more blood, so it will be positive in a fairly mild case, while the thin smear might still be negative. However, it is difficult or impossible to tell the kind of malaria on a thick smear. A thin smear will reveal the kind of malaria, but the person has to be much sicker before it is positive, because it involves looking at less blood. Sometimes the percentage of infected red cells in the blood is determined. In an expatriate adult or a child, 5% infected cells is life-threatening. But an adult national might tolerate as many as 20% infected cells and still survive.

Antibody tests involve putting a drop of blood on a small stick or card or in a tiny plastic well, washing it off and then looking at the color. These must be used carefully according to directions. They must not be used after their expiration dates. The dipstick and card tests for falciparum malaria become positive with the first high fever; they will be negative for non-falciparum malaria. The test labelled PfLDH turns negative quickly after the malaria is treated; PfHRP2 remains positive, possibly for as much as a month. Patients with some kinds of severe ARTHRITIS may have false positive tests, and there may be false negatives in some geographic areas. Some new antibody tests are being developed which detect all kinds of malaria.

Facilities: expert nursing care, IV fluids, a blood bank and transfusion facilities, a monitored bed, level 3 or above.

Practitioner: tropical/travel experience is essential.

VI. HIGHER-LEVEL CARE IN WESTERN COUNTRIES[2]

THE BAD NEWS

Most American doctors will not treat malaria unless they have a lab report stating that there is malaria on the blood smear. If you can find a doctor trained in India or a former missionary doctor, he might treat you without a positive smear.

Most lab techs and pathologists don't know how to do malaria smears properly. Most of them would not recognize malaria on a properly done smear unless it was an overwhelmingly severe infection.

The United States has the highest case fatality rate in the world for malaria. There are not many cases, so doctors don't know about it. Treatment is delayed, inadequate or both, and proper drugs are hard to find. Older ages and Asian or European ethnicity are risk factors for a fatal outcome.

Severe falciparum malaria may be present even with a properly done negative malaria smear. In Bangkok, Thailand, 30% of autopsy-proven cases of cerebral malaria had repeatedly negative malaria smears done by experienced technicians. Technicians in the USA are generally not experienced, and there are only few in Europe. All the malaria parasites get stuck in the tiny blood vessels, so the blood that is examined appears to be free of malaria. With blackwater fever, the malaria smear is almost always negative; with cerebral malaria it is commonly negative.

The most common misdiagnosis in severe malaria is HEPATITIS. The second most common misdiagnosis is MENINGITIS. American doctors, once they diagnose malaria, may want to use injectable QUININE, but it is not available in the States, except from CDC. In the past the CDC required a positive malaria smear in order to release it.

---

1 Seven or below assumes a low altitude. At 2000 meters or above the lowest permissible hemoglobin is 8.

---

2 This section concerns typical care in the USA, Canada and most locations in Europe. Competent tropical medical expertise is available in London, Liverpool and Tubingen (Germany). See Appendix 13 of Volume 1 for recommended treatment locations.

TOC   SYMPTOMS   DIFFERENTIALS   CONDITIONS   DRUG INDEX   REGIONAL NOTES   INX

A REASONABLE RESPONSE

If you are dealing with a malaria problem when making travel plans, try to route your trip through London. The travel clinic there is particularly good.

When returning to the West on furlough, take your own medicines with you; include some oral and intravenous QUININE which can be bought over the counter in tropical developing countries, but is hard to find in the States. An alternative is injectable artemisinin-type medication; however, that is commonly fake or substandard. It is good to have two kinds. If you come down with malaria, and it is not too bad, treat yourself with oral medicines. Take a course of PRIMAQUINE after you are done with your preventive. This may prevent your becoming ill again.

Try to choose a doctor of tropical ethnic origin. In most places a South Asian is best, but it must be one who took most of his training in South Asia.

If you do end up in a hospital, ask your doctor to have the lab tech do a hematocrit. This is a thin disposable tube of blood that is spun to separate the red cells from the watery part. If the lab tech breaks the hematocrit tube by the buffy coat and smears out the red cells from right underneath the buffy coat, making and staining it like an ordinary thin blood smear, the malaria parasites will be concentrated there, and they are more likely to be seen.

If a family member has a spinal tap for meningitis but he actually has cerebral malaria, the spinal tap will either be normal, or it might indicate a viral meningitis. Sometimes the lactate content of the spinal fluid is elevated, but this is not a routine lab test; it must be specially ordered.

Severe malaria should be treated on suspicion of the diagnosis, without waiting for confirmation. Anyone who has been in a malarious area and is seriously ill should be treated for malaria plus whatever else he has. The heart drug, QUINIDINE, is a very close relative (stereo-isomer) of the anti-malarial QUININE. It works just fine for severe malaria, but the person must be on a monitor in an intensive care unit to watch his heart rhythm. Eli Lily Company (800-821-0538) and/or Center for Disease Control malaria hotline (770-488-7788) in the USA might help with procurement. Oral medication may be substituted when the patient improves. Since oral quinine is absorbed rapidly, if vomiting can be prevented a feeding tube can be used even in unconscious patients to give quinine, although IV is better.

The blood sugar might drop during an episode of severe malaria, from the malaria or from the QUININE or QUINIDINE. Pregnant women and children are particularly prone to this complication. The patient should have a glucose solution running intravenously and his blood sugar should be monitored. This is particularly problematic for diabetics.

If you are truly desperate, go to a liquor store and buy quinine water over the counter. Drinking a liter or two may buy you some time to get yourself to an appropriate place. However, it will make your malaria blood test false-negative, so you may be refused treatment.

MALNUTRITION[3]

Regional Notes: F, I, N, O, R, S, U.

Entry category: syndrome cluster.

Includes: kwashiorkor, marasmus, vitamin deficiencies.

Definition: malnutrition is the failure to take in, process or absorb enough food stuffs to sustain life and development.

Mildly to very ill; class 1–2; worldwide, frequency variable and related to the culture. Use of alcoholic beverages aggravates malnutrition.

Kwashiorkor (malnutrition with swelling) occurs mainly in cool, humid areas. These are generally cultures with diets of manioc-tuber, millet-sorghum or wheat. Marasmus (skinny malnutrition) occurs in areas that are hot and dry.

Age: any; children are most susceptible. Marasmus is most common under 1 year of age; kwashiorkor, after 1 year old. Either type can occur in adults. **Who:** babies, especially bottle-fed; an older baby when a younger one has taken his place at the breast; any poor diet. It is more likely with severe diarrhea. Kwashiorkor is very common after MEASLES or diarrhea. **Onset:** usually slow unless an illness tips the balance in a marginally nourished child.

Clinical

GENERAL MALNUTRITION

Necessary: children fail to grow normally. The upper arms are thin; black hair turns reddish or blond, but blond hair turns dark. Some ethnic groups develop straight and brittle hair rather than a color change. Dark skin becomes paler than normal. Europeans may have darkening of skin. Measure the circumference of the upper arm, half way between the shoulder and the elbow. (See the illustrations and standard measurements in Volume 1, Chapter 5.) The smaller the arm measurement, the greater the child's risk of dying. Malnourished children never smile. If you can get a child to smile, he is probably not malnourished.

Frequently: malnourished children are lethargic, with big bellies so that they look pregnant. They may have swollen feet which can be dented with pressure from a finger.

Maybe: he has a sore tongue. His sexual and mental development is delayed. Menstruating females may stop menstruating.

Sometimes: they are just skinny without any swelling. The skin of their lower legs may peel. They may have open sores. Their eyes may be affected by XEROPHTHALMIA. Vertical cracks in lips are common. They may have a glue-like body odor. Their appetites may also decrease, so that they refuse food when it is offered.

---

3 See Chapter 5 in Volume 1, and the malnutrition *lecture* at www.villagemedicalmanual.org.

A sore tongue is common, so that eating is painful. They may have sharp, shooting or chewing pains in their lower legs. Some children have swellings by their ears, similar to MUMPS and/or HIV INFECTION.

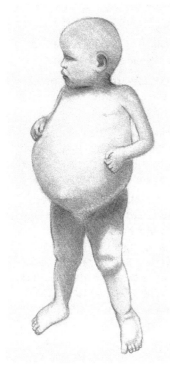

This child is malnourished, not fat. Note his upper arms that are skinny. If you press a thumb on his feet, you will leave dents. OW

Complications: ANEMIA, BRAIN DAMAGE, chronic diarrhea or MALABSORPTION (See Protocol B.14), HYPOGLYCEMIA, DIABETES, MILK INTOLERANCE, susceptibility to infections. PNEUMONIA is a common cause of death.

Vitamin deficiencies

- Deficiency in B vitamins, folate or vitamin B12 can cause a disease very similar to tertiary SYPHILIS. The symptoms develop slowly over months. They begin with severe aching in the feet. Then sharp pains develop in the foot, followed by shooting pains up and down the leg. Pressure on the legs or feet aggravates the pain. Problems with vision and hearing may follow. The patient becomes uncoordinated, and he cannot tell where an arm or leg is without looking. The tongue is sore.

- A deficiency of niacin causes PELLAGRA: rough scaly skin, abdominal pains, diarrhea and irrational behavior.

- Deficiency in vitamin D causes RICKETS. Infant formula is not fortified enough to prevent this. Infants on formula need additional vitamin D. Adults with RICKETS have bone pain, and their bones are fragile, fracturing easily.

- Deficiency in vitamin E can cause incoordination.

Causative diseases: ASCARIASIS, GIARDIASIS, TUBERCULOSIS, MALABSORPTION (Protocol B.14) and all the causative diseases of that, MEASLES, BRUCELLOSIS.

Similar conditions: see Protocols B.6: Limb Swelling and B.7: Liver/Spleen Problems. In any arable area, first treat for GIARDIASIS (diarrhea) and ASCARIASIS (no diarrhea). If the patient consents to eat thereafter, just feed him and don't worry about similar diseases. If he refuses to eat or if he has general body swelling, see the appropriate protocols in the Symptom Index. Deficiency of the B vitamins resembles tertiary SYPHILIS that affects the spinal cord.

Bush laboratory: usually ANEMIA. Urine usually shows ketones.

Treatment

Prevention: agricultural development, nutrition education. Provide supplementary feeding for children after any diarrhea (especially watery) and after any serious illness. See Volume 1, Chapter 5 to ascertain what deficiency diseases are likely to be prevalent in your area and what locally available foods are needed. Then routinely advise parents to give their children these foods.

Referrals: a refeeding program run by an NGO, if locally available, is ideal.

Patient care: see the detailed instructions in Volume 1, Chapter 5. It is essential to distinguish between marasmus (skinny malnutrition) and kwashiorkor (swollen malnutrition) since the initial treatments of the two conditions differ.

With kwashiorkor, the child's weight in kg x 30 is the number of ml of milk a child should consume in 24 hours; start with a high-carbohydrate diet and work up to this milk consumption gradually.

When giving antibiotics initially, be sure not to use any for which LIVER DISEASE is listed as changing the dosage. A malnourished liver doesn't handle these antibiotics well.

Results: with kwashiorkor there will be initial weight loss for a couple weeks. With marasmus there should be significant weight gain within 7 days. Length or height should increase over 2 months.

Mansonellosis perstans

See Regional Notes F, M.

MASTITIS

Cause: bacteria.

Clinical

Mastitis is CELLULITIS or ABSCESS of the breast, most common in nursing women. It occurs after 2 weeks following delivery and is usually related to missed feedings which stagnate the milk. Usually there is a moderate to high fever, pain, redness or warmth and swelling. There may be a pus discharge from the nipple or the mass, and the nipple may be inverted.

Similar conditions: FILARIASIS and TUBERCULOSIS are similar, as well as some types of breast CANCER.

Treatment

Treat for CELLULITIS or ABSCESS first; consider alternatives if no better in 3–4 days. Keep the breasts empty after draining pus. Milk will normally leak for a while through the drainage incision.

MASTOIDITIS

Cause: bacteria.

Definition: mastoiditis is an infection of the bony bump behind the ear.

Age: usually children. **Who:** those with ear infections. **Onset:** usually gradual.

Clinical

This is an infection of the bone behind the ear. It is a complication of an untreated EAR INFECTION. The swelling pushes the ear forward. There may be local redness, drainage and a fever. If left untreated, it may cause MENINGITIS.

Treatment

The same as for EAR INFECTION, MIDDLE, but continue for at least 2 weeks. Surgery may be necessary, level 4 or 5.

MEASLES

Regional Notes: E, F, I, S, U.

Cause: virus.

Synonyms: hard measles, morbilli, red measles, rubeola, ten-day measles.

Definition: measles is a viral infection of the body, most common in children.

Moderately to very ill; class 2; contagious, highly; worldwide, common except where there are immunizations. Occurs in epidemics.

Age: over 4–5 months, mostly before 4 y.o., occasionally adults. **Who:** unimmunized; far worse in malnourished children; both worse and more common with overcrowding. **Onset:** 9–14 days after exposure; then over a day or two.

Clinical

Necessary: the patient has a high fever, a cough, runny nose and red eyes. His eyes are painful, and light makes the pain worse. A rash breaks out about the third day of illness. It is red spots on fair skin, sandpapery on black skin, sandpapery-red on intermediate skins. It starts on the head, then spreads to the rest of the body. By the third day of the rash, it is heavy all over.

Sometimes: there may be sneezing initially. The patient may have raised white spots on a red base in his mouth early in the disease. These spots may be painful. Babies may stop nursing because of them. In severe measles the rash darkens and the skin peels after 4–11 days. HIV patients may have no rash with measles.

Commonly: the patient develops diarrhea (which may be bloody), vomiting and DEHYDRATION. A couple of days after the rash breaks out, the patient may develop PNEUMONIA or EAR INFECTION, MIDDLE. He may become short of breath. There is a 50% mortality with PNEUMONIA.

Complications: KERATITIS (sometimes due to HERPES), BRAIN DAMAGE, MALNUTRITION, EYE INFECTION, XEROPHTHALMIA, GANGRENE of the limbs, blindness, deafness, SEIZURES, aggravation of TUBERCULOSIS and death. Death is particularly likely in children under 1 year old. After measles the patient may develop POST-MEASLES CACHEXIA, a condition of lethargy, refusal to eat, MALABSORPTION and weight loss, resulting in death. Measles is not severe in immunized patients.

Similar conditions: see Protocols B.8, B.10 and B.12. Consider RUBELLA, SPOTTED FEVER, DENGUE FEVER, SCARLET FEVER, MONONUCLEOSIS. Before the measles rash breaks out, epidemic INFLUENZA is indistinguishable.

Treatment

Prevention: immunize all children six months old or older, except those with BURKITT LYMPHOMA, TUBERCULOSIS or severe MALNUTRITION. Check with a local M.D. to find out at what age to give it in your area. There is a heat-stable vaccine available. It can be held at room temperature (70's **O**F) for 2 days and at body temperature for 7 hours.

Referrals: facilities and practitioners: IV fluids, antibiotics, nutritional support, a general practitioner or a pediatrician might be helpful, at level 2 or more.

Patient care:

- Right at first, before anything else, give VITAMIN A to prevent blindness. ZINC (egg yolks) is also helpful.

- Check vital signs every 4 hours.

- Diet: sugar initially, then milk, as much as tolerated. Pass a stomach tube if necessary. Use soy milk if diarrhea is severe. Empty the mother's breasts during the illness; insist on nursing for 2 months after, or use a high-protein diet. The refeeding mixture used in MALNUTRITION is excellent. Encourage fluid intake.

- Treat the fever with ACETAMINOPHEN and cooling.

- Use no antibotics unless and until there is PNEUMONIA.

- Watch the respiratory rate, listen to the lungs and watch for signs of EAR INFECTION daily. If EAR INFECTION or PNEUMONIA develops, treat with PENICILLIN. If that does not seem to work, use CLOXACILLIN or a CEPHALOSPORIN.

- Use BISMUTH SUBSALICYLATE for diarrhea, PROMETHAZINE for vomiting.

- Treat DEHYDRATION.

- Treat POST-MEASLES CACHEXIA just like MALNUTRITION from any other cause.

Results: 90% death rate in malnourished Africans; rare deaths in previously healthy Europeans. The darker the skin, the worse the prognosis.

Mediterranean tick typhus

See SPOTTED FEVER. Mediterranean tick typhus and African tick typhus are both listed under SPOTTED FEVER. Mediterranean tick typhus tends to be less severe than African tick typhus. The geographic distributions overlap.

MELIOIDOSIS

Regional Notes: O, S, U.

This is a kind of SEPSIS that occurs in Southeast Asia and aboriginal Australia, but it may occur elsewhere. It may be associated with severe weather or with near-drowning. It most commonly starts with PNEUMONIA or URINARY INFECTION. Patients frequently have had previous poor health, and the death rate is high. The best drugs are Ceftazidime, Imipenem or Meropenem, all listed under CEPHALOSPORIN. The patient needs 12 weeks of antibiotics to eradicate the problem, once he feels better.

MENINGITIS

Regional Notes: E, F, I, O, R.

Entry category: disease cluster.

Synonym: cerebrospinal meningitis.

Definition: meningitis is an infection of the meninges which is the covering over the brain and spinal cord.

Cause: usually bacteria or virus.

Always very ill; class 3; contagious usually; worldwide, quite uncommon, easily confused with cerebral MALARIA, which is not contagious. TB meningitis occurs wherever TUBERCULOSIS is common; it is not contagious.

Age: any. **Who:** anyone, especially those with previous EAR INFECTION (ear pain) and SINUSITIS (headaches or face pain), also those with previous head injury or PNEUMONIA or active TB. **Onset:** hours to days. If the onset is over a week or more, it is probably due to TUBERCULOSIS or BRUCELLOSIS.

Clinical

ORDINARY MENINGITIS
Necessary: patients are always very ill; adults stay in bed and children are never alert and playful. Adults have a high fever and a severe headache, frequently going down the neck to the back. Exceptions: elderly patients, diabetics, newborns and HIV-infected patients may present without fevers. Meningitis caused by TUBERCULOSIS might not cause a fever.

Usually: a conscious patient over 2 y.o. has a stiff neck; he cannot put his chin on his chest; trying causes pain, but he can turn his head from side to side without pain. The neck stiffness may be subtle; look for it. Shaking the head increases pain. A baby will cry harder rather than being comforted when held by his mother. The patient prefers to lie on his side, back arched.

Sometimes: vomiting occurs in adults; it is almost invariable in children. Those under 18 months may have a bulging soft spot on the top front scalp, but this occurs late in the disease. Failure to find this is no argument against the diagnosis. Initially babies and children may be irritable; confusion, lethargy, loss of consciousness are common if the problem has persisted for some time. There may be irregular respiration. There are sometimes abnormal pupils (do not get smaller in the presence of light) or SEIZURES. Sometimes the patient has a rash which may be red spotted. The covering over the white of the eye may be swollen. The patient may have eye pain in the presence of light. There may be diarrhea.

Occasionally: the first symptom is bizarre behavior. ARTHRITIS may develop during treatment. Large dark blisters may form on the skin. These blisters resemble second-degree burns and are treated similarly.

TUBERCULOUS MENINGITIS
Necessary: there is a slow onset, an abnormal mental state and some abnormality of the face, the eyes or the pupil response to light, e.g. a new-onset "lazy eye" or unequal pupils. The patient may be dizzy.

Complications of either type: STROKE (especially when due to TUBERCULOSIS). Stroke causes floppy weakness of a limb, usually just on one side, which later becomes stiff. Other complications: deafness, BRAIN DAMAGE, SEPSIS and death. With SEPSIS the skin might turn black, blistered or both; there may be abnormal bleeding; loss of consciousness; GANGRENE; ARTHRITIS; BRAIN DAMAGE.

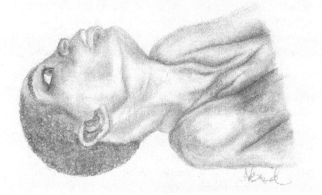

Meningitis causes the neck to be stiff; the patient is most comfortable with the head thrown back. AB

Causative diseases: meningitis may be caused by ordinary bacteria, SYPHILIS or TUBERCULOSIS; rarely by ENTERIC FEVER, BRUCELLOSIS or PLAGUE.

Similar conditions: see Protocols B.8, B.10 and B.13. *Indistinguishable:* cerebral MALARIA, HEAT STROKE, ENCEPHALITIS, NEUROLEPTIC MALIGNANT SYNDROME, RELAPSING FEVER. Patients with secondary SYPHILIS who harbor the HIV virus might appear to have meningitis when they, in fact, have SYPHILIS. *Slow-Onset:* BRUCELLOSIS and LEAD POISONING. Also consider TRICHINOSIS (swollen muscles), POLIO (limb paralysis), TETANUS (general muscle spasms), RABIES (spasms with swallowing water or a breeze on the face), SPOTTED FEVER (rash beginning on limbs).

Treatment

Prevention: the kind of meningitis that is very contagious and occurs in epidemics has a sudden onset; a healthy person becomes extremely ill within hours. You can prevent the disease with RIFAMPIN or vaccine. Other antibiotics that work are CIPROFLOXACIN, OFLOXACIN, ceftriaxone (CEPHALOSPORIN), AZITHROMYCIN. Vaccines are available for the epidemic types: meningococcal vaccine for types A, C, Y and W135. There is now also a vaccine for type B.

Referrals: speedy referral to at least a level 2 facility is mandatory. See Volume 1, Appendix 13. Consider that public transport may be inadvisable because of contagion if the onset was over hours rather than days. Laboratory; a blood count and examination of the spinal fluid obtained with a spinal tap might be useful. For a spinal tap, sterile equipment, good technique and a very clean environment are essential. This might be available at a level 2 facility. At a level 3 or 4 facility, there might be cultures available as well as other more sophisticated tests. Facilities: IV equipment and fluids, injectable antibiotics, at least level 2. Practitioner: pediatrician, internist or general practitioner. An infectious disease specialist is ideal.

Patient care: begin immediately! Arrange transport. Until the patient departs treat as follows.

- Record vital signs every 2 hours.

- Give fluids to prevent DEHYDRATION. (See Appendix 1 for using a stomach tube.) MULTIVITAMINS are helpful for nutritional support.

- Use antibiotics: use them IV if you are able. IM is second-best and oral is third-best. If the onset was slow, use drugs appropriate for TUBERCULOSIS and/or BRUCELLOSIS rather than the antibiotics listed below. In an area where there is much HIV INFECTION, try to use medication that is also appropriate for SYPHILIS.

- AMPICILLIN for 14 days. Do not substitute ERYTHROMYCIN. PENICILLIN might work but not benzathine PENICILLIN.

- Give CHLORAMPHENICOL for 14 days in addition; use CHLORAMPHENICOL alone if the patient has PENICILLIN allergy, adding an appropriate[1] CEPHALOSPORIN if possible. If you will not be able to treat for 14 days, a single large dose of IM long-acting CHLORAMPHENICOL is about 95% effective.

- An alternative to AMPICILLIN plus CHLORAMPHENICOL but expensive is CEPHALOSPORIN; use a kind that is listed for meningitis.

- Add DEXAMETHASONE. This reduces the long-term bad consequences in many cases. PREDNISONE or PREDNISOLONE may substitute. Treat for cerebral MALARIA in malarious areas.

- In breast-fed babies, empty mother's breasts at least four times a day. Give the milk down a stomach tube if you can do so without making the child vomit.

- For vomiting, use PROMETHAZINE.

- For SEIZURES, use PARALDEHYDE, PHENYTOIN or PHENOBARBITAL. If you use anti-seizure medications, increase the dosage of CHLORAMPHENICOL by 10 to 15%.

Results: improvement should be evident within 72 hours; the stiff neck may take weeks to resolve.

MENOPAUSE

Regional Notes: F.

Definition: menopause is the cessation of a woman's monthly periods anywhere from age 40 to 55.

There may be episodes of sweating, heavy menstruation, personality changes and drying of the vagina, making intercourse uncomfortable. Hormonal therapy is available under a physician's supervision. CALCIUM plus estrogen and exercise can help prevent the bone thinning that occurs with menopause. Contraceptive cream helps with vaginal dryness.

MENSTRUAL CRAMPS

Definition: menstrual cramps are low abdominal pains during menstruation. The problem is responsive to IBUPROFEN. If severe, try BIRTH CONTROL PILLS for three months.

MENTAL ILLNESS

Definition: mental illness is illness caused by emotional problems.

Clinical

There may be depressed, hyperactive or bizarre behavior. Diagnose this only when other causes of the problem have been excluded. This is easily confused with ATTENTION DEFICIT DISORDER, DEMONIZATION and some physical illnesses such as cerebral MALARIA and BRUCELLOSIS. Also see STRESS and DEPRESSION.

---

1 *Appropriate in this case means one that is listed as suitable for meningitis.*

It may be confused with, cause or be caused by drug ADDICTION. It may be associated with increased or decreased appetite and weight gain or loss.

Similar conditions: it is important to distinguish mental/spiritual causes from physical causes. The following factors indicate a physical (infectious or toxic, usually) cause for the illness; you should observe all three characteristics.

- Either the problem started suddenly, or it changes markedly over hours or days.
- The patient cannot pay attention.
- He talks nonsense, is lethargic or hyperactive.

Treatment

Some medications that are useful to control behavior over the short term are: DIAZEPAM, PHENOBARBITAL, CHLORPROMAZINE.

MIGRAINE HEADACHE

Regional Notes: F.

Synonym: vasospastic headache.

Definition: a recurrent throbbing headache, usually one-sided, due to spasm of the blood vessels in the brain.

Cause: heredity.

Mildly to moderately ill; class 1; worldwide, culturally variable, common in Westerners.

Age: 15–50 y.o. for the first episode; not common in elderly Westerners. **Who:** anyone, especially relatives of those with migraines, recurrent. **Onset:** minutes to hours.

Clinical

Necessary: severe eye pain or headache, aggravated by light, sound or shaking of the head. It may last 1 hour to 4 days. It never causes a fever.

Usually: one-sided headache or one side worse than the other; vomiting is common. It is always throbbing initially, but it may be constant later.

Occasionally: the patient complains of numbness and tingling or weakness of one side of the body and there may be temporary paralysis or double vision.

Similar conditions: if the headaches are of increasing severity or are consistently on one side rather than variable, then the patient may have a brain tumor. ALTITUDE SICKNESS (altitude over 8000 feet), HEAT ILLNESS (hot environment) and MALARIA may appear similar.

Treatment

Prevention: at times NIFEDIPINE, PROPRANOLOL or VERAPAMIL might be helpful. A diet avoiding chocolate, cheese and wine sometimes decreases the frequency and severity.

Patient care: dark, quiet and pain medicines, injectable if necessary; TRAMADOL works fine. DIPYRONE works okay, but there are occasional deaths from using it; do not use it unless you are truly desperate and the family agrees to the risk. Try to get the patient to sleep. Use PROMETHAZINE or HYDROXYZINE for vomiting and sedation.

MILK INTOLERANCE

Synonyms: lactase deficiency; lactose intolerance, milk allergy.

Definition: milk intolerance is abdominal distress (diarrhea, gas pains, vomiting) due to one of the sugars in milk which the body is unable to digest.

Cause: heredity, complication of some illnesses.

Not ill to mildly ill; class 1; worldwide.

Age: children after weaning; adults. It may occur for the first time in an adult after some illness. **Who:** anyone, especially Asians, South Americans, Africans and those who have had MALNUTRITION or any intestinal disease. Many women with milk intolerance before pregnancy become tolerant during pregnancy. **Onset:** over hours to weeks.

Clinical

The patient has watery diarrhea, possibly with abdominal cramps and gas whenever he drinks milk. He may vomit.

Similar conditions: see Protocol B.14. The treatment for milk intolerance will not help any other diarrhea.

Bush laboratory: collect some of the diarrhea and let it sit for an hour or two. Test the watery part with a urine dipstick. It will show an acid pH (5 or 6) and a negative dipstick test for sugar. The sugar test, however, will be positive with Clinitest tablets. See Volume 1 Appendix 2.

Treatment

LACTAID replaces the missing enzyme for digesting milk. Otherwise a milk-free diet is helpful. Diluting milk 50:50 with clean water may help. Fermented milk products such as YOGURT can usually be used. Soy milk is always tolerated. Sometimes the problem lasts only a week or two, but usually it is lifelong. See Chapter 5 for milk-free granola and grape-nut recipes, both high-protein foods.

Miscarriage

See ABORTION. Miscarriage is a spontaneous (unintentional) abortion.

MOLLUSCUM CONTAGIOSUM

Definition: a viral skin infection causing skin bumps.
Cause: virus.
Not ill; class 1; contagious; worldwide.

Age: any. **Who:** anyone, but most common in the developing world in people with HIV. It can be transmitted sexually and also by non-sexual direct contact. **Onset:** over days to weeks.

Clinical

The patient develops little fleshy skin bumps of nearly uniform size, usually 2–200 of them but sometimes huge numbers, about 2–4 mm diameter with flat or slightly rounded tops, some with center holes. In children they are mostly on the face, trunk and limbs. In adults they are mainly in the genital area. They neither itch nor hurt.[1] Their color is like fair skin, even in dark-skinned people. The patient is not ill because of them. The insides are cheesy, not watery.

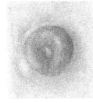

This is a magnified molluscum contagiosum bump. AB

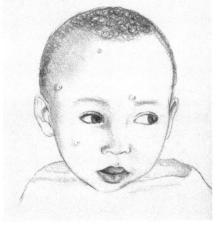

This is the appearance of a child with molluscum contagiosum on his face. OW

Similar conditions: ordinary genital WARTS turn white after 3–5 minutes if they are painted with vinegar.

Treatment

It sometimes works to disrupt the bumps with a sharp blade or sterile needle. Reassure an otherwise-healthy patient that they will go away by themselves in 8 weeks or sooner. In a patient with HIV, many bumps indicate that the patient will die shortly. They may not go away.

---

1 *In patients with immune deficiency such as AIDS or CANCER, they might itch.*

MONGOLIAN SPOT

Entry category: normal variant.

Definition: mongolian spot is a darker colored area of skin on the lower back or buttocks of a baby.

Not ill; class 1; worldwide.

Age: children. **Who:** those with intermediate skin color, neither fair nor dark black. **Onset:** usually pres15sent since birth.

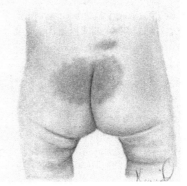

This is a small Mongolian spot; the spot may be extensive. AB

Clinical

Necessary: the patient has what looks like a black and blue spot over the back or buttocks. It is roughly symmetrical. The skin is never broken, and it never itches or hurts. It does not change color over several days like a bruise does.

Treatment

None. This is a normal skin color variation. It is included with conditions so it will not be mistaken for abuse or illness.

Mongolism

See DOWN SYNDROME.

Monkeypox

See Regional Notes F.

Monkey fever

See Kyasanur Forest disease in Regional Index I, entered under ARBOVIRAL FEVER.

MONONUCLEOSIS

Regional Notes: F, R.

Synonyms: Epstein-Barr virus infection, glandular fever, mono, kissing disease.

Definition: mononucleosis is a viral infection of the lymphatic system.

Cause: virus.

Mildly to moderately ill; class 1–2 depending on severity; contagious; worldwide, neither common nor rare.

Age: teenagers in Western cultures, children in tropics. **Who:** anyone; a person cannot get it twice, but relapses are common. **Onset:** 1–2 days.

Clinical

Necessary: the patient has a fever and complains of extreme fatigue.

Usually: the lymph nodes in the front of his neck are swollen and possibly those in back also. The swollen nodes are tender to touch.

Sometimes: he may have a sore throat, but the pain is not severe. He has large, red tonsils (provided they were not previously removed) with white blotches. His spleen and liver may enlarge, causing some upper abdominal pain. If he takes AMPICILLIN, he will get a red spotted rash that resembles MEASLES. (Stop the AMPICILLIN.) He may get the rash even without taking AMPICILLIN.

Diagnostic criteria: fever plus fatigue and at least 1 of the following: abnormal throat, abdominal pain, large lymph nodes in the neck, large spleen.

Similar conditions: see Protocols B.7, B.9 and B.12. "Mono" with a severe headache may be Q FEVER. Consider TULAREMIA, especially in southern Europe. Consider also chronic fatigue as a result of GIARDIASIS or MANSONELLOSIS PERSTANS.

Treatment

Referrals: laboratory: there is a reasonably simple blood test for this; it is likely to be found in a level 3 hospital.

Patient care: bed rest only. Antibiotics do no good. Allow no contact sports or rough-housing. If the spleen is bruised, it may rupture and kill the patient.

Results: 2 weeks to 12 months with frequent relapses.

MOSSY FOOT

Regional Notes: F, I, M, R, S.

Synonyms: endemic elephantiasis; podoconiosis.

Definition: mossy foot is foot swelling cause by silica particles.

Cause: soil particles that work their way into bare feet.

Age: usually older teen-agers and adults. School-aged children may show early symptoms. **Who:** those who walk barefoot in certain geographical areas. These places are all at more than 1000 meters (3000 feet) elevation, with rainfall over 1000 mm (40 inches) per year; near old volcanoes with red clay soil. Not everyone gets it. **Onset:** slowly over years.

Clinical

The swelling of mossy foot usually starts on one side (left or right) and then affects the other side. The first symptom is burning pain in the feet and up the inside of the lower leg. Then there is itchy swelling, starting on the feet and progressing to the trunk. The swelling is not pitting (see Chapter 1, Volume 1). As it progresses, the foot swells and the skin becomes thickened and rough, like an elephant's skin. Breaks in the skin develop which become infected. The swelling always begins in the feet, not the legs, distinguishing it from FILARIASIS.

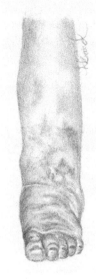

This leg and foot have comparable swelling. The foot swelled first, then the leg. In advanced cases you will see innumerable tiny bumps, all close together, resembling moss. These areas are hard and rough to the touch. With FILARIASIS, the leg swells first and eventually the foot catches up. AB

Similar conditions: see Protocol B.6.B.

Treatment

Prevention: wearing shoes from childhood prevents the problem; shoes keep it from getting worse in those already affected. Commonly the swelling decreases after wearing shoes for some years.

Referrals: in severe cases, surgical removal of the roughened skin and tissue is possible, but the results of the surgery are often poor. Much can be accomplished by the procedures described below without surgery.

Patient care

- Wash three times a day with soap and water.

- Soak the feet, up to the ankles, in a bleach solution for 20 minutes once a day. This helps kill infections and will help stop the oozing of fluids, which often occurs. The bleach solution is made by adding one teaspoon of ordinary bleach to 3 liters of clean water. The use of topical antibiotic salves is also helpful.

- After soaking and drying the feet, apply WHITFIELD'S OINTMENT once a day. This will help soften the rough, hardened skin.

MUMPS

Synonyms: infectious parotitis, parotitis.

Definition: mumps is a viral infection of the salivary glands and sometimes the testicles and pancreas.

Cause: virus.

Mildly to moderately ill; class 1; contagious; worldwide, common.

Age: any, especially children. **Who:** usually those not immunized. **Onset:** 12–25 days incubation.

Clinical

Necessary: first the patient has general achiness, loss of appetite and fever. Then he develops swelling of the glands in front of and below his ears. The swelling is neither red nor warm.

Maybe: It may be painful with eating certain foods, but it is not tender to the touch. He may complain of ear pain. It is difficult to talk or eat.

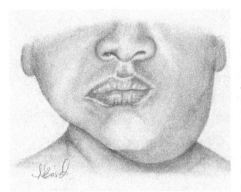

This is a severe case of mumps; one cannot see the angle of the jaw on the affected side. In this case the mumps is only on the patient's left; usually mumps affects both sides. AB

Sometimes: he may have abdominal or ear pain. The gums by the molars may swell. Adults may have painful swelling of the testicles. Symptoms of ENCEPHALITIS and eye problems are rare.

Complications: infertility is a rare complication in sexually mature males. Patients with mumps ENCEPHALITIS usually recover fully.

Similar conditions: see Protocol B.8 if the eyes are red and painful. Consider ABSCESS of a tooth (decayed tooth visible). If very ill, consider TYPHUS. BURKITT LYMPHOMA may be similar in children. ALCOHOLISM (generally only adults), LIVER DISEASE or LIVER FAILURE (bilirubin in the urine), PELLAGRA (rash on sun-exposed skin), VINCENT STOMATITIS. A similar kind of swelling is present in young children with MALNUTRITION and/or HIV INFECTION.

Treatment

Prevention: immunization is 70% effective.

Patient care: treat the fever with cooling and ACETAMINOPHEN. Place ice packs on swollen areas. Antibiotics do no good.

MUSCLE STRAIN

Synonyms: pulled muscles, myositis.

Definition: muscle strain is muscle damage caused by unaccustomed exercise.

Cause: injury.

Not ill to mildly ill; class 1; worldwide, very common everywhere.

Age: mostly older children and adults. **Who:** those engaging in unaccustomed physical activity. Those whose bodies have been jolted. **Onset:** sometimes immediately, worse 1–2 days after the activity or accident.

Clinical

The patient has sore muscles. He may have chest or abdominal pain if he exercised those muscles. The pain of a neck strain may radiate to the shoulder and arm. Low back strain is similar to SLIPPED DISC. It may cause painful pelvic muscles. The two are frequently indistinguishable at first; both may cause sudden onset of pain and shooting pains in the legs. Muscle strain never causes fever.

Similar conditions: the pain of a fractured bone is maximum immediately after the accident. It does not get worse over a couple of days. Consider BRUCELLOSIS (fevers off and on), TUBERCULOSIS of the bone (specific bone tenderness), SCIATICA (may be indistinguishable), POLIO (limb weakness or paralysis). PYOMYOSITIS may appear similar, but the tenderness and swelling are in one local place only, and there is usually a fever. TENDINITIS is indistinguishable.

Treatment

Referrals: facilities: x-ray may be helpful to exclude other diagnoses. Practitioner: general practitioner, internist.

Patient care: rest, heating pads, IBUPROFEN and pain medicines. Patients with back strain must lie on a very firm surface, on the back (with a pillow under the knees) or on either side, for 4 days, 24 hours a day. Meals and bathroom duties should be done lying down. If there is still pain after 4 days, extend the time to 2 weeks. If the patient has difficulty urinating, numb feet or persistent pain, he must be sent to a hospital. *Results:* 1–7 days, longer if the patient does not rest.

MYCETOMA

Regional Notes: F, I, M, R.

Present worldwide in tropical and subtropical areas, more arid than humid, from 15° south to 30° north.

Entry category: disease cluster.

Synonyms: madura foot, maduromycosis, deep mycosis, mycosis.

Definition: mycetoma is a fungal or bacterial infection of the soft tissues of the body: the muscle, skin or lungs. The bacterial kind predominates in India and Mexico; the fungal kind predominates elsewhere.

Cause: fungus or bacterium.

Not ill to moderately ill; class 2–4; worldwide.

Age: any; mainly older children and young adults.
Who: anyone; poor hygiene; minor wounds in hands and feet, especially from acacia trees and cacti; males more than females, mainly farmers and herders. **Onset:** slow, fungal kind over weeks to years; incubation also over years. The bacterial kind progresses more rapidly.

TOC

SYMPTOMS

DIFFERENTIALS

CONDITIONS

DRUG INDEX

REGIONAL NOTES

INX

Clinical

This may affect either the lungs or the skin.

LUNG FORM

This is a slowly progressive disease, resembling TUBERCULOSIS and indistinguishable without lab facilities.

SKIN FORM

This commonly starts on the foot (rarely the hand, face or thigh) with painless swelling. Then a bump, ABSCESS, ulcer or IMPETIGO-like sore, about 1 cm in diameter, begins. There are small amounts of an oily substance with some dry grains like chalk, yeast or coal dust coming out of the wounds. The grains are off-white, yellow or black; rarely red, orange or brownish. They may be hard or soft. Pain is usually minimal, but there may be deep itching. The patient may develop pain after some time if there is secondary infection of the wound. Then there may be ordinary pus in large amounts. There may be destruction of the underlying bones and muscles, but the pain is surprisingly little, considering how bad the swelling and open sores look. There may be multiple holes connecting the various wounds so that the whole area looks like a sponge. The foot may become shorter. The patient is likely to complain of foot heaviness rather than pain. In some areas this may cause ulcers which destroy the nose.

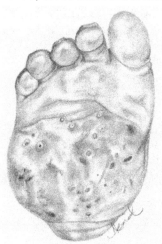

This is the appearance of mycetoma on the bottom of a foot. AB

Similar conditions: *skin form:* CANCRUM ORIS (on the face); tertiary SYPHILIS; tertiary YAWS; IMPETIGO (which is seldom on the feet); ABSCESS (tender to touch); TROPICAL ULCER. Also consider ACTINOMYCOSIS, CUTANEOUS LEISHMANIASIS and BURULI ULCER. The dry grains are specific for mycetoma.

Treatment

Referrals: laboratory; lab with a microscope may be able to examine the grains or culture the wounds to determine the type of mycetoma and suggest a likely treatment. It is not difficult to distinguish fungal and bacterial types and thus to suggest a helpful treatment.

Patient care: it varies with the form. Local medical lore may help. The kind with black grains requires surgery, but you can try KETOCONAZOLE; those with white, yellow or red grains (caused by bacteria), can sometimes be cured with medicines: (DAPSONE plus STREPTOMYCIN) for a month or (CO-TRIMOXAZOLE plus RIFAMPIN) for 3–4 months (more expensive). ITRACONAZOLE may work for the kind with white grains. IODINE applied locally might be helpful in the early stages.

MYIASIS

Regional notes: F, M, R.

Entry category: infestation.

Synonyms: maggot infestation, maggots.

Includes: screw worm.

Definition: a wound in the skin or moist surface caused by fly larvae (maggots) that penetrate intact skin or caused by larvae that invade an open wound or body cavity.

Cause: fly larvae.

Mildly ill; class 1; regional: mostly tropical areas although temperate areas also have wound myiasis. It is present nearly worldwide. The type of myiasis varies from place to place. Local lore is helpful in this regard. Nasal and ear myiasis are found in Asia and Africa.

Age: any. **Who:** those who are exposed to certain kinds of flies; especially those with open wounds, sleeping unprotected, sick, crippled or not motivated to chase flies away. **Onset:** variable, usually soon after exposure.

Clinical

The symptoms vary according to the body part affected:

- **Wound myiasis:** open wounds get maggots in them; they look like little worms. They enlarge wounds and cause infection.

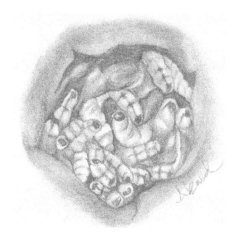

This wound is full of maggots; they look like small worms, but they are really larval forms of flies. AB

- **Eye myiasis**: same kinds as wound myiasis, plus some others which are common where sheep and goats are raised. These may produce severe eye infections (pain, redness, swelling, pus) and blindness.

- **Ear, nose, throat myiasis**: same kinds as eye and wound get into ears, nose and throat, producing infection (pain, redness, swelling, inability to hear, inability to smell, inability to swallow.)

- **Intestinal myiasis**: many different kinds of flies deposit eggs on food. The larvae then are passed in the stool. They are harmless.

- **Genitourinary myiasis**: flies lay their eggs in the genital area. The maggots may cause urinary, vaginal or rectal injury; pain with urination, sexual relations or bowel movements. They may be seen during childbirth or sexual encounters.

- **Skin myiasis**: some maggots can penetrate intact skin; see regional notes for the specific type(s), if any, for your area. Usually there are red, swollen spots on the skin.

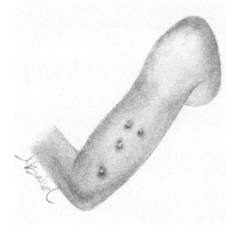

This is myiasis of a left arm. The larvae have burrowed under the skin. AB

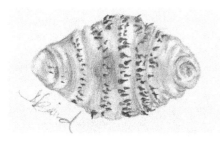

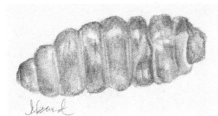

Shown on the left are magnified views of maggots. The different kinds vary in appearance. In both cases, the view is looking down from above. Looking from the side, they resemble short/fat worms. Note the segments. Note the length/width proportions. The actual length is about a centimeter. AB

Complications: secondary infection (CELLULITIS, ABSCESS); TETANUS.

Similar conditions: nothing else has visible, short, fat creatures. The worms of GUINEA WORM are very long and skinny. LOIASIS (only rain forest Africa) worms are larger than myiasis larvae; they are the size and shape of small earthworms. STRONGYLOIDIASIS and LARVA MIGRANS cause itchy lines underneath the skin, which myiasis larvae do not.

Treatment

Prevention: insect repellent might be helpful. IVERMECTIN, a deworming medication, dissolved in skin cream and rubbed on the skin, works for animals and is harmless for humans.

Referrals: this condition may require surgery, at level 3 or higher.

Patient care: varies with the type of fly. Remove maggots if they can be removed easily. If you place petroleum jelly (Vaseline) over them they may be easy to remove as they come up for air. In the case of the Tumbu fly, the petroleum jelly makes the diagnosis. If you watch the little hole carefully, you will note little air bubbles rising through the petroleum jelly. The development of the larva is over 6 days; you must wait at least until day 4 before removing it. Use ANTIBIOTIC EYE DROPS rather than the eye ointment for eye myiasis. If maggots are in eyes, ears, throat and genital areas,and cannot be removed easily, they must be removed at a hospital. After removing the maggots, treat all myiasis wounds like TROPICAL ULCER.

Nairobi eye

See Regional Notes F.

NECROTIZING FASCIITIS

This is a type of CELLULITIS or GANGRENE. It may be called "flesh-eating bacteria". First there are fever and chills, then hours or days later, an area of skin develops redness, blisters and drainage, along with a general whole body illness. Blisters progress rapidly and the area turns bluish. Pain is extreme, much worse than one would expect. There is swelling and tenderness beyond the discolored skin. Fever is high, pulse is rapid and blood pressure is low; there may be a bad smell, numbness of the affected area, loss of consciousness and little urine production. The patient will die without surgery. Give antibiotics as for GANGRENE only if evacuation is imminent. Otherwise prepare the patient for death.

NEURALGIA, NEURITIS, NEUROPATHY

These terms refer to a variety of problems causing pain, weakness, loss of sensation and other symptoms of nerve dysfunction. Generally there are no viable options other than referral to higher-level facilities. See Symptom Protocols A.8.B, A.10.B, A.33.B and A.60.B, Protocol B.13 and SPINAL NEUROPATHY.

NEUROLEPTIC MALIGNANT SYNDROME

This is a rare reaction to drugs used for anesthesia, vomiting, and for emotional upset. There is a high fever and general muscle stiffness. It can kill. Treat the fever with medications and cooling.

OLD AGE

When medical care is offered in developing areas, uneducated nationals may not understand the limits of such care. They may see no reason why anyone with a stethoscope cannot make an 80 year-old feel like a 20 year-old again. They present with multiple complaints, the following being the most common:

- Poor vision, sometimes due to cataract (which may be corrected with surgery) and sometimes due to other factors. Consider XEROPHTHALMIA.

- Poor hearing; consider tertiary SYPHILIS if recent onset.

- Aching bones, muscles and joints.

- Insomnia, fatigue, day/night reversal.

- Difficulty swallowing, usually due to a deficient number of teeth.

- Trembling.

- Constipation.

Rather than chasing down each of these symptoms, it is appropriate to simply inform the patient that he or she is not 20 years old, and these symptoms are to be expected with advancing age. A single dose of multivitamins may be helpful, since elderly people commonly are malnourished.

ONCHOCERCIASIS

Regional Notes: F, M, R.

Synonym: river blindness.

Includes: sowda.

Definition: onchocerciasis is an infection with the worm *Onchocerca volvulus,* the larvae of which damage the eyes and the skin. It is a tropical disease.

Cause: worm larvae.

Not ill to very ill; class 2 or 3

Age: any, but serious problems with eyes are generally seen only in adults. **Who:** bitten by simulium (black) flies which breed in fast-flowing water, males more than females. **Onset:** several months after the bite, nodules develop and grow slowly over 3–4 years.

Clinical

Necessary Initially: a national complains of itchy skin but does not have a rash other than scratch marks.

Usually: expatriates present differently[1.] Common symptoms in expatriates are back pain; enlarged lymph nodes; a generalized, spotted red rash with itching; and joint pains with swelling.

1 *In expatriates, symptoms which are common to a number of diseases may develop in the homeland; they are frequently ignored or treated with symptomatic medication which may help for a while.*

Sometimes: the patient describes a feeling of creatures moving around within his skin. He may have KERATITIS with eye pain, tearing and light avoidance. IRITIS may develop. This disease causes blindness, sometimes by clouding the cornea, and sometimes by destroying the inside or back of the eye. When it causes opaque scars on the cornea, the process starts at the outer rim at 4 and 8 o'clock and moves inward. It always affects both eyes, though one may be worse than the other. The entire cornea(s) may be covered with "snowflakes". The eyes are painful at first; later they lose sensitivity. There may be decreased vision which is apt to be worse in bright light.

Usually: bumps form right underneath the skin, mainly in areas where the skin normally lies right over bone, such as scalp, breast bone and shin. Nodules may range in size from a pea to a small egg. They feel bumpy inside, not smooth like LOIASIS. They are painless, not tender to touch and not particularly itchy. When the nodules are on or near the head it is important that they be surgically removed. Twenty percent of affected patients have white spots or irregular areas on their skin where the pigment is gone. There may be bags of skin in the groin, with big lymph nodes in the folds.

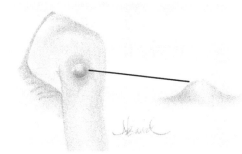

The skin bumps of onchocerciasis have peaks. They feel lumpy inside, as if the skin covered a bunch of small raisins. AB

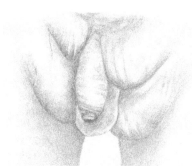

The groin lymph nodes are enlarged. The skin loses its elasticity, so the lymph nodes in the groin hang down in big folds of skin. It looks like the patient has an extra 4 scrotum. AB

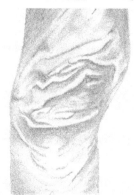

Young people develop wrinkled skin resembling the normal skin of very old people. AB

Occasionally: onchocerciasis may cause ELEPHANTIASIS of the limbs like FILARIASIS does. It may cause general darkening of the skin or may cause skin changes so that the skin surface resembles orange peel or becomes very wrinkled. There may be swelling of the skin with scaly bumps in patients living in the arid Sahel (Africa). There may be EPILEPSY, IRITIS, blindness. HIV INFECTION makes the symptoms worse.

Similar conditions: *eye symptoms:* see Protocol B.8: Red Painful Eyes. *Itching all over:* distinct from HEPATITIS and JAUNDICE in that the whites of the eyes are not yellow, and onchocerciasis does not cause bilirubin in the urine. *Nodules:* CYSTICERCOSIS nodules are smaller. HYDATID DISEASE nodules might look similar but they are soft; onchocerciasis nodules are firm. SYPHILIS and YAWS might cause similar firm nodules, but there will be other symptoms also, as well as a different history. *Skin changes:* VITILIGO might look similar, but it is not itchy. LEPROSY also involves sharp shooting pains, and it is never itchy. FILARIASIS also causes skin changes and limb swelling. *Back and joint pains* are similar to other causes of ARTHRITIS. Also consider BRUCELLOSIS and bone TB. In Westerners, suspect onchocerciasis if there is ARTHRITIS with a high eosinophil count.

Treatment

Prevention: control of fly population; wear trousers and hats, put screens on houses. Avoid building houses near fast-flowing streams. Find out what time of day the flies bite and avoid visits to a river during those hours. Inquire about the WHO control project.

Referrals: laboratory: many hospitals can take a little piece of skin and examine it under the microscope to make a definite diagnosis. A blood count will probably show increased eosinophils (other diseases do also). In the absence of eye symptoms, a definite diagnosis may be made by giving 25 mg of DIETHYLCARBAMAZINE (DEC). This will provoke a tremendous itching response with onchocerciasis. A cream made of ordinary hand lotion and crushed DEC, rubbed on the skin, will give an itching response within 48 hours. This is safer but more time-consuming.

Patient care: the current treatment of choice is DOXYCYLCINE for 6 weeks plus a single dose of IVERMECTIN, if there is no LOIASIS or FILARIASIS in the area (i.e. the patient is not likely to have one of these diseases). The DOXYCYCLINE destroys bacteria on which the worms depend. It does not directly kill the worms. If it is used for 4–6 weeks before one of the treatments listed below, the patient is not so likely to have a bad reaction.

- Treatment of everyone in an area is safe and results in a decreased incidence of eye problems. It should be done every 6 months. IVERMECTIN is better than DEC.

- DIETHYLCARBAMAZINE (DEC) is the older, traditional drug. Do not treat severe cases with it as you may cause fatal ANAPHYLAXIS.

- **With eye symptoms:** use maximum doses of DIPHENHYDRAMINE along with the DEC, and use PREDNISOLONE EYE DROPS for the first five days of therapy in the presence of eye symptoms.
  No eye symptoms: eye drops, PREDNISONE and

DIPHENHYDRAMINE may be used only as needed. In either case, do not use the DIETHYLCARBAMAZINE unless you have EPINEPHRINE and DIPHENHYDRAMINE on hand. DIETHYLCARBAMAZINE does not kill adult worms in nodules. The patient needs repeated treatments over a long period of time or should be sent to a hospital for suramin treatment or nodule removal.

- MEBENDAZOLE plus LEVAMISOLE may destroy the adult worms safely.

There is a lot of money being put into onchocerciasis eradication (Jimmy Carter project). Probably new treatment protocols will be developed.

Complication of treatment: DRUG ERUPTION may be seen with DIETHYLCARBAMAZINE. Before treating your patient, become familiar with this.

Onyalai

See Regional Notes F.

OSTEOMYELITIS

Cause: bacteria.

Definition: osteomyelitis is a bacterial infection of the bone, usually due to staphylococcus (Gram-positive, but needs special antibiotics).

Moderately to very ill; class 2–3; worldwide; in Africa and Saudi Arabia it is more common than elsewhere because of SICKLE CELL DISEASE being prevalent. It is generally common where sanitation is poor.

Age: any; most common in 7–25 age range. **Who:** those with wounds or TROPICAL ULCERs, especially the malnourished. BURULI ULCER and DONOVANOSIS can cause this. Patients with SICKLE CELL DISEASE or HIV INFECTION are particularly prone. **Onset:** over weeks to months**.**

Clinical

Necessary: this causes fever, general fatigue and deep bone pain. Lightly tapping or rolling a pencil along the bone aggravates the pain. There is always pain, tenderness and swelling in the affected area.

Usually: it is a dull pain at first which becomes worse over 2–3 months. When it affects the leg there is a limp. It is commonly either above or below a large joint (e.g. elbow or knee), though it may be anywhere: back, pelvis, jaw, shoulder. The skin is usually pulled inward, shaped like a sink hole.

Maybe: there are muscle cramps or spasms. When it affects the back, there may be sharp shooting pains. There may be holes in the skin which drain pus. In advanced cases the bones may be so weak that they fracture from very slight trauma, as in turning over in bed. Except in SICKLE CELL DISEASE or multiple injuries, it almost always affects only one part of the body.

If it is a patient who has SICKLE CELL DISEASE, the site is usually the hands in those under 5 y.o.; it is anywhere on the limbs in those who are older. In this case it may be symmetrical rather than one-sided.

Similar conditions: see Protocol B.6 for limb(s), B.13 for the back. If the onset is slow, consider bone TUBERCULOSIS, BRUCELLOSIS and DONOVANOSIS.

Treatment

Referrals: laboratory: level 3 or above might be able to do cultures to determine the correct antibiotic. Facilities: if the symptoms have been for only a short while (a matter of days), x-rays might not show anything; in any case, plain x-ray will not distinguish bone death (in SICKLE CELL DISEASE) from osteomyelitis. Osteomyelitis is likely if the patient's fever is high, and he has a whole body illness. Practitioners; a general practitioner, internist or pediatrician is essential; a surgeon might be needed.

Patient care: treatment should be started on the basis of clinical assessment, because the condition can advance very rapidly.

- If the illness is of recent onset (within less than a week), use antibiotics: 6 weeks minimum with CLOXACILLIN, AUGMENTIN, a CEPHALOSPORIN, CLINDAMYCIN or CIPROFLOXACIN. CHLORAMPHENICOL or GENTAMYCIN might work.

- If you cannot tell if it's due to TUBERCULOSIS or not, use RIFAMPIN, CIPROFLOXACIN and two other TB drugs for a minimum of 18 months. RIFAMPIN is also the best drug if there is a foreign object (e.g.bullet) lodged in the area.

- If the patient has SICKLE CELL DISEASE, then first try a CEPHALOSPORIN or CIPROFLOXACIN. CIPROFLOXACIN is not supposed to be used in children, but this illness is so very serious and disabling that it may be worth the risk. If the illness has been for more than a week or if he becomes worse while on treatment, the patient must be sent to a hospital immediately; his bone must be drilled open to release pus.

- Without surgery advanced disease will not respond to antibiotics over the long term.

OVALOCYTOSIS / ELLIPTOCYTOSIS

Includes: elliptocytosis (a related hereditary defect), spherocytosis.

Definition: ovalocytosis is a hereditary defect in the structure of red blood cells.

Not ill to very ill; class 2–4; regional. Ovalocytosis mainly occurs in Malaysia and New Guinea, but it affects some families throughout the world.

Elliptocytosis is common in North Africa and West Africa; for your purposes the two conditions are indistinguishable. Spherocytosis occurs in Europeans; this is also indistinguishable.

Age: 3 months and older. **Who:** those from affected families; the gene is dominant. **Onset:** variable.

Clinical

Ovalocytosis is similar to THALLASEMIA but not as serious. There may be ANEMIA and a large liver and spleen. Ovalocytosis protects against MALARIA and thus is a survival advantage.

Complications: it sometimes causes crises with viral illnesses, when the spleen suddenly destroys many red cells, causing large amounts of urobilinogen in the urine with sudden ANEMIA, JAUNDICE, and possibly KIDNEY DISEASE or SHOCK. Persons with this disease are prone to GALLBLADDER DISEASE.

Similar conditions: see Protocols B.3 and B.7. TROPICAL SPLENOMEGALY is indistinguishable in your situation, except that it does not run in families.

Treatment

Referrals: see ANEMIA. If the anemia is severe, then speedy referral is important. See Volume 1, Appendix 13. Laboratory; a blood smear and some other tests can help with diagnosis, level 3 facility or above. Facilities; a blood bank and transfusion facilities with HIV testing. Practitioner; a hematologist is ideal; an internist or pediatrician might be helpful. Sometimes surgery (spleen removal) is necessary.

Patient care: mild cases are treatable with FOLATE.

Overdose

See Symptom Protocol A.11.

Palpitations

See Symptom Protocol A.3.D.

PANCREATITIS

Regional Notes: F, I.

Definition: pancreatitis is an inflammation of the pancreas, a gland in the upper abdomen.

Cause: variable.

Very ill, usually; class 4; worldwide.

Age: adults, usually. **Who:** usually a complication of ALCOHOLISM, MUMPS, childhood MALNUTRITION, GALLBLADDER DISEASE, EBOLA VIRUS DISEASE or ASCARIASIS. Sometimes due to injury. **Onset:** over minutes to hours.

Clinical

There is intense central or upper-central abdominal pain going through to the back and severe vomiting. The abdomen may be swollen. It may cause MALABSORPTION, DIABETES or both; it may result in death.

In Africa, Malaysia and India, there is a type of pancreatitis that is not associated with the conditions listed. It affects mostly males, starting in their teens. It also leads to DIABETES and/or MALABSORPTION.

Similar conditions: see Protocol B.7: Liver/Spleen Problems if appropriate. *Abdominal pain:* consider ACUTE ABDOMEN, GALLBLADDER DISEASE (pain more right than central), PEPTIC ULCER (pain more burning), AMEBIASIS (pain more burning and usually right-sided). *Diarrhea:* see Protocol B.14.

Treatment

Referrals: speedy referral is important; see Volume 1 Appendix 13. Laboratory: various blood tests are helpful to confirm the diagnosis. Facilities: level 3 or above: stomach tubes, suction, IV's, surgical theatre. Practitioner: at least an internist; a gastroenterologist is ideal. A surgeon may be required.

Patient care: treat like ACUTE ABDOMEN and send the patient to a hospital. He will die in your care.

PARAGONIMIASIS

Regional Notes: F, I, M, O, S, U.

Synonyms: lung fluke disease, pulmonary distomiasis.

Definition: paragonimiasis is an infection of the lung with the lung fluke, *Paragonimus westermani.* It is a tropical disease.

Cause: worm.

Mildly to moderately ill; class 1–2; regional.

Age: any. **Who:** anyone living in an affected area who eats raw or poorly cooked shellfish. It may also be acquired from game meat that is infected, from contaminated hands or from utensils used to prepare such foods. **Onset:** 6–8 weeks incubation; symptoms develop over days.

Clinical

Necessary: the patient has a cough which is worse in the mornings and after exertion, producing brownish or reddish sputum.

Usually: this does not cause weakness as TB does; patients may have bloody sputum for 20 years without diminished capacity for work.

Sometimes: there are night sweats, shortness of breath or chest pain that is worse when breathing in. There is fever in 1/4 to 1/2 of patients.

Occasionally: patients have diarrhea resembling DYSENTERY and abdominal pain. The patient may develop finger clubbing similar to that of HEART FAILURE. The parasites may go to the brain causing BRAIN DAMAGE, STROKE or SEIZURES.

Complications: uncommonly STROKE, BRAIN DAMAGE, SEIZURES, blindness, paralysis, lumps under the skin; more common in children than in adults.

Similar conditions: cough: TUBERCULOSIS. *Diarrhea:* see DYSENTERY and similar diseases.

Treatment

Prevention: do not eat raw shellfish. Wash hands and utensils used in preparing shellfish.

Referrals: laboratory; a hospital laboratory can examine sputum for the eggs. They are quite large and not hard to find, but the test is not sensitive. You must have several negative tests before you believe it. In some places there are blood tests available. There are always a lot of eosinophils in the blood count.

Patient care: PRAZIQUANTEL is 80–90% effective. BITHIONOL is an older drug. TRICLABENDAZOLE may be helpful.

PARAPHIMOSIS

Cause: poor hygiene.

Definition: paraphimosis is a condition in an uncircumcised male in which the foreskin is pulled back and then swells so it cannot be replaced over the pink part of the penis. The condition may be painful.

The foreskin should be cut immediately to prevent GANGRENE. See Appendix 1 in Volume 1 for the procedure. Then the patient can be sent for circumcision when it is convenient.

PARKINSON'S DISEASE

Regional Notes: F, I.

Definition: Parkinson's disease is a type of brain damage that causes a particular type of trembling and incoordination.

Mildly to very ill; class 3; worldwide, uncommon.

Age: elderly; younger people on certain tranquilizing drugs. **Who:** anyone, especially those on tranquilizers (CHLORPROMAZINE, METOCLOPRAMIDE and similar drugs). Reportedly this can also be caused by repeated exposures to insecticides. **Onset:** slow, over weeks to months.

Clinical

Initially: there may be a loss of the sense of smell.

Thereafter: the patient's hand(s) tremble(s), especially when at rest. The trembling improves if he tries to do something, and it usually starts on the dominant side before affecting the other side also. There are few or no spontaneous body movements. The face is expressionless (symmetrically droopy); the voice soft, slurred and difficult to understand. Because of not swallowing, the patient may begin to drool. The gait is peculiar. He looks as if he is falling forward and moving his legs to keep up with his body. His limbs appear to be stiff. He may "freeze" when turning or going through a doorway.

TOC

SYMPTOMS

DIFFERENTIALS

CONDITIONS

DRUG INDEX

REGIONAL NOTES

INX

Sometimes: there is imbalance and difficulty in recovering from a stumble. Later there may also be problems with urine and bowel functions and loss of intelligence.

Similar conditions: *with a fever or history of fevers:* consider RELAPSING FEVER, ENTERIC FEVER. *Trembling:* withdrawal (see ADDICTION), LIVER DISEASE and LIVER FAILURE (also yellow eyes or distended abdomen), KIDNEY DISEASE (also flaky skin and urine-like body odor), BRAIN DAMAGE from any cause, PELLAGRA (also rash). *Droopy face:* LEPROSY that affects both sides of the face, BELL'S PALSY, LYME DISEASE.

Treatment

Referrals: there are good drugs available in the West; a level 3 or above hospital may help. The side-effects and dosages of the drugs need to be monitored carefully. A neurologist might be helpful to confirm the diagnosis.

Patient care: if the problem has not been going on for long, stopping tranquilizer drugs may bring improvement. In the West there are drugs both to retard the development of the disease and to treat symptoms. Drugs for treatment are generally not available in developing countries. Consult a local physician.

PARONYCHIA

Definition: a paronychia is a small abscess that sometimes forms on the side of a fingernail. See the section on Wound Infection, Chapter 10 in Volume 1 for instructions on how to treat this.

Parovirus

See FIFTH DISEASE.

PELLAGRA

Regional Notes: E, I, O, R.

Synonyms: NIACIN deficiency.

Includes: ariboflavinosis.

Definition: pellagra is a deficiency of the B vitamin niacin (niacinamide, nicotinamide).

Mildly to moderately ill; class 1; worldwide.

Age: mostly middle-aged. In some areas, children and infants also. **Who:** those eating a diet deficient in NIACIN; corn, sorghum or starch-only diets. The TB drug ISONIAZID is sometimes associated with this. **Onset:** symptoms get better and worse over weeks to months.

Clinical

Necessary: at least two of the following: diarrhea; a symmetrical, roughened skin rash; difficulty swallowing; and mental changes. Pellagra does not cause fevers.

Initially: pellagra causes indigestion, mental changes and diarrhea; occasionally it causes constipation. Upper abdominal pains are worse with food; he is likely to complain of gas. The patient has little or no stomach acid, so his vomit does not taste sour like it normally would. He may have MALABSORPTION and ANEMIA.

Then: his urine has a pH of more than 7. He is pale, listless, has large pupils, headaches and vague pains. The whites of his eyes look bluish. He is irritable and depressed. He is likely to become irritated with bright lights, colors and noises. The symptoms are seasonal, changing with diet.

Usually: a symmetrical rash appears, first on the areas of the skin exposed to the sun or subject to friction, such as the knees, elbows or scrotum. It does not extend to the fingertips. The skin may be swollen. First it is like a sunburn which burns, itches and blisters. The burning and itching are worse with sun exposure. Then it flakes and peels. In Africans the color is black or purplish; in Asians it is reddish or brown. Over time the skin thickens.

Later: he is rambling and disoriented. Children stop growing and gaining weight; they are mentally slow.

Sometimes: the patient also has burning, tingling and aching of the palms, soles or both. He may develop trembling, stiff muscles, incoordination or stiff weakness. There may be a sore tongue which looks beefy red, cracks by the sides of the mouth and a poor appetite. This is due to the coexistence of a deficiency of other B vitamins.

Maybe: the rash may affect the inside of his mouth, decreasing his sense of taste and making it difficult to swallow. There is excessive saliva.

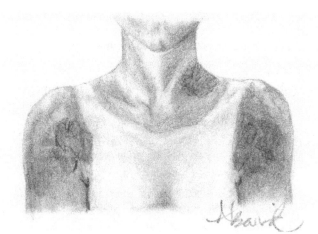

This is an intermediate case of pellagra. There are definite borders between sun-exposed and unexposed skin. The exposed skin is darkened in color and roughened. There is sparing of the skin that is normally shaded from the sun, such as the upper neck. In advanced cases all of the skin is affected. AB

Similar conditions: see Protocols B.10 and B.14.

Trouble swallowing: POLIO, RABIES, CHAGA'S DISEASE.

Diarrhea: there is excessive saliva in pellagra but not in SPRUE. *Skin changes:* ONCHOCERCIASIS has more itching, and it is similar all over the body; ECZEMA and TINEA might appear similar, but they are not worse in sun-exposed skin. *Mental changes:* ATTENTION DEFICIT DISORDER, tertiary SYPHILIS, mental BERIBERI, ALCOHOLISM, LEAD POISONING, tuberculous MENINGITIS, TROPICAL SPASTIC PARAPARESIS. Try the treatment for pellagra and see if it works. *Pains in limbs:* BERIBERI.

Treatment

Prevention: soaking corn in lime before using it prevents pellagra in corn-only diets.

Patient care: NIACIN, NIACINAMIDE. Use MULTIVITAMINS since other vitamin deficiency diseases either coexist or else are indistinguishable. An alternative is feeding the patient a diet including whole grains other than corn and sorghum.

Results: within 1–2 months.

PELVIC INFECTION (PID)

Regional Notes: E, F, R.

Entry category: disease cluster.

Synonyms: pelvic inflammatory disease, PID.

Includes: tubo-ovarian abscess.

Definition: pelvic infection is a bacterial infection of the female genital organs.

Moderately to very ill; class 2; contagious; worldwide, related to sexual activity and hygiene.

Age: mostly sexually mature. **Who:** any sexually active female, especially promiscuous. Post-menopausal women are vulnerable to tuberculous pelvic infection. **Onset:** variable; slow with TB, rapid with GONORRHEA or CHLAMYDIA although the incubation period is long.

Clinical

Necessary: after a long symptom-free interval, there is lower abdominal pain and pain with intercourse. If the patient pushes a tampon deep into her vagina, she will aggravate the pain.

Usually: the pain is centered, not markedly worse right or left. The onset of the pain is during menstruation.

Maybe: there is fever and rectal pain. The patient may have pus flowing from her vagina. There may be ARTHRITIS, a rash or both.

Occasionally: pain is more right or left, especially if there is an abscess.

Complications: infertility, liver pains.

Bush laboratory: use your urine dipsticks to check vaginal secretions for leukocytes. If there are no leukocytes, there is no PID from gonorrhea or chlamydia. The test will be negative with PID due to TB.

Similar conditions: see Protocol B.1: *Sexually Transmitted Diseases* and also B.9: *Fever and Abdominal Pain*. Check carefully for TUBAL PREGNANCY. Consider ENDOMETRIOSIS. Consider SEPSIS if the patient just delivered or miscarried. ACUTE ABDOMEN Type 2 may be indistinguishable. Consider HEPATITIS (bilirubin in urine) and KIDNEY INFECTION (leukocytes in urine). Female genital SCHISTOSOMIASIS HEMATOBIUM may be indistinguishable; treat for it if you are in an affected area.

Treatment

Prevention: discourage promiscuity, treat partner(s), treat TUBERCULOSIS.

Referrals: laboratory; a hospital lab can do a smear or culture for GONORRHEA, CHLAMYDIA and TB; they can check urine for the eggs of SCHISTOSOMIASIS HEMATOBIUM. Facilities and practitioners: an abstinence-based sexually transmitted disease clinic is ideal.

Patient care: if the pain is localized more right or left, if pain is severe, or if there is a high fever, send the patient to a hospital. Sexually active patients and babies born to infected mothers may have EYE INFECTION; it must be treated to prevent blindness, using both injected or oral antibiotic plus ANTIBIOTIC EYE OINTMENT.

Drug options:[1]

Option #1: ceftriaxone (see CEPHALOSPORIN), a single dose IM plus DOXYCYCLINE plus [either METRONIDAZOLE or CHLORAMPHENICOL], continuing the two oral medications for 14 days.

Option #2: CO-TRIMOXAZOLE plus DOXYCYCLINE plus METRONIDAZOLE, continuing all for 14 days.

Option #3: [either OFLOXACIN or LEVOFLOXACIN] with METRONIDAZOLE for 14 days.

Option #4: AZITHROMYCIN plus FLUCONAZOLE plus SECNIDAZOLE, single dose. Otherwise AZITHROMYCIN must be used over 5 days, and it is expensive.

In the regimens above, one can substitute CLINDAMYCIN for 14 days of the other drugs once the patient's pain is gone.

Option #5: use TB drugs if you suspect the cause as TB: failed treatment with the first 4 options, TB exposure, negative leukocytes on dipsticks or other symptoms consistent with TB.

---

1 *Recommendations are always changing due to the development of resistance to antibiotics. It is best to follow the advice of local health authorities. It is essential to keep records of dates, drugs given, duration of treatment and results so you have an idea what works in your particular area. If two treatment regimens don't work, consider that the cause could be either TB or fake or substandard drugs. Don't buy drugs made in India or China. Buy from an expensive location or a Western hospital.*

TOC   SYMPTOMS   DIFFERENTIALS   CONDITIONS   DRUG INDEX   REGIONAL NOTES   INX

PEPTIC ULCER

Regional Notes: F, N, U.

Includes: duodenal ulcer, stomach ulcer.

Definition: peptic ulcer is a spontaneous wound of the inside of the stomach or duodenum.

Cause: stress, heredity, bacteria.

Mildly to very ill; class 1 unless vomiting blood, "coffee grounds" or passing black, tarry stool; then class 2–3; worldwide.

Age: anyone, even children. It is especially common in South Asian children who usually present with upper abdominal pains. **Who:** those under stress; alcoholics are especially prone. **Onset:** usually gradual, occasionally sudden.

Clinical

Peptic ulcer does not cause fever. It is possible that this may be entirely without symptoms.

Usually: the patient complains of central or upper-right abdominal pain 2–3 hours before meals, followed by relief after eating. It is bad enough to awaken him at night.

Sometimes: there is indigestion or pain after meals. The patient may suddenly vomit blood or "coffee grounds," which is digested blood. He may pass blood by rectum as foul-smelling, black tarry diarrhea. He may pass a lot of gas by rectum. There may be nausea and vomiting.

Complications: if the ulcer perforates the patient has sudden onset of ACUTE ABDOMEN, with pain going straight through to his back. If it suddenly bleeds vigorously, he may develop SHOCK. If he consistently vomits all his food right after he eats, then his upper intestine is blocked, and he needs surgery.

Similar conditions: TUBERCULOSIS involving the stomach can be indistinguishable. GASTRITIS is a minor form of the same thing and is treated the same. GALLBLADDER DISEASE, PELLAGRA, and BERIBERI are usually worse rather than better with food. AMEBIASIS may be very similar with burning upper abdominal pains, but there are usually night sweats and at least occasional fevers. PELLAGRA and IRRITABLE BOWEL usually involve more vague symptoms.

Treatment

Referrals: laboratory: a level 3 lab to check for anemia and a bacterial cause might be helpful. Facilities: x-ray with contrast material; endoscopy might be available at level 3 or above. A stomach tube and suction might be available at level 2. Practitioner: gastroenterologist or general practitioner; a surgeon might be helpful.

Patient care: in many areas this problem is caused by bacteria. Treatment with AMOXICILLIN plus [either CLARITHROMYCIN, METRONIDAZOLE or OFLOXACIN] plus [BISMUTH SUBSALICYLATE, CIMETIDINE, RANITIDINE or OMEPRAZOLE] may be curative. TINIDAZOLE can substitute for METRONIDAZOLE.

The English drug Tripotassium dicitratobismuthate is similar to BISMUTH SUBSALICYLATE. DOXYCYCLINE may be a useful substitute for one of the other drugs. Avoid using a drug that has recently been used for another reason. Treat for 14 days. Do not allow him to use ASPIRIN or IBUPROFEN. Tell him to avoid spicy-hot foods, coffee, tea and colas. If the patient has significant weight loss, the problem may be due to CANCER. If he is vomiting blood send him to a hospital, especially if he has a large spleen. (See Volume 1 Appendix 13) Otherwise:

MANAGING VOMITING BLOOD

- Keep the patient in bed and check his vital signs frequently; watch for SHOCK.

- Place a large-diameter stomach tube if you have one, larger than the one made from IV tubing. Put a vial or two of EPINEPHRINE in a liter or two of clean ice water. Use a large syringe to empty the stomach through the tube. Then put your cold EPINEPHRINE-water solution into the syringe and squirt it down the tube. Immediately pull it back out into the syringe, and empty it into a waste bucket. Repeat this process until the returning water is clear. Take the stomach tube out as soon as you are done emptying the stomach.

- Give the patient ANTACID hourly while awake, every 4 hours at night. Do this for a week and then treat like a regular ulcer.

- Keep the patient on a bland diet without milk or milk products for a week. Milk relieves pain immediately, but it makes the ulcer worse over time.

- In some areas special medications may be used which decrease the production of stomach acid: CIMETIDINE, OMEPRAZOLE and RANTIDINE are most common. They should not be used routinely in developing areas, because they decrease resistance to TB.

Results: relief in a week; treat for a month.

PERICARDITIS

Regional Notes: F.

Includes: restrictive pericarditis, pericardial effusion.

Definition: pericarditis is inflammation of the sack that the heart lies in.

Moderately to severely ill; class 3–4; worldwide.

Cause: variable.

Age: any. **Who:** those with KIDNEY DISEASE, PNEUMONIA or other RESPIRATORY INFECTIONS. Common with LASSA FEVER and some other viral infections. Not common but may occur with RHEUMATIC FEVER, FAMILIAL MEDITERRANEAN FEVER and REITER SYNDROME. It is common with TB, but if it is painless; you may not recognize it. It will look like ordinary HEART FAILURE. **Onset:** variable.

Clinical

Necessary: one or both of the following two symptom-groups:

1. HEART FAILURE (restrictive type) with nearly inaudible heart sounds. Usually there is a large, tender liver and a very small difference between the two blood-pressure numbers (e.g., 100/96). The veins on the patient's neck may be swollen.[1]

2. The patient may have chest pain, either like PLEURISY or else worse with leaning back, improved with leaning forward. With swallowing there may be pain over the lower breastbone and/or straight back from there. The pain may go to the ridge of muscles on top of his shoulder, near his neck on the right, left or both sides.

Maybe: he may have a harsh, murmur-type sound audible with a stethoscope. There may be a fever, but it is usually not high. Pulse may be rapid.

Similar conditions: the pains of ANGINA, HEART ATTACK and PLEURISY are not affected by swallowing or leaning forward. COSTAL CHONDRITIS might give similar pain but the chest wall is tender to touch; it is not tender with pericarditis. AMEBIASIS, if it occurs on the left side of the liver, might cause similar pain and may cause true pericarditis. Rarely, in specific geographical areas only, consider HYDATID DISEASE.

Treatment

Referrals: see Volume 1 Appendix 13. Laboratory; a microscopic examination of fluid taken from the pericardium might be helpful, as well as examining sputum for evidence of TUBERCULOSIS. This requires a level 3 lab. Facilities: x-ray, electrocardiogram or ultrasound, level 3. Practitioner; a cardiologist is ideal.

Patient care: check for the diseases that may cause this, and treat accordingly. If TB is most likely also give PREDNISONE along with the anti-TB drugs. Do not give PREDNISONE instead of or before the anti-TB drugs! Keep the patient in bed, sitting. Use IBUPROFEN for pain. COLCHICINE as used for GOUT is a second option. Send the patient out if at all possible.

PERTUSSIS / WHOOPING COUGH

Regional Notes: E, F, N, S, U.

Includes: parapertussis.

Definition: pertussis is a specific bacterial infection of the airways causing prolonged cough.

Very ill but may not appear ill; class 2; contagious; worldwide, epidemics among unimmunized.

Age: children, especially infants. Adults, especially the elderly. **Who:** those in contact with another case; unimmunized or immunized a long time ago. **Onset:** 6–12 days after exposure; initially a 1–2 week period of "cold" symptoms before the cough develops.

Clinical

Necessary: there is no fever. Children have severe coughing spells, frequently turning blue, choking and vomiting. The cough sounds dry but he produces thick, sticky white sputum. He looks perfectly healthy between coughing spells. Adults have a chronic cough which may last for weeks to months.

Sometimes: at the end of each coughing spell, the patient takes a deep, fast breath, giving a "whoop" sound. He may cough up or vomit blood. The whites of his eyes may become blood-red. The eyes and face may swell, and he may be short of breath. This will resolve in time. The younger the patient, the more severe the disease.

Occasionally: he may have SEIZURES and become unconscious. The severe coughing may cause RECTAL PROLAPSE, or HERNIA. If he has teeth, check below his tongue. Children who cough hard with their tongues out frequently cut the little tab of tissue that secures the underside of the tongue to the bottom of the mouth in the midline. (This does not need treatment.)

Babies less than 6 months old, the elderly and those who are malnourished are most likely to die. They may have coughing spells without the "whoop".

Complications: PNEUMONIA, HERNIA, SEIZURES, BRAIN DAMAGE, RESPIRATORY FAILURE, death.

Similar conditions: usually the type of cough is distinctive in babies. In older children it may resemble any other chronic cough. Consider TUBERCULOSIS. See Protocol B.4 if the patient is short of breath.

Treatment

Prevention: immunize children as soon as possible, preferably before 2 months old. A safe immunization, dTap, is now available for older children and adults. Isolate and treat contacts with ERYTHROMYCIN.

Referrals: laboratory; a sophisticated hospital lab can do a culture. Facilities: IVs and nutritional support are very important, a level 3 or 4 facility. Practitioners: pediatrician or internist.

Patient care: it is useless to give antibiotic to patients who have been ill for a week or more. It does not shorten the over-all illness, and it is a waste of antibiotic.

Patient care in severe cases

- Keesp the patient near you, lying on his side, head down.

- Place a stomach tube if the patient will not take food on his own.

---

1 It is normal for neck veins to be swollen in anyone lying down. What you are looking for here is swollen veins with the patient sitting up or semi-reclining.

TOC

SYMPTOMS

DIFFERENTIALS

CONDITIONS

DRUG INDEX

REGIONAL NOTES

INX

- Empty the mother's breasts every 3-4 hours. Put the milk (or a refeeding mixture) down the tube: 20 ml/kg every 3 hours or 150 ml/kg daily.
- If the patient vomits, put the milk or food right back down. Do not use anti-nausea medication for vomiting. It will not help.
- Keep the humidity high; use steam in an enclosed space or hang wet sheets around the bed.
- Use ERYTHROMYCIN or CHLORAMPHENICOL for 14 days, ONLY if you can begin the drug during early "cold" symptoms. ERYTHROMYCIN is by far the better. CO-TRIMOXAZOLE may work also. Otherwise PREDNISONE may be helpful.
- Use PARALDEHYDE or DIAZEPAM for repeated SEIZURES.
- Watch the patient's weight closely. Give MULTIVITAMINS; MALNUTRITION is a common consequence of pertussis.

Results: 10 weeks, with mild relapses up to a year. 50% of infants will die. Deaths are rare in older children.

PHIMOSIS

Regional Notes: F, R.

Definition: phimosis is a condition in an uncircumcised male in which the foreskin is stuck to the pink tip of the penis.

Cause: poor hygiene.

Mildly ill; class 2; worldwide, related to hygiene.

Age: any. **Who:** uncircumcised males with poor hygiene. **Onset:** gradual, over weeks.

Clinical

The foreskin is stuck to the pink part of the end of the penis. The penis is usually painful and sometimes swollen. This may be caused by CHANCROID. Be sure to check the penis well for ulcers, including under the foreskin after you coax it back.

Similar Condition: PARAPHIMOSIS.

Treatment

Soak the penis in warm water, gradually coaxing the foreskin back by hand. LIDOCAINE ointment may help. The patient needs circumcision. See Volume 1, Appendix 1 if you can't send him.

PIG-BEL

Regional Notes: F, O, S, U.

Synonyms: enteritis necroticans, necrotizing enteritis, necrotizing jejunitis.

Definition: pig-bel is a bowel malfunction due to a bacterial toxin in malnourished children.

Mildly to severely ill; class 1–4 depending on how sick the patient is; regional, especially in New Guinea (both sides).

Age: children and teens, not nursing infants. **Who:** poorly nourished children who suddenly overindulge in protein, especially pork. Especially common where the staple food is sweet potatoes or yams. **Onset:** fairly sudden, 24 hours to 1 week after the overindulgence.

Clinical

Necessary: crampy abdominal pain, bloating and vomiting.

Frequently: bloody diarrhea and fever. Symptoms may vary between a mild gastroenteritis, a chronic malabsorption (prompt diarrhea anytime the patient eats anything) and an overwhelming acute abdomen (type 2) that results in death.

Similar conditions: many. In most cases only the historical setting of a pig feast after chronic MALNUTRITION will cause you to consider this diagnosis. *In mild cases* consider GASTROENTERITIS and/or FOOD POISONING. *With MALABSORPTION* see Protocol B.14. *In severe cases* consider FOOD POISONING, ACUTE ABDOMEN and HEMORRHAGIC FEVER.

Treatment

Prevention: before a pig feast restrict the use of sweet potatoes. Offer children an alternative carbohydrate with small protein supplements. Treating ASCARIASIS might also help.

Immunization is available, but it is not safe; a small percentage of children die from the immunization. It should be used only in areas where this disease kills large numbers of children, and people will not change their habits.

Referrals: speedy referral is important. See Volume 1 Appendix 13. Surgery at level 2 or 3 might be helpful. It is important that the surgeon be familiar with the condition. Laboratory and imaging are not helpful.

Patient care: empty the stomach with a large-diameter stomach tube. Correct DEHYDRATION. Give PENICILLIN, AMPICILLIN or CHLORAMPHENICOL. Surgery is frequently helpful.

PINGUECULA

Definition: a pinguecula is a fleshy, white bump which grows on the white of the eye, close to the edge of the cornea. It is a common problem in the tropics. Since it sticks out a little, it may become irritated as the upper lid moves over it. It looks quite similar to CHICKEN POX or TB that has affected the eye. Treatment is referral only, and it is not urgent.

Pinta

See Regional Notes M.

PLAGUE

Regional Notes: E, F, I, K, M, O, R, S, U.

Synonyms: black death, peste, Yersinia pestis infection.

Includes: bubonic plague.

Definition: plague is an infection with the bacterium *Yersinia pestis.*

Moderately to severely ill; class 3; some forms are contagious; potentially worldwide, largely tropical, reported from the southwestern United States; Uganda; Kazakhstan (related to gerbils rather than rats); Madagascar; central, east and southern Africa; India; mountainous South America; Southeast Asia (especially Burma); Mongolia; western China; and the former USSR.

Plague is spread by fleas of rodents (rats, mice, prairie dogs and ground squirrels). At present it is mostly a rural disease but does, at times, become urban. If and when this is used as a biological weapon, it will most certainly be urban. Cats are often the link between the rodents and humans. Plague occurs sporadically and also in epidemics. It is likely to occur when people move into a rodent-infested area or when rodents move into populated areas as, for example, when an area is temporarily evacuated so that untended food is left. If the rodent population spontaneously dies or is killed, an epidemic is likely. Cats get sick with plague, but dogs do not. A flea from a sick cat or a healthy dog might transmit the disease.

Age: any; those over 40 are particularly prone to the septicemic form of plague. **Who:** those bitten by animal insect parasites (especially fleas) or exposed to humans or animals with plague. **Onset:** rapid, over hours. Incubation 2–15 days**.**

Clinical

PNEUMONIC, MENINGITIC, SEPTIC PLAGUE
Death occurs within hours, too soon for treatment. With PNEUMONIC plague there is cough and shortness of breath early, with rapid shallow respiration and much watery sputum, which then becomes blood-stained.

BUBONIC (LYMPH NODE) PLAGUE
Necessary: there is an irregular fever and (beginning the 2nd– or 3rd day) extremely painful, swollen lymph nodes, most often in the groin in adults, sometimes in the armpit(s) or neck (especially in children). Pain precedes the swelling by at least 2 days. The skin over the nodes is darkened; the darkening may be slight or obvious. The nodes rapidly increase in size, and they are firm. They become soft over about a week and may then break open. The patient is very ill. Without treatment, the fever lasts 6–12 days.

Usually: he will have a headache and back pain. After some initial anxiety, the patient is mentally abnormal: agitated, lethargic or bizarre. The sizes of the lymph nodes vary from the size of an almond to the size of a child's head. There is no relationship between the size of the nodes and how sick the patient is. There may be a tiny scab where the patient was bitten by the flea that infected him. There may be incoordination of hands or gait; speech may be garbled.

Frequently: the skin around the node(s) is inflamed. The skin may die, turn black, peel or break open. There may be spontaneous black and blue areas on the skin. The spleen and liver may be large and tender. Vomiting and constipation are common. The eyes may be reddened, causing confusion with LEPTOSPIROSIS.

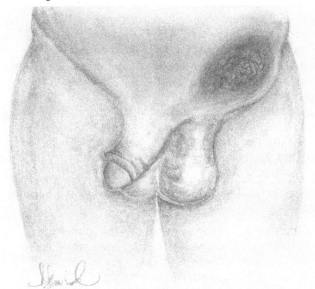

This boy has large lymph nodes in his groin. The blackness is obvious in this case; it may be subtle. The skin may be either smooth or disrupted. Usually the nodes are extremely painful and tender. AB

Occasionally: the disease may have minimal symptoms, and recovery may be spontaneous. Don't discount a report of plague that presents that way.

Complications: pregnant women abort and then usually die.

Similar conditions: see Protocol B.10 for lethargy, B.11 for a skin ulcer plus "flu" and B.12 for large lymph nodes. This looks like a rapid-onset AFRICAN SLEEPING SICKNESS; the mental changes are prominent. *Pneumonic and meningitic plague* are indistinguishable from PNEUMONIA and MENINGITIS, respectively. Death is almost inevitable. *Septic plague* is a rapidly fatal SEPSIS.

TOC   SYMPTOMS   DIFFERENTIALS   CONDITIONS   DRUG INDEX   REGIONAL NOTES   INX

Bubonic plague: TULAREMIA may also cause dark-discolored, large lymph nodes, but there are no mental changes. Plague apathy is similar to ENTERIC FEVER, but the black, discolored lymph nodes should distinguish the two diseases. TYPHUS usually has a rash associated with it. If in doubt, treat for both. If the large lymph nodes are in the groin, consider one of the SEXUALLY TRANSMITTED DISEASEs. However, with SEXUALLY TRANSMITTED DISEASEs there is usually normal skin color, and the patient is not as ill. Also consider CAT-SCRATCH DISEASE and ANTHRAX.

Bush laboratory: bloody urine indicates a bad prognosis.

Treatment

Prevention: do not kill rats or other rodents in quantity without first spraying insecticide in their habitats. Do not handle a dead rodent without first spraying it with insecticide. In areas with plague an epidemic may begin with the spontaneous death of rodents. Fleas leave the dying and dead rodents to bite humans. Immunization is available, but it only works for bubonic plague, not pneumonic or septicemic plague. It is better to take daily DOXYCYCLINE than to be immunized. Burn contaminated cloth; treat any other contaminated objects with lysol, or heat. The dead must be buried immediately, with only one person handling the corpse; that person must be treated.

Give DOXYCYCLINE for 10 days to anyone who had contact with a patient, even children and pregnant women, because of the big risk in not treating.

Referrals: only evacuate by means of a towed trailer. Treatment should not be delayed to seek a hospital unless it is very nearby. Laboratory: hospitals can do smears and cultures, but the procedures are dangerous for the technicians and one should not wait for results before treatment. Facilities: IV's and injectable antibiotics. Practitioners: general practitioner or infectious disease specialist with tropical/travel expertise.

Patient care: wearing gloves and mask and using a disposable 10 ml syringe, withdraw the pus from the abscessed node(s). Then thoroughly heat the syringe and contents in a covered container to destroy them. Immediately start high-dose antibiotics, preferably by injection. GENTAMYCIN or STREPTOMYCIN is best. (CHLORAMPHENICOL plus AMPICILLIN) or DOXYCYCLINE may work also. STREPTOMYCIN may make the person sicker at first. If there is a severe headache or signs of MENINGITIS, use (CHLORAMPHENICOL plus AMPICILLIN). CEPHALOSPORIN and RIFAMPIN are no good. CIPROFLOXACIN might work but is unproven. LEVOFLOXACIN is good, given IV.

Results: this usually responds well. Death occurs in under 5 days for untreated bubonic, in 1–2 days for untreated pneumonic or septicemic plague.

PLANT POISONING

Plants and plant products listed here

Ackee	Gallbladder of	Mantakassa
Aflatoxin	raw fish	Margosa oil
Argemone oil	Ginger jake	Miraa
Atriplicism	Ginseng	Miscara
Ava	Heliotropium	Muiragi
Betel nut	Hypericum	Muscarine
Botulism	perforatum	Mushrooms
Cassava	Impila	Nicotine
Castor beans	Jequirity beans	Outers
Claviceps	Jimson weed	Panax
Comfrey	Kava kava	Ricin
Coral plant	Kawa	Senecio
Crotalaria	Khasari	St. John's wort
Datura	Khat	Strychnine
Djenkol bean	Konzo	Uppers
Downers	Lathyrism	Valerian
Ephedra	Lolism	Water hemlock
Ergot	MaHuang	
Ginkgo biloba	Manicheel	

Regional Notes: F, O, R, S, U.

Cause: plant toxins.

Entry category: syndrome clusters.

Not ill to severely ill; class 1–4; worldwide.

(ARSENIC POISONING and LEAD POISONING are listed separately. If the patient has taken drugs, check the Drug Index. See FOOD POISONING if meats are involved. The division is sometimes arbitrary.)

Age: any. **Who:** those eating the offending substance, having skin contact or inhaling fumes. **Onset:** extremely variable, from within less than a minute to possibly after years of habitual consumption.

General treatment

If the patient is alert, if he has taken the poison within the past two hours, and if the specific type of poisoning does not prohibit it, give him several bottles of ACTIVATED CHARCOAL. This is best, and it eliminates the need to induce vomiting. If you don't have enough charcoal, then make him vomit. IPECAC[1] is ideal; it causes violent stomach spasms, thus emptying the stomach completely. Afterward settle his stomach with DICYCLOMINE, PROMETHAZINE, HYDROXYZINE or similar medication.

---

1 These directions contradict the current standard of care in the States which discourages the use of ipecac. However, they are useful for remote rural areas in developing countries. If Western medical care is available, it should be used, rather than these directions. The general treatment should be used in addition to the specific antidote unless there is a contraindication.

TOC   SYMPTOMS   DIFFERENTIALS   CONDITIONS   DRUG INDEX   REGIONAL NOTES   INX

In either case, give him something to induce diarrhea; this will decrease the chance of his absorbing more poison. If the poison he took causes diarrhea treat him with ORS instead.

Plants, toxins and treatments

ACKEE

This is present in West Africa and the West Indies. Also known as vomiting sickness, it is due to eating unripe ackee fruit from the Irsin tree. (Only unripe fruit is toxic; the ripe fruit is good to eat.) There is a 90% death rate if it is not treated. About 2 hours after eating the patient has abdominal pain and vomiting; Then he seems to recover. Then he becomes sweaty and shaky, and falls unconscious from low blood sugar. He has persistent forceful vomiting and SEIZURES. His temperature will be low or normal. He may develop LIVER FAILURE.

Treatment: empty the stomach and give alcoholic beverage when the patient first becomes ill (see ALCOHOL in the Drug Index). If he is unconscious, give sugar whatever way you can, preferably IV. If you cannot give it IV, give ALCOHOL, ACTIVATED CHARCOAL and sugar by stomach tube. Do not make the patient vomit any more than he already has.

AFLATOXIN

This is a mold found in peanuts and grains; it is a purplish color. It is one of the most powerful liver toxins known to man. Sausages are also a source of the toxin since they usually contain moist grains. Exposure to small doses over a long time causes liver CANCER. Exposure to large doses rapidly causes immediate toxicity: LIVER FAILURE, swelling of the lower limbs, abdominal pain and vomiting. Treatment may be available at level 3 or higher hospitals.

ARGEMONE OIL

This occurs in southern Africa, India, Mauritius and the Pacific Islands. Also known as epidemic dropsy, argemone oil poisoning is due to cooking oil made from the seeds of Mexican poppy. The death rate is about 5%. The patient develops swelling of his lower limbs, his face or his whole body, for about two weeks. He has fever, diarrhea and vomiting. This lasts about 6 weeks. Usually there are patches of darker skin on the faces of South Asians. Bumps appear on the skin. They vary greatly in size and appearance; they are full of blood vessels which bleed readily. The calf muscles are very sensitive to pressure. Later, HEART FAILURE (dilated type) develops. ANEMIA, KIDNEY DISEASE (nephrotic type), severe weakness and eye problems may occur. Pregnant women frequently abort. **Treatment:** DIPHENHYDRAMINE is helpful, as are MULTIVITAMINS and a high-protein, high-fat diet.

ATRIPLICISM

Caused by eating the leaves of a plant in China. About 15 hours after eating the leaves the patient's hands itch and then swell. His face and eyelids may swell and look bluish. The swollen parts may develop blisters, ulcers and GANGRENE. **Treatment:** use only the routine treatment for any poisoning.

AVA

See *kava kava* below.

BETEL NUT

Asians commonly chew this with lime and areca nut. It is a mild stimulant, producing flushing of the face. It stains the teeth black and the lips red. Used routinely it causes mouth CANCER. **Treatment:** none.

BOTULISM

A kind of FOOD POISONING which causes symptoms 6 hours to 6 days after eating the offending food, usually badly preserved cooked beans or sausage. It is present worldwide. The sequence of symptoms is as follows: abdominal pain, nausea or vomiting, diarrhea, difficulty swallowing or speaking, difficulty opening the eyes, double vision, weakness in limbs (after the head symptoms), inability to urinate and difficulty breathing. The pulse and blood pressure fluctuate. The mouth may be very dry. There is no numbness or tingling. Also see FOOD POISONING.

Similar conditions: RABIES, POLIO, DIPHTHERIA, TICK PARALYSIS. **Treatment:** not feasible in a rural setting. Send the patient out. He may require help with breathing. Some hospitals also can give antitoxin which is most helpful. Antibiotics don't work.

CASSAVA

Also known as manioc, tapioca or mantakassa, it is a common source of carbohydrate throughout the tropics. (There is sweet cassava and ordinary cassava; sweet cassava does not require special preparation, but ordinary cassava does. Both the solid food and the cooking water contain the toxin.) Hungry people sometimes shorten the preparation, eating the plant material insufficiently processed. This causes cyanide poisoning. High doses cause sudden onset of SEIZURES, loss of consciousness, cessation of breathing and death. This occurs within a minute or two after drinking cooking water. Medium doses cause dizziness, increased respiration, flushed face, headache, big pupils, low blood pressure and rapid pulse. This occurs within an hour or so. Patients who take in low doses over extended periods of time may develop pains in their limbs, stiff weakness of the limbs, slurred speech, fevers, headache, dizziness, GOITER, DIABETES and MALABSORPTION. It may cause blindness or deafness. **Treatment:** unless you have access to a cyanide poison kit, you cannot treat the problem. There are some reports that large doses of VITAMIN B$_{12}$ may help.

TOC   SYMPTOMS   DIFFERENTIALS   CONDITIONS   DRUG INDEX   REGIONAL NOTES   INX

CASTOR BEANS

Castor beans are the source of the toxin ricin. They are brown with black streaks, tear-drop shaped, about 1 cm in length, with a slight nipple-type bulge on the sharp end. The leaves have 6 lobes—the plants are about 30 cm high and are common along the roadside. The beans, used for making castor oil (used in brake and hydraulic fluid), cause ordinary diarrhea. As few as 8 beans, if chewed, are potentially fatal. Symptoms start in 8–24 hours with nausea, vomiting, diarrhea, LIVER FAILURE, KIDNEY DISEASE and death. See the separate entry for ricin. The two poisonings overlap.

CLAVICEPS

Poisoning is due to a fungus that grows on grains. It causes abdominal pain, diarrhea, vomiting and sometimes hallucinations. The blood vessels shrink, cutting off circulation to the limbs, producing paleness, coolness and pain in the fingers and toes, possibly the chest also. This may cause GANGRENE and HEART ATTACK. The patient may have a headache, a slow pulse, low blood pressure, SEIZURES, coma and death. **Treatment:** nitroglycerin, used for heart trouble, may be helpful, but you probably will not have this.

COMFREY

This is used as an ethnic medicine for fractures, tendon injuries, internal ulcers and lung congestion. There is a major problem with liver toxicity and subsequent LIVER FAILURE.

CORAL PLANT

This is present in Africa, the Americas and the Mediterranean. It is a traditional medicine for constipation, made from the nuts. It causes abdominal cramps, thirst, vomiting and diarrhea. **Treatment:** not necessary as the poison is eliminated with the vomiting that it causes.

CROTALARIA

Poisoning is from a variety of plants present worldwide, used to make bush teas. It causes LIVER FAILURE by making the veins in the liver narrow so blood cannot pass as it should. Within 10 days the patient develops abdominal pain, a large liver and fluid in his abdomen. **Treatment:** bed rest and a low-salt, high-protein diet.

DATURA

This is a criminal's poison used to make a victim unconscious or kill him; a similar poison is present in the leaves and in green skin of potatoes that have been exposed to light. There is loss of consciousness with large pupils, possibly nausea, vomiting, incoordination and hallucinations. **Treatment:** there are drugs available to treat this, but they are not feasible to keep or use in the village situation. Many insecticides, however, contain compounds similar to these drugs. In a desperate situation, you can try spraying some insecticide on a cloth and holding it near the patient's nose. If he improves in a few minutes, repeat this as needed until the poison wears off, using just enough to keep him conscious.

DJENKOL BEAN

Mainly in Indonesia and Malaysia, it is used as a food after being buried in the ground for 10 days and eaten when it sprouts. It is poisonous when eaten fresh. Sharp crystals form in the urine producing bloody urine, kidney pain (flanks), pain with urination and sometimes KIDNEY DISEASE. The poisoning can be recognized by the very strong disagreeable odor of the urine and the patient's breath. **Treatment:** empty the stomach, giving baking soda (sodium bicarbonate) in addition to ACTIVATED CHARCOAL. Watch for KIDNEY DISEASE. Usually the patient survives.

DOWNERS

See *ADDICTION*.

EPHEDRA

This is an "upper" or stimulant. It can cause sudden death, HEART ATTACK, HEART FAILURE, STROKE and LIVER FAILURE. It is similar to the drug EPINEPHRINE and to caffeine.

ERGOT

This is a fungus that grows on rye. It makes the blood vessels contract, thus causing poor circulation to the limbs and heart. It is associated with severe pain. Symptoms may be similar to claviceps poisoning. It may result in blood clots that go to the lung (see PULMONARY EMBOLISM). It may also cause ABORTION and GANGRENE. **Treatment:** like claviceps (see above).

GINKGO BILOBA

This is an herbal product that is used to reverse normal aging; reportedly it improves memory, helps ringing in the ears, impotence and age-related visual problems. The usual symptoms associated with this are stomach upset, headache and various rashes with stinging and burning sensations. It may also be associated with seizures and abnormal bleeding.

GINGER JAKE

This is caused by mixing a lubricating oil with cooking oil. It occurs in outbreaks when many people eat together. It first causes floppy weakness of the lower legs and later of the hands. About two years later, the weak muscles become stiff rather than floppy. **Treatment:** nothing helps.

GINSENG

This is supposed to increase one's sense of health. It is used to treat sexual problems, HEART FAILURE, low immunity and CANCER. Adverse effects are irrational behavior, vaginal bleeding and LIVER FAILURE.

HELIOTROPIUM

See *crotalaria*, above.

HYPERICUM PERFORATUM

See St. John's wort, listed below. It is another name for the same thing.

IMPILA
A plant in southern Africa which causes KIDNEY DISEASE, nephrotic type.

JEQUIRITY BEANS
These are red, oval, with a black cap on one end, length about 1 cm. The beans are used to make rosaries and are also used in rattle-like noise-makers. The poison is the same as castor beans, but symptoms are delayed for about 3 days; then there is LIVER FAILURE and death.

JIMSON WEED
This is a poisonous plant, present worldwide, with effects similar to the drug ATROPINE and the plant datura. Bizzare behavior is prominent. **Treatment:** send the patient out to a major medical facility if he is very ill. If he is not very ill, it is feasible to just let the effects wear off. This should happen within 24 hours.

KAVA KAVA
This is used in the South Pacific to make an intoxicating drink. The roots and leaves of the plant are chewed by humans, then spit out and mixed with coconut milk. The effects are sedative. A roughening of the skin occurs in those who take this routinely.

KAWA
See *kava kava*, above.

KHASARI
See *lathyrism*.

KHAT
A traditional drug used as a stimulant, it is widespread in the Middle East and eastern Africa. The leaves and twigs of a Miraa tree are chewed, smoked or used for teas. It is chemically and physiologically similar to amphetamines. It causes a rapid pulse. Some people become happy and gregarious, others become mellow. Repeated use may lead to ADDICTION. **Treatment:** none.

KONZO
African term for poisoning due to cassava. Refers to the sudden onset of stiff weakness. Resembles TROPICAL SPASTIC PARAPARESIS.

LATHYRISM
This occurs in the Mediterranean, East Africa and India where "khasari" is eaten. The problem is caused by a plant that grows wild, looks similar to the edible variety and contaminates food when the plants are harvested together. The patient develops muscle spasms in his legs which pull his left leg to the right and his right to the left. As a result, he walks cross-legged, as if he had a full bladder and was trying not to wet his pants. The arm and trunk muscles are not affected.

The patient's mental state does not become abnormal. Sexual impotence and incontinence of urine occur frequently. The condition is permanent. **Treatment:** nothing helps, though some claim that MULTIVITAMINS and a high-protein diet help.

LOLISM
Common in Africa and the Middle East; due to moldy wheat. Within 15 minutes the patient becomes dizzy, has a headache, slurred speech, trembling and staggering. There may be diarrhea, vomiting and abdominal pain. The patient may become unconscious or nearly so and remain that way about 10 hours. **Treatment:** empty the stomach and then give ACTIVATED CHARCOAL.

MAHUANG
See *ephedra*.

MANICHEEL
In the Western Hemisphere a kind of large tree produces a corrosive resin. All parts of the tree are poisonous; even sleeping under it or breathing its sawdust can cause problems. Eating its fruit may be fatal. Bumps resembling blisters form on the skin; they produce intense pain, and the face swells. Eaten, the fruit burns the mouth and esophagus, and may cause abdominal pain, vomiting, diarrhea, paralysis and death. **Treatment:** treat skin problems like burns. Give ACTIVATED CHARCOAL if any part is eaten. PREDNISONE may be helpful also.

MANTAKASSA
See *cassava*, above.

MARGOSA OIL
This is a traditional medicine used in India and by Asians elsewhere. It is a deep yellow extract of the seeds of the Neem tree; the darker the oil, the more poisonous it is. It has a bad smell and a bitter taste. Within hours it causes vomiting, frantic behavior, loss of consciousness, possibly SEIZURES and death. **Treatment:** the only effective treatment is in a hospital. In the meantime sugar may help. Give the patient sugar until he arrives at a hospital.

MIRAA
See *khat*.

MISCARA
See *lolism*.

MUIRAGI
See *khat*.

TOC

SYMPTOMS

DIFFERENTIALS

CONDITIONS

DRUG INDEX

REGIONAL NOTES

INX

MUSCARINE

This is a poison found in some mushrooms and insecticides. Symptoms begin in less than an hour. There is a general outpouring of body fluids: sweat, tears, diarrhea, saliva and fluid in the lungs causing ASTHMA, choking and coughing. Also there may be blurred vision, small pupils, cramps and slow pulse. **Treatment:** ATROPINE; this may require very large doses, as much as 5–10 times the usual dose. Give repeatedly, but only until symptoms are relieved. DIPHENHYDRAMINE, DICYCLOMINE and other medications that give the side effect of a dry mouth may be helpful.

MUSHROOMS

There are many kinds. Muscarine mushroom poisoning is described above. Most poisonous mushrooms cause GASTROENTERITIS. Some are used in animistic rituals to produce hallucinations. The deadly mushrooms have a long latent period, more than 6–8 hours and cause LIVER FAILURE, KIDNEY DISEASE, coma and death. **Treatment:** use the general treatment listed above, and send the patient to a hospital.

NICOTINE

Present in tobacco; children sometimes eat it. Poisoning causes nausea, excess saliva, abdominal pain, diarrhea, sweating, headache, temporary loss of hearing and eyesight and mental changes. The patient then becomes dizzy, faint and short of breath. He may die. **Treatment:** give ACTIVATED CHARCOAL.

OUTERS

See *ADDICTION*.

PANAX

See *ginseng*.

RICIN

If ricin is inhaled it causes fever, nausea, vomiting, cough, congestion, shortness of breath and death within 72 hours. Ricin swallowed causes belly pain, vomiting, diarrhea, bleeding, death of liver, spleen and kidneys. Ricin injected causes local pain and swelling. Later death of the tissues occurs in that area and adjacent body organs. Ricin comes from castor beans, a common shrub that grows beside roads in tropical areas. See castor beans, above.

SENECIO

Similar to crotalaria (above); it affects children 2–5 years old. It occurs in southern Africa, India, the West Indies and Ecuador. It causes painless enlargement of the liver. **Treatment:** bed rest and a high-protein diet.

ST. JOHN'S WORT

This is an herbal supplement used as a sedative and to treat various kinds of pains. It causes sensitivity to sunlight and sometimes irrational behavior. The herb interferes with many medicines. It causes toxicity of some and negates the effects of others.

STRYCHNINE

Used as a criminal's poison worldwide, it produces spasms of all muscles and small pupils. Effects are immediate. The patient dies because he cannot breathe due to the muscle spasms. He may have SEIZURES. It resembles TETANUS except that the onset is much faster. It resembles NEUROLEPTIC MALIGNANT SYNDROME which is treatable. **Treatment:** hopeless. The patient will die.

TOBACCO-COW'S URINE

This is a folk medicine, mixed and used in western Africa. It causes paralysis and blindness. See PLANT POISONING due to nicotine. The cow's urine component is harmless; the main effect is the nicotine. **Treatment:** send the patient to a major medical facility. If this is impossible, VITAMIN B_{12} may possibly help.

UPPERS

See *ADDICTION*.

VALERIAN

Used as a sedative. See the "downers" section of drug ADDICTION.

WATER HEMLOCK

Some kinds have edible fruits and leaves; in all kinds the roots are poisonous. Some symptoms are seizures and muscle weakness. It is the muscle weakness that makes the patient stop breathing and experience visual loss. Death is almost inevitable.

Similar conditions: too many to list; see the appropriate B protocols. In cases where multiple people take the same thing at the same time, the onset of symptoms is within hours of each other.

Referrals: this is generally helpful if the patient is quite ill. Familiarity with the particular ethnic situation is more important than paper credentials on the part of the practitioner. A level 3 or above facility is desirable. A consult with a toxicologist is most desirable, even if he has no tropical/travel experience. A consultant toxicologist can be accessed through the internet.

PLEURISY

Entry category: syndrome.

Synonyms: devil's grippe, pleurodynia, Bournholm disease.

Definition: pleurisy is an inflammation of the membrane between the lungs and the chest wall.

Cause: variable.

Not ill to severely ill, depending on cause; class 1–3; worldwide, causes vary with region.

Age: mostly adults. **Who:** anyone. **Onset:** usually sudden.

Clinical

Necessary: the patient has sharp chest pains[1], worse with deep breathing. The chest wall is not tender to touch.

Usually: in temperate climates most pleurisy is caused by a virus and is not serious; it lasts about a week. If it lasts longer or if the patient has a fever, you should find the cause. In the tropics, most pleurisy is due to one of the diseases listed.

Causative diseases: PNEUMONIA, TUBERCULOSIS, AMEBIASIS (especially in nationals), PERICARDITIS, HYDATID DISEASE.

Similar conditions: COSTAL CHONDRITIS (tenderness to touch over the joints next to the breast bone), chest injury, RHEUMATIC FEVER, FAMILIAL MEDITERRANEAN FEVER.

Treatment

For simple pleurisy, treat with pain medication such as DICLOFENAC, CODEINE or TRAMADOL. DIPYRONE is frequently available, but there are occasional deaths from it; it should not be used under these circumstances. If the problem persists, use ASPIRIN or IBUPROFEN in the doses for ARTHRITIS. ACETAMINOPHEN is not helpful. Identify and treat the underlying disease, if any.

PNEUMONIA

Regional Notes: E, F, M, N, R, S, U.

Entry category: disease cluster.

Synonym: pneumonitis.

Definition: pneumonia is a lung infection.

Cause: bacteria, viruses, fungi.

Moderately to very ill; class 1–3 depending on severity; contagious; worldwide, very common.

Age: any. **Who:** anyone, especially those with poor immunity. **Onset:** usually rapid, over 12–24 hours; occasionally slow.

Clinical

Necessary: cough and at least one of the following: shaking chills; chest,[1] shoulder or upper abdominal pain; shortness of breath; rapid respiration; abnormal sounds heard through the stethoscope. The patient's oxygen saturation will be low unless he is also anemic.

Usually: fever in patients over 6 months old, none in those who are malnourished, small infants or elderly.

SIMPLE PNEUMONIA

This occurs in previously healthy children, adults or ones who have had, at most, a prior cold or EAR INFECTION. Initially the patient has a shaking chill and then develops a fever. His chest is congested. He has a cough with sputum which may be white, yellow, green, bloody or rusty.

His respiration is rapid, and he may feel short of breath. Chest pain is common. As the patient improves he may have drenching sweats. Africans may have JAUNDICE. Children may have diarrhea or vomiting. This kind of pneumonia responds to PENICILLIN; use AMOXICILLIN or AMPICILLIN in children under 6 y.o.

COMPLICATED PNEUMONIA

This does not respond to PENICILLIN. It occurs in infants, in children under 5 y.o., in those with prior illnesses that have left them weak and after SEIZURES, head injuries or alcoholic binges. Symptoms are similar, but chills and fever may be absent. In infants who are short of breath, the fronts of their abdomens, just below the ribs, pull in with every breath. They will not nurse or eat well because they are too short of breath. They may nod or grunt with each breath. Their sputum may smell foul.

ANY PNEUMONIA

You may be able to hear rales: fine, high-pitched, crackly sounds like hair rubbed between two fingers by the ear. (See also Chapter 1 in Volume 1.) Rales usually occur first at the end of inspiration. Instead of rales you may hear a longer expiration than inspiration; this indicates a particularly severe pneumonia. In severe cases, there is grunting with each breath, and those with fair skin look blue around the mouth. In dark-skinned children, the bluish coloration may be seen by comparing the tongue color to that of a sibling. The patient will have a fast respiratory rate, lethargy or both.

Normal Respiratory Rates (breaths per minute):	
Newborn	30–60
1 y.o.	20–40
2–3 y.o.	20–30
5 y.o.	20–25
10 y.o.	17–22
Adults	12–20

Complications: if the patient is not getting better with treatment, he may have pus in his chest which will require drainage at the hands of a surgeon. In this case the patient will have continuing chest pain, chills or fever and night sweats. Send the patient to the nearest hospital, treating for complicated pneumonia meanwhile.

---

1 The location of the chest pain is usually in a line straight down (with the patient standing) from the skin fold on the front of the armpit. The patient will choose to lie on the affected side.

Causative and associated diseases: RESPIRATORY INFECTION, ASCARIASIS, HOOKWORM, TUBERCULOSIS, ENTERIC FEVER, rarely PLAGUE.

Similar conditions: this is one type of RESPIRATORY INFECTION; see that entry for a description of related diseases. Also see Protocols B.4, B.5, B.9 and B.13 if applicable. *Recent-onset pneumonia* is indistinguishable from early HOOKWORM, STRONGYLOIDIASIS or ASCARIASIS as these worms migrate through the lungs. PULMONARY EMBOLISM may also involve a fever and be indistinguishable. If the patient acts mentally abnormal, consider ENTERIC FEVER, TYPHUS, RELAPSING FEVER, rarely PLAGUE. In the presence of *abdominal pain* consider ACUTE ABDOMEN and AMEBIASIS. In areas where *dogs live close to people* and lick children's faces, consider HYDATID DISEASE. If the patient has *recently handled newborn animals*, he may have Q FEVER, a form of pneumonia that responds to DOXYCYCLINE or RIFAMPIN.

Treatment

Referrals: speedy referral is important if the patient is short of breath. See Volume 1, Appendix 13. Laboratory; a blood count and sputum for Gram stain and culture might be available at a level 3 or above. Most hospital labs can do smears and stains of sputum to determine which antibiotic will be best. Facilities: chest x-ray, IVs with fluids and injectable antibiotics, oxygen, expert nursing care and respiratory therapists. Practitioners: pediatricians, general practitioners and internists.

Patient care: if the patient cannot tolerate oral medicines, you should use injectable. High humidity is also helpful. Prop the patient in the sitting position and have him drink large amounts of water.[1] If an infant will not nurse empty the mother's breasts at least every 4 hours and give the milk to the child, using a stomach tube if you can do so without making him more short of breath. Be careful for MALNUTRITION and for DEHYDRATION.

Initial choice of antibiotics:

Modify these choices per local information and your own experience with previous patients.

Patients under two months old, those malnourished or HIV-infected: use a CEPHALOSPORIN initially, second- or third-generation.

Patients over two months but less than 6 months old and previously healthy: use ERYTHROMYCIN or AZITHROMYCIN if possible, otherwise AMOXICILLIN; do not use CEPHALOSPORIN.

Preschool patients, previously healthy, without HIV INFECTION: AMOXICILLIN initially; if that doesn't work go to CEPHALOSPORIN

School-aged children: initially use ERYTHROMYCIN, AZITHROMYCIN or CLARITHROMYCIN, and if that doesn't work, try CHLORAMPHENICOL.

Sputum with a putrid odor: send the patient out or failing that, use PENICILLIN plus (METRONIDAZOLE or TINIDAZOLE).

Simple pneumonia: give PENICILLIN by mouth for 10 days. Under 6 y.o. but previously healthy, use AMOXICILLIN. You may substitute ERYTHROMYCIN.

Previously healthy with sudden-onset pneumonia, high fever, bloody or rusty sputum: use PENICILLIN, AZITHROMYCIN, CLARITHROMYCIN or ERYTHROMYCIN, **not** CIPROFLOXACIN.

With initial sore throat, achiness or chest pain: try ERYTHROMYCIN first.

Pneumonia after a chest wall injury: use CLOXACILLIN. Send the patient out soon if he is not rapidly improving.

Complicated pneumonia: use CHLORAMPHENICOL alone or AMPICILLIN plus CHLORAMPHENICOL.

Pneumonia in HIV patients: when a patient with HIV acquires ordinary PNEUMONIA, he must be treated with CHLORAMPHENICOL plus AMPICILLIN. CIPROFLOXACIN, OFLOXACIN or CO-TRIMOXAZOLE may work. Standard treatment with PENICILLIN or AMOXICILLIN is inadequate for someone HIV-positive, even if he does not have full-blown AIDS. There is a peculiar type of pneumonia that tends to affect AIDS patients. PENTAMIDINE, CO-TRIMOXAZOLE or ATOVAQUONE might be useful.

Results: improvement in 12–24 hours. If not, switch to CHLORAMPHENICOL in a previously healthy person. In patients with HIV INFECTION, switch to PENTAMIDINE, CO-TRIMOXAZOLE or ATOVAQUONE. In other previously ill patients add METRONIDAZOLE. Consider TUBERCULOSIS if the patient does not improve after two or three different antibiotics.

PNEUMOTHORAX

Regional Notes: M, O, S.

Definition: pneumothorax is a collapse of a lung, a condition in which there is air between the chest wall and the lung surface. This air pushes down on the lung, preventing the lung from expanding as it should.

Cause: variable.

Moderately to very ill; class 2–3; worldwide.

Age: mostly teens and young adults. **Who:** anyone, especially Asians. **Onset:** usually instantaneous.

---

1 *The high humidity and hydration help to make the secretions moist and therefore easier to bring up. If the patient becomes dehydrated, his secretions are thick and sticky, and they tend to stay in the lungs for a longer time, thus delaying recovery.*

Clinical

Necessary: there is sharp chest pain and shortness of breath due to the collapse of a lung in a previously healthy young person or as a result of TB or some other lung problem. You will not be able to hear breath sounds on the side of the collapsed lung.

Similar conditions: see Protocol B.4.

Treatment

Referrals: speedy referral by ground transport is important. Air transport can kill the patient. See Volume 1, Appendix 13. The patient will need a chest tube with suction. A surgeon is most appropriate, but many general practitioners can manage this condition. X-ray is desirable, but many physicians can manage without; the physical exam is diagnostic.

Patient care: if the patient appears to be dying, passing a long, sterile hypodermic needle into his chest on the side where you hear no breath sounds may be life-saving. Put it in below the armpit. Feel where there is a rib and put the needle in over top of the rib. (Nerves and blood vessels run along the lower edge of each rib, and it is best to avoid these.) You will hear a rush of air as the needle enters. Leave the needle in until the patient arrives at a hospital. With the needle in, air transport at low altitude is okay.

Poisoning

See Symptom Protocol A.11: POISONING; see also ARSENIC POISONING, LEAD POISONING, PLANT POISONING and FOOD POISONING, in this index.

POLIO

Regional Notes: F, I, K, O, R, S, U.

Synonyms: infantile paralysis, poliomyelitis.

Definition: polio is a viral infection affecting the nerves that control movement; it does not affect the nerves that control feeling.

Mildly to very ill; class 2–4 depending on how well the patient is breathing; contagious; worldwide, related to immunization, most common in the tropics.

Age: anyone; usually less than 6 y.o.; commonly under 2 y.o. **Who:** not immunized. Fatigue, pregnancy, trauma, surgery and injections of any sort predispose to paralysis in someone who is developing polio. **Onset:** 6–48 hours for the illness. The onset of paralysis is sudden.

Clinical

Necessary: after a "cold", diarrhea or burning eye pain (see EYE INFECTION) the patient develops a fever, stiff neck, sharp and crampy muscle pains in his limbs, severe back pain, or headache and weakness. The weakness begins within the first 14 days. The muscles closer to the body are affected more than those further out; it is easier to move fingers and toes than hips and shoulders. There is no loss of feeling. Limb paralysis is floppy.

Maybe: paralysis of the face, throat, breathing and neck muscles may also occur. Muscle pain is not aggravated but may be relieved by someone else moving the patient's limbs.

Usually: there is heightened skin sensitivity. The pain may persist for weeks, even though the paralysis does not worsen. The weakness is in the lower limbs only; upper limb weakness is unusual in developing countries. The paralysis is not absolutely symmetrical, i.e., the right or left may be affected more than the other. The patient has trouble walking. He becomes as paralyzed as he will be in 3–5 days. Once the fever drops, the patient will not usually become more paralyzed.

Sometimes: the patient is not able to urinate on his own. He may be constipated also. There may be high-frequency muscle spasms. Full recovery occurs in about half the patients within 18 months.

Complications: RESPIRATORY FAILURE, PNEUMONIA, URINARY INFECTION, URINARY OBSTRUCTION, constipation, IMPACTION.

Similar conditions: *pains* may be similar to those of DIPHTHERIA (sore throat), PELLAGRA (rash or mental symptoms), ARSENIC POISON (horizontal white line on fingernails), BERIBERI (poor diet) and tertiary SYPHILIS (stiff weakness). See Protocol B.13 if there is back pain. *Spasms* may be similar to TETANUS (face and arm spastic also), RICKETS (no sunlight exposure) and PLANT POISON due to strychnine (more sudden onset).

Floppy weakness may be similar to TICK PARALYSIS, PORPHYRIA, PLANT POISON due to botulism (indistinguishable), BERIBERI (poor diet) and DIPHTHERIA (throat or skin infection). Polio is a kind of SPINAL NEUROPATHY; other causes of that condition may be indistinguishable. ARBOVIRAL FEVER due to WEST NILE VIRUS is indistinguishable. RABIES can be similar, but the patient is always dead within a week.

Treatment

Prevention: immunize. The polio immunization called IPV is safest. The most recent immunizations are single, not triple, because one of the three original kinds of polio has been eliminated. Immunization does not protect against the kind that begins with burning eye pain. If there is any possibility of RABIES, see the precautions for that disease.

Referrals: speedy referral is important; see Volume 1, Appendix 13. Facilities of at least level 3 or 4 are required, preferably Western-run. Laboratory and imaging are occasionally helpful, but oxygen and professional respiratory therapy are essential. A high-tech facility might have an antiviral drug that reportedly works for this.

TOC SYMPTOMS DIFFERENTIALS CONDITIONS DRUG INDEX REGIONAL NOTES INX

Patient care: first entirely undress the patient and check him for ticks, especially in his hair, including pubic hair and armpits. TICK PARALYSIS can mimic this and is easily remedied by removing the tick.

Avoid all IM injections in a patient for whom you suspect a polio diagnosis; IVs are okay.

The patient may require assistance to breathe. Watch for PNEUMONIA and URINARY INFECTION. If you cannot send the patient to a hospital:

- Keep the patient near you and at bed rest for a week. Keep him lying on either side, head down, so he will not choke on his tongue or his saliva. Watch his airway.

- Diet: give whatever he will take. Be sure to check to see if the patient can swallow water before giving each meal. Give a liquid diet by stomach tube if the patient cannot swallow.

- Check twice daily to make sure the patient urinated; if not, put in a urinary catheter. See Volume 1 Appendix 1. Check vital signs every 4 hours.

- Check breathing by asking the patient to shout. If he can't shout, he's not breathing adequately.

- Give no sedatives, CODEINE or other narcotics for pain. Use ACETAMINOPHEN or IBUPROFEN instead. Moist heat is useful for muscle pains.

- Move each limb daily as far as it can be moved in every direction; you will not injure the patient with this. Do not allow him to exercise with his own power at all until a week after paralysis begins.

Results: recovery is very slow. If eye pain was the initial illness, recovery will be complete. With ordinary polio, recovery varies from slight to complete. It may result in RESPIRATORY FAILURE. As long as the patient can speak or cry loudly, his respiration is adequate. If he can speak or cry only very softly, he is breathing inadequately. A paralyzed limb will not grow normally.

PORPHYRIA

Clinical

This is an inherited disease which presents variably with skin manifestations (especially sensitivity to light) or recurrent abdominal pains, together with mental illness and/or weakness. The abdominal/mental symptoms seldom start before puberty. The weakness affects the muscle groups closest to the trunk, i.e. the shoulders and hips. Attacks may occur spontaneously or as a result of taking some drug. The drugs listed in the Drug Index have notes if they should not be used in the presence of porphyria. Discontinue any of the drugs that might have caused the crisis. Send out for further treatment; there is not much else you can do besides offering pain relief.

POST-MEASLES CACHEXIA

Definition: post-measles cachexia is the refusal to eat that often occurs when a child is recovering from MEASLES. Also see the chart under MALNUTRITION in this index for similar diseases. It may result in kwashiorkor (malnutrition with general body swelling) or in MALABSORPTION (prompt, watery diarrhea whenever the patient eats). See Protocol B.14 for similar conditions. Treatment consists of nourishing the patient by means of a stomach tube, splinting his elbows to keep him from pulling the tube out. He will develop an appetite in a week or two. Properly managed, deaths should be rare.

POSTPARTUM SEPSIS

Definition: postpartum sepsis is SEPSIS after an ABORTION, miscarriage or childbirth. See Chapter 7 in Volume 1.

PREMENSTRUAL TENSION

Synonym: PMS.

Definition: premenstrual tension is emotional distress, frequently DEPRESSION, occurring a few days to a week before menstruation. It can be mild or severe. Use sedation or IBUPROFEN if necessary.

PROCTITIS

Regional Notes: F, R.

Entry category: syndrome.

Definition: proctitis is inflammation of the rectum.

Cause: variable.

Proctitis causes rectal pain (especially right before bowel movements), along with the symptoms of DYSENTERY. Bleeding is bright red but not large amounts. The patient passes much mucus or pus, and has little warning before defecating. There may also be crampy abdominal pain. It may be due to SCHISTOSOMIASIS HEMATOBIUM, SCHISTOSOMIASIS MANSONI, DYSENTERY due to amebae, HERPES, LYMPHOGRANULOMA VENEREUM (mainly in females and homosexual males) or GONORRHEA. It is particularly common in homosexuals but may occur in anyone. Treat the underlying disease as well as DYSENTERY. If the causative disease might be LYMPHOGRANULOMA VENEREUM, then treat for a full 21 days.

TOC   SYMPTOMS   DIFFERENTIALS   CONDITIONS   DRUG INDEX   REGIONAL NOTES   INX

PROSTATITIS

Regional Notes: F, R.

Synonyms: enlarged prostate, prostate trouble.

Definition: prostatitis is an inflammation of the prostate, a gland that lies between the rectum and the base of the penis.

Cause: bacteria, usually.

Age: adults; **Who:** males only, usually sexually active. **Onset:** minutes to hours.

Clinical

This is a type of URINARY INFECTION in males which causes rectal pain or a heavy feeling or aching between the base of the penis and the rectum. It is a common complication of TUBERCULOSIS, SCHISTOSOMIASIS MANSONI, and/or SEXUALLY TRANSMITTED DISEASE, in particular GONORRHEA and CHLAMYDIA. It can occur for an unknown cause.

Commonly: there are fever, chills, fatigue, joint and muscle pain and genital pain. The patient may have a discharge from his penis.

Maybe: the patient has to bear down to urinate. He might urinate small amounts frequently and have pain in doing so. If the condition is severe he may develop URINARY OBSTRUCTION.

Similar conditions: TUBERCULOSIS of male genitals may be indistinguishable.

Treatment

Treat it like any other URINARY INFECTION. CO-TRIMOXAZOLE is particularly good for this. OFLOXACIN is also okay; If you use CEPHALOSPORIN it should be second- or third-generation since the problem is usually Gram-negative. Treat for a minimum of 21 days.

PTERYGIUM

Definition: a pterygium is an opaque white area on the cornea, prevalent in those living outdoors in sunny areas.

Clinical

The white area grows from the edge of the cornea of the eye to the center, like a slice of pie, at the 3 or 9 o'clock position.

Treatment

It can be prevented by wearing dark glasses. Eye drops may be useful, but they should not be used without a physician's guidance. Surgery may also be helpful.

PULMONARY EMBOLISM (PE)

Includes: pulmonary infarct.

Definition: pulmonary embolism is a crisis caused by a blood clot which formed somewhere in the body and then broke loose and went to the lungs.

Age: mostly adults; **Who:** it usually happens in ill or sedentary people, or it is related to PLANT POISONING: ergot. **Onset:** usually sudden, over seconds to minutes.

Clinical

It causes sudden shortness of breath, chest pain and maybe HEART FAILURE and death. There may be fever, and the patient is likely to cough up frothy pink sputum.

Treatment

Not feasible in developing areas. Either send the patient out or prepare him for death.

PYODERMA

See IMPETIGO.

PYOMYOSITIS

Regional Notes: F, M, U.

Definition: pyomyositis is a deep muscle ABSCESS.

Cause: bacteria.

Mildly to moderately ill; class 2–3; worldwide, related to level of medical care, may be due to injections or arise spontaneously.

Age: any, mostly 5–25 y.o. **Who:** anyone, especially those with poor immunity. It is related to non-sterile injections. **Onset:** over days, maybe longer.

Clinical

Necessary: there is a warm tender swelling of the muscles in the patient's back, buttock(s) or one of his limbs. The tenderness and swelling are always worse over muscle than over a joint. The swelling is always firm, never soft. It is not symmetrical.

Usually: fever, chills. It most often affects the hip, thigh or lower leg. It is difficult to tell the difference between this and a bone infection. If the muscles involved are essential for walking, the patient will limp or refuse to walk.

Similar conditions: see Protocol B.6 [limb(s)]or B.13 [back]. If the warmth and swelling are worse over a joint, consider various causes of ARTHRITIS.

Treatment

Referrals: speedy referral is necessary; See Volume 1, Appendix 13. Laboratory: hospital labs can do a smear and culture of the pus to determine which antibiotic to use. Facilities: IV's and injectable antibiotics are helpful, as is x-ray and/or ultrasound. Practitioner; a surgeon is ideal.

Patient care: first give a large dose of antibiotic (CEPHALOSPORIN is best). Then send out unless the abscess is near the surface so you can drain it; don't dig around deep. After draining the abscess, continue the antibiotic. If you cannot drain it, antibiotics will do no good. If it drains but then does not heal well, it may need to be drained again.

Results: improvement in a matter of weeks with proper nursing care.

Q FEVER (QF)

Regional Notes: E, F, I, K, R, S, U.

Synonyms: Balkan grippe, Red River fever, Nine Mile fever.

Definition: Q fever is a bacterial illness, caused by the bacterium *Coxiella burnetti.*,

Not ill to very ill; class 1; contagious from infected animals and insects, from humans in the context of childbirth. It occurs worldwide except for New Zealand; it is not only tropical.

Age: any. **Who:** those exposed to infected domestic animals (especially newborns) or the dust thereof, meat or milk. The sex ratio is 1 before puberty; after puberty there are many more females than males affected. It may be sexually transmitted. **Onset:** mostly gradual, possibly sudden; incubation 2–4 weeks.

Clinical

Necessary: fever with chills, sweats, fatigue, headache, cough or bilirubin in the urine.

Maybe: muscle pains, loss of appetite, lasting a few days to a few weeks if there are no complications. There is rarely a rash. The liver is large and tender.

Complications: PNEUMONIA, HEPATITIS (common), HEART FAILURE (uncommon) due to the infection entering the heart valves (valvular type).

Similar conditions: MONONUCLEOSIS except for the severe headache. TYPHUS which can be treated with some of the same drugs. See Protocol B.2 (for fever and body pains) and B.4 (if the patient is short of breath).

Treatment

Prevention: a vaccine is available.

Referrals: laboratory diagnosis is useless unless a person is at a high-tech laboratory and specimens are taken within a couple days of onset of illness, before any antibiotics have been taken. Facilities: with very sick patients IVs and injectable antibiotics might be useful.

Patient care: it responds well to ERYTHROMYCIN, CIPROFLOXACIN, DOXYCYCLINE or RIFAMPIN. DOXYCYCLINE is best, because many similar diseases respond to this. Fever should drop within 3 days. PENICILLIN and CEPHALOSPORIN are no good for this.

RABIES

Regional Notes: F, I, N, O, S, U.

Synonyms: hydrophobia, lyssa.

Definition: rabies is a kind of viral encephalitis.

Very ill; class 1; nearly 100% death rate in anyone's care; maybe contagious if the patient bites someone; virus is present in saliva, urine and tears. Present in all regions, although some islands are free of it.

Age: any. **Who:** those bitten by a rabid animal and not immunized. Occasionally exposure to the droppings of rabid bats will cause rabies. **Onset:** usually sudden, frequently after a 2–3 day period of just not feeling well. Incubation period is 4 days to years, usually weeks to months; shorter with head, neck and hand wounds; shorter with severe bites or bites from wild animals.

Clinical

ORDINARY (FURIOUS) RABIES
This accounts for 75% of all cases. Initially the patient has pain, tingling or itching at the site of the bite, which then spreads. He becomes very sensitive to light and sound. The onset of symptoms may include episodes of excitability, crazy behavior and incoherent speech.

PARALYTIC RABIES
This accounts for 25% of all cases; it is usually from bats. Initially it begins like POLIO with simple paralysis which progressively becomes worse. The paralysis moves from limb toward trunk. There is always muscle twitching, urine incontinence early and muscle weakness, mainly closer to the trunk (shoulder/hip more than hands/feet). There is no loss of sensation with this—the patient can still feel touch and pain. It may also resemble MENINGITIS with SEIZURES and a stiff neck.

BOTH KINDS
When fully developed, the most common symptom is painful spasm of the throat with attempts to swallow liquids. Sometimes a breeze blowing over the skin will also trigger spasms.

Usually: the patient has a fever and a general influenza-like illness.

Sometimes: he has back pain, arching of the back and an erection that will not go away. The patient develops muscle spasms of his throat, paralysis of his limbs or both. When the disease causes paralysis, the paralysis starts at the bite and moves toward the head. Vital signs may change rapidly; thus one might see either a rapid or slow pulse and respiratory rate, a high or low temperature and an erratic blood pressure.

Similar conditions: POLIO must be differentiated from paralytic rabies. Polio usually involves lower limbs only and the patient does not have spasms from a breeze blowing over his skin or from drinking water (as is true for rabies). Rabies may also resemble other forms of ENCEPHALITIS, of which this is one kind. DEMONIZATION may be similar, as may TETANUS and occasionally ALCOHOLISM. See Protocol B.13 if there is back pain.

TOC   SYMPTOMS   DIFFERENTIALS   CONDITIONS   DRUG INDEX   REGIONAL NOTES   INX

Treatment / prevention

Referrals: only a level 5 facility has any hope of saving the patient. However, a lower level facility might help keep him comfortable until he dies. Facilities: IV fluids to prevent dehydration; major sedative and pain medication; an air-conditioned room free of breezes; spiritual counsel.

Pre-exposure prevention

If you are in an area of high rabies incidence or delayed evacuation, you should be immunized. Human Diploid Cell Vaccine is very safe. To immunize before exposure, give 0.5 ml IM on each of days 0, 7 and 21 or 28. Alternatively, give 0.l ml intradermal (ID), like a TB skin test, on each of these days. The intradermal is not as reliable as the IM, but it is far cheaper. It does not work reliably in the presence of CHLOROQUINE. In Western countries, a blood test is available to determine if the immunization was effective. Antiserum and vaccine are still needed after a bite, though in fewer doses. A previously unimmunized person should have the vaccine within 48 hours of a bite, but later immunization is better than none.

Post-exposure ID immunization

On day zero (when the patient presents), inject 0.1 ml ID in each of these 8 places: the right and left upper arms, below the right and left shoulder blades in back, the right and left thighs and on the right and left lower abdomen. On day 7 do the same at 4 sites: the upper arms and the thighs. On days 28 and 90, do the same at one site, on one upper arm.

Treatment of a rabid animal bite

- Thoroughly cleanse and rinse out wounds with alcohol, iodine or both. Open puncture wounds with a scalpel blade. Provide a tetanus shot if necessary. Do not suture wounds!

- If the bites were provoked[1] and made by a domestic animal that had rabies shots, no further prevention is necessary.[2] If bites were unprovoked or made by an unimmunized or wild animal, the patient should have one dose of hyperimmune rabies antiserum or hyperimmune rabies globulin IM. (These are blood products with immune proteins.) Inject some around the wound. Give the rest IM in the upper arm, not in the buttocks. Follow the directions with the product. If the product is animal serum, you must check for sensitivity first. You should have EPINEPHRINE on hand and review the treatment of ANAPHYLAXIS. Draw 0.1 ml of serum into a 1 ml syringe. Then draw 0.9 ml of saline into the same syringe so you have a total of 1 ml. Mix this by tipping the syringe back and forth. Drop 0.1 ml of this diluted solution inside one lower eyelid. A little bit of redness is normal.

- A strong allergic reaction to the eyedrop test within 15 minutes indicates you should not proceed with the serum or globulin injection. Only vaccinate. If you can send the patient to a doctor or nurse for desensitization, then he might be able to take the serum or globulin.

- 24 hours after the globulin or antiserum or immediately if the patient had an allergic reaction, vaccinate the patient. Follow the directions with the product. Two older, cheaper types of vaccine are available in developing countries: Semple and Duck Embryo. ALLERGY can be a problem. Read the package inserts carefully. The Semple type may cause redness, swelling, itching and pain at an injection site. Stop the vaccination if this happens. You may continue with a different type and use PREDNISONE. Human Diploid Cell Vaccine (HDCV), RVA and PCEC are more expensive, safer (as regards allergy) and not as available.

Patient care in human rabies

There have been occasional reports of survivals with long-term intensive care at level 5. There has only been one survival of a patient who had symptoms before any immunization; she had profound brain damage. Send the patient out for this care promptly if the family so chooses. Otherwise use high doses of sedatives and pain medicines until death. Inform the family that the patient will die. The virus is present in saliva and tears, so use a mask and exam gloves. Rabies patients are prone to bite, so avoid putting your hands near his face.

Results: the patient is not unconscious until late in the illness. Death occurs within a week in furious rabies, within 3 weeks in paralytic rabies.

RADIATION ILLNESS

Regional Notes: E.

Definition: radiation illness is an illness due to the damaging effects of ionizing radiation.

Not ill to very ill; class 1–4; worldwide, but rare in nations that have no nuclear history. Some developing areas may have a problem if they are used as nuclear waste dumps or if there are natural deposits of radioactive minerals.

Age: any. **Who:** those exposed to a source of radiation; those who drink contaminated water, eat contaminated food or ingest radioactive materials. **Onset:** within hours for major exposures; after years or possibly in the next generation for small-dose, chronic exposures.

---

1 *Provoked means that one can understand that the animal's attack was defensive. Examples would be a child trying to pull a bone out of the mouth of a dog or coming between a mother animal and her young one.*

2 *Be sure to check the origin of the rabies vaccine. There have been counterfeit vaccines on the market.*

TOC SYMPTOMS DIFFERENTIALS CONDITIONS DRUG INDEX REGIONAL NOTES INX

Clinical

There are two classes of effects: acute effects occur with exposure to large doses, and chronic effects occur with multiple exposures to small doses.

ACUTE EFFECTS

Within a couple of hours there is loss of appetite. Thereafter there is nausea, vomiting and diarrhea; anemia; susceptibility to infection; weight loss; loss of hair; sterility; apathy alternating with agitation; incoordination; seizures; coma and death. Death, if it occurs, almost always is within 30 days.

CHRONIC EFFECTS

With exposures during very early pregnancy (from conception until 8 weeks), either the baby will die, or he will grow normally. Exposures after that time are likely to cause retarded growth, mental retardation or significant disabilities such as blindness or deafness. Exposures may cause CANCER later in life: leukemia and bone tumors appear after 2–4 years and other CANCER (especially thyroid, lung, skin and breast) after 10–40 years. Radiation may also cause CATARACT.

Similar conditions: acute effects: GASTROENTERITIS, ANEMIA from other causes, HIV, TUBERCULOSIS and BRAIN DAMAGE from other causes. Prenatal effects may be similar to the prenatal effects from RUBELLA, TOXOPLASMOSIS or HERPES.

Treatment

Prevention: if you live in an area where this is likely to be a problem, obtain a radiation counter to check your water and food. There is no way to reliably purify contaminated water although some systems may work under some circumstances. Contaminated food must be discarded. If someone has ingested contaminated food, others should be protected from him. How long depends on the substance ingested.

Referrals: don't use public transport if the patient consumed a radioactive substance; use a towed trailer. Symptomatic care only is generally available: IVs, transfusions and the like at a level 3 or above

Patient care: there is no effective treatment for the problem. Persons who have been exposed to radiation should be watched so that early treatment of CANCER can be initiated.

RADICULOPATHY

This is a syndrome also known as "pinched nerve". It is due to a nerve irritation in or beside the spinal cord, causing sharp shooting pains, numbness or heaviness in the arms (if it affects the neck); or the legs (if it affects the lower back). It may be caused by SLIPPED DISC, FLUOROSIS, LYME DISEASE (in eastern Europe), TUBERCULOSIS, BRUCELLOSIS and possibly other diseases also.

RAT BITE FEVER[1]

Regional Notes: I.

Entry category: two nearly indistinguishable diseases.

Includes: Haverhill fever, Sodoku.

Definition: rat bite fever is caused by a bacterium (*Actinobacillus muris*) or a spirochete (*Spirillum minor*) transmitted by the bite of a rat.

Mildly to very ill; class 1–3; worldwide, but rare in Africa and the Americas, common in Asia. It is tropical.

Age: any, but mostly children. **Who:** those bitten by rats or rat-eating animals; those who consume food contaminated by rat urine. **Onset:** over about 3 days, after an incubation of 3–30 days.

Clinical

Necessary: there are chills and fevers, headache, nausea and weakness. With one type the bite wound heals and then breaks open; with the other type it stays healed but there is a rash. Without treatment, the fever falls on its own at about 4–6 days, stays down for a few days and then comes back.

Sometimes: there are joint pains (a migrating multiple-joint ARTHRITIS which relapses at 2 week intervals), general muscle aching and a rash. The joint pains involve the large and small joints of the limbs, mostly away from the trunk. The rash consists of purplish spots or lumps, mostly on the chest and arms. The pulse is not slow relative to the fever. There may be dizziness, insomnia, headache, ringing in the ears, blurred vision and delirium. If left untreated, the fever and other symptoms come back repeatedly over months. There may be a large liver.

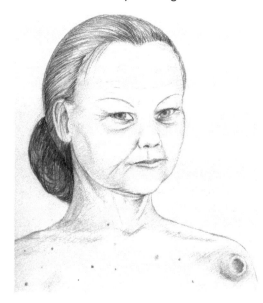

This is a woman with the rash. Note the wound. OW

1 *See the Powerpoint lecture entitled* Intermediate Organisms *at* www.villagemedicalmanual.org.

TOC   SYMPTOMS   DIFFERENTIALS   CONDITIONS   DRUG INDEX   REGIONAL NOTES   INX

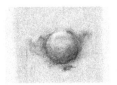

This is a close-up of one of the rash bumps. AB

Complications: HEART FAILURE.

Similar conditions: see Protocols B.2, B.6 and B.11. RELAPSING FEVER is the main one; the treatments are similar.

Treatment

Referrals: see Volume 1, Appendix 13. Laboratory: only level 4 and above in a specialty center for tropical/travel medicine. Facilities: IVs and injectable antibiotics, level 3 or above.

Patient care: use PENICILLIN as for STREP INFECTION, DOXYCYCLINE or STREPTOMYCIN. DOXYCYCLINE is best since it covers many similar diseases.

RECTAL PROLAPSE

Regional Notes: M.

Definition: rectal prolapse is the rectum falling out of the anus, so the moist, pink part that should be inside sticks out.

Cause: variable.

Clinical

The rectum turns inside out so it is hanging out with some of the moist pink surface visible on the outside. It may be a tiny bit or a large amount. The problem mostly affects women and children. There may be incontinence.

Causative conditions: this is usually due to chronic diarrhea, PERTUSSIS, KIDNEY DISEASE (nephrotic) or TRICHURIASIS. It can also be related to constipation, MALNUTRITION or GIARDIASIS.

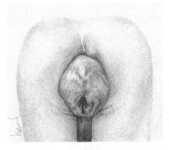

This is a rectal prolapse. There are obvious circumferential lines around it, usually more prominent than shown. There is a center hole. This one is large; most are smaller. AB

Similar conditions: HEMORRHOIDS usually affects adults, but the bulge is never larger than the patient's little toe; they have smooth surfaces whereas a prolapse has a wrinkled surface. Also see Volume 1, Chapter 6, for uterine prolapse.

Treatment

Referrals: a hospital that has experience in treating this might be helpful, level 2 or above.

Patient care: gently push the rectum back in with your gloved hands **if and only if the rectal surface** is still pink. (A little dark color right around the anus itself is normal in dark-skinned people.) If a significant portion of the part that should be pink is black instead, the patient must be sent to a hospital if he is to survive.

If you have trouble pushing it back in, then sprinkle table sugar on the moist pink part, covering the entire surface with sugar. This will reduce the swelling which will allow you to successfully push it in. After the rectum is all the way back in, the buttocks must be taped together. Take the tape off for bowel movements only, and then replace it after pushing the prolapse back in again. Treat the patient for TRICHURIASIS. Treat for other conditions as appropriate. He will heal in a couple weeks if his nutrition is adequate.

REITER SYNDROME / REACTIVE ARTHRITIS

Entry category: disease.

Definition: Reiter syndrome[2] is an autoimmune disease that follows after venereal CHLAMYDIA infection or some other diseases.

Moderately to very ill; class 2–3; worldwide, related to sexually transmitted diseases and sometimes other diseases.

Age: usually young adults. **Who:** those who have had bacterial DYSENTERY or CHLAMYDIA INFECTION, males more commonly than females. There may also be a predisposing genetic factor. This kind of arthritis may be caused by HIV INFECTION. It is very commonly associated with HIV in Africa, with GONORRHEA worldwide. **Onset:** incubation 1–3 weeks for some causes; onset over hours to days for others.

Clinical—one or more of the following, possibly with a fever:

- Pain with urinating and/or pus in the urine (dipstick is positive for leukocytes).

- EYE INFECTION or IRITIS.

- Chest pain consistent with PERICARDITIS.

- Pain and swelling in 1–4 joints, mainly the large joints of the spine, pelvis or the lower limbs, made worse with rest, not symmetrical. There may be morning stiffness.

- Pain and swelling of one tendon, most commonly in back of the heel, in front of the heel, by an elbow; or one digit—usually a toe rather than a finger.

- Pain and swelling of one finger or toe, so the digit looks like a sausage.

- Spontaneous wounds: the wounds must be searched for; they may be relatively painless.

- Mouth ulcers, which are painless or APHTHOUS STOMATITIS which is painful.

- Raw red areas around the base of the penis tip in uncircumcised males. The same problem in a circumcised male causes crusts rather than raw red areas.

- Rough scaly changes in the skin of the soles, palms and nail beds.

---

2 Reactive arthritis or Reiter syndrome, is almost the only cause of asymmetrical multiple-joint arthritis with a fever. Reiter syndrome is the older name. The disease was first described by a Dr. Reiter who later participated in the Holocaust. The scientific community therefore boycotts using his name. I use it here because of the confusion of "arthritis" causing eye symptoms, mouth sores and other non-joint manifestations.

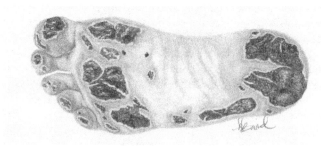

The appearance of the sole of the foot in Reiter syndrome. The darkened areas have thick scaly skin on them. Tertiary YAWS may look similar, as may ARSENIC POISONING. AB

Complications: severe symptoms and progression of symptoms in patients who are HIV-positive.

Treatment

Referrals: referral to a sexually transmitted disease clinic is desirable. A level 3 or above hospital might have some alternative treatments.

Patient care: re-treat the underlying infection. If there were genital symptoms initially, then use DOXYCYCLINE. If there were abdominal symptoms initially, then use a Gram-negative antibiotic. Then use IBUPROFEN or a similar medication. A short course of PREDNISONE may be helpful.

Results: about half these patients have a total cure and the other half develop a chronic ARTHRITIS.

RELAPSING FEVER[1] (RF)

Regional Notes: E, F, I, K, M, O.

Synonym: borreliosis.

Includes: tick-borne relapsing fever, louse-borne relapsing fever.

Definition: relapsing fever is an illness caused by a spirochete, either *Borrelia recurrentis* or *Borrelia duttoni*. The fever is sustained rather than relapsing. In the pre-antibiotic era, it was indeed relapsing, the relapse occurring after days to a week. There were no antibiotics, so patients suffered long enough to endure multiple spectacular relapses.

Mildly to severely ill; class 2; louse-borne: may occur wherever there are body lice, historically at high elevations. Tick-borne: mountainous areas of Asia and the Middle East; Horn of Africa and Africa south of the equator; scattered areas in the western half of South America; northern Mexico. This is not known to occur in the islands of Southeast Asia or in the Pacific area.

Age: any. **Who:** infection is caused by crushing head or body lice or by being bitten by ticks. In the tick-borne fever, the ticks are soft ticks (See Volume 1, Appendix 10). Soft ticks act like bedbugs, biting people at night. Very likely the person is not aware of having been bitten. **Onset:** sudden, over minutes to hours; incubation 2–14 days.

---

1 *See the Powerpoint lecture:* Intermediate Organisms *at www.villagemedicalmanual.org.*

Clinical

BOTH KINDS

Necessary: the patient has chills; sweats; fevers; headache (forehead or back of the head); fatigue; and general bone, joint and muscle pains. It involves both large and small joints. The shaking chills last about 30 minutes as the temperature rises. During a crisis (after a matter of days), there is an additional chill followed by severe sweating within minutes to hours, weakness and low blood pressure, during which time death is common.

Usually: the pulse is rapid relative to the fever. He has a dry cough and abdominal pain. The patient commonly acts "spacy", as in ENTERIC FEVER. The liver may also be large and tender, as well as the spleen.

Sometimes: there is JAUNDICE (especially with louse-borne disease) and a rash over the upper body with tiny black and blue marks (also more common with louse-borne). The patient may vomit. He may be dizzy or have trouble swallowing. He is likely to have a dry mouth and seek darkness.

Occasionally: there is abnormal bleeding with a drop in blood pressure which may result in coma or death.

TICK-BORNE

In tick-borne relapsing fever there are joint pains which involve both large and small joints. The pain may be severe, but the joints are not red or swollen. Tick-borne fever may cause lethargy and weight loss. Onset to first crisis is less than 7 days, each episode similar to the previous ones.

LOUSE-BORNE

Louse-borne fever commonly causes vomiting. Onset to first crisis is less than 10 days, each episode shorter and milder than the previous ones. Convalescence is prolonged; see Volume 1, Appendix 8, on the care of the seriously ill patient.

Complications: nosebleed and visual problems, loss of consciousness, BELL'S PALSY, SEIZURES, STROKE, MENINGITIS, HEMORRHAGIC FEVER (louse-borne), PNEUMONIA, trembling like PARKINSON'S DISEASE, paralysis like POLIO, mental symptoms like cerebral MALARIA, SEPSIS, ARTHRITIS, IRITIS, LIVER DISEASE or LIVER FAILURE, HEART FAILURE, ABORTION, death.

Similar conditions: see Protocols B.2, B.7, B.8, B.9, B.10. In DENGUE FEVER the headache is felt more in the eyes. In YELLOW FEVER and TYPHUS the pulse is slow relative to the fever and they both have distinctive body odors. RAT-BITE FEVER may be similar, but there is a history of a bite or consuming contaminated food. In no other disease do chills and sweating follow this closely. In other diseases the episodes of sweating are separated from the chills and fever by at least 12 hours. LEPTOSPIROSIS may be indistinguishable, but it also responds to DOXYCYCLINE.

LYME DISEASE may be similar, but it has a slower onset and slower progression. Also, fevers above 101.3°/38.5° are common in relapsing fever but uncommon in LYME DISEASE.

Bush laboratory: there is usually protein in the urine with louse-borne relapsing fever.

Treatment

Prevention: avoid ticks and body LICE. Remove ticks and treat the bites with IODINE. See Volume 1, Appendix 10 for dealing with body lice.

Referrals: see Volume 1 Appendix 13. Laboratory; a thick blood smear done during a fever (the same as is done for malaria) may show the spirochetes; they are easier to find in louse-borne than in tick-borne relapsing fever. They look like skinny cork-screws. Failure to find them does not exclude the diagnosis. The white cell count will be high. Practitioner: tropical/travel medicine expertise is desirable, but speed is more important.

Patient care: PENICILLIN, DOXYCYCLINE or ERYTHROMYCIN. A single dose is sufficient for louse-borne; seven days is necessary for tick-borne. If there are psychological changes it is important to treat for 21 days. Sometimes the treatment makes the patient sicker or causes SHOCK for a few hours; have him lie down for 6 hours after he takes his first dose. Give the patient fluids, but do not stop treatment for shock. It will not recur after the first one or two doses.

RESPIRATORY[2] FAILURE

Entry category: syndrome.

Synonym: ventilatory failure.

Definition: respiratory failure is a condition of breathing inadequately.

Age, Who, Onset: anyone, fast or slow onset.

Clinical

Symptoms are blueness around the mouth (check the color of the tongue in those with dark skin), an abnormally fast or slow respiratory rate and finally, progressive lethargy leading to loss of consciousness and death. A sign that is both sensitive and specific is an abnormally low reading on a pulse oximeter; an alternative is to ask the patient to shout. If he cannot, then he is deteriorating.

Causative conditions: it may be due to muscle weakness as in POLIO; to fatigue when breathing requires excess work as in ASTHMA, HEART FAILURE and ANTHRAX; or to diseased lungs as in TUBERCULOSIS or PNEUMONIA. IRIS, a complication of AIDS treatment, may cause this.

Treatment

Referrals: almost any level 2 or above facility can be helpful; send the patient to the highest level possible. Oxygen, a chest x-ray, IV fluids and injectable antibiotics or DIURETICS might all be helpful.

Patient care: when this occurs in a previously healthy adult who has PNEUMONIA, treat with large doses of ERYTHROMYCIN. Decrease his fluids to 75% of what you calculate he needs, as long as he is making the minimum amount of urine (Symptom Protocol A.58); he will recover better if he is slightly dehydrated. Have him rest in a sitting position.

---

2 *Medical purists will point out that this should be ventilatory failure. True. This work is intended for non-medical people who find this technically correct terminology confusing.*

RESPIRATORY INFECTION

Regional Notes: I, M.

Entry category: disease cluster.

Includes: bronchitis, cold, croup, emphysema, sinusitis, chronic obstructive lung disease.

Definition: respiratory infection is an infection of the airway from the nose and lips down to the lungs.

Cause: viruses, bacteria, fungi, worms.

Mildly to severely ill; class 1–4; some contagious; worldwide, related to crowding and nutrition.

Age: any, especially children. **Who:** anyone, especially malnourished, crowded conditions, smoke and/or dust exposure and some genetic factors. **Onset:** usually over days; occasionally minutes.

Clinical

Necessary: any of the following: nasal congestion; plugged ears with hearing loss; runny nose; cough; shortness of breath; fast respiratory rate; face pain, swelling, or headache; sore throat; red eyes; large lymph nodes in the neck; loss of smell; foul breath; loss of taste. In severe cases, fair-skinned patients may look bluish around the lips. (The bluishness may be seen on the tongue in those with dark skin.)

Maybe: there may be appetite and weight loss.

COLD
Congestion, plugged ears, runny nose, cough, white sputum.

BRONCHITIS
Lingering cough after a cold; green, yellow or bloody sputum; maybe chest pain.

SINUSITIS
Congestion, face pain, or headache, sometimes pus in nose or throat, maybe upper teeth pain.

CROUP
Barking, dry cough in a child less than 6 y.o.; sudden onset; low or no fever; short of breath; and hoarse.

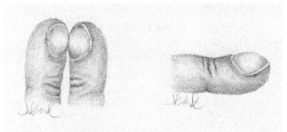

With chronic respiratory infection the tops of the fingernails become dome-shaped, rather than being like a section of a cylinder. This indicates either a chronic respiratory condition or a heart condition, though on occasion it may be a family trait. AB

CHRONIC RESPIRATORY INFECTION

This is also known as emphysema or chronic obstructive lung disease. It consists of cough, shortness of breath and wheezing which is present most, if not all, of the time. The patient may sleep sitting up and have a severe cough when awakening each morning. He will be short of breath when exercising. He may have a barrel-shaped chest. His fingernails may have a peculiar rounded appearance, as with HEART FAILURE. The patient may have an irregular pulse.

Similar and overlapping conditions: Epidemic INFLUENZA is almost indistinguishable from a common cold except for the higher fever and the epidemic context. PNEUMONIA; PERTUSSIS; DIPHTHERIA; TUBERCULOSIS; and FILARIASIS, which may cause something resembling ASTHMA. HEART FAILURE may present this way. See Protocols B.4 for shortness of breath and B.10 for lethargy. Another cause of bloody sputum is early ASCARIASIS. TUBERCULOSIS is a frequent cause of adult-onset wheezing. If and when a cough has lasted for over 3 months, consider the diseases listed for chronic cough. Epidemic INFLUENZA is like a cold with a high fever.

Treatment

Referrals: laboratory; a smear and culture of the sputum, done in a hospital lab, might be helpful, level 3 or more. Facilities: x-ray and/or ultrasound might be helpful. Surgery may be helpful on occasion; seek a level 3 or higher facility.

Patient care:

With wheezing, use THEOPHYLLINE, ALBUTEROL or METAPROTERENOL. Do **not** use antihistamines. **Do not use antibiotics unless there is a fever.**

With croup (a tight or barking cough), use steam or high humidity, but **not decongestants or antihistamines.**

With any other cough, use COUGH SYRUP.

With adults: first check the description of PNEUMONIA; if it fits well, follow those directions rather than the ones below. Also check HEART FAILURE.

With nasal congestion or a runny nose, give VITAMIN C and fluids. You may also use PSEUDOEPHEDRINE tablets or EPHEDRINE NOSE DROPS provided there is no tight or barking cough or wheezing. **Do not use antibiotics unless there is a fever or pus.**

With a cough and a fever of more than 38.5°C (101.3°F), pus coming from the nose or back of the throat or yellow-green sputum, treat with antibiotic. PENICILLIN, AZITHROMYCIN, CLARITHROMYCIN or ERYTHROMYCIN are best; DOXYCYCLINE, SULFA, AMPICILLIN or CO-TRIMOXAZOLE are acceptable. If wheezing is present, use THEOPHYLLINE or METAPROTERENOL additionally.

With a chronic cough, first check for TUBERCULOSIS. If he has no TB, he may need to be on THEOPHYLLINE continually. You may add PREDNISONE for short periods. He should sleep sitting up. Once a day put him in the head-down knee-chest position and beat on his back with your open hand while he breathes in steam. This loosens stuck mucus and enables the patient to cough it up.

Treatment of coughs in children

A simple but reliable system is as follows.

Severity of illness	Rapid Breathing[1]	Chest Suction[2]	Treatment
Mild	No	No	No antibiotic
Moderate	Yes	No	Antibiotic
Severe	Maybe	Yes	Hospitalize

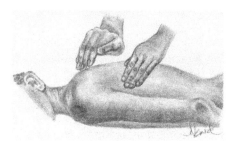

Hitting the back of the chest with cupped hands helps to loosen secretions. AB

RHEUMATIC FEVER (RF)

Regional Notes: E, F, I, K, M, N, O, R, S, U.

Definition: rheumatic fever is a disease caused by a misguided immune reaction against strep infection which ends up damaging the heart and the joints.

Mildly to severely ill; class 1–4; worldwide, especially in the 10–40 window of the Eastern Hemisphere. It is related to the level of available health care.

Age: usually children for a first episode; HEART FAILURE is most common at 10–15 y.o., sometimes younger. The disease is more severe in older children and adults than in younger children. **Who:** those who have had inadequately treated STREP INFECTION or prior rheumatic fever. Malnourished children and South Pacific Islanders are particularly prone. **Onset:** hours to a day or two. The problem tends to recur. The HEART FAILURE usually develops slowly, over weeks to months, but it may develop rapidly, causing death within days to weeks.

Clinical

Necessary: the patient is tired, loses his appetite, and has at least one pair of swollen joints. To diagnose the disease, the patient must have had a sore throat 1–6 weeks earlier or have current evidence of a STREP INFECTION. In addition, he must have at least two of the following:[3]

---

1 *Rapid breathing is a rate more than 50 if less than 12 months old, over 40 if 1–3 years old, over 30 if over 3 years.*

2 *Chest suction means that the child's lower chest and abdomen pull way in with each breath. Nodding or grunting with each breath is equivalent.*

3 *Criteria for the diagnosis of rheumatic fever are more stringent in the States, but some of the symptoms and findings seen there just do not occur in the tropics. Hence, only one additional criterion is needed to make a diagnosis.*

- Previous rheumatic fever.
- A fever with no other obvious cause.[1]
- Pain and swelling in two or more joints, usually large joints and the lower limbs before the upper limbs. The pain is maximal at 12–24 hours and lasts about a week, never more than 3 weeks. RF acquired in developing countries may manifest with migrating joint pains without visible swelling.
- Either a heart murmur, HEART FAILURE or an enlarged heart.[2]
- A red, non-itchy rash with borders that move, more visible with heat. It starts early and lasts for a long time.

> **Distinctive rash of rheumatic fever**
> On occasion there is a rash which makes the diagnosis of rheumatic fever quite certain. It is a reddened area of skin with distinct edges that move over a matter of hours or days. If you will mark the edges with an indelible marking pen, then you can observe the movement. There is no other rash that looks quite like this.

Usually: the fever is sustained and high; it never returns to normal during an episode. The pulse is rapid. The sore, swollen joints are usually at least one pair of the same joints on the two sides (e.g., both ankles) unless the joints are in the midline (e.g., the spine). The pain moves from one set of joints to another. There is no morning stiffness which improves with exercise. Usually with the first episode there are mainly joint pains; with subsequent episodes there are heart problems.

Occasionally: the fingernails have a scooped-out appearance, and the patient has heavy chest pains which may go to the shoulder, arm or jaw. He may have large lymph nodes in the front of his neck. He may have a skin rash which consists of either raised doughnut-type rings on the skin or else tender red bumps over the hairy surface of the arms, the front of the legs, and/or the spine in back.

Complications: STROKE, HEART FAILURE, PERICARDITIS, PLEURISY.

Similar conditions: see Protocol B.6: Limb Swelling or B.13: Back Pain. *Joint pains:* BRUCELLOSIS involves fever and joint pains also, but the joints are never red or warm as they are in rheumatic fever, and the onset is slower. RUBELLA has joint pains and fevers, but there is also a red spotted rash. GONORRHEA can cause a single swollen red joint. If the patient is sexually active, give enough antibiotic to take care of that possibility. *Heart problems:* HEART FAILURE from other causes may be similar. *Skin rash* may be similar to AFRICAN SLEEPING SICKNESS (parts of Africa only).

Treatment

Prevention: treat all patients with STREP INFECTION for a full 10 days, preferably using long-acting injectable PENICILLIN.

Referrals: speedy referral; see Volume 1, Appendix 13. Laboratory: an electrocardiogram, blood tests and throat culture may be helpful. Seek a level 4 facility, preferably with a cardiologist. Facilities: in severe cases a level 4 or 5 facility with advanced injectable drugs, a monitored bed and advanced surgical capabilities might be appropriate.

Patient care: in areas where rheumatic fever is common, any sudden-onset arthritis plus fever merits treatment for rheumatic fever.

- Confirm the diagnosis by noting the dramatic, immediate response of the condition to ASPIRIN.[3]
- Absolute bedrest until the patient has recovered from this episode: no fever and no hot swollen joints for 5 days.
- Treat HEART FAILURE, valvular type, if necessary.
- Use ASPIRIN (high dose) initially and PENICILLIN. In allergy to PENICILLIN, try to find independent advice; failing that, use a first-generation CEPHALOSPORIN.
- After the patient is done with PENICILLIN, give CLINDAMYCIN to eliminate strep from the throat.
- The patient must have PENICILLIN monthly for the rest of his life if he has any evidence of heart trouble. Without heart trouble, monthly PENICILLIN for 5–10 years might suffice.
- Females with loud heart murmurs, or HEART FAILURE should be cautioned against becoming pregnant. Pregnancy may be fatal.

RHEUMATOID ARTHRITIS (RA)

Definition: rheumatoid arthritis is a chronic joint inflammation wherein the body's immune system attacks the joints, both large and small. See ARTHRITIS. It is a type of ARTHRITIS, usually with low or no fever and with morning stiffness that improves during the day.

Age: it may affect children as well as adults. **Who:** mostly Westerners; it is not common in poor nationals from tropical areas. **Onset:** any one episode over hours; recurs.

Treatment

It is treatable with high doses of ASPIRIN. Advanced, level 4 Western facilities have more helpful medications. Sometimes surgery is helpful.

RHINITIS

In areas other than Africa this refers to a runny nose caused by a cold. For Africa see Regional Notes: F, which describe another kind of disease altogether.

---

1 Be sure to use the corrected temperature. See Volume 1, Chapter 1.C.
2 See Volume 1 Chapter 1 to learn how to determine heart size.

3 Many different kinds of ARTHRITIS respond to ASPIRIN, but only rheumatic fever responds dramatically within hours rather than days. The test is both sensitive and specific.

TOC

SYMPTOMS

DIFFERENTIALS

CONDITIONS

DRUG INDEX

REGIONAL NOTES

INX

RICKETS

Cause: vitamin D deficiency, usually resulting from inadequate exposure to sunlight.

Regional Notes: I, N, O, R.

Mildly to moderately ill; class 1; worldwide, related to clothing and housing which eliminate exposure to sun; especially common in urban, Muslim and Arctic areas.

Age: nursing babies with affected mothers; other children are usually 1–2 y.o. **Who:** those whose skin is not exposed to sun. It tends to occur in adults where there are high-rise buildings and/or air pollution, in women with a first pregnancy and in Muslim women. Dark skin requires more sun exposure than fair skin. Rickets may also be caused by lack of calcium in the diet. Good sources of calcium are: fish; leafy green vegetables; rhubarb; milk and milk products. Rickets may also be due to KIDNEY DISEASE or cereal diets. **Onset:** slowly.

Clinical

INFANTS AND CHILDREN

In infants, the forehead is very prominent. The soft spot on the head stays open for a long time. (Normally it closes before 18 months.) The child's head sweats excessively. In babies, the joints beside the breast bone are swollen. The lower ribs may be pulled in on the sides, like a second waist above the normal one; this lasts into adulthood. They have a delay in teething. They are likely to be floppy and irritable, have stiff muscle weakness and spasms. They may have SEIZURES. There is loss of appetite and failure to gain weight. Children refuse to use their legs.

Frequently: the bones at the ankles and wrists look swollen; the increased size is bony, not soft. They develop a hunchback appearance along with either knock-knees or bowed legs. They may be able to bend their joints abnormally.

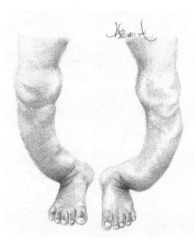

This is a spectacular example of rickets. The bowing of the legs might be subtle instead.
AB

ADULTS

Frequently: patients with rickets develop thin bones, resulting in deep bone pain.

The spine, pelvis, legs and ribs are particularly affected, causing back, pelvic or chest pain. The pain is worse with movement, weight bearing and any pressure on the affected area. The back bone may curve abnormally either forward or backward, causing a stooped or pot-belly appearance. Bowed legs may develop later. In patients with thin bones minor injuries may result in fractures. The gait becomes waddling as muscles weaken.

Similar conditions: see Protocol B.6: Limb Swelling.

Small children: SCURVY in infants is almost identical; if you suspect either, treat for both. However, in rickets the swellings beside the breast bone are rounded rather than angular. Consider MENINGITIS due to TUBERCULOSIS, LEAD POISONING and congenital SYPHILIS. TETANUS can appear similar, but the spasms become obvious quite soon. Many of the symptoms are similar to HIV INFECTION, including the teething delay and delay in the closure of the soft spot on the head.

In older children and adults: also consider ARTHRITIS, TB of the spine, BRUCELLOSIS and BERIBERI.

Treatment

Referrals: a level 4 hospital lab might be able to do some helpful blood tests.

Patient care: VITAMIN D, either in capsule form or by injection or (preferably and more cheaply) exposure of the skin to sun without intervening glass. This may be difficult for females in Muslim cultures. Milk to which vitamin D has been added may be helpful. Milk naturally does not contain much vitamin D. MULTIVITAMINS which contain vitamin D might also be useful. (Most MULTIVITAMINS include vitamin D.)

Results: 2–3 months.

Rickettsial pox

See SPOTTED FEVER; this is one form.

Rickettsiosis

This is a general term that is covered in this manual by TYPHUS and SPOTTED FEVER. See the Powerpoint lecture entitled Intermediate Organisms.

ROSEOLA

Synonym: exanthem subitum.

Definition: roseola is a general viral infection that affects mostly children.

Mildly ill; class 1; contagious; worldwide.

Age: 6 months to 3 years. **Who:** any child. **Onset:** 10–15 days incubation.

Clinical

Necessary: there is a sudden fever of 39.5°–41°C (103°–106°F) which lasts 3–5 days, then leaves as a fine red rash appears over the neck and trunk for 1–2 days and the child feels better.

Sometimes: there are cold symptoms (nasal congestion and cough), fussiness and vomiting.

Complications: FEBRILE SEIZURE.

Similar conditions: *fever:* MALARIA. *Rash:* SCARLET FEVER in which case there is always a fever as long as there is a rash.

Treatment

Cool the patient and give ACETAMINOPHEN, but the fever responds poorly to this. Use no antibiotics.

ROTAVIRUS INFECTION

Cause: virus.

Mildly to very ill; class 1–3; contagious; worldwide.

Age: mostly 3 months to 2 years; nearly every child in the world has had an episode before age 5. It also occurs in adults. **Who:** those who consume infected water, especially the immune deficient. **Onset:** sudden after an incubation of 1–3 days.

Clinical

Necessary: there is a milky-smelling, watery, severe diarrhea. If the disease is untreated, it lasts 5–7 days.

Sometimes: there is a mild fever, abdominal pain, and/or symptoms of a common cold.

Treatment

Prevention: boil drinking water during an epidemic. A vaccine is available that works well.

Referrals: facilities; a level 3 or above hospital may be helpful. There are some specific laboratory determinations for this, as well as IV fluids to prevent dehydration.

Patient care: treat DEHYDRATION. *Lactobacillus casei GG* might also be helpful. Reportedly the drug NITAZOXANIDE is helpful.

RUBELLA

Regional Notes: F, S.

Synonyms: German measles, three-day measles.

Definition: rubella is a viral infection that affects mostly children.

Mildly to moderately ill; class 1; contagious; worldwide, epidemics are common.

Age: any, most common in children. **Who:** anyone not immunized. **Onset:** incubation 12–23 days.

Clinical

In adults: there is initially fever, fatigue and cold symptoms for 4–10 days before the rash. Adults may have joint pains starting with the rash or within 3 days thereafter. The pains last for up to 4 weeks. When pregnant women have the disease, their babies may be born with CATARACT, HEART FAILURE, deafness, mental retardation or any combination of these.

In older children, after the initial symptoms as described for adults, the patient has a red, spotty rash for 3 days with enlarged lymph nodes in front and back of his neck.

Young children develop the rash and fever together.

In all patients: on the first day the rash is heaviest on the face and trunk. By the third day it has cleared on the face and trunk and is heaviest on the limbs. There may be aching all over and a peculiar body odor, like fresh feathers.

Similar conditions: *fever and rash:* MEASLES, (rash progresses without clearing rapidly), ARBOVIRAL FEVER, LEPTOSPIROSIS, SPOTTED FEVER, DENGUE FEVER and diseases similar to these. *Joint pains:* RHEUMATIC FEVER and check similar diseases under that. Also consider BRUCELLOSIS (slower onset) and other causes of ARTHRITIS.

Treatment

Prevention: immunize with MMR or rubella alone. Do not immunize pregnant women!

Patient care: cool the patient and give ACETAMINOPHEN. Antibiotics are not helpful; do not use them.

SAND FLY FEVER

Regional Notes: E, F, I, K, R.

Cause: virus.

Moderately ill to very ill; class 2.

Age: any. **Who:** those bitten by sand flies. (This kind of sand fly feeds mostly on chickens, less on cows and horses and only occasionally on humans.) **Onset:** very sudden, over hours, with a short incubation of 3–6 days, maximum fever within the first 24 hours.

Clinical

Necessary: an initial fever with headache and/or eye pain and general muscle pains, lasting 2–4 days. The liver and spleen are normal size and non-tender. There may be a rash.

Usually: the patient's eyes are red, the face is flushed and the patient avoids light and eye movement because it causes more pain. There may be nosebleed. There may be depression.

Commonly: the worst pain is in the low back.

Sometimes: there is also nausea, vomiting, abdominal pains and diarrhea. There may be mental changes. The neck may be stiff. The worst of the disease is over in a few days, but the patient does not feel healthy for weeks.

Complications: none.

Similar conditions: see Protocol B.2.

Treatment

Keep the patient hydrated and well fed. Use ACETAMINOPHEN for pain. RIBAVIRIN may be helpful. Do not use antibiotics.

SCABIES

Regional Notes: F, I, M, U.

Synonyms: sarcoptic itch, acariasis.

Definition: scabies is a skin infestation with a mite.

Entry category: infestation.

Miserable but not ill; class 1; very contagious. worldwide, common everywhere.

Age: any, especially children. **Who:** those in contact with someone who has the disease, by touch, sexual contact, shared clothing or bedding. See Volume 1, Appendix 10, for a picture of the scabies mite. **Onset:** over hours to days, after an incubation of 6-8weeks.

Clinical

Itching red spots like MEASLES spots, but it may be possible to see little lines between the spots. With a magnifying glass you might see the causative mites, although the mites are not necessarily where the rash is present. Just a few mites will make a whole body rash. It frequently starts in the web spaces of the fingers or toes, or on the wrists, waist or ankles. For diagnosis, apply a little watery ink to the skin and then wash it off. SCABIES will show little ink-colored lines remaining between the red spots. If it involves the face, it looks like whitish dry crusts, not red spots. Facial scabies is always in children less than 5 years old. In infants 0–1 year old, the buttocks and genital area may be most severely affected. After the disease has progressed the spots may turn into a generally rough, scaly skin area. In HIV patients, scabies may not itch.

Complications: IMPETIGO or CELLULITIS which may, in turn, cause KIDNEY DISEASE. If there is secondary infection it should be treated with antibiotics.

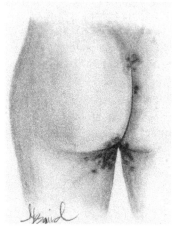

Scabies causes rough spots, first and worst in the web spaces of the hands. Itching is severe. There are satellite spots. The buttocks and genital areas are also commonly affected. AB

Similar conditions: IMPETIGO, which may also be a complication. Ordinary IMPETIGO doesn't itch, but if it is due to scabies it will itch. Also consider TINEA, ECZEMA or CONTACT DERMATITIS, none of which itch as badly as scabies. CANDIDIASIS may be indistinguishable. With early STRONGYLOIDIASIS and LARVA MIGRANS a red, wormy-type line is visible under the skin. The lines of scabies are very short.

Treatment

Wash all clothing, towels and bedding while being treated, and treat all members of a family at once, regardless of whether they have symptoms. Use 0.5% MALATHION if and only if, the skin is intact; apply it to the whole body (skipping the face if that is not affected) and repeat a week later. Itching may persist for 1–2 weeks; this does not imply treatment failure. An alternative is povidone IODINE OINTMENT, which heals both the scabies and the secondary IMPETIGO.

Alternatives are PERMETHRIN, 1% LINDANE, 10% CROTAMITON (Eurax)[1] and 25% BENZYL BENZOATE (Ascabiol).[2] 6% SULFUR in petroleum jelly for two days may also be used. LINDANE and SULFUR have been taken off the market in England. Oral IVERMECTIN reportedly also works well. IVERMECTIN is effective for both scabies and LICE, but it should not be used in geographical areas with LOIASIS (humid central and west Africa).

Scarlet fever

STREP INFECTION with a rash. See STREP INFECTION.

Schistosomiasis

SCHISTOSOMIASIS HEMATOBIUM. See Regional Notes F, R.

SCHISTOSOMIASIS INTERCALATUM. See Regional Notes F.

SCHISTOSOMIASIS JAPONICUM. See Regional Notes O, S.

SCHISTOSOMIASIS MEKONGI. See Regional Notes O, S.

SCHISTOSOMIASIS MANSONI (SM)

Regional Notes: F, M. R.

Cause: worm.

Synonyms: intestinal bilharziasis, snail fever, bilharzia.

Not ill to very ill; class 3; regional, only in scattered areas of Africa, the Middle East and the Americas. It is a tropical disease.

Age: any, especially boys 5–15 y.o. who like to swim. **Who:** skin exposed to water with infected snails. **Onset:** sometimes immediate itching; other symptoms in 4–13 weeks.

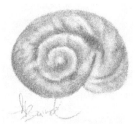

Snails that carry schistosomiasis Mansoni are flat-shaped. The center swirls on both sides are indented. Diameters are 1–2 cm. AB

---

1   *Apply nightly for 2 nights, bathing 24 hours after the second application.*
2   *Apply daily for 2 days while wearing the same clothing. On the third day, bathe, change clothes and bedding and launder them.*

TOC   SYMPTOMS   DIFFERENTIALS   CONDITIONS   DRUG INDEX   REGIONAL NOTES   INX

Clinical

Initially: there may be itching where the organisms entered the body. Expatriates especially may begin with KATAYAMA DISEASE. Nationals frequently skip this stage.

30–90 days after exposure (development stage): regardless of whether or not there was itching or KATAYAMA DISEASE, the patient develops fever, fatigue, abdominal discomfort, nausea and cough. Expatriates are particularly likely to develop fatigue and indigestion. There may be refusal to eat with weight loss. This stage can resemble ENTERIC FEVER, but the mental status is normal.

Later: when the disease is fully developed, there is either chronic DYSENTERY with MALABSORPTION or else symptoms of LIVER FAILURE with a large liver and spleen. The liver enlarges before the spleen. Many times it is the left lobe of the liver that is primarily enlarged; this may, to the inexperienced, appear to be spleen rather than liver. There might be sharp shooting pains, weakness of the limbs and numbness or tingling. This might also cause urinary symptoms like SCHISTOSOMIASIS HEMATOBIUM, including pain with intercourse and infertility in females.

Much later: LIVER FAILURE occurs. The patient has thin limbs and an abdomen full of fluid so he looks pregnant. He may have JAUNDICE. He may bleed very easily, coughing up blood or developing major bruises from minor injuries. At this stage his liver may be very small.

Complications: SPINAL NEUROPATHY occurs mostly in young males. It is a devastating complication causing numbness, weakness and loss of bladder and bowel functions. A common consequence is ANEMIA due to either blood loss or destruction of blood cells by the spleen. The growth of children is slowed. Adolescents may have delayed sexual maturity. It may cause RECTAL PROLAPSE, HEART FAILURE or vomiting blood. Rarely this may cause STROKE, BRAIN DAMAGE, MALABSORPTION, SHOCK or death.

Similar conditions: see Protocol B.7: Liver/Spleen Problems.

Initially: consider other causes of KATAYAMA DISEASE and SERUM SICKNESS. *Development stage***:** consider ENTERIC FEVER and the initial stages of other worms: TRICHURIASIS, STRONGYLOIDIASIS or HOOKWORM. *Late-stage:* MALABSORPTION, see Protocol B.14. If there is LIVER FAILURE, check other causes in the Condition Index. There may be VAGINITIS-type symptoms. It may resemble PROCTITIS or KIDNEY INFECTION.

Bush laboratory: there may be protein, urobilinogen, blood or bilirubin in urine. It is possible to hatch the worm eggs and see the larvae with simple equipment. See Volume 1, Appendix 2. In an infected area, any abdominal symptoms and any large liver or spleen merits a hatching test. The formol gel test may be positive.

Treatment

Prevention: use latrines. Avoid exposure to water with infected snails. Let a bucket of water without snails stand overnight before washing with it. ARTEMISININ prevents the disease if used the first 21 days after exposure; use PRAZIQUANTEL after 21 days. For repeated exposures (as in fishermen), use ARTEMISININ and PRAZIQUANTEL together. Seek local lore.

Referrals: laboratory: hospital laboratories can examine stool for the worm eggs, but they may be hard to find. There will be increased eosinophils evident in a blood count during the initial stages in about half of the infected expatriates. Blood tests may not turn positive until 6 weeks after the exposure. Practitioners: tropical/travel expertise is desirable. A surgeon may be necessary.

Patient care:

- Treat with PRAZIQUANTEL. OXAMNIQUINE works also, and MEBENDAZOLE may work. NIRIDAZOLE is a dangerous old drug that should no longer be used. In acute schistosomiasis (see KATAYAMA DISEASE) the symptoms can become worse with the first dose of PRAZIQUANTEL. One should use PREDNISONE or another STEROID for two days before giving PRAZIQUANTEL plus 3 days after the PRAZIQUANTEL.

- In advanced liver disease PROPRANOLOL might be helpful. Seek professional medical advice.

- Reportedly adding MEFLOQUINE and some form of ARTEMISININ increases the cure rate.

- If a patient is treated early in the course of his disease, he should have a second treatment after 6–12 weeks to eliminate the newly matured worms.

Results: good prognosis in an otherwise-healthy person. You should evaluate whether the patient is cured by doing lab determinations at 1, 3 and 6 months after treatment. The prognosis is poor when a patient has both schistosomiasis and HEPATITIS.

SCIATICA

Entry category: syndrome.

Synonyms: sciatic nerve irritation.

Definition: sciatica is an inflammation of the right or left sciatic nerve, the nerve that runs from the lower back, across the buttock and down the back side of the leg.

Cause: variable.

Mildly ill; class 1–4; worldwide.

Age: usually adults. **Who:** anyone, especially those with prior back trouble. Those with BRUCELLOSIS are prone to developing this. **Onset:** hours to days.

Clinical

There is no fever with this in and of itself, but there may be with BRUCELLOSIS or TUBERCULOSIS, two possible causes.

Necessary: the patient has pain in the low back, buttocks, down the back of one or both legs or any combination of the above. Pushing the center of the buttock aggravates the pain in that leg. With the patient lying flat on his back, raising his leg at the ankle with the knee held straight aggravates the pain in the back of the thigh. The pain may be sharp-shooting, and there may also be pains of muscle cramps. The pain is worse on movement, with coughing and with straining to have a bowel movement.

Causative diseases: if BRUCELLOSIS causes this, the episodes of pain are accompanied by fevers, general fatigue and joint pains. TUBERCULOSIS affecting the bones of the spine may cause it.

Similar conditions: if it lasts a long time, consider SLIPPED DISC.

Treatment

Referrals: facilities at level 3 or above may be most helpful. X-ray, MRI and lab can help with the diagnosis of the specific cause.

Patient care: treat like MUSCLE STRAIN.

SCOLIOSIS

Synonym: curvature of the spine.

Definition: scoliosis is sideways curvature of the spine so that instead of being dead center in the back, it curves toward the right or the left.

Cause: usually unknown.

Mildly to moderately ill; class 2–4; worldwide.

Age: usually teens and older. **Who:** anyone. **Onset:** gradual, over weeks to months.

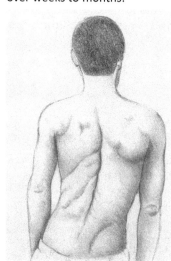

This is a moderate case of scoliosis. It will probably require surgery. OW

Clinical

Scoliosis usually begins in the teen years unless it is due to TUBERCULOSIS, BRUCELLOSIS, POLIO or DIPHTHERIA. One shoulder and hip are higher than the other, and the bone on the back of the higher shoulder or hip is more prominent than the other, giving a lop-sided appearance.

Treatment

Patient care: if the curvature is due to TUBERCULOSIS or BRUCELLOSIS, then medication is essential. If it is due to unknown causes but is diagnosed early, it may be correctable by exercises alone. If it is allowed to continue, it may be correctable only with surgery or not at all. Seek professional advice at level 4 or 5; send a picture by email.

SCRUB TYPHUS[1]

Regional Notes: I, O, S, U.

Synonym: Tsutsugamushi disease.

Excludes: tick typhus which is listed under SPOTTED FEVER; murine typhus and louse-borne typhus which are described under TYPHUS in this index.

Definition: scrub typhus is a disease caused by *Orientia tsutsugamushi;* it affects the whole body.

Mildly to very ill; class 2–3; This occurs from the northeast coast of Australia, on north throughout Asia, as far as the northern border of Mongolia. It is quite rare in the north.

Age: any. **Who:** bitten by a mite carrying the disease. These mites live in grasses and bite those walking by. Agricultural exposure is most common. **Onset:** variable; incubation about a week. The chronology and symptoms vary by geographic area. Seek local lore.

Clinical

Necessary: there is headache, light avoidance, red eyes, nasal congestion, enlarged spleen and constipation.

Usually: there is a gradual onset of fever which begins on the first day and rises each day thereafter until the fifth day. When the fever falls, it does so abruptly. There is swelling around the eyes.

Sometimes: there are one or more tiny, painless black scab(s) with a red halo where the mite bit (commonly on or near the genital area) and large, painful tender lymph nodes nearby or closer to the trunk. Other nodes may also be enlarged but less so. The mite scabs are painless and hard to find; they are frequently missed.

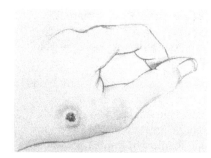

This is a typical scab from a mite that carried scrub typhus. Other diseases may cause similar scabs. With scrub typhus there is usually only one such scab. It may be difficult to find, frequently being in the genital area. AB

---

1 *See the Powerpoint lecture:* Intermediate Organisms *at www.villagemedicalmanual.org.*

Commonly: the pulse may be slow relative to the fever. About the seventh day, the patient develops a red spotted rash which starts on the trunk or face and then spreads to the limbs. A dry cough is common. The liver and spleen may be large. There may be hypersensitivity to sound followed by deafness.

Sensitive	Specific
Red eyes	Tender lymph nodes
Progressive onset	Tiny crusted scab(s)

Complications: in 98% of the patients, blind spots develop as a result of the disease. MENINGITIS or ENCEPHALITIS may occur. Death may occur during the second week. Untreated pregnant women and older patients frequently die. The disease makes HIV worse.

Similar conditions: see Protocols B.8, B.9, B.11 and B.12. TYPHUS is similar, but other symptoms precede the fever. Also see similar diseases listed under ARBOVIRAL FEVER. PLAGUE can appear similar, but then the enlarged lymph nodes are black, extremely painful and tender. LEPTOSPIROSIS, SPOTTED FEVER and Q FEVER may be indistinguishable.

Bush laboratory: protein is in the urine.

Treatment

Prevention: one dose of DOXYCYCLINE or CHLORAMPHENICOL can prevent the disease. However, it is better to use bug repellents.

Referrals: see Volume 1, Appendix 13. Laboratory: ordinary labs are useless. Very advanced laboratories with specific tropical/travel medical capabilities may be helpful. A test called PCR is specific but not sensitive; don't believe a negative result. Facilities with IVs and injectable antibiotics might also be helpful—level 2 or above. Practitioners: tropical/travel medical expertise is most helpful.

Patient care: follow the general treatment for TYPHUS. DOXYCYCLINE and CHLORAMPHENICOL work fine for this, but CHLORAMPHENICOL does not work well for Q FEVER which may be indistinguishable. In pregnancy the treatment is a single dose of AZITHROMYCIN. Do not use CIPROFLOXACIN or any CEPHALOSPORIN. Treat the patient until 7 days after the fever has entirely disappeared.

Results: fever may drop within 3 days, but in about 20% of patients the fever will continue longer.

SCURVY

Regional Notes: F, I, N, R. .

Definition: scurvy is a disease caused by a deficiency of vitamin C (ascorbic acid).

Mildly to moderately ill; class 1; worldwide, related to diet, common in tropical refugee camps. It is also common in the Arctic.

Age: any; infants develop symptoms from 6–12 months of age, earlier if breast fed. **Who:** diet low in vitamin C. Most common in hot/dry areas and Arctic. **Onset:** gradual.

Clinical

Necessary: a history of a diet lacking fresh fruits and vegetables or an infant breast fed by a vitamin C-deficient mother. Scurvy does not cause fever.

Usually: there is weight loss; weakness; stiff leg muscles; swollen and bleeding gums resulting in loosened teeth which fall out easily; large tongue; enlarged lymph nodes; and rough dry skin with tiny black and blue spots, like halos, around the bases of the hairs on the legs. There is swelling of the ankles and excessive bleeding: nosebleeds, blood-red spots on the whites of the eyes, heavy menses, bloody urine, bloody stool, bloody vomit and bleeding from minor wounds. There may be a putrid-sweet body odor and foul breath. This can cause headaches. There may be swelling of the joints in the front of the chest, between the ribs and the breastbone, resembling rosary beads under the skin. This is similar to RICKETS, but the bumps beside the breastbone are angular rather than round.

Sometimes: there is HEART FAILURE with an irregular pulse and abnormal heart sounds. There may be bleeding by the bones and joints causing bone and joint pains.

Infants refuse to use their legs; they lie in a frog-leg position. The legs are stiff. Their gums bleed with teething. They are irritable and fail to gain weight.

Complications: occasionally sudden death or severe pain in the long leg bones.

Similar conditions: *weakness, stiffness and weight loss:* MENINGITIS due to TUBERCULOSIS, HIV and LEAD POISONING might be similar in children. *Swollen joints:* see Protocol B.6. RICKETS is almost identical; if you suspect either, treat for both. *In infants* consider congenital SYPHILIS. Other types of MALNUTRITION (PELLAGRA, BERIBERI) may be similar and may coexist. Usually the bleeding gums are distinctive. *Bruising* might also be caused by LIVER FAILURE.

Bush laboratory: diagnosis can be made with a blood pressure cuff. Inflate the cuff above the upper number of the patient's blood pressure, leave it there for 30 seconds and then let it down. In scurvy this will result in a fine blue-red rash on the skin beyond the cuff. (The other diseases in which this test will be positive are HEMORRHAGIC FEVER, some MENINGITIS and SEPSIS.) Urine and stool may be positive for blood. Urine will be positive for protein.

Treatment

Vitamin C is present in citrus fruits, papaya and most fresh green vegetables, as well as in most ordinary vitamin tablets.

Results: with treatment improved in a few days, healthy in several weeks.

SEABATHER'S ERUPTION

Definition: seabather's eruption is an infestation with jellyfish larvae.

Age: any; **Who:** those who swim in the sea, particularly in the Caribbean area. **Onset:** rapid, right after bathing.

Clinical

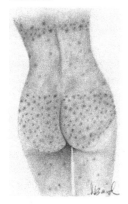

The spots are most dense on parts of the body covered with elastic fabric, in this case a tight bikini. AB

This is a very itchy spotted rash after swimming in salt water, mainly under clothing pressure points. With severe infestations the patient may develop a fever. The spots may become inflamed; blisters and secondary infection are common.

Treatment

Frequent washing with soap and water; use DIPHENHYDRAMINE for the itching. Gentle electrical zapping as for snakebite might help the itching. See Volume 1, Chapter 9.

SEIZURES

Regional Notes: F, I, O, S, U.

Entry category: syndrome.

Synonyms: convulsions, fits.

Definition: seizures are rhythmic movements caused by abnormal spontaneous electrical activity in the brain.

Very ill during seizure, variable thereafter; class 1–3; worldwide, common, related to local illnesses.

***This is a syndrome, not a diagnosis; it gives a general approach to the problem. You must figure out the cause of the seizures. See Symptom Protocol A.7.A if you have not done so already.

Age: any. **Who:** anyone, especially with FEBRILE SEIZURE (children), DIABETES, after severe head injury, ALCOHOLISM, TOXEMIA (pregnant), MALARIA, MENINGITIS, ENCEPHALITIS, KIDNEY DISEASE, RESPIRATORY FAILURE, CYSTICERCOSIS, HEAT ILLNESS, side effect or overdose of certain medications, withdrawal from some drugs or STROKE. Some people have seizures from time to time for no apparent reason. Either they are just prone to them, or seizures may result from a previous severe illness or injury. This is called EPILEPSY. There are medicines to prevent the seizures. **Onset:** suddenly, within seconds.

Clinical

Necessary: if both right and left are affected, the patient is unconscious. Some or all muscles jerk or twitch rhythmically. Trembling or fluttering motions are not seizures. Pelvic thrusting is not seizure.

Frequently: the patient is arched back. He is incontinent of urine, stool or both. His eyes are rolled back. He may slow or stop his breathing and turn blue. He will be lethargic for a few minutes to an hour after such an episode.

Sometimes: the patient may have movement in just one body part, or he may have a brief period of staring and lack of awareness of his environment.

Complications: sometimes BRAIN DAMAGE.

Causative diseases: many diseases can cause seizures; almost anything that can cause unconsciousness can also cause seizures. *With no fever:* consider HYPOGLYCEMIA, HYPERVENTILATION, TOXEMIA, EPILEPSY, ALCOHOLISM (withdrawal), SYPHILIS, STROKE, CYSTICERCOSIS, PLANT POISONING, DEMONIZATION (seizures tend to occur selectively during worship services) and ADDICTION (withdrawal from downers). Injuries, especially head injuries, can also cause seizures. *With a fever:* HEAT ILLNESS, FEBRILE SEIZURE, MENINGITIS, ENCEPHALITIS, MALARIA, TRICHINOSIS, SCHISTOSOMIASIS JAPONICUM, SEPSIS and RELAPSING FEVER.

Similar conditions: TETANUS (almost continual spasms, not as much movement); PLANT POISONING (strychnine), SCURVY, POLIO, RHEUMATIC FEVER, RABIES and RICKETS (general muscle spasms without loss of consciousness). See Protocol B.10 if the patient is merely unconscious.

Treatment

Referrals: laboratory; a large hospital lab may be able to do an electroencephalogram and blood tests which may determine the cause of the problem. Facilities: level 4 or 5. Practitioners; a neurologist is most helpful. For simple seizures a pediatrician or internist might suffice.

Patient care

• Use ACETAMINOPHEN to decrease fevers.

• Time the seizure with a clock or watch. If it lasts over five minutes by the clock or if the patient has a second one before becoming conscious, he must be treated. If the patient has or might have MALARIA or treated DIABETES, put a stomach tube in to give sugar water. Be sure to position him on his side, head down. Sugar may also be given by rectum.

• Use PHENYTOIN, PARALDEHYDE, DIAZEPAM or PHENOBARBITAL to prevent more seizures. If the seizure is due to alcohol withdrawal, use only DIAZEPAM, not the other drugs.

• If a patient with a fever has a second seizure or if his seizure will not stop, he probably has cerebral MALARIA, MENINGITIS, or HEAT ILLNESS.

• Give PHENYTOIN SODIUM for EPILEPSY.

• Treat for ONCHOCERCIASIS in areas where that occurs.

SEPSIS

Regional Notes: F, I, N, O, R, S, U.

Entry category: disease cluster.

Synonyms: septicemia, septic shock.

Definition: sepsis is an overwhelming whole body bacterial infection in which blood, which should be sterile, has bacteria in it. It usually results from an inadequately treated local infection.

Cause: bacteria.

Includes: endocarditis.

Very ill: class 4; some forms may be contagious; worldwide, related to level of medical care. MELIOIDOSIS is a particular type of sepsis that occurs in SE Asia and aboriginal Australia; it is tropical.

Age: any; especially newborns and reproductive women.
Who: prior or current infection; injury or childbirth under unclean conditions; rupture of the bag of waters 18 hours or more before birth; HIV; LEPROSY; MALARIA; CANCER; pregnancy; elderly; those who have had their spleens removed; laboratory workers who handle infective material; patients with other diseases that decrease immunity.
Onset: few hours to a day or two; this frequently starts out as a localized infection, such as PNEUMONIA or URINARY INFECTION, which then becomes a whole body infection.

⚠ SEPSIS EMERGENCIES

Agitation, confusion, coma.
Pulse >120 or respiration > 24/minute in an adult.
Low blood pressure.

Clinical

Necessary: the patient is unconscious or nearly so. His pulse and respiration are fast or irregular. He has an infection of some sort or had one recently. Either he has a high fever, or he is cold and clammy. Infants, elderly and those malnourished may not have a fever.

Maybe: the source of the original infection may or may not be obvious. He may have abdominal pain with evidence of ACUTE ABDOMEN. He may have a musty body odor. His blood pressure may be low. He may have a red spotted rash. If the original infection was PNEUMONIA, he will be short of breath. Vomiting is usual. There may be ANEMIA or a large spleen.

Occasionally: there are little flecks of blood beneath his fingernails resembling splinters. These change color over days, like ordinary bruises.

Women: those who have just delivered or miscarried may have pus coming from the vagina and pain in the genital area. See Chapter 7 in Volume 1 regarding treatment.

Newborns: they will be lethargic and suck poorly; they may have a fever or a low body temperature. They vomit. They may have diarrhea, a swollen abdomen, an infected umbilical cord and SEIZURES. They will have a weak cry and JAUNDICE. There may be signs of PNEUMONIA or MENINGITIS which will resemble or precede sepsis.

Complications: HEART FAILURE, SEIZURES, SHOCK and death, which may occur rapidly.

Causative diseases: any disease for which an antibiotic is ordinarily prescribed.

Similar conditions: see Protocols B.2, B.4, B.9 and B.10.

Bush laboratory: there may be blood in the urine.

An easy way to diagnose the problem is to draw some of the patient's blood into a glass (not plastic) syringe or test tube. Draw some blood from a healthy person into a similar syringe or test tube. Let both blood specimens clot with the syringes or tubes in an upright position (about an hour). With sepsis, the blood clot will form mostly on the bottom of the tube or syringe; a normal blood clot will form mostly along the side of the tube.

Treatment

Prevention: treat minor infections promptly and adequately. Drain all ABSCESSes. A patient who has a heart murmur (see Volume 1, Chapter 1) should have antibiotics before any dental or surgical procedure and after any dirty injury or animal bite.

Referrals: don't send an unconscious patient to a level 2 hospital. The mortality rate is about 50% in good, level 5 Western ICUs. Laboratory; a level 3 or 4 hospital lab can do blood cultures to determine which antibiotic is best. Facilities: IVs and injectable antibiotics are very important. The patient may require a monitored bed at level 4 or 5. Practitioners: infectious disease with tropical/ travel expertise is most helpful.

Patient care: if the sepsis occurred in the context of childbirth, see Volume 1, Chapter 7.

- Keep the patient in bed on his side, head down if unconscious. Check his airway.

- Use PROMETHAZINE or HYDROXYZINE to prevent vomiting. Place a stomach tube and give as much rehydration fluid as the patient will tolerate until his blood pressure and pulse are reasonably normal. See Volume 1, Appendix 1, for directions on how to make and use stomach tubes. See the first page of Volume 2, Symptom Index, for a list of normal pulse and blood pressure numbers.

- Give a liquid diet by stomach tube as soon as possible.

- Check vital signs every 2 to 4 hours.

- Use IBUPROFEN and ACETAMINOPHEN alternately every 2 hours, plus cool bathing for fever.

- Try to find the source of infection and treat that. Drain any ABSCESS. See Volume 1, Appendix 1.

- Antibiotics should be injectable.

- With visible pus: without a bad odor, use CLOXACILLIN or a first generation CEPHALOSPORIN.

TOC   SYMPTOMS   DIFFERENTIALS   CONDITIONS   DRUG INDEX   REGIONAL NOTES   INX

TOC

SYMPTOMS

DIFFERENTIALS

CONDITIONS

DRUG INDEX

REGIONAL NOTES

INX

- *Visible pus with a bad odor:* add METRONIDAZOLE.
- *Animal bite context:* with visible pus, use CO-TRIMOXAZOLE; with localized redness and swelling, no pus, use PENICILLIN, AMOXICILLIN or CIPROFLOXACIN.
- *Ordinary sepsis:* use (PENICILLIN plus CHLORAMPHENICOL) or an appropriate CEPHALOSPORIN. Intravenous OFLOXACIN is also good. You may substitute AMPICILLIN for PENICILLIN or CO-TRIMOXAZOLE for CHLORAMPHENICOL. Add METRONIDAZOLE or TINIDAZOLE if the patient just gave birth, if this is due to PNEUMONIA, if the bowel is involved or if it occurs after an injury.
- *In infants use* [ACYCLOVIR plus (high-dose AMPICILLIN & GENTAMYCIN)] or else [ACYCYLOVIR plus (CHLORAMPHENICOL or a third-generation CEPHALOSPORIN)].
- *Melioidosis:* in Southeast Asia and aboriginal tropical Australia, in sepsis that started with PNEUMONIA or KIDNEY INFECTION, use ceftazidine or one of the carbapenems (both under CEPHALOSPORIN) for 3 months followed by at least 3 months of CO-TRIMOXAZOLE.

Results: 48 hours improved.

Septic abortion

See SEPSIS and ABORTION.

SERUM SICKNESS

Entry category: syndrome.

This is a complex type of ALLERGY, originally described when an animal or human was injected with the serum of a dissimilar creature. It can also be caused by certain drugs, particularly ASPIRIN, ALLOPURINOL, IBUPROFEN, FUROSEAMIDE, PENICILLIN, PHENYTOIN, STREPTOMYCIN and SULFA drugs. It can also be caused by some diseases: LARVA MIGRANS, MENINGITIS, STREP INFECTION (causing RHEUMATIC FEVER), LIVER FLUKE, DENGUE FEVER, MALARIA, HEPATITIS and HIV INFECTION, for example. KATAYAMA DISEASE is one form of serum sickness.

Age: any **Who:** those exposed to certain drugs or diseases. Onset is usually about 10 days for the first exposure; it is 1–2 days for subsequent exposures.

Clinical

Necessary: at least two of the following:
- fever.
- prominent rash, usually hives.
- headache or body pains: muscles, bones and joints.

Initially: there may be nausea, vomiting, shortness of breath with wheezing, fever, chills, HIVES. After 2–16 days there may be protein in the urine and in about half of the patients, a large-joint ARTHRITIS. In the skin there is first redness (warmth in dark skin), then a rash like MEASLES or HIVES. The lymph nodes and spleen may be enlarged.

Complications: KIDNEY DISEASE, HEART FAILURE, ARTHRITIS.

Similar conditions: see Protocol B.12.

Treatment

This must be medically determined and supervised.

SEXUALLY TRANSMITTED DISEASE: (STD)

(Also see this index for the individual diseases.)

Synonyms: STD, venereal disease.

Entry category: disease cluster.

Regional Notes: F, I, M, N.

Definition: sexually transmitted diseases are those diseases acquired through direct contact of the warm moist surfaces of the body.

Clinical

These diseases, in this work, are GONORRHEA, CHANCROID, SYPHILIS, CHLAMYDIA, LYMPHOGRANULOMA VENEREUM, HERPES and DONOVANOSIS, which are all described separately. HIV INFECTION and other diseases may also be transmitted sexually; they are not included in this list if their major manifestations are non-genital. If you suspect any one of these STD's, you should not try to diagnose but to treat according to Protocol B.1, unless the particular diagnosis is obvious from the history. An example would be a spouse diagnosed in a laboratory as having one of these.

The symptoms of sexually transmitted diseases are as follows. For these purposes, the rectum and anus are considered to be part of the genital area.

- Spontaneous sores, bumps or ulcers (in either sex) on the skin of the genital region or any body part that had sexual contact. These are skin ulcers.
- Large lymph nodes in the groin (in either sex) in the absence of sores on the legs and feet.
- Burning with urinating (in either sex) or pus from the penis in a male.
- Vaginal pain, itching or discharge in a female, possibly with some bleeding.
- Swollen scrotum in a male.
- Low abdominal or genital pain in a female; pain with intercourse.

Similar conditions: see Protocols B.1, B.11 and B.12.

Skin bumps and ulcers: see the chart in B.1. Consider AMEBIC SKIN ULCER and DIPHTHERIA most urgently. Consider WARTS. Skin bumps due to VISCERAL LEISHMANIASIS (PKDL) have an affinity for the face, genitals and warm, moist, pink surfaces. LEPROSY never affects the genital areas.

Treatment

Prevention: faithfulness or abstinence.

Patient care: see Protocol B.1. Refer to the descriptions of the particular diseases for which drugs to use. An expensive but effective shotgun treatment is AZITHROMYCIN as it is used for MALARIA. This covers all the bacterial STDs except for tertiary SYPHILIS and SYPHILIS in a newborn; use PENICILLIN additionally.

SHINGLES

Synonym: varicella zoster infection.

Definition: shingles is a nerve infection with *varicella zoster*, the causative virus of chicken pox. It secondarily affects the skin.

Mildly to moderately ill; class 2; contagious in that children can get CHICKEN POX from an adult with shingles. Adults do not get shingles from children; worldwide.

Age: older adults; children with DIABETES or HIV.
Who: almost anyone, but especially those with poor immunity.
Onset: over several days.

Clinical

There is a painful rash[1] (sometimes also itchy) in a band, usually on one side of the trunk, sloping down from the back and around to the front. The rash breaks out after several days of pain in that area of skin. The rash never crosses the center line more than an inch. It may be on the face or the shoulder, in which case it is in an area rather than a band. It may also affect the inside of the mouth and the white of the eye. Usually there are blisters at first which then break and crust.

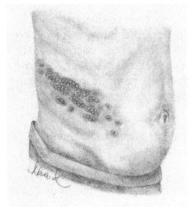

There are innumerable tiny blisters in a band around one side of the trunk. The band is always higher in the back, sloping down to the front. There are satellite spots. AB

Similar conditions: see Protocol B.8 if the eyes are involved. CHICKEN POX blisters are scattered and itchy. HERPES may appear similar. TRENCH FEVER causes a whole body illness with general aching. SPINAL NEUROPATHY causes similar pains, usually also numbness, tingling, weakness or bladder/bowel problems.

Treatment

Prevention: immunization.

Patient care: cool wet-to-dry compresses (see Volume 1, Appendix 1) and pain medicines may be helpful. The rash lasts 2–3 weeks and the pain at least 6 weeks. ACYCLOVIR may work for treatment. It is helpful to use PREDISONE additionally.

SHOCK ⚠ Life-threatening-threatening emergency!

Entry category: syndrome.

Definition: shock is a crisis in which the circulation of blood is inadequate to sustain life. (This refers to physiological shock, not to someone's being emotionally upset. Emotional upset is not shock in the medical sense, even if the patient faints.)

Very ill; class 4; worldwide.

If this is from an insect sting or an injection, treat for ANAPHYLAXIS with EPINEPHRINE.

Age: any. **Who:** those with ANAPHYLAXIS, severe DEHYDRATION, blood loss, SEPSIS, some injuries, ACUTE ABDOMEN, THALLASEMIA, HEMORRHAGIC FEVER and treatment of RELAPSING FEVER. **Onset:** within minutes with bleeding and ANAPHYLAXIS; variable otherwise.

Clinical

Necessary: the patient's skin is ashen, cool and moist. His pulse is fast. His blood pressure is low. He is not urinating much unless he had a full bladder beforehand. He is weak and lethargic. If you try to raise him to a sitting or standing position, he will lose consciousness. Anyone who can stand upright and remain conscious is not in shock.

Usually: respiration is rapid.

Similar conditions: someone who is upset or excited may pass out, but it lasts only a minute, and does not need treatment. Other similar diseases: SEPSIS, HYPOGLYCEMIA, sudden drop in blood pressure or temperature during MALARIA, RELAPSING FEVER and a reaction to medication for RELAPSING FEVER can both mimic and cause shock.

Treatment

Referrals: treatment in a facility that has IVs with fluids and injectable drugs is essential. Closeness is more important than level of care.

Patient care:

- If you can start an IV, do so. Give a salt solution (normal saline, Darrow's solution or lactated Ringer's) as quickly as possible until the patient is more alert, or he has had 20 ml/kg, whichever comes first. In the absence of ACUTE ABDOMEN, intraperitoneal fluids may substitute.

- If you do not have IVs, position the patient on a slanted board, head down and legs up. If you have elastic bandages, put them on the legs, rolling them snugly from the ankles up to the thighs. Be sure to start at the ankles. This squeezes the blood out of the leg veins so it goes into the trunk.

- Give fluids if the patient can drink. Position him on his side and watch his airway continually.

- If the shock is due to infection or ACUTE ABDOMEN, treat that also.

---

1 Children do not commonly get shingles, but when they do get it, it may be painless.

TOC

SYMPTOMS

DIFFERENTIALS

CONDITIONS

DRUG INDEX

REGIONAL NOTES

INX

SIBERIAN TICK TYPHUS

See SPOTTED FEVER. This is one type of spotted fever that occurs in eastern Europe and throughout Asia. It is a temperate and Arctic problem.

SICKLE CELL DISEASE (SCD)

Regional Notes: F, I, M., R

Synonyms: sickle cell anemia, SS hemoglobinopathy.

Definition: sickle cell disease is an abnormal hemoglobin. Hemoglobin is the red stuff in the blood that captures oxygen in the lungs and releases it in the rest of the body. The abnormal hemoglobin causes the red blood cells to break apart easily. This, in turn, plugs the blood vessels; the usual symptoms of this disease follow from this.

Mildly to extremely ill; class 2–3; Found worldwide, mainly in persons of African genetic heritage; a mild form occurs in some Greeks, Arabs and South Asians.

Age: begins 3–6 months old, occasionally older. **Who:** offspring of two parents, both of whom carry the gene for the condition. Both parents must be of one of these genetic heritages: African, Arab, South Asian or Greek. It affects both sexes equally. **Onset:** individual episodes over a few hours; recurrent crises.

Clinical

HISTORY

There is almost always a family history of an illness consistent with sickle cell disease: episodes of severe pain, large spleen, anemia, jaundice and infections. The spleen and liver swelling cause a continual ANEMIA and make the patient prone to infections. African spleens stay large until age 3–5 y.o.; then they shrink. Spleens may remain large in other ethnic groups.

There are two other problems with spleens swelling

- If it suddenly enlarges, then the patient develops sudden ANEMIA. This tends to happen between ages 4 months and 3 years. The patient needs a blood transfusion the first time this happens. If it happens repeatedly the spleen should be removed.

- If it is very large after age 5 (most common in eastern Saudi Arabia and in India), then children stop growing. The spleen may be removed.

GROWTH AND DEVELOPMENT

There is short height before puberty, a growth spurt afterwards, and normal final height. Puberty is delayed. There are very long limbs, narrow pelvis and shoulders. BMI is usually low throughout life.

ACUTE CHEST SYNDROME

In children over 2 years old this is the most common cause of death: shortness of breath, chest pain that is worse with deep breathing, fever and turning bluish from lack of oxygen. Infection in the upper lungs is common. This may cause the chest to become barrel-shaped. The lung changes can lead to HEART FAILURE, causing swelling of the liver and of the legs and feet.

Patients over 20 years old tend to have more pain and shortness of breath but less fever. There is less often infection. The pain is usually in the lower chest rather than the upper chest. There may be sudden death from PULMONARY EMBOLISM.

PREGNANCY

During the last trimester of pregnancy and immediately after childbirth there is risk of acute chest syndrome for the mother; however with severe disease most patients don't live long enough to become pregnant.

BONE CRISIS

When blood clots travel to bones there is severe bone pain—deep pains that never let up and are worse at night. There may be permanent bone damage. Children less than 5 y.o. commonly have swollen hands, feet, fingers and toes; older children and adults (especially pregnant women) have bone crises in their long limb bones, backs and pelvises. If there is infection in the bone(s), there will be a high fever; see OSTEOMYELITIS.

KIDNEY CRISIS

There may be blood, protein or urobilinogen in the urine and maybe large quantities of urine. With nephrotic KIDNEY DISEASE there is much protein in the urine, and the patient has swelling of his/her legs and feet; prognosis is poor. With nephritic KIDNEY DISEASE there will be blood in the urine and shortness of breath; prognosis is better.

SKIN RASH

When clots lodge in the skin they may cause little bruise marks, the size of the heads of pins.

NEUROLOGICAL CRISIS

When clots go to the brain there may be symptoms of BRAIN DAMAGE or STROKE. The patient may have SEIZURES, coma, vomiting and headache. He may become blind.

APLASTIC CRISIS

Aplastic means that the bone marrow suddenly stops functioning. This causes sudden ANEMIA. Blood transfusion is life-saving.

LEG ULCERS

These are most common in the Americas and between 10–30 y.o. First there is pain, then a color change and hardening of the skin. The ulcers are deep and painful. They heal slowly and frequently break open again, lasting a long time (a matter of years). They heal first around the edges and then fill in the center. The skin around the ulcers is darker than normal, whereas the skin of the healed area is lighter than normal.

GALLSTONES

Gallstones develop in older patients.

ABNORMAL SUSTAINED ERECTIONS

These are persistent and painful; they occur in children over 4 y.o. and in adults. There is no sexual arousal associated. There are two kinds: 1. come-and-go: recurrent at night, lasting 3–6 hours, with normal function otherwise; 2. major: lasting 24 hours or more, mostly in adults, frequently resulting in impotence. Usually people with major attacks have had episodic attacks before. DEHYDRATION can contribute to the problem.

Complications: SCD may cause STROKE (even in children), ANEMIA, HEART FAILURE, KIDNEY DISEASE, OSTEOMYELITIS, GALLBLADDER DISEASE and SEPSIS.

Similar conditions: see Protocols B.3, B.4, B.5, B.6, B.7, B.9 and B.13. The most common are listed below: *hot, swollen body parts:* CELLULITIS, ARTHRITIS or SCURVY. *Shortness of breath:* see Protocol B.4. *Failure to grow* well may look like ordinary MALNUTRITION, SCURVY, RICKETS or HIV.

ANEMIA with large spleen and fatigue: Protocols B.3 and B.5. *Frequent fevers and infections:* may resemble HIV INFECTION, MALARIA, ACUTE ABDOMEN, HEPATITIS and RHEUMATIC FEVER. *Swelling of the hands:* LOIASIS (Africa only) can cause similar swelling; congenital SYPHILIS may cause swelling, but then the fingertips are spared.

Bush laboratory: if you measure hemoglobin, you will find ANEMIA. During a crisis urine may contain excessive urobilinogen.

Treatment

Prevention: advise healthy parents of a child with SCD that with each pregnancy their chances of having another child with SCD are one in four. They should consider adopting rather than conceiving.

Referrals: see Volume 1, Appendix 13. Laboratory: level 3 or 4 hospitals can do blood tests to show the sickle-shaped red cells under a microscope, but these tests are unreliable if the patient has had a recent transfusion. They are also unreliable on babies under 3 months of age. A sophisticated lab can test normal people to see if they carry the gene and thus advise them concerning a marriage partner. Sometime the problem is evident on an ordinary blood smear. Facilities: there are many facilities at a level 3 or 4 that are useful: IV fluids, oxygen, transfusion capabilities and respiratory therapy. These facilities are so essential to survival that patients, once diagnosed, should make every effort to live near such a place. Practitioners; a hematologist is most helpful or a general practitioner, pediatrician or internist with SCD experience.

Ordinary patient care:

Symptomatic treatment: CHOLESTYRAMINE helps for intolerable itching.

- All patients should take FOLATE, ZINC and medication to prevent MALARIA. (MALARIA is a common cause of death in patients with SCD.) The diet should contain animal products, or the patient should receive injections of VITAMIN B$_{12}$. MULTIVITAMINS might also be helpful.

Crisis patient care:

- Give a large amount of fluid by mouth or stomach tube. Even slight DEHYDRATION can cause major problems. Use HYDROXYZINE or PROMETHAZINE to prevent vomiting.

- Keep the patient warm; cold tends to aggravate the problem.

- Give extra FOLATE or feed the patient fresh, raw or only slightly cooked leafy vegetables. Daily folate is critical in reproductive women.

- Children with this problem should be checked for blood in their stools and should be questioned as to diet. If there is blood in the stool or the patient eats a diet low in IRON or VITAMIN C, you should give IRON supplements, but only if he has not had multiple transfusions. Daily oral PENICILLIN from the time of initial diagnosis until age 5 improves chances for survival. Pregnant women should all get IRON, VITAMIN C and FOLATE.

- If you have pain medications use these freely.

Leg ulcers: treat with packing and ointments (see TROPICAL ULCER). Sprinkling PHENYTOIN in the ulcers helps healing. If there is not a prompt response to local treatment, use oral antibiotics: PENICILLIN plus CHLORAMPHENICOL.

Large spleen: give daily PROGUANIL as a MALARIA preventive; this may decrease the spleen size within 6 months.

Bone pain with fever should be treated as OSTEOMYELITIS with CHLORAMPHENICOL plus CLOXACILLIN.

Respiratory symptoms require PENICILLIN plus (ERYTHROMYCIN or AZITHROMYCIN).

Treatment of abnormal erections: there are some hormone treatments. One can try sedatives, exercise, pain relievers, cold showers or cold compresses to the penis. Use hydration with drinking or IV fluids; some blood pressure lowering medicines (but NOT DIURETICS); oxygen inhalation; and blood transfusion. Surgery may be helpful.

Results: pain should improve within 24 hours.

TOC   SYMPTOMS   DIFFERENTIALS   CONDITIONS   DRUG INDEX   REGIONAL NOTES   INX

SLIPPED DISC

Synonyms: herniated disc.

Definition: slipped disc is a nerve irritation caused by the spinal cartilage pushing on the nerves where they come out between the back bones.

Cause: unknown, injury or overweight condition.

Moderately ill: class 2–3; worldwide, frequency depends on heredity and culture. Not generally common; MUSCLE STRAIN and SCIATICA are similar and much more common.

Age: adults, usually. **Who:** anyone, sometimes hereditary or may be due to FLUOROSIS, BRUCELLOSIS or TUBERCULOSIS. **Onset:** usually sudden, possibly gradual.

Clinical

Necessary: the patient has excruciating neck or back pain.

Usually: the pain is sharp, and it shoots down the arm(s) or leg(s). In the case of back and leg pain, holding the leg straight at the knee and raising it by bending it at the hip causes severe pain in the back of the thigh. The patient cannot walk well if at all.

Sometimes: he may have weakness, numbness or tingling in one or both legs, and he may not be able to walk or urinate. If the slipped disc is in the neck, then the pain goes down one or both arms with weakness or numbness in the arm or hand.

Causative diseases: BRUCELLOSIS, BURKITT LYMPHOMA, FLUOROSIS (neck only) or TUBERCULOSIS. It might happen for no good reason at all.

Similar conditions: many. The most common similar disease is ARTHRITIS that affects the lower spine. Also consider SCIATICA and MUSCLE STRAIN. With a very gradual onset and stiff weakness, consider TROPICAL SPASTIC PARAPARESIS. With slipped disc, straight leg raising (see Volume 1, Chapter 11) on the good side may worsen the pain on the bad side.

Treatment

Referrals: see Volume 1, Appendix 13. This is essential, at a level 3 or higher facility with an orthopedic surgeon or a neurosurgeon.

Patient care if unable to send out: six weeks of absolute bed rest except that the patient may get up to move his bowels. Urination should be into a urinal. Use pain medication. He may lie on either side or on his back (with a pillow under his knees) but not belly down. If the problem is in the neck rather than the lower back, the patient should wear a collar as for a whiplash injury. A beanbag chair used as a pillow may be helpful. Seek outside advice concerning how long to continue this. Other treatment is not feasible in remote areas. Check for numbness and weakness of the limbs. If the patient has either, send him within a day. If he has trouble urinating use a urinary catheter until you can send him. See Appendix 1 in Volume 1. Treat BRUCELLOSIS or TUBERCULOSIS if necessary.

SMALLPOX

This is a devastating viral disease that was eliminated worldwide in the 1970s, However, some stocks of the virus have disappeared, so there is a terrorist concern. It is temperate as well as tropical. It is highly contagious. First there is a fever and rapid pulse, headache and back pain. On the third day the rash breaks out, first on the wrists and the face, spreading within hours to the rest of the body, including the palms and the soles. The rash is blistery; the blisters remain for up to a week before starting to dry, whereas with CHICKEN POX the blisters start drying immediately. About 1/3 of the patients die; 1/3 are badly scarred for life; 1/3 survive without scarring. There is a good immunization, but there are no good medications for treatment. There are pictures in the CDC Public Health Image Library.

SMOKE INHALATION

Definition: smoke inhalation is a malfunction of breathing due to the irritant effects of smoke. Symptoms range from a slight cough to moderate shortness of breath to sudden RESPIRATORY FAILURE. This can develop suddenly up to 72 hours after exposure. High humidity and THEOPHYLLINE may be helpful. Use no CODEINE for the cough unless a physician approves. A similar disease is ASTHMA. Also see Protocol B.4.

SPINAL NEUROPATHY

Entry category: syndrome.

This term refers to nerve problems in the spinal cord, sometimes from injury, other times from diseases.

Causative diseases are: DONOVANOSIS, SCHISTOSOMIASIS (mostly MANSONI but may be one of the others), TUBERCULOSIS, HERPES, MENINGITIS, SYPHILIS, ENTERIC FEVER, CANCER, LYME DISEASE, some viral infections, some immunizations or any tumor or injury of the spine. The onset can be sudden or gradual. It may be symmetrical or asymmetrical, frequently with back pain which wraps around the trunk like a band, somewhat higher in the back and lower in the front. (This is similar to SHINGLES.)

There is numbness and/or tingling and/or weakness of one or both limbs. This may also affect the saddle area. The patient may have trouble starting to urinate or passing stool, or he may be incontinent or impotent. If the underlying disease is diagnosed and treated promptly, there may be recovery. Otherwise the prognosis is poor. In any case, if you consider this diagnosis, promptly seek care at a level 4 or 5.

There are three kinds of spinal neuropathy.

A. If the spinal cord is being squeezed, this is called a **compressive neuropathy.** It may be due to tumor, abscess or abnormal bone. TB is the most common cause. First there is pain in the center line of the back or neck. Usually numbness and tingling occur before weakness. The symptoms may be asymmetrical. Bladder and bowel function may be affected. *Referral* must be to a surgical facility.

B. The alternative to compressive is **non-compressive neuropathy.** If the cause is infection, this has a rapid onset over hours to days. It may be due to SYPHILIS, SCHISTOSOMIASIS, BRUCELLOSIS, CHLAMYDIA or some viral infections. Usually the symptoms are first asymmetrical. Referral should be to a neurologist or a medical facility, not to a surgical facility. You can try treatment for whatever infectious disease is common in your area.

C. Spinal neuropathy due to **COBALAMIN DEFICIENCY** is of slow onset with no prior back and neck pains. Numbness and tingling come first, then weakness and incoordination. There may be mental symptoms or bladder and bowel dysfunction. Symptoms will improve but may not totally reverse with injections of VITAMIN B$_{12}$ or with the patient consuming raw liver. (Consuming raw liver is dangerous.)

SPLENIC CRISIS

This is a problem that happens to people who have very large spleens for whatever reason. There are three possibilities.

SPLENIC INFARCT
This means that a bit of the spleen dies. There is spleen pain and tenderness, but the problem takes care of itself with simple pain relief.

SPLENIC ABSCESS
This means that there is a pocket of pus. There is probably a fever. This requires surgical drainage at a hospital. Antibiotics alone are not helpful.

SPLENIC RUPTURE
This is usually rapid onset, with internal bleeding and SHOCK. You will not likely have time, but if you can get him out, it must be to a surgeon.

SPOTTED FEVER[1]

Regional Notes: E, F, I, K, M, N, O, R, S, U.

Synonyms: Rickettsiosis, Boutonneuse fever, African tick typhus, Mediterranean tick typhus

Includes: tick typhus and Rickettsial pox. In many places there are place names attached, such as Mediterranean tick typhus and African tick typhus.

Excludes: Rocky Mountain spotted fever, see the SPOTTED FEVER entry in the M Regional Notes.

Definition: spotted fever is a fever plus rash that is caused by various species of Rickettsiae.

Moderately to very ill; class 2–3.

Age: any. **Who:** tick-bitten for tick typhus. Dog contact in the Mediterranean area. Rickettsial pox is transmitted by mites or by consuming contaminated food and drink. It is mainly urban, in South Africa and north-eastern Asia. Flea-borne spotted fever comes from flea bites. **Onset:** incubation less than 12 days for tick typhus; 1–2 weeks for Rickettsial pox; unknown for flea-borne spotted fever.

1 *See the Powerpoint lecture:* Intermediate Organisms *at www.villagemedicalmanual.org.*

Clinical

TICK TYPHUS
Necessary: moderately or very ill after a few days. There is sudden onset of a high fever with headache, stiff neck and red eyes. A rash breaks out by day 4 or 5. It begins on the limbs and may involve the palms and soles. The rash is heaviest on the wrists and ankles. It is not itchy. There may be scar(s) from a tick bite.

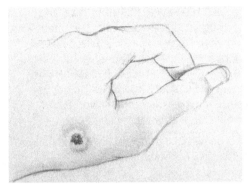

This is the scab from a tick bite on the hand. There may be one or many. The scab is likely to be tiny and hard to find. OW

Maybe: severe muscle pains and vomiting. The patient may become delirious and may develop GANGRENE. Lymph nodes are likely to be large.

Complications: KIDNEY DISEASE, STROKE, RESPIRATORY FAILURE, internal bleeding.

RICKETTSIAL POX
First there is a bump on the skin which grows to 0.5–1.5 cm. It becomes a blister which dries, scabs and heals. About a week after the initial bump, there is sudden onset of fever. The rash, consisting of tiny blisters which resemble CHICKEN POX, starts on day 1 or 2 of the fever; it does not involve the palms or soles. The blisters dry and heal without scarring. Headache and eye pain are common. There are muscle pains and large lymph nodes. There may be vomiting, a stiff neck, dizziness and an enlarged spleen.

FLEA-BORNE SPOTTED FEVER
There is a worldwide distribution except for the Arctic. The patient has a fever, fatigue, headache and rash. There may be a small scab where the infected flea bit. The patient may have large lymph nodes and a large spleen.

Complications: sometimes a mild MENINGITIS.

Similar conditions: Rickettsial pox may be similar to CHICKEN POX. For tick typhus consider ARBOVIRAL FEVER and the similar diseases. See Protocols B.2, B.8, B.10, B.11 and B.13. The distinctions between many of these diseases can be subtle. If tick typhus is a possibility treat for it. It can be rapidly fatal if not treated, especially in Africa.

Treatment

Prevention: avoid tick bites: exclude dogs from houses, protect arms and legs when pushing through brush; do not sleep on the ground. Wash your floors weekly with malathion-water to eliminate fleas.

Referrals: laboratory; a blood test, the Felix-Weil, is useless, being neither sensitive nor specific. Practitioners: tropical/travel medical expertise is essential.

Patient care: since SPOTTED FEVER, SCRUB TYPHUS and murine TYPHUS are not distinguishable, early treatment with DOXYCYCLINE improves outcome. For Rickettsial pox, use only DOXYCYCLINE or RIFAMPIN. For other types of spotted fever: DOXYCYLINE, CHLORAMPHENICOL, [RIFAMPIN plus ERYTHROMYCIN], possibly CLARITHROMYCIN. Do not use CIPROFLOXACIN since it makes the problem worse. You should treat until 3 days after the fever is gone.

Results: fever will drop within 4 days, usually. Rickettsial pox response to DOXYCYCLINE is 2–4 days.

SPRUE

Regional Notes: F, I, O, R, S, U.

Synonyms: tropical enteropathy, tropical sprue, post-infectious malabsorption.

Definition: sprue is a malfunction of the bowel, due to some unknown factor associated with residence in certain tropical areas.

Moderately ill; class 1–2; nearly worldwide. It occurs mainly in Asia south of the 40th parallel, in the Pacific islands and northern Australia, in West Africa and Africa south of the DRC, in South America north of the Amazon valley and throughout Central America and the Caribbean.

Age: usually adults. **Who:** anyone, especially expatriates, but nationals can get it also. **Onset:** usually slow, within 6 months of arriving in an area; the onset might also be rapid on occasion, and the diarrhea always lasts at least 3–4 months.

Clinical

Necessary: continual or recurrent severe diarrhea which is foul, greasy and floating. There is no fever from this. The patient has much gas; loud, rumbling bowel sounds; and a bloated abdomen (gas, not water).

Usually: there is sensitivity in the mouth; alcohol and acidic or spicy foods cause pain. Then the patient complains of fullness in the upper central abdomen. The diarrhea may at first alternate with constipation. Temperature and blood pressure tend to be low.

Later: the tongue becomes red and shiny; blisters or ulcers form within the mouth. There may be vertical cracks in the lips. The patient develops ANEMIA,[1] has loss of appetite, weight loss, weakness and is likely to become apathetic and irritable with DEPRESSION and inability to concentrate. Physical exam shows a large, non-tender liver; there may be mild JAUNDICE. The skin becomes a pale muddy color, sometimes with dark spots.

Similar conditions: MALNUTRITION or ANEMIA from other causes. PELLAGRA is similar, but it also causes excessive saliva production which sprue does not. See Protocol B.14.

Bush laboratory: urine dipsticks used on the watery part of the stool show a stool pH of 6 or less.

Treatment

Referrals: see Volume 1, Appendix 13. A level 4 or 5 facility with a gastroenterologist experienced in tropical/travel medicine is most appropriate.

Patient care: DOXYCYCLINE and MULTIVITAMINS are essential, as well as a low-fat, high-protein diet. There should be rapid improvement if your diagnosis is correct. Give a shot of VITAMIN B_{12} if you can. If you are not able to and the patient does not improve within a week, minced raw beef liver taken orally is a substitute for the B_{12} injection. B_{12} by mouth is not adequate for treatment, nor is cooked liver. Be sure that the raw liver comes from a healthy animal; even so, this is dangerous as it may transmit other diseases. The only permanent solution may be residence in a temperate climate. About 50% of patients relapse if they return to the tropics.

STD

See SEXUALLY TRANSMITTED DISEASE and also Protocol B.1.

STREP INFECTION; STREP THROAT

Regional Notes: F, I.

Synonyms: tonsillitis, bacterial pharyngitis.

Includes: scarlet fever.

Excludes: RHEUMATIC FEVER

Definition: strep infection is an infection with group A beta-hemolytic streptococci. Scarlet fever is a strep infection with a rash.

Cause: bacteria.

Mildly ill: class 1 usually, occasionally Class 4; contagious; worldwide, common everywhere.

Age: any. **Who:** anyone. **Onset:** sudden. Incubation for scarlet fever is 1–4 days

---

1 Anemia is due to vitamin deficiencies, both B_{12} and folic acid. Give B_{12} either with or before folic acid when treating the patient.

Clinical

Necessary: adults have a sore throat and pain with swallowing; children have abdominal pain, a sore throat or both.

Usually: the patient has a fever. His breath may have a foul odor. He has no cough and no stuffy nose. The patient's tonsils are red and swollen with white pus spots on them. His tongue is finely spotted like a strawberry, either white on red or red on white. Neck lymph nodes in front are swollen and tender.

Sometimes: if the patient has a fine red rash except for a pale circle around his mouth, he has SCARLET FEVER. This will be invisible on black skin. The rash appears smooth and lobster-color at first, being worse in the skin folds. Then it appears like a sunburn. Finally it has a sandpapery texture. It may eventually peel. It begins on the lower body and moves up. There may be vomiting, fatigue and whole body pains. The rash lasts 5–7 days without treatment.

Complications: RHEUMATIC FEVER and KIDNEY DISEASE, usually nephritic type. An ABSCESS may form on a tonsil which must be treated in a hospital facility. It can be fatal. If it is compromising the patient's breathing, withdrawing pus with a large needle on a large syringe may be helpful.

Similar conditions: the most common confusion is between strep throat and a viral infection. With a viral infection the onset is gradual; pain is not severe; there are watery eyes and a runny nose; the throat may be red with tiny blisters and ulcers. With a strep throat the onset is sudden; pain is severe; the nodes in the neck are large and tender; the eyes and nose are normal; the throat is red, possibly with white pus on the tonsils.

Large lymph nodes: see Protocol B.12; note that TULAREMIA comes from eating infected food or drinking infected water.

Abnormal tonsils: TULAREMIA, MONONUCLEOSIS and DIPHTHERIA can look identical; the only reliable distinction in most areas is that with MONONUCLEOSIS and TULAREMIA the patient still has a fever and fatigue after 3 days of the usual antibiotic. DIPHTHERIA causes additional symptoms such as double vision and muscle weakness.

Fever and abdominal pains: ENTERIC FEVER (apathetic), PNEUMONIA (rapid respiration), MALARIA (more than one chill), TULAREMIA (no response to the usual antibiotic). Protocol B.9.

Fever and rash: see Protocol B.2.

Treatment

Referrals: laboratory; a hospital, level 3, can culture the bacteria or do a rapid test for strep. Facilities: if the patient is very ill, then IV fluids and injectable antibiotics may be appropriate.

Patient care: PENICILLIN or ERYTHROMYCIN for a full 10 days. Taken for less time it does not prevent the development of RHEUMATIC FEVER. AZITHROMYCIN is a very good alternative since it is eliminated from the body very slowly. Use this treatment for ANY sore throat in a patient with prior RHEUMATIC FEVER, with RHEUMATIC FEVER in the family or with a heart murmur.

Results: 2–3 days. The patient is no longer contagious 48 hours after beginning antibiotics.

STRESS

Entry category: syndrome.

Definition: stress is physical illness due to emotional causes.

Each person has his own peculiar pattern of response to stress. Some have increased or decreased appetite with weight gain or loss. Some people develop abdominal pain with vomiting or diarrhea. Some get headaches, neck pain, or heavy chest pain. The patient may urinate frequently. Children may start bed-wetting after having been dry. They may have insomnia or day-night reversal and may sigh frequently. Adults and older children may be short of breath. See DEPRESSION also as these are frequently associated.

If a person under stress has physical symptoms which he has had before and if, in addition, his vital signs are reasonably normal, he probably has another stress reaction. Therapy is directed toward the symptoms (for example, ASPIRIN for the headache) and relieving the stress. It may be difficult for achievers to withdraw from a situation when they think this is giving up. An authority should encourage or order them to withdraw, thus removing moral responsibility. See Protocol B.10.B for other similar conditions.

STROKE

Regional Notes: F, O, R, S.

Synonyms: apoplexy, cerebrovascular accident (cva)

Definition: stroke is brain damage caused by interruption of the circulation to the brain.

Cause: variable.

Very ill: class 3; worldwide.

Age: any; mostly adults but sometimes children, particularly those with SICKLE CELL DISEASE or SYPHILIS. **Who:** varies with the cause. In tropical areas, this is usually due to some infectious disease; in Africans, frequently HYPERTENSION, prior HEART FAILURE (valvular) or RHEUMATIC FEVER. It may be due to head injury. **Onset:** variable but usually sudden.

Clinical

Necessary: the patient has one or more of the following: slurred speech, drooping of half of his face, weakness or paralysis on one side of his body, lethargy, loss of consciousness or SEIZURE.

TOC · SYMPTOMS · DIFFERENTIALS · CONDITIONS · DRUG INDEX · REGIONAL NOTES · INX

Usually: the weakness or paralysis is initially floppy and becomes stiff within a couple days or weeks. Because of the weakness, the patient may appear uncoordinated.

Sometimes: the patient understands speech and knows what he wants to say, but cannot say it. Confusion and trouble swallowing are common.

Occasionally: there may be dizziness, numbness and tingling, fainting, irregular or slow respiration or incontinence of urine. If there is a severe headache at onset, the patient may have a stiff neck like MENINGITIS.

Causative diseases: *without fevers:* SYPHILIS is a major consideration. This is likely if a relatively young person has a general, whole body illness with headache and mental changes before the onset of the stroke symptoms.

Also consider TOXEMIA (if pregnant), head injury, HYPERTENSION, CYSTICERCOSIS, SICKLE CELL DISEASE, SYPHILIS, HYDATID DISEASE, SCHISTOSOMIASIS JAPONICUM, ALTITUDE SICKNESS, CHAGA'S DISEASE. *With fevers:* RELAPSING FEVER, DIPHTHERIA, TYPHUS, RHEUMATIC FEVER, LARVA MIGRANS, AMEBIASIS, ENCEPHALITIS or MENINGITIS.

Similar conditions: POLIO (onset slower, usually lower limbs only), RABIES and BERIBERI. See Protocol B.10.B.

Treatment

Referrals: see Volume 1, Appendix 13. A level 4 or 5 hospital with a neurologist and rehabilitation facilities is most appropriate. If the patient is having trouble swallowing a level 2 or 3 hospital might help.

Patient care: treat whatever disease (if any) caused this. See Volume 1 Appendix 8 for instructions in caring for a very sick patient.

Results: recovery is unpredictable; it ranges from none to complete.

STRONGYLOIDIASIS

Regional Notes: E, F, I, M, O, R, S, U.

Synonyms: pinworm (British), threadworm (American). swollen baby syndrome (Pacific area).

Definition: strongyloidiasis is a bowel or whole body infection with the worm *Strongyloides stercoralis.*

Not ill to very ill; class 1 (usual) or 4 (with SEPSIS); widespread in tropical climates, especially those with sandy soil. It is especially common in the Pacific area, Southeast Asia and the Western Hemisphere.

Age: any. **Who:** anyone with skin touching infected soil, anyone eating soil-contaminated foods. Once a person has it, he will reinfect himself. Whole body disease is most common in those of African or Caribbean genetic heritage. **Onset:** variable.

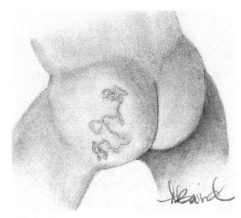

This picture of strongyloides shows a very large area. In real life, this may be more subtle. Any itchy, red or warm, swollen line on the buttocks or by the anus is likely to be strongyloides or LARVA MIGRANS. AB

Clinical

BOWEL INFECTION

Necessary: either there are no symptoms at all or the patient has abdominal pain plus ANEMIA or an itchy rectal-genital area.

Maybe: there may be an itchy red rash (raised spots or lines) where the worm larvae penetrated the skin. The lines may be on the buttocks or lower back, radiating up from the anus; otherwise they are on parts of the body that contacted soil. These lines last for a few hours to a few days and then disappear; they are less definite than for LARVA MIGRANS. They recur multiple times. The larvae migrate through the lungs causing a fever and a cough similar to ASCARIASIS, but it is usually not as severe.

Maybe: after the worm enters the bowel the patient may develop diarrhea, possibly with MALABSORPTION and weight loss. If you look carefully, you may see the worms in the stool. They are the size and shape of a comma in small print. This disease may cause constipation, cravings, DYSENTERY, MALABSORPTION, MALNUTRITION and ANEMIA.

WHOLE BODY INFECTION

Necessary: there are always some abdominal complaints: nausea, vomiting, diarrhea, pain or bleeding. There are also respiratory complaints: cough or shortness of breath.

Complications: this may cause SEPSIS in the presence of PREDNISONE and related drugs or in the presence of the following conditions which decrease natural immunity: HIV INFECTION, LEPROSY, pregnancy, chronic MALARIA and TUBERCULOSIS.

Similar conditions: *abdominal pain plus ANEMIA:* HOOKWORM, TRICHURIASIS, DYSENTERY and SICKLE CELL DISEASE. *Itchy anus and/or buttock:* LARVA MIGRANS, TAPEWORM, ENTEROBIASIS, ALLERGY, CANDIDIASIS and SCABIES. *Severe diarrhea:* see Protocol B.14.

Bush laboratory: strongyloides hatching test, Volume 1, Appendix 2.

Treatment

Referrals: speedy referral is necessary if the patient is very ill. See Volume 1, Appendix 13. Laboratory: hospitals can do stool tests, but the best tests done by good technicians still detect only 1/4 to 1/2 of all cases. The hatching test is better. Whole body disease does not cause increased eosinophils. Facilities: if there is SEPSIS, IV fluids and injectable antibiotics at a level 3 or above facility are essential. Practitioner: someone experienced in tropical/travel diseases.

Patient care: THIABENDAZOLE, IVERMECTIN and ALBENDAZOLE were the only drugs that worked before; now TRIBENDIMADINE seems to work well. IVERMECTIN by injection is the drug you should use if the patient has a whole body infection. MEBENDAZOLE and PYRANTEL PAMOATE have a much lower cure rate. LEVAMISOLE kills only the larval stage of the worm. The patient will reinfect himself if there are any worms left at all. If the first treatment fails, give a second treatment for double the time. CAMBENDAZOLE is a veterinary drug which reportedly works well with no side effects. NITAZOXANIDE may work.

SWIMMER'S ITCH

Synonyms: cercarial dermatitis.

Definition: swimmer's itch is an allergic reaction to penetration of the skin by larval schistosomes.

Cause: larval form of human or animal schistosomes; see SCHISTOSOMIASIS.

Age: any; **Who:** those swimming or bathing in fresh water inhabited by human or animal schistosomes. **Onset:** suddenly, within minutes of exposure.

Clinical

Sudden onset of severe itching, redness and swelling of the skin. The problem will last 2–3 days without treatment and resolve itself. The symptoms are much worse with animal (usually water bird) schistosomes than with human schistosomes. In areas with human SCHISTOSOMIASIS, see KATAYAMA DISEASE to know what to look for 3–6 weeks hence.

Treatment

Prevention: immediate rubbing alcohol on the skin, as soon as the problem is first noticed. Take along a bottle of alcohol whenever swimming in a lake where there are water birds.

Patient care: use DIPHENHYDRAMINE or steroid creams. Using PRAZIQUANTEL at this stage is not helpful. ARTEMISININ should be used in areas with human SCHISTOSOMIASIS. This may prevent the development of human SCHISTOSOMIASIS. With water bird schistosomes, the parasites cannot develop anyway.

SYPHILIS (venereal)[1]

I   Introduction

II Clinical

    Primary

    Secondary

    Tertiary

    Pregnancy

    Congenital

    With HIV

III Similar diseases

IV Treatment

I Introduction

Regional Notes: E, F, I, K, M, O, R, S, U.

Synonyms: lues, treponematosis pallidum infection.

Definition: syphilis is an infection with the spirochete *treponema pallidum.*

Includes: venereal syphilis only in this entry.

Not ill to very ill; class 1–3; stage 2 is contagious; transmission 50%. In developing countries, about 40% of prostitutes have it. With no medical care, the rate is about 10% –15% among middle class, 20% among impoverished. Where there is medical care the rate is 4–5% among blood donors.

Note: venereal syphilis is almost always sexually transmitted; endemic syphilis is transmitted non-sexually. There are three kinds of endemic syphilis: PINTA (Americas only; see M Index), TREPONARID (arid areas only; see this Index and Regional Notes) and YAWS (humid areas only; see this Index and Regional Notes). Venereal syphilis, PINTA, TREPONARID and YAWS are all closely related diseases; each gives partial immunity to the others. SYPHILIS (i.e., venereal syphilis) is described here; see the separate entries for the three kinds of endemic syphilis.

Age: adults; sexually abused children; babies of infected mothers. **Who:** those who have had a sexual relationship outside of faithful marriage; partners of an unfaithful spouse; children born to infected mothers, health workers who handle infected children or adults in the secondary stage of the disease.

Onset in adults, no HIV: incubation: 9–90 days from infecting contact until the primary ulcer. Incubation: 2 weeks to 6 months until symptoms of secondary syphilis. Usually there are no symptoms at all for the next two years; incubation: 1–20 years until symptomatic tertiary syphilis.

Onset in adults with HIV: the symptoms of primary and secondary syphilis may occur at the same time and progression of the disease to tertiary is much faster. The latent period may be abolished; the patient may have symptoms of secondary and tertiary at the same time.

Onset in congenital infection: it may manifest for the first time from birth up to 30 years.

---

1 See the PowerPoint lecture lecture entitled Syphilis at www.villagemedicalmanual.org.

II Clinical kinds of syphilis

PRIMARY SYPHILIS

This starts with a (usually) single, round or oval ulcer on the contact area, 0.3–3 cm in diameter; it is relatively painless (but possibly tender), and it is swollen on the rim and underneath. With some sexual practices the mouth, buttocks, anus or fingers might have the primary chancre which is usually painful but not swollen underneath.

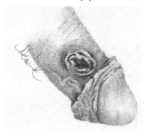

A genital syphilis chancre is usually roughly round or oval. There is swelling around the rim. AB

Usually there is only one ulcer unless the patient also has HIV INFECTION. Usually there is no visible pus; the ulcer looks clean, and it does not bleed readily. It persists for at least 2 weeks before starting to heal. Painless enlargement of the groin (or the neck) lymph nodes starts a week later, usually on both sides for genital ulcers, possibly one side elsewhere. The enlarged nodes are firm, and they are not stuck to the flesh around them. The skin over top has a normal appearance. They persist for weeks or months after the primary ulcer heals.

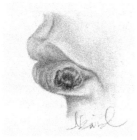

Chancres on other sites vary as regards pain and appearance. They last 3–7 weeks. There are always large lymph nodes. AB

SECONDARY SYPHILIS

The healing primary ulcer or its scar may still be present. This develops about 6 weeks after primary syphilis, but it may develop at the same time in patients who are HIV-infected. Secondary syphilis may occur without the ulcer of primary syphilis or primary syphilis without the symptoms of secondary. In the latter case, primary syphilis advances directly to tertiary. The secondary stage happens, but the patient is not aware of it.

These are the most common scenarios for secondary.

- On fair or light brown skin, a symmetrical, red or brown spotted rash (which may be subtle) develops mainly on the trunk and face; it may also include the limbs, palms and soles.[1] Most often the spots can be seen but not felt; they may be hard to see. There may be few or many. They are not itchy in fair Europeans, but they may itch and appear dark-colored or white in those with dark skin. The rash, if it occurs, arises over a week or two, not hours or days. The patient is not ill to mildly ill. These are some appearances:

- A measles-type rash, few or no spots on the face.

- Circles, irregular shapes or targets, sometimes with rims, usually in groups rather than single; common in those with dark skin.

- Like acne, but more bumps than scars. With acne there are more scars than bumps.

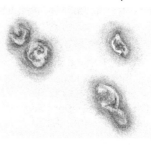

These are irregular shapes with rims. The size and appearance may vary. AB

- The patient may have fever, headache, enlarged and tender lymph nodes, weight loss, loss of appetite and fatigue. Usually headache is prominent. The enlarged nodes are those near the primary ulcer plus the nodes by the elbow(s) and the back of the neck.

- The patient may have slightly raised, round, relatively painless patches on moist pink surfaces of the mouth and genitals, silver-gray in color, with red halos. These may ulcerate. Usually they are toward the front of the mouth and on one side only.[2] He may have splits in the skin by the side of his mouth or long grooves or an ulcer on his tongue. He may have bleeding gums so the condition resembles SCURVY.

- He may have flat-topped, pale moist "warts" near the site of the primary ulcer,[3] sometimes elsewhere, usually on warm moist body parts. Genital warts are common. The warts are flat, without stems. These are common in females and those of African genetic heritage.

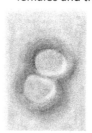

There are usually a countable number (in the absence of HIV INFECTION) and they are widely spaced, with normal skin present between the warts. See Volume 1, Chapter 6 for an illustration of their distribution on female genitals. AB

In some patients patches of hair on his head or elsewhere may fall out symmetrically. The scalp has a moth-eaten appearance. The affected areas have fine hairs in them; the patient is not totally bald in these areas. There is no visible scarring. There is no predilection for one part of the scalp or another.

- There may be joint pains and even ARTHRITIS. The pain is not worse with movement and may thus be relieved. Often several joints are affected the same time. Stiffness, if any, is minimal.

---

1 *Some Africans have sole spots without palm spots. This is normal. Sole spots due to syphilis are always accompanied by palm spots at the same time.*

2 *Thus they can be distinguished from similar patches due to DIPH-THERIA, which usually occur on both sides and tend to be toward the back of the mouth.*

3 *Not all genital warts are due to syphilis. Some are viral. Warts due to syphilis are usually moist and they have a broad rather than narrow base.*

TOC   SYMPTOMS   DIFFERENTIALS   CONDITIONS   DRUG INDEX   REGIONAL NOTES   INX

- Secondary syphilis may cause spontaneous ABORTION. Rarely there is HEPATITIS, IRITIS, STROKE or MENINGITIS. Secondary syphilis is prone to relapse; the same symptoms may occur a second and third time.

TERTIARY SYPHILIS

This may be totally without symptoms. When there are symptoms, they occur 5–30 years later in about 2/3 of those who have had primary or secondary syphilis. **In tertiary syphilis, 2/3 of the patients have no history of primary or secondary disease.** Tertiary syphilis is common in children with untreated congenital syphilis. This may affect many different parts of the body, as follows, listed from most common to least common. It is not unusual for tertiary syphilis of the heart and the nervous system to occur together. Bone and skin tertiary syphilis tend to occur together.

Skin

A patient may have lumps under his skin. The lumps may break open to become ulcers resembling TROPICAL ULCERS, which heal very slowly if at all.

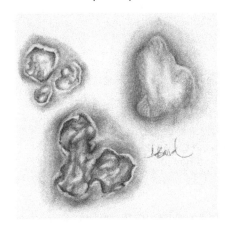

Tertiary syphilis ulcers start out with swelling below. First a group of ulcers form (upper left). Then the ulcers coalesce to make a large, scalloped ulcer (lower left) Finally (upper right) the ulcer heals, leaving wrinkled, thin scar with scalloped raised edges. The whole process is totally painless. AB

Bones and joints

Slow-growing lumps may form in the bones. The amount of pain and tenderness varies between patients, but swelling is more prominent than pain or tenderness. The pain is worse at night. Movement does not aggravate the pain and there is no symmetry. The most common sites are head and face, front of the chest and shin.[4]

Large joints may be swollen symmetrically (usually knees, maybe ankles, elbows, shoulder, wrist and small joints) and move abnormally. Swelling is more prominent than pain. There may be skin changes with this. There may be lightning pains from trunk to limb.

Heart

There may be an irregular pulse and ANGINA (chest pain), or HEART FAILURE. His pulse pressure may be high. He may be dizzy because of this. He cannot tolerate exercise. This is most common in developing countries and in those with African genetic heritage.

Head, brain, mental

There is an off-and-on or slow onset of symptoms with episodes of improvement even without treatment, usually beginning age 35–50 in acquired syphilis beginning in young adults in the case of congenital syphilis. Irritability, poor judgment, trembling, seizures, one-sided headaches and abnormal pupils are evident first. A relatively young patient might have a STROKE. Usually the stroke is preceded by headaches, mental changes and fatigue (in contrast to ordinary strokes). There may be day-night reversal. Then the patient becomes either stupid or maniacal, maybe with delusions of grandeur. He has slurred speech, fainting spells and weakness or paralysis. Usually the patient is not aware of his poor functioning. Finally he becomes bedridden and dies with BRAIN DAMAGE. This, as well as spinal cord syphilis (see below), are most likely to occur with European genetic heritage.

Spinal cord (rare)

At first there are lightning pains. Then there is loss of pain and temperature sensation. Eye symptoms (see below), loss of bladder control, deafness and speech problems may follow. After that the patient becomes uncoordinated; he cannot tell where his limbs are in space. He has to look at his hands or feet in order to move them in a coordinated manner. Finally, the patient becomes paralyzed and bed-ridden. He dies from some other infection.

Eyes

He may not be able to fully open his eyes. He may have trouble with eye movements so he sees double or has crossed eyes. He may have unequal pupils, KERATITIS or IRITIS, see flashes of light and have distorted vision. This is particularly common in the presence of HIV INFECTION. A common problem is that the pupils do not respond to light, but they do change size with looking near or far.

Mouth and nose

A painless bump may form on the tongue in the midline. This may break down to become an ulcer. There may be longitudinal cracks in the tongue or holes in the roof of the mouth. It may destroy the cartilage so the bridge of the nose is sunken.

Pelvic area

Painless lumps may form in the testicles. The bladder might not empty all the way, so the patient retains urine. This is likely to become infected, leading to KIDNEY DISEASE. He is likely to have impotence and a leaky bladder.

Abdomen

There are recurrent, severe abdominal pains, episodes of vomiting or both. They come on suddenly, last days and then vanish, leaving the patient exhausted.

SYPHILIS DURING PREGNANCY

Syphilis acquired in pregnancy causes miscarriage, stillbirth or illness in the newborn. Syphilis acquired late in pregnancy may cause symptoms of primary or secondary syphilis at or shortly after birth. Sometimes a baby is born healthy but becomes ill during childhood or young adulthood. If there is latent syphilis (without symptoms, between secondary and tertiary syphilis), the woman has a 70% chance of having an infected baby.

---

4 With saber shins, the middle 1/3 of the shin is thicker in the front-back direction than the upper and lower thirds. Hence the shin bows forward so its shape resembles a saber. See the website www.villagemedicalmanual.org.

TOC SYMPTOMS DIFFERENTIALS CONDITIONS DRUG INDEX REGIONAL NOTES INX

CONGENITAL SYPHILIS

Most symptoms occur after 4 months of age and many after years. The early and late-onset symptoms are listed separately here, but in real life there is no definite dichotomy.

SYMPTOMS AT BIRTH LOOK LIKE NEONATAL SEPSIS

Prognosis is poor. There may be low birth weight, an enlarged liver and spleen, a blistery rash, JAUNDICE, ANEMIA, and/or general whole body swelling. The placenta may be abnormally large. His bowel may be obstructed. He may have a rash like secondary syphilis.

CONGENITAL: BIRTH TO 2 YEARS LOOKS LIKE SECONDARY SYPHILIS

General

The baby may fail to nurse well or gain weight. vigorously.

Developmental milestones may be delayed.

He may appear like a tiny wrinkled old man.

He may have anemia and abnormal bleeding.

He may have KIDNEY DISEASE with whole body swelling.

He may have enlarged lymph nodes.

Skin structures

He develops shiny red, possibly peeling skin on his palms and soles, splits in his skin or skin bumps that look like warts. The skin changes may involve parts or the whole body. They may be red spots, blisters or both. There may be cracks around the mouth, nose or anus. He may have no eyebrows or brittle hair.

Head

The soft spot on the head will stay open for a long time. The soft spot may bulge out, as the head becomes progressively larger, causing hydrocephalus.

Face

Sore red eyes with decreased vision.

He may have a continually runny nose, possibly with blood, as if he has a cold. The lips tend to split.

There may be white patches in his mouth or throat, hoarseness, abnormal growths or holes on the pink moist surfaces.

There is delayed eruption of the baby teeth (similar to HIV INFECTION and RICKETS).

He may snore or have noisy breathing.

Abdomen

His liver and spleen may be large.

He may vomit.

He may have a distended abdomen with fluid in it.

Limbs

He may have swollen fingers, like sausages, sparing the end portions. Other causes of sausage fingers involve entire fingers.

His limbs may become tender, swollen or both. They may be fragile, fracturing with slight movement.

Summary of diagnosis of syphilis in an infant in the absence of laboratory support. The patient should have either two major criteria or one major and one minor.

Major criteria

- an enlarged liver, with or without an enlarged spleen.

- limb problems which are usually symmetrical: swelling, refusal to move or tenderness.

Minor criterion

a generalized rash on the skin or abnormal white patches within the mouth. If the rash involves the palms and soles, then this becomes a major criterion.

CONGENITAL: 2–30 YEARS OLD LOOKS LIKE TERTIARY SYPHILIS

Face

Sunken bridge of the nose with small cheek bones, a wide forehead and a protruding lower jaw.

Mouth

There may be a delay in eruption of the first teeth. Upper front permanent teeth have single notched cutting edges, curved sides, and are smaller than normal. They are susceptible to decay.

Eyes

Clouding of the cornea with redness around, pain, tearing jerky eye movements.

Ears

Deafness: sudden or gradual onset, usually ages 5–25, commonly with ringing in the ears, dizziness or both beforehand. The patient may have trouble maintaining balance.

Skeleton

Shins are thickened in the middle third; the front is sharp and bowed forward.

Collar bones are thickened in their entirety or else only the joint near the breast bone. This may be one or both sides.

Symmetrically swollen large joints, particularly the knees.

Nervous system

Numbness and tingling with loss of feeling on limbs

Incoordination, mainly or only with eyes closed. This may cause the patient to stamp hard with each step as he walks.

Any symptom of tertiary syphilis, such as paralysis, heart disease or insanity may occur, up to age 30 from congenital infection.

TOC   SYMPTOMS   DIFFERENTIALS   CONDITIONS   DRUG INDEX   REGIONAL NOTES   INX

Syphilis and HIV

There may be multiple primary ulcers.

The rash of secondary syphilis may be asymmetrical and look different than usual.

There may be tender, spontaneous swellings in the bones.

There is usually no latent period; syphilis jumps directly from primary or secondary to tertiary.

Relapses are common, and genital warts are common with relapses.

Syphilis commonly affects the nervous system and eyes. It can cause stroke, blindness, insanity and other nervous system problems. Of those who develop insanity because of syphilis, about 25% are children.

III. Similar conditions

Very many, too many to list all.

Primary syphilis: this is similar to other SEXUALLY TRANSMITTED DISEASEs. Usually the ulcer is single, swollen and painless. The lymph nodes of syphilis are not stuck together, and ulcers do not break down and bleed or drain.

Secondary syphilis: see Protocol B.2. Syphilis can be confused with INFLUENZA, MEASLES or any other illness with a fever, but the rash of syphilis develops slowly, over weeks. FIFTH DISEASE rash may involve the palms and soles (as the fever drops), but it is most prominent on the cheek, which syphilis is not.

Syphilitic warts do not resemble ordinary WARTS since they have moist, flat, light-colored surfaces. Ordinary genital warts turn white after being soaked for 3–5 minutes in vinegar; syphilis warts do not.

They differ from the wart-like skin bumps of DONOVANOSIS in that they are skin color or pale, whereas those caused by DONOVANOSIS are red. The warts of syphilis clear within a week with PENICILLIN but those of DONOVANOSIS require more than two weeks with any antibiotic.

Tertiary syphilis affecting the heart may be similar to HEART FAILURE due to bad valves. BERIBERI causes leg weakness also, but the trouble walking is no worse in the dark, and the pains of BERIBERI are more burning. The lightning pains are similar to SHINGLES. The bone problems can be similar to the other diseases listed in Protocol B.6. Some MALNUTRITION can be nearly identical, but it is reversed (slowly) with MULTIVITAMINS, or VITAMIN B_{12} injections. Tertiary syphilis is one of many causes of BRAIN DAMAGE. See Protocol B.10.

Congenital syphilis: RICKETS, SCURVY, HIV INFECTION, THALLASEMIA.

IV Treatment

Prevention: find and treat sexual contacts. Wash your hands well. Wear gloves while doing physical exams on high-risk patients or touching anyone with a rash.

Referrals: speedy referral for syphilis in a newborn and tertiary syphilis is very desirable.

Laboratory: fairly simple blood tests are available. These tests (RPR and VDRL) are not sensitive in primary and tertiary syphilis, but they are sensitive in secondary syphilis. The primary ulcer must be present for at least a week before the test turns positive. There are occasional false-positives in old age or in the presence of some other diseases, most notably LEPROSY and some kinds of ARTHRITIS.

More reliable tests are more expensive and less available. The blood tests for syphilis should become negative a year after treatment for primary syphilis, two years after treatment for secondary syphilis, and five years after treatment for tertiary syphilis. They may remain positive in the presence of HIV. If the patient has syphilis involving his brain or spinal cord, then the same test (RPR or VDRL) must be done on spinal fluid taken out of the backbone with a needle. Sterility is of utmost importance when the fluid is taken.

Since ordinary syphilis and the various forms of endemic syphilis (PINTA, YAWS, TREPONARID) are all closely related, all laboratory tests will be positive regardless of which form (venereal or endemic) of the disease the patient has. This should be kept in mind when expatriate parents are confronted with a question of childhood sexual abuse in their home countries. **A positive blood test for syphilis can readily be acquired non-sexually in developing areas. Venereal syphilis can also readily be acquired non-sexually in cultures where congenital syphilis is both common and commomly unrecognized. It needs treatment.**

Practitioner: an abstinence-based sexually transmitted disease clinic is ideal for primary and secondary. A pediatrician should treat a newborn. An infectious disease specialist should manage tertiary syphilis.

Patient care: for primary syphilis, unless you are very sure of the diagnosis, treat according to Protocol B.1 rather than for syphilis alone. PENICILLIN is still the drug of choice for this. Some authorities recommend AZITHROMYCIN for primary and secondary.

> ***Caution:*** with the first dose of PENICILLIN the patient may become sicker with a fever, a drop in blood pressure and shortness of breath. Do not stop the medication for that.
>
> An hour before the first dose, give one dose of DIPHENHYDRAMINE. Then give PENICILLIN. Syphilis requires continual treatment without missing doses. Many of the effects of tertiary syphilis will not change in spite of treatment, but treatment may prevent their worsening. DOXYCYCLINE, ERYTHROMYCIN, CEPHALOSPORIN or CHLORAMPHENICOL may also be effective. Because of the problems with keeping people on medicine, WHO recommends benzathine PENICILLIN; one injection replaces 10 days of drug by mouth. Infants born with the disease should have weekly benzathine penicillin injections for 4 weeks. However, benzathine penicillin does not adequately treat syphilis that has affected the brain.

TAPEWORM

Regional Notes: E, F, I, K, M, N, O, R, U.

Includes: diphyllobothriasis (fish), hymenolepiasis (rat), taeniasis (beef and pork).

Definition: tapeworm is a bowel infestation with one of the worms listed above.

Not ill to mildly ill; class 2; some contagious; worldwide, related to diet. Beef and/or pork tapeworm is found almost worldwide. Fish tapeworm is found in temperate and Arctic climates, in fish from fresh or slightly brackish water, 4°–25°C (39°–77°F), having vegetation and not fast flowing. There must be some (but not gross) contamination by raw sewage. Currently it is found almost exclusively across northern Russia and in parts of South America. It used to be prevalent in Scandinavia and eastern Europe. Rat tapeworm is common in Sicily, Argentina, Southeast Asia and the southern areas of the former Soviet Union.

Age: anyone. **Who:** anyone eating insufficiently cooked pork, beef or fish. Rat tapeworm is from direct contact with human or rat stool or from eating grain with insects in it. **Onset:** 2–3 months after eating the offending food.

Clinical

Necessary: either no symptoms, worm segments seen in the stool, rectal itching or increased appetite plus weight loss. Children fail to grow properly. Rat tapeworms cause itching of the anus.

Sometimes: there is abdominal pain. Segments of pork or beef tapeworm are flat and quadrangular, measuring about 0.2–0.5 x 0.5–1 cm.; thus they can be seen and identified with a magnifying glass.

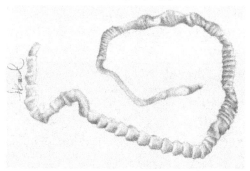

This is a full tapeworm, about a third normal size. Usually people pass just small segments, not whole worms. A segment of a tape worm looks like a piece of confetti. Sometimes people feel these segments moving around their anuses. AB

Complications: CYSTICERCOSIS is caused by pork tapeworm eggs in the stool getting back into the mouth. It is essential, therefore, to be very careful in handling contaminated stool. Give medication to cause diarrhea after a worm treatment; be sure this stool is properly disposed of and the patient well washed afterward. Fish tapeworm can cause severe ANEMIA, nutritional type, but reportedly only in the Arctic.

Similar conditions: abdominal pain: IRRITABLE BOWEL may be similar. *Itchy anus:* STRONGYLOIDIASIS, LARVA MIGRANS, ENTEROBIASIS, SCABIES or food allergies. *Weight loss with increased appetite:* DIABETES may cause weight loss with increased appetite, but also thirst and increased urination which are not found with tapeworm. Also consider THYROID TROUBLE, high-thyroid.

Treatment

Referrals: laboratory; a hospital lab can check stool for tapeworm eggs or pieces of the worms. This test is specific but not sensitive. Practitioner: tropical/travel medicine is helpful.

Patient care: treat ASCARIASIS first if the patient was exposed. For tapeworm: PAROMOMYCIN, PRAZIQUANTEL or NICLOSAMIDE. PRAZIQUANTEL is best if you have it, but it requires special precautions with pork tapeworm. MEBENDAZOLE is useful for pork tapeworm only. NICLOSAMIDE is unsafe with pork tapeworm. ALBENDAZOLE reportedly works fine for both beef and pork tapeworm. TRIBENDIMIDINE or NITAZOXANIDE may work.

TB

See TUBERCULOSIS.

TENDINITIS

Definition: tendinitis is inflammation of tendons which are the bands connecting muscles to bones. Tendons are adjacent to joints.

Age: mainly adults. **Who:** those who engage in unaccustomed exercise. It may occur as a side effect of CIPROFLOXACIN and other -oxacin drugs. **Onset:** over hours to days.

Clinical

There is pain and tenderness adjacent to a joint, with painful motion of that joint. Volume 1, Chapter 9 H, describes and illustrates the common sites of tendinitis.

Treatment

Rest the joint and use IBUPROFEN or similar medications. If this does not work there may be a torn tendon which needs surgical repair.

TETANUS

Regional Notes: E, F, I, R, S.

Synonyms: lockjaw.

Definition: tetanus is a spastic muscle disease caused by the toxin produced by the bacterium *Clostridium tetani*.

Very ill; class 3; worldwide, related to immunization.

Age: any. **Who:** injured but (usually) not immunized. The injury may be so minor that the patient does not remember it. In newborns, the mother was not immunized, and the cord was cut with a dirty knife. The disease is particularly common in areas where there are livestock and where hygiene is poor. **Onset:** 4–20 days after injury. The disease may start rapidly, over 1–2 days or slowly, over a week. In newborns it occurs within 10 days of birth.

Clinical

Initially the patient is irritable and restless, feverish, aching in all his muscles and complaining of a headache. Newborns first stop sucking. Then they develop spasms similar to adults.

Later: he has muscle spasms and cannot open his mouth. He has excessive secretions such as saliva. He has a stiff back, neck, limbs and abdomen with spells of muscle spasms all over which are painful and exhausting. He remains conscious. Spasms are triggered by any disturbance. Spasm of the face muscles produces a peculiar grimacing expression.

Spasm of the respiratory muscles may slow respiration and eventually prevent breathing, causing death. The patient may have drenching sweats. His blood pressure is apt to rise and fall unpredictably.

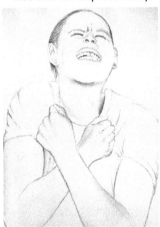

This is the typical appearance of a patient with tetanus. The arms may be extended rather than flexed as is shown here. OW

Similar conditions: see Protocol B.13.

Initial fever and headache may resemble INFLUENZA or diseases similar to that If the muscle spasms start in the neck, it may resemble early MENINGITIS.

Muscle spasms: PLANT POISONING due to strychnine (symptoms begin within 30 minutes of eating), RABIES, POLIO. MENINGITIS can look similar, but then the abdomen is not rigid, whereas it is rigid with tetanus. Similar to NEUROLEPTIC MALIGNANT SYNDROME (rapid onset). Do not confuse the side effects of CHLORPROMAZINE and similar drugs (causing spasm of facial muscles) with this disease. If this may be the cause, try to treat the jaw spasms with DIPHENHYDRAMINE. If the treatment works the problem is not tetanus.

Bush laboratory: with the long handle of a spoon, touch the back of the patient's throat. Normally the patient will gag and try to eject the blade. If he has tetanus he will bite down instead.

Treatment

Prevention: immunize everyone you can, especially pregnant women. Give wrapped, clean or sterile razor blades to each midwife to use for cutting umbilical cords. Replace each used blade with a clean one when it is returned. For immunization, children should get DPT and adults (including pregnant) dT or Tdap. Give an initial injection, a booster 6 weeks later, and another at one year. Immunizations last for 5–10 years. Clean wounds well and bandage them.

Referrals: advanced lab is useless for diagnosis; it might be helpful for management. IV fluids and advanced drugs are helpful. A level 4 or 5 hospital will be helpful. Practitioners: anesthesiologists, emergency doctors or pediatricians.

Patient care: send to a hospital. Until then—

- Keep the patient in bed in dark and quiet, positioned on his side. Turn him every 2 hours during the day and every 4 hours during the night.
- Put a stomach tube in place.
- For babies, empty the mother's breasts every 4 hours and put the milk down the tube. (See the instructions below for others.)
- Keep a bulb syringe handy and suck out saliva when the patient cannot swallow. There will be excessive secretions; the patient may develop DEHYDRATION and KIDNEY DISEASE.
- Medication is given as adult doses; reduce dose according to weight for children. First give MAGNESIUM SULFATE. This will minimize the need for other sedatives and will make it easier to keep the patient stable.
- Then give DIAZEPAM 20 mg by stomach tube; 2 hours later, give CHLORPROMAZINE 50 mg. Continue alternating DIAZEPAM and CHLORPROMAZINE, giving one or the other every 2 hours. With the DIAZEPAM, give 150 ml of water. With the CHLORPROMAZINE give 250 ml of refeeding mixture followed by water to rinse the tube.

- Additionally, give PARALDEHYDE by rectum, as often as spasms occur. PROMETHAZINE may substitute for CHLORPROMAZINE; PHENOBARBITAL may substitute for DIAZEPAM. Check doses and precautions in the Drug Index.

- Initially, also give TETANUS IMMUNE GLOBULIN: 3,000 units adult dose. Give it in 3 injections in 3 sites, a one-time dose only, IM, never IV. Try to obtain this, but it may not be available.

- There is increased need for fluids; patients tend to become dehydrated. MILK OF MAGNESIA by stomach tube may be helpful for constipation.

- If there is a wound, however minor, open it, clean it out and give METRONIDAZOLE, TINIDAZOLE (preferably) or PENICILLIN for infection, even if the wound looks good.

- Check daily for PNEUMONIA; use PENICILLIN if this develops.

- When the patient has had no spasms for the past 2 days, then every other day lower the dose of DIAZEPAM by 5 mg at a time and lower the dose of CHLORPROMAZINE by 10 mg at a time. If spasms recur, return to the previous doses.

- Start the patient on a liquid diet through a straw when he is able to swallow.

Results: 1–3 weeks; 75% death rate at least. Recovery may take months but it will be complete. If the wound was a quinine injection, if the incubation was 4 days or less, or if the time from first symptom to spasms was less than 48 hours, the prognosis is poor.

THALLASEMIA

Regional Notes: F, I, M, O, S, U.

Includes: alpha thallasemia, beta thallasemia and a variety of other abnormal hemoglobins.

Definition: thallasemia is an inherited abnormality of the hemoglobin (red pigment) in the blood. Thallasemia is labeled alpha or beta; alpha thallasemia is not very severe; this entry focuses on beta thallasemia.

Not ill to severely ill; class 3; worldwide, it affects some of Mediterranean, Asian and African genetic heritages. Consider migrations in previous centuries; Hispanics in the Western Hemisphere, Irish (because of migration from Spain) and Jews worldwide are at risk.

Age: symptoms start at age 6–12 months in severe cases; occasionally they are delayed until 5 years. In minor cases first symptoms might be a crisis in later childhood or in adulthood. **Who:** certain families and ethnic groups. **Onset:** gradual.

Clinical

Necessary: ANEMIA and family history of a similar problem. There are three kinds of beta thallasemia corresponding to three levels of severity.

BETA THALLASEMIA MINOR

is without symptoms and can be ignored.

Beta thallasemia intermedia

causes occasional problems requiring transfusion, but the patient is healthy most of the time. The patients usually have no symptoms at all until adult life when eating some food or taking some medicine causes sudden ANEMIA due to destruction of red cells. The patient develops JAUNDICE. With this episode, KIDNEY DISEASE, HEART FAILURE, SHOCK and death may occur.

BETA THALLASEMIA MAJOR

causes severe anemia and requires frequent blood transfusion. With transfusion, there is a danger of getting too much iron in the body which can cause other problems. Western-type medical facilities can both transfuse and deal with the excess iron.

The patient may be born healthy, but during the first year he may develop feeding problems, fevers, diarrhea and failure to grow properly. He has a prominent forehead similar to RICKETS, wide set eyes and a low bridge of the nose. He might look similar to a child with DOWN SYNDROME, but he is not retarded. He has a large liver and spleen. If the spleen enlarges rapidly during a crisis, there will be left upper abdominal pain. The patient may have ANEMIA of the nutritional type, frequent infections, dental problems and brittle bones, with bone and joint pains.

Complications: there may be a tendency to bleed easily: nosebleeds, bloody urine, bloody stool, bloody vomit, heavy menstruation and excessive bleeding from minor wounds. Patients may develop TROPICAL ULCERS. Most will die between 6 and 12 years old from HEART FAILURE or infection. Those who reach their teens may have delayed sexual maturity, MALABSORPTION or DIABETES. Thallasemia may cause GALLBLADDER DISEASE or KIDNEY DISEASE.

Similar conditions: *ANEMIA and large spleen:* see Protocols B.3 and B.7. *Failure to thrive* in an infant: see the chart under MALNUTRITION in this index; also consider RICKETS, CRETINISM and DOWN SYNDROME if the facial appearance is peculiar. *Yellow whites of the eyes* in a crisis in an adult: see JAUNDICE.

Treatment

Referrals: laboratory; a well-equipped, level 3 or above hospital laboratory can do a blood test (hemoglobin electrophoresis) for this. The diagnosis can be surmised from an ordinary blood smear if a competent pathologist or technician reviews it. Facilities; a hospital can prolong life with blood transfusions and expensive medicines. Practitioner: if the patient has a very large spleen, it might be appropriate for a surgeon to remove it. Otherwise a hematologist is most appropriate.

Patient care: in the village, use FOLATE, VITAMIN C and ZINC regularly. Make sure the patient eats animal products or else give VITAMIN B$_{12}$. Treat infections and HEART FAILURE. If they have not been transfused, pregnant women from affected families should take FOLATE and IRON throughout pregnancy. Do not treat ANEMIA with IRON in patients that have had transfusions recently; reproductive females who have not had transfusions and who eat a low-iron diet may receive IRON for a month.

THYROID TROUBLE

Entry category: disease cluster.

Includes: hypothyroidism, thyrotoxicosis.

Definition: thyroid trouble is malfunction of the thyroid gland of the lower front of the neck. The gland regulates the rate at which the body produces energy. Thyroid hormone may be excessive or deficient.

Mildly to severely ill; class 3–4; worldwide, varying frequency; generally uncommon.

Age: usually adults. **Who:** anyone; some ethnic groups are more susceptible than others. **Onset:** usually gradually over weeks or months.

Clinical

There are two types: low-thyroid and high-thyroid.

BOTH TYPES
There may be hoarseness, GOITER or eyes that appear to pop out at you because you can see the whites above the corneas when the patient looks at you. In both types the patient has little stamina with exercising. Beyond that the two types differ.

LOW-THYROID

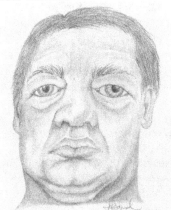

Low-thyroid causes a sleepy appearance as shown. This is a mild case. AB

The patient is always tired, gains weight in spite of a decreased appetite, has thin brittle hair, low body temperature, slow pulse and constipation. He will not tolerate being cold. He may have loss of the outer 2/3 of the eyebrows. He may have a floppy weakness of his limbs, particularly the upper legs and arms. He may sleep excessively and be depressed. His heart size may be enlarged (see Volume 1, Chapter 1.) Women are likely to have heavy periods. This is very common with GOITER and with CRETINISM.

HIGH-THYROID
The patient is nervous, trembles, has insomnia and loses weight. His appetite is increased; he moves his bowels frequently. He may have a sustained fever, fast pulse, high blood pressure. Males may develop breasts. Females have light menses. This may be a complication of GOITER, of treatment for GOITER or of treatment for low-thyroid.

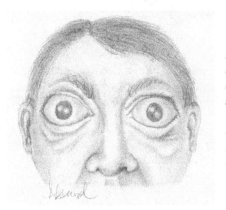

High-thyroid causes a wide-eyed appearance as shown above. The drawing is of an extreme case; it might not be this obvious. AB

Similar conditions: *high-thyroid* may be similar to ATTENTION DEFICIT DISORDER (present since childhood), ADDICTION to uppers or withdrawal from downers (drug usage history), TOXEMIA of pregnancy, BERIBERI (poor diet), some kinds of MENTAL ILLNESS and occasionally DEMONIZATION. *With a fever:* consider cerebral MALARIA and TYPHUS. *Low-thyroid* may resemble DEPRESSION; ADDICTION to downers or withdrawal from uppers; PELLAGRA and RADIATION ILLNESS. See Protocol B.10.B: Confusion/Lethargy.

Treatment

Referrals: see Volume 1, Appendix 13. Laboratory; a well-equipped hospital lab can do blood tests to confirm the diagnosis and determine the appropriate medicine or surgery. Facilities: at least a level 3 hospital, probably level 4 is necessary to treat this. There are good treatments for both, but the labs and medicines are expensive.

Patient care: do not try to treat high-thyroid yourself. If your patient has symptoms of low-thyroid and GOITER and you are in an area where both GOITER and CRETINISM are common, then treat with IODINE. Check the patient twice a week for the first two months. If he develops thyroid trouble of the high-thyroid type, stop the IODINE treatment and send him to a hospital.

TICK PARALYSIS

Some ticks, mainly the Americas and the Pacific area, inject a poison which make the patient weak and paralyzed, possibly numb also. The weakness is symmetrical and there is no pain. It starts away from the trunk and moves toward the trunk. The patient may stop breathing. In the Pacific area, there may be changes in the pupils, or the paralysis may involve only one part of the body.

TOC | SYMPTOMS | DIFFERENTIALS | CONDITIONS | DRUG INDEX | REGIONAL NOTES | INX

Any unexplained weakness or paralysis should prompt you to totally undress the patient and check his entire body surface for ticks, especially in his hair (including armpits and pubic hair).

Similar diseases: POLIO, DIPHTHERIA, RABIES PLANT POISONING due to botulism. Polio causes no changes in sensation (numbness or tingling), but this is common with tick paralysis.

Treatment

Remove the tick either by spraying it with insecticide first or else injecting LIDOCAINE around its mouth parts. The patient may get worse before improving. Improvement is rapid in the Americas, but it may be delayed up to two weeks in the Pacific area. Don't fail to look for other ticks after removing one. The one you removed might not be the one injecting the toxin.

Tick typhus

See SPOTTED FEVER.

TINEA

Regional Notes: F, I, M, O, R, S, U.

Entry category: disease cluster.

Includes: ringworm, athlete's foot, mycosis, dermatomycosis, dermatophytosis, epidermophytosis, trichophytosis.

Definition: tinea is a class of fungus infections of the skin.

Not ill; class 1; contagious; worldwide, especially humid and poor hygiene; common.

Age: any, especially children. **Who:** anyone. Tinea versicolor is most common in warm humid areas where it may affect most of the population. **Onset:** slowly, usually.

Clinical

SCALP TINEA

This is otherwise known as ringworm; it causes circular or oval bald spots.

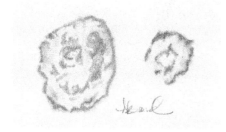

This is one appearance of tinea spots. The appearance varies. AB

ATHLETE'S FOOT

On the feet this manifests with itching, burning, cracking and peeling of the skin between the toes.

TINEA VERSICOLOR

Otherwise known as body tinea, this causes a rash consisting of raised red rings with clear centers or little scattered patches of skin that are lighter, darker or redder than the surrounding skin. Wiping the area results in scales of dirty skin coming off on a damp washcloth.

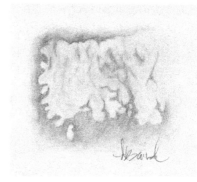

This shows a close-up of one of the patches of tinea versicolor. AB

Tinea imbricata

Tinea imbricata occurs only in the humid tropics. It consists of concentric circles and swirls of tiny flakes. It is itchy.

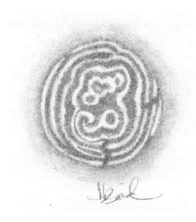

The drawing shows a circle, but swirls are actually more common. AB

Similar conditions: LEPROSY is never itchy which this usually is. Tinea never causes sharp shooting pains or numbness which LEPROSY usually does. PELLAGRA rash is mainly on sun-exposed skin. The rash of secondary SYPHILIS can look similar, as also (rarely) ARSENIC POISONING.

Treatment

Referrals: laboratory; a level 3 hospital laboratory or a dermatologist's office lab can examine scrapings and advise on appropriate medication.

Patient care: try local treatment first: NYSTATIN, TOLNAFATE, MICONAZOLE, WHITFIELD'S OINTMENT, CLOTRIMAZOLE or GENTIAN VIOLET. Sometimes painting the skin with tincture of IODINE is helpful. Stubborn cases can usually be cured with GRISEOFULVIN or KETOCONAZOLE. If you use KETOCONAZOLE, have the patient swallow it with citrus juice or a cola soft drink. After that have him exercise until he sweats and not shower until several hours later. The drug in the sweat helps the skin. With these drugs the patient may have a DRUG ERUPTION with the first dose. Do not stop the medication for this. (But do stop medication in the case of a true drug ALLERGY or SERUM SICKNESS.)

TORTICOLIS (spontaneous)

Entry category: syndrome.

Synonym: wry neck.

Definition: torticolis is spontaneous spasm of the muscles of the neck, usually on one side only.

Cause: unknown.

Not ill; class 1; worldwide, very common.

Age: usually teens and adults; when it occurs in newborns, it is very serious. **Who:** anyone. When it occurs after trauma, it is very serious. **Onset:** usually sudden but may be gradual.

Clinical

Necessary: after sleeping or relaxing, the patient finds that his neck is painful. He holds his head tipped to one side and will not straighten it because of pain. There is no fever, and the patient is not ill otherwise. His arms, legs and back are not affected. There is no history of trauma.

Similar conditions: TRICHINOSIS (also swollen muscles and fever), TETANUS (also other pains and spasms), side-effect of CHLORPROMAZINE or similar medications. Slow onset torticolis may be due to TUBERCULOSIS or CANCER. Torticolis in the context of neck injury is potentially devastating. It is an entirely different condition from that described here, though it may look similar.

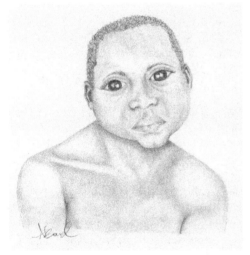

This man has spasms on the right side of his neck, pulling his head to that side. AB

Treatment

Referrals: send those with torticollis due to trauma and newborns out for higher-level care promptly. Do not use the instructions below.

Patient care: for spontaneous torticolis; pain medicines, a neck collar, bedrest and local heat for 3–4 days. *Results:* 3 days with a neck collar for simple torticolis not due to another disease.

TOXEMIA

Regional Notes: F, I, O.

Synonyms: pregnancy-induced hypertension, PIH.

Includes: eclampsia, pre-eclampsia.

Definition: toxemia is a disorder of late pregnancy, of unknown origin, that causes failure of the regulation of body water.

Cause: unknown.

Mildly to very ill; class 2, mild; class 3–4, severe; worldwide, more frequent amongst poor, at high altitudes and young women.

Age: any reproductive female. **Who:** pregnant, usually during the last 3 months of pregnancy. Previous toxemia increases the chance the problem will recur. Overweight is a risk factor, as is having relatives with the condition. Toxemia may also occur up to 7 days after delivery. **Onset:** days to weeks.

Clinical

Note that there is no fever connected with this.

Necessary: high blood pressure (a rise of 30 points or more or a pressure over 130/80 in non-Westerners, 140/90 in Westerners); swollen feet, protein in urine or both.

Usually: initially there is headache and swelling of legs and feet, particularly at the end of the day. There is a decrease in the amount of urine produced. A crisis may occur at the time of delivery; she may have SEIZURES, become unconscious or have a STROKE. Agitation is common at this stage. She may die. Some warning signs that this crisis is coming are abdominal pains (especially upper-right), itching of the face, decreased vision, seeing flashing lights, headache and increased blood pressure.

Complications: STROKE, KIDNEY DISEASE, HEART FAILURE, LIVER FAILURE[1] or BRAIN DAMAGE. In spite of a decrease in blood pressure after delivery, the patient may develop HYPERTENSION as a life-long problem. The baby may suffer from prematurity and/or low birth weight.

Similar conditions: high blood pressure: HYPERTENSION of other causes. *Swelling of legs and feet:* HEART FAILURE, KIDNEY DISEASE, LIVER DISEASE, LIVER FAILURE, VARICOSE VEINS, FILARIASIS or MOSSY FOOT. See Protocol B.6.B. *Mental symptoms:* BERIBERI (poor diet), DEMONIZATION; see Protocol B.10.B.

Bush laboratory: protein in the urine, 1+ or more. A bedside test is helpful. Have the patient lie on her left side for 15 minutes. Then take her blood pressure. Have her roll onto her back. In 5 minutes, take her pressure again. If the second pressure is 20 points or more higher, she is very likely to develop toxemia.

---

1 There will be pain and tenderness in the right upper abdomen; the patient may have abnormal bleeding and bruising.

TOC   SYMPTOMS   DIFFERENTIALS   CONDITIONS   DRUG INDEX   REGIONAL NOTES   INX

Treatment

Prevention: good diet. Watch every pregnancy you can in order to diagnose and treat this early and prevent complications.

Referrals: laboratory: there are no nifty diagnostic tests. Facilities: IVs and fluids; facilities for rapid delivery or surgery; oxygen; injectable medications, at least level 3. This is essential if the problem develops before 5 months. Practitioner: general practitioner or obstetrician.

Patient care: if the problem is mild or just threatening, treat the patient with CALCIUM and ASPIRIN. If a crisis is occurring, send the patient to a hospital if possible. If this is not possible—

- Keep the patient in bed, lying on her left side.

- Use PHENOBARBITAL for sedation and to prevent SEIZURES.

- Use HYDRALAZINE or NIFEDIPINE to lower blood pressure.

- Use FUROSEAMIDE or HYDROCHLOROTHIAZIDE to make the patient urinate and get rid of fluid.

- Check the patient at least twice weekly. Send out for delivery, for SEIZURES and if symptoms do not improve. If you cannot possibly send out, try to contact a physician or midwife for instructions on how to use MAGNESIUM SULFATE IM. If no instructions are available and the situation is critical, use the directions in the Drug Index. There should be improvement within a couple of days.

TOXOPLASMOSIS

Regional Notes: F, I, K, M, N, O, R, S, U.

Definition: toxoplasmosis is an infection with the protozoa *Toxoplasma gondii.*

Not ill to severely ill; class 2–3; worldwide, travel-associated and common in developing countries, related to cats and the eating of rare meat, especially lamb. It is generally less prevalent than average in arid regions and at high altitude. Slaughterhouse workers are particularly prone to infection.

Age: any. **Who:** travelers are prone to get this, especially those with decreased immunity due to HIV, TB, MALARIA or CANCER. This comes from ingesting cysts in undercooked meat (especially pork and lamb), or from contaminated soil or water. **Onset:** variable. Incubation 1–3 weeks.

Clinical

This may be without symptoms.

Sometimes: there is a fever plus enlarged lymph nodes in the neck; severe fatigue; a large spleen. The symptoms are like MONONUCLEOSIS, except the tonsils usually appear normal. There may be a red sore throat. The patient sleeps almost all day every day for 2–10 weeks if untreated, and usually recovers. In those with poor immunity, it may cause ENCEPHALITIS which usually results in death. A woman who has the disease during pregnancy may have a baby who is mentally retarded, has other abnormalities or dies. Sometimes the baby looks normal but later becomes blind.

Similar conditions: see Protocols B.10 and B.12.

Treatment

Prevention: cook all meat well. Pregnant women must avoid cats and anything that may be cat-contaminated.

Referrals: refer quickly in the presence of pregnancy or HIV. See Volume 1, Appendix 13. Laboratory: sometimes a hospital lab can do a smear for diagnosis. Sophisticated labs can do blood tests. Practitioners: infectious disease specialist, pediatrician, internist, general practitioner.

Patient care: be sure the patient eats and drinks enough. Use PYRIMETHAMINE and SULFAMETHOXAZOLE in combination. FANSIDAR or [PYRIMETHAMINE plus CLINDAMYCIN] work well. CO-TRIMOXAZOLE, CLARITHROMYCIN, AZITHROMYCIN, ATOVAQUONE and DAPSONE are reportedly alternatives. ARTEMISIA in some form may work. Treat for a month. Treat pregnant women with SPIRAMYCIN until delivery.

TRACHOMA

Regional Notes: E, F, I, M, O, R, S, U.

Definition: trachoma is an eye infection with the bacterium *Chlamydia trachomatis.*

Not ill to mildly ill; class 1–2; contagious; worldwide, especially common in hot, dry, low-income areas with dirt, flies and overcrowding; less common amongst nomads and in sparsely populated areas.

Age: any. **Who:** anyone, especially close personal contacts of infected persons. Females are more susceptible than males. **Onset:** over days initially; it takes years from first symptoms to blindness.

Clinical

Initially: no symptoms at all or else a mild, irritated-type eye discomfort. If there are no symptoms initially, you probably will not recognize the problem until the advanced stage when the eyelid scars.

Usually: bubbles underneath the upper eyelid, with or without symptoms of an EYE INFECTION (red, scratchy, weeping eyes). Turn the eyelid inside out. (See Appendix 1 in Volume 1.) Underneath the lid you will find whitish, bubbly, pimple-like spots, sometimes few and hard to see, sometimes obvious like cobblestones.

Later: as these spots heal they scar; the scarring contracts the under side of the upper lid, which makes the lashes turn inward. The lashes scratch the cornea whenever the patient blinks. These scratches heal with scarring, causing the cornea to become opaque starting from the top and always worse on top than on the bottom. The eyelid may droop. There may be little gray pits around the edge of the cornea. This may also affect the lower lid, scratching the bottom of the cornea.

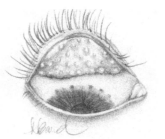

The bubbles under this eyelid are obvious; they may be subtle. The pits around the cornea are also obvious; they may be subtle. AB

Complications: blindness. In areas where this is common, 10% of the older population may be blind from this.

Similar conditions: see Protocol B.8. ALLERGY (vernal conjunctivitis) can cause similar bubbles underneath the upper eyelid. The opacities in the cornea always start on the top with trachoma of the upper lid; they start on the bottom, middle or sides with other diseases.

Treatment

Prevention: for mass treatment of a village, treat all children twice daily with eye ointment for five consecutive days once a month for 6 months. In those with obvious disease, also give DOXYCYCLINE by mouth daily for 5 consecutive days each month for 6 months. If you can teach mothers to wash children's faces frequently, this will do much to decrease the incidence of blindness in the community.

Referrals: laboratory: ordinary smears are useless. Cultures may be helpful. Practitioners: an ophthalmologist with experience in treating this is best. Many nurses who have been personally instructed can do the surgery necessary to correct the problem of eyelashes scratching the cornea.

Patient care: ANTIBIOTIC EYE DROPS or OINTMENT as in EYE INFECTION; sulfa, tetracycline or chloramphenicol ointment is the best, used together with oral medicines: CHLORAMPHENICOL for 10 days is best in places where it has not been abused by over-prescription. Otherwise SULFADIAZINE or CO-TRIMOXAZOLE as in URINARY INFECTION, continued for 10 days. DOXYCYCLINE and ERYTHROMYCIN also work; ERYTHROMYCIN is better.

Some people prevent the corneas' being scratched by plucking eyelashes. This practice should be encouraged. In advanced cases surgery may be helpful, but only if the patient can perceive light and tell what direction it is coming from. It is quite feasible for a non-medical person to learn to do this eyelid surgery, but he must be personally tutored.

AZITHROMYCIN will cure trachoma infection with one dose. It will not, however, heal a damaged cornea. It can be used for mass treatment of whole communities; one should treat at least 80% of the people for it to have a good effect. It is similar to ERYTHROMYCIN.

Results: improvement 3–6 weeks; continue drops or ointment for 2 months total.

TRENCH FEVER[1]

Regional Note: E.

Definition: trench fever is a whole body infection with the bacterium *Bartonella quintana,* which is a type of Rickettsia.

Moderately to very ill; class 1–4; contagious through body lice; worldwide in times of war, mainly in temperate climates.

Age: any; **Who:** those with body lice: usually soldiers in trenches and the urban homeless, maybe refugee camps; **Onset:** usually sudden; after a 4–36 day incubation. There may be a few days of not feeling well before the major symptoms begin.

Clinical

Necessary: fever. The fever pattern varies greatly.

Usually: there is sudden onset of a severe flu-like illness with a high fever, a headache mostly behind the eyes and severe back and leg pain, especially the shins. Damp weather increases the pains. Symptoms increase over 2–3 days, then decrease over 2–3 days. The patient usually stays in bed.

Maybe: there may be sensitivity to touch in bands around the chest, back and abdomen, similar to SHINGLES. There may or may not be a red rash or an enlarged spleen. The rash spots are 2–6 mm in diameter, pink, and the color fades with pressure. There are less than 200 of them. They disappear within a day. Recovery takes a long time, frequently 2 months.

Specific symptoms are these.
- *Fever of sudden onset.*
- *Headache focused behind the eyes.*
- *Headache worse with eye movement.*
- *Red eyes.*
- *Dizziness.*
- *Shin pain with tenderness.*

Complications: blindness, HEART FAILURE (valvular type).

Similar conditions: ARBOVIRAL FEVER, INFLUENZA, LEPTOSPIROSIS, RELAPSING FEVER (which causes calf, not shin pain), SHINGLES and DENGUE FEVER. See Protocols B.2 and B.13. DENGUE FEVER is similar except that shin pains are not more prominent than other bone pains.

Treatment

Prevention: discourage body lice by frequent washing and delousing. Insecticides will kill living lice, but many of them do not kill the eggs. Boiling clothing or ironing might be necessary.

---

1 *See the Powerpoint lecture:* Intermediate Organisms *at www.villagemedicalmanual.org.*

TOC   SYMPTOMS   DIFFERENTIALS   **CONDITIONS**   DRUG INDEX   REGIONAL NOTES   INX

Referrals: see Volume 1, Appendix 13. Laboratory: there are blood cultures and various antibody tests, but they are not simple and routine. You will not find them in most level 3 hospital labs. Facilities: IV fluids and injectable antibiotics might be helpful. Practitioners: tropical/travel expertise is best for initial treatment, a cardiologist and/or expert nursing for complications.

Patient care: antibiotics should be given for 4–6 weeks; there are many relapses with shorter courses. Use DOXYCYCLINE, CHLORAMPHENICOL, ERYTHROMYCIN or AZITHROMYCIN. If the patient has HEART FAILURE, that should be treated with ceftriaxone (a type of CEPHALOSPORIN) plus GENTAMYCIN.

Results: without treatment trench fever symptoms usually last for 5 days. Treatment should shorten this.

TRENCH FOOT

See IMMERSION FOOT. Trench foot is similar, but cold is more of a factor than wetness.

TREPONARID

Regional Notes: F, K, M, O, R, U.

Synonyms: endemic syphilis, bejel, dichuwa, njovera (Zimbabwe).

Definition: this is a non-sexually transmitted disease found in arid areas, caused by *Treponema pallidum*, the same organism that causes SYPHILIS (which is sexually transmitted).

Not ill to very ill; class 1–3; contagious; common in arid areas, especially during the (relatively) rainy season. TREPONARID, PINTA, YAWS and SYPHILIS are all related diseases; each gives partial immunity to the others.

Age: any age, but especially children. **Who:** this is spread by direct contact, flies and shared drinking vessels. It is found mainly in poor, rural areas with overcrowded housing. **Onset:** days to weeks.

Clinical

PRIMARY
This begins with white patches on the pink inside of the mouth, splits on the corners of the mouth, or sores on the breasts of a mother who nurses an affected child.

SECONDARY
Moist warts appear on the warm areas of the body: the armpits and folds of skin. These may be itchy. See the illustration of the warts of secondary SYPHILIS. The lymph nodes may be enlarged. There may be "split peas" under the skin of the fingers. There may be pains in the limb bones, especially at night, with misshapen bones. There may be thick, possibly peeling skin of the palms and the soles, with ulcers.

TERTIARY
The patient may develop big holes where the disease has eaten away the nose, the roof of the mouth or the skin elsewhere. See the SYPHILIS lecture which shows the appearance of tertiary SYPHILIS.

Similar conditions: initial skin problem: the disease is quite similar to YAWS and the treatment for either will cure the other. *Moist warts* may be indistinguishable from secondary SYPHILIS; the treatments are the same. *Skin bumps* may be similar to those with RHEUMATIC FEVER and SYPHILIS. *Facial skin ulceration:* CANCRUM ORIS, CUTANEOUS LEISHMANIASIS and tertiary SYPHILIS.

Treatment

Prevention: wash your hands well. Discourage flies and the sharing of drinking cups. Treat existing cases.

Referrals: laboratory; any blood test for SYPHILIS will be positive in this, since the organisms that cause the two are indistinguishable. See the laboratory paragraph under SYPHILIS. Practitioners: tropical/travel experience may be helpful.

Patient care: same as described for SYPHILIS.

TRICHINOSIS

Regional Notes: E, F, I, K, M, N, O, R, S, U.

Synonyms: trichinellosis, trichiniasis.

Definition: trichinosis is a whole body infection with the larval worm *Trichinella spiralis*.

Mildly to very ill; class 1–3; usually occurs in small epidemics; it is rare worldwide except for eastern Europe, the Arctic and Southeast Asia.

Age: any but nursing babies. **Who:** eating poorly cooked pork or wild carnivore meat. Usually there are groups of cases. **Onset:** begins 1–7 days after eating infected meat.

Clinical

Initially (necessary): the patient has nausea, vomiting, abdominal pain and headache.

Later (necessary): muscle stiffness, swelling, an aching pain (especially of the chest wall), fever and facial swelling (including eyes) develop 9–28 days after eating the infected meat. The fever is high, and it always develops after the muscle swelling.

Maybe: the patient has trouble chewing, breathing and swallowing. A thin man may look muscular because of the muscle swelling, but weight loss is evident later on. In the Arctic it may cause chronic diarrhea.

Sometimes: there are mental problems. There may be little lines of blood in the fingernails resembling splinters. The whites of the eyes may be blood-red. Finally the patient may become very lethargic and lapse into a coma.

Complications: HEART FAILURE, blindness, deafness and PNEUMONIA. Occasionally symptoms resemble MENINGITIS.

Similar conditions: initial symptoms: INFLUENZA, FOOD POISONING, ENCEPHALITIS, STRONGYLOIDES or multiple other minor illnesses. *Fever and muscle stiffness* resemble TETANUS, RABIES (faster progression) and TROPICAL SPASTIC PARAPARESIS (much slower progression). Also see Protocols B.2 and B.13.

Trichinosis causes prominent muscle swelling early on. *Body swelling:* MALNUTRITION, HEART FAILURE, KIDNEY DISEASE. See Protocol B.15. *Mental problems,* lethargy and coma: check BRAIN DAMAGE of other causes. See Protocol B.10.

Treatment

Prevention: cook all meat very well. Freezing meat at very low temperatures for at least 2 weeks may help.

Referrals: laboratory: blood test or biopsy at a hospital. The blood count shows many eosinophils, but this is also present with other diseases. The test is sensitive but not specific; a negative result means the person does not have the disease. Facility; a tropical/travel facility is most appropriate.

Patient care: use MEBENDAZOLE or ALBENDAZOLE initially. They may not help later on. These drugs are useful for the abdominal symptoms, not for muscle pains, or heart problems, though it may keep them from becoming worse. PREDNISONE may be helpful when the disease is advanced, but it must be used with either MEBENDAZOLE or ALBENDAZOLE.

TRICHURIASIS

Note: do not confuse this with trichiasis, which is a complication of TRACHOMA. Trichuriasis is a disease that causes abdominal symptoms. Trichiasis is an eye condition, causing the lashes to grow downward and scratch the cornea.

Regional Notes: E, F, I, M, O, R, S, U.

Synonyms: whipworm, trichocephaliasis.

Definition: trichuriasis is a bowel infestation with the worm *Trichuris trichuris.*

Not ill to mildly ill; class 1; worldwide, related to hygiene and clay soil in warm humid areas. It is generally extremely common, with 10–70% of the population being infected in some areas of the world. It is tropical.

Age: any, especially children. **Who:** consumers of contaminated food, water or soil. **Onset:** slowly, usually.

Clinical

Usually: the patient has one or more of the following: general abdominal pains, diarrhea, ANEMIA, blood in his stool and slow growth. Trichuriasis does not cause a fever. It might cause MALABSORPTION: prompt diarrhea that occurs whenever the patient eats anything.

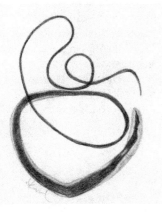

This shows an extended, magnified trichuris worm. Normally the worm is coiled up on one end; it resembles a miniature, coiled spring. One end of the worm is much fatter than the other; thus it is called whipworm. The actual size is like the head of a pin. AB

Sometimes: this causes RECTAL PROLAPSE; little worms will be visible on the moist pink rectal surface that sticks out between his buttocks. The worms may also be visible in the stool. The patient passes large amounts of gas by rectum. Children who have this develop a craving for eating dirt, and they stop growing. The craving will disappear after treatment, and the child will have a growth spurt.

Complications: RECTAL PROLAPSE, ACUTE ABDOMEN, Type 2 and GANGRENE. If there are many worms, the patient may have swollen feet, the ends of his fingers may grow wider than normal giving them a clubbed appearance and his abdomen may be distended with fluid so that he waddles when he walks.

Similar conditions: RECTAL PROLAPSE may also be caused by PERTUSSIS, KIDNEY DISEASE (nephrotic type), or it may happen for no good reason at all. *Bloody diarrhea with no fever* may also be caused by DYSENTERY, STRONGYLOIDIASIS, HOOKWORM and rarely ARSENIC POISONING. *MALABSORPTION:* see Protocol B.14. *Swollen feet and abdomen* may resemble MALNUTRITION (kwashiorkor) or abdominal TUBERCULOSIS. *Swollen finger tips* resemble those due to HEART FAILURE or chronic RESPIRATORY INFECTION.

Treatment

Prevention: encourage the use of outhouses. Discourage the use of human waste as fertilizer. Keep barn yard animals from eating human waste. Keep flies off food. In mass treatment campaigns it is most important to treat the 2–10 y.o. children.

Referrals: laboratory: worm eggs may be found in stool with a microscope. It is a reasonably simple and reliable test. Two negative results eliminate the diagnosis.

Patient care: see RECTAL PROLAPSE if that is a problem. Use MEBENDAZOLE, ALBENDAZOLE, IVERMECTIN or FLUBENDAZOLE to kill the worms. In severe cases with rectal prolapse, enemas containing MEBENDAZOLE may be necessary in addition to oral medicine. Oxantel pamoate or NITAZOXANIDE may work.

TROPICAL SPASTIC PARAPARESIS (TSP)

Regional Notes: F, I, M, U.

Definition: tropical spastic paraparesis is a manifestation of a viral infection causing stiff weakness of the lower body. The virus is related to HIV.

Mildly to moderately ill; class 2–3; widespread, probably worldwide; most common where HIV INFECTION is common, mainly tropical.

Age: over 30 y.o mainly, rarely an onset after age 50. **Who:** females more than males, mainly those who are promiscuous or have a promiscuous partner. **Onset:** over months to years.

TOC

SYMPTOMS

DIFFERENTIALS

CONDITIONS

DRUG INDEX

REGIONAL NOTES

INX

Clinical

Necessary: the patient initially has back pain, and over time he develops leg spasms and inability to use his lower limb(s).

Usually: this affects right and left similarly. It affects the muscles closer to the trunk more than those away from the trunk. The patient walks cross-legged, as if he has a full bladder and is trying not to wet himself. Problems controlling urine in anyone and impotence in males occur early in the course of the disease.

Maybe: there may be loss of sensation, but the stiff weakness is much more prominent than the sensory loss. The patient may have burning pains. The patient may be constipated.

Similar conditions: see SPINAL NEUROPATHY. *Stiff weakness* might also be caused by BRAIN DAMAGE of any sort. Back pain and stiff weakness of lower limbs may resemble tertiary SYPHILIS. Also consider PLANT POISONING due to konzo or cassava. *Inability to tell where a limb is in space* may resemble either tertiary SYPHILIS or COBALAMIN DEFICIENCY. Most other causes of lower limb weakness result in floppy weakness rather than stiff weakness. *Burning pain* may be similar to BERIBERI, but in this case the weakness is floppy and bowel/bladder function is not affected.

Treatment

Prevention: discourage promiscuity.

Referrals: a physical therapist might be helpful. Other than that, there is nothing to do.

Patient care: you can try treating the patient with ARTEMISININ; add moringa if you can find it. It might or might not help. There is nothing else to do.

TROPICAL SPLENOMEGALY (TSS)

Regional Notes: F, I, M, O, R, S, U.

Entry category: syndrome.

Synonyms: TSS, HSS, hyper-reactive malarial splenomegaly .

Definition: tropical splenomegaly is an abnormally large spleen caused by chronic malaria plus some other unknown factor.

Not ill to severely ill; class 1–2.

Age: older children and adults. **Who:** those who have had MALARIA repeatedly. Pregnant women are especially vulnerable to sudden crises from this. It occurs in some geographical areas and not in others. See the Regional Notes. **Onset:** very slow, over months. There may be a sudden crisis.

Clinical

Necessary: the patient has a large spleen. (Normally the spleen is the size of the fist, cannot be felt and is tucked under the lower ribs on the left side.) As it enlarges, the patient has a heavy achiness in his upper-left abdomen.

Maybe: the spleen may become the size of a full-term pregnancy, filling the entire abdomen and extending down into the pelvis. Large spleens cause ANEMIA, susceptibility to infection and easy bleeding (nosebleed; bloody urine, stool and vomit; heavy menstruation; excessive wound bleeding). Other symptoms are cough, fatigue, a large liver, difficulty swallowing, poor appetite and JAUNDICE.

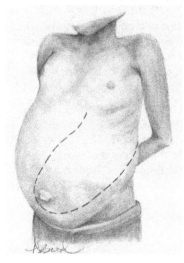

This boy has a moderately large spleen. It is firm and not tender to touch. AB

Complications: a crisis with sudden ANEMIA, SEPSIS, KIDNEY DISEASE and death. See SPLENIC CRISIS.

Similar conditions: see Protocol B.3. In TSS the swelling is more left and upper than right or lower, thus differing from pregnancy and LIVER DISEASE.

Bush laboratory: the patient has urobilinogen in his urine without bilirubin. Draw some blood and put it in an ordinary tube. It will clot and (over a few hours) the clot and serum will separate. Draw off some of the (slightly yellowish) serum. Put half of it in a cold place overnight and the other half at room temperature. In the morning the room temperature serum will still be clear, but the refrigerated serum will be cloudy.

Treatment

Prevention: malaria prophylaxis.

Referrals: laboratory: at level 3 or above, blood tests might be helpful in order to exclude primary liver disease that is making the spleen swollen as a result. Facilities: x-ray, CT scan, ultrasound might all be helpful. The patient might need surgery to remove the spleen, especially if he has a spleen ABSCESS. Practitioners: tropical/travel esperience is most appropriate. A hematologist will be helpful.

Patient care: MALARIA-preventive medicines are most important. PROGUANIL is the best. These medicines must be given over at least 6 months. (See MALARIA in the Condition Index.) Some surgeons may remove such spleens. If they are removed, however, the patient must have access to MALARIA medicines and antibiotics without fail for the rest of his life. Otherwise simple infections will become life-threatening.

TROPICAL ULCER

Regional Notes: F, I, R, S, U.

Definition: tropical ulcer is a spontaneous wound of the skin that grows into a crater; it occurs in warm climates.

Cause: variable.

Mildly to moderately ill; class 1–2; widespread in the tropics, related to poor hygiene. It is mostly a rural problem.

Age: any. **Who:** anyone, especially the malnourished and dirty; common when flies land on open sores. **Onset:** over days, occasionally slowly.

Clinical

Necessary: there is an open sore on the lower body with a scooped-out center, like a crater.

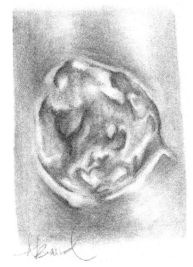

Tropical ulcers are roughly round or oval. They have slightly raised, rolled edges. The inside part is usually not smooth; there may or may not be pus AB

Usually: there is visible pus and large groin lymph nodes. The ulcer is painful.

Sometimes: he has a fever, or he is very ill. Tropical ulcers may have raised red edges and may be very large; part or all of a toe, finger or calf may be eaten away. There may be maggots in the ulcer, in which case the patient should be treated for MYIASIS also.

Complications: SEPSIS, GANGRENE, loss of limb and death.

Similar conditions: see Protocol B.11. *Abdominal or genital ulcers:* AMEBIC SKIN ULCERS and SEXUALLY TRANSMITTED DISEASEs. *Ulcerated part raised up with a cauliflower surface*: DONOVANOSIS, CANCER, YAWS. *Painless ulcer*: TB, ANTHRAX, DIABETES, SYPHILIS and BURULI ULCER (the edges of the ulcer are flat rather than raised and the edge overhangs the ulcer). *Excessive swelling around the ulcer:* ANTHRAX. *Doughnut-edged, very painful* ulcer: DIPHTHERIA.

Treatment

Prevention: frequent bathing. Clean and cover all cuts and scrapes, no matter how minor they are. Eating fish or using bag balm may prevent the formation of ulcers.

Referrals: laboratory; a smear or culture in a hospital laboratory may be helpful. Facilities: with very large ulcers plastic surgery might be helpful.

Patient care; any ulcer more than 5 cm in diameter probably will not heal in your care unless you can do skin grafting. To grraft the ulcer, it must first be free of infection. See Chapter 9, Volume 1. No ulcer will heal unless the patient eats a high-protein diet.

- Check the patient for DIABETES.

- Clean the ulcer daily with a dilute antiseptic in water, rinsing it out well. Soap and strong antiseptics kill the healing cells. Then pack it with either sugar, papaya fruit or papaya leaves; cover it with a bandage. Change the bandage daily, checking for fly larvae and picking out those you find. Keep the area covered continually. Cool wet-to-dry compresses are an alternative for removing debris. See Volume 1, Appendix 1. Once the worst of the debris has been removed, sprinkle the ulcer daily with powdered PHENYTOIN. This will aid healing. ANTIBIOTIC OINTMENT is also helpful.

- Give MULTIVITAMINS and extra dietary protein.[1] ZINC is also helpful as a nutritional supplement.

- Antibiotics: treat the patient for AMEBIC SKIN ULCER if the ulcer is on the trunk or near the genitals. PENICILLIN or DOXYCYCLINE might be helpful for other ulcers. If you do not see improvement within a week use a CEPHALOSPORIN instead. CIPROFLOXACIN or CHLORAMPHENICOL might work. If the pus is bluish the patient must be sent to a hospital.

- As soon as the pus and dead tissue are gone so you can see healthy pink flesh, stop the antibiotic and packing treatment. Just wash the ulcer daily with normal saline (see Volume 1, Appendix 1), adding a half-teaspoon of bleach to each liter. Keep it covered with a clean bandage, preferably with ANTIBIOTIC OINTMENT on it. Continue this until it is totally healed. ZINC by mouth or a zinc paste may also help.

Results: begin 1 week, complete 2 months.

TUBAL PREGNANCY

Regional Notes: F, R.

Synonyms: ectopic pregnancy.

Definition: tubal pregnancy is a pregnancy that implants and grows in the tube that leads from an ovary to the uterus. This is one kind of ectopic pregnancy, 'ectopic' referring to its not being in the right place.

Cause: variable.

---

1 *An egg a day or a glass of milk daily is appropriate.*

TOC   SYMPTOMS   DIFFERENTIALS   CONDITIONS   DRUG INDEX   REGIONAL NOTES   INX

Mildly to very ill; class 4: nearly 100% deaths unless sent out. Worldwide, common with PELVIC INFECTION and TUBERCULOSIS.

Age: any reproductive female. **Who:** anyone, especially someone with prior PELVIC INFECTION. **Onset:** hours to a few days.

Clinical

Necessary: the patient is a reproductive female who complains of lower abdominal pain.

Usually: the pain is localized to the right or left. She has a history of an irregular, late or light period. She may have had some bleeding since and may be bleeding when you see her. There is pain either with intercourse or with pushing a tampon deep inside. There may be shoulder pain.

Maybe: the patient had previous symptoms of pregnancy: nausea, fatigue, and/or sore breasts.

The pain worsens over hours or days until the tube ruptures. The rupture causes SHOCK: fast pulse; low blood pressure; cool, clammy skin; and fainting. It is usually less than one week from the first pains until rupture.

Causative diseases: this may be caused by TUBERCULOSIS, FILARIASIS, CHLAMYDIA, GONORRHEA or another PELVIC INFECTION. It may occur by itself.

Similar conditions: an ABSCESS due to PELVIC INFECTION may be indistinguishable, as may a twisted ovarian cyst or a twisted fibroid. Surgery is necessary regardless. ENTERIC FEVER and DYSENTERY due to amebae may have similar localized pain. ACUTE ABDOMEN may be indistinguishable, but the management is the same.

Treatment

Prevention: treat PELVIC INFECTION and TUBERCULOSIS.

Referrals: laboratory; a blood test for pregnancy may be helpful; urine tests are not reliable. Facilities; a surgeon, anesthesia and operating theatre are essential, as are IV fluids. A blood bank and facilities for transfusion are highly desirable.

Patient care: send the patient to a hospital for surgery. She will certainly die otherwise, and a surgeon can save most patients. Treat for SHOCK meanwhile. Check the patient's blood pressure every half hour, at least; never leave her unattended. If sending out is impossible, prepare her to die.

TUBERCULOSIS (TB)[1]

Section Outline

I	Introduction
II	Clinical: childhood form
III	A. Clinical: adults, lung
	B. Clinical: adults, non-lung
IV	HIV + TB
V	Similar diseases
VI	Prevention
VII	Referrals
VIII	Treatment principles
IX	Treatment programs
X	Results

I. Introduction[2]

Regional Notes: E, F, I, K, M, N, O, R, S, U.

Synonyms: TB, consumption, phthisis.

Includes: Pott's disease (spine), mesenteric lymphadenitis (abdomen); lupus vulgaris (skin); scrofula (neck lymph nodes).

Definition: tuberculosis is an infection with *Mycobacterium tuberculosis* or a related organism.

Not ill to very ill; class 2–3; adult-type lung TB is contagious; TB occurs worldwide, but reportedly it is not common in the Caribbean.

Age: any, but onset is uncommon in 5–10 year olds. **Who:** family of infected adults with lung TB, especially those who are malnourished or have poor immunity; those who drink unpasteurized milk from infected cattle; nursing babies of untreated mothers. Children are especially vulnerable in the year following an episode of MEASLES. Children under 5 y.o. get the childhood form, while those over 10 y.o. get the adult form of lung TB. Children between 5 and 10 usually do not get TB, but when they do, it may be either form. Persons with HIV INFECTION are most susceptible and often get non-lung forms of TB. People of South Asian ethnic origin are more susceptible than other ethnic groups. Elderly people commonly get TB, but they may not have typical symptoms. **Onset:** slowly, over weeks or months; more rapidly in the presence of HIV INFECTION.

---

1 See the PowerPoint lecture entitled Tuberculosis at www.villagemedicalmanual.org.

2 The descriptions given here are only a general summary. If tuberculosis is common in your area, it is essential that you obtain more complete information. The best book available is Clinical Tuberculosis by Crofton, Horne and Miller, ISBN 0-333-56690; published by Health Books International, in the UK.

II. Clinical childhood form

TB in children is hard to detect. Frequently in infants there is merely failure to thrive. It is rare for babies to be born with TB; it is almost always acquired from a tuberculous mother in early infancy. When they are born with it they have large livers, fevers and failure to gain weight. They may have yellow whites of the eyes and difficulty breathing. The most common symptom in older children is a disinclination to play. It usually affects the middle and lower lungs, not the upper lung as in adults. Young children are apt to have abnormal sounds throughout their chests. Non-lung TB is common in children, affecting about 25% of 1–5 year olds.

The table below will enable you to rationally make a decision to treat or not to treat; you should treat right away with the absolute criterion, with two majors and one minor, or with one major and three minor criteria.

Absolute criterion
New-onset midline spine bump, no history of trauma
Major criteria
Definite family history of TB
Malnutrition not improved in one month, food available
Cough over 1 month, not improved with antibiotic or dewormers
Abnormal breath sounds entire chest
Minor criteria
Probable family history of TB
Refusal to eat
Ill more than 4 weeks
Night sweats
Firm, non-tender large joint swelling, not symmetrical

III. Clinical adult forms

The manifestations of TB vary with what organ or organs are involved. Frequently lung TB coexists with other forms, though any single organ or any combination of organ involvement may occur. With some forms of TB there may be fevers, night sweats, loss of appetite, weight loss, failure to gain weight in children and delayed sexual development. Patients may feel feverish without having an objective, measurable fever.

III.A Clinical, adults, lung

Lung TB is by far the most common in the West and in most of the world it accounts for at least half the cases. In adults there may be no symptoms whatsoever, or the patient may have general weakness and fatigue, with loss of appetite, a cough (which may be mild) and weight loss. In some areas, lung TB may present with wheezing like ASTHMA; this is especially common amongst elderly patients.

Commonly: there are abnormal lung sounds but the patient does not appear to be very short of breath. The abnormal sounds are best heard during the patient's first inspiration after coughing. The chest x-ray looks worse than what one would expect from the few symptoms observed. This being the case, it is important to readily refer patients for x-ray, including ones with few symptoms. Patients with obvious symptoms plus very abnormal sounds can be treated without a chest x-ray.

Sometimes: the patient may have a subnormal temperature in the morning and fever in the late afternoon (or perhaps all day) and be unaware of this. The fever comes and goes gradually; it is not obvious as in MALARIA; lack of fever is no argument against the diagnosis. The patient may have night sweats, hiccups, hoarseness or chest pains. In advanced lung disease the patient has a chronic cough and white, yellow, green or bloody sputum. He loses weight and may become short of breath.

Occasionally crackles or noisy breath sounds can be heard over the upper lungs (adults) or any part of the chest (children and those HIV+). His windpipe in his lower neck may be pulled to one side rather than being dead center. There may be muscle pains and spasms in the shoulder on the affected side. The patient's voice may be abnormal. Those with dark skin may have a skin color fairer than normal This is common with malnutrition of any cause, including TB.

Similar conditions to lung TB are these.

See Protocol B.4. *Mild cough* is also found in many diseases, including ALLERGY, RESPIRATORY INFECTION, WORMS and SMOKE INHALATION; it may occur for no good reason at all. *Loss of appetite and weight loss* are prominent features of HIV INFECTION which may be indistinguishable and commonly coexists with TB. *Wheezing*: consider FILARIASIS and ASTHMA. *Chronic cough:* in adults with night sweats and/or weight loss, the presence of abnormal breath sounds in the upper lungs but not the lower makes TB the most likely diagnosis. Failure to respond to a course of antibiotic and failure to gain or maintain weight in spite of adequate food supply makes the diagnosis of TB likely. *Shortness of breath*: see the table in B.4. *Bloody sputum* is also found in the initial stage of ASCARIASIS as well as in PARAGONIMIASIS and RESPIRATORY INFECTION.

III.B Clinical adults, non-lung

This may coexist with lung TB or occur alone. In children and young adults ordinary lung TB progresses to involve other parts of the body. In older adults it is usually due to previous lung TB which has healed or gone dormant and then started up again. Most patients with non-lung TB have no feverishness, fatigue or loss of appetite. Most of them also have no active lung TB at the time.

TOC SYMPTOMS DIFFERENTIALS CONDITIONS DRUG INDEX REGIONAL NOTES INX

CHEST WALL TB

Sometimes TB breaks out on the chest wall so the patient has soft, painless, cool swellings over his ribs. These swellings may break open and crust over, resembling IMPETIGO. Chest wall TB might cause a lung to collapse, a pool of pus to accumulate in the chest or both. High fevers, severe chest pains with deep breathing and shortness of breath are common. It can look very similar to PNEUMONIA that does not respond to the usual antibiotics.

BREAST TB

Breast TB may present with a painful and tender lump. It looks just like breast CANCER, except that cancer is not initially painful, whereas breast TB sometimes is. The pain and tenderness are present in about half of the patients. The patient may or may not have TB in the lung adjacent to that breast. Do not allow a woman to have a mastectomy for CANCER unless she has both a chest x-ray and biopsy. A biopsy, even without a pathology report, may reveal the diagnosis. The inside of a tuberculous lump looks like cheese. Cancer does not.

DISSEMINATED TB (WIDESPREAD)

This refers to many organs being affected at the same time. It used to be called miliary TB. It is most common in children, in patients 65 or older and in Africans. Most of the patients have whole body symptoms such as fatigue, feverishness, weight loss and night sweats, along with cough in 2/3 of the patients. Usually there is objective fever though it might not be high. Be sure to use a corrected temperature; see Volume 1, Chapter 1. Chest x-ray might be normal, or it may show white dots all over. Usually other symptoms reflect the involvement of one or more other organ systems, the most common being the lungs, liver, spleen, kidney and bone marrow. See Protocol B.3: Fever with Anemia. **Treatment** should begin on the suspicion of the diagnosis, since delay in treatment can be disastrous.

LYMPH NODE TB (SCROFULA)

TB of the lymph nodes is most common in females and in those of Asian/Pacific genetic heritage. It causes the nodes in the neck (by far the most common), armpit (rare) or groin (rare) to be painlessly and gradually (over weeks to months) enlarged. At first they are not tender to touch, they are separate from each other and they are moveable. Later they may become tender and stick together. They are not warm to the touch. They may drain through a spontaneous hole in the overlying skin. The fluid drainage will have a faint odor of stale beer. You must put your nose close to perceive this. The large nodes may push against the windpipe, causing a dry cough similar to PERTUSSIS. This is especially common in older children and teenagers.

Similar conditions to lymph node TB: see Protocol B.12: Large Lymph Nodes.

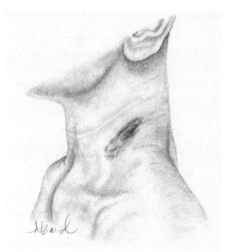

Scrofula presents with multiple, firm, non-tender neck lymph nodes, stuck together. They may be much bigger than pictured here. In this drawing there is a spontaneous wound in the skin. The skin may be intact. AB

EYE TB

TB of the eye causes painful, 1–2 mm diameter, white or yellow bumps on the border between the white and the cornea with some redness nearby. This may start rapidly. There may be itching or pain; there is tearing and light avoidance. The condition is most common in girls 5–10 years old. There may be ulcers on the cornea. Sometimes the back of the eye is affected, decreasing vision.

HEAD/NECK TB

Patients may have chronically draining ears that do not clear with treatment for ordinary EAR INFECTION. They may have ear pain; ringing or roaring in their ears; dizziness (spinning or off-balance sensation); hoarseness with or without pain; a moist whispering voice; difficulty swallowing; or tiny, painful crater-like ulcers on their tongues. The patient may develop BELL'S PALSY. The symptoms are always of gradual onset except for the BELL'S PALSY. In these cases there is almost always lung TB also.

BONE TB

TB of the bone is of two types. It may be in the bone itself, especially the spine (most common). This is a kind of slow-onset OSTEOMYELITIS. Alternatively it may be in a joint, usually a large, weight-bearing joint such as a hip, knee, spine or foot. Occasionally the elbows are affected. Children (but not adults) might develop TB of the fingers, with whole-finger swelling.

The patient has mild to moderate pain, stiffness or both in the affected area but usually no tenderness. The symptoms start slowly, over months. Any single-joint, slow-onset arthritis in a weight-bearing joint or in the spine should be treated as if it were TB. Most often there are NOT accompanying symptoms of night sweats, weight loss and chronic cough. On examination, the joint may feel a bit spongy, different from other joints. Sometimes holes develop in the skin and release watery pus. Bone TB preferentially affects women and the elderly. It is worthwhile to send patients for x-rays.

Bone TB has a fairly distinctive appearance for someone who is used to reading films. The picture can be sent by email.

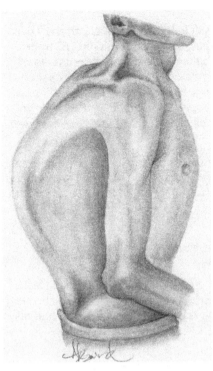

The backbone sticks out in back. This is a severe case; the condition might be subtle with nothing more than a slight midline bump. There is no relationship between the size of the lump and the extent of the nerve damage. AB

Spinal TB: in the chest area, pain comes first, then back stiffness, then abnormal shape. The area may be tender to touch. In the neck area, the patient refuses to turn his head from side to side. His neck may be stiff with his head tilted to one side; see TORTICOLIS. His shoulders or arms may hurt. The patient may have floppy weakness with walking or with using his arms. The affected area of the spine usually sticks out if the disease is advanced. Spinal TB may benefit from surgery. Rapid diagnosis and treatment are essential—treat on the mere suspicion—because any delay might cause paralysis. Spinal TB responds to medication only, provided there is no weakness or paralysis. The curved backbone probably won't straighten.

Hip TB: the patient limps, and has thin, wasted thigh muscles compared to his other side. His mid-thigh circumference will be less than the other side. He may have pain, and the affected leg may be shorter than the other. The patient has trouble swinging his leg out to the side.

Knee TB: there is swelling followed by pain and thin thigh muscles.

Joint TB other than spinal requires early surgery in addition to medication.

Similar conditions to bone TB: ARTHRITIS from other causes, LYME DISEASE, HEPATITIS, RUBELLA and ordinary TORTICOLIS. In these cases the symptoms usually start over hours to weeks at the most. With BRUCELLOSIS the onset may be gradual like TB, i.e., over weeks to months or years. BRUCELLOSIS invariably has more whole body symptoms. FLUOROSIS may also appear similar, but it gives a dark discoloration of the teeth. See Protocol B.13 if the problem is in the back.

Consider also DONOVANOSIS and OSTEOMYELITIS. Bone TB is a kind of osteomyelitis, but the term osteomyelitis is used in this work to indicate a non-tuberculous causative germ.

ABDOMINAL TB

TB of the abdomen has several forms: about 1/3 of the patients with abdominal TB have loss of appetite, lethargy and weight loss. The others will have one of the symptom groups listed below without loss of appetite or lethargy.

Big belly or TB peritonitis: a distended abdomen full of fluid. Onset is less than a month usually. When the person lies down, he bulges out on both sides, just below his ribs. The books claim that this affects mostly middle-aged people. In the author's experience, this is a common presentation in children with failure to thrive. On physical exam, multitudinous tiny nodes can be felt within the abdomen, a "bean-bag belly". Response to anti-tuberculous drugs is rapid—within a week an observant parent will notice improvement. The size of the abdomen decreases over months.

Upper abdominal pain and vomiting: this mimics PEPTIC ULCER DISEASE; there may be prompt vomiting of an entire meal soon after eating.

Upper right abdominal pain with distension and a large, tender liver, similar to HEPATITIS. There may be a large spleen, fluid in the abdomen and occasionally JAUNDICE.

Cramps: the patient has crampy central abdominal pains off and on with loud bowel sounds, and he is sometimes constipated. He might vomit. This problem has not responded to treatment for ASCARIASIS. It may turn into ACUTE ABDOMEN type 3.

Lump and/or diarrhea: there is a painful, slowly developing lump in the abdomen, commonly the lower right, either not tender or mildly tender. The texture is like bread dough or foam rubber. Maybe the patient has off-and-on diarrhea with lower central abdominal cramping and fevers. The diarrhea may be bloody or have mucus in it. It may become MALABSORPTION—see below.

MALABSORPTION: severe, immediate diarrhea whenever the person eats anything. It causes MALNUTRITION, usually in adults.

ACUTE ABDOMEN Type 2.

Similar conditions to abdominal TB: see Protocol B.7: Liver/Spleen Problems. *A distended abdomen with fluid* may also be due to HEART FAILURE, LIVER DISEASE, LIVER FAILURE or TRICHURIASIS. Try to distinguish this from other causes of abdominal distension due to gas or an enlarged abdominal organ. *Crampy central abdominal pain* is most likely due to WORMS; treat for that first. IRRITABLE BOWEL might also appear similar, but then there is usually diarrhea also, at least off and on. *An abdominal lump plus diarrhea* might also be due to AMEBIASIS. The lump might be due to an ovarian cyst, and the diarrhea might be due to DYSENTERY.

TOC SYMPTOMS DIFFERENTIALS CONDITIONS DRUG INDEX REGIONAL NOTES INX

TOC

SYMPTOMS

DIFFERENTIALS

CONDITIONS

DRUG INDEX

REGIONAL NOTES

INX

A large, tender liver might be due to HEPATITIS, ASCARIASIS, AMEBIASIS, or HEART FAILURE. In most cases the onset will be much faster than in TB. In some areas of the world, consider the various forms of SCHISTOSOMIASIS which may also be of slow onset. In this case it will take a hospital to sort out the possibilities, or you can try the hatching test for schistosomes—see Volume 1, Appendix 2. MALABSORPTION: see Protocol B.14.

MALE GENITAL/RECTAL TB

TB causes swelling of the testicles which might be painful. Sometimes a hole forms in the skin and drains. This makes the diagnosis easy. In advanced cases there may be bloody semen. This may cause PROSTATITIS, URINARY INFECTION or incidental blood found on urinalysis. When this involves the rectum, there may be rectal bleeding and/or FISTULA by the anus.

Similar conditions to male genital TB: CANCER of the testicle (mainly in young men) might be similar. Other causes of EPIDIDYMITIS and PROSTATITIS have a more rapid onset.

FEMALE GENITAL/PELVIC TB

PELVIC INFECTION in females may be due to TB. It is treated like TB rather than like ordinary PELVIC INFECTION. It causes pain with intercourse, and it is a common cause of infertility. There may be no menstruation or excessive menstruation. It may be a cause of slow-onset ACUTE ABDOMEN. In areas where there is much TB, it should be treated when the ordinary PELVIC INFECTION treatment fails.

URINARY TB

As in other forms of non-lung TB, patients usually do not have fever, fatigue, night sweats and loss of appetite. Urinary TB is most common in older people. Initially there is frequent urination without pain or urgency. Although white cells in the urine are visible with a microscope, the urine will test negative for leukocytes with the urine dipstick. In the more advanced disease there is blood, back pain, (usually just one side) or lower center-front abdominal pain. When this happens there is likely to be urgency (the need to go RIGHT NOW!!) and pain with urination. Abnormal holes may form between the bladder and the rectum or vagina. See FISTULA. In this case, the patient may be incontinent, with mixed gas, urine and stool coming out of the anus, penis or vagina.

Similar conditions to urinary TB: ordinary KIDNEY INFECTION and SCHISTOSOMIASIS HEMATOBIUM (Africa and Middle East only); CANCER; also consider the various SEXUALLY TRANSMITTED DISEASEs. If the patient has a plain abdominal x-ray, it may show calcium in the kidney(s), similar to KIDNEY STONEs.

PERICARDIAL TB

TB pericarditis may result in HEART FAILURE with a low pulse pressure.[1] It is indistinguishable from PERICARDITIS from other causes, but the patient usually has some other form of TB also. It is more common in Africans than in others. Symptoms include cough, chest pain (relieved by sitting up and leaning forward), shortness of breath with lying down and night sweats, as well as a large liver and swollen ankles.

ADRENAL TB

TB infection of the adrenal glands causes hormone problems. The patient may have a low blood pressure and may develop a craving for salt. The craving should be indulged rather than discouraged.

SKIN TB

Ulcers: skin TB that presents as a skin ulcer is described under BURULI ULCER.

Sores: skin TB can also present as redness (warmth in black skin); lumps; flat, raised areas; or cracks in the skin. It may destroy cartilage. This is known as lupus vulgaris. It usually, but not always, occurs in patients with lung TB

Lumps: another form, known as ERYTHEMA NODOSUM, consists of tender red lumps along the shins. TB is just one cause of ERYTHEMA NODOSUM.

Abscesses: this can also cause ABSCESSes; the pus is usually watery rather than thick. It does not smell bad.

Similar conditions to skin TB: see Protocol B.11: consider LEPROSY, CUTANEOUS LEISHMANIASIS, tertiary SYPHILIS and CANCER for lupus vulgaris. ERYTHEMA NODOSUM can be caused by STREP THROAT, MONONUCLEOSIS, LEPROSY, CHLAMYDIA and various kinds of CANCER.

Choosing drugs to use

Notes: on the chart following.

1 *Streptomycin can cause irreversible hearing loss if it is given in excessive dosage. If a person is already hard of hearing, even a slight hearing loss can cause a major disability.*

2 *Fluid in the abdomen causes the abdomen to be distended. When the patient lies flat on his back, his waist bulges out on both sides. See Volume 1, Chapter 1.*

3 *Ethambutol can cause irreversible blindness if it is used for more than 2 months. If the patient reports visual difficulties as soon as they occur and the drug is stopped right away, then usually vision will be recovered. If the drug is given to children too young to report visual problems, they might be permanently blinded.*

Note: the chart is only a summary. It is important to look up each intended drug in the Drug Index in order to be sure that the drug is used correctly.

---

1 *See Vol. I, Chapter 1 for a description of pulse pressure.*

TABLE OF DRUGS: ADVANTAGES, DISADVANTAGES AND WHEN TO AVOID USING THEM

Drug	Advantages	Side effects/Disadvantages	Patients to avoid using
Isoniazid	Cheap. Works well. Oral.	Requires using pyridoxine.	Liver disease. Allergic reactions to this are rare.
Rifampin	Works well. Low dose. Oral.	Expensive, stomach upset.	Liver disease. HIV+ patients taking HAART medications.
Rifabutin	Stronger, requires a lower dose.	Expensive, relatively new.	Same as rifampin; it is a related drug. May be used in HIV+ patients taking HAART medications.
Rifampentine	Can be used weekly for Rx.	Expensive, relatively new.	Same as rifampin; this is a related drug.
Thiacetazone	Cheap. Oral.	Weak, belly pain.	HIV-positive patients. Caucasians and Asians. Liver disease.
Streptomycin	Cheap.	Injectable only. Dizziness. Cost of syringes.	Pregnant women. Hard of hearing.[1] Fluid in abdomen,[2] bone TB.
Ethambutol	Works well. Oral.	Expensive, decreased vision.	Kidney patients. Visual problems.[3] Very young children.
Ethionamide	Gets into the brain and thus useful for meningitis.	Relatively new on the market.	Same as ethambutol; this is a related drug.
Pyrazinamide	Works well. Oral.	Expensive, requires high dose.	Liver disease, patients with abdominal TB from milk.
Ciprofloxacin	Oral.	Expensive, should take 2–3x daily.	Not for children or pregnant women. Should be taken in the morning. Sometimes abdominal distress.
Moxifloxacin	Oral, works for MENINGITIS.	Like ciprofloxacin New on the market.	The dosage of RIFAMPIN must be increased; seek advice.
Linezolid	Oral, new.	Expensive, problems unknown.	Seek other information. This is a new Gram-positive antibiotic that reportedly also works for TB.

1 *Streptomycin can cause irreversible hearing loss if it is given in excessive dosage. If a person is already hard of hearing, even a slight hearing loss can cause a major disability.*

2 *Fluid in the abdomen causes the abdomen to be distended. When the patient lies flat on his back, his waist bulges out on both sides. See Volume 1, Chapter 1.*

3 *Ethambutol can cause irreversible blindness if it is used for more than 2 months. If the patient reports visual difficulties as soon as they occur and the drug is stopped right away, then usually vision will be recovered. If the drug is given to children too young to report visual problems, they might be permanently blinded.*

OUTLINE FOR CALCULATING THE TOTAL COST FOR TREATING ONE PATIENT FOR TUBERCULOSIS

First two months (Initial Phase):

Drug #1 _____ per month x 2 months = _____

Drug #2 _____ per month x 2 months = _____

Drug #3 _____ per month x 2 months = _____

Drug #4 _____ per month x 2 months = _____

Syringes _____ per month x 2 months = _____

Subsequent months (Continuing Phase):

Drug #1 _____ per month x __ months = _____

Drug #2 _____ per month x __ months = _____

Drug #3 _____ per month x __ months = _____

Total cost for treatment = _____ **(Sum of 8 items above, plus wages, transportation costs, etc.)**

EXAMPLE COST ESTIMATE (in British Pounds) FOR TB DRUGS

Drug	Adult usual dose	Unit size	Cost per bottle	Daily x 30 d	Thrice Weekly	Twice Weekly
Rifampin plus isoniazid	2 tablets daily	300 mg rifampin + 150 mg isoniazid	17.65£ per 1000 tablets	0.99£	0.42£	0.28£
Rifampin	2 tablets daily	300 mg	2.75£ per 100 tablets	15.40	6.60	4.40
Isoniazid	1 tablet daily	300 mg	2.80£ per 1000 tablets	0.08	0.10	0.07
Ethambutol	3 tablets daily	400 mg	8.45£ per 1000 tablets	0.47	0.36	4.08
Pyrazinamide	4 tablets daily	500 mg	12.35£ per 1000 tablets	0.87	0.56	6.20
Streptomycin	1 vial daily	1 gram, injectable vials	4.15£ per 50 vials	2.32	1.00	0.26
Ciprofloxacin	3 tablets daily	500 mg	1.95£ per 100	1.65	—	—
Syringes, disposable	1 syringe daily for streptomycin	—	3.30£ per 100	0.92	0.40	0.26

Note that this only gives relative cost. The numbers for the prices are not recent.

Meningeal TB

Meningitis due to TB occurs much more commonly in children than in adults. It may be one manifestation of disseminated TB. It requires Western subspecialty diagnosis and treatment which must be initiated early in the course of the illness. There is almost always a history of TB or of contact with a coughing adult. There are three stages.

First, a non-specific illness of fever, fatigue, loss of appetite, headache and backache, frequently with vomiting, lasting over 5 days, usually a matter of weeks.

Second, there is a severe headache, changes in personality and a decrease in mental functioning, along with fever. Older patients may present to psychiatrists at this stage.

Third, seizures, abnormal eye movements, stiff neck and markedly decreased mental functioning to the point of coma.

Referral: you should not do a spinal tap, but if someone else does one, request a little spinal fluid in a tube. If the patient has TB meningitis, a little web or clot may form on its own within an hour or two. This is specific but not sensitive for TB meningitis.

Similar Conditions to meningeal TB: see Protocol B.14. LEAD POISONING; BRUCELLOSIS that affects the central nervous system, CYSTICERCOSIS and some slow-onset ARBOVIRAL FEVERs which have a component of ENCEPHALITIS.

IV. HIV infection + TB

HIV plus TB is very common. Half or more of dually infected patients have non-lung TB and around half of these have lung TB also. There is a slow onset. TB is always progressive (continually becoming worse), never staying stable as it frequently does in non-HIV infected patients.

Clinical diagnosis

With HIV infection, the presence of a dry cough for longer than 3 weeks with chest pain, enlarged neck lymph nodes and shortness of breath suggests tuberculosis rather than pneumonia. HIV makes the chest x-ray abnormalities different than the usual tuberculous appearance. There may be finger clubbing with HIV + TB. See the illustration under RESPIRATORY INFECTION.

Treatment

- In theory it would be desirable to treat both diseases simultaneously, but there are nasty drug interactions between RIFAMPIN and some of the HIV drugs. You should get professional advice on dosages. You can get into trouble fast with these drug interactions.

- There is commonly a reaction within the immune system when the two diseases are treated together. It is called IRIS: immune reconstitution inflammatory syndrome. See *IRIS* in this index.

- Treatment should be extended well beyond the 6 months required if the patient were HIV-negative. The patient should be isolated1 for life; he will probably always be contagious.

---

1 *That is, he must live in a separate location where his food is brought to him and no one is near him any more than necessary. He should wear a mask whenever he is out in public.*

V. DISEASES SIMILAR TO TB IN GENERAL

An unexplained fever lasting a week or more is probably TB, MALARIA, BRUCELLOSIS or ENTERIC FEVER. If the fever varies by more than 2°F on most days, it is probably not ENTERIC FEVER; if it is continually high, it is probably ENTERIC FEVER in a national or MALARIA in an expatriate. If the patient became ill over 2–5 days, it is most likely ENTERIC FEVER. With severe joint pains in multiple joints and a slower onset, BRUCELLOSIS is most likely. With a more rapid onset, MALARIA is more likely. Consider COCCIDIOMYCOSIS if the patient is from the arid Americas.

VI. Prevention

Germs are carried by water droplets exhaled by an older child or adult patient with lung TB. Hoarse patients are very contagious. Children under 5 years old and patients with only non-lung TB are almost never contagious.

Examine all patients from behind. Treat all children who have had contact with an active case. As long as they do not have HIV INFECTION, contagious patients become non-contagious after about 2 weeks on medication. Patients with both HIV INFECTION and TB remain contagious for a very long time. They should be housed separately.

BCG is an immunization for tuberculosis. It is anywhere between 5% and 80% effective in preventing the disease, according to different studies.

VII. Referrals

See Volume 1, Appendix 13, remembering that lung TB in older children and adults is contagious; other forms are not.

Laboratory tests for tuberculosis are these.

- Skin testing is useless in developing countries. There are so many sources of false negatives and false positives that it really doesn't give any information at all.

- *Sputum **smear***: positive in 50% to 70% of proven TB; occasional false-positives, particularly if there is dust or dirt mixed in with the sputum or contaminating the slide. A level 3 or 4 hospital laboratory can do a sputum smear or culture for lung TB. The sputum specimen must be stained within 24 hours. If the lab uses a cold method (does not heat the slide), the only positives they will report have overwhelming infections. The hot method is much more sensitive.

  Bleach treating the sputum specimen before staining it improves sensitivity. It also protects the person transporting the specimen and the technician staining it. Just mix the specimen with an approximately equal amount of household bleach.

- *Sputum **culture***: positive in 85% to 90% of lung TB; occasional false-negatives; no false-positives.

- *Chest x-ray* becomes positive later in the disease; after a year or more it is reliably positive with lung TB.

- *Blood tests:* the sedimentation rate is useless. In Western facilities a new test is available, called quantiferon. Authorities differ as to how reliable it is. Another test called GenX is likewise difficult to evaluate.

TOC · SYMPTOMS · DIFFERENTIALS · CONDITIONS · DRUG INDEX · REGIONAL NOTES · INX

- *Biopsy* is necessary for non-lung TB; if this is not possible try treating the patient for a month. Improvement is evidence that the problem was indeed TB rather than something else. An exception is lymph node TB; this may become worse at first, then it improves very slowly.

Facilities: facilities for injections may be helpful. Also a surgical theatre for biopsy or removal of diseased organs.
Practitioner: an infectious disease specialist is most appropriate.

VIII. Treatment general principles

Whom to treat, factors in deciding this.

Interpreting lab results: don't believe a negative result on a sputum test done with the cold method. Do believe a positive result. Don't believe a negative result on a sputum test done with the hot method if the patient has symptoms consistent with TB and if he has not responded to ordinary antibiotics.

Reliability: if your patient defaults (he stops taking his drugs), this will cause drug resistance in the community. The patient will die anyway and many others will die also, because their disease will not respond to the drugs.

Drug supply: evidence has shown that it is best to start with 4 drugs and then reduce to 3 drugs after 2 months. Giving two drugs or less causes resistance in the community. The patient will die anyway if you give less than the prescribed number of drugs.

Prognosis: don't treat any patient who is dying. It is a waste of precious medication, and it fosters distrust of TB treatment in the community. If the patient can either walk (with help) or sit up on his own, he has potential to recover.

Drug resistance: MDR: multi-drug resistant TB. If the patient has been treated before unsuccessfully or if he caught his TB from someone who was treated unsuccessfully, he may have resistant TB. TB bacteria that are resistant to RIFAMPIN and ISONIAZID are called MDR or multi-drug resistant. You cannot treat such patients, but you might refer them to a major TB treatment center in a large city. If you cannot do that, at least keep them isolated from other people so they cannot spread the germs. Everybody who becomes infected with such germs will die unless he can be treated in a specialty location. Involve community leaders, so everyone understands how dangerous these people are. Institute programs to teach people to cover their mouths when they cough and not to share eating or drinking utensils with those who are ill.[1]

Compliance: getting patients to comply with treatment programs is difficult. Many will stop treatment when they feel better. It is a good idea to have patients leave a deposit at the start of treatment and get their deposit back when they finish. This increases compliance.

If the patient has large lymph nodes, they may enlarge further at the beginning of treatment; do not allow the patient to stop treatment because of this. The problem will resolve.

Nutrition is extremely important. It is throwing money away to treat for TB when the patient has a low-protein diet that is devoid of vitamins. Give protein supplements and MULTIVITAMINS if this is the case.

Drugs

There are some antibiotics that seem to work fine for TB. They are expensive when bought commercially. You may substitute one or more of these for one or more of the usual TB medications listed below. It is essential to independently confirm the appropriate dosage.

Do not give RIFAMPIN or RIFABUTIN together with HAART (the medicines for HIV INFECTION). The RIFAMPIN decreases the effect of the HAART and thus the precious HAART medicines are wasted. Either delay the HAART drugs until after the TB is treated, or treat the TB with drugs other than RIFAMPIN (and related drugs). There are so many problems with HIV and TB together; you should not be treating both diseases at the same time in any case. Do not let a TB patient start on HAART unless he is supervised by a medical professional. Do not give TB medications to someone already on HAART.

RIFABUTIN is a new drug that is useful for TB. It is related to RIFAMPIN, but is used at half the RIFAMPIN dosage. Do not use RIFABUTIN and RIFAMPIN together. Rifampentine is another rifampin-related drug that stays in the body for a much longer time. It can be used weekly rather than twice or thrice weekly.

CIPROFLOXACIN, CLARITHROMYCIN, OFLOXACIN and PEFLOXACIN are also antibiotics that seem to be active against TB. Do not use more than one of the "-oxacin" drugs at the same time.

PAS (para-aminosalicylate) is an old drug that is very cheap and is sometimes used for TB. The problem is that it requires swallowing huge numbers of pills (10–20) each day so that compliance is a problem. The table on page 202 uses old cost data, but it reflects the relative cost of drugs. Recently the cost of all TB drugs, particularly rifampin, has been increasing rapidly. Also, the more expensive drugs are commonly counterfeited.

• Corruption

There may be corruption in association with national TB treatment programs. For example:

"All TB treatment is free" is equivalent to "Only the rich are treated." With donated medicines, if NGO's cannot recover part of their costs, they just will not offer treatment. If the government says, "It has to be free," NGO's will say, "Then it won't be given." Governments may discourage corruption by having very few treatment centers in large cities. This works, but it adds transportation and accomodation costs for the patients who cannot be treated in their own locations. The patients cannot do their usual jobs either.

---

1 *The author has found that in developing areas few people believe the germ theory of disease and there is no innate sense of sanitation.*

Even when treatment is absolutely free, it might be necessary for patients to bribe the NGO employees to do the job they are already salaried to do, to dispense the medicine.

Patients will take some of their meds and then sell the rest on the black market when they start to feel better. A solution to this problem is to grind all TB meds, since only intact pills can be sold. Find some readily available, small, uniform measuring devices (such as the caps off the backside of plastic syringe holders or baby spoons) to measure. You can tell if patients are selling their medicines on the black market: patients who swallow their medicines are glad to finish the course of treatment. Those who sell their pills will ask for more when told they are finished.

Healthy people will bribe a lab tech to issue a false positive sputum smear in order to obtain the TB meds to sell on the black market. Such people usually report a chronic cough. Have the patient sit and wait for an hour before you listen to his chest. While he waits observe if he actually coughs or not. If he reports coughing up bloody sputum, ask him to do so while you watch (from a distance). It is possible to tell a real cough from a fake cough by the sound. Check the sputum for blood with your urine dipstick if (and only if) he has no evidence of sores or bleeding in his mouth. Genuine sputum from the lungs is gooey, not frothy. Saliva from the mouth is frothy, not gooey.

- **Clinical factors: whom and how to treat:**

Children without symptoms, living with a TB patient: use ISONIAZID as a single daily dose for 6 months.

For a child with symptoms, living with a TB patient, then give antibiotic for 7 days. If there is no response, try another antibiotic for 7 days. If there is still no response, then start treatment for non-lung TB. Choose a protocol according to the list below.

Pregnant women who have TB should be treated, even in very early pregnancy, but do not use STREPTOMYCIN before delivery since it might cause the baby to be deaf. After delivery STREPTOMYCIN is okay since the little that appears in the breast milk will not be absorbed into the baby's blood stream.

Lymph node TB: treat for an extended period of time, at least 9 months and preferably a whole year. Don't treat young people who are only concerned with looking nice; they will default. Only treat those who feel rotten. Asssure them that if they default they will feel rotten again, and you will not treat them a second time.

*Meningitis TB and pericardial T*B: initially use DEXAMETHASONE, PREDNISONE or PREDNISOLONE in addition to the other medications to decrease the long-term disability.

Bone TB: follow the directions below for general TB treatment, but treat the patient with at least 4 drugs for 18 months.

- **Logistical factors**

First decide which drugs you cannot use. This might be due to unavailability, inability to sterilize syringes (STREPTOMYCIN), a high prevalence of HIV INFECTION (THIACETAZONE) or a high cost (PYRAZINAMIDE). Check his urine with a dipstick. If there is protein or blood avoid drugs that are toxic for kidneys (ETHAMBUTOL). If there is bilirubin avoid drugs that are toxic for liver (ISONIAZID, RIFAMPIN and PYRAZINAMIDE).

Then decide which medications you can use. See the above table, "Choosing drugs to use for TB". List alternatives that you might be able to use if the primary medications fail. If you use ISONIAZID you should also use PYRIDOXINE unless the patient eats a healthy diet. The protocols below do not include CIPROFLOXACIN, but you can substitute that for another medication. You can even convert a partly injectable protocol to an all-oral protocol by substituting CIPROFLOXACIN for STREPTOMYCIN.

Then consider what personal, logistical, geographical and cultural factors will influence how you will give the TB medications.

- If your patient is responsible, you will more likely succeed in using the cheaper options that require treatment over a year or more. You can increase motivation by bonding with the patient socially—having tea with him and affirming his worth.

- What is the financial condition of your patient? Patients who are extremely poor may not even be able to afford the cheaper treatment options. For most patients cost is an important factor. But if you choose an option solely on the basis of finances, you may end up with defaulters and consequent deaths or re-treatments. It can be false economy.

- How feasible is it to have a community worker supervise the treatment of your TB patient? If your patient can have good supervision, you are more likely to be able to use twice-weekly and thrice-weekly options. Religious authorities and anthropologists are particularly good for this, since it gets them into the local homes. You must pay them if you expect them to be honest. However, even with paying, it is unwise to trust the ethics of such a person unless you have independent evidence. Make surprise visits to determine if a patient has been given his medication that day or week.

- If RIFAMPIN was given the person's urine must be orange an hour or two later. If it is not orange the RIFAMPIN was not swallowed. Try to talk to your patients privately and ask them if the supervisor requires additional payment from them.

- How far away from your location does your patient live? Does he live near a road that you travel regularly? If he lives far away he will need a local temporary residence for starting treatment or else your treatment options will be very limited. If he lives near a road that you travel, it works well to have him meet you by the roadside at a specific time and place.

IX. Treatment programs

• Choice of initial schedule

Is it better to (A) treat daily for a long time; (B) treat intermittently (2 or 3 times weekly); or (C) treat with a combination of daily and intermittent schedules? First read the paragraphs below. Then consult the section below, entitled "Treatment Schedule Options." It gives a list of optional schedules along with relative prices.

Daily dosages of oral medications only are good to use with reliable patients. The patient can take his own medication daily without supervision. However, if he forgets, it is harder to ascertain that he has, in fact, forgotten; his forgetting leads to wasted medication, relapses and drug resistance. At first it is best to give a patient only one weekly packet of medication at a time in order to get him in the habit of taking it responsibly. Soon after he starts, show up at his house in the middle of the week to check if he took the correct number of pills. Require him to return the empty envelopes or other containers as evidence that he took the medication. As you form a relationship with him, and he learns to take it each morning, you can start giving medication for 2–4 weeks at a time. Daily dosages including injectable medication are only feasible if the patient is staying at or very near a clinic facility. This is an advantage with very sick patients if you have a place for them to stay. It keeps their contagious sputum out of their home, and it gives a time of bonding during the initial phase of their treatment.

Intermittent dosages of oral medications may be used with semi-reliable patients, preferably with supervision. Even illiterate supervisors are fine; ethics are more important than smarts. You can put a picture of each patient on his bag of medication and have the volunteer make a check mark whenever the patient gets his medication. It is easy to find out quickly if a patient has defaulted and this eliminates some medication wastage. The patient receives encouragement several times a week, and he feels accountable to his supervisor and to you.

Intermittent dosages, including injectable medications, can be used for patients living within less than a 30-minute walk of a health professional qualified to give injections. Provision must be made for the patient to receive his oral medications anyway, even if the health professional is out sick, on holiday or does not show up.

Getting started

Weigh the patient and decide on the dosage of each medication. See the Drug Index. Consider contraindications and precautions.

Give the medication for a month and re-examine the patient. Ask him if he has taken his medication. If he says "no", find out why not. If he has had intolerable side effects, offer to change the medication. If he chokes and gags coach him on a better technique for swallowing.[1] If he has no good excuse discharge him from treatment so as not to develop drug resistance in the community. To confirm an affirmative answer ask him about how many pills he takes, when he takes them and what their colors and sizes are. If he says he took the medicine but doesn't know what it looks like, he's lying (assuming he is not blind or mentally slow). If he claims to have taken RIFAMPIN within the last 12 hours, his urine should be an orange color.

Evaluate improvement. Weigh him and see if he has gained weight. Ask him if he feels any better. If he is a child, ask the parent or sibling if he runs and plays now or if he helps with chores. If he says he is not improved, try to evaluate if this is an honest answer or if there is some cultural reason why he is denying improvement. (In some cultures, people think that they will get their money back or get injections which they desire.) If he has gained weight, he has improved.

• Continuation

Decide whether and how to continue. If he has taken his medication and feels better, then continue the same medication. If he truly does not feel any better, then you have two options: either send him to a center for drug-resistant TB or stop treatment.

Suspect drug resistance if either the patient or others in the community have had inadequately treated TB. This commonly happens when a TB treatment program runs out of drugs for a time. If the patient has to buy his own medication each month, he will stop buying the medication as soon as he feels better.

Consider the possibility of HIV INFECTION. Arguments against treating HIV-positive patients are the risk of developing resistant TB in the community, the expense and the poor prognosis. If donors are supplying the funds for the drugs they should have a voice in this decision. If the patient or his family can pay the cost of the drugs, then it is feasible to treat, provided they can pay up front for the entire treatment.

Treatment schedule options

Note that these recommendations are simplified from standard sources because the typical reader is not medically trained. They are also modified for developing areas where the only patients diagnosed are those with advanced disease. The assumption is that there are no reliable sputum or blood tests to confirm or deny the patient's response to treatment. There are second-line drugs which may substitute for these; seek independent information: amikacin, kanamycin, PAS or capreomycin.

---

1 For capsules, take a full glass or cup. Put one capsule in your mouth and looking down at the floor, take a generous mouthful of liquid. The capsules, being lighter than water, will float to the back of the throat. For tablets, throw the head back, looking at the ceiling as you swallow. Tablets, being heavier than water, will sink toward the back of the throat and go down easily.

Option #1: ordinary patients

For patients with:

- no LIVER DISEASE (urine negative for bilirubin).

- no bone TB (no bone pain or joint swelling).

- no signs of MENINGITIS (headache, stiff neck, weakness or paralysis).

- no HIV INFECTION (negative blood test).

- no previous treatment; this is the first time he is being treated for TB.

Choose four of the following seven drugs to use for the first two months. Your choice should include isoniazid, rifampin or both:

> RIFAMPIN, ISONIAZID, ETHAMBUTOL, PYRAZINAMIDE, CIPROFLOXACIN, OFLOXACIN, STREPTOMYCIN.

- avoid any —OXACIN in children, pregnancy and breast-feeding.

- don't use two —OXACIN drugs.

- avoid STREPTOMYCIN during pregnancy; there is no problem with breast-feeding. Avoid this or reduce the dose in the elderly.

- avoid ETHAMBUTOL and STREPTOMYCIN in the presence of KIDNEY DISEASE.

- avoid ETHAMBUTOL in children who are too young to report loss of vision; if this is difficult, use it for 2 months only.

Choose three of the same four drugs to use for the next 7 months, making a total of 9 months of treatment. (Under some circumstances the total treatment duration must be increased to 12, 18 or 24 months, mainly for non-lung TB or in the presence of HIV INFECTION.)

Choose how to give them: the options are:

- intermittent: three times weekly for an entire 9 months.

- two months of daily treatment, followed by twice-weekly for the next 7 months.

Option #2: drug or liver problems

The patient has LIVER DISEASE, his TB is resistant to both ISONIAZID and RIFAMPIN, or he has severe side effects to both and thus cannot take them. Seek independent advice. But if this is not possible:

- use four of the other drugs (beside ISONIAZID and RIFAMPIN) for an entire 18 months, watching the patient carefully to see if his liver disease worsens.

- if the liver disease worsens, stop PYRAZINAMIDE and continue with the other three for 24 months in all.

Option #3: bone or meningeal TB

The patient has evidence of TB in his bones, or he has TB meningitis: treat as above for 18 months, using four drugs for two months followed by three drugs for 16 months. With meningitis, only ISONIAZID, PYRAZINAMIDE, MOXIFLOXACIN and ethionamide get into the brain and thus work well. Tuberculosis of the spine responds to drugs only if there is no paralysis. Spinal TB with paralysis and any TB of the limb joints require early surgery.

Option #4: HIV infection or AIDS present

With AIDS, you must isolate the patient whether you treat him or not; he is contagious and will remain so, even with optimal treatment. It is best not to treat him since the drugs are precious, you will prolong his suffering, and he will infect more people during the added time. If you do treat, follow the recommendations below.

With no AIDS but an HIV-positive blood test, treat as an ordinary patient for a minimum of 12 months. The books say to treat until the sputum is free of TB bacteria for 6 months; at the very least the patient should be free of a cough productive of sputum with blood for a minimum of 6 months. If the patient is taking HAART (the anti-AIDS drugs), then do not use RIFAMPIN since that makes HAART ineffective.

Option #5: second time around

Relapse or recurrence of previously treated tuberculosis:

If the patient defaulted after a matter of months, ascertain why this happened. If he is likely to default again, then do not treat him. Arrange for him to live in isolation until he dies, using the legal system to enforce this. He is dangerous.

If he did not default the first time or if he is unlikely to default again, then use five of these drugs initially for 3 months, followed by four drugs for the next 5 months, to make a total of 8 months of treatment.

X. Results

Sometimes the patient feels better within 2 weeks. Observable improvement is seen within 2–3 months usually. Lymph nodes may initially swell more with treatment before they begin to decrease in size. TB in the presence of either VISCERAL LEISHMANIASIS or AIDS is usually fatal.

TULAREMIA

Regional Note: K.

Definition: tularemia is an infection by the bacterium *Pasteurella tularensis* or related species, Gram-negative.

Moderately ill; class 3; contagious; regional: Northern Hemisphere only: N America, Europe, central Asia, China, Scandinavia, Turkey, the Balkans, north coast of Africa.

Age: any. **Who:** those exposed to small wild animals; to arthropods that feed on them; to water, grain or dust that is affected by them; to pus; or to a coughing patient. There is bioterrorist potential. **Onset:** suddenly, after an incubation of 1–14 days.

Clinical

Necessary: a high fever, chills, headache, fatigue and generalized muscle pains. The fever may be constant or up and down. The person becomes bed-ridden early.

Commonly: vomiting and abdominal pain. The fever may leave for 1–3 days and then return.

Maybe: a rash which changes to a small skin ulcer may appear at the site of the animal or tick bite, usually within 3 days after the onset of the fever. The rash may become blistery, resembling HERPES. The lymph nodes will be enlarged and painful. In adults it is usually the groin lymph nodes that are enlarged; in children it is usually the armpit, elbow or neck lymph nodes. The enlarged nodes persist for months. There may be little lumps underneath the skin between the skin ulcer and the enlarged lymph nodes. They are tender to touch. There may be large red tonsils which may have pus on them.

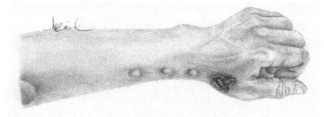

There is an open wound which develops from an insect bite. There may be lumpy red streaks from the wound toward the trunk. The case pictured is obvious; in real life this may be subtle. AB

Rarely: the disease may cause symptoms that resemble PNEUMONIA, EYE INFECTION (pus and painful, yellow bumps on the white of the eye) or STREP THROAT. There may be ERYTHEMA NODOSUM.

Similar conditions: ANTHRAX, PLAGUE, STREP INFECTION, DIPHTHERIA, MONONUCLEOSIS. See also Protocols B.2, B.11 and B.12.

Treatment

Prevention: avoid small wild animals in affected areas. If you are caring for a patient, be careful about hand-washing, eye protection, wearing gloves and masks and disposing of pus and body secretions carefully. There is an immunization available for those at high risk.

Referrals: this is probably not worthwhile unless it is at a location like London or Tubingen. See Volume 1, Appendix 13. Laboratory: there is no simple and reliable test. Blood tests don't turn positive until almost 2 weeks after the onset of the disease. Facilities: IV fluids and injectable antibiotics may be helpful.

Patient care: STREPTOMYCIN or GENTAMYCIN is best. CIPROFLOXACIN, DOXYCYCLINE, RIFAMPIN or CHLORAMPHENICOL may work. Reportedly relapses are common with CIPROFLOXACIN and DOXYCYCLINE. Do not use CEPHALOSPORINs, PENICILLIN, ERYTHROMYCIN or related drugs. Treat for at least 10 days. Do not drain abscessed lymph nodes until the patient has been on antibiotic for at least a few days.

TUNGIASIS

Regional Notes: I, M.

Entry category: infestation.

Synonyms: sand flea, jigger, chigoe, chica, pico, pique, suthi.

Definition: tungiasis is a skin infestation of the sand flea *Tunga penetrans.*

Not ill; class 1; widespread in Africa, India and the Americas, with a spotty distribution.

Age: any. **Who:** exposed to a particular kind of sand flea. **Onset:** soon after exposure.

Clinical

The flea penetrates the skin causing swelling and a white or black bump the size of a split pea on or beneath the skin. These are usually beneath toenails or fingernails, between toes or where skin touched bare ground. The swellings are painful, at times itchy and there may be many of them. This may contribute to MOSSY FOOT.

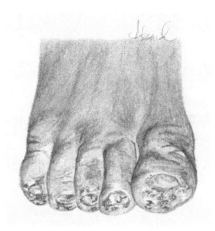

Note the black spots near and underneath the toenails. AB

TOC   SYMPTOMS   DIFFERENTIALS   CONDITIONS   DRUG INDEX   REGIONAL NOTES   INX

Similar conditions: MYCETOMA might look similar, but that does not preferably affect the tips of the toes.

Treatment

Prevention: wear enclosed shoes. Sweep floors. Avoid exposure of skin to dirt. Wear gardening gloves.

Patient care: remove the surface of the skin with a sterile needle (hypodermic or sewing needle) or a sharp pointed scalpel blade, and take the flea out with forceps. Then treat these holes like any other open wound. For fleas under the toenails, shave off the nail. Then use the directions in Volume 1, Chapter 9 for removing a splinter embedded underneath the nail. Prevent further problems by wearing enclosed shoes always, not flip-flops or sandals.

TURISTA, TRAVELER'S DIARRHEA

Regional Notes: E, F, I, M, R, S, U.

Entry category: syndrome

Synonym: travelers' diarrhea.

Cause: variable, but usually virus or Gram-negative bacteria.

Mildly ill; class 1–2; contagious; worldwide, very common everywhere, cause is regional. See also Protocol A.56: Diarrhea, in the Symptom Index, this volume.

Age: any. **Who:** anyone, especially travelers. These are the risk factors:

- a developing environment.
- an adventuresome spirit.
- arrival within the past two weeks
- using ice in soft or alcoholic drinks.
- consuming moist or wet food.
- consuming undercooked hamburgers.
- history of HIV INFECTION, CANCER or taking medicine for GASTRITIS or PEPTIC ULCER.
- swimming in untreated water.

Onset: few hours to a day or two after an incubation of 1–2 days.

Clinical

Necessary: the patient has watery diarrhea.

Maybe: he may have lower-right or lower-left abdominal pain or both. He may also have loss of appetite, vomiting and cramps. To distinguish this ordinary diarrhea from other problems, see the chart in Symptom Protocol A.56.

Treatment

Prevention: boil water before drinking, or filter with a good filter (e.g., Katadyne). All foods (e.g. salads) that will not be cooked should be soaked in iodine-water; see Volume 1, Chapter 2. Avoid consuming food or drink from street vendors. At restaurants buy hot foods; don't eat cold food or salads. It doesn't matter how up-scale the restaurant is. Up-scale restaurants may buy foods from street vendors parked in the alley behind the establishment. Order hot tea or coffee, bottled soft drinks, carbonated water or pre-packaged bottled water.

Don't accept water served in a glass. Drink from bottles that you see opened. Long-term residents (e.g. aid workers) should avoid treating diarrhea with antibiotics as much as possible, in order to develop immunity to the local germs.

Referrals: it is important to send out the following patients: those dehydrated, passing obviously bloody or black stool, severe vomiting, severe abdominal pain, high fever, diarrhea still severe after 1–2 days. See Volume 1, Appendix 13. Laboratory; any hospital lab with a microscope can check the stool for white cells, which indicate whether or not the problem is due to bacteria. You can shake up stool with a little water and check it with your urine dipsticks. A positive leukocyte test indicates that the cause of the diarrhea is bacteria, which should respond to antibiotics. A lab report of bacteria in the stools is meaningless since all stool is 50% bacteria. A check for parasites and cultures for bacteria can also be done. Facilities: IV fluids and injectable antibiotics might be helpful.

Patient Care:

Follow the treatment flow diagrams in the Symptom Index.

Diarrhea in infants which is persistent but does not qualify as MALABSORPTION can be treated with colostrum, the fluid from the breast of a mother who has just given birth but does not yet have milk. Alternatively, give GENTAMYCIN orally (ordinarily an injectable drug) and CHOLESTYRAMINE; give each of these by mouth or stomach tube 4 times a day, but NOT at the same time. Do this until the diarrhea stops plus a few extra doses.

Results: 2–3 days.

TYPHUS[1]

Regional Notes: E, F, I, M, O, R, S, U.

Entry category: disease cluster.

Synonyms: louse-borne typhus, murine (flea-borne) typhus, shop typhus (murine), typhus fever.

Includes: murine typhus, louse-borne typhus, Brill-Zinsser disease.

Excludes: tick typhus, Rocky Mountain spotted fever and Rickettsial pox which are all included under SPOTTED FEVER. Also excludes SCRUB TYPHUS and Q FEVER, which are listed separately.

Definition: typhus is a whole body infection caused by certain Rickettsiae.

Mildly to very ill; class 1–3; regional; louse-borne typhus is found anywhere there is crowding and body LICE: Central America, South America, Africa, Europe, Russia and the Himalayan area. It also occurs in epidemics following social, economic or political instability. It is directly contagious from patients since louse droppings become aerosols. Murine typhus occurs on coasts and along transportation routes from the coast. It is also in areas of grain storage where there are rats, more during the summer than the winter. Neither disease is exclusively tropical.

---

1 *See the Powerpoint lecture:* Intermediate Organisms *at www.villagemedicalmanual.org.*

TOC

SYMPTOMS

DIFFERENTIALS

CONDITIONS

DRUG INDEX

REGIONAL NOTES

INX

Age: any. **Who:** bitten by a louse or flea, depending on the type of typhus. Louse-borne typhus tends to be epidemic; Murine typhus tends to show up in sporadic cases with a history of rat contact. **Onset:** variable. Louse-borne typhus incubation is about 12 days, and the onset is rapid. Murine typhus incubation is 6–14 days. The initial symptom onset is slow and mild, but the fever and chills develop suddenly after a few days.

Clinical

BOTH KINDS

Necessary: a severe flu-like illness, with the headache and general pains coming before the fever. The patient is somewhat giddy initially.

Frequently: the patient is constipated and has sores in his mouth with a dry black tongue. A red rash which lasts 2–10 days appears between the third and seventh days in 90% of cases in fair skin; it may not be visible on black skin. It itches. It starts in the armpits, and it spreads rapidly from there to the trunk and limbs. It affects the face least, if at all. In murine typhus it does not affect the palms and soles. In louse-borne it is heaviest on the back, but in murine, on the front. The patient is unable to stick his tongue out because of swelling below it.

Maybe: the patient has painful swelling of his face in front of his ear(s), similar to MUMPS. He may have large lymph nodes. There may be a slow pulse relative to the fever[1] and low blood pressure. The disease may be very mild in children.

Without treatment, the temperature remains elevated for 12–14 days. When it finally falls it does so very rapidly. Fingers may be painful, pale and cold; the palms may peel. The patient may become short of breath or have a STROKE, deafness, loss of hair or GANGRENE. He may become unconscious or exhibit crazy behavior. He may be incontinent of urine or stool and have abnormal bleeding: nosebleed; bloody urine, stool or vomit; excessive menstruation; or excessive bleeding from minor wounds. Death is usual during the second week of untreated louse-borne illness. The death rate is high for older people (about 50% at age 50) and exceedingly high in pregnancy. Survivors have a long convalescence, frequently complicated by BEDSOREs. There are frequently profound emotional problems also.

LOUSE-BORNE TYPHUS

The symptoms of louse-borne typhus develop over 2 days. Initially the patient has chills, headache, pains in his back and limbs (especially the shins), vomiting and giddiness. There are always mental changes. Patients tend to crouch to relieve the pain. There is a sudden fever after several days of illness. The face and eyes are red and there is increasing headache. The spleen is usually large. After 8 or 9 days he becomes stuporous, delirious, trembling and awake but unresponsive. He might have day-night reversal. His body odor is musty, like wet leather boots forgotten in a plastic bag for a month. His urine also has a musty odor and may test positive for blood.

Louse-borne typhus may relapse years after the primary episode. This is called Brill-Zinsser Disease. It is usually mild and responds well to antibiotics.

MURINE (FLEA-BORNE) TYPHUS

Symptoms are fairly constant. Abdominal pains are present in almost all patients. The main murine typhus symptoms are headache, a cough, nausea and vomiting. Painful eye movements and painful muscles are prominent. Muscle and joint pains are mainly in the trunk and the limbs near the trunk. Respiratory distress is very common. There may or may not be mental changes like louse-borne.

Complications: PNEUMONIA, HEPATITIS, HEART FAILURE, MENINGITIS, ABORTION and RESPIRATORY FAILURE.

Similar conditions: see Protocols B.2, B.8, B.9, B.10 and B.13. LEPTOSPIROSIS, SCRUB TYPHUS, Q FEVER and SPOTTED FEVER may be indistinguishable from this. Early treatment with DOXYCYCLINE is prudent, since it covers them all. The rash of MEASLES is severe on the face, whereas with typhus it is not. TRENCH FEVER may be very similar but then there is fever from the beginning. IN LEPTOSPOROSIS and RELAPSING FEVER, the muscles are tender to touch. SCRUB TYPHUS is treated similarly. ENCEPHALITIS and ARBOVIRAL FEVER(s) may be indistinguishable. Those treatments are merely supportive, which you will do with typhus anyway. Consider HEMORRHAGIC FEVER if there is abnormal bleeding.

Treatment for both kinds

Prevention: be very careful when handling a patient, so you are not bitten by his lice or fleas. Use a face mask. Make every effort to distinguish the two types of typhus; you should know whether to address body lice or rats when pursuing public health measures.

Referrals: laboratory; a Weil-Felix blood test is useless. It is neither sensitive nor specific. Facilities: IV fluids, injectable antibiotics and expert nursing care are most helpful, level 3 or above. Practitioners: tropical/travel medical experience may be helpful.

Patient care:

- Keep the patient near you.

- Shave the patient completely and delouse him. Put his clothes into very hot water. Delouse everyone who had contact with him. Wash floors daily with malathion water to suppress the flea population.

- Give food and water as tolerated; supplement his diet with MULTIVITAMINS.

- Give ACETAMINOPHEN for the fevers.

- Bathe him and change sheets at least daily to prevent BEDSOREs. Turn him at least every 2 hours during the day and every 4 hours at night.

- For antibiotics, DOXYCYCLINE is best. Use CHLORAMPHENICOL if it is uncertain whether you are dealing with typhus or ENTERIC FEVER. PREDNISONE may be helpful in very ill patients; use it as recommended for ENTERIC FEVER. Do not use CIPROFLOXACIN, since this is associated with a poorer prognosis. Treat until 3 days after the fever is gone.

---

1 *See Symptom Protocol A.3 in this volume.*

Results: 3–4 days a little improved; long convalescence, over 2–3 months for murine typhus, possibly faster in louse-borne. Mortality rate may be as high as 60% for louse-borne, but it is less than 5% for murine typhus. Adequate nursing during this time is very important. See Volume 1, Appendix 8.

ULCERATIVE COLITIS

This is an inflammation of the bowel, indistinguishable from DYSENTERY with your facilities and expertise. Treat it like DYSENTERY; send the patient to a hospital if his problem persists or recurs.

ULCERS

Definition: an ulcer is a structural defect of a body surface, either external or internal.

See KERATITIS (corneal [eye] ulcer), PEPTIC ULCER (stomach pain), TROPICAL ULCER (skin ulcer, usually on the leg), TUBERCULOSIS of the skin (Buruli ulcer on limb[s]), SEXUALLY TRANSMITTED DISEASE (genital ulcers) and AMEBIC SKIN ULCER (on the lower trunk or genital area).

UMBILICAL HERNIA

Entry category: structural defect.

Definition: umbilical hernia is a weak spot in the abdominal wall at the navel, allowing the bowel to pass through the deeper layers of the wall until it lies right under the skin.

Not ill; class 1; worldwide.

Age: mainly children. **Who:** anyone, especially Africans. **Onset:** over days to weeks.

Clinical

This is a large, soft, bulging navel common amongst some children. It is only rarely of consequence and then only when it is small. Large ones look funny, but they cause no trouble. A paraumbilical hernia (identical appearance) in adults might cause ACUTE ABDOMEN, Type 3.

Treatment

None or surgery, the difference being if there is significant abdominal pain and/or tenderness of the hernia.

URETHRAL STRICTURE

Regional Notes: F, R.

Entry category: syndrome.

Definition: a urethral stricture is a narrowing of the tube that passes urine from the bladder to the outside of the body.

Mildly to very ill; class 3–4; worldwide.

Age: usually adults. **Who:** anyone, especially promiscuous males; rarely females. Usually due to illness in those over 30 y.o.; injury, under 30 y.o. **Onset:** usually slowly with illness.

Clinical

Necessary: the patient is unable to urinate normally. At first he bears down to urinate; subsequently he may not be able to urinate at all. His bladder becomes distended. This is called URINARY OBSTRUCTION.

Sometimes: he will dribble a little with a very full bladder, but he is unable to empty himself.

Complications: if left untreated KIDNEY DISEASE will result.

Causative diseases: GONORRHEA, CHLAYMIDIA, MYIASIS, URETHRITIS, BLADDER STONE, TUBERCULOSIS, SCHISTOSOMIASIS MANSONI, SCHISTOSOMIASIS HEMATOBIUM and injuries.

Similar conditions: PROSTATITIS may be indistinguishable but usually occurs in those over 50 years old. URINARY INFECTION is more common in females.

Treatment

Referrals: at a level 3–4 hospital, it is possible with an instrument to enlarge the urethra under anesthesia. This may need to be done multiple times.

Patient care: attempt to pass a urinary catheter twice only. If you are unable to pass it in two attempts, empty the bladder with a needle. See Volume 1, Appendix 1. This may be repeated. Send the patient out for further care; you can do nothing more.

URETHRITIS, MALES

Entry category: syndrome.

Definition: urethritis is an inflammation of the tube that passes urine from the bladder to the outside of the body.

Cause: bacteria.

Mildly ill; class 1–2; worldwide, common.

Age: teens and older, sexually abused children. **Who:** anyone; usually sexually active and promiscuous. It is sometimes associated with a SEXUALLY TRANSMITTED DISEASE. REITER SYNDROME is one cause. **Onset:** frequently sudden but may be gradual.

Clinical

Necessary: there is burning pain with urination, erection or both.

Usually: pus drips from the penis. Groin lymph nodes are large and tender. There may be frequent urination of small amounts of urine. The urine may be bloody, and the stream may be poor.

Complications: PROSTATITIS, EPIDIDYMITIS, KIDNEY INFECTION or KIDNEY DISEASE.

Treatment

Prevention: treat all sexual contacts.

Referrals: laboratory: hospital and clinic labs can examine a smear of the pus with a microscope to determine the cause. Facilities; a sexually transmitted disease clinic is ideal.

Patient care: if the patient or his partner has been unfaithful, see Protocol B.1. If unfaithfulness is unlikely, treat with SULFADIAZINE or CO-TRIMOXAZOLE as for a KIDNEY INFECTION. OFLOXACIN is a drug that may be useful. If this fails, follow Protocol B.1.

URINARY INFECTION (UTI)

Entry category: disease cluster.

Synonyms: urinary tract infection, bladder infection, cystitis.

Definition: urinary infection is a bacterial infection of the bladder.

Mildly ill; class 1–2; worldwide, very common in females of all ages and in infant boys.

See KIDNEY INFECTION. A urinary infection is the same except the patient has abdominal instead of back pain. It is treated the same way. Symptoms may be fever; frequent painful urination of foul cloudy urine; incontinence; and low abdominal pain. The urine test will be positive for leukocytes and/or nitrites in about 90% of patients. If you suspect it, treat it; treatment is safe and inexpensive. If the problem has been of slow onset, has been going on for more than a month, and does not respond to two drugs, it is probably due to TUBERCULOSIS. In this case leukocytes and nitrites will be negative on urine dipstick. White blood cells will show up under a laboratory microscope. If the treatment does not work see Protocol B.9 for similar diseases. ENDOMETRIOSIS is a similar condition and may be indistinguishable.

URINARY OBSTRUCTION

Regional Notes: F, R.

Entry category: syndrome.

Synonyms: urinary retention, obstructive uropathy.

Definition: urinary obstruction is blockage of the outflow of urine. It may be due to mechanical obstruction of the flow or to nerve damage that prevents initiating urination.

Mechanical causes: it may be due to STD (see Protocol B.1), URETHRAL STRICTURE, SYPHILIS, FILARIASIS, SCHISTOSOMIASIS, KIDNEY STONE or CANCER.

Nerve causes: sometimes it is associated with back pain, numbness and tingling or paralysis of the legs. It may be associated with SPINAL NEUROPATHY.

If it develops rapidly, there is severe pain like that of KIDNEY STONE. It may be painless if it develops slowly.
If the blockage is below the bladder, the bladder becomes big and hard, like a pregnancy; it can be drained by a needle or a catheter. (See URETHRAL STRICTURE.) If the blockage is further up, the pain will be only or mainly on one side. The patient will probably be able to urinate normally when his bladder fills with urine from the healthy side. See Volume 1, Appendix 1 for draining a full bladder. Refer to a urologist.

UTERINE PROLAPSE

This is a condition in which the uterus, rather than being suspended within the pelvis, descends through the vagina and hangs out between the woman's legs. See Volume 1, Chapter 6.

VAGINITIS and VAGINOSIS

Regional Notes: F, R.

Entry category: syndrome

Definition: vaginitis is an inflammation of the birth canal. Vaginosis is infection without inflammation.

Mildly ill; class 1; contagious; worldwide, very common.

Age: puberty and older. **Who:** any female, especially those with poor hygiene, sexually active or on antibiotics, but anyone can get it. **Onset:** hours to weeks.

Clinical

See the chart on next page, *Kinds of Vaginitis*. Vaginitis may also be caused by MYIASIS, ENTEROBIASIS or SEXUALLY TRANSMITTED DISEASE.

Similar conditions: check SCHISTOSOMIASIS HEMATOBIUM also in regions F and R. Female schistosomiasis causes pelvic discomfort, an abnormal discharge with itching and pain with urinating. It can easily be mistaken for ordinary vaginitis. See HERPES also, especially if the pain is burning or there are blisters. See the illustrations in Volume 1, Chapter 6.

Referrals: laboratory: hospital labs can examine the vaginal discharge to determine the cause. You can check the pH with a urine dipstick. Facilities: referral to a sexually transmitted disease clinic is ideal.

1. 0.3% boric acid is 3 grams or 2.5 ml of boric acid/liter water. Trichomonas increases risk of HIV. It can cause PROSTATITIS in men and male infertility, as well as cervical CANCER in females. In pregnancy, use METRONIDAZOLE, not TINIDAZOLE.

Treatment

Use the drug(s) listed in the chart. Also, it is important to use ERYTHROMYCIN in addition, for 7 days, to eliminate mycoplasma, a kind of bacteria that causes premature labor.

KINDS OF VAGINITIS

	Bacteria	Trichomonas	Candidiasis	Pelvic Infection
Itch/pain	Neither or little	Some itching	Severe itching	Pain
Odor	Strong, fishy, foul	Some, little	None	None or putrid
Reddened moist parts?	No	Yes	Yes	Maybe
Discharge	White or gray, runny or creamy, pH = 5 or more	Much, foamy, greenish, pH = 5 or more	White, thick, sticky, pH = 4.5 or less	Pus, positive leukocytes on urine dipstick
Treatment	SULFA, METRONIDAZOLE, TINIDAZOLE	METRONIDAZOLE, TINIDAZOLE, CLOTRIMAZOLE, 0.3% boric acid douche[1]	NYSTATIN or YOGURT used as a douche	Antibiotic, see PELVIC INFECTION, may be due to TB
Treat partner?	No need	Yes	Yes	Yes

VARICOSE VEINS

Cause: unknown.

Definition: varicose veins are swollen veins on the surface(s) of the lower limb(s).

Entry category: structural defect.

Mildly ill; class 1; Widespread, culturally related.

Age: adults. **Who:** those who stand in one place, women who have had babies or are currently pregnant. **Onset:** usually gradual.

Clinical

Big, soft, lumpy, bluish veins are visible beneath the skin of the patient's legs. Frequently the patient complains of an aching pain in his legs and swelling in his feet while standing. The big veins collapse and become invisible if the patient lies down with his feet up above the level of his heart.

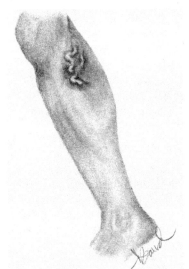

These are fairly subtle varicose veins. They may be very large, the diameter of one's little finger. They may cover almost the entire lower leg. AB

VINCENT STOMATITIS

This is an infection of the moist pink surfaces of the mouth, gums and/or tonsil area. The area is bright red with some white, black or both on it. The breath may have a very foul odor. There is accompanying swelling of the face. It is indistinguishable with your facilities from DIPHTHERIA, except that it does not cause muscle weakness. It is responsive to PENICILLIN.

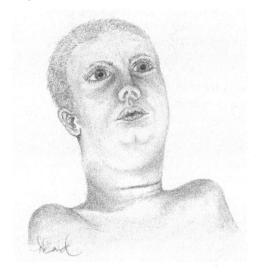

Note the swelling, mostly below the chin, more center than right or left. AB

TOC

SYMPTOMS

DIFFERENTIALS

CONDITIONS

DRUG INDEX

REGIONAL NOTES

INX

VISCERAL LEISHMANIASIS (VL)

Regional Notes: E, F, I, K, M, O, R.

Synonyms: kala-azar, black sickness, dum-dum fever.

Definition: visceral Leishmaniasis is an infection with protozoa of the Leishmania family, usually *Leishmania donovani*. It affects mostly the lymphatic system (spleen, liver, lymph nodes).

Includes: post kala-azar dermal Leishmaniasis, PKDL.

Cause: protozoa.

Mildly to severely ill; class 2–3. not directly contagious. Regional, not found in Southeast Asia or in the Pacific areas. See the maps in the Regional Notes.

Age: affected ages vary by region. It frequently affects infants in the Mediterranean area.

Who: those living in affected areas and bitten by sand flies. Sand flies bite particularly at dusk, but they feed throughout the night. In South Asia and Africa the disease is maintained in humans. In the Mediterranean, Middle East and Brazil, dogs get the disease and humans get it from sand flies that bite both humans and dogs. Patients do not get the disease a second time, but relapses are common. People with poor immunity are particularly vulnerable. **Onset:** incubation 10 days to 2–3 years; As a rule, in Europeans and at the beginning of epidemics, the onset is sudden; where the disease is common nationals have slow onsets.

Clinical

ORDINARY VISCERAL LEISHMANIASIS

Necessary: patients have fevers off and on (possibly with chills), weight loss and very large spleens. Initially, the patient is likely to feel reasonably healthy, walking around and eating normally, even with a fever of 101.3O/38.5O. The spleen is always down to the navel by the third month, and the liver is obviously large by the sixth month. The spleen and liver are non-tender[1] and smooth; the spleen is the larger of the two. There is always ANEMIA after the first month, and it is usually severe.

Usually: night sweats, fatigue, loss of appetite, cough, nosebleeds, bleeding gums and ANEMIA occur. PNEUMONIA and diarrhea are common.

Sometimes: the lymph nodes in the groin are enlarged. The appetite is good, but the patient loses weight anyway. Children do not grow normally. Teen-agers have delayed sexual development. There is some JAUNDICE. The fever rises and falls 2 to 4 times in each 24 hours.[2] Newborn babies of pregnant women with VL might have large livers and spleens. In severe cases the patient may lose his hair or have swollen ankles. There may be abnormal darkening of the skin, mostly on the head in nationals, but this does not occur in pure-blooded Europeans. The skin becomes dry and rough.

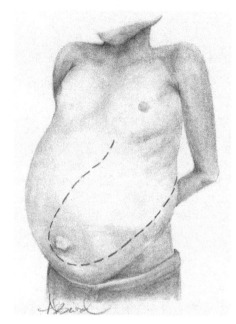

This boy has a moderately large spleen. It is firm and not tender to touch. AB

Complications: SPLENIC CRISIS, CANCRUM ORIS, PNEUMONIA, ANEMIA, SEPSIS, PKDL and death. Patients are vulnerable to other infections.

VL WITH HIV INFECTION

There may be symptoms which are not at all typical, such as lack of fever and no enlarged spleen. Commonly there is watery diarrhea, sore throat, difficulty swallowing, abdominal and rectal pains. These patients usually do not respond well to drugs; the prognosis is poor.

POST-KALA-AZAR DERMAL LEISHMANIASIS (PKDL)

Uncommonly, after the original illness has passed, the patient develops lighter patches of skin, 1 cm or less, which then become bumps, mainly on his face and genitals. These may occur on moist pink surfaces. He may have a fever. Bumps range in size from peas to grapes, may be red and neither itch nor hurt. The appearance is similar to ACNE but it's harder to tell where one bump stops and another one starts. There is no loss of feeling and they never occur below the knees. The skin on top is thin and shiny. It may be indistinguishable from lepromatous LEPROSY.

Similar conditions: see Protocols B.3, B.5, B.7 and B.12.

The fever pattern is distinctive: it rises 2–4 times a day rather than once a day as in ENTERIC FEVER and most other fever-causing illnesses. The fever pattern is similar to BRUCELLOSIS, with the fever going away for as much as 2–4 days at a time. However, VL does not cause the joint pains and sharp shooting pains of BRUCELLOSIS.

---

1 It may be tender in children and with rapid onsets.
2 This is quite distinctive for VL.

Likewise, the pulse is rapid all the time; it does not become slower as the fever decreases. Chills may cause confusion with MALARIA. Large groin lymph nodes may cause confusion with SEXUALLY TRANSMITTED DISEASEs. The very large spleen might resemble TROPICAL SPLENOMEGALY. The weight loss and liver swelling might resemble abdominal TB, some CANCER or LIVER FAILURE of other causes. The loss of hair, general fatigue and loss of appetite resembles secondary SYPHILIS. If the whites of the eyes are yellow, see JAUNDICE.

Bush laboratory: there is sometimes protein, urobilinogen or both in the urine. The formol gel test is easy to do, but it does not turn positive until the patient has been ill for 3 months. One drop of 37% formalin added to a drop of serum on a microscope slide turns milky white and congeals within a few seconds. See Volume 1 Appendix 2. The only other diseases for which this is positive are HIV INFECTION and a certain rare CANCER (multiple myeloma). If the patient was malnourished before falling ill, the test may give a false negative.

Treatment

Prevention: the sand flies that cause this are weak fliers; they have trouble biting in a breeze. A fan is protective. Use insecticide on dogs and in rodent burrows. Use insect repellent or insecticide on clothing. Fine-mesh mosquito net is helpful, especially if it is sprayed with insecticide or insect repellent.

Referrals: laboratory: in South Asia the parasites can sometimes be found in blood stained for malaria parasites. High-tech labs may have two serological (blood) tests: DAT is harder to perform and requires frozen chemicals. K39 is easier to perform, and does not require refrigeration. There may be false negatives in people with AIDS, so it is probably useless to spend the money. The tests will be positive in people without full-blown AIDS (who have the HIV virus but are not yet sick). There will also be positive results in those who have been treated and have recovered, staying positive for a couple of years. Another test, the latex agglutination, uses urine rather than blood and turns negative after successful treatment. *Facilities:* there are a number of different injectable drugs that must be given under physician supervision. It is essential to find a facility in a large city of a developing country where the disease is common, even if this involves international travel. *Practitioner:* physicians can make a definitive diagnosis by doing a spleen or bone marrow biopsy; the organisms appear under the microscope. Western-trained physicians abhor the idea of a spleen biopsy, but it can be done safely. Previous experience with spleen biopsy is helpful. See Volume 1, Appendix 13.

Patient care:

- Anti-VL drugs: STIBOGLUCONATE, PENTAMIDINE, ALLOPURINOL, SITAMAQUINE, maybe TAFENOQUINE, PAROMOMYCIN or AMPHOTERCIN B. VERAPAMIL, KETOCONAZOLE or ITRACONAZOLE might be useful. Give IRON with the other drug(s), but do not give it alone if you are not able to treat the disease.

- MILTEFOSINE is a drug which can be given by mouth for both VL and PKDL. It is safer than STIBOGLUCONATE in the presence of HIV INFECTION, but relapses are more likely.

- ASPIRIN should never be used in someone with this disease. Do not treat the fevers at all, since they are beneficial.

- Treat PKDL the same as ordinary visceral Leishmaniasis.

- Check for and treat TUBERCULOSIS; patients with both VL and TUBERCULOSIS commonly die.

Results: the patient usually feels somewhat better within the first week after starting treatment. The spleen size will decrease dramatically during the first few days with STIBOGLUCONATE injections.

Vitamin A deficiency

See XEROPHTHALMIA.

VITILIGO

Regional Notes: F, M.

Entry category: disease.

Definition: vitiligo is a defect in pigmentation of skin, of unknown cause.

Not ill; class 1; worldwide, more common in the tropics.

Age: any. **Who:** any but the fairest skin. **Onset:** gradual.

Clinical

Areas of normally dark skin become light, usually on the hands, feet or face first. It usually starts out with a few small areas which then enlarge and blend into each other. The areas involved are symmetrical,[3] except for the face. There is no fever, no rash, no scaly texture and no numbness. The skin in the affected areas resembles the skin of a normal European.

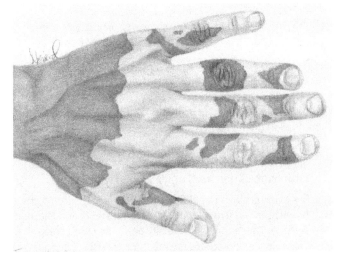

Note that the light-colored skin is like normal fair skin. The borders between the brown and white skin are definite lines and the lines are wavy. AB

---

3 *Symmetrical means that the pattern of affected skin is roughly (though not exactly) the same on the right and left halves of the body.*

Similar conditions: scarring in dark skin; LEPROSY (light skin color is never both flat and symmetrical); maybe TINEA (which usually itches).

Treatment

Referrals: nobody can do anything about this.

Patient care: dark cosmetic cream. The condition causes a social stigma connected with its similarity to LEPROSY. Protect affected areas from sunlight; they are vulnerable to developing skin CANCER.

WARTS

Regional Notes: F, M.

Includes: condyloma acumminata, papilloma venereum, verruca vulgaris.

Excludes: condyloma lata (the "warts" of secondary SYPHILIS)

Definition: warts are bumpy swellings on the skin caused by viruses.

Not ill; class 1–4; worldwide, common.

Age: any. **Who:** anyone. **Onset:** variable.

Clinical

NON-GENITAL WARTS
The patient has roughened dry bumps on the skin, less than 1 cm in diameter, painless and not itchy. There is no fever with this. They may be flat-topped or rounded.

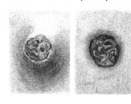

Ordinary warts have rough tops and they look dry. Other than that, they vary a lot in appearance and number. They may or may not be countable. These are two appearances of ordinary warts, magnified 4 times There may be others. AB

GENITAL WARTS
There are three distinct appearances; in all cases the warts are multiple, painless and not itchy. They have a dry appearance. If you soak ordinary genital warts for 3–5 minutes in plain vinegar, they turn white.

- Dome-shaped with smooth tops, skin-colored or slightly pinkish, a few millimeters in diameter. These usually form on the drier areas of the genital skin.

- Irregular, grainy or cauliflower-like surfaces, either with or without a narrow stem between the wart and the skin surface. These may grow in either dry or moist areas. The color is skin-colored, whitish or grayish.

- Giant warts may be irregular and grainy, multiplying and blending together. This usually happens when immunity wanes, such as in HIV INFECTION, pregnancy, OLD AGE or DIABETES. They are hard to get rid of. The color may change from skin-colored to bright red or dark-colored (brown or black).

Complications: there may be secondary infection or ulceration. Giant warts may obstruct the birth canal. There may be bleeding. Wart viruses can cause CANCER.

Similar conditions: MYCETOMA (check geography); MOSSY FOOT; FILARIASIS (geography). TREPONARID, YAWS and SYPHILIS all cause moist warts. MOLLUSCUM CONTAGIOSUM looks like warts, but the surfaces are smooth and there is a tiny center hole in some of the bumps; true warts do not have center holes.

Treatment

On the outer skin, not in the genital area, do nothing. A surgeon can remove them or they may disappear by themselves. In the genital area there are various local treatments that can help with symptoms and improve appearance. These treatments do not get rid of the virus and they do not prevent malignancies. You should send the patient for a firm diagnosis because of the possibility of malignancy.

WEST NILE VIRUS

This is an ARBOVIRUS which has emerged within the past decade. It is present on all continents except Antarctica. It occurs during the summer months, and is indistinguishable from POLIO except that there may be mental changes. Prolonged fatigue is common after the acute illness. Treatment is merely supportive in developing areas. Western medical care may be helpful.

Worms

This is a general term covering HOOKWORM, STRONGYLOIDIASIS, ASCARIASIS, TRICHURIASIS and ENTEROBIASIS. These worms all travel through the lungs, causing a cough. (TAPEWORM, GUINEA WORM, FILARIASIS, SCHISTOSOMIASIS, LARVA MIGRANS and TRICHINOSIS are in different categories.) It is useful to give a worm treatment twice a year to all children; use PYRANTEL PAMOATE, ALBENDAZOLE or MEBENDAZOLE. ALBENDAZOLE is the best general dewormer. This probably will not cure STRONGYLOIDIASIS.

XEROPHTHALMIA

Regional Notes: F, I, M, O, R, S.

Definition: xerophthalmia is a defect in the outer surface of the eye caused by a deficiency of VITAMIN A.

Mildly ill to very ill; class 1; occurs worldwide; widespread and many times seasonal—when fruits are not available. It is most common in southern India, Bangladesh and Indonesia.

Age: any. **Who:** those eating a diet deficient in vitamin A, fat or both. Nursing babies of mothers with marginal vitamin A consumption are also susceptible, especially babies with WORMS, diarrhea, MEASLES and general MALNUTRITION. Refeeding malnourished children may cause blindness if vitamin A is not provided initially. **Onset:** usually gradual but may be very rapid, especially in the presence of other diseases or when refeeding a malnourished child.

TOC

SYMPTOMS

DIFFERENTIALS

CONDITIONS

DRUG INDEX

REGIONAL NOTES

INX

Clinical

Initially necessary: initially there are roughened, whitish, foam blobs which form beside the outer edge of the cornea or on the lid margins. These areas look like bits of meringue or soapsuds. Then the same thing happens along the edge closest to the nose and finally along the lower part of the cornea. Night blindness develops.

Initially frequently: there are tears and light avoidance.

Later usually: in more advanced disease, there is dryness and haziness of the cornea. Areas of the whites of the eyes may look wrinkled and brownish, like white nylon ironed with a too-hot iron. Finally the cornea is totally destroyed. During all this, the eye is surprisingly pain-free, but there is tearing. The dry eyes are not from lack of tears, but rather from the change in the surface of the eye, so tears don't stick to the surface.

Sometimes: the final stage is associated with EYE INFECTION. A dry rash may appear over the outer parts of the upper arms and forearms. At times a small hole develops in the cornea. The iris moves forward and a little piece gets caught in the hole, giving the pupil an irregular shape. The skin and the bowel are also affected. The skin is rough and dry; there may be diarrhea.

ZINC, IRON, protein and fats are necessary for the body to use vitamin A. If these are missing from the diet the disease will advance more rapidly.

Complications: in all cases of xerophthalmia and in some cases of marginal vitamin A intake, there is a profound immune deficiency.

Similar conditions: see Protocol B.8. With TRACHOMA, the destruction of the cornea starts at the top and works down. In xerophthalmia it starts in the central and lower cornea first. IRITIS can look similar, but it is painful. RUBELLA in a newborn can cause similar eye changes. Many diseases cause immune deficiency, as also does pregnancy and OLD AGE. ZINC DEFICIENCY will also cause night blindness. Zinc is necessary to process vitamin A. Hence night blindness should be treated with both ZINC and VITAMIN A.

Treatment

Prevention: urge the consumption of foods containing vitamin A (see below). Cooking, especially frying in oil, aids the absorption of the vitamin. Try to give the vitamin to breast-feeding mothers and women of childbearing age. However, during pregnancy high doses might be toxic to the fetus.

Patient care: in areas where this is common it is reasonable to treat all sick children. In the presence of eye symptoms it is vital to start treatment immediately. Even a few hours may save vision. Give the patient VITAMIN A by mouth or by injection (oral is as good as injectable); give ZINC also. Use water-based VITAMIN A, not oil-based initially; the water-based form is absorbed more rapidly. Then give a diet rich in the vitamin. Vitamin A is found in liver, eggs, dairy products and green and yellow fruits and vegetables. Red palm oil contains large amounts of the vitamin.

Results: start in 1–3 days; complete in 2 weeks.

Yanonga

See Regional Notes U.

YAWS

Regional Notes: F, I, M, O, R, S, U.

Synonyms: endemic treponematosis, endemic syphilis, bouba, frambesia, parangi, pian.

Definition: yaws is an infection closely related to SYPHILIS but not sexually transmitted. It is caused by the spirochete *Treponema pertenue.*

Includes: gangosa—which refers to a gangrene-like ulcer caused by yaws, and gondou—which refers to the enlargement of the bones of the face caused by yaws.

Not ill to very ill; class 1; contagious; widespread in undeveloped, humid areas. YAWS, PINTA, SYPHILIS and TREPONARID are all related; each gives partial immunity to the others.

Age: primary and secondary yaws are mostly in children and mothers. In areas where the disease had been eradicated and then came back, it may be epidemic in adults. Tertiary yaws occurs mostly in people in their 20's and 30's, males more than females. **Who:** anyone living in an affected area, especially those with exposed minor wounds. It is commonest in arable rural areas where there is poverty and overcrowded housing. Tertiary is more common during the rainy season. **Onset:** over weeks.

Clinical

The disease occurs in 3 stages: primary, secondary and tertiary.

PRIMARY YAWS
This causes an ulcer or a lump at the site of a previous minor injury. It starts small and enlarges to 3–5 centimeters. It usually itches. If it is a lump it looks like a blob of dried pus on the skin; the surface is similar to a cauliflower or an irregular wart. Frequently the patient also has aching limbs, fever and enlarged lymph nodes. He may have splits by the corners of his mouth or general swelling of his fingers.

SECONDARY YAWS
This begins 2–16 weeks after the primary. Similar ulcers or lumps form around the primary site or spread out over the body. Ulcers may be round or crescent-shaped. On any one person and between people they vary greatly in size and shape. They can always be felt on the skin. Some are raised, some are craters with rims and some are depressed below the skin surface. Some of the rims may be interrupted. Some are like targets with raised rims and centers. They are most common on the face, armpits and the pelvic area. They may be itchy, but they are painful if they are on the palms or soles. Palm and sole yaws tend to be ulcers rather than bumps.

As some heal, others form. Sometimes there are bone changes: painful swellings along the lower legs, fingers (especially close to the palms) and nose, not affecting joints specifically as ARTHRITIS does. The painful swellings may be tender to touch.

TOC SYMPTOMS DIFFERENTIALS CONDITIONS DRUG INDEX REGIONAL NOTES INX

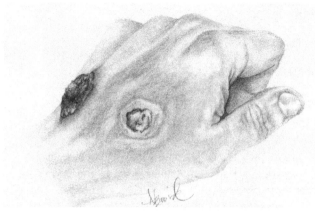

Yaws here is on the hand. It is most commonly on the trunk of children. There are both bumps and ulcers. The bumps look like blobs of dried pus, usually off-white. The ulcers are not deep. AB

TERTIARY YAWS

You should be able to find scarring from old primary or secondary yaws. Tertiary may take any one of these forms.

- Bumps under the skin which break open, causing ulcers. These are identical to those caused by tertiary SYPHILIS.

- Swelling of the lips, at times massive.

- Lumps along the long bones of a limb, right under the skin, at first very tender.

- Bone pain with inflammation on the top; when on the nose or in the mouth this may form an ulcer that eats away like CANCER. This is called gangosa. Bone pain is a deep aching pain, worse at night, in high humidity and with weight bearing.

- Painless little hard bumps next to joints.

- Swelling of the bones in the middle of the face, the bridge of the nose and adjacent cheek bones, called gondou. It is symmetrical. This starts out as a persistent headache, then causes discharge from the nose, then swelling.

- Difficulty in articulate speaking.

- Extremely dry, thick skin on palms and soles which develop painful cracks and ulcers.

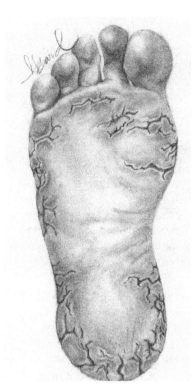

This is the appearance of a sole affected by tertiary yaws. AB

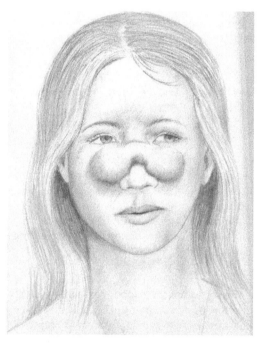

This is a young woman with gondou on her face. OW

TOC   SYMPTOMS   DIFFERENTIALS   CONDITIONS   DRUG INDEX   REGIONAL NOTES   INX

Similar conditions: primary and secondary yaws resemble CUTANEOUS LEISHMANIASIS (check geography), WARTS (dry surface), TREPONARID (arid areas) or LEPROSY. Also check other causes of skin ulcers. *Swollen fingers* are like TUBERCULOSIS, congenital SYPHILIS and SICKLE CELL DISEASE.

IMPETIGO involves confluent areas of skin. Yaws skin lesions are discreet and involve both ulcers and bumps. CUTANEOUS LEISHMANIASIS lesions are discreet, and there are usually either ulcers or bumps, not both. *Bone changes* resemble other bone diseases: TUBERCULOSIS, OSTEOMYELITIS, BRUCELLOSIS, SICKLE CELL DISEASE and CANCER. *Tertiary yaws* resembles tertiary SYPHILIS. The distinction is unimportant since the diseases are related and the treatments are the same. *The painless little hard bumps* might resemble those of RHEUMATIC FEVER or TUBERCULOSIS, diseases which are in other ways quite different. *Gangosa* resembles CANCER, CANCRUM ORIS, GANGRENE and some forms of CUTANEOUS LEISHMANIASIS, tertiary SYPHILIS and skin TUBERCULOSIS.

Treatment

Prevention: teach parents to use the cultural equivalent of band-aids and ANTIBIOTIC OINTMENT for minor cuts and scrapes. Treat existing cases.

Referrals: laboratory: some level 3 hospital labs can do darkfield microscopic examination of scrapings from the wounds. See the laboratory note under SYPHILIS also.

Patient care: use PENICILLIN, DOXYCYCLINE or ERYTHROMYCIN. Long-acting, injectable PENICILLIN is helpful. Single dose AZITHROMYCIN may work.

In a promiscuous culture, if you do mass treatment of yaws, venereal SYPHILIS will run rampant. SYPHILIS is more destructive than yaws.

Results: some results in 48 hours; complete in one week in primary and secondary; healing may take weeks with tertiary, and it may never be complete. Sometimes surgery is necessary.

Yellow fever

See Regional Notes F, M.

ZINC DEFICIENCY

Cause: nutritional and environmental.

Mildly to moderately ill; class 1; worldwide, tropics.

Age: any. **Who:** anyone, especially expatriates not acclimatized to the tropics, those with diarrhea and those exercising. **Onset:** days to 2 weeks.

Clinical

Necessary: night blindness, lethargy, apathy and general weakness.

Usually: there is a decreased sense of taste and smell, behavioral problems, diarrhea, skin rashes, loss of hair, decreased growth in children, delayed sexual development in teenagers, impotence, abnormal menstrual cycles, delayed wound healing and susceptibility to infections.

Similar conditions: night blindness is just like XEROPHTHALMIA. Failure to grow in children resembles other causes listed in the chart under MALNUTRITION, in this index.

Susceptibility to infection is also seen in HIV INFECTION, TUBERCULOSIS, VISCERAL LEISHMANIASIS, XEROPHTHALMIA, OLD AGE, and DIABETES.

Treatment

Patient care: ZINC may be taken as tablets. Zinc is eliminated mostly in sweat and stool, so the hotter the weather and the more diarrhea, the more zinc is needed. The average adult needs a minimum of 10 mg of zinc for each liter of fluid he drinks during the day to a maximum of 50 mg. Someone zinc-deficient to begin with should have more for about a week. High-zinc foods are whole grains, meats other than fish and sausage, eggs, low-fat milk products, shellfish and leafy and root vegetables.

INDEX D: DRUG INDEX

ALPHABETICAL LISTING OF DRUGS

Generic names are listed except in a few places where the brand name is more commonly used. UPPER CASE words refer to entries in the Condition Index or the Drug Index.

SAFETY NOTATION

Safety class: 1: very safe if used according to directions.

Safety class: 2: requires special precautions.

Safety class: 3: relatively unsafe in non-professional hands

STABILITY NOTATION

A: will not decompose under ordinary circumstances; keep it at room temperature in tropical or temperate climates.

B: the dry drug is stable but the liquid must be refrigerated and used within less than a week.

C: the drug may be stored at room temperature in temperate climates but should be kept in a cool place or refrigerated in the tropics. Sometimes there is a notation as to maximum temperature. If there is no notation, drug companies generally state 30° C or 85O F as the maximum storage temperature.

D: needs refrigeration

Dark: prolonged exposure to light ruins the drug; store it in the dark, taking it out only to use it.

Unknown: no data could be found for this characteristic of the drug.

ABBREVIATIONS

Gm	gram
Mg	milligram = .001 gram
Mcg	microgram = .001 mg
Meq	milliequivalents, the unit of measure for potassium and some other drugs
ML	milliliters
Unit	the measure of penicillin, insulin and some other drugs
IM	intramuscular
SQ	subcutaneous
IV	intravenous

PREGNANCY DESIGNATIONS

A	Good evidence of no harm in humans
B	Good evidence of no harm in animals, no evidence either way in humans
C	May cause harm in animals; unknown if there is harm in humans; benefits may outweigh the risk.
D	There is some evidence of harm in humans, but benefits may outweigh the risk.
X	Don't even consider using this in pregnancy. It does terrible things to unborn babies.

ABACAVIR

Anti-HIV drug; nucleoside reverse transcriptase inhibitor

Safety class: 3 Stability unknown Pregnancy unknown Breast-feeding unknown.

Brand names: Ziagen, 300 mg and 20 mg/ml injection. Also comes combined with LAMIVUDINE and ZIDOVUDINE. The combination brand name is Trizivir.

Indications: HIV INFECTION.

Contraindications: ALLERGY to this drug. Do not give this to patients weighing less than 40 kg or to children under 12 years old.

Precautions: the patient must not drink alcohol while using this. Seek advice before using this together with CO-TRIMOXAZOLE. Abacavir might cause fatal ALLERGY reactions after it is stopped and then started again. Seek independent advice for LIVER DISEASE and if contemplating prolonged usage. Stop the drug for fever, rash, fatigue, abdominal symptoms or shortness of breath.

Side-effects: unknown; see side-effects for LAMIVUDINE and ZIDOVUDINE.

Dosage: for older children and adults: 300 mg two times a day.

ACETAMINOPHEN

Antipyretic, Analgesic

Safety class: 1 Stability: A Pregnancy: B

Brand names: Febrinol, Liquiprin, Panadol, Paracetamol, Tempra, Tylenol. Supplied, usually, as 325, 500, 650 or 1000 mg tablets. Sometimes available as liquid for children.

Indications: fever, mild pain relief, pain relief after head injury.

Contraindications: ALLERGY to the drug, ENTERIC FEVER.

Precautions: if you use this at the same time as CHLORAMPHENICOL, see the precautions listed under that drug. Avoid prolonged use with ALCOHOLISM. May cause false blood glucose results in DIABETES.

Overdose and prolonged use: LIVER FAILURE (see Protocol B.7); KIDNEY DISEASE.

Dosage: 650–1000 mg every 4 hours as needed for adults; reduce dose for children. Overdose: see Protocol A.11 in the Symptom Index.

Alternatives: ASPIRIN, IBUPROFEN.

ACETAZOLAMIDE

Diuretic, Water pill

Safety class: 2 Stability: C Pregnancy: C

Brand name: Diamox.

Indications: ALTITUDE SICKNESS, GLAUCOMA, adaptation to high-altitudes.

Contraindications: ALLERGY to the drug, LIVER FAILURE, KIDNEY DISEASE, chronic RESPIRATORY INFECTION, pregnancy, SULFA allergy.

Precautions: if the patient develops a skin rash, stop the drug. This may provoke KIDNEY STONES. In a patient on PHENYTOIN SODIUM, any heart medicine or other diuretics (water pills) use this only at a physician's direction. This drug interferes with many lab tests—don't believe lab results drawn while the patient is taking this.

Side-effects: sleepiness, numbness, tingling. This occurs with only a small percentage of patients. Sometimes there is nausea, vomiting and weight loss. If used in a patient with LIVER FAILURE, it may cause confusion.

Overdose and prolonged use: KIDNEY DISEASE, LIVER FAILURE (see Protocol B.7).

Dosage: reduce dose in the elderly.

ALTITUDE SICKNESS, altitude adaptation: 250 mg daily from 2 days before ascent until 2 days after ascent.

GLAUCOMA: 125–250 mg by mouth every 8 hours, which must be continued for the patient's whole life.

ACICLOVIR

See ACYCLOVIR; this is the British spelling for the same drug.

ACT (Artemisinin Combination Therapy)

ACT stands for artemisinin combination therapy. It is a combination of ARTEMISININ plus some other anti-microbials that work against malaria. Now that so much malaria is chloroquine-resistant, older drugs and newer ones both have been combined with artemisinin, giving the advantages of both immediate response and sustained repression of malaria. Some of the drugs thus combined are: ATOVAQUONE, PIPERAQUINE, MEFLOQUINE, PYRONARIDINE, AZITHROMYCIN and LUMEFANTRINE.

ACTIVATED CHARCOAL

General antidote for poisoning

Safety class: 1   Stability: A

Supplied as generic powder to mix with liquid.

Indication: to neutralize any swallowed drug or poison.

Contraindications: lack of a secure airway;. more than two hours elapsed since the poisoning.

Precautions: if the patient is vomiting, give him something to settle his stomach first so he does not vomit the charcoal. Do not give this at the same time as IPECAC. It will neutralize the IPECAC. Charcoal does not taste bad, but it looks like black slime. Disguise it with a cola drink or have the person drink it through a straw out of a covered container. Use a water-mix, not capsules.

Dosage: children: 0.5–1gm/kg; Adults get 25–100 grams. Modify the dose according to how much poison the patient took.

ACYCLOVIR, ACICLOVIR (British)

Antiviral

Safety class: 1   Stability: C   Pregnancy: C

Brand names: Zovirax. Supplied as cream and tablets.

Indications: HERPES, SHINGLES.

Contraindications: pregnancy, prior ALLERGY to the drug, DEHYDRATION, other drugs that may cause KIDNEY DISEASE.

Precaution: if taken by mouth, avoid DEHYDRATION.

Side-effects: headache, diarrhea, nausea, dizziness, joint pains, skin pain. These effects occur in only a small percentage of patients.

Overdose and prolonged use: stomach upset, LIVER FAILURE (see Protocol B.7); KIDNEY DISEASE, dizziness, trembling, confusion, agitation.

Dosage: reduce the dose in the presence of KIDNEY DISEASE.

Initial episode of HERPES: 200 mg by mouth every 4 hours, five times a day for 7 days. For very severe cases, 800 mg every 4 hours, five times a day for 7–10 days.

Recurrent HERPES may also be treated with 800 mg twice daily for 5 days.

Initial episode of SHINGLES: 800 mg five times a day for 7–10 days. Some authorities say to use it with PREDNISONE.

Available in a 5% cream to be used every 4 hours for 5 days.

Alternatives: Valaciclovir and Famciclovir and Cidofovir are newer drugs that do about the same thing.

ALBENDAZOLE

Dewormer, anthelmintic

Safety class: 2   Stability: C   Pregnancy: C

Supplied as 200 mg and 400 mg tablets.

Brand names: Albenza, Albazine, Alben, Valbazen, Zentel, Eskazol.

Indications: ASCARIASIS, CAPILLARIASIS, CYSTICERCOSIS, ENTEROBIASIS, FILARIASIS, GIARDIASIS, HOOKWORM, HYDATID DISEASE, LARVA MIGRANS, LOIASIS, MANSONELLOSIS PERSTANS, STRONGYLOIDIASIS, TAPEWORM, TRICHINOSIS, TRICHURIASIS, diarrhea due to HIV INFECTION.

Contraindications: ALLERGY to the drug; maybe pregnancy

Precautions: if used in large doses for HYDATID DISEASE, it may cause HEPATITIS. Stop the drug if this occurs.

Avoid pregnancy during treatment and for one month afterward. In the presence of CARBAMAZEPINE or PHENYTOIN, the dose may need to be increased. If this drug is taken with CIMETIDINE, there will be a larger amount in the blood, so it might become toxic. If it is taken with a fatty meal or with grapefruit (or its juice), there will be a larger amount in the blood, so if you are giving a high dose, it might be toxic.

Overdose and prolonged use: LIVER FAILURE (see Protocol B.7).

Dosage: unspecified doses are for adults. Reduce dose in the presence of LIVER DISEASE or LIVER FAILURE. Reduce dose according to weight for children. This is safe to use with IVERMECTIN and PRAZIQUANTEL.

ASCARIASIS: adults and children over 2 years old or 10 kg get a single dose of 400 mg. Those under 2 years old or 10 kg get 200 mg.

CAPILLARIASIS: 400 mg twice daily for 10 days.

CYSTICERCOSIS: 400 mg twice a day for 28 days. Use DEXCHLORPHENIRAMINE and PREDNISONE with this.

Diarrhea due to HIV INFECTION: 800 mg twice daily for 14 days.

ENTEROBIASIS: same as ASCARIASIS. Repeat in 2 weeks. Treat the whole family at the same time.

FILARIASIS: 400–600 mg, single dose.

GIARDIASIS: 400 mg daily for 5 days.

HOOKWORM: 400 mg twice a day for 1–2 days.

HYDATID DISEASE: 400 mg twice a day for 28 days. Give this treatment 4 times, with 15–day rest periods between treatments. If the disease recurs the patient will need surgery.

LARVA MIGRANS: cutaneous: 200 mg twice a day for 5–7 days. Deep: 400 mg daily for 21 days (eye). In Asia extend this time to 28 days, both eye and other. Non-Asia, non-eye, 5 days may be okay.

LOIASIS: 200 mg twice daily for 21 days.

MANSONELLOSIS PERSTANS: 400 mg twice daily for 10 days.

STRONGYLOIDIASIS: 400 mg twice a day for 10–14 days.

TAPEWORM, beef or pork: 400 mg daily for 3 days.

TRICHINOSIS: 400 mg twice a day for 14 days.

TRICHURIASIS: 400 mg daily for 3–7 days.

Alternatives: MEBENDAZOLE, THIABENDAZOLE, PYRANTEL PAMOATE.

ALBUTEROL

Anti-asthmatic, Bronchodilator

Safety class: 2   Stability: C   Pregnancy: C

Supplied as tablets, as injectable liquid and as inhaler. The drug might be labeled in micrograms (mcg): 1000 mcg = 1 mg.

Synonym: salbutamol.

Brand names: Proventil, Ventolin.

Indications: ASTHMA, chronic RESPIRATORY INFECTION, premature labor.

Contraindications: heart problems, HEART FAILURE, pregnancy (except for use in premature labor), age under 6.

Precautions: not used in children under 6 y.o. It is very toxic in children; a small overdose can kill. Seek physician advice before using this together with any heart medications or antidepressants.

Side-effects: if the patient develops a pressure-like chest pain (ANGINA), then stop the drug. Other side-effects: nervousness, trembling, rapid heart rate, headache, muscle cramps, insomnia, nausea, weakness, dizziness. These effects occur in only a small percentage of patients.

Dosage: children 6–12 y.o.: 0.1 mg/kg every 6–8 hours. Adult dose: 2 mg to 6 mg tablet, every 6–8 hours, as needed, maximum daily dose 32 mg. The inhaler may be used as 2 puffs inhalation every 4 hours. For premature labor, give 0.1–0.25 mg IM every 5–10 minutes until contractions have stopped; then give 4 mg by mouth every 6–8 hours. An alternative is terbutaline, similar dosage.

Alternatives: METAPROTERENOL, THEOPHYLLINE

ALCITABINE

This is an anti-AIDS drug.

ALCOHOL

Sedative, muscle relaxant

Synonyms: ethanol, ethyl alcohol.

Safety class: 2   Stability: A

Indications: muscle relaxation to put a dislocated shoulder in place; antidote for PLANT POISONING: ackee; antidote for poisons found in home-brewed alcohol and wood alcohol.

Contraindications: loss of consciousness, inadequate breathing. Do not use this together with DIAZEPAM or with other sedatives. Do not give this to someone with a family history of PORPHYRIA.

Precautions: try to avoid using this during pregnancy. An intoxicated patient may become combative; be prepared to deal with this. If the patient passes out, be sure he has an adequate airway and is lying belly down so vomit will run out of his mouth. Always use alcoholic beverage for this; never use rubbing alcohol or wood alcohol.

Overdose and prolonged usage: LIVER FAILURE.

Dosage: 80 proof alcoholic beverage is 40% alcohol. The adult dose of 80 proof is 6 ml/kg or 360 ml for a 60 kg person. It may be given by mouth or stomach tube. For 40 proof, double the number of ml given; or for 160 proof divide the ml dose in half. (For 160 proof, dilution may be desirable to prevent throat irritation.) Calculate the adult dose, then reduce it according to weight for children.

Table of alcohol dosages for muscle relaxation: number of milliliters vs. body weight and proof of the product.

It is best not to use anything weaker than 60 proof.

Proof	60 kg	40 kg	30 kg	20 kg	10 kg
160	180 ml	120 ml	90 ml	60 ml	30 ml
120	240 ml	160 ml	120 ml	80 ml	40 ml
80	360 ml	240 ml	180 ml	120 ml	60 ml
60	480 ml	320 ml	240 ml	160 ml	80 ml

ALLOPURINOL

Xanthine oxidase inhibitor

Safety class: 3   Stability: C   Pregnancy: C

Brand names: Lopurin, Zyloprim.

Indications: CUTANEOUS LEISHMANIASIS (only the simple Mexicana type and must be used with another drug also), GOUT, VISCERAL LEISHMANIASIS.

Contraindications: ALLERGY to the drug, KIDNEY DISEASE, pregnancy, breast-feeding.

Precautions: this may bring on an episode of GOUT in those predisposed if the initial dose is too high for that person. Continue the drug at a reduced dosage. If it causes rash, stop the drug. Rashes occur mainly with KIDNEY DISEASE. A rash may also appear if this is used with AMPICILLIN. If this is used at the same time as THEOPHYLLINE, it increases the amount of THEOPHYLLINE in the blood, possibly to toxic levels. Reduce the dose of THEOPHYLLINE. It may cause cataracts. Take this with a lot of water. It may cause drowsiness.

Dosage:

CUTANEOUS LEISHMANIASIS: 5 mg/kg four times daily for 28 days or 10 mg/kg twice daily for 18 days, perhaps combined with sodium STIBOGLUCONATE. Seek local confirmation.

GOUT prevention: begin at 100 mg daily for one week. The second week, increase it to 200 mg daily; if this dose is not adequate to prevent a recurrence, increase to 300 mg daily for the third and subsequent weeks.

VISCERAL LEISHMANIASIS: 5–10 mg/kg every 8 hours for 10 weeks. This must be combined with sodium STIBOGLUCONATE, and it must be used in a hospital setting.

ALOE VERA

This is a common native plant with thick leaves. The gel, obtained by cutting a leaf and squeezing it, is useful for treating all kinds of skin problems, especially burns. Otherwise cut the leaf open and lay it on the wound. Reportedly an oral form of this works for HIV INFECTION. The oral form may be toxic.

AMIKACIN

Aminoglycoside, second-line anti-TUBERCULOSIS drug and Gram-negative antibiotic

Safety class: 3   Stability: C   Pregnancy: D

Supplied as 100mg/2ml; 500mg/2ml; 1gm/4ml

Brand name: Amikin.

Indication: TUBERCULOSIS, staphylococcus infection

Contraindications: ALLERGY to this drug or any aminoglycoside (STREPTOMYCIN, GENTAMYCIN), KIDNEY DISEASE.

Precautions: don't use with other aminoglycosides. Don't use it with PENICILLIN, any CEPHALOSPORIN, AMPHOTERCIN B or diuretics such as HYDROCHLORTHIAZIDE or FUROSEAMIDE. Watch for insufficient respiratory effort (stop the drug), hearing loss or dizziness (stop the drug). Don't use in patients with any muscle weakness. Should not be given for a long time but temporarily is okay.

Side-effects: muscle weakness, KIDNEY DISEASE.

Dosage: no oral form; 7.5 mg/kg IM twice daily, maximum of 500 mg. Begin daily, then decrease to 2–3 days per week. In obese patients, calculate what his weight would be, given his height and a BMI of .2. Use that weight for his dosage. If you can't calculate this, don't use the drug.

AMODIAQUINE

Antimalarial

Safety class: 3   Stability: C

Brand names: Basoquin, Camoquin, Flavoquin, Myaquin. Available in Kenya, Colombia and Pakistan.

Same uses, same side-effects, same doses as CHLOROQUINE for MALARIA; do not use it for amebic DYSENTERY. It may or may not be useful for CHLOROQUINE-resistant MALARIA, depending on the area. It can cause a severe skin reaction resembling a burn. Stop the drug immediately if this occurs. Rarely it kills the bone marrow and hence the patient. It can also cause HEPATITIS.

AMOXICILLIN AMOXYCILLIN (British)

Antibiotic, Gram-positive and Gram-negative

Safety class: 2   Stability: B   Pregnancy: B

Brand name: Amoxil.

Caution: do not use amoxicillin in patients with PENICILLIN ALLERGY.

Supplied as 250 and 500 mg tablets and oral liquid. The injectable form is AMPICILLIN. Amoxicillin is an oral, long-acting ampicillin, causing less diarrhea.

Indications: ACUTE ABDOMEN, ANTHRAX prevention, BARTONELLOSIS, CELLULITIS, CHLAMYDIA, DYSENTERY (except for Shigella), middle EAR INFECTION, ENTERIC FEVER, EPIDIDYMITIS, GONORRHEA, valvular HEART FAILURE, KIDNEY INFECTION, LEPTOSPIROSIS, LYME DISEASE, MENINGITIS, PELVIC INFECTION, PEPTIC ULCER, PIG-BEL, PLAGUE, PNEUMONIA, RESPIRATORY INFECTION, SEPSIS, URETHRITIS, URINARY INFECTION. It may be used as a substitute for PENICILLIN.

Contraindications: ALLERGY to PENICILLIN or any "cillin" drug; MONONUCLEOSIS.

Precautions: if the patient has MONONUCLEOSIS, ampicillin will cause a rash; stop the drug,

Diarrhea may occur. Treat the diarrhea with ORS, but do not stop the drug unless the diarrhea is severe and you have an alternative antibiotic. When given with ALLOPURINOL, a rash may develop. Oral contraceptives might not work when taken along with this.

If there is allergy, the patient may never again take any penicillin-type drug for the rest of his life.

Dosage: reduce dose in the elderly and for KIDNEY DISEASE. Adult doses are given; reduce dose according to weight for children. The oral and injectable doses are the same. When it is used as a substitute for PENICILLIN, it must be used in the same dose as PENICILLIN.

ACUTE ABDOMEN: 500 mg three times a day for 14 days.

ANTHRAX prevention—use only if the organism is sensitive to PENICILLIN: 500 mg every 8 hours for 60 days.

BARTONELLOSIS: same as ACUTE ABDOMEN.

CELLULITIS: 250–500 mg, depending on severity, every 8 hours for 10 days.

CHLAMYDIA: 500 mg three times a day for 10 days.

DYSENTERY: 500 mg three times a day for 5 days.

EAR INFECTION: same as CELLULITIS.

ENTERIC FEVER: same as ACUTE ABDOMEN.

EPIDIDYMITIS: 250–500 mg every 8 hours for 3 days.

GONORRHEA exposure: 3500 mg by mouth, one dose.

TOC

SYMPTOMS

DIFFERENTIALS

CONDITIONS

DRUG INDEX

REGIONAL NOTES

INX

GONORRHEA disease: 3500 mg by mouth in a single initial dose, then 500 mg 3 times a day for 10 days.

HEART FAILURE: 3000 mg an hour before a medical or dental procedure; 1500 mg 8 hours later.

KIDNEY INFECTION: same as CELLULITIS.

LEPTOSPIROSIS:[1] 500 mg every 8 hours for 7 days.

LYME DISEASE: same as CELLULITIS.

MENINGITIS: initially use AMPICILLIN, ideally 50–60 mg/kg IM or IV every 6 hours for 14 days. The usual adult dose is 3000 mg every 4 hours. If injections are not an option, try the same dose orally. Use this together with GENTAMYCIN (injectable) or CHLORAMPHENICOL (oral or injection).

PELVIC INFECTION: same as GONORRHEA disease.

PEPTIC ULCER: 1000 mg twice a day for 14 days, used together with [CLARITHROMYCIN or LEVOFLOXACIN] and [CIMETIDINE or a similar drug].

PIG-BEL: same as ACUTE ABDOMEN.

PLAGUE: same as MENINGITIS.

PNEUMONIA: same as CELLULITIS.

RESPIRATORY INFECTION: same as CELLULITIS.

SEPSIS: same as MENINGITIS, together with GENTAMYCIN.

URETHRITIS: same as GONORRHEA disease.

URINARY INFECTION: same as EPIDIDYMITIS.

Alternatives: in ALLERGY, it is best to use an alternative drug specific for the disease. Otherwise use CHLORAMPHENICOL or CO-TRIMOXAZOLE. In severe infections such as SEPSIS and MENINGITIS, an alternative is a CEPHALOSPORIN.

AMOXICILLIN + CLAVULANIC ACID

Antibiotic, Gram-positive and Gram-negative

Safety class: 1–2   Stability: A

Brand names: Augmentin (USA), Co-amoxiclav (UK).

This is supplied as chewable tablets of 125 mg amoxicillin with 31.25 mg of clavulanic acid or 250 mg amoxicillin with 62.5 mg clavulanic acid. It is also available as adult film-coated tablets with 125 mg clavulanic acid for each 250 mg of amoxicillin.

Indications: ABSCESS, some CELLULITIS, CHANCROID, EXFOLIATIVE DERMATITIS, OSTEOMYELITIS, PYOMYOSITIS.

Contraindications: ALLERGY to any penicillin plus the same contraindications and precautions as AMPICILLIN and AMOXICILLIN. Do not use this in the presence of CIRRHOSIS or any significant LIVER DISEASE.

Side-effects: upset stomach with higher doses.

Dosage: reduce the dose in the elderly.

OSTEOMYELITIS: 500 mg (amoxicillin) every 8 hours for a minimum of 6 weeks.

Everything else: 250 mg (amoxicillin) every 8 hours until better plus three days.

---

1 *It is useless to give antibiotic for leptospirosis if the patient has been ill for 4 days or more.*

AMPHOTERCIN B

Anti-fungal, anti-Leishmania. It is expensive. If the word "liposomal" is attached the drug is safer and even more expensive.

Safety class: 3   Stability: C   Pregnancy: B

Supplied as vials of 50 mg.

Brand names: Fungilin, Fungizone, Abelcet, AmBisome, Amphool.

Indications: COCCIDIOMYCOSIS, MYCETOMA, VISCERAL LEISHMANIASIS, CUTANEOUS LEISHMANIASIS.

Contraindications: maybe pregnancy; breast feeding, allergy or previous bad reaction to the drug.

Precautions: this drug is dangerous and must only be used with physician supervision in a hospital context. If the blood pressure drops the drug must be stopped. The drug is a kidney poison so it must not be given together with other drugs that affect the kidneys. Liposomal amphotercin B is more expensive but safer to use.

Side-effects: nausea, vomiting, diarrhea, abdominal pain, loss of appetite, headache.

Overdose and prolonged use: KIDNEY DISEASE.

Dosage: seek current information and local lore, since the best dosage schedule varies from place to place. Usually a test dose is necessary. Reduce the dose if there is KIDNEY DISEASE.

AMPICILLIN

Antibiotic, Gram-positive and Gram-negative

Safety class: 2   Stability: B

Brand names: Omnipen, Polycillin. Supplied as 250 and 500 mg tablets. Liquid supplied as 125 or 250 mg per 5 ml (1 tsp). Generic and injectable forms are available.

Caution: do not use ampicillin in patients with PENICILLIN ALLERGY.

This is a previous form of what is now AMOXICILLIN. It may still be found in oral form in developing areas. There is no injectable form of amoxicillin, so ampicillin must be used if injections are required. The mg dosage of ampicillin is the same as amoxicillin, but it is eliminated from the body more quickly. Hence, it must be given 4 times a day rather than 3 times.

AMPICILLIN + SULBACTAM

This is like AMOXICILLIN plus CLAVULANIC ACID, used the same way but injectable. The dosage refers to the AMPICILLIN component. If that is correct, the sulbactam dosage will also be correct.

AMPRENAVIR

This is an anti-AIDS drug.

ANESTHETIC EYE DROPS

Topical anesthetic

Safety class: 2   Stability: C, dark

Brand names: Ophthaine (0.5% proparacaine hydrochloride), Pontocaine (0.5% tetracaine), Dorsacaine (0.4% benoxinate hydrochloride). Many generic preparations exist. Use only drops labeled "ophthalmic".

Indications: examination of an injured eye and removal of a foreign body from the eye.

Contraindications: ALLERGY to any "-caine" drug.

Precautions: all of these drops burn as they go in the eye. Warn the patient not to squeeze his eye shut; blinking is okay.

Caution: do not send the patient out with a bottle of eye drops to keep comfortable. Used more than once, these drops retard healing of an eye injury and may cause blindness. Use HOMATROPINE ophthalmic drops to keep the patient comfortable longer.

Dosage: 1 or 2 drops in the affected eye about 20 seconds before you begin examination or removal of the foreign body from the eye. You may use another drop or two if the first dose wears off during the examination.

ANTACID

Stomach acid neutralizer

Safety class: 1   Stability: A

Brand names: Maalox and others.

Supplied as liquid or tablets, usually containing Magnesium Hydroxide or Aluminum Hydroxide. Some Calcium-containing compounds are also available but these should not be used as they, over the long term, aggravate the problems they are intended to treat.

Indications: GASTRITIS, PEPTIC ULCER, vomiting blood.

Contraindications: ACUTE ABDOMEN, KIDNEY DISEASE.

Precautions: stomach acid protects against bacteria. When stomach acids are neutralized by antacids, bismuth preparations or histamine antagonists (e.g. RANITIDINE) this protection is lost so that bacteria are more likely to cause problems.

Maalox may give mild diarrhea. If the patient has HEART FAILURE, give him more DIURETIC if you use Maalox or any sodium-containing antacid.

Do not give this at the same time as DOXYCYCLINE, PHENYTOIN or KETOCONAZOLE.

Dosage: reduce the dose during pregnancy. Adults, severe symptoms: 30 ml by mouth every hour while awake, every 2 to 4 hours at night. A patient may keep a bottle with him and just take a swallow hourly. Reduce dose for children according to weight.

Alternatives: Amphojel, Gelusil, Mylanta; all are nearly equivalent, except some tend to give diarrhea and others tend to constipate.

ANTIBIOTIC CREAM

Topical antibiotic

Safety class: 1   Stability: A

Supplied as tubes of 15gm or 30gm, some varieties being Neosporin, Bacitracin, Polymixin.

Indications: IMPETIGO; various infected wounds. For EAR INFECTION, EXTERNAL, use only preparations labeled "ophthalmic" or "otic".

Contraindications: ALLERGY to any of the components of the particular product.

Dosage: wash the affected area and apply a small amount of the cream daily.

ANTIBIOTIC EYE DROPS / OINTMENT

Topical antibiotic

Safety class: 1   Stability: A

Synonym: ophthalmic drops/ointment

Brand names: Achromycin Ophthalmic (a tetracycline), Chloromycetin Ophthalmic (chloramphenicol), Erythromycin Ophthalmic, Garamycin ophthalmic, Sodium Sulamyd Ophthalmic (a sulfa drug). Many generic preparations are available.

Indications: treatment of an eye injury; treatment after removal of a foreign body; treatment of EYE INFECTION, KERATITIS, TRACHOMA and cuts near the eyes. For severe infections, eye drops are more reliable. Ointment is more convenient. 1% sulfadiazine ointment should be used for KERATITIS due to a fungus. These preparations may also be used for EAR INFECTION, external.

Contraindications: ALLERGY to the antibiotic in the drops or ointment. Do not use ointment if the patient may have a cut or hole in his eyeball. Drops may be used in this case. Do not use any old or contaminated drug; sterility is absolutely essential.

Precautions: gentamycin ophthalmic drops or ointment do not work for TRACHOMA. Note that ophthalmic drops or ointment can be used in ears, but not antibiotic creams or ointments that are not ophthalmic.

Caution: ointment blurs vision for about 10 minutes. Use only products labeled "ophthalmic"; other antibiotic ointments should not be used. Avoid neosporin ophthalmic ointment; allergic reactions are common.

Dosage:

Drops: use 2 drops in affected eye(s) every hour until the condition improves, then every 2 hours.

Ointment: place about 1/4 inch of ointment anywhere inside the lower lid; repeat every 6 hours. Use for 2 weeks in TRACHOMA; until healed plus 2 days for other problems. You must use oral antibiotics also for TRACHOMA.

Alternatives: IODINE EYE DROPS; using human milk as eye drops works fine in some places. It's harmless to try it.

ANTIBIOTIC OINTMENT

Topical antibiotic

Safety class: 1   Stability: A

Includes: Neosporin ointment, Bacitracin ointment, Povidone Iodine Ointment.

Do not use this on the eyelids or in the eyes and ears. For these uses, small tubes labeled "ophththalmic" should be used. If needed for eyes or ears, see the previous entry!

Povidone Iodine Ointment: see Procedures 9 and 10 in Appendix 1 of Volume 1 for preparation of this.

Indications: IMPETIGO, TROPICAL ULCER; put on any wound, open or sewn, to prevent infection.

Contraindications: ALLERGY to ingredient(s) of specific preparation.

Dosage: use sparingly for economic reasons. The amount used does not matter medically. Use until the wound or rash is healed.

ANTIBIOTICS/ANTIMICROBIALS

These are medicines that either kill germs or inhibit their growth. See AMOXICILLIN, AMPICILLIN, CEPHALOSPORIN, CHLORAMPHENICOL, CIPROFLOXACIN, DOXYCYCLINE, ERYTHROMYCIN, GENTAMYCIN, METRONIDAZOLE, NEOSPORIN, PENICILLIN, RIFAMPIN, SPECTINOMYCIN, STREPTOMYCIN, SULFA, TINIDAZOLE, CO-TRIMOXAZOLE. Antibiotic refers to those that counteract bacteria; antimicrobials refer to those that counteract any germ.

ANTIVENIN SERUM / ANTIVENOM SERUM

Safety class: 3   Stability: D

See Snake Bite, Volume 1, Chapter 9.

Artemisinin Combination Therapy (ACT)

See the explanation of this under ACT.

ARTEMISININ

Antimalaria, antischistosome, anti-HIV, possibly anti-cancer

Includes: artemether, artesunate, qinghasou, artemison, dihydroartemisinin.

Safety class: 1

Brand names: Alaxin, Artequik

Stability: varies; Artemether: stability: A. Pregnancy: should be avoided because in early pregnancy, in animals it is toxic to embryos. However, there is no evidence of its being problematic in humans. Also, malaria causes miscarriage, so the risk may be worthwhile. Co-artem has been shown to be safe in pregnancy.

Artemisia is the name of the plant from which the drug, artemisinin, is derived. Some artemisia plants have very little active ingredient, whereas others have a lot. The plants that grow to be about 2 meters tall before they go to seed have adequate active artemisinin. Plants that go to seed at 1 meter are no good. Special seeds, directions and growing conditions are required. The plant is fastidious; it requires moist, cool, high-altitude. Find ANAMED in Germany on the internet for more information.

Artemisinin and qinghasou are synonyms for the active ingredient of the original natural product, a folk medicine from China. Artemisinin is available as oral, suppository and IM injectable forms.

Artemether and artesunate are related medicines that were manufactured from artemisinin. They are expensive. Artemether is available in capsules for oral use and in a stable form for IM injection. Artesunate is available in oral tablets. It is also available in suppository form and for IM and IV use. The brand name of the suppositories is Plasmotrim Rectocaps; they come in 50 mg and 200 mg sizes. It is difficult to make up and use the injectable forms. A good combination is AZITHROMYCIN 750 mg plus artesunate 100 mg, AZITHROMYCIN is a Gram-positive antibiotic that is also active against malaria. It is expensive.

Artemether is sometimes combined with benflumetol, an anti-malarial that lasts for a long time in the blood stream. This seems to be safe and to work well against falciparum malaria. Usual adult tablets contain 20 mg of artemether and 120 mg of benflumetol. Half-sized tablets for children are available.

Artemether-lumefantrine is another drug combination. Brand names are Coartemether, Co-artem, Riamet. There are no significant additional side-effects. Tablet size: 20 mg artemether plus 120 mg lumefantrine. It is safe and effective to use in children. It is frequently counterfeited.

Dihydroartemisinin-piperaquine is another combination. The brand name is Artekin. One tablet contains 40 mg of DHA and 320 mg of piperaquine. There are minimal side-effects.

Artemison is a derivative of artemisinin.

Indications: MALARIA, especially that originating in Southeast Asia. The drug suppresses but does not cure SCHISTOSOMIASIS HEMATOBIUM and SCHISTOSOMIASIS MANSONI. If taken within 21 days after exposure to any SCHISTOSOMIASIS, it decreases the likelihood of KATAYAMA DISEASE. Reportedly the tea, combined with dried moringa leaves, reverses the symptoms of advanced HIV INFECTION, enabling bed-ridden patients to return to work. Reportedly it is active against some CANCERs: melanoma, colon, breast, squamous cell (skin) and endometrial. Reportedly means there is anecdotal, not controlled experimental evidence.

Contraindications: prior ALLERGY to this drug. Pregnancy is no longer a contraindication, though it should be avoided in early pregnancy. When used to treat chloroquine-resistant vivax malaria, particularly in the Pacific area, there are many treatment failures.

Precautions: when used daily, the blood levels drop to about 20% within 5 days. It takes a week for the body to recover, so the stuff starts working again. This effect is due to liver enzymes which can be blocked with ticlopidine, clopidogrel, KETOCONAZOLE or ITRACONAZOLE.

Use it with another anti-malarial drug unless it can be used for a full 7 days without missing any doses. AZITHROMYCIN is a good drug to use with this.

Note that the artemisinin-based drugs are commonly fake and substandard. Don't seek the best price.

Pay attention to expiration dates; it goes bad quickly.

Side-effects: nausea and vomiting at higher doses, sometimes at ordinary doses when using the tea made from the dried leaves. The tea has a wretched taste. Reportedly there can be some adverse effects on hearing and coordination with prolonged usage at high doses. Caffeine-induced insomnia in those otherwise caffeine-tolerant indicates an adequate blood level.

Dosage: if the patient is vomiting, artesunate (and possibly also other forms) may be used rectally at twice the usual oral dose. The dose may have to be increased if used in pregnancy, because pregnant women eliminate the drug faster than non-pregnant patients.

Artemisia-leaf tea: if using good quality dry-leaf artemisia, 1% is artemisinin. Measure out 5 grams (2 tablespoons or 30 ml) of ground dried leaves. Make this up as a tea in a liter of water, using water that is hot but not yet boiling. MALARIA: add a lot of sugar since the taste is terrible. Take 250 ml (one cup) of this tea every 8 hours for 4 doses. HIV INFECTION: 1 liter of tea daily in divided doses for one month. In addition a high-protein diet and 10 grams of Moringa olifiera dried leaves should be given daily. Dried leaf artemisia can be combined with peanut butter or honey (equal volumes, the ground dried leaves being packed) to give a paste that is tolerable to swallow. Used this way the dose is 5 ml a day. Since the artemisia leaf powder, taken this way, is not exposed to heat, the dose of the dry leaf powder is 1 gram per day. Tablets of 250 mg dry leaf powder may be available. Gelatin capsules negate the effects of artemisinin.

The doses below are for MALARIA only; probably the processed drug from pharmaceutical companies does not work for HIV INFECTION.

Artemisinin: use DOXYCYCLINE, MEFLOQUINE or another antimalarial along with this. Oral dose of artemisinin is 10–20 mg/kg daily for 3 days; Adult dose by suppository is 600 mg at 0 and 4 hours, followed by 400 mg at 24, 36, 48 and 60 hours after the initial dose. Reduce dose according to weight for children.

Artesunate suppositories adult dosage is one 200mg suppository at 0, 4, 8, 12, 24, 36, 48 and 60 h; Oral artesunate dosage is 5–6 mg/kg single daily dose x 3 days.

For repeated SCHISTOSOMIASIS exposures, use 6 mg/kg weekly along with PRAZIQUANTEL. IV dosage is 2.4 mg/kg at 0, 12 and 24 hours and then daily.

IV artesunate may be hard to obtain. You should not delay treatment in order to obtain it. All forms are effective; they should be used with MEFLOQUINE, FOSMIDOMYCIN, QUININE or AZITHROMYCIN, possibly with other anti-malarials.

Combination: artesunate plus dapsone plus proguanil— brand name and correct dosage not available— reportedly works well in Thailand where there is much resistant malaria. Observe the contraindications for all three drugs.

Artemether IM injectable dosage is 3.2 mg/kg initially, followed by 1.6 mg/kg daily, for two more days. It is probably less effective than IV artesunate.

Combination: artemether-benflumetol: the usual adult dose is 4 tablets per dose at 0, 8, 24 and 48 hours.

Combination: artemether-lumefantrine. Dose for adults: 4–6 tablets initially followed by 4–6 tablets at 8 hours and then 4–6 tablets twice daily for 2 more days.

Combination: Dihydroartemisinin-piperaquine. Give one tablet for every 20 kg of patient daily for 3 days. Thus a 60 kg adult would get 3 tablets daily for 3 days. The dose is not fussy.

For severe MALARIA:

Day 1 Artemether 3.2 mg/kg IV or IM Otherwise artesunate, 2.4 mg/kg IV at 0, 12 and 24 hours.

Subsequent days: 1.6 mg/kg daily artemether or artesunate 2.4 mg/kg daily until oral therapy is possible. Then use one of the other options to complete 10 days of treatment.

For ordinary MALARIA:

Day 1: oral artesunate 5 mg/kg or oral artemesinin 25 mg/kg

Days 2 &3: MEFLOQUINE 15–25 mg/kg + (either 2.5 mg/kg of artesunate or 12.5 mg/kg artemesinin)

Rectal dosage: rectal dose is 10–20 mg/kg artemisinin initially, after 12 hours, then daily until awake and able to take oral medication.

TOC SYMPTOMS DIFFERENTIALS CONDITIONS DRUG INDEX REGIONAL NOTES INX

TOC   SYMPTOMS   DIFFERENTIALS   CONDITIONS   **DRUG INDEX**   REGIONAL NOTES   INX

ARTIFICIAL TEARS

Wetting agent for ophthalmic use

Safety class: 1   Stability: A

Brand names: Tears Naturale, many others

Indications: dry eyes due to lack of tears, XEROPHTHALMIA, BELL'S PALSY, LEPROSY, OLD AGE.

Contraindications: none

Precautions: be sure not to contaminate the bottle by touching an infected eye with the tip and then touching another eye. Don't use the same bottle for more than 90 days.

Dosage: two drops as often as necessary to keep the eye moist. Patching at night may help.

Alternative: place a hot, wet towel over the eyes for 10 minutes at a time, several times a day.

ASPIRIN

Analgesic; anti-inflammatory; antipyretic

Synonym: acetylsalicylic acid.

Safety class: 2   Stability: A   Pregnancy: undetermined

Brand names: many. Supplied as 325 and 500 mg adult tablets and in 80 mg (USA) and 100 mg (Europe) children's tablets. There is no liquid form.

Indications: fever, mild pain relief, blood clot prevention, ARBOVIRAL FEVER (Ross River fever and SAND FLY FEVER only), ARTHRITIS, CATARACT, fever, HEART FAILURE, KATAYAMA DISEASE, LEPROSY reaction, PLEURISY, RHEUMATIC FEVER, TOXEMIA. Some recommend that anyone over 50 years old should take daily low-dose aspirin.

Contraindications: previous ALLERGY to the drug, previous PEPTIC ULCER or vomiting of blood, any bleeding tendency. Should not be used along with QUININE. Should not be used with any viral illness in children or young adults. It should not be used in any ARBOVIRAL FEVER which potentially could become HEMORRHAGIC FEVER. It should not be used in AFRICAN SLEEPING SICKNESS, ENTERIC FEVER, GOUT, EBOLA VIRUS DISEASE or VISCERAL LEISHMANIASIS.

It should generally not be used in children, breast-feeding mothers or in the presence of G6PD DEFICIENCY.

Precautions: patients with ASTHMA which began in adulthood frequently have aspirin ALLERGY.

Aspirin may provoke internal bleeding. BISMUTH SUBSALICYLATE (Pepto-Bismol) may cause an overdose. Do not take these two drugs together.

Take aspirin with food or milk rather than on an empty stomach.

Aspirin may aggravate hyperactivity in some hyperactive people.

Aspirin interferes with many lab tests; don't believe lab results drawn while the patient is taking this.

Watch the tablet size carefully. The usual tablet size in western countries is 325 mg. Some countries have 500 mg tablets. 5 grains is 325 mg; 7.5 grains is 500 mg.

Side-effects: ringing in the ears.

Overdose and prolonged usage: see Symptom Index, Protocol A.11 for overdose. In severe overdose there is a change in mental functioning: nervousness, hallucinations, confusion, shortness of breath.

Dosage: adult doses are listed; reduce dose according to weight for children.

Pain and fever: 650–1000 mg every 4 hours as needed.

Age over 50 years old: 80–100 mg daily for stroke and blood clot prevention.

ARBOVIRAL FEVER: like ARTHRITIS

ARTHRITIS: begin with 750–850 mg every 6 hours. Give it faithfully on time, not only when symptoms are severe. Increase the dose every 4 days by 150–175 mg per dose until the patient starts to have ringing in his ears; then drop back to the previous dose. **The idea is to give as high a dose as possible, without causing ringing in the ears.** Give this amount until the problem is entirely cleared up and then for another week. Some people must take the drug for years.

CATARACT prevention: one 325 or 500 mg tablet daily.

HEART FAILURE: one 100 or 325 mg tablet daily.

KATAYAMA DISEASE: like ARTHRITIS.

LEPROSY reactions: like ARTHRITIS.

PLEURISY: like ARTHRITIS.

RHEUMATIC FEVER: like ARTHRITIS.

TOXEMIA: 60 mg daily, adult dose.

Alternatives: ACETAMINOPHEN is not as good for ARTHRITIS. IBUPROFEN is an alternative for other ARTHRITIS but not for RHEUMATIC FEVER.

ATOVAQUONE

Anti-protozoa

Safety class: 2   Stability: C   Pregnancy: C

Supplied as 250 mg tablets

Brand name: Mepron; brand name of Atovaquone + PROGUANIL is Malarone. It is very expensive. The usual adult tablets are 250 mg atovaquone plus 100 mg proguanil. Pediatric tablets are 62.5 and 25 mg respectively.

Indications: MALARIA, TOXOPLASMOSIS, occasionally PNEUMONIA in HIV INFECTION, when the patient cannot tolerate CO-TRIMOXAZOLE.

Contraindications: ALLERGY to the drug. If a patient has taken this drug for malaria prevention but he gets malaria anyway, he should not also take it for treatment.

Precautions: it is unknown if there are problems with this in children, during pregnancy or in elderly people. Use cautiously, if at all, in breast-feeding women; in animal studies there was much drug in breast milk. Use only with physician supervision if the person has DIABETES. It may make the diabetes worse. The drug should be taken with food, since more drug gets into the blood stream that way. Do not use this together with ZIDOVUDINE, TETRACYCLINE, METOCLOPRAMIDE RIFAMPIN or RIFABUTIN.

Side-effects: burning upper abdominal pain, nausea, vomiting, diarrhea, insomnia, headache, rash, itching.

Dosage: the drug should be taken with fatty foods for best effect. The dose may need to be decreased in the presence of LIVER DISEASE (see Protocol B.7), LIVER FAILURE or KIDNEY DISEASE.

PNEUMONIA: 750 mg three times a day for 21 days.

MALARIA prevention: 1 adult tablet daily for adults.

Children 10–20 kg get 1 pediatric tablet daily.

Children 21–30 kg get 2 pediatric tablets daily.

Children 31–40 kg get 3 pediatric tabletits daily.

Children 41 kg or more get 1 adult tablet daily.

MALARIA treatment 1000 mg daily for 3 days; this must be used with PROGUANIL. It does not work well alone.

TOXOPLASMOSIS: 750 mg with food for 21 days.

Alternatives: CHLOROQUINE plus CHLORPHENIRAMINE; MEFLOQUINE; FANSIDAR; QUININE; HALOFANTRINE.

ATROPINE

Anticholinergic

Safety class: 3   Stability: C   Pregnancy: C

Supplied as generic drug in ampules and syringes for IM injection. There is no oral form. Use drops labeled "ophthalmic" for eyes.

Indications: some scorpion bites, INSECTICIDE POISONING, PLANT POISONING: muscarine. (These all cause much saliva, abdominal cramps, diarrhea, sweating, paralysis, slow pulse, small pupils and vomiting.) Also used in eye drops to dilate the pupil and relieve the pain of KERATITIS.

Contraindications: do not use this drug if the patient has less than three of the symptoms listed above. Infants are very sensitive to the drug—be particularly careful with dosages and stop if the child becomes excitable or any of his vital signs (pulse, respiratory rate, temperature) becomes grossly abnormal. Do not give in the presence of GLAUCOMA. Should not be used in the presence of myasthenia gravis, a type of muscle weakness. It may aggravate difficult urination in older men.

Side-effects of this class of drugs (anti-cholinergics): constipation, inability to pass urine (especially in older men), susceptibility to HEAT ILLNESS, dry mouth, decrease in sweating, rapid pulse, sensitivity to light, blurred vision.

Give ONLY enough to relieve the symptoms; how much will vary greatly from one patient to the next. Check the pulse. Unless the patient is very seriously ill do not allow the pulse to go above 1.5 times the upper limit of normal for his age. See the listing of normal vital signs in front of the Symptom Index.

Dosage: the following are the doses that you should start with. As long as the patient is very ill, give this amount subcutaneously repeatedly as needed: 10–20 micrograms/kg:

50 kg = 1 mg maximum;

30 kg = 0.6 mg maximum

10 kg = 0.2 mg maximum

The drug should start taking effect in 5 minutes or less.

As eye drops, use 1 drop in the eye as often as necessary to keep the pupil dilated and the eye pain-free. Vision will be blurred. The effects of one drop last up to a week. Assure the patient that it will wear off. Use HOMATROPINE EYE DROPS for shorter duration.

AUGMENTIN

See AMOXICILLIN + CLAVULANIC ACID

AZITHROMYCIN

Antibiotic, Gram-positive and some Gram-negative; macrolide-type

Safety class: 1   Stability: C   Pregnancy: B

Brand name: Zithromax; generic drug is available. Comes in 250 mg capsules and 200 mg/5 ml liquid. There is also an injectable form.

Indications: may be used like ERYTHROMYCIN, but it is more expensive. Also: BARTONELLOSIS (either type); CELLULITIS; CHANCROID; CHLAMYDIA; CRYPTOSPORIDIOSIS; DONOVANOSIS; mild to moderate DYSENTERY; ENTERIC FEVER; GONORRHEA; LYMPHOGRANULOMA VENEREUM; MALARIA; PNEUMONIA; Q FEVER; RESPIRATORY INFECTION; SCRUB TYPHUS; SPOTTED FEVER; STREP INFECTION; SYPHILIS (early); TRACHOMA; TOXOPLASMOSIS; TRENCH FEVER; YAWS.. Some sources say this can be used for PELVIC INFECTION. and others say it should not be used. Seek independent advice.

Contraindications: prior ALLERGY to this drug or to related drugs such as ERYTHROMYCIN or CLARITHROMYCIN; LIVER DISEASE; infants under 3 months old.

Precautions: makes the skin sensitive to the sun; might cause nausea and stomach pain; safety in pregnancy is uncertain. Do not take with antacids because it is then not well absorbed. Do not use this with THEOPHYLLIN, DIGOXIN or any blood thinners.

TOC   SYMPTOMS   DIFFERENTIALS   CONDITIONS   DRUG INDEX   REGIONAL NOTES   INX

The drug should not be combined with other drugs that cause abnormal heart rhythms. The medical jargon is that it prolongs the QT interval.

Side-effects: nausea, vomiting, diarrhea, abdominal pain, loss of appetite, constipation, HEPATITIS, headache, dizziness, mental changes, joint pains, SEIZURES. Rarely it might cause LIVER FAILURE.

Dosage: reduce dose with LIVER DISEASE. For most indications for most adults the usual dose is 500 mg once daily for 3 days unless listed otherwise. Reduce the dose according to weight for children.

BARTONELLOSIS: seek information elsewhere.

CELLULITIS: 250 mg twice daily for 5–10 days.

CHANCROID and CHLAMYDIA: 1 gram single dose

CRYPTOSPORIDIOSIS: 600 mg daily for 28 days, used together with PAROMOMYCIN.

DONOVANOSIS: 1 gram weekly for 6 weeks or 5–10 mg/kg every 8 hours IV for 5–7 days.

DYSENTERY: 1 gram, single dose

ENTERIC FEVER (only mild to moderate, not severe): 500 mg once daily for 7 days.

GONORRHEA: 2 grams, single dose.[1]

LYMPHOGRANULOMA VENEREUM: the dose is uncertain. Seek local advice. In any case it is essential to withdraw pus from the buboe (large, soft lymph node) in addition to giving the antibiotic.

MALARIA: 750 mg twice daily or 1000 mg daily for 3 days, used with ARTEMISININ (artesunate) or with QUININE; don't use this alone. For malaria prevention the dose is 750 mg initially, then 250 mg daily.

PELVIC INFECTION: 1 gram single dose, given with FLUCONAZOLE and SECNIDAZOLE also in single doses. Some protocols call for using this daily for 5 days.

PNEUMONIA: 500 mg on day 1; 250 mg daily on days 2–5— for moderate pneumonia in patients under 60 years old. In those over 60 years old, also use CO-TRIMOXAZOLE for 10 days.

Q FEVER: 10 mg/kg initially, then 5 mg/kg every 6 hours for 4 days

RESPIRATORY INFECTION: 250 mg twice a day for 5–10 days.

SCRUB TYPHUS: 500 mg single dose; this is the drug of choice in pregnancy.

SPOTTED FEVER: 500 mg daily until 3 days after the fever drops.

STREP INFECTION: 500 mg daily x 10 days.

SYPHILIS: 500 mg daily for 10 days. (This may not work as well as PENICILLIN, and there is resistance in some areas.)

TOXOPLASMOSIS: in the presence of AIDS, give 500 mg every 8 hours for 3–6 weeks. In the absence of AIDS, give 500 mg on the first day, then 250 mg daily for the next 4 days.

TRACHOMA: 20 mg/kg to a maximum of 1000 mg, single dose, for mass treatment.

TOXOPLASMOSIS: 500 mg daily, length of time unknown.

TRENCH FEVER: 500 mg daily for 4–6 weeks.

YAWS: 20 mg/kg single dose.

BENZNIDAZOLE

Anti-trypanosome; available in Brazil

Safety class: unknown   Stability: unknown

Brand name: Rochagan

Indication: CHAGA'S DISEASE

Contraindications: unknown; pursue local information on this. The information currently available is inadequate for you to use this for treatment.

Precautions/side-effects: skin rashes occur in half of the patients and nerve inflammations in many later during the course of treatment. Pursue further information before using the drug.

Dosage: seek dosage from another source.

BENZOIC ACID OINTMENT

Topical anti-fungal ointment

Safety class: 1   Stability: A

Supplied as Whitfield's ointment when the benzoic acid is combined with salicylic acid. It inhibits fungal growth and causes the surface layer of skin to shed. See WHITFIELD'S OINTMENT.

BENZOYL PEROXIDE

Anti-acne

Safety class: 1   Stability: A

Brand names: Clearasil and others.

Indications: ACNE.

Contraindications: previous ALLERGY to the drug.

Precautions: discontinue if there is an allergic reaction.

Side-effects: local irritation may occur; stop the drug temporarily. Resume using it in smaller amounts and less frequently.

Dosage: apply 1–3 times daily.

---

1 *This large a dose may cause distressing side-effects, but the alternatives, CIPROFLOXACIN and related drugs, are no longer any good for GONORRHEA in homosexuals or that acquired in urban areas.*

BENZYL BENZOATE

Scabicide

Safety class: 1   Stability: C

Brand names: Ascabiol, Benylate, Demodek, NBIN, Scabanca, Temedex, Tenutex, Vanzoate, Venzonate. Many veterinary forms. Supplied as 50% and 28 % solutions, liquid, in bottles.

Indications: SCABIES. May also help for LICE, but this is questionable.

Contraindications: previous ALLERGY to the drug. The American literature permits usage during pregnancy and infancy, but the British literature says that it is contraindicated. The manufacturer says it should not be used on the head and neck, but other sources say it may be needed there. Some sources say it should not be used in children but these are the main ones that need it. In any case, it is much less toxic than the alternative, LINDANE.

Precautions: this may occasionally cause CONTACT DERMATITIS. Do not use the drug again if this occurs. The patient may still itch for 1–3 weeks after treatment; this does not imply that the treatment failed; it is normal. Do not apply this to the hands of babies and young children who will put their hands in their mouths; it is intended for external use only.

Dosage: have the patient bathe first. Then apply the 28% lotion. If you have 50% lotion, first dilute it with water, 50:50. Apply it while the skin is damp, avoiding the pink, moist areas of genitals and mouth. Be sure to scrub the fingernails and be sure there is medication beneath them. Fingernails commonly transmit scabies. Let the first application dry. Then apply a second layer and let that dry. Bathe 48 hours later. Repeat the treatment in 7–10 days if there are new scabies spots. Launder clothing and bedding, putting them out in the sun to dry.

Alternatives: Crotamiton; LINDANE (which may not be used during pregnancy or infancy); Malathion 0.5%; SULFUR in petroleum jelly.

BEPHENIUM HYDROXYNAPHTHOATE

Dewormer, anthelmintic; available in Kenya

Safety class: 1   Stability: A

This is an old dewormer, expensive and not very good. If you are forced to use it, read the directions with the product.

Alternatives: ALBENDAZOLE, FLUBENDAZOLE, MEBENDAZOLE, PIPERAZINE plus TETRACHLOROETHYLENE, PYRANTEL PAMOATE.

BIRTH CONTROL PILLS

Hormone

Safety class: 2   Stability: C

Brand names: Demulen, Enovid, Loestrin, Modicon, Norinyl, Ortho-Novum, Ovulen, many others.

Indications: abnormal menstruation, prevention of pregnancy.

Contraindications: heavy cigarette smoking, HYPERTENSION, family history of blood clots or STROKE, artificial heart valve, age over 40, CANCER of the breast or genital or urinary area. The birth control pills with two drugs in them (progesterone and estrogen) are contraindicated in breast-feeding mothers since they dry breast milk. They should not be used in persons who have PORPHYRIA, a hereditary disease.

Precautions: the stronger kinds (those with higher numbers after the name) and to a lesser extent the others, are associated with an increased risk of STROKE and blood clots, especially for patients who eat a Western diet, are heavy cigarette smokers or have HYPERTENSION. The pills may aggravate MIGRAINE headaches. Use no-estrogen tablets in breast-feeding women. Many different drugs interfere with the contraceptive function of BCP's. Use another form of contraception additionally while taking any other medication or seek independent information concerning the status of the particular drugs that you must take.

Dosage: one tablet daily according to directions.

BISMUTH SUBCITRATE

This is another form of bismuth, used the same as BISMUTH SUBSALICYLATE. The usual adult dose is 120 mg four times a day. Sometimes the word "colloidal" is attached to the name.

BISMUTH SUBSALICYLATE

Anti-diarrhea; anti-nausea

Safety class: 1   Stability: A

Brand names: Pepto-bismol, Pink bismuth.

The English drug tripotassium dicitratobismuthate is basically the same as BISMUTH SUBSALICYLATE, but it should not be used in KIDNEY DISEASE. Also see colloidal BISMUTH SUBCITRATE (previous entry).

Indications: TURISTA, nausea, PEPTIC ULCER. The crushed tablets may be made into a paste and used on HERPES as well as the rash of MEASLES.

Contraindications: easy bleeding from any cause. Prior ALLERGY to the drug; do not use at the same time as ASPIRIN or IBUPROFEN or medication to lower the blood sugar in DIABETES. Do not use this along with medication for GOUT. If used along with DOXYCYCLINE or TETRACYCLINE, separate the times by at least 2 hours. Even then, the bismuth may bind to the doxycycline or tetracycline so it does not work. Do not use it by mouth in the third trimester of pregnancy or in children or young adults with any viral illness. This drug may interfere with the test for urine glucose.

Side-effects: temporary darkening of stool and tongue. It may aggravate hyperactivity. The medication is visible on x-ray.

Dosage: reduce the dose in the elderly.

PEPTIC ULCER: 1 tablet or 1 teaspoon (5 ml) of liquid every 6 hours for 14 days.

TURISTA (traveler's diarrhea) preventive: 2 tablets or 2 teaspoons of liquid 4 times a day. Tablets should be chewed.

Everything else: 2 tablets or 2 teaspoons of liquid every hour as needed to a maximum of 8 daily doses.

Alternatives: RANITIDINE for PEPTIC ULCER. Attapulgite is an aluminum silicate clay preparation that works similarly and is useful for mild diarrhea.

BITHIONOL

Anthelmintic, specifically for the flukes. Not available in the USA or in Canada; available in Turkey and many other places.

Safety class: 2   Stability: unknown

Brand names: Actamer, Bitin, Lorothidol; veterinary.

Indications: LIVER FLUKE [fasciola (very good), clonorchis (helps somewhat)], PARAGONIMIASIS, TAPEWORM.

Contraindications: prior ALLERGY to this drug.

Precautions: it may cause abdominal distress, hives and some protein in the urine. It is essential to give a laxative after treatment for pork TAPEWORM. Dispose of the stool carefully since it is infectious—will cause CYSTICERCOSIS.

Dosage: seek confirmation locally.

LIVER FLUKEs: 30–50 mg/kg by mouth every other day for 20–30 days.

PARAGONIMIASIS: same as LIVER FLUKE.

TAPEWORM: dosage unknown

Alternative: PRAZIQUANTEL.

CALCIUM

Mineral

Safety class: 1, oral   Stability: A

Brand names: too numerous to mention.

Indications: TOXEMIA, MENOPAUSE, EBOLA VIRUS DISEASE, some hormonal problems. IV calcium gluconate is useful for the spasms associated with CHOLERA.

Contraindications: rarely some hormonal problems. Do not use without independent advice along with any heart medicines as it may alter the functioning of these.

Precautions: in people who have PEPTIC ULCER, this may make the condition worse. It may lessen the absorption of other nutrients. Calcium lactate tablets should be chewed.

Side-effects: constipation.

Dosage: 500 mg four times a day.

CAMBENDAZOLE

Dewormer, anthelmintic, mainly veterinary

Safety class: 2 or 3   Stability: unknown

Pregnancy: unknown; suspected of causing harm.

Brand names: Ascapilla, Bonlam, Camben, Camvet, Equiben, Novazole, Noviben, Porcam. Available in the USA, Brazil.

Indications: STRONGYLOIDIASIS. It is probably also effective for other worm problems.

Contraindications: ALLERGY to the drug, pregnancy.

Precautions: as of this writing, this is a veterinary drug which is gradually being approved for human use.

Dosage: a single dose of 5 mg/kg; 300 mg is the usual adult dose.

CARBAMAZEPINE

Safety class: 3   Stability: C   Pregnancy: D

Brand names: Tegretol, Epitrol.

Indications: SEIZURES, EPILEPSY, maybe ATTENTION DEFICIT DISORDER.

Contraindications: this is useful for some kinds of seizures only; it is contraindicated for other kinds. Thus it should not be used without professional advice, especially for Asians. It is contraindicated in pregnancy and breast feeding.

Precautions: this sometimes damages the bone marrow, an effect that may be fatal. It interacts badly with some other drugs, including BIRTH CONTROL PILLS, Do not use this with ISONIAZID. Stop if the patient develops a rash. Caution with LIVER DISEASE or LIVER FAILURE.

Dosage: adults: 200 mg daily to start out; this may be increased to twice, thrice or four times daily. Over time the required dosage increases somewhat. Don't take any more than 400 mg at one time.

CARBAPENEMs

This is a class of antibiotics closely related to and described under CEPHALOSPORINs. Examples are imipenem with cilastatin, meropenem, ertapenem. Seek independent information before using these.

CEPHALOSPORINs

Safety class: 2   Stability: variable, many B

Includes: cefalexin, cefotaxime, ceftazidine, ceftriaxone, cefuroxime (and others).

Note that this is a large class of drugs; as listed below. Closely related classes such as monobactams and carbapenems are listed herein also.

Cephalosporins are divided into four groups

First-generation cephalosporins are best for Gram-positive infections; they may work for some Gram-negative.

Second-generation work for Gram-positive and negative, but are ideal for neither.

Third-generation are good mainly for Gram-negative but they also work for some Gram-positive.

Cephalosporin-related drugs cover most Gram-positive and Gram-negative.

Indications: ABSCESS, ACUTE ABDOMEN, CAT-SCRATCH DISEASE (third generation), CELLULITIS, CHANCROID, DONOVANOSIS, EAR INFECTIONS, ENTERIC FEVER, EXFOLIATIVE DERMATITIS, GALLBLADDER DISEASE, GONORRHEA,[1] KIDNEY INFECTION, LYME DISEASE, MEASLES complications, MENINGITIS, OSTEOMYELITIS, PELVIC INFECTION, PNEUMONIA, PYOMYOSITIS, SEPSIS, STREP THROAT, SYPHILIS, URINARY INFECTION, wound infections.

Contraindications: prior ALLERGY to any cephalosporin is a contraindication to all cephalosporins and related drugs for the rest of the patient's life.

Precautions: check the internet for additional and more recent precautions. Sometimes people who have an ALLERGY to PENICILLINs are also allergic to cephalosporins. Don't use these drugs in penicillin-allergic patients unless you have EPINEPHRINE on hand and you have reviewed what to do in an allergic emergency (see Volume 1, Chapter 4).

Some of these drugs are toxic for those with KIDNEY DISEASE. (If your patient has a normal blood pressure [apart from pressure-lowering medications] and a normal urine dipstick, he does not have kidney disease.) In the presence of kidney problems, use these drugs only with expert medical advice.

Do not use higher doses with PROBENECID; the amounts in the blood might increase to the point of making the patient toxic.

Stop the drug for any of these:

- new-onset SEIZURES
- new-onset severe diarrhea
- new-onset skin condition
- new-onset KIDNEY DISEASE
- new-onset LIVER FAILURE
- SERUM SICKNESS due to the drug (this is rare except for cefachlor, in which it is common.)
- new-onset bleeding problems, rare except for cefoperazone and cefotetan, in which it is common.

Some of these can cause falsely positive tests for sugar in the urine.

Dosages and uses: see the following tables.

The duration of therapy should be until the problem is completely gone plus another 2–3 days, unless specified otherwise. MENINGITIS must be treated for 2 weeks; OSTEOMYELITIS must be treated for 6 weeks. Any disease that makes the patient sick enough to be bedridden should be treated for a minimum of 10–14 days. If current product information is available, believe that rather than the dosages given here. In particular, lower doses might be useful for less serious infections. Nationals in developing countries frequently respond well to low doses. The doses given are for the more serious conditions.

Choosing a specific drug

If you have one of these drugs, check if it is good for the disease you intend to treat with it. If you don't have any of these, make a list of which might be helpful and which generation each of these is. Then go to a pharmacy and ask for one of them. If the pharmacist doesn't have any of those listed, ask him for another cephalosporin of the same generation. Look at the package insert to check if it is useful for the purpose you have in mind.

If a drug that you have on hand is not listed, find out if it is a first, second or third generation cephalosporin. Many drugs of the same generation will be useful for the same sorts of things. Exceptions are: for MENINGITIS, LYME DISEASE, GONORRHEA and CHANCROID, only use drugs listed for these diseases. Most cephalosporins are useful for OSTEOMYELITIS, skin and soft tissue infections, URINARY INFECTIONS and PNEUMONIA, unless listed otherwise.

First-generation cephalosporins are good for Gram-positive infections mostly.

Second-generation cephalosporins cover both Gram-positive and Gram-negative, but neither very well.

Third-generation cephalosporins are good for mostly Gram-negative infections.

---

1 Although these drugs work for gonorrhea, they do not generally work for CHLAMYDIA which is frequently clinically indistinguishable and is very common in the developing world.

First-generation cephalosporins

Abbreviations used in the tables:

A = abdominal infections; Bj = bone/joint; Ch = chancroid; Ef = enteric fever; Ent = ear/nose/throat; G = gonorrhea; M = meningitis; O = other; P = pneumonia; Se = sepsis; Sk = skin/soft tissue*; U = Urinary tract

* *This includes ABSCESS, CELLULITIS, EXFOLIATIVE DERMATITIS, PYOMYOSITIS, IMPETIGO (severe), wound infections. CAT SCRATCH DISEASE involves the skin and soft tissue but it reportedly should be treated only with third-generation cephalosporins.*

generic Brand names	Route	Good for:[1]	Not for:	Cautions[2]	Kinds of bacteria	Usual dosage in adults
cephalexin **Keflex Panixine**	oral, empty stomach	Bj, Ent, Sk, P, U	G, Ef, M	usual	Gram-pos, some Gram-neg	250–500 mg every 6 hours
cefadroxil **Duracef, Ultracef, Baxan**	oral	P, Sk, U; ?A	Ent, M, G	usual	Gram-pos, some Gram-neg	0.5–1 gm every 12–24 hours
cephradine **Anspor, Velosef**	oral	Ent, Sk, P, U	M, Ef	usual	Gram-pos, some Gram-neg	0.25–1 gm every 6–12 hours
cefazolin **Ancef, Kefzol**	IM/IV	Bj, P, U, Sk, Se	M, Ef	usual	Gram-pos, some Gram-neg	0.25–1.5 gm every 6–12 hours

1 A drug still might not work for these conditions if the particular disease is caused by bacteria that are resistant to it.

2 That is, in addition to the general cautions listed in the text under Cephalosporins in the Drug Index.

Second-generation cephalosporins

generic Brand name	Route of Admin.	Good for:[1]	No	Cautions[2]	Kinds of bacteria	Usual dosage in adults
cefachlor **Cechlor**	oral, empty stomach	Ent, P, S, U, ? A	M	SERUM SICKNESS	Gram-pos, Gram-neg	250–500 mg every 8 hours
cefamandole **Mandole**	IM/IV	A, Bj, Ent, Sk, U	Ef, M	usual and like antabuse[3]	Gram-neg, some Gram-pos	1–2 gm every 4-8 hours
cefoxitin **Mefoxin**	IM/IV	A, Bj, C, G,[4] P, Sk, Se, U,	M	low blood pressure	Gram-neg anaerobes[5]	1000–2000 mg IM or IV every 6 hours
loracarbef **Lorabid**	Oral	Ent, Sk, P, U	M, Se	usual	Gram-pos, some Gram-neg	200-400 mg every 12 hours
cefuroxime **Ceftin[6]** **Zinacef**	oral IM/IV	Bj, Ent, G, M, P, Sk, O[7]		take orally with food; occasional bleeding	Gram-neg, some Gram-pos	Bj, Sk: 0.25–1.5 gm every 12 hours inj.; G: 1 gm single dose; M: 60 mg/kg IV, 3 g max, every 8 hours; Ent, P: 250 mg twice daily oral

1 A drug might not work for these conditions if the particular disease is caused by bacteria that are resistant to it.

2 That is, in addition to the general cautions listed in the text under Cephalosporins in the Drug Index.

3 The patient becomes very ill if he drinks any alcohol or even gets alcohol on his skin.

4 2000 mg IM single dose with 1000 mg of probenecid.

5 These are infections that occur in wounds, in the context of surgery, and/or those that have foul-smelling pus.

6 This is cefuroxime axetil, the oral drug, which should be taken with food. Zinacef is the injectable form.

7 Early LYME DISEASE.

TOC SYMPTOMS DIFFERENTIALS CONDITIONS DRUG INDEX REGIONAL NOTES INX

Third-generation cephalosporins

Abbreviations used in the tables:

A = abdominal infections; Bj = bone/joint; Ch = chancroid; Ef = enteric fever; Ent = ear/nose/throat; G = gonorrhea; M = meningitis; O = other; P = pneumonia; Se = sepsis; Sk = skin/soft tissue*; U = Urinary tract

* *This includes abscess, CELLULITIS, EXFOLIATIVE DERMATITIS, PYOMYOSITIS, IMPETIGO (severe), wound infections. CATSCRATCH DISEASE involves the skin and soft tissue but it reportedly should be treated only with third-generation cephalosporins.*

Names	Route	Good for	Not for	Cautions	Kinds of bacteria	Usual dosage, adults
cefixim Suprax	oral	Ent, P, G	Sk, Bj, Se, M, Ef, U	usual	Gram-neg mostly and LEPTOSPIROSIS	G: 400 mg single dose Other: 400 mg, daily
ceftriaxone Rocephin	IM/IV	Bj, Ch, Ent,[1] Ef, G,[2] M, O,[3] Sk, U	Chlamydia	not in newborns with jaundice; not with calcium solutions[4]	Gram-pos Gram-neg LEPTOSPIROSIS	A, M, U, Sk: 1–2 gm, 1–2 x daily; IM in children: 100 mg/kg daily for 14 days. Ch, G: 250 mg single dose Ef: 2 gm daily x 10 days

1 *Ear infections in children: 50 mg/kg single dose.*

2 *Dosage for GONORRHEA eye infections in newborns: 50 mg/kg single dose. Does not work for chlamydia which may be indistinguishable with your facilities.*

3 *LYME DISEASE (1-2 gm every 12-24 hours x 14 days), SYPHILIS (1 gm IM daily x 10 days for early disease, x 14 days for secondary and tertiary disease), MENINGITIS prevention (125 mg IM once).*

4 *Also this, more than the other cephalosporins, is apt to cause KIDNEY FAILURE.*

Non-cephalosporin, related drugs

generic Brand name	Type	Route	Good for[1]	Not for:	Cautions	Kinds of bacteria	Usual dosage in adults
aztreonam Azactam	monobactam	IM/IV	Se, P, Sk, U, A, G	M, Bj	usual	Gram-neg	0.5–2 gm every 8 hours; G 1 gm single dose
meropenem Merrem	carbapenem	IV	A, M, Sk, M[2]		usual	Gram-pos Gram-neg	0.5–1 gm every 8 hours
Imipenem Primaxin	carbapenem	IM/IV	A, P, U, Se, Sk, Bj	M	usual, decrease dose if less than 70 kg	Gram-neg Gram-pos	0.5–1 gm every 12 hours
Cefotetan Cefotan	cephamycin	IM/IV	A, G	M, Eye	bleeding with large doses	Gram-neg anaerobes	1–2 gm every 12 hours

1 *A drug still might not work for these conditions if the particular disease is caused by bacteria that are resistant to it.*

2 *Only in patients more than three months old.*

CHAMOMILE TEA

This is an herb tea, widely available, which is useful for COLIC in babies and for abdominal cramps due to dietary indiscretion in adults. It is a useful alternative to DICYCLOMINE to help distinguish between belly pain that needs a surgeon and belly pain that will run its course and go away. Reportedly in large amounts it is toxic to the liver.

CHLORAMPHENICOL

Antibiotic (mostly Gram-negative)

Safety class: 2+   Stability: C

Pregnancy: C, don't use near delivery time

Brand names: Chloromycetin, Mychel-S; generic veterinary drug available. Supplied as 250 and 500 mg capsules. There is a long-acting injectable form called Tifomycine. The nearly identical drug, thiamphenicol, which is good for GONORRHEA and some MENINGITIS, is included here.

Indications, usual: ABSCESS, ACUTE ABDOMEN, DONOVANOSIS, EAR INFECTION, ENTERIC FEVER, EYE INFECTION with fever, GONORRHEA, MENINGITIS, PLAGUE, SEPSIS, SPOTTED FEVER, TRACHOMA, TYPHUS.

Indications, occasional: BARTONELLOSIS, BRUCELLOSIS, CHOLERA, DYSENTERY, LEPTOSPIROSIS, OSTEOMYELITIS, PERTUSSIS, PIG-BEL, PNEUMONIA, TREPONARID, TROPICAL ULCER, TULAREMIA, wound infections.

Indications, rare: KIDNEY INFECTION, LYME DISEASE, PERTUSSIS, skin ulcers due to SICKLE CELL DISEASE, SYPHILIS, URINARY INFECTION.

Contraindications: previous ALLERGY or other reaction to this drug, necessitating stopping it. Do not use during labor and delivery, or the baby may die shortly after birth; see Volume 1 Chapter 6. Do not use it in nursing mothers. Do not use this in diabetic patients who are taking oral medication to lower their blood sugar. Do not use it in non-African patients who have G6PD DEFICIENCY. It is generally tolerated in those of African genetic heritage.

Precautions: many physicians are afraid of this drug because of rare fatal reactions due to bone marrow suppression. Such reactions are rarer than fatal reactions to PENICILLIN; they do occur in 1/30,000 patients. They are extremely rare in those of African genetic heritage. If a patient develops a new infection or ANEMIA while on this drug, stop it immediately. Be sure the patient really needs it before giving it. Do not use it for any viral illness. If a newborn stops nursing, develops a swollen abdomen and looks bluish, starting 2–9 days after beginning the drug, stop the drug immediately. ACETAMINOPHEN increases the amount of chloramphenicol in the blood stream and may cause toxicity.

Side-effects: rashes and fevers due to the drug; nausea; vomiting; an unpleasant taste in the mouth; diarrhea; irritation in the private parts.

These effects occur in only a small percentage of patients. Infants may have a decrease in appetite. When giving this drug for SYPHILIS, BRUCELLOSIS or ENTERIC FEVER, the patient may get sicker before he begins to get better.

Dosage: reduce doses for infants, in LIVER DISEASE and in KIDNEY DISEASE.

The following doses are for adults except where stated otherwise. Reduce dose according to weight for children. For ordinary chloramphenicol, injectable IM dose equals oral.

Long-acting, injectable chloramphenicol is one dose IM for any and all diseases:

Adults and children over 40 kg.: 3 grams IM

Patients 25–39 kg.: 2 grams IM

Children 10–24 kg.: 1 gram IM

ABSCESS: 250 mg by mouth every 6 hours until healed plus 2 days or for 10 days, whichever comes first.

ACUTE ABDOMEN: adult dose is 25 mg/kg IM every 6 hours for 14 days. Children get 17 mg/kg every 6 hours. Newborns over a week old (full term) get 8 mg/kg every 6 hours; those under a week old (full term) get 4 mg/kg every 6 hours. See precautions for newborns. For premature babies, use the dose for those under a week old until they weigh 4 kg or more.

BARTONELLOSIS: 500 mg by mouth every 6 hours for 14 days.

BRUCELLOSIS: 250 mg by mouth every 6 hours; use this with two other antibiotics.

CHOLERA: 500 mg by mouth every 6 hours until the diarrhea has decreased.

DONOVANOSIS: 500 mg three times daily until entirely healed plus another week.

DYSENTERY: same as CHOLERA.

EAR INFECTION: 250–500 mg by mouth every 6 hours for 10 days. Begin at the higher dose and decrease the dose as the patient feels better.

ENTERIC FEVER: same as BARTONELLOSIS.

EYE INFECTION: same as ACUTE ABDOMEN.

GONORRHEA: 500 mg of thiamphenicol 5 times a day for 2 days.

KIDNEY INFECTION: 500 mg by mouth every 6 hours for 5 days.

LEPTOSPIROSIS:[1] 2000–3000 mg IM or by mouth initially, then 250–500 mg every 6 hours until the temperature is normal plus 3 more days.

LYME DISEASE: same as EAR INFECTION.

MENINGITIS: same as ACUTE ABDOMEN.

OSTEOMYELITIS: 500 mg by mouth every 6 hours for 6 weeks minimum. Use it with another antibiotic.

PERTUSSIS: same as BARTONELLOSIS; not useful after the first week of symptoms.

PIG-BEL: same as ACUTE ABDOMEN.

---

1 *It is useless to give any antibiotic for leptospirosis if the patient has been ill for 4 days or more.*

PLAGUE: 500 mg oral, IM or IV, every 6 hours for 5 days.

PNEUMONIA: same as EAR INFECTION

SEPSIS: same as ACUTE ABDOMEN.

SICKLE CELL DISEASE skin ulcers: same as ABSCESS.

SPOTTED FEVER: same as LEPTOSPIROSIS.

SYPHILIS: same as BARTONELLOSIS.

TRACHOMA: same as EAR INFECTION.

TREPONARID: same as BARTONELLOSIS.

TROPICAL ULCERS: same as ABSCESS.

TULAREMIA: same as BARTONELLOSIS.

TYPHUS: same as LEPTOSPIROSIS; treat for 7 days.

URINARY INFECTION: same as KIDNEY INFECTION.

Wound infection: same as ABSCESS.

Alternatives: nothing else cheap is as good, but use AMPICILLIN for MENINGITIS, TYPHUS, ENTERIC FEVER, PIG-BEL, KIDNEY INFECTION or ACUTE ABDOMEN. CEPHALOSPORINs and CIPROFLOXACIN are more expensive alternatives.

CHLOROQUINE

Antimalarial

Safety class: 2   Stability: C   Pregnancy: used routinely without any problem; no formal classification

This is very toxic in overdose for children; a small overdose can kill, especially on an empty stomach.

Brand names: Aralen, Avlochlor, Nivaquine, Resochin. Supplied as tablets with 125, 250 or 500 mg chloroquine phosphate of which 60% is chloroquine base. IM chloroquine usually comes as 40 or 50 mg base per ml.

Includes: Hydroxychloroquinesulfate (Plaquenil). Same actions, precautions and dosage as Chloroquine.

Indications: MALARIA prevention and treatment, amebic DYSENTERY if used with DOXYCYCLINE, LEPROSY reaction, ARTHRITIS.

Contraindications: ALLERGY to this drug. If given at the same time as oral cholera vaccine, the vaccine will not work properly. It is better to delay giving one or the other. Do not give it to persons with severe G6PD DEFICIENCY or to those with PORPHYRIA (a hereditary problem). Do not use in patients who have EPILEPSY. Do not use this along with METHYLENE BLUE. Do not use it in severe LIVER DISEASE.

Side-effects: headache, blurred vision, abdominal pain, temporary emotional problems (such as nightmares) with each dose (an effect that seems to be more prominent with old drug). Itching is common in black skin; it may respond to vitamin B complex or MULTIVITAMINS. Sometimes there is nausea, vomiting, diarrhea and abdominal pain.

Cautions:

- Used over the long term, chloroquine sometimes damages vision. The safe upper limit for long-term use is 2.5 mg/kg chloroquine base per day or 4 mg/kg chloroquine phosphate tablets.

- It is acceptable to use larger amounts for a few days now and then, as long as the average over a month is no more than the amounts stated above.

- An early sign of eye problems is seeing halos around lights. Check vision when using chloroquine at higher doses and discontinue if vision decreases.

- Neurological problems are apt to become worse with this drug.

- The drug is sometimes associated with altered heart rhythms which may cause sudden death. Thus it should not be combined with other such drugs. The medical jargon is that it prolongs the QT interval.

- Falciparum MALARIA is usually resistant to this drug.

Dosage: the dose is particularly fussy in children; be sure to weigh a child rather than estimating weight. A small overdose can kill.

Reduce the dose in those with mild LIVER DISEASE.

When determining dosage, keep in mind that the dose is usually given in terms of base. Base refers to chloroquine itself. Chloroquine is always attached to other substances. For example, chloroquine phosphate comes as 125 and 250 mg tablets, of which 60% is base. (The rest is phosphate.) Therefore these tablets contain 75 and 150 mg of base respectively.

Amebic DYSENTERY: adults get 150 mg base by mouth, twice a day for 20 days. Reduce dose according to weight in children. The patient must get DOXYCYCLINE also.

ARTHRITIS: 250 mg (one tablet) daily or 500 mg twice a week. This helps about 75% of patients. Stop it if it doesn't help. Stop it if eyesight worsens.

LEPROSY reaction: adult dose is 200 mg base twice a day for 14 days.

MALARIA prevention: adults take 300 mg base by mouth, once a week. Reduce dose according to weight for children. Begin 2 weeks before going and continue for 6 weeks after leaving.

MALARIA treatment Mild attack: adults get 600 mg of base by mouth initially, 300 mg base 6 hours later, then 300 mg base 12 hours after the second dose, 300 mg base 24 hours after the third dose and daily for a week total. Children get 10 mg/kg base by mouth initially, then 5 mg/kg at 6 hour, 12 hour and 24 hour intervals, same schedule as for adults. The children's dose is not to exceed the adult dose.

If the patient is vomiting first try to use PROMETHAZINE and oral chloroquine. If this does not work give adults 200 mg base IM every 6 hours for 2 doses; children get chloroquine base: 5 mg/kg IM initially, 6 hours later, then daily for 2 days.

Alternatives: adding CHLORPHENIRAMINE reverses chloroquine resistance of falciparum MALARIA in the Eastern Hemisphere. Alternatively, use FANSIDAR, QUININE, MEFLOQUINE or an ACT drug.

CHLORPHENIRAMINE / CHLORPHENAMINE

Antihistamine

Safety class: 1   Stability: A   Pregnancy: B

Supplied as tablets with 4 mg.

Brand names: Chlortrimeton, Piriton, Calimal.

Indications: ALLERGY, MALARIA

Contraindications: simultaneous treatment with a type of antidepressant called MAOI which stands for monoamine oxidate inhibitors.

Side-effects: sleepiness, worsening of GLAUCOMA, constipation, inability to pass urine (especially in older men), susceptibility to HEAT ILLNESS, dry mouth, decrease in sweating, rapid pulse, sensitivity to light, blurred vision, seizures in children, agitation in elderly.

Dosage: reduce dose in elderly and in patients with chronic RESPIRATORY INFECTION. Adult dose is 4 mg every 6 hours; reduce dose according to weight for children.

Alternatives: DEXCHLORPHENIRAMINE is a similar drug. The usual dose is half that listed above. It is unknown if this works for malaria or not.

CHLORPROGUANIL

Malaria preventive.

Safety class: 1   Stability:A

Brand name: Lapudrine

Indications: MALARIA prevention.

Contraindications: ALLERGY to the drug.

Side-effects: occasional nausea and loss of appetite which decreases with continued usage.

Dosage: adult dose is 20 mg by mouth twice weekly. Reduce dose according to weight for children.

CHLORPROMAZINE

Sedative, anti-nausea.

Safety class: 2   Stability: C   Pregnancy: no assigned category; animal studies show fetal toxicity.

Brand names: Largactil, Thorazine. Comes in 10, 25 and 50 mg tablets and in IM injectable.

Indications: CHOLERA, emotional upset, MENTAL ILLNESS, HICCUPS, pain, vomiting, in a cream for CUTANEOUS LEISHMANIASIS, used to decrease shivering when treating a person for HEAT ILLNESS, TETANUS, used to relieve suffering in terminal illness.

Contraindications: ALLERGY to this drug; KIDNEY DISEASE, CIRRHOSIS, LIVER FAILURE, EPILEPSY. Do not give to those with PARKINSON'S DISEASE, LIVER DISEASE, or HEART FAILURE. Do not give this to patients who are already sedated for some other reason. Do not give it to those on antidepressants. Do not give to nursing mothers.

Precautions: this can cause loss of muscle control, particularly of the jaws. It makes the skin sensitive to sunburn. It also makes patients sensitive to HEAT ILLNESS. Patients should not drink alcoholic beverages while taking this. ANTACIDs should not be taken within two hours.

Rarely a patient may develop a high fever, stiff muscles and widely variant vital signs. Stop the drug, cool the patient and never use this or related drugs on him or her again. See NEUROLEPTIC MALIGNANT SYNDROME.

Do not crush or chew tablets. Wear gloves when using liquid forms; do not get the medication on your hands.

This drug interferes with many laboratory tests, including pregnancy tests. Don't believe lab tests drawn while the person is on this drug.

Warn the patient not to engage in any dangerous activity while taking this drug.

Side-effects: the most common one is a fall in blood pressure when the patient suddenly stands. Other effects are faintness, rapid heart rate, a stuffy nose, a dry mouth, blurred vision and worsening of URINARY OBSTRUCTION. These effects occur in only a small percentage of patients.

Overdose and prolonged usage: if given routinely for weeks or months, this can cause PARKINSON'S DISEASE with involuntary movements and trembling. It can also cause LIVER FAILURE; see Protocol B.7.

Dosage: reduce the dose in the elderly and, those with KIDNEY DISEASE, GLAUCOMA or URINARY OBSTRUCTION. It is very toxic; an overdose can kill.

The dose by IM injection is the same as that by mouth.

CHOLERA: 10 mg every 6 hours adult dose; reduce dose by weight for children.

CUTANEOUS LEISHMANIASIS: grind 1000 mg (twenty 50 mg tablets) and mix with 50 grams (a little less than 1/4 cup) of methylsalicylate cream. Use this three times a day for a month, applying it directly on the affected skin area.

Emotional upset, HICCUPS, pain, vomiting, shivering: 10–25 mg every 6 hours.

TETANUS: see TETANUS in the Condition Index.

Terminal care: start with 25 mg every 6 hours and increase the dose as necessary. A probable maximum would be 200 mg every 6 hours. Don't be rigid. Use as much as necessary to relieve suffering.

CHOLESTYRAMINE

Absorbent

Safety class: 1   Stability: C   Pregnancy: C

Brand names: Colestid, Questran. Similar, related drugs are colestipol and colesevelam. Supplied in packets of 4 grams each.

Indications: a powder used in the West for high blood cholesterol; in the tropics it is used to treat persistent diarrhea in babies. It is also useful to treat the itching caused by JAUNDICE, KIDNEY DISEASE and SICKLE CELL DISEASE. It may be used for TURISTA: traveler's diarrhea.

Contraindications: constipation, LIVER FAILURE; ALLERGY to the drug.

Precautions: this will inactivate other drugs given at the same time. Stagger the times given; give other drugs at least an hour before or 4–6 hours afterward. Also be aware that the other drugs may fail to work properly.

This interferes with many lab tests—do not believe lab results of blood drawn while the patient was taking this drug.

Side-effects: nausea and excessive gas.

Dosage: for the itching of JAUNDICE: 4 grams 1–3 times daily as needed. For other problems adult dose is 4 gram by mouth before meals and at bedtime. Reduce dose according to weight for children.

CIMETIDINE

Histamine receptor antagonist.

Safety class: 1–3   Stability: C   Pregnancy: B

Brand name: Tagamet, Dyspamet. Supplied as 200, 400 and 800 mg tablets; in liquid it is 300 mg/5ml.

Indications: ANAPHYLAXIS, GASTRITIS, PEPTIC ULCER; used to counteract the abdominal side-effects of steroids such as PREDNISONE and DEXAMETHASONE.

Contraindications: if the patient has LIVER FAILURE or KIDNEY DISEASE, check with a physician about how much to lower the dosage.

Precautions: stomach acid is a defense against bacteria that are taken in by mouth. With this type of medication as well as with ANTACIDs, this barrier is lowered or destroyed. Therefore sanitary food preparation is essential. Patients become vulnerable to TUBERCULOSIS.

Use this only under professional advisement in patients on any other medication. There are interactions with many other medications.

Do not believe lab tests on blood drawn while the patient is taking this drug. The drug interferes with many different tests.

Side-effects: this may cause breast development in males.

Dosage: reduce the dose in the elderly, in those with LIVER DISEASE or KIDNEY DISEASE.

ANAPHYLAXIS: adult dose is 300 mg by any route, every 6 hours for 5 days; reduce dose for children.

PEPTIC ULCER: 400 mg twice daily for 14 days, given along with antibiotics.

For other indications use an adult dose: 400 mg twice a day or 800 mg at night only. Reduce this to 400 mg at night once the symptoms are totally gone.

CIPROFLOXACIN

Quinolone-type antibiotic (Gram-negative and Gram-positive, mostly Gram-negative)

Safety class: 3   Stability: C   Pregnancy: C

Brand names: Cipro, Ciproxin.

Indications: ABSCESS, ANTHRAX, BARTONELLOSIS, BRUCELLOSIS, CHANCROID, EAR INFECTION, ENTERIC FEVER, It can be used to prevent MENINGITIS after an exposure. It is sometimes used for the prevention of traveler's diarrhea: TURISTA. Stubborn infections, not responsive to other medications, especially CHANCROID, CHOLERA, CYCLOSPORIASIS, DONOVANOSIS, bacterial DYSENTERY, GONORRHEA, KIDNEY INFECTION, OSTEOMYELITIS, PNEUMONIA, PROSTATITIS, PYOMYOSITIS, Q FEVER, TUBERCULOSIS, TULAREMIA, TURISTA. Do not use this for PELVIC INFECTION.

Contraindications: EPILEPSY; pregnancy and breast-feeding; age less than 20 if the problem is not life-threatening. Do not use in the presence of psychiatric problems, KIDNEY DISEASE, LIVER FAILURE, with STEROIDS or with blood thinners. Do not use it if LEPTOSPIROSIS, SPOTTED FEVER or TYPHUS is a possible diagnosis (red eyes and/or muscle pains). Seek approval before using this in elderly.

Precautions

If the patient has SEIZURES while on this drug, stop it. If the patient develops numbness, tingling or weakness while taking this, stop it.

Avoid using the drug in the elderly and those on STEROIDS; they may develop tendinitis.

Do not give the drug with ANTACIDs, or it will not work.

If given at the same time as THEOPHYLLINE, reduce the dose of THEOPHYLLINE.

BRUCELLOSIS may relapse after being treated with this.

The drug damages the growth centers of bones in some animals and might do so in humans.

If the patient has a blood test in a hospital laboratory, the test might falsely show liver or kidney abnormalities. Ciprofloxacin in the blood interferes with the blood test.

It is best to give the drug in the morning since it might cause insomnia.

Side-effects: children frequently have joint pains with using this, but the pains disappear when the drug is discontinued. It is apt to cause insomnia.

TOC

SYMPTOMS

DIFFERENTIALS

CONDITIONS

DRUG INDEX

REGIONAL NOTES

INX

Dosage: reduce the dose to 1/2 the usual dose in the presence of KIDNEY DISEASE. For most diseases the usual dosage is 250–750 mg every 12 hours.

ANTHRAX: if the patient is very sick, give 400 mg IV every 12 hours until improved; then change to oral, 500 mg every 12 hours for 60 days. For prevention, 500 mg every 12 hours for 60 days.

BARTONELLOSIS (Oroya form): 500 mg three times daily for 14 days; This will also cure ENTERIC FEVER which frequently coexists.

BRUCELLOSIS: 250–750 mg by mouth every 12 hours for 6 weeks.

CHANCROID: 500 mg every 12 hours for 3 days.

CHOLERA: 250–500 mg every 12 hours until the problem is improved.

CYCLOSPORIASIS: 500 mg every 12 hours for 7–10 days.

DONOVANOSIS: 500 mg every 12 hours for 2 weeks.

DYSENTERY: a single dose of 750 mg is enough.

EAR INFECTION: for a draining ear, make up ear drops using injectable drug in normal saline, 0.2% to 0.5%. In 10 ml of saline put 20–50 mg of drug.

ENTERIC FEVER: 500 mg every 12 hours for 14 days.

GONORRHEA, genital or sore throat: 500 mg single dose.

GONORRHEA, disseminated (skin and/or joint) 500 mg twice daily for at least 3 days.

KIDNEY INFECTION: 500 mg every 12 hours for 5–7 days.

MENINGITIS prevention: 750 mg single dose.

OSTEOMYELITIS: 250–750 mg every 12 hours for 6 weeks.

PNEUMONIA: 500 mg every 12 hours for 10 days.

PROSTATITIS: 500 mg every 12 hours for 10 days.

PYOMYOSITIS: 500 mg every 12 hours for 10 days—the pus must also be drained out.

Q FEVER: 500 mg every 12 hours for 14 days.

TUBERCULOSIS: adult dose is 1500 mg daily.

TULAREMIA: 750 every 12 hours for 10 days; expect relapses in about half of the patients.

TURISTA prevention: 500 mg daily.

Alternatives: other fluoroquinolones such as NORFLOXACIN = Utinor; OFLOXACIN = Tarivid, Pefloxacin. NORFLOXACIN 400 mg or OFLOXACIN 300 mg is equivalent to CIPROFLOXACIN 500 mg.

For treatment of diarrhea, Bicozamycin, aztreonam and rifaximin are non-absorbed (they do not enter the bloodstream but stay in the bowel) antibiotics that might work okay, avoiding side-effects.

For TULAREMIA, alternatives are STREPTOMYCIN, GENTAMYCIN or DOXYCYCLINE.

CLARITHROMYCIN

Macrolide antibiotic, Gram-positives, some others.

Safety class: 1–2   Stability: C   Pregnancy: C

Brand name: Klaricid, Clarosip, Klaricid XL.

Comes in 250 mg tablets.

Indications: BURULI ULCER, CELLULITIS, EAR INFECTION, LEPROSY, sometimes PEPTIC ULCER, PNEUMONIA, RESPIRATORY INFECTION, Mediterranean SPOTTED FEVER, TOXOPLASMOSIS, TUBERCULOSIS.

Contraindications: prior ALLERGY to this or to related drugs such as AZITHROMYCIN or ERYTHROMYCIN. Do not use at the same time as astemizole or terfenadine, two antihistamines without the side-effect of sleepiness. Possibly contraindicated in KIDNEY DISEASE, LIVER DISEASE, pregnancy and breast-feeding.

Precautions: consult a physician before using at the same time as warfarin, THEOPHYLLIN, drugs for HIV INFECTION or CARBAMAZEPINE (Tegretol).

The drug sometimes alters electrical activity in the heart which might cause sudden death. Thus it should not be combined with other such drugs. The medical jargon is that it prolongs the QT interval. See the back cover.

Side-effects: nausea, vomiting, abdominal pain, problems with taste and smell, loss of appetite, HEPATITIS, headache, dizziness, mental changes, KIDNEY DISEASE, joint pains, SEIZURES, skin sun sensitivity. Rarely it might cause LIVER FAILURE. Side-effects occur in a small percentage of patients.

Dosage: do not give in patients with KIDNEY DISEASE unless you consult a physician about dose reduction. For most uses, 250 mg every 12 hours for 7 days; in severe cases 500 mg every 12 hours for 14 days except as listed below.

BURULI ULCER: 7.5mg/kg daily for 8 weeks.

PEPTIC ULCER: 250 mg every 12 hours for 7–14 days.

SPOTTED FEVER: 250–500 mg every 12 hours until 3 days after the fever has dropped.

TUBERCULOSIS: 250–500 mg every 12 hours.

LEPROSY: 500 mg daily

TOXOPLASMOSIS: 2 grams (2000 mg) daily

Alternatives: AZITHROMYCIN for most indications.

CLINDAMYCIN

Antibiotic, Gram-positive/anaerobic/staph

Safety class: 3   Stability: B   Pregnancy: B

Brand names: Dalacin C, Cleocin.

Indications: ABSCESS (if the pus smells foul or not), ANTHRAX, CELLULITIS, DIPHTHERIA, MALARIA, OSTEOMYELITIS, RHEUMATIC FEVER, TOXOPLASMOSIS. It is sometimes used with CIPROFLOXACIN or GENTAMYCIN for treating PELVIC INFECTION. It might be used for some other infections under physician direction.

Contraindications: diarrhea of any sort. If diarrhea develops while the patient is on the drug, it must be discontinued immediately. It should not be used with any anti-diarrhea medications (aside from ORS which is okay) or with ERYTHROMYCIN. It is also contraindicated in CIRRHOSIS and LIVER FAILURE.

Precautions: it is better to use safer antibiotics. Be sure to tell the patient to discontinue the drug if he develops diarrhea while on it. Do not use this for MENINGITIS.

Side-effects: nausea, vomiting, gas.

Dosage: reduce dose in the presence of LIVER DISEASE.

ABSCESS: recommended dosage unknown.

ANTHRAX: 900 mg IV every 8 hours until improved; then change to oral medication. Treat for a total of 60 days.

CELLULITIS: 150–450 mg every 6 hours until better, plus 3 days.

DIPHTHERIA: uncertain but other antibiotics are to be used for 14 days.

MALARIA: this should be used with a second drug. The adult dose is 900 mg by mouth two times a day for 5 days, used with another anti-malarial drug, usually FOSMIDOMYCIN.

OSTEOMYELITIS: 150–300 mg every 6 hours for 6 weeks.

PELVIC INFECTION: 450 mg four times a day for 14 days. If the patient is very ill and if you have IV facilities, you should start with 600 mg IV every 8 hours, (along with GENTAMYCIN) until she is improved, then switch to the oral.

RHEUMATIC FEVER: used after PENICILLIN to thoroughly eliminate the strep: 7 mg/kg three times daily for 10 days.

TOXOPLASMOSIS: 600 mg every 6 hours for 6 weeks, taken along with PYRIMETHAMINE.

CLOFAZAMINE

Anti-leprosy

Safety class: 2   Stability: unknown   Pregnancy: C

Brand names: B663, Lamprene.

Indications: LEPROSY, lepromatous type, maybe BURULI ULCER.

Contraindications: prior ALLERGY to the drug, breastfeeding.

Side-effects: it discolors light-colored skin, possibly permanently and thus should not be used in fair-skinned patients. It turns urine red. It causes nausea, vomiting, abdominal pain and/or diarrhea. It makes skin sensitive to sunburn.

Overdose and prolonged usage: LIVER DISEASE.

Dosage: you may need to reduce the dose in LIVER DISEASE or avoid using this.

BURULI ULCER: dosage unknown; seek alternative advice.

LEPROSY: 50 mg by mouth daily, plus 300 mg once a month. Some authorities recommend a higher dose at first. Do not give over 100 mg daily for more than three months. If the patient is having a LEPROSY reaction, Type 2, use a high dose while decreasing the dose of PREDNISONE. Then reduce the dose of clofazamine.

CLOTRIMAZOLE

Anti-fungal

Safety class: 1   Stability: A

Brand names: Canesten, Empecid, Lotrimin, Mycelex, Mycosporin, Trimysten. Available in creams and lozenges.

Indications: CANDIDIASIS, TINEA, VAGINITIS due to trichomonas.

Contraindications: prior ALLERGY to this drug.

Side-effects: may cause burning and itching.

Dosage:

Skin: apply cream twice a day until the problem is gone plus 2 more days.

Vagina: use the cream daily for 7 days.

Mouth: suck on a lozenge 5 times a day for 14 days.

CLOXACILLIN

Antibiotic, Gram-positive, anti-staph penicillin.

Safety class: 2   Stability: C   Pregnancy: B

Brand names: Cloxapen, Tegopen Available as capsules (250 and 500 mg) and as powder for liquid at 125 mg/5 ml.

Indications: ABSCESS with a fever; ARTHRITIS, if it develops suddenly in one joint only; PYOMYOSITIS; OSTEOMYELITIS; PNEUMONIA, after MEASLES. It is only good for staph.

Contraindications: ALLERGY to any PENICILLIN. Try not to use with DOXYCYCLINE, ERYTHROMYCIN or CHLORAMPHENICOL.

Precautions: observe the patient for ALLERGY: HIVES, swelling or redness of the skin, difficulty breathing, a feeling of faintness. This drug can cause ANAPHYLAXIS just like ordinary PENICILLIN and must be treated accordingly. If there is allergy, the patient may never again take any PENICILLIN-type drug for the rest of his life.

Don't believe lab tests for protein or glucose, taken while the patient is on this drug. The drug interferes with the lab test.

Overdose and prolonged usage: LIVER FAILURE; see Protocol B.7.

Dosage: reduce the dose with KIDNEY DISEASE, possibly also with LIVER FAILURE. Standard dose is 250–500 mg every 6 hours for adults; reduce dose according to weight for children. Give this until the problem is resolved plus for 2 more days. Give it for at least 3 weeks in ARTHRITIS.

Alternatives: flucloxacillin which is better absorbed and thus preferable when and where it is available. An alternative is NITAZOXANIDE.

TOC

SYMPTOMS

DIFFERENTIALS

CONDITIONS

DRUG INDEX

REGIONAL NOTES

INX

CO-ARTEM

A combination antimalarial drug: LUMEFANTRINE plus ARTEMISININ (artemether): fixed combination of 120 mg of lumefantrine with 20 mg of artemether. See the entries for the individual component drugs. The dosage is under ARTEMISININ. This has been shown to be safe in early pregnancy. Because it is expensive, in developing countries it is the most commonly substandard or fake drug. If it doesn't work, that is probably why. Seek drug of European or American origin, which will be expensive

CODEINE

Narcotic, pain medicine, cough medicine.

Safety class: 2   Stability: C, dark.   Pregnancy: C

Brand names: comes combined with other drugs which are labeled with numbers such as Empirin #3, Tylenol #2, etc. Generally #1 contains 7.5 mg, #2 contains 15 mg, #3 contains 30 mg and #4 contains 60 mg of codeine per tablet.

Indications: pain, severe cough.

Contraindications: head injury, shortness of breath, PERTUSSIS, POLIO, ALLERGY to codeine, diarrhea due to antibiotic usage, ASTHMA, chronic RESPIRATORY INFECTION, concurrent usage of other sedative drugs.

Precautions: this simply doesn't work in some people. Codeine decreases the urge to breathe; people who must struggle to breathe lose their incentive.

It causes constipation; consider giving a laxative (MILK OF MAGNESIA). Patients may feel nauseated from codeine, but the nausea usually is not severe enough to cause a problem.

Be very careful when traveling with this drug. It is a narcotic, and you may get a jail term if you are caught carrying it.

Addiction occurs rarely after long continual usage. There may be psychiatric effects similar to uppers or downers (see ADDICTION).

Overdose and prolonged usage: ADDICTION, LIVER FAILURE; see Protocol B.7.

Dosage: reduce the dosage with LIVER DISEASE. Be very careful of the dosage in children; a small overdose can kill. Children: 0.8–1.5 mg/kg/dose by mouth or IM injection, to maximum of the adult dose. Adults: 15, 30 or 60 mg by mouth or IM injection. This dose may be repeated every 3 hours as needed for pain. For cough, start with the lowest dose and increase it as necessary. Response: 20–30 minutes.

Alternatives: dosage given comparable to 30 mg codeine (dosage range for adult given in parenthesis): Darvon 65 mg by mouth (50–100); Demerol 25 mg by mouth or IM (25–100); Nalbuphine 5 mg IM. TRAMADOL 50 mg IM.

Withdrawal symptoms after addiction: abdominal pain, diarrhea, tearing of eyes, agitation, desperation for drug.

COLCHICINE

Anti-gout

Safety class: 3   Stability: B   Pregnancy: D

Supplied as tablets

This is very toxic to children; a small overdose can kill.

Indications: GOUT; FAMILIAL MEDITERRANEAN FEVER.

Contraindications: pregnancy, breast-feeding, any disease of the stomach or bowels, any heart disease, KIDNEY DISEASE, LIVER FAILURE, any disease of the blood. Should not be taken at the same time as any drug that has psychiatric effects.

Precautions: the drug interferes with one lab test to measure a hormone. Other lab tests should be okay.

Side-effects: nausea, vomiting, abdominal pain, a decrease in immunity, ANEMIA.

Overdose and prolonged usage: KIDNEY DISEASE.

Dosage: reduce dose in LIVER DISEASE and/or KIDNEY DISEASE—seek professional advice.

GOUT: the final dose is 0.5 mg every 12 hours. If the patient has not taken it before, give 0.5 mg every hour for 4 doses, then every 2 hours for 2 doses, then twice a day. An alternative regimen: 1 mg initially followed by 0.5 mg every 2–3 hours until relief of pain or vomiting and diarrhea. Maximum: 10 mg.

FAMILIAL MEDITERRANEAN FEVER: 0.5–2 mg/day

CORTISONE CREAM/OINTMENT

Topical steroid

Safety class: 1   Stability: A

Synonyms: similar products will be marked hydrocortisone, triamcinalone or any of several other "-one" drugs, as cream or ointment. You should use cream on rashes that look moist, ointment on those that look dry.

Includes: hydrocortisone cream/ointment

Indications: CONTACT DERMATITIS, external EAR INFECTION, any rash that itches, NAIROBI EYE.

Contraindications: none, but any products that contain the syllable "fluro" should not be used on the face.

Precautions: not to be used on pink moist areas such as lips, vagina, tip of penis, in or around eyes. Where this is applied leave the part unbandaged at least 8 hours a day.

Dosage: use sparingly four times a day as needed.

CO-TRIMOXAZOLE

Antibiotic, Gram-negative; sulfa drug plus folate antagonist

Safety class: 2   Stability: B

Synonyms: trimethoprim/sulfamethoxazole, SMZ/TMP, Sulfatrim, TMP/SMZ.

Brand names: Bactrim, Cotrim, Septra, others.

Indications: ABSCESS, ANTHRAX, BRUCELLOSIS, CELLULITIS, CHANCROID, CHLAMYDIA, CHOLERA, CYCLOSPORIASIS, DONOVANOSIS, DYSENTERY, EAR INFECTION (middle), ENTERIC FEVER, EPIDIDYMITIS, GIARDIASIS, GONORRHEA, KIDNEY INFECTION, LYMPHOGRANULOMA VENEREUM, MYCETOMA, PERTUSSIS, PELVIC INFECTION, PNEUMONIA, PROSTATITIS, Q FEVER; RESPIRATORY INFECTION, SEPSIS, TOXOPLASMOSIS, TRACHOMA, TURISTA, URETHRITIS, URINARY INFECTION, occasionally for VAGINITIS. It may be used to prevent pneumonia in the infants of HIV-infected mothers. In this case it also prevents malaria. It works if it is prescribed for another reason; it should not be used purposely as a malaria preventive.

Contraindications: ALLERGY to this or any SULFA drug. Newborns, early pregnancy (unless the patient takes FOLINIC ACID), maybe HIV INFECTION, ANEMIA, elderly. Do not give this in G6PD DEFICIENCY, with other drugs that are liver-toxic, with oral drugs for reducing blood sugar or with the drug, methenamine (also used for URINARY INFECTION).

Side-effects: nausea, vomiting, diarrhea, abdominal pain, dizziness, headache, fatigue.

Precautions

Do not allow the patient to become or remain dehydrated (see DEHYDRATION) while on the drug.

If the patient develops HEPATITIS, stop the drug.

The drug may cause sun sensitivity in fair skin. If a sunburn-like or a blistering or peeling rash develops, stop the drug immediately (see EXFOLIATIVE DERMATITIS).

Because it kills normal vaginal bacteria, females may develop VAGINITIS due to CANDIDA.

Overdose and prolonged usage: LIVER FAILURE; see Protocol B.7.

Dosage: reduce the dose with KIDNEY DISEASE.

The regular drug contains 80 mg of trimethoprim and 400 mg of sulfamethoxazole. This is known as single strength or SS. The double strength drug, labeled DS or DF, contains twice these amounts. The given doses are for adults; reduce dose according to weight for children.

ABSCESS: 1 DS or 2 SS tablets every 12 hours until healed plus 2 more days.

ANTHRAX: no good

BRUCELLOSIS: 1 DS or 2 SS tablets every 12 hours for 21 days. Use with other antibiotics.

CELLULITIS: same as ABSCESS.

CHANCROID: 2 SS twice daily for 7 days

CHLAMYDIA: no good

CHOLERA: same as ABSCESS.

CYCLOSPORIASIS: 1 DS or 2 SS tablets every 12 hours for 7 days with no HIV INFECTION; for 14 days in the presence of HIV INFECTION.

DONOVANOSIS: 1 DS or 2 SS tablets every 12 hours until entirely healed plus one more week. Repeat the entire treatment as soon as there is any evidence of relapse.

DYSENTERY: same as ABSCESS.

EAR INFECTION: 1 DS or 2 SS tablets every 12 hours for 10 days.

ENTERIC FEVER: same as BRUCELLOSIS.

EPIDIDYMITIS: 1 DS or 2 SS tablets every 12 hours for 3 days.

GIARDIASIS/cyclosporosis: 1 SS tablet every 12 hours for 7 days.

GONORRHEA: 2 DS or 4 SS tablets twice a day for 10 days.

KIDNEY INFECTION: same as EAR INFECTION.

MYCETOMA: 2 SS or 1 DS tablet twice daily for 6–9 months.

Q FEVER: 1 DS or 2 SS tablets every 12 hours for 2 weeks.

PELVIC INFECTION: same as GONORRHEA.

PERTUSSIS: 1 DS or 2 SS tablets, twice daily for 5 days.

PNEUMONIA: same as EAR INFECTION.

PNEUMONIA prevention in infants: ½ of a single-strength tablet three times weekly.

PROSTATITIS: same as EPIDIDYMITIS.

RESPIRATORY INFECTION: same as ABSCESS.

SEPSIS: same as BRUCELLOSIS.

TOXOPLASMOSIS: dosage unknown., duration 1 month

TRACHOMA: same as BRUCELLOSIS.

TURISTA: same as ABSCESS. It should not be used for prevention since it is not much better than BISMUTH SUBSALICYLATE, and has significant side-effects.

URETHRITIS: same as GONORRHEA.

URINARY INFECTION: same as EPIDIDYMITIS; extend the time to 7 days for children and elderly.

VAGINITIS: same as ABSCESS.

Alternatives: other Gram-negative antibiotics. For CHANCROID use ERYTHROMYCIN. For PNEUMONIA in a patient with HIV INFECTION, use ATOVAQUONE.

TOC

SYMPTOMS

DIFFERENTIALS

CONDITIONS

DRUG INDEX

REGIONAL NOTES

INX

COUGH SYRUP

Used for RESPIRATORY INFECTION, this is usually a combination of two or more of the following classes of drugs:

Antihistamine, the most common being CHLORPHENIRAMINE. This type of drug dries secretions and is most helpful for runny noses and eyes. It should not be used if the patient is short of breath; it will aggravate croup, wheezing and ASTHMA.

Decongestant, the most common being PSEUDOEPHEDRINE. This shrinks swollen membranes and so helps to open nasal passages. It may raise the patient's blood pressure.

Expectorant, the most common being guaifenesin, liquefies phlegm so it is easier to cough up. It is likely to make the patient cough more, but it will help him recover sooner.

Cough suppressant, the most common being dextromethorphan hydrobromide, keeps the patient from coughing. If the patient does not cough up what he should, he may develop PNEUMONIA. It is best to use a cough suppressant only at night and let the patient cough during the day.

CROMOGLYCATE

Non-steroid ophthalmic anti-inflammatory

Brand name: Opticrom. Supplied as a 4% solution; expensive.

Indications: prevention of eye irritation from ALLERGY (vernal conjunctivitis).

Contraindications: do not use with soft contact lenses.

Dosage: 1–2 drops in each eye every 4–6 hours, without missing any doses.

CROTAMITON

Scabicide, insecticide

Safety class: 1   Stability: C

Brand names: Crotamitex, Eurax, Euraxil, Veteusan. The human form of the drug is a 10% cream or lotion; if the product you buy is stronger, dilute it with hand lotion or hand cream before using it. For example, if it is 20%, dilute it 50:50 to make it 10%.

Indications: SCABIES, itching after treatment thereof.

Contraindications: prior ALLERGY to the drug.

Precautions: this may cause irritation over inflamed skin or if it is applied for too long a period of time. Do not apply this to the hands of babies and young children who will put their hands in their mouths. If you splint their elbows, they will be able to play, but they cannot put their hands in their mouths.

Dosage: apply to the entire body from the chin down. Apply it while the skin is damp, avoiding the pink moist areas of the genitals. Leave it on for 24 hours; then wash it off and apply it again. Change clothing and bed linen at that time. Wash off the second application after 24 hours; change clothing and bed linen again.

CURCUMIN

This is a useful herb which is being developed as a drug. It is found in turmeric, the major ingredient of curry powder. 50mg/kg twice daily for 6 days improves the prognosis in cerebral malaria. It may be useful for some cancers in which case it is given as 7 consecutive daily doses every 3 weeks. It is a useful addition to ARTEMISININ when it is used for CANCER. It is a general anti-inflammatory medication.

CYCLOSERINE

Anti-TUBERCULOSIS, second-line

Safety class: 3   Stability: C   Pregnancy: C

Brand name: Seromycin.

Indication: TUBERCULOSIS.

Contraindications: ALLERGY to this drug, mental illness, epilepsy, KIDNEY DISEASE, ALCOHOLISM, any neurological problem.

Precautions: not to be taken with alcohol or with ISONIAZID. Discontinue the drug for ALLERGY, mental changes, new ANEMIA, new neurological symptoms

Side-effects: mainly neurological symptoms; stop the drug for these kinds of side-effects. If ANEMIA develops, it can be treated with VITAMIN B_{12} and FOLIC ACID.

Dosage: 250–500 mg by mouth twice daily; Children 10–20 mg/kg by mouth twice daily. The amount of this drug in the blood should be checked regularly with blood tests.

DAPSONE

Sulfone, anti-LEPROSY, MALARIA-preventive

Safety class: 3;   Stability: C, dark; Pregnancy: C

Brand names: Avlosulfon, Croysulfone, DDS, Diphenasone, Diphone, Disulone, Dumitone, Eporal, Novophone, Sulfadione, Sulfona-mae, Udolac. Combination drug with PYRIMETHAMINE is MALOPRIM; it is used for MALARIA prevention.

Indications: CUTANEOUS LEISHMANIASIS, LEPROSY, MALARIA prevention, MALARIA treatment in combination with PROGUANIL and ARTEMISININ (artesunate); MYCETOMA, TOXOPLASMOSIS prophylaxis. Sometimes useful for recluse spider bites (see Appendix 10 in Volume 1).

Contraindications: breast feeding. ALLERGY to dapsone. People who are allergic to SULFA drugs can usually take dapsone, but they should be watched for ALLERGY. Probably it is unwise to give in the presence of LIVER DISEASE. Do not give to patients with PORPHYRIA (a hereditary disease).

Precautions: there is a 0.1% chance of serious side-effects which may be fatal. Stop the drug if the patient develops a new fever, JAUNDICE, ANEMIA, blistering or peeling of the skin (see EXFOLIATIVE DERMATITIS), any new rash or crazy behavior. (The peeling skin is quite common in the South Pacific, so the drug should probably not be given to Pacific Islanders.) Check the description of the complications of the treatment of LEPROSY before using the drug for that.

Serious side-effects may occur in persons with G6PD DEFICIENCY. Check the patient's urine just before the second dose. If it has turned quite dark or has more urobilinogen than previously, discontinue the drug. This is especially important in those of Mediterranean origin and some East Asians. It is best if such persons use this drug only at the recommendation of a physician and in as low a dose as possible.

Side-effects: loss of appetite, nausea and vomiting. These effects occur in only a small percentage of patients. Rarely, headache, nervousness, insomnia, blurry vision, numbness, weakness and fever may occur. Very rarely and unpredictably this drug may destroy the bone marrow, causing ANEMIA and making the person susceptible to new infections.

Overdose and prolonged usage: LIVER FAILURE; see Protocol B.7.

Dosage:

CUTANEOUS LEISHMANIASIS: consult an M.D. for dosage and directions.

LEPROSY: 100 mg daily for adults. This must be given for 6 months for tuberculoid and indeterminate leprosy, for 2 years minimum for other types. Reduce dose according to weight for children.

MALARIA prevention: two 100 mg tablets of Maloprim initially, then one weekly for adults.

MALARIA treatment: ARTEMISININ (artesunate) 4 mg/kg, dapsone 2.5 mg/kg, PROGUANIL 8 mg/kg, all daily for 3 days. Works well in Thailand.

MYCETOMA: 100 mg twice daily for six to nine months.

TOXOPLASMOSIS prophylaxis: 50 mg/day, used with PYRIMETHAMINE.

Spider bites: 100 mg twice daily.

DELAVIRDINE

This is a drug active against AIDS.

DEXAMETHASONE

A drug closely related to PREDNISONE but stronger, frequently used in CYSTICERCOSIS, severe ENTERIC FEVER and in MENINGITIS. See the description of PREDNISONE and use it similarly, noting that the comparable dosage is much lower (0.75 mg of dexamethasone is equivalent to 5 mg of PREDNISONE or PREDNISOLONE). It is good to use CIMETIDINE along with this to decrease side-effects.

Do not use this in the presence of PORPHYRIA, HIV INFECTION, at the same time as any vaccines, during pregnancy and breastfeeding. It causes problems with many different drugs and diseases and thus should only be used at the recommendation of a physician.

The usual dose of dexamethasone for MENINGITIS due to TUBERCULOSIS is 12 mg/day for adults; for children use 0.1 mg/kg daily. Continue this dosage for 3 weeks and then taper it gradually, reducing the dose every other day until it is stopped.

ENTERIC fever dosage is 6 mg initially, followed by 3 mg every 6 hours for 2 additional doses. Physicians may prescribe higher doses.

ALTITUDE SICKNESS: 4 mg every 8 or 12 hours.

DEXCHLORPHENIRAMINE

Antihistamine

Safety class: 2   Stability: C, dark   Pregnancy: B

Brand name: Polaramine.

Indications: used with ALBENDAZOLE in the treatment of CYSTICERCOSIS. It may also be used as an ordinary antihistamine for ALLERGY.

Contraindications: prior bad reaction to the medication. Must not be used in newborns. Do not use this during an acute ASTHMA attack. Do not use it with antidepressants.

Precautions: it should not be used with alcohol.

Side-effects: drowsiness, worsening of GLAUCOMA, constipation, inability to pass urine (especially in older men), susceptibility to HEAT ILLNESS, dry mouth, decrease in sweating, rapid pulse, sensitivity to light, blurred vision.

Dosage: reduce the dose in children and the elderly.

CYSTICERCOSIS: 2 mg by mouth every 4 hours around the clock when used with ALBENDAZOLE.

ALLERGY: 4 mg every 4–6 hours.

Alternatives: CHLORPHENIRAMINE is a similar drug.

DIAZEPAM

Sedative, Muscle relaxant

Safety class: 2–3   Stability: A, dark; it is a controlled substance in the West   Pregnancy: D

Brand name: Valium. Supplied as tablets and injectable for IM or IV. IM = oral dose.

Indications: emotional upset, SEIZURES, muscle relaxation for putting a dislocated joint back in place, TETANUS, sometimes to assist in withdrawing from ALCOHOL. (See ALCOHOLISM.)

Contraindications: prior ALLERGY to the drug, any difficulty breathing, POLIO. It should not be used in the presence of KIDNEY DISEASE or in a person who is very lethargic or unconscious. Do not use it during breast-feeding or in patients less than 6 years old.

Precautions: should not be used for more than a day or two because it is potentially addictive. When using higher doses, watch to be sure the person does not stop breathing. If the person has ALCOHOL in his blood stream, he will absorb more diazepam than he would otherwise. Therefore cut the dose by 1/3 to 1/2. If he frequently drinks alcohol but has none in his blood stream right now, you may have to use higher-than-normal doses.

The drug causes people to breathe less than usual. In some it may make them stop breathing altogether.

Used routinely, this drug causes DEPRESSION.

TOC
SYMPTOMS
DIFFERENTIALS
CONDITIONS
DRUG INDEX
REGIONAL NOTES
INX

Warn the patient not to engage in any potentially hazardous activity while taking this. Do not give it to women who are breastfeeding.

This drug interferes with various lab tests; don't believe lab results of blood drawn while the patient was taking this.

Side-effects: sun sensitivity, drowsiness.

Dosage: reduce the dose in patients who are elderly or sickly.

Adult dose: 2mg–20mg by mouth or IM injection, every 4 hours as needed. Reduce dose according to weight for children. Control of SEIZURES and fixing a dislocated joint requires IV administration; watch breathing. Rectal dosage for control of seizures is 0.5 mg/kg (usual adult dose is 35 mg). Do not use tablets for this. Use the injectable form, or else dissolve tablets in water and give as an enema. For TETANUS follow the dosage given under TETANUS treatment in the Condition Index.

DICLOFENAC

This is a NSAID similar to IBUPROFEN. It works reasonably well for pain.

DICYCLOMINE

Antispasmodic, anticholinergic.

Safety class: 1–2   Stability: C   Pregnancy: B

Brand name: Bentyl; generic drug is available. Supplied as 10 mg capsules and 20 mg tablets. Injectable drug also available. IM = oral dose.

Indications: abdominal pain; TURISTA; FOOD POISONING; GALLBLADDER DISEASE; GASTROENTERITIS; IRRITABLE BOWEL; nausea and vomiting; PLANT POISONING, muscarine.

Contraindications: newborns, breastfeeding, prior ALLERGY to the drug; PROSTATITIS; difficulty urinating: a full bladder that will not empty, except with dribbling. (Usually this occurs in older men and in women who have just given birth.) Do not use this with bacterial DYSENTERY or poisonings. It will make the patient sicker. Do not use it if you suspect ACUTE ABDOMEN type 3: abdominal pains that come in waves with pain-free intervals between.

Side-effects: worsening of GLAUCOMA, constipation, inability to pass urine (especially in older men), susceptibility to HEAT ILLNESS, dry mouth, decrease in sweating, rapid pulse, sensitivity to light, blurred vision.

Overdose and prolonged use: LIVER FAILURE; see Protocol B.7.

Dosage: reduce the dose for elderly patients. Adult dose is 20 mg by mouth or IM injection, every 6 hours as needed. Reduce dose according to weight for children.

Alternative: CHAMOMILE TEA.

DIDANOSINE

This is a drug that is used for HIV INFECTION.

DIETHYLCARBAMAZINE (CITRATE) DEC Anti-filarial

Synonym: DEC

Safety class: 2+   Stability: A

Brand names: Banocide, Ethodryl, Filarizan, Hetrazan, Notezine and many others; generic diethylcarbamazine is available as a veterinary drug. Supplied as 50 mg and 200 mg tablets. It is an old drug that has largely been replaced by IVERMECTIN.

Indications: FILARIASIS (wuchereria), LOIASIS, MANSONELLOSIS PERSTANS, ONCHOCERCIASIS, ASTHMA due to FILARIASIS.

Contraindications: pregnancy, HEART FAILURE, KIDNEY DISEASE.

Precautions: an allergic reaction (see ALLERGY) when this drug is used probably is not a reaction to the drug itself, but to the dead worms. This is not a problem when it is given after several weeks of DOXYCYCLINE. If it should occur, use the slow-start schedule given below.

Side-effects: headache, tiredness, joint pain, appetite loss, nausea and vomiting. There may be enlargement of the lymph nodes with pain. Patients with recent MALARIA may relapse unless they are treated for that at the same time. DRUG ERUPTION sometimes occurs.

Dosage: all doses are oral. Reduce all doses according to weight for children. The slow-start schedule is given in italics below: it must be used for ASTHMA due to filariasis.

Use DIPHENHYDRAMINE and PREDNISONE for allergic reactions (see ALLERGY). It is essential to have both EPINEPHRINE and DIPHENHYDRAMINE or another antihistamine available when you start the drug. If you use PREDNISONE, give it six hours before the first daily dose for the first five days.

FILARIASIS treatment:

Slow-start, 21-day schedule for adults

Day 1: 50 mg once.

Day 2: 50 mg every 8 hours.

Day 3: 100 mg every 8 hours

Days 4–21: 2 mg/kg, max 150 mg, every 8 hours.

Thereafter:

Option #1: 6 mg/kg once a week for 12 weeks. Patient compliance and effectiveness is better with this schedule than with the other.

Option #2: 6 mg/kg in a single dose, given along with IVERMECTIN after a slow start as above.

Fast-start and final dosage schedule:

FILARIASIS treatment: 100–150 mg three times a day for 21 days. It is good to use ALBENDAZOLE along with this to kill the adult worms.

FILARIASIS prevention: 300 mg in one dose once a month. If the patient had previous exposure to the disease, start out using small doses weekly along with DIPHENHYDRAMINE, building up to 300 mg. Beginning preventive therapy when entering the area avoids this problem.

LOIASIS treatment: seek local advice before using DEC for this; it might be dangerous. Adult dose: 50 mg three times a day for 10 days. Then give no drug for 2 weeks. Follow this by 200 mg three times a day for 21 days.

LOIASIS prevention: seek local advice before using DEC for this; it might be dangerous. Adult dose is 300 mg daily for 3 consecutive days once a month or 300 mg weekly.

MANSONELLOSIS PERSTANS: 200 mg daily for 21 days, used along with MEBENDAZOLE.

ONCHOCERCIASIS: 25 mg daily for 1 week, then 50 mg daily for I week, then 100 mg daily for 1 week, adult dose. Repeat the treatment after the patient has had a month off the drug and a third time after another month off the drug. If the patient has not had previous DOXYCYCLINE or if he has an allergic reaction anyway, then use the slow-start schedule.

Alternatives: IVERMECTIN is safer than DEC for FILARIASIS and ONCHOCERCIASIS.

DIGOXIN

Heart medicine, digitalis.

Safety class: 3   Stability: A, dark   Pregnancy: C

Brand name: Lanoxin; generic drug is available, but it is best not to use generic or veterinary drug. Supplied as tablets of 0.125 and 0.25 mg.

Indications: HEART FAILURE, some kinds but not all kinds; seek higher-level advice.

Contraindications: present or recent severe diarrhea or vomiting, MALNUTRITION with swelling of the abdomen or ankles, unreliable patient, inability to keep away from children, KIDNEY DISEASE, prior ALLERGY to the drug, pulse less than 60. This interacts badly with a variety of other drugs and conditions.

Precautions: use only when and as an M.D. directs. Doses must be exact. Never give extra. Check the pulse before each dose and do not give it if the pulse is less than 60.

Side-effect: breast development in males. Overdose and prolonged usage: extremely toxic. Twice the recommended dose may be fatal. Some of the early symptoms of too much drug are loss of appetite, nausea and vomiting. Diarrhea and abdominal discomfort may also occur. Headache, fatigue, dizziness and sleepiness as well as mental symptoms or blurred vision also indicate too much drug. Stop the drug completely if any of these occur. Start it again after these symptoms are gone, using only half the prior dose.

Dosage: reduce the dose in the elderly, in KIDNEY DISEASE and in THYROID TROUBLE. The adult dose is 0.25 mg by mouth daily in one dose for adults of average size. Use 0.125 mg daily in small adults. Children get 0.005 mg/kg daily. This must be continued for a long time, perhaps for life.

DILOXANIDE FUROATE

Amebicide

Safety class: 1   Stability: C

Not available in the USA or in Canada.

Brand names: Ame-boots, Entamide, Furamide; combination with METRONIDAZOLE is called Entamizole. Supplied in 500 mg tablets.

Indications: AMEBIASIS, DYSENTERY due to amebae; used to clear the bowel of amebae after the person has been treated for AMEBIASIS.

Contraindications: previous ALLERGY to this drug.

Precautions: the drug enters the blood poorly and thus has little or no whole-body effect. It may cause hives, vomiting, itching or excessive gas passage by rectum. These effects occur in only a small percentage of patients.

Dosage: 500 mg by mouth every 8 hours for 10 days for adults. Reduce dose according to weight for children.

DIPHENHYDRAMINE

Antihistamine

Safety class: 1   Stability: A   Pregnancy: B

Brand name: Benadryl; generic drug is available. Supplied as 25 and 50 mg capsules.

Indications: this is useful to counteract the muscle spasm side-effects of METOCLOPRAMIDE and phenothiazines (PROCHLORPERAZINE, CHLORPROMAZINE); It is also used for ALLERGY, ANAPHYLAXIS, CHICKEN POX, FILARIASIS, insomnia, motion sickness, ONCHOCERCIASIS, PLANT POISONING: argemone oil or muscarine, SEABATHER'S ERUPTION, SWIMMER'S ITCH.

Precautions: causes sleepiness and may make ASTHMA worse. The patient should not drink alcoholic beverages while taking this.

Side-effects: worsening of GLAUCOMA, constipation, inability to pass urine (especially in older men), susceptibility to HEAT ILLNESS, dry mouth, decrease in sweating, rapid pulse, sensitivity to light, blurred vision. On occasion it may cause SEIZURES, dizziness, ringing in the ears, loss of appetite, nausea, abdominal pain. These effects occur in only a small percentage of patients.

Overdose and prolonged usage: LIVER FAILURE (see Protocol B.7); KIDNEY DISEASE.

Dosage: adults: 25–50 mg by mouth or IM injection, every 4 hours as needed. Reduce dose according to weight for children. Reduce the dose for the elderly.

Alternatives: CHLORPHENIRAMINE, DEXCHLORPHENIRAMINE, dramamine, histadyl, PROMETHAZINE, tripelennamine.

DIPYRONE

This is a pain medication, commonly available orally as well as by injection in developing countries. It has been taken off the market in the West, because of rare fatal reactions.

It works nearly as well as narcotics, but it is non-addicting, and it is cheap. It should not be used for ordinary pain, but it is useful under emergency conditions and also for routine care of terminally ill patients. It should not be used in patients with PORPHYRIA. The IM or oral dosage is 1000 mg for adults.

DIURETICS

This refers to a class of drugs.

Synonym: "water pill".

This is a class of drugs that make a patient urinate a lot. They cause DEHYDRATION which is sometimes desirable. They harm patients who have swelling due to infection, LIVER FAILURE or MALNUTRITION. See Symptom Protocol A.61.

DOXYCYCLINE

Antibiotic, Gram-negative.

Safety class: 2   Stability: A, dark   Pregnancy: D

Brand names: Tanamicin, Tecacin, Tetradox, Vibradox, Vibramycin, Vibra-Tabs, Vibravenos and others. Generic drug is available. This drug has replaced TETRACYCLINE.

Indications: ACNE, ANTHRAX, BARTONELLOSIS, BRUCELLOSIS, CANCRUM ORIS, CAT-SCRATCH DISEASE, CELLULITIS, CHANCROID, CHLAMYDIA, CHOLERA, DONOVANOSIS, DYSENTERY, FILARIASIS, FOOD POISONING, GONORRHEA, LEPTOSPIROSIS, LYME DISEASE, LYMPHOGRANULOMA VENEREUM, MALABSORPTION, MALARIA prevention and treatment, MANSONELLOSIS PERSTANS, ONCHOCERCIASIS, PELVIC INFECTION,[1] PEPTIC ULCER, PINTA, PLAGUE exposure and treatment, Q FEVER, RAT BITE FEVER, RELAPSING FEVER, RESPIRATORY INFECTION, SCRUB TYPHUS, SPOTTED FEVER (Rocky Mountain and Mediterranean, possibly other types), SPRUE, SYPHILIS, TRACHOMA, TRENCH FEVER, TREPONARID, TROPICAL ULCER, TULAREMIA, TURISTA, TYPHUS, URETHRITIS, YAWS. This will work for ACNE, but it is dangerous if the patient has not had his appendix removed. It is rarely used for KIDNEY INFECTION. It might possibly work for GIARDIASIS.

Contraindications: ALLERGY to any TETRACYCLINE-type drug; old drug, past expiration date.

Pregnancy and breastfeeding are normally contraindications but when the drug is necessary for something potentially life-threatening (e.g. prevention of PLAGUE after a significant exposure) this may be violated since the benefit outweighs the risk. Do not use this in patients with PORPHYRIA (a hereditary disease)

---

1 *Recent information indicates that this is not useful for pelvic infection because of widespread resistance, especially in disease acquired in urban settings and/or amongst homosexuals. Seek local advice. Even if it locally effective, it should always be used with another drug, usually LEVOFLOXACIN.*

Precautions: this drug stops the growth of bacteria but does not kill them; its effect depends on the body's own ability to kill the germs. Therefore it is not usually the best drug if the patient is very seriously ill or if his immunity is poor. It is also not the best drug to use if the disease progresses rapidly e.g. ANTHRAX, CANCRUM ORIS, CHOLERA, PLAGUE, some SPOTTED FEVER. These diseases are listed as indications only because, in developing areas, one's options are limited. Doxycycline causes sun sensitivity in fair skin.

Oral contraceptives may fail with this.

It makes patients prone to CANDIDIASIS, masks the signs and symptoms of appendicitis and theoretically causes dark staining of teeth in children under 7 and the offspring of pregnant women who take the drug. Recent medical literature disputes this.

Watch expiration dates; do not use expired drug.

If you use this together with milk, any ANTACIDs or BISMUTH SUBSALICYLATE; separate the times of taking the medications by at least 2 hours.

Side-effects: abdominal pains, nausea, vomiting, diarrhea. Stop the medication for DYSENTERY that appears to be due to the medication.

Overdose and prolonged usage: LIVER FAILURE (see Protocol B.7); pregnant women are particularly prone to this.

Dosage: these are adult doses; reduce the dose for children; reduce the dose with LIVER DISEASE.

ACNE: 50–100 mg daily until better.

ANTHRAX exposure: 100 mg daily for 60 days plus immediate immunization.

ANTHRAX treatment 100 mg IV every 12 hours for 10 days, then switch to oral for 60 days total.

BARTONELLOSIS: 100 mg twice daily for 6 weeks.

BRUCELLOSIS: 200 mg each evening; use this with other antibiotics.

CANCRUM ORIS: 100 mg twice daily until the problem is getting no worse, then for another 4 days.

CAT-SCRATCH DISEASE: 100 mg daily for 14 days.

CELLULITIS: 100 mg twice daily until healed plus 4 days.

CHANCROID: 300 mg single dose

CHLAMYDIA (without LGV): 100 mg twice daily for 2 weeks.

CHOLERA: 300 mg in a single dose.

DONOVANOSIS: 100 mg twice daily until entirely healed and then for another week; repeat this as necessary for relapses.

DYSENTERY: 100 mg daily for 10 days.

FILARIASIS: 200 mg daily for 6–8 weeks, before using other drugs such as DIETHYLCARBAMAZINE, ALBENDAZOLE or IVERMECTIN; 3 weeks works but not as well.

FOOD POISONING: 100 mg daily until better, plus one more day.

GONORRHEA: 100 mg twice daily for 7 days.

LEPTOSPIROSIS:[2] 100 mg twice daily for 7 days.

LYME DISEASE: 100 mg daily for 60 days   With headache and movement problems, 200 mg daily for 14 days. Prevention after a tick bite is a single dose of 200 mg.

LYMPHOGRANULOMA VENEREUM: 100 mg twice daily for 3 weeks.

MALABSORPTION: 100 mg daily for 3 weeks.

MALARIA prevention: 100 mg daily.

MALARIA treatment 100 mg twice daily for 10 days.

MANSONELLOSIS PERSTANS: 200 mg daily x 6–8 weeks.

ONCHOCERCIASIS: 100 mg twice daily x 6–8 weeks before other drugs.

PELVIC INFECTION: 100 mg twice daily for 14 days; use this with LEFOFLOXACIN or another drug. There is much resistance to this; it may not work.

PEPTIC ULCER: 100 mg daily for 10–14 days, with other antibiotics.

PINTA: same as SYPHILIS according to the stage of the disease.

PLAGUE exposure: 100 mg every 12 hours for two days.

PLAGUE treatment 100 mg IV every 12 hours until improved, then switch to oral for 14 days total.

Q FEVER: 100 mg twice daily for 15 days.

RAT BITE FEVER: 100 mg twice daily for 7–10 days.

RELAPSING FEVER: 100 mg, single dose.

RESPIRATORY INFECTION: 100 mg daily until better, then for another 2–3 days.

SCRUB TYPHUS: 100 mg twice daily for 3 days.

SPOTTED FEVER: this is the drug of choice, even in children. 100 mg twice daily until fever is gone plus 3 more days. (Note that this does not work for all kinds of SPOTTED FEVER! It does work for Mediterranean SPOTTED FEVER and Rocky Mountain SPOTTED FEVER. It also works for flea-borne spotted fever. Seek local lore.)

SPRUE: 100 mg single dose

SYPHILIS, primary and secondary: 100 mg every 12 hours for 15 days.

SYPHILIS, tertiary: 100 mg twice daily for 28 days, being sure to not miss any doses. (Note that this does not work for tertiary syphilis that has gone to the brain.)

SYPHILIS, tertiary that has gone to the brain: reportedly (not on good authority) 200 mg twice daily for 28 days works.

TRACHOMA: 100 mg daily for 3 weeks.

TRENCH FEVER: 200 mg daily x 28 days, used with GENTAMYCIN.

TREPONARID: same as SYPHILIS, according to the stage of the disease.

2 It is useless to give antibiotic for leptospirosis if the patient has been ill for 4 days or more.

TROPICAL ULCER: 100 mg daily until healed.

TULAREMIA: 100 mg twice daily for 2 weeks.

TURISTA: 100 mg, single dose.

TYPHUS: same as SPOTTED FEVER.

URETHRITIS: same as GONORRHEA.

YAWS: same as SYPHILIS according to the stage.

EFAVIRENZ

This is an anti-AIDS drug.

EFLORNITHINE

Anti-trypanosome

Safety class: 2   Stability: unknown

Supplied as oral and injectable drug for AFRICAN SLEEPING SICKNESS; supplied as a cream in the West for removing facial hair in females. The cream is pregnancy category C. The category is unknown for the oral/injectable.

Synonyms: DFMO, difluoromethylornithine

Brand name: Ornidyl.

Indications: AFRICAN SLEEPING SICKNESS, Gambian type. It does not work reliably for Rhodesian type but it might work in some patients.

Contraindications: ALLERGY to this drug, severe ANEMIA, uncorrected.

Side-effects: fatigue, sore throat, fever, diarrhea, abdominal pain, nausea and vomiting, loss of appetite, easy bleeding, occasionally hair loss. It may damage hearing, damage bone marrow (causing ANEMIA, abnormal bleeding or susceptibility to infection) or cause SEIZURES. It may reduce the effectiveness of vaccines.

Precautions: the drug is hard to obtain, but reportedly is available through the WHO. The loose chemical is a white powder resembling cocaine in appearance, so carrying it across borders could cause trouble. Severe diarrhea caused by the drug necessitates stoping the drug. Wait until the diarrhea goes away and then begin the drug again at the same dose. Injectable drug causes less diarrhea than drug given by mouth. and relapse is less likely. The doses are the same both ways.

Dosage:

AFRICAN SLEEPING SICKNESS, early: 50 mg/kg every 6 hours (average adult dose is 3000 mg per dose, 12,000 mg daily) for 6 weeks.

AFRICAN SLEEPING SICKNESS with mental symptoms: 200 mg/kg every 12 hours for 7 days if given with NIFURTIMOX; for 14 days if given without NIFURTIMOX, IV if possible. Follow this by 75 mg/kg by mouth every 6 hours for 21 to 28 days.

AFRICAN SLEEPING SICKNESS relapse: 100mg/kg every 6 hours for 7 days only.

Results should be evident in 1–2 weeks.

TOC   SYMPTOMS   DIFFERENTIALS   CONDITIONS   DRUG INDEX   REGIONAL NOTES   INX

EMETINE

This and its less-toxic cousin, dehydroemetine, are old drugs that previously were used for amebae, both DYSENTERY and other kinds of AMEBIASIS. Emetine is very toxic for heart and muscles. It is still used for LIVER FLUKE when safer alternatives are not available. It should be used only with a physician's supervision. Keep the patient at absolute bedrest until a week after the treatment. The dose for either emetine or dehydro-emetine is 1 mg/kg IM daily to a maximum of 65 mg daily.

EPHEDRINE NOSE DROPS (1%)

Topical decongestant

Safety class: 1   Stability: A, dark

Indications: RESPIRATORY INFECTION, stuffy nose.

Contraindications: high blood pressure, current use of antidepressants.

Precautions: using too many drops, may cause congestion when the drug is stopped. Babies should have the drops diluted 1:7 or 1:15 as they are particularly sensitive to them.

Dosage: one drop in each nostril.

Alternatives: croyban, neo-synephrine, otrivin, privine hydrochloride, tyzine, all essentially the same as ephedrine.

EPINEPHRINE

ASTHMA and ALLERGY medicine

Safety class: 2   Stability: C, dark

Synonym: adrenalin (British)

Supplied as glass vials and preloaded syringes with 1 mg in 1 ml; labeled 1:1000. Also 10 ml bottles, same strength. Preparations labeled 1:10,000 should not be used.

Indications: ALLERGY if severe; ANAPHYLAXIS; ASTHMA; FILARIASIS maybe; bleeding PEPTIC ULCER (class 1 used thus.)

Contraindications: none when used for ANAPHYLAXIS or severe ASTHMA. Contraindicated in HEART FAILURE and HYPERTENSION when used for mild ASTHMA or ALLERGY. Do not use during pregnancy unless the situation is life-threatening.

Precautions: when given by injection, this drug aggravates HYPERTENSION and makes the pulse fast. Some patients become very shaky and agitated; reassure the patient and wait for it to wear off.

Dosages for ANAPHYLAXIS, assuming normal body size for age:

Adults	0.5 ml
8–12 y.o.	0.4 ml
5–7 y.o.	0.3 ml
2–5 y.o.	0.2 ml
6 mo–2 y.o.	0.1 ml
Infant	0.05 ml

HIVES and other ALLERGY: use half the doses listed above.

ASTHMA, moderate to severe and ANAPHYLAXIS: repeat the dose every 5–10 minutes until the patient shows some improvement. Then repeat every 30 minutes until the patient is very much improved.

ASTHMA, mild to moderate: repeat every 20 minutes. Use a maximum of 3 doses.

ERGONOVINE MALEATE

Oxytocic

Safety class: 3   Stability: D, dark   Pregnancy: X

Alternative names: ergometrine maleate, methergine, methylergonovine maleate, methylergometrine maleate.

Brand name: Methergine. Supplied as 0.2 mg tablets and IM vials with 0.2 mg/ml. It may be unnecessary to refrigerate some forms. Check with your pharmacist.

Indications: severe bleeding after childbirth or after a spontaneous miscarriage.

Contraindications: during delivery do not use this if the patient has not yet delivered both baby and placenta. If she is miscarrying, do not use this if she has not yet passed the tissue (baby and placenta) and the bleeding is not severe. (If the bleeding is severe, more than a pint, in a miscarriage you may give the drug in spite of her not having passed the contents of her uterus.) Other contraindications in the States are HYPERTENSION and TOXEMIA. Do not use this in patients with PORPHYRIA, (a hereditary disease).

Precautions: ordinarily you should use one dose only. It may, however, be used more often if the patient is developing signs of SHOCK. The drug causes severe cramping.

Side-effects: if a person is particularly sensitive to this drug, it may cause her hands or feet to become cold, pale and numb. Pulses will diminish. GANGRENE may occur if the dose is large enough. ANGINA may develop. Other symptoms are headache, nausea, diarrhea, dizziness, weakness and inability to think right. It may raise the blood pressure to dangerous levels.

Dosage: 0.2 mg by mouth or IM injection.

Results: bleeding should be decreased in half an hour.

ERYTHROMYCIN

Antibiotic (mostly Gram-positive)

Safety class: 1   Stability: B   Pregnancy: B.

Brand names: E-Mycin, Ilosone, Wyamycin, Bristamycin. Supplied as 250 and 500 mg tablets.

Indications: ABSCESS, ACNE, BARTONELLOSIS (Verruga type), CAT-SCRATCH DISEASE, CELLULITIS, CHANCROID, CHLAMYDIA, DIPHTHERIA, DONOVANOSIS, DYSENTERY due to amebae, middle EAR INFECTION (but not in young children), FOOD POISONING, GASTROENTERITIS, LEPTOSPIROSIS, LYMPHOGRANULOMA VENEREUM, PELVIC INFECTION not due to GONORRHEA, PERTUSSIS, PINTA, PNEUMONIA, Q FEVER, RELAPSING FEVER, RESPIRATORY INFECTION, SPOTTED FEVER; STREP THROAT, SYPHILIS, TRACHOMA, TRENCH FEVER, TREPONARID, rarely

TURISTA, VAGINITIS, YAWS. It may be used for a tooth infection for any tooth except the third molar. It may substitute for PENICILLIN in someone who is allergic to PENICILLIN, but *not* with MENINGITIS, *nor* tertiary SYPHILIS, *nor* SEPSIS, *nor* GONORRHEA!

Contraindications: previous ALLERGY to the drug or any similar drug. Do not use with KETOCONAZOLE or with medication for SEIZURES. Do not use in the presence of LIVER DISEASE; see Protocol B.7. Do not give this with antihistamines (allergy pills) that do not cause sleepiness.

Precautions: this drug frequently gives stomach pain and upset. Taking it with food minimizes this. Try only a single tablet as the first dose. Try to avoid using erythromycin estolate (use a form with another last name). Erythromycin can cause pain resembling GALLBLADDER DISEASE.

When giving this drug along with THEOPHYLLINE, the dose of the latter should be decreased; toxicity may develop from ordinary doses.

Do not give this to patients with PORPHYRIA (a hereditary disease).

This alters the electrical activity of the heart which might cause sudden death. Thus it should not be combined with other such drugs. The medical jargon is that it prolongs the QT interval. See the back cover.

Dosage: the following doses are for adults; reduce the dose according to weight for children. Reduce the dose with LIVER DISEASE. Do not crush the tablets.

ABSCESS: 250 mg every 6 hours until better, plus 2 more days.

ACNE: 250 mg three times a day continuously.

BARTONELLOSIS: 250 mg four times daily for 14 days.

CAT-SCRATCH DISEASE: 250 mg four times daily for 14 days.

CELLULITIS: 250–500 mg every 6 hours for 10 days. Start at the higher dose and decrease the dose as the patient improves.

CHANCROID: 500 mg every 6 hours for 7 days

CHLAMYDIA: 500 mg every 6 hours for 14 days

DIPHTHERIA: same as CELLULITIS.

DIPHTHERIA prevention: 500 mg every 6 hours for 7 days.

DONOVANOSIS: 500 mg 4 times daily until entirely healed, plus another week.

DYSENTERY: 250 mg 4 times daily for 10 days.

EAR INFECTION: same as CELLULITIS.

FOOD POISONING: 250 mg every 6 hours until the symptoms are gone, plus another 1–2 days.

GASTROENTERITIS: same as ABSCESS.

LEPTOSPIROSIS:[1] same as CELLULITIS.

LYMPHOGRANULOMA VENEREUM: 500 mg every 6 hours for 21 days.

PELVIC INFECTION: 250 mg every 6 hours for 21 days.

---

1 *It is useless to give antibiotic for leptospirosis if the patient has been ill for 4 days or more.*

PERTUSSIS: 250 mg every 6 hours for 14 days.

PERTUSSIS prevention: same as DIPHTHERIA prevention.

PINTA: 500 mg twice daily for 5 days.

PNEUMONIA: same as CELLULITIS.

Q FEVER: 1000 mg every 6 hours for 14 days.

RELAPSING FEVER: 500 mg, one dose.

RESPIRATORY INFECTION: same as CELLULITIS.

RESPIRATORY FAILURE: 1000 mg every 6 hours until much improved, then the same as for CELLULITIS.

SPOTTED FEVER: used with RIFAMPIN; 500 mg every 6 hours until the fever is gone plus 3 days.

STREP THROAT: same as CELLULITIS.

SYPHILIS, primary and secondary: 500 mg every 6 hours for 14 days.

TRACHOMA: same as PELVIC INFECTION.

TRENCH FEVER: 500 mg 4 times daily for 3 months.

TURISTA: same as ABSCESS.

TREPONARID: same as SYPHILIS.

VAGINITIS: 500 mg 4 times daily for 7 days.

YAWS: 500 mg every 6 hours for 14 days.

As a PENICILLIN substitute: same dose, same duration as PENICILLIN.

Tooth infection: 250–500 mg every 6 hours until the symptoms are gone plus another 2 days. The affected tooth should be pulled.

Alternatives: AZITHROMYCIN (Zithromax), CLARITHROMYCIN (Klaricid), SULFADIAZINE, CHLORAMPHENICOL. PENICILLIN is preferable in non-allergic patients.

ETHAMBUTOL

Anti-tuberculosis, first-line drug

Safety class: 1   Stability: C   Pregnancy: C

Brand name: Myambutol; generic available.

Indications: TUBERCULOSIS.

Contraindications: do not use with KIDNEY DISEASE. Do not use this with anyone unable to report visual loss. Do not use it in someone with optic neuritis. Do not use this with any other neurotoxic drug: one that causes SEIZURES or problems with movement or numbness and tingling in side-effects or overdose.

Precautions: patient may become color blind to green (rare); he may become totally blind with an overdose and occasionally with normal doses.

Side-effects: decreased vision (stop the drug), decreased ability to distinguish red and green, also rash or fever due to the drug. These effects occur in only a small percentage of patients. Check vision every 2 weeks in patients on the drug. This may make GOUT worse.

Overdose and prolonged usage: KIDNEY DISEASE.

TOC SYMPTOMS DIFFERENTIALS CONDITIONS DRUG INDEX REGIONAL NOTES INX

Dosage: reduce the dose with KIDNEY DISEASE.

Daily dosage for first 8 weeks
11–14 kg: 0.5 400-mg tablet daily.
15–20 kg: 1 400-mg tablet daily.
21–29 kg: 1.5 400-mg tablets daily.
30–35 kg: 2 400-mg tablets daily.
36–44 kg: 2.5 400-mg tablets daily.
45–55 kg: 3 400-mg tablets daily.
Subsequent daily dosage
Under 11 kg: don't use this.
11–19 kg: 0.5 400-mg tablet daily.
20–34 kg: 1 400-mg tablet daily.
35–44 kg: 1.5 400-mg tablets daily.
45–55 kg: 2 400-mg tablets daily.
Subsequent twice weekly dosage
Under 11 kg: don't use this.
11–19 kg: 1.5 400-mg tablets twice weekly.
20–34 kg: 3 400-mg tablets twice weekly.
35–44 kg: 4.5 400-mg tablets twice weekly.
45–55 kg: 6 400-mg tablets twice weekly.
Subsequent thrice weekly dosage
Under 11 kg: don't use this.
11–19 kg: 1 400-mg tablet thrice weekly.
20–34 kg: 2 400-mg tablets thrice weekly.
35–44 kg: 3 400-mg tablets thrice weekly.
45–55 kg: 4 400-mg tablets thrice weekly.

If you want to calculate more accurately, the formula is 25 mg/kg daily for the first 8 weeks only; for an average adult this is 1400 mg. Then reduce to 30 mg/kg thrice weekly or 45 mg/kg twice weekly. (See TUBERCULOSIS in the Condition Index for the duration of therapy.)

Alternatives: PAS, RIFAMPIN, STREPTOMYCIN (injectable only), PYRAZINAMIDE, CIPROFLOXACIN.

ETHIONAMIDE

Anti-TUBERCULOSIS, second-line drug

Brand name: Trecator-SC.

Supplied as 250 mg tablets.

Safety class: 3   Stability: C   Pregnancy: C

Indication: TUBERCULOSIS

Contraindication: ALLERGY to this drug, LIVER DISEASE.

Precautions: liver problems are likely when used with RIFAMPIN. Management of DIABETES may be more difficult.

Stop the drug if HEPATITIS develops. Get frequent blood tests to check for liver damage.

Side-effects: decreased blood pressure, sore joints, decreased vision, low blood sugar. Take PYRIDOXINE with this in order to prevent numbness, tingling and weakness.

Dosage: adults: 250–750 mg by mouth twice a day; start at the lower dose. Chilcren get 15–20 mg/kg by mouth twice a day. Give this with PYRIDOXINE.

FAMCICLOVIR

Stability: C   Pregnancy: B

Antiviral, similar to ACYCLOVIR. The usual dose is 250 mg every 8 hours for 7 days. Recently this has been used to prevent the development of HERPES: it is given as 1000 mg twice in one day when the patient first notices that a new episode is starting. It prevents the full-blown disease from developing.

FANSIDAR

Antimalarial

Safety class: 1.5   Stability: B, dark   Pregnancy: C.

No longer available in the USA; available in the UK.

Brand name: Fansidar; (Composition: PYRIMETHAMINE 25 mg + sulfadoxine 500 mg.)

Also supplied in ampules for IM use.

Indications: TOXOPLASMOSIS; prevention and treatment of CHLOROQUINE-resistant MALARIA. In many areas MALARIA is resistant to this also. Fansidar does not work well for malaria in South America.

Contraindications: infants less than 2 months old; nursing mothers; ALLERGY to this drug or any SULFA drug or PYRIMETHAMINE (Daraprim). Early pregnancy. Do not give this to someone with ANEMIA due to a deficiency of FOLATE. Do not give this to patients with PORPHYRIA or to those with G6PD DEFICIENCY.

Side-effects: nausea, vomiting, diarrhea, loss of appetite; these effects will pass. There is rarely ANEMIA due to the bone marrow dying (this is commonly fatal) or SEIZURES. The drug must be stopped immediately for these.

Some persons develop a skin reaction to this drug, resembling a burn (see EXFOLIATIVE DERMATITIS). If this happens, stop the drug immediately! There is a 0.1% chance of serious side-effects, some of them fatal.

Precautions: if the patient is pregnant, also give FOLINIC ACID, if you can.

Avoid using this with ZIDOVUDINE or NEVIRAPINE, both anti-AIDS drugs.

Note that for MALARIA treatment, it takes 24–48 hours for Fansidar to start to work. Therefore for cerebral MALARIA or other severe forms, it is necessary to use QUININE or ARTEMISININ also for at least the first few days.

Dosage: the dose may need to be increased in the presence of HIV INFECTION but these patients more often have serious side-effects also.

TOXOPLASMOSIS: 2 tablets daily for 6 weeks.

MALARIA prevention: adult dose is 1 tablet weekly. Reduce dose according to weight for children. Begin when entering a malarious area and continue for 6 weeks after leaving. (Not recommended.)

MALARIA treatment 1 ampule IM or 3 tablets by mouth, one dose only, for adults. Children 9–14 y.o. get 2 tablets; 4–8 y.o. get 1 tablet and less than 4 get 1/2 tablet. This assumes a normal (Western) weight for age.

FILICIN

An extract from a male fern plant, used to treat TAPEWORM. It works well but is dangerous, causing blindness, HEART FAILURE and occasionally death.

FLUBENDAZOLE

Be sure not to confuse this with the following entry.

Dewormer, anthelmintic

Safety class: 2   Stability: C   Pregnancy: X

Brand names: Flubenol, Flumoxal, Flumoxane, Fluvermal, Flutelmium, Frommex, others; mostly veterinary. Available in Europe, Egypt, Israel and South America.

Indications: HYDATID DISEASE, ASCARIASIS, CYSTICERCOSIS, HOOKWORM, TRICHURIASIS.

Contraindications: pregnancy.

Precautions: this drug is a veterinary drug; its use for humans is unproven; side-effects are largely unknown.

Dosage:

CYSTICERCOSIS: 20 mg/kg twice a day for 10 days. This is an average adult dose of 1200 mg per dose.

Everything else: 300 mg daily for 3 days. (But HYDATID DISEASE dosage not known.)

FLUCONAZOLE

Be sure not to confuse this with the previous entry.

Brand name: Difulcan   Pregnancy: C for VAGINITIS; D otherwise.

This alters the electrical rhythm of the heart and thus might cause sudden death. Thus it should not be used with other such drugs. The medical jargon is that it prolongs the QT interval. See the back cover.

It is used in a dosage of 150 mg once, for VAGINITIS due to yeast. You should seek further information elsewhere before using it. It has been also used for CUTANEOUS LEISHMANIASIS, 200 mg daily x 6 weeks, but it is expensive, and does not work well. It is sometimes used in a dose of 150 mg, together with AZITHROMYCIN and SECNIDAZOLE, to treat PELVIC INFECTION. It is worth trying if you can get it free. It needs dosage adjustment in KIDNEY DISEASE. Side effects are headache, nausea and abdominal pain.

FLUROQUINOLONE

This refers to a class of drugs; see CIPROFLOXACIN. Other examples are LEVOFLOXACIN, OFLOXACIN and PEFLOXACIN. There is some recent evidence that the latter two drugs work well for LEPROSY. CIPROFLOXACIN does not work for LEPROSY. All of these drugs should be avoided in the elderly and those on STEROIDS. They should not be used in Asia where there has been prior medical care, since there is a lot of resistance to them.

FOLATE, FOLIC ACID

Vitamin

Synonyms: folic acid; folinic acid is a closely related compound.

Safety class: 1   Pregnancy: A (okay.)

Stability: B; liquid preparations are very unstable.

Brand names: many; usually available by generic name. Folinic acid = Leukovoran. It is expensive.

Indications: ANEMIA due to folic acid deficiency; ANEMIA caused by MALABSORPTION, MALARIA, OVALOCYTOSIS, SPRUE, SICKLE CELL DISEASE, TURISTA, THALLASEMIA.

Contraindications: a vegan diet (no milk, eggs or meat ever); MALABSORPTION; SPRUE. In all these cases, it may be given if some VITAMIN B_{12} is given by injection first. Do not give to a patient with COBALAMIN DEFICIENCY or to someone on PHENYTOIN.

Precautions: dose on bottles is frequently in mcg (microgram). 1 mcg is 1/1000 of a mg. Therefore 100 mcg is 0.1 mg, and it will take 10 tablets of 100 mcg each to make 1 mg. Since VITAMIN A and VITAMIN D are harmful in large amounts, it is important not to take large amounts of MULTIVITAMINS containing these in order to obtain enough folate.

Dosage:

MALABSORPTION: 5 mg daily.

SPRUE: 5 mg daily for 30 days.

Pregnancy: 1 mg daily for 30 days.

Everything else: 1 mg by mouth daily, adults and children both; continue until the patient feels better and then for another week.

Alternatives: diet with fresh vegetables, MULTIVITAMINS containing sufficient folate or folic acid (most do not).

FOLINIC ACID

See FOLATE. This is a form that is used by pregnant women who take PYRIMETHAMINE, FANSIDAR, PROGUANIL or CO-TRIMOXAZOLE for an extended period of time. It provides FOLATE in a form that humans can use, but bacteria cannot use. Folinic acid counteracts the negative effects of the other drugs on the baby. It is expensive.

FOSMIDOMYCIN

This is a new anti-malarial drug used in combination with CLINDAMYCIN or artesunate (ARTEMISININ). It should not be used alone. Seek independent information concerning contraindications, side-effects and precautions. The usual dose is 900 mg every 12 hours for 7 days.

FURAZOLIDONE

This is a new medication that is used for some protozoal diseases: GIARDIASIS, amebic DYSENTERY. It has some nasty psychiatric side-effects; avoid using it!

FUROSEMIDE

Water pill, diuretic

Safety class: 2   Stability: B, dark   Pregnancy: C

Synonym: frusemide (UK)

Brand name: Lasix; generic drug is available. Supplied as 40 mg tablets, sometimes other sizes.

Indications: HEART FAILURE, HYPERTENSION; sometimes KIDNEY DISEASE, TOXEMIA.

Contraindications: ALTITUDE SICKNESS, DEHYDRATION, previous diarrhea or vomiting lasting a week or more, ALLERGY to any SULFA drug, CIRRHOSIS, LIVER FAILURE. Do not give this together with aminoglycoside-type antibiotics (e.g. GENTAMYCIN or STREPTOMYCIN) or with medication for HYPERTENSION unless it is prescribed for the particular patient. Don't use this for swelling other than that caused by HEART FAILURE or KIDNEY DISEASE.

Precautions: this drug wastes POTASSIUM from the body. If you give more than just a few doses, the patient should consume food high in potassium (apricots, avocados, bananas, citrus fruits, coconut water, dates, papaya, potatoes, pumpkin, spinach) unless he has KIDNEY DISEASE. If he does have KIDNEY DISEASE, he should not consume high-potassium foods.

This drug interferes with several lab tests; don't believe lab tests on blood drawn while the person was on this drug.

Side-effects: nausea, abdominal pain, rashes, tingling. These effects occur in only a small percentage of patients. Deafness is a very rare side-effect; stop the drug if this occurs. The drug may make the skin sensitive to sunburn.

Overdose and prolonged use: LIVER FAILURE; see Protocol B.7.

Dosage: reduce the dose in the elderly, in LIVER FAILURE and in KIDNEY DISEASE.

Adults: 40–80 mg by mouth; reduce dose for children. Repeat this every half hour until the patient has to urinate. (The drug increases urine production.) Then give the drug once or twice a day, forever with HYPERTENSION, only as long as there are symptoms for other conditions.

GAMMA GLOBULIN

This is a human blood product which is given by injection every 3–6 months to prevent HEPATITIS. The ordinary American product prevents HEPATITIS A only. The ordinary French product prevents HEPATITIS A and HEPATITIS E. A special product is available to prevent HEPATITIS B in those who are exposed but have not been immunized. The usual dose in all cases is 0.06 ml/kg, injected IM, one time only.

GANCICLOVIR

This is an anti-HIV INFECTION drug.

GATIFLOXACIN

Antibiotic: Gram-positive and Gram-negative

Safety class: 3   Stability: unknown   Pregnancy: C

This has been taken off the market in many places because it unpredictably lowers blood sugar. It is safety class 1 when used in eye drops. See ANTIBIOTIC EYE DROPS.

Pregnancy: related drugs are contraindicated.

Brand name: Tequin, Zymar, Zymaxid

Indication: ANTHRAX, possibly other indications similar to CIPROFLOXACIN.

Contraindication: prior ALLERGY to this or to any "-oxacin" drug; age under 18 years old.

Precautions: don't give this with ANTACID, IRON, ZINC, CIMETIDINE, PHENYTOIN, THEOPHYLLIN, DIGOXIN or any blood thinners.

Dosage: reduce the dose with KIDNEY DISEASE. Usual adult dose is 200–400 mg daily, by mouth or IV.

GENTAMYCIN

Antibiotic, Gram-negative, aminoglycoside

Safety class: 3   Stability: B   Pregnancy: D

Brand names: Garamycin, G-mycetin, Cidomycin, Genticin. Supplied as injectable, cream, ointment and eye drops only; not available in an oral form.

Indications: used by injection at the direction of a physician for a whole-body infections, also ACUTE ABDOMEN, BRUCELLOSIS, ENTERIC FEVER resistant to other drugs, GALLBLADDER DISEASE, MENINGITIS in a newborn, OSTEOMYELITIS, PLAGUE, PYOMYOSITIS, SEPSIS, TRENCH FEVER, TURISTA or TULAREMIA. The injectable form of the drug (there is no oral form) may be given by mouth for severe, persistent diarrhea in infants. It counteracts the bacteria in the bowel, but is not absorbed into the blood stream. (The eye drops or ointment may be used for EYE INFECTION, see ANTIBIOTIC EYE DROPS/OINTMENT.)

Contraindications: ALLERGY to the drug or to any other aminoglycoside such as STREPTOMYCIN. The injectable form is contraindicated in pregnancy and in KIDNEY DISEASE. Do not use this with other drugs that may cause KIDNEY DISEASE or in patients who have muscle weakness or trembling. Do not use it in patients with CIRRHOSIS or LIVER FAILURE; see Protocol B.7.

Precaution: this drug is given orally with CHOLESTYRAMINE for diarrhea, but the two drugs must not be given at the same time of day; stagger the times they are given by two hours or more.

Side-effects: SEIZURES, BRAIN DAMAGE or a drop in the blood pressure when given by injection. With excessive IM doses, deafness and KIDNEY DISEASE may develop. This is not a problem with topical usage.

Overdose and prolonged usage: KIDNEY DISEASE, deafness.

Dosage: reduce the dose in the elderly and in the presence of KIDNEY DISEASE or hearing loss.

ACUTE ABDOMEN: same as MENINGITIS.

BRUCELLOSIS: 1mg/kg IM every 8 hours for 6 weeks.

ENTERIC FEVER: 1 mg/kg IM every 8 hours for 10 days.

GALLBLADDER DISEASE: same as MENINGITIS.

MENINGITIS: 1 mg/kg IM every 8 hours for 14 days.

OSTEOMYELITIS: 1 mg/kg IM every 8 hours for 6 weeks minimum.

PLAGUE: 2 mg/kg IV loading, then 1.7 mg/kg IV every 8 hours for 7 days.

PYOMYOSITIS: same as MENINGITIS.

SEPSIS: same as MENINGITIS.

TRENCH FEVER: 1 mg/kg every 8 hours IV x 14 days, used with DOXYCYCLINE.

TULAREMIA: same as PLAGUE.

TURISTA:[1] 8 mg/kg by mouth every 4 hours for 3 days.

Other uses: see ANTIBIOTIC EYE DROPS or ANTIBIOTIC OINTMENT.

Alternatives: in SEPSIS, use a third-generation CEPHALOSPORIN.

GENTIAN VIOLET

Topical disinfectant.

Safety class: 1   Stability: A

Synonym: crystal violet

Brand names: Aksuris, Oxiuran, Viocid.

Indications: most commonly used for any and every skin problem. It gives a brilliant bluish-purple color to the skin which, with repeated use, may become permanent. May be used for CANDIDIASIS or TINEA when better treatments are not available.

Note that this is not very effective for preventing infections of the skin. Unsophisticated people love its brilliant color and prefer to use this to washing with soap and water. Soap and water are much more effective in preventing infection.

GRISEOFULVIN

Anti-fungal

Safety class: 3   Stability: C   Pregnancy: X

Brand names: Fulvicin U/F, Grifulvin V, Grisactin. Supplied as 125, 250 and 500 mg tablets. Available in the United States and in India.

Indication: FAVUS, TINEA.

Contraindications: pregnancy (causes fetal deformities). Avoid pregnancy while taking the drug and for one month afterward. A man should not father a child within 6 months of treatment. Also contraindicated while breast feeding and in any kind of liver disease (see LIVER FAILURE). Do not give with oral contraceptives (they may not work), to patients who have PORPHYRIA or with alcoholic drinks.

Precautions: rarely the patient may develop a swollen face: STOP THE DRUG. Griseofulvin may cause ANAPHYLAXIS like PENICILLIN. Be sure you can recognize this. See Volume 1, Chapter 4. Some people who are allergic to PENICILLIN are also allergic to this. (See ALLERGY.) Watch carefully.

Side-effects: headache, which will disappear with continued use. There is sun sensitivity. Other side-effects include pains in the limbs, lethargy, confusion, nausea, diarrhea, gas. The blood count may drop (causing ANEMIA and susceptibility to infection) as the drug damages the bone marrow. It may cause protein in the urine. It may cause breast development in males. There may be a DRUG ERUPTION.

Overdose and prolonged usage: LIVER FAILURE; see Protocol B.7.

Dosage: this should be given with a fatty meal.

Infants: 2.5 mg/kg every 6 hours; Children (30–50 lb): 30–62 mg every 6 hours; Children (over 50 lb.): 62–125 mg every 6 hours.

Adults: 125–250 mg every 6 hours; Treat for 3 weeks if palms, soles and nails are not affected. Treat for 6–25 weeks if these are affected.

Results: begin in 2–3 days.

---

1 Used orally, you can ignore pregnancy as a contraindication. It only kills bacterial within the bowel; it is not absorbed into the blood stream and thus cannot harm the baby.

HAART

This is an acronym for "highly active anti-retroviral therapy"—a combination of drugs to treat HIV INFECTION. Detailing the treatment plan is beyond the scope of this book, but some individual drugs are listed.

HALOFANTRINE

Antimalarial, British only, not used much anymore

Safety class: 3   Stability: C   Pregnancy: C

Brand name: Halfan. Supplied as a liquid of 100 mg/ml and 250 mg tablets. Not available in the United States.

Indications: CHLOROQUINE-resistant and FANSIDAR-resistant MALARIA.

Contraindications: ALLERGY to the drug; pregnancy, nursing mothers, any personal or family history of heart disease involving abnormal heart rhythms, an abnormal EKG, usage of other drugs that cause LIVER FAILURE, current or recent usage of MEFLOQUINE.

Precautions: this is a dangerous drug. It should only be used on the advice of a physician. Never give it at the same time or shortly after MEFLOQUINE, QUININE or CHLOROQUINE, any psychiatric medications, any heart medications or any ALLERGY medications. It can cause life-threatening heart problems even in otherwise-healthy patients. It alters the electrical rhythm of the heart and thus might cause sudden death. Thus it should not be used with other such drugs. The medical jargon is that it prolongs the QT interval. See the back cover.

Side-effects: transient nausea, vomiting, diarrhea and stomach cramps. Itching may occur in black skin. Try vitamin B complex to treat the itching. It is dangerous if taken with fatty foods. It can cause LIVER FAILURE; see Protocol B.7.

Dosage: take on an empty stomach. 500 mg by mouth every 6–8 hours for 3 doses; repeat this after 7–14 days if this is the first time the person has ever had MALARIA. Children get 8–10 mg/kg per dose; give 3 doses, 6 hours apart.

Alternatives: CHLOROQUINE plus CHLORPHENIRAMINE.

HEXADECYLPHOSPHOCHOLINE

See MILTEFOSINE. This is an alternative generic name.

HIB

This is an immunization which prevents some middle EAR INFECTIONs and one form of MENINGITIS in infants and young children.

HOMATROPINE EYE DROPS

Pupil dilator; Mydriatic

Safety class: 2   Stability: C

Brand names: Isoptohomatropine; tropicamide is a generic equivalent.

Indications: KERATITIS, treatment of a scratched cornea, pain after removal of a foreign object.

Contraindications: GLAUCOMA; check for this!

Precautions: unless the eye is numb, these drops burn as they go in; it is a normal effect which will pass after 10 minutes or so.

Dosage: one drop in the affected eye every 5 minutes for 2 doses. Then use ANTIBIOTIC EYE OINTMENT in it and patch it for at least 12 hours. You may repeat the drops as needed for pain. The patch may be removed after the pupil becomes small in response to light.

HYDRALAZINE

Blood pressure medicine, antihypertensive

Safety class: 2   Stability: A   Pregnancy: C

Brand name: Apresoline; generic drug is available. Supplied as 10, 25, 50 and 100 mg tablets.

Indications: HYPERTENSION, TOXEMIA, maybe KIDNEY DISEASE.

Contraindications: ALLERGY to the drug, prior severe HEART FAILURE, ANGINA or RHEUMATIC FEVER. Do not give this at the same time as IBUPROFEN or similar medications. Do not give to patients that have PORPHYRIA (a hereditary disease).

Precautions: discontinue this drug if any of the following occur: joint pains, fever, chest pains like ANGINA.

Side-effects: common side-effects are headache, heart pounding, loss of appetite, nausea and vomiting, diarrhea, fast pulse. Less common are constipation, anxiety, sleep disturbances and a stuffy nose. Sometimes there is fluid retention, with swelling of the feet and ankles toward the end of the day.

Overdose and prolonged usage: LIVER FAILURE; see Protocol B.7.

Dosage: 10 mg to 50 mg by mouth every 6 hours. Start at the lower dosage and work up, increasing every 3 or 4 days until the blood pressure is normal. Reduce the dose for the elderly and possibly also for LIVER FAILURE. Reduce the dose according to weight in children. Continue throughout life in HYPERTENSION, until after delivery in TOXEMIA. In a crisis in TOXEMIA, a physician or nurse can give 10 mg slowly IV every 30 minutes until the pressure comes down.

Alternatives: NIFEDIPINE, HYDROCHLOROTHIAZIDE.

HYDROCHLOROTHIAZIDE

Water pill, diuretic

Safety class: 2   Stability: A   Pregnancy: B

Brand names: Hydrodiuril; generic drug is available. Supplied as 25 and 50 mg tablets.

Indications: HEART FAILURE, HYPERTENSION, mild KIDNEY DISEASE, TOXEMIA.

Contraindications: DEHYDRATION, diet-controlled DIABETES, ALLERGY to any SULFA drug, severe KIDNEY DISEASE. Do not give this to diabetics who use oral medication for blood sugar. Do not give this to women who are breastfeeding, to patients who have PORPHYRIA or to those with G6PD DEFICIENCY, CIRRHOSIS or LIVER FAILURE.

Precautions: unless this is used for KIDNEY DISEASE, the patient must take POTASSIUM or consume food high in POTASSIUM (apricots, avocados, bananas, citrus fruits, coconut water, dates, papayas, potatoes, pumpkins, spinach, tomatoes). With KIDNEY DISEASE, give no POTASSIUM.

Side-effects: weakness, sun sensitivity, low blood pressure, a feeling of faintness.

Overdose and prolonged use: KIDNEY DISEASE.

Dosage: reduce the dose for the elderly and possibly with KIDNEY DISEASE. Adults get 25–50 mg by mouth once or twice daily. Reduce dose according to weight for children. Continue the drug throughout life in HYPERTENSION, just until the problem is past in other conditions. It may be necessary to continue long-term in HEART FAILURE.

Alternatives: FUROSEAMIDE, hygroton; the patient needs POTASSIUM as above.

HYDROCORTISONE

Steroid

Safety class: 3   Stability: C   Pregnancy: C

Brand names: Cortef, Hydrocortone, others. Supplied as tablets and as short-acting and long-acting injections. Eye drops are usually made out of a similar, related drug, PREDNISOLONE.

Indications: ALLERGY; ANAPHYLAXIS; ANTHRAX; ASTHMA; CONTACT DERMATITIS; CYSTICERCOSIS; ECZEMA; ENTERIC FEVER; EXFOLIATIVE DERMATITIS; FILARIASIS; HEART FAILURE; KATAYAMA DISEASE; KIDNEY DISEASE; LEPROSY reactions; ONCHOCERCIASIS.

Contraindications: HIV INFECTION, ANGINA, some infections. Used in a patient with STRONGYLOIDIASIS it may cause SEPSIS and death. If this is a possibility, treat for STRONGYLOIDIASIS before using this drug. Probably should not be used in pregnancy because it may cause cleft palate in the baby. The drug may activate TUBERCULOSIS which is dormant. With a history of TB or in an area where TB is common, the drug should be used only with a physician's supervision. Do not use in the presence of CHAGA'S DISEASE. Don't use it if there is any history of MENTAL ILLNESS or HYPERTENSION.

Precautions: unless directed otherwise by a physician for the particular illness, it is important not to use this drug for more than 5 days at a time before stopping it for at least a week. When using it for a longer time, one usually gives it only every other day. If the patient has already been on the drug for more than 5 days, stop it gradually, not abruptly. If the patient has an emotional breakdown, stop the drug gradually. The drug may activate amebae, causing AMEBIASIS or complications thereof. Regard any diarrhea as amebic DYSENTERY. It impairs wound healing and may cause DIABETES.

Side-effects: MENTAL ILLNESS, increased appetite, an illusory sense of well-being, brittle bones that fracture easily, failure to grow in children, with long-term usage, CATARACTS. Overdose and prolonged usage: CATARACTS, KIDNEY DISEASE, LIVER FAILURE, (see Protocol B.7).

There are bad long-term side-effects of the drug: muscle weakness, brittle bones, PEPTIC ULCER, DIABETES, SHOCK, death, to name a few. These never occur if the drug is used for 5 days or less. The dose of the drug is not nearly as critical as the length of time it is used.

Dosage:

Oral adult dose is 5–30 mg, 2–4 times daily for a maximum of 5 days unless ordered otherwise by a physician. Use the higher doses in very ill patients. Reduce dose according to weight for children.

IM adult dose is 100 mg in a single injection, which causes an anti-inflammatory action for 30–48 hours.

When this is used as an alternative to PREDNISONE, the usual dose is four times that of PREDNISONE; i.e., give 20 mg of HYDROCORTISONE in place of each 5 mg of PREDNISONE.

IBUPROFEN

Analgesic, anti-inflammatory, NSAID

Safety class: 2   Stability: C   Pregnancy: B

Brand names: Pediaprofen, Motrin, Rufen, Advil. Comes as 200, 400 and 600 mg tablets and in liquid for children. The 200 mg tablet is available without a prescription in the United States.

Indications: fever (reduction of any fever), ARTHRITIS, COSTAL CHONDRITIS, headaches, menstrual cramps, MUSCLE STRAIN, PERICARDITIS, PLEURISY, sprains.

Contraindications: ALLERGY to ASPIRIN, ibuprofen or any NSAID (non-steroidal, anti-inflammatory drug). Don't use this at the same time as ASPIRIN, ALCOHOL, HYDROCORTISONE, PREDNISONE, CIPROFLOXACIN or related drugs. Do not use in the presence of CIRRHOSIS or LIVER FAILURE.

Precautions: may cause abdominal pain, nausea and vomiting. Use carefully if at all if your patient has a PEPTIC ULCER or a history of one.

Side-effects: dizziness, headache, nausea, vomiting, diarrhea.

Overdose and prolonged usage: KIDNEY DISEASE, LIVER FAILURE (see Protocol B.7).

TOC | SYMPTOMS | DIFFERENTIALS | CONDITIONS | **DRUG INDEX** | REGIONAL NOTES | INX

Dosage: give the drug with food. Adult dose is 200–600 mg by mouth every 6 hours as needed. Child dose is 5–10 mg/kg every 6 hours.

IMODIUM

See LOPERAMIDE.

INDINAVIR SULFATE

Anti-HIV drug; protease inhibitor

Safety class: 3   Stability: dry, room temperature

Pregnancy: C

Brand name: 200 mg, 400 mg

Indication: HIV INFECTION

Contraindications: prior ALLERGY to this drug.

Precautions:

Don't use St John's wort while taking this.

Indinavir interacts badly with many different drugs

Don't consume grapefruit (or its juice) while taking this.

Seek independent advice before giving this in the presence of LIVER DISEASE or DIABETES.

Stop for worsening ANEMIA or abnormal bleeding.

Side-effects: KIDNEY STONES in children, nausea/vomiting/diarrhea/abdominal pains, mental changes, skin changes, JAUNDICE.

Dosage: adult dose: 600–800 mg every 8 hours.

IODINE

Mineral; antiseptic

Safety class: 2–3. Stability: varies. Pregnancy: this is a necessary nutrient; use products intended as supplements.

Synonym: Lugol's Solution (an iodine solution).

Brand names: Lipiodol is iodine-oil to be taken by mouth. Ethiodol is iodine-oil for injection; it is used for taking x-rays, to show certain body parts clearly. Lugol's solution is 5% iodine and 10% potassium iodide; tincture of iodine is 2.5% iodine and 2.5% potassium iodide, made up in alcohol. Povidone iodine is iodine attached to an organic compound to stabilize it. It is available as a powder in 1 kg plastic tubs.

Indications: CANDIDIASIS, IMPETIGO, MYCETOMA, sometimes TINEA, CUTANEOUS LEISHMANIASIS. Also used to purify water for drinking and for soaking fruits and vegetables before eating. It may be used for goiter due to iodine deficiency, but there is conflicting information in the literature, so you should not use this without professional advice.

Povidone iodine is dissolved in normal saline to make ANTIBIOTIC EYE DROPS (actually, antiseptic) which can be used for KERATITIS and EYE INFECTIONS. Mixing povidone iodine with petroleum jelly makes a good ANTIBIOTIC OINTMENT for wounds. (This is also available commercially.) See Volume 1 Appendix 1, Procedures 9 and 10.

Contraindications: older people with lumpy goiters—it will not help these and may harm them; ALLERGY to iodine; GOITER not due to iodine deficiency. (This will generally be in areas where most of the diet is from the sea, and there is no CRETINISM.) Pregnant women with GOITER need iodine to prevent their babies being born with CRETINISM. On the other hand, large doses of iodine for prolonged times can cause fetal problems during pregnancy.

Precautions: keep this out of reach of children. See the Symptom Index, Protocol A.11 if it is taken in large doses. When treating patients for GOITER or THYROID TROUBLE (low-thyroid), watch for symptoms of THYROID TROUBLE (high-thyroid). If this occurs, stop the iodine. Iodine preparations with 7% available iodine should not be used in wounds. First dilute them 1:3 with water.

Side-effects: rash, discoloration of the skin and nails.

Dosage:

GOITER: one drop of tincture of iodine in a liter of drinking water weekly for 4 weeks, then monthly. Ethiodol: recommended dose is a single IM injection of 950 mg. Lipoidol dose is 2 ml in one dose yearly.

IMPETIGO, CUTANEOUS LEISHMANIASIS: smear the tincture of iodine or iodine ointment over the affected area daily.

MYCETOMA: use only on direction of an M.D.

THYROID TROUBLE: same as GOITER.

TINEA: apply the tincture of iodine to the skin (excluding the nipples in nursing women).

Drinking water purification: 5 drops of tincture of Iodine per liter and wait for 15 minutes for everything but GIARDIASIS. If there is GIARDIASIS, use 12 drops and wait an hour. The water will not taste good.

Food purification: put iodine of any sort in water, enough to make a solution the color of weak tea. Soak the food for 30 minutes, and then rinse with clean drinking water.

IODOQUINOL

Amebicide

Safety class: 3   Stability: C

Brand Name: Yodoxin

This is a compound that is sometimes used to clear the bowel of amebae. DILOXANIDE FUROATE is safer than this. Excessive doses are associated with loss of vision. Dosage is 650 mg three times daily for 20 days.

IPECAC, SYRUP OF

Emetic

Safety class: 1   Stability: C, dark   Pregnancy: C

Supplied as generic drug in 30 ml bottles.

Indication: to cause vomiting after poisoning.

Contraindications: do not use this if the patient appears as if he may become unconscious or if he took anti-depressant medication. Do not use for acids, lye, gasoline- or kerosene-type poisons. Check for mouth burns if you are not sure what the patient took; do not give ipecac in the presence of mouth burns. Instead, give PROMETHAZINE to prevent vomiting and give milk or water, ACTIVATED CHARCOAL and MILK OF MAGNESIA.

Precautions: this description applies only to syrup of ipecac. Do not use the fluid extract.

Dosage: 5 ml from 6 months to a year; 15 ml (1 tablespoon) in children up to 2 y.o.; 30 ml (2 tablespoons) in children over 2 y.o. and adults, both followed by 2 glasses of warm liquid, any kind except milk.

Results: 15–30 minutes.

Alternatives: put a large-diameter stomach tube down, empty the stomach, then rinse with large amounts of water (see Volume 1 Appendix 1). If the patient is alert but refuses to swallow the ipecac, get enough people to help hold him down, put a stomach tube down and pour the ipecac and warm water down the tube. Then remove the tube and stand back.

IPRATROPIUM

Safety class: 2   Stability: A   Pregnancy: B

Available as dry powder for inhalation and as an aerosol for inhalation. Available as 20 micrograms per inhalation or 40 micrograms per inhalation. The drug is related to ATROPINE.

Indications: ASTHMA, ALLERGY

Contraindications: previous bad reaction to this medication, currently a severe asthma attack. (The drug is used for asthma but it should not be given in the context of a severe attack going on—only for a mild attack or to prevent an attack.) Do not give this to anyone with GLAUCOMA.

Precautions: try not to use this in pregnancy or in older men who have difficulty urinating. Counsel patients not to exceed the recommended dosage. If the patient develops a rash with using this stop the drug. With eye exposure there will be pain and blurring of vision. This will wear off.

Side-effects: worsening of GLAUCOMA, constipation, inability to pass urine (especially in older men), susceptibility to HEAT ILLNESS, dry mouth, decrease in sweating, rapid pulse, sensitivity to light, blurred vision.

Dosage: note that the dose is micrograms, not milligrams. One microgram is 0.001 milligram. Adults: 20–80 micrograms at a time, 3–4 times daily. Children 6–12 y.o. 20–40 micrograms 3 times daily. Children under 6 y.o. 20 micrograms 3 times daily.

Alternatives: ALBUTEROL, THEOPHYLLIN, EPINEPHRINE by injection.

IRON

Safety class: 1 (oral) or 3 (IM).

Stability, oral: A; IM, C   Pregnancy: A

Synonym: ferrous sulfate, ferrous with another last name such as gluconate.

Includes: imferon and iron dextran as injectable iron. Ferrous fumarate, ferrous gluconate and ferrous sulfate are generic names for oral iron. Ferrous sulfate is by far the best and cheapest. Some people tolerate one kind of iron better than another.

It is essential to get enough into a person. Equivalent doses are as follows:

    ferrous sulfate: 300 mg = 60 mg iron

    ferrous sulfate anhydrous: 200 mg = 65 mg iron

    ferrous fumarate: 200 mg = 65 mg iron

    ferrous gluconate: 300 mg = 35 mg iron

Indications: ANEMIA, mild MALNUTRITION, pregnancy, occasionally VISCERAL LEISHMANIASIS.

Contraindications: any history of multiple blood transfusions, HEMOCHROMATOSIS. ALLERGY due to iron injection means you must not give another iron injection. Oral iron is still acceptable.

Precautions: be sure to treat the patient for a minimum of 3 months in order to build up his/her iron stores. Iron may be constipating in older people. ANEMIA due to MALARIA or SICKLE CELL DISEASE should be treated mainly with FOLATE; iron may be useful in some cases (see the Condition Index and the lecture entitled *Anemia* at www.villagemedicalmanual.org). Detain the patient for 30 minutes after injection: watch for ANAPHYLAXIS. Use a long needle and make sure the injection is into muscle; if it goes into the fatty layer it will permanently stain skin. Oral iron will turn stools black and may give a false-positive test for blood in the stool. Recheck after the patient has been off iron for a week.

Side-effects: nausea, vomiting, abdominal pain.

Dosage:

Oral: ferrous sulfate is better than ferrous with any other last name; it is absorbed the best. Children: 10 mg/kg ferrous sulfate three times a day to a maximum of 900 mg daily. Adults: 300 mg ferrous sulfate three times a day. Use this for a minimum of three months. In case of overdose, see the Symptom Index, Protocol A.11.

Injection: a single dose of 100 mg/ml Iron dextran is used. Determine the volume to be used as follows: for a hemoglobin above 6, (or if the hemoglobin level is unknown), divide the child's weight (in kg) by 3 in order to get the dosage volume in ml (of 100 mg/ml solution) that you should give.

For a hemoglobin below 6(45%), divide the child's weight (in kg) by 2, to get the volume in ml (of 100 mg/ml solution) that you should give.

If your Iron dextran solution is only 50 mg/ml, double the volume calculated above.

Dosage of injectable iron at 100mg/ml

TOC   SYMPTOMS   DIFFERENTIALS   CONDITIONS   **DRUG INDEX**   REGIONAL NOTES   INX

Weight	Hemoglobin > 6	Hemoglobin < 6
10 kg/22 lb	3.3 ml	5.0 ml
20 kg/44 lb	6.7 ml	10.0 ml
30 kg/66 lb	10.0 ml	15.0 ml
40 kg/88 lb	13.3 ml	20.0 ml
50 kg/110 lb	16.7 ml	25.0 ml

Each single injection should be a maximum of 5 ml. Larger patients will need multiple injections to reach the proper final dose. Give the injections in the buttocks only.

ISONIAZID

Anti-tuberculous

Safety class: 2   Stability: C, dark   Pregnancy: C

Brand names: INH, Niconyl, Nicozide, Nydrazid, Rimifon, Tyvid.

Indications: suspected or proven TUBERCULOSIS.
All household contacts of patients with the adult-type of lung TB, especially spouse/children/parents.

Contraindications: previous HEPATITIS which was the result of isoniazid therapy; current HEPATITIS or other liver disease; CIRRHOSIS, LIVER FAILURE; ALLERGY to the drug; current use of NIRIDAZOLE; unreliable patient who will not take the drug regularly. (If you give such a person the drug, it will not help him, and it will cause resistant TUBERCULOSIS to develop in your community.) Do not give this at the same time as ALCOHOL, PHENYTOIN or CYCLOSERINE.

Precautions: give this with food. Check patients monthly. Check the whites of eyes for yellow; stop the drug if this develops. (Normally there is slight yellow around the edges of the whites. This is not significant.) Check the urine for bilirubin (urine dipstick) and stop the drug if this turns positive.

Give the patient a PYRIDOXINE tablet at least twice weekly while on isoniazid (1/4 or 1/2 tablet daily is okay also), more frequently if he develops numbness in his legs or feet.

Decrease the dose of isoniazid if a patient develops nausea, headache, loss of appetite, dry mouth, incoordination or drowsiness, if this appears to be due to the drug.

Stop the drug immediately if the patient develops crazy behavior or JAUNDICE. Advise the patient not to drink alcoholic beverages.

The drug gets into breast milk, but that is probably not a problem.

The drug interferes with a test for sugar in the urine.

Side-effects: numbness and tingling of the limbs, nausea, vomiting, diarrhea, abdominal pain.

Overdose and prolonged usage: KIDNEY DISEASE, LIVER FAILURE (see Protocol B.7).

Dosage: reduce the dose in those more than 35 years old and in the presence of KIDNEY DISEASE.

To calculate accurately for your patients, adults get get 5 mg/kg to a maximum of 300 mg single daily dose. Infants and children get 10 mg/kg to a maximum of 300 mg. For TB

MENINGITIS all patients get 10 mg/kg daily and you must be sure to use two other anti-tuberculous drugs with it. Give it for 6 months except with bone and joint TB and with TB MENINGITIS; in those cases use it for 12 months.

For any age, you may switch to 15 mg/kg (maximum of 900 mg) twice or thrice weekly after 2–8 weeks (preferably 8) on the above dosage. Results should be evident in 3–4 weeks.

Daily dosage	
Under 6 kg	0.5 of a 100 mg tablet
6–11 kg	One 100-mg tablet
12–29 kg	0.5 of a 300 mg tablet
30–50 kg	One 300 mg tablet
Twice or thrice weekly dosage	
3–4 kg	0.5 of a 100 mg tablet
5–8 kg	One 100 mg tablet
9–14 kg	0.5 of a 300 mg tablet
15–25 kg	One 300 mg tablet
26–34 kg	1.5 of a 300 mg tablet
35–45 kg	Two 300 mg tablets
46–52 kg	2.5 of 300 mg tablets
> 52 kg	Three 300 mg tablets

Alternatives: ETHAMBUTOL, RIFAMPIN, STREPTOMYCIN, CYCLOSERINE, CIPROFLOXACIN, PYRAZINAMIDE, PARA-AMINOSALICYLIC ACID.

ISOQUINE

This is an antimalarial drug, related to AMINODIAQUINE and CHLOROQUINE.

ITRACONAZOLE

Anti-fungal, anti-Leishmania, other uses

Safety class: 3

Brand names: Sporanox, Onmel.

Indications: usually used for FUNGAL INFECTION, but in the context of the Third-World, it is more often used for LEISHMANIASIS, MYCETOMA or CANCER.

Contraindications: HEART FAILURE, KIDNEY DISEASE, LIVER FAILURE.

This alters the electrical rhythm of the heart and thus might cause sudden death. Thus it should not be used with other such drugs. The medical jargon is that it prolongs the QT interval. See the back cover.

Similar to KETOCONAZOLE; used in simple CUTANEOUS LEISHMANIASIS, Mexicana type, 200 mg twice daily for 28 days. It may also be useful in MYCETOMA and VISCERAL LEISHMANIASIS. Do not give the capsule form with medicines for PEPTIC ULCER. Itraconazole must be taken with a full meal. Used for CANCER, the dose is 100 mg daily, taken at the same time as dried artemisia annua leaf powder. Seek independent information elsewhere before using this.

IVERMECTIN

Dewormer, anthelmintic

Safety class: 1   Stability: C   Pregnancy: C

Brand names: Cardomec, Heartguard 30, Ivomec, Mectizan, Oramec, Stromectol, Zymectin. Supplied in 6 mg tablets, 1 mg capsules and 1% liquid (10 mg/ml). It is also available as a 1.87% cream, veterinary form, brand name Equalan. It may be fake or substandard since it is hard to obtain.

Indications: ASCARIASIS, ENTEROBIASIS, FILARIASIS treatment and prevention, LARVA MIGRANS prevention, LICE, MANSONELLOSIS PERSTANS prevention, ONCHOCERCIASIS, SCABIES, STRONGYLOIDIASIS, TRICHURIASIS.

It is not useful for HOOKWORM. Dangerous for LOIASIS; seek advice. It is safe to give with ALBENDAZOLE and PRAZIQUANTEL.

Contraindications: pregnancy; children under 5 y.o. or 15 kg; ALLERGY to the drug; any serious illness, especially MENINGITIS. In areas with LOIASIS, it can cause BRAIN DAMAGE.

Precautions: the drug causes miscarriages as well as developmental problems in animals. When used for FILARIASIS or ONCHOCERCIASIS, it should not be used before a course of DOXYCYCLINE. The drug appears in breast milk and should not be used in nursing mothers with infants less than 7 days old. Keep the patient lying down for an hour or two after he takes the drug or his blood pressure may drop, causing him to faint. Adverse effects are much more common in expatriates than in nationals.

Side-effects: occasionally there is headache and general achiness, fever and chills, swelling, painful lymph nodes and itching. Rarely a patient may develop severe low blood pressure and fainting. This should be treated by having him lie flat for a couple of days until he feels better. Patients with prior ASTHMA may get an attack; treat that like any other attack of ASTHMA. If the patient also has ASCARIASIS, he will pass the worms.

Dosage: adults get 12 mg as one single dose for most purposes except TRICHURIASIS, STRONGYLOIDIASIS and FILARIASIS. Reduce the dose according to weight for children.

FILARIASIS treatment: 12–24 mg every 3 months until the problem has resolved. Alternatively, 0.4 mg/kg in a single dose, given with a single dose of DIETHYLCARBAMAZINE.

FILARIASIS prevention: 0.1 mg/kg (average adult dose would be 5–7 mg) in a single dose once or (preferably) twice a year. There is some evidence that even lower doses may work.

LARVA MIGRANS: cutaneous: give 0.2mg/kg in a single oral dose. Deep: same dose, daily x 2 days.

LICE: 0.2 mg/kg in a single oral dose.

MANSONELLOSIS PERSTANS prevention: 15 mg/kg every 3 months.

ONCHOCERCIASIS: repeat the treatment every 6–12 months.

SCABIES: the veterinary cream is applied to affected areas weekly for 4 weeks or else 0.2 mg/kg in a single oral dose.

STRONGYLOIDIASIS: 12 mg daily for 2 days. If not clear, give this daily until 1–2 weeks after the symptoms clear.

TRICHURIASIS: 12 mg daily for 3 days.

KAOPECTATE

Anti-diarrhea

Safety class: 1   Stability: A

Indications: mild to moderate diarrhea.

Contraindications: ACUTE ABDOMEN.

Precautions: try not to give this at the same time as any antibiotics; it cancels the effect of antibiotics.

Dosage: adults: 15–30 ml after each loose bowel movement. Children: 5–15 ml as above.

Alternatives: BISMUTH SUBSALICYLATE, Lomotil (diphenoxylate hydrochloride), Paregoric, Imodium.

KETAMINE

General anesthetic

Safety class: 3   Stability: A   Pregnancy: A

Brand name: Ketalar and generic veterinary drug. Supplied in a variety of strengths: 10 mg/ml, 50 mg/ml, 100 mg/ml. Be sure to check your supply. **This is a controlled substance.**

Indications: gives 30–45 minutes (IM) of unconsciousness needed for a painful procedure such as straightening a fractured limb or cleaning a dirty wound. IV the duration is 15–20 minutes, sometimes longer.

Contraindications: do not use this if the patient has eaten within the past 6 hours. Do not use this if you have not had instruction on how to maintain an airway in an unconscious patient. Do not use this if your patient has had an allergic reaction to this drug. (See ALLERGY.) The drug raises blood pressure, so do not give it to someone with uncontrolled HYPERTENSION. Do not use this in early pregnancy unless you are truly desperate. Late pregnancy and during delivery are okay.

Precautions: possession of this drug can cause major legal problems in the States and the UK since it is tightly controlled. Awakening may take hours. Adults commonly have very bad dreams while awakening. They may become violent. Patients should be warned about this and sedative medication such as PROMETHAZINE should be available, as well as a quiet, soothing environment and someone to calm the patient if he should become agitated. Reportedly if the patient is calm before being given the drug, he is less likely to be agitated upon awakening. It will be worth your time to sedate and reassure the patient before putting him to sleep with this. Be sure that fractures are well-splinted. Terrifying dreams may recur days or weeks later.

Side-effects: MENTAL ILLNESS, HYPERTENSION.

Dosage: the IV anesthetic dosage is 2 mg/kg. Light sedation: 4 mg/kg IM. Anesthesia: 6–10 mg/kg IM, one dose. Be extremely careful with the dose. The following table gives ml at 100mg/ml for IM injection. Give twice this ml volume if you have 50 mg/ml. **Don't use this table if you will give it IV.**

Weight	Sedation	Anesthesia
10 kg	0.4 ml IM	0.6–1.0 ml IM
20 kg	0.8 ml IM	1.2–2.0 ml IM
30 kg	1.2 ml IM	1.8–3.0 ml IM
40 kg	1.6 ml IM	2.4–4.0 ml IM
50 kg	2.0 ml IM	3.0–5.0 ml IM

You may repeat the full dose when the patient is fully awake or a half dose when he awakens just enough to object to pain. It can be renewed repeatedly.

KETOCONAZOLE

Anti-fungal and other uses

Safety class: 3   Stability: C   Pregnancy: C

Brand name: Nizorol.

Indications: CANDIDIASIS; CUTANEOUS LEISHMANIASIS, simple Mexicana type; MYCETOMA; TINEA; possibly VISCERAL LEISHMANIASIS. It may be added to TRICLABENDAZOLE to increase the cure rate in LIVER FLUKE disease.

Contraindications: ALLERGY to the drug or any other – azole drug, CIRRHOSIS, LIVER DISEASE, current use of ERYTHROMYCIN or astemizole or terfenadine (newer antihistamines). Contraindicated in pregnancy, breast-feeding. Don't use this at the same time as DIAZEPAM or other sedative medication.

Precautions: this drug will not work if taken by mouth with DICYCLOMINE, ANTACIDs, medicines for PEPTIC ULCER or with RIFAMPIN. If it causes HEPATITIS, the drug must be stopped. Never use it for more than 2 weeks without physician approval. Warn the patient not to drink alcohol while on this; it may make him very ill. The drug causes falsely abnormal liver function blood tests. It also may damage the liver.

The drug is sometimes associated with altered electrical activity in the heart which may cause sudden death. Thus this should not be combined with other such drugs. The medical jargon is that it prolongs the QT interval. See the back cover.

Side-effects: nausea and vomiting are most frequent; taking the drug with food helps. Less common effects are headache, sensitivity to light, numbness and tingling in limbs, a rash and a bleeding tendency. It can cause DRUG ERUPTION.

Overdose and prolonged usage: LIVER FAILURE; see Protocol B.7.

Dosage:

For adults, 200–400 mg by mouth daily. Children's daily dose is 3.3–6.6 mg/kg:

CANDIDIASIS 1–4 weeks.

LIVER FLUKE: adding this (200 mg daily) to TRICLABENDAZOLE increases the cure rate.

TINEA of skin: 1–2 months.

TINEA of nails: 6–12 months.

For CUTANEOUS LEISHMANIASIS, it only is helpful in the type that rapidly cures itself. Given that the drug is expensive and dangerous, the wisdom of using it for this is questionable. The dosage for this is 600 mg daily for 4 weeks. Alternatively, use the commercial 2% cream or else grind 1000 mg of the drug and mix it with 50 ml of dimethyl sulfoxide cream, obtained from your pharmacist. Other creams do not work as well. Apply this 3 times a day for a month.

MYCETOMA Seek a physician's advice before using.

VISCERAL LEISHMANIASIS: seek independent sources on dosages.

Alternatives: itraconazole (Sporanox), fluconazole (Diflucan).

LACTAID, LACTASE, LACTRASE

Lactase enzyme

Safety class: 1   Stability: C

Brand name: LACTAID

Indication: MILK INTOLERANCE

Contraindication: ALLERGY to this medication.

Dosage: 1 tablet before each glass of milk. The dosage is according to the amount of milk, not according to the patient's size. Do not reduce the dosage for children, but do reduce it for lesser amounts of milk.

Alternatives For some people, using fermented milk products such as yogurt or cheese eliminates the need for this medication.

LACTOBACILLUS GG

This is a bacterium used to make YOGURT. It is available in powdered form in health food stores. It is helpful in treating diarrhea in infants. An alternative is to use yogurt itself.

LACTRASE

See LACTAID above.

LAMIVUDINE

Anti-viral; nucleosidase analog

Safety class: 3   Stability: C   Pregnancy: C

Brand name: Epivir

Indication: HIV INFECTION, HEPATITIS B.

Contraindication: ALLERGY to this drug

Precautions: CO-TRIMOXAZOLE increases the amount of this drug in the blood and therefore might cause toxicity. Don't use in children who have had PANCREATITIS

Side-effects: abdominal distress, flu-like illness, abnormal bleeding, many others.

Dosage: decrease the dose with KIDNEY DISEASE. Usual adult dose is 150 mg twice daily or 300 mg daily.

LEVAMISOLE

Dewormer, anthelmintic

Not available in the USA or in Canada.

Safety class: 2   Stability: unknown   Pregnancy: C

Brand names: Anthelpor, Aviverm, Cevasol, Cyverm, Dilarvon, Ketrax, Levipor, Nemacide and others. Supplied as 40 mg and 150 mg tablets.

Indications: ASCARIASIS, possibly HOOKWORM, STRONGYLOIDIASIS. Used with MEBENDAZOLE for MANSONELLOSIS PERSTANS and ONCHOCERCIASIS. Also useful in MALNUTRITION, to boost immunity.

Contraindications: previous ALLERGY to this drug. Seek independent information before using this in anyone who has an autoimmune disorder or HIV INFECTION.

Precautions: side-effects are headache, nausea, dizziness and confusion. If the patient develops a flu-like illness, then stop the drug.

Overdose and prolonged usage: LIVER FAILURE (see Protocol B.7), KIDNEY DISEASE

Dosage:

ASCARIASIS: 50–150 mg

HOOKWORM: does not work well; dosage like ascariasis

STRONGYLOIDIASIS: does not work well; dosage like ascariasis

MANSONELLOSIS PERSTANS: adult dose is 300 mg daily for 1 week, used with MEBENDAZOLE or ALBENDAZOLE.

ONCHOCERCIASIS: 2.5 mg/kg twice weekly the week before MEBENDAZOLE, plus the same dose continued for the 3 weeks the MEBENDAZOLE is given. Repeat every 6 months.

MALNUTRITION: 2.5 mg/kg daily for 2–5 days.

Everything else: 5 mg/kg, single dose.

LEVOFLOXACIN

Antibiotic, Gram-negative mostly, a second-generation quinolone related to CIPROFLOXACIN.

Safety class: 3   Stability: C   Pregnancy: C

Brand name: Levaquin

Indications: same as CIPROFLOXACIN and GATIFLOXACIN; also PELVIC INFECTION, if given IV, reportedly works for PLAGUE.

Contraindications: prior ALLERGY to any drugs in this class; age under 18 years old.

Precautions and Side-effects: the same as other drugs in this class; see CIPROFLOXACIN. Occasionally there are problems with high or low blood sugar in those who take this. It is best not to use this in elderly people or those taking STEROIDs.

This alters the electrical rhythm of the heart and thus might cause sudden death. Thus it should not be used with other such drugs. The medical jargon is that it prolongs the QT interval. See the back cover.

Dosage: reduce the dosage in KIDNEY DISEASE.

Usual adult dose is 500 mg by mouth or IV daily. For PELVIC INFECTION, give this for 14 days. For PEPTIC ULCER, give 250 mg twice daily. Since OFLOXACIN (a related drug) is used with METRONIDAZOLE, it is reasonable to try to use this drug with METRONIDAZOLE also, albeit this is not standard treatment. Seek local advice.

LIDOCAINE

Local anesthetic

Safety class: 1   Stability: A

Brand name: xylocaine; generic drug is available. Supplied in 10 ml and 50 ml bottles of 1% and 2%. See next entry for ointment. The drug is very stable, so "expired" drug may be used as long as it is still sterile. It tolerates heat well so it can be resterilized.

Indications: inject around a cut to numb the area for suturing. May be used intravenously for a regional block (see Chapter 8). Swab in the mouth for burns. Smear over scrapes to numb while cleaning, used for FISSURES and PHIMOSIS.

Contraindications: ALLERGY to any "-caine" drug except for procaine.[1] If the patient has had recent SEIZURES or a history of frequent SEIZURES, use a maximum of 2 cc of 1% or 4 cc of 0.5% at a time for adults, reduce this according to weight for children.

Precautions: do not use lidocaine containing EPINEPHRINE on fingers, penis, nose, toes or IV. Have EPINEPHRINE handy for rare allergic reactions. If lidocaine goes down the throat, do not let the patient eat or drink until the numbness wears off (about 30–60 minutes).

Plain EPINEPHRINE should be used for allergic reactions to lidocaine (see ALLERGY), but it should be injected in the arm rather than at the site where the lidocaine was used.

Side-effects: confusion, seizures, trembling, breathing problems, low blood pressure, slow pulse rate.

Dosage: not specific, but use no more than 10 ml of 1% or 5 ml of 2% on an adult at any one time if the patient has never had a SEIZURE. (See contraindications if he has.) Takes effect immediately when injected alongside a cut, and it lasts for 20 minutes. You may re-inject. It takes effect in 10–20 minutes for a nerve block. (See Volume 1, Chapter 8 or Chapter 10 for directions on how to inject.)

Alternatives: procaine[1] 1% is like 1% lidocaine; it may be used in lidocaine ALLERGY. Marcaine 0.25% is used like 1% lidocaine, except it should not be used IV. It must not be used in lidocaine ALLERGY. It lasts longer than lidocaine.

---

1 Procaine is unrelated chemically to lidocaine. Most other -caine drugs are related to lidocaine rather than procaine and therefore will cause similar allergy problems.

LIDOCAINE OINTMENT 4% or 5%

Topical anesthetic

Safety class: 1   Stability: A

Indications: same as LIDOCAINE, but in semi-solid form and therefore more convenient for putting on cuts and scrapes and around rectum. It is useful in FISSURES and PHIMOSIS as well as injuries. A low-tech alternative is to thicken 2% lidocaine with cornstarch, as if you were making gravy, then simmer it for a while until the volume is about half what it had been. Lidocaine is heat-stable. It never truly expires.

LINDANE

Insecticide

Synonyms: hexachlorocyclohexane, gamma benzene hexachloride.

Safety class: 3   Stability: A, dark   Pregnancy: C

Supplied as a 1% lotion, cream or shampoo.

This is very toxic for children if it is swallowed or used in excess. Very toxic for cats. Off the market in the UK.

Brand names: Gamene, Kwell, Lindatox, Scabene, Scabisan, many others. Veterinary lindane is cattle dip.

Indications: FLEAS, LICE, SCABIES, any other insect that inhabits the surface of the human body.

Contraindications: infancy or pregnancy, raw skin or open cuts where the medication is to be applied. Don't use in anyone less than 50 kg body weight. In pregnant women and small infants, use PERMETHRIN instead.

Precautions: it is never to be taken internally. This is never to be applied to pink, moist areas of the body. Do not apply this right after a warm bath.

Side-effects: SEIZURES, nervousness, irritability, insomnia, dizziness, double vision, sleepiness, irregular heart rate. These effects occur in only a small percentage of patients. If used excessively, it can damage the bone marrow.

Dosage: wash well. Then apply the lindane sparingly over all affected parts and adjacent areas. In SCABIES it must be applied over the whole body from the chin down. Be sure to clean fingernails well and treat them. Leave on for 24 hours and then shower. If you are treating more than just a few small areas, the treatment may not be repeated until a week after the first treatment and then only if fresh new spots appear. Itching may continue for several weeks after a successful treatment. Wash all clothing and bedding while the drug is on the skin, before washing it off. Use very hot water.

Alternatives: BENZYL BENZOATE, 10% crotamiton, SULFUR in petroleum jelly (off the market in Britain), 0.5% MALATHION, PERMETHRIN.

LINEZOLID

This is a new antibiotic, mostly Gram-positive. It also happens to work for TUBERCULOSIS. Seek detailed information elsewhere. It is safety class 3; only use it on the advice of a physician.

LISINOPRIL

Anti-hypertension; ACE inhibitor

Safety class: 3   Stability: C

Pregnancy: D, contraindicated

Brand names: Carace, Zestril.

Indication: HYPERTENSION

Contraindications: ALLERGY to this drug, pregnancy, DIABETES if the patient is on oral medication.

Precautions: concurrent use of diuretics, advanced age, KIDNEY DISEASE, seek advice before using this with any other drugs.

Side-effects: loss of a sense of smell, a dry cough, cold symptoms. If the patient develops swelling of the face and/or the throat, stop the drug immediately and don't restart it.

Dosage: usually 10 mg in a single dose each morning.

LOPERAMIDE

Antimotility agent

Safety class: 2   Stability: C   Pregnancy: C

Brand names: Imodium, Arret, Diasorb, Normaloe. Usually 2 mg tablets.

Indications: TURISTA, GALLBLADDER DISEASE due to ASCARIASIS, IRRITABLE BOWEL.

Contraindications: do not use this in developing countries. Bacterial DYSENTERY, particularly that caused by Shigella; any diarrhea with a fever; diarrhea due to antibiotics; ACUTE ABDOMEN; children under 4 y.o. (except by physician recommendation). Do not give to women who are breastfeeding.

Precautions: if the patient develops abdominal distension while on this medication, stop it immediately.

Side-effects: worsening of GLAUCOMA, constipation, inability to pass urine (especially in older men), susceptibility to HEAT ILLNESS, dry mouth, decrease in sweating, rapid pulse, sensitivity to light, blurred vision.

Dosage: adults: 4 mg initially, then 2 mg after each loose stool, maximum 16 mg daily. Reduce dose according to weight for children.

LOPINAVIR + RITONAVIR

Anti-HIV INFECTION; protease inhibitor

Safety class: 3   Stability: C   Pregnancy: C

Brand name: Kaletra.

Indication: HIV INFECTION

Contraindications: ALLERGY to this drug; Current usage of any sedative such as DIAZEPAM.

Precautions: try not to use this together with QUININE, QUINIDINE or RIFABUTIN. Be aware that CARBAMAZEPINE, PHENOBARBITAL, DEXAMETHASONE, PHENYTOIN and RIFAMPIN will decrease the amount of this in the body. Stop the drug for severe abdominal pain. Don't use it with LIVER DISEASE. The drug will worsen DIABETES.

Side-effects: unknown

Dosage: for 15–40 kg: 10 mg/kg lopinavir twice a day (together with the ritonavir)

For 7–15 kg: 12 mg/kg lopinavir twice a day (together with the ritonavir)

LUMEFANTRINE

Anti-malarial, similar to BENFLUMETOL, related to CHLOROQUINE-type drugs, combined with ARTEMISININ.

Safety class: 1   Stability: A   Pregnancy: A

Brand names: Riamet, Co-artem, Coartemether. This is expensive and thus commonly fake or substandard.

Tablet size is 2.0 mg artemether plus 12 mg lumefantrine.

Indications: MALARIA, used in combination with some form of ARTEMISININ, usually artemether.

Contraindications: previous ALLERGY; current use of RIFAMPIN, CARBAMAZEPINE, PHENYTOIN, St. John's wort (see PLANT POISONING).

Precautions: avoid using this in the presence of any heart disease, LIVER DISEASE, KIDNEY DISEASE. Avoid using this with anti-HIV drugs, with antidepressants, anti-fungal medications, other antimalarial medications, CIMETIDINE, grapefruit or grapefruit juice, ERYTHROMYCIN-type drugs, heart medications, CIPROFLOXACIN and similar drugs. Don't use this after its expiration date; the ARTEMISININ component is very unstable.

Side-effects: dizziness (warn the patient against hazardous activities), nausea, vomiting, diarrhea, abdominal pains, headache, insomnia, sore joints and muscles, itching, rash.

Dosage: be sure to give the drug with a meal of fatty foods to increase its effect. Standard adult dose (over 35 kg) is 4 tablets initially, 8 hours later, then twice daily for 2 more days. For 25–35 kg, give as above, using only 3 tablets per dose.

MAGNESIUM SULFATE, IM or IV

Anti-toxemia, mineral, muscle relaxant

Safety class: 3   Stability: C   Pregnancy: okay

Supplied as generic drug.

Indications: TOXEMIA of pregnancy; SEIZURES or threatened SEIZURES during later pregnancy, labor or within a week after delivery. It is also useful in TETANUS as it decreases the amount of sedative that must be given. Sometimes it is used in ALCOHOLISM and in LEPTOSPIROSIS with mental symptoms (lethargy or craziness). It may be useful in treating EBOLA VIRUS DISEASE.

Contraindications: some kinds of heart disease; KIDNEY DISEASE. Don't use this along with sedative drugs. It is contraindicated in severe HEPATITIS, CIRRHOSIS and LIVER FAILURE.

Precautions: note that this listing is for the drug by injection. Oral magnesium sulfate is not absorbed into the blood stream and thus has no whole-body effects. When given by injection, you should check the patient's respiratory rate and urine production continually. If respirations are less than 16 per minute or urine production is less than 100 ml for the last 4 hours, withhold the next dose until these become normal.

IM Injections are painful.

Watch the blood pressure; stop the drug and then resume at a reduced dose if the pressure becomes lower than normal or if the patient feels faint.

Overdose: RESPIRATORY FAILURE, KIDNEY DISEASE. Antidote for overdose is calcium gluconate, 10%, 10–20 mg IV.

Dosage: the following are adult doses. Contact a physician or midwife for instructions. Use the following instructions only if this is not possible:

Readers with no experience with IV's should use a 50% solution, IM. For an average-sized woman, give 10 grams (20 ml) IM initially, 10 ml in each buttock. Then give 5 grams (10 ml) IM every 4 hours. Reduce the dose according to weight for small women. Stop the drug 2 hours before the anticipated time of delivery.

Readers with experience in IV medications: give 4–6 grams (4000–6000 mg) IV over 20 min with maintenance of 1–2 g/h thereafter, being sure that the patient still has reflexes. Pediatric dose is 20–100 mg/kg/dose. If you can't test reflexes, then use the IM instructions.

MALATHION

Insecticide

Safety class: 2   Stability: C, dark

Brand names for dilute product: Derbac-M, Prioderm, Quellada M, Suleo-M. The concentrate (50%) is frequently available in markets that serve farmers. It is very toxic in full strength, but it can be diluted.

Indications: FLEAS, LICE, SCABIES; eliminates bedbugs.

Contraindications: ALLERGY to this substance; inability to accurately dilute and use it. Prior bad reaction to this product. Seek physician approval before using this on children under 6 months old or on anyone who is quite ill.

Precautions: be sure that you buy malathion. There are products with similar names that a clerk will assure you can be used the same, but many of them are more toxic. Make up small batches frequently since malathion decomposes in water.

DO NOT ALLOW THE CONCENTRATED (50%) PRODUCT TO TOUCH YOUR SKIN! If you accidentally spill it on yourself, wash it off immediately. Malathion smells bad but the smell does not last for long. Be sure to keep this out of reach of children, as it is very toxic if taken by mouth.

Toxic symptoms: a general outpouring of fluid from everywhere: salivation, urination, diarrhea, tears, shortness of breath because of respiratory secretions. Antidote is ATROPINE.

Dosage: use the prediluted product according to the product directions. Dilute the concentrated (50%) malathion to 0.5%. This is a 100-fold dilution, e.g., 10 ml (2 teaspoons) per liter (1000 ml) of plain water. The diluted solution may be used on the skin or hair; it also decontaminates louse-infected clothing. It kills the lice but not the eggs.

If you dilute the concentrated malathion (10 ml per liter) with kerosene and use this to paint the legs of your bed frame (some morning, because of the smell), it will eliminate bedbugs within 1 or 2 nights.

Washing your floors once a week with a teaspoon of the concentrate in a bucket of water will eliminate most insect-type creatures from your house. The smell will leave in less than an hour.

MALOPRIM

Anti malarial; contains DAPSONE (100 mg) and PYRIMETHAMINE (12.5 mg).

Used for prevention of MALARIA especially in children.

Dosage: 2 tablets initially, then 1 tablet weekly for adults, reduced according to weight for children. Check precautions and contraindications of the individual drugs.

MEBENDAZOLE

Dewormer, anthelmintic

Safety class: 1   Stability: A   Pregnancy: C

Brand names: Equivurm, Fugacar, Mebenvet, Mebutar, Multispec, Nemasole, Ovitelmin, Pantelmin, Parmeben, Phardazone, Rumatel, Sirben, Telmin, Telmintic, Vermirax, Vermox. Supplied as 100 mg tablets.

Indications: ASCARIASIS, CAPILLARIASIS, ENTEROBIASIS, GIARDIASIS, HOOKWORM, HYDATID DISEASE, LOIASIS, MANSONELLOSIS PERSTANS, ONCHOCERCIASIS, TRICHURIASIS.

Possibly: TURISTA, GUINEA WORM, MALABSORPTION, STRONGYLOIDIASIS and pork TAPEWORM.

Contraindications: ALLERGY to this, early pregnancy.

Side-effects: nausea, vomiting, diarrhea, abdominal pain.

Dosage: give the drug with a fatty meal. Reduce the dose in the presence of LIVER FAILURE.

ASCARIASIS: 100 mg twice a day for 3 days, regardless of age. Cure rate is 98%.

CAPILLARIASIS: 400 mg daily for 20 days; if the patient relapses, use the same dose for 30 days.

ENTEROBIASIS: 100 mg, single dose, same amount regardless of body weight. Give a dose now and one in 10 days; treat all family members. Cure rate is 95%.

GIARDIASIS: 200 mg three times a day for 3 days.

GUINEA WORM: 200 mg three times a day for 6 days.

HOOKWORM: 600 mg, single dose (not so good) or 100 mg twice a day for 3 days. Cure rate is 96%.

HYDATID DISEASE: 200 mg/kg daily (120 tablets daily for a 60 kg person) for 6 months.

LIVER FLUKE (fasciola): 500 mg three times a day x 21 days.

LOIASIS: 2000 mg (20 tablets) daily for 21–28 days.

MANSONELLOSIS PERSTANS: 100 mg twice a day for 1 week, used with LEVAMISOLE. 100 mg twice a day for 14–21 days used with DIETHYLCARBAMAZINE.

ONCHOCERCIASIS: 1000 mg (10 tablets) twice a day for 28 days, plus LEVAMISOLE.

STRONGYLOIDIASIS: 100 mg every 8 hours for 14–21 days.

Pork TAPEWORM: 300 mg twice a day for 3 days.

TRICHURIASIS: like HOOKWORM; cure rate is 68%.

All other worms, deworming, MALABSORPTION, TURISTA: 100 mg twice daily for 3 days. 500 mg in a single dose usually works, but not quite as well; patients may vomit. Repeat this treatment every six months while living in a worm-infested area.

Alternatives: ALBENDAZOLE, CAMBENDAZOLE, FLUBENDAZOLE. These are better absorbed than mebendazole and thus require lower doses for diseases such as HYDATID DISEASE.

MEFLOQUINE

Antimalarial

Safety class: 2   Stability: A   Pregnancy: B

Brand names: Lariam, Laricur. Combined with FANSIDAR in Fansimef and MSP. May be combined with ARTEMISININ.

Usually supplied in 250 mg tablets. In the States the drug has 250 mg total of which 228 mg is base. In many countries overseas one tablet has 274 mg of which 250 mg is base. The amount of drug and base is so close that one need not distinguish or calculate closely.

Indication: MALARIA, especially falciparum, both treatment and prevention. It may not work well for preventing non-falciparum MALARIA.

Contraindications: ALLERGY to this drug, simultaneous use of PROPRANOLOL or similar drugs. Do not use this in patients with a history of EPILEPSY, MENTAL ILLNESS, DEPRESSION, CIRRHOSIS or LIVER FAILURE. It also should not be used in some kinds of heart disease. Do not use it at the same time as CHLOROQUINE, in anyone who is on medication for heart problems or with valproic acid.

Precautions: when used with PHENYTOIN SODIUM or PHENOBARBITAL (SEIZURE medicines), it may lower the blood levels of those drugs, thus provoking SEIZURES.

Mefloquine ought to be combined with another drug, since resistance to it is developing in many areas.

Warn the patient not to engage in hazardous activity while taking this medication.

The drug is sometimes associated with altered electrical activity in the heart; this, in turn, is sometimes associated with sudden death. Thus this should not be combined with other such drugs. The medical jargon is that it prolongs the QT interval. Do not use it with other drugs that have this same notation. See the back cover.

Do not use HALOFANTRINE with mefloquine or within 15 weeks of using mefloquine.

Side-effects: nausea, vomiting and dizziness, especially in young children. These effects occur in only a small percentage of patients. Serious mental disturbances, hallucinations or SEIZURES may occur. This is rare in males who take it for prophylaxis. It is more common in females and very common in anyone who takes the larger dose required for treatment. Nightmares are common, especially in Europeans, even at the lower prophylactic doses. This may also cause burning, numbness, tingling, weakness and incoordination in fine movements.

Dosage:

MALARIA treatment 750–1250 mg by mouth, one dose only. It is absorbed better if the tablets are crushed and dissolved in a liquid. The dosage for children is 15 mg/kg initially followed by 10 mg/kg 12 hours later. It is well tolerated and there are less adverse side-effects than in adults.

MALARIA prevention: 250 mg weekly, from one week before entering a malarious area until 4 weeks after leaving the area. Alternatively, 1 tablet daily for 3 days before travel, then 1 weekly. If you are short of medication, a tablet every other week might (or might not) be sufficient.

MELASOPROL

Trypanosomicide; anti-African sleeping sickness

Safety class: 3+   Stability: unknown

Pregnancy: unknown, probably not safe.

Brand names: Melarsen Oxide-BAL, Mel-B, RP 3854.

This is an arsenic compound. See ARSENIC POISONING.
Indication: AFRICAN SLEEPING SICKNESS, late stage, except where there is resistance to the drug.

Contraindication: previous ALLERGY or adverse response to this drug.

Precautions: the drug is fatal in 4–6% of the patients to whom it is given. It works for late-stage AFRICAN SLEEPING SICKNESS for which there are few if any options. It is given intravenously in a hospital setting only. It is a dangerous drug, not to be used in a village setting.

Don't use this in the presence of KIDNEY DISEASE, HEART FAILURE or LIVER DISEASE without independent physician recommendation.

Use PREDNISONE or PREDNISOLONE, 40 mg/day adult dose for several days before starting this drug.

Dosage: in all cases where there is a dosage range, start at the lower end and work up gradually. Although it is given IV, it must be given on an empty stomach.

Adult dose is 1–3.6 mg/kg IV daily for 3 days. After 1 week without the drug, 3.6 mg/kg IV daily for 3 days. After 10–21 days, repeat this cycle.

Children: 0.36 mg/kg IV initially, increased gradually to a maximum of 3.6 mg/kg IV at intervals of 1–5 days, for a total of 9–10 doses.

MELATONIN

Sleeping pill. Available without prescription at health food stores in the States, not in the UK.

Supplied as 5 mg tablets intended to be swallowed. The 1 mg tablets labeled "cherry flavor" are intended to be dissolved under the tongue. They work much better for some people.

Indication: this is a natural sleep-producing substance that is marketed by natural food stores It is very useful for counteracting JET LAG.

Side-effect: it may cause incoordination.

Dosage: for eastern travel, take 3–5 mg at 6–7 p.m. local time on the day of departure, even if that means during a flight. If this will interfere with an airline meal, eat your own bag lunch before so that you will be able to sleep as soon as you take it. After arrival, take 3–5 mg at bedtime for the first 3 nights.

For western travel, take 3–5 mg at bedtime for the first 4 nights after arrival. In both cases, you may take another dose before 4 A.M.

METAKELFIN

Antimalarial

Almost the same as FANSIDAR; used the same.

METAPROTERENOL

Bronchodilator

Safety class: 2   Stability: C   Pregnancy: C

Brand names: Alupent, Metaprel. Supplied as tablets or inhaler.

Indications: ASTHMA, chronic RESPIRATORY INFECTION.

Contraindications: HYPERTENSION, excessively fast pulse, pregnancy, age under 6, HEART FAILURE, DIABETES. Don't use it with drugs for depression, or heart drugs.

Precautions: may cause trembling, nervousness, high blood pressure and a fast pulse.

Dosage: reduce the dose for the elderly. Adults get 20 mg three to four times a day or 2 inhalations every 4 hours. Children (6–9 y.o.) get 10 mg or (over 9 y.o.) 20 mg three to four times a day.

Alternatives: ALBUTEROL, THEOPHYLLINE, SALBUTAMOL.

METHYLENE BLUE

An alternative name is methylthioninium blue, available in the UK. This is an antimalarial drug that is used for other medicinal purposes and as a stain in the laboratory. The commercial product used as a stain has toxic contaminants in it. It should not be used as a medicine.

The pharmaceutical product (brand name Proveblue) is being rediscovered as an antimalarial. It should not be used alone since it starts working slowly; it should be combined with some ARTEMISININ-type drug. A big advantage is that it eliminates the form of the malaria parasite that is transmitted to mosquitoes, thus decreasing the amount of malaria in the community. The disadvantages are that it turns the urine blue-green, turns the whites of the eyes blue, and it tastes terrible. It also sometimes causes vomiting and pain with urination. It interacts badly with some other drugs and thus should not be used with just anything. It should not be used in persons with G6PD DEFICIENCY. The usual dose is 10mg/kg twice daily, for 7 days if used alone, for 3 days if used in combination with other drugs.

METOCLOPRAMIDE

Anti-vomiting medication

Safety class: 2   Stability: C   Avoid in pregnancy

Supplied as: 5mg/ml injection, 5 mg & 10 mg tablets.

Brand names: Reglan, Vominorm, Maxolon. Supplied as oral tablets and injectable solution.

Indications: upper abdominal pain due to gastritis, or heartburn; nausea; vomiting.

Contraindications: pregnancy, previous bad reaction to the drug.

Precautions & Side-effects: this may make diarrhea worse. Some people get neck muscle spasms, involuntary limb movements, grimacing, trembling and abnormal eye movements. Depression is also a side-effect. Use this for a maximum of 12 weeks. Watch for NEUROLEPTIC MALIGNANT SYNDROME.

Dosage: adults 5–10 mg orally, by IM injection or very slowly IV, to a maximum of 60 mg/day. Reduce dose according to weight for children.

METRIFONATE

Anti-schistosome, anthelmintic

Safety class: 2   Stability: unknown   Pregnancy: unknown

Brand names: Anthon, Bilarcil, Combor, Difrifon, Dipterex, Dylox, Dyrex, Mastotem, Neguvon, Tugon.

Indications: SCHISTOSOMIASIS HEMATOBIUM. (This is a cheap alternative to PRAZIQUANTEL which is very expensive.) This drug also helps for HOOKWORM although it is not intentionally used for it. It may work for FILARIASIS.

Contraindications: recent (within the last few days) exposure to insecticides or planned exposure within a day after taking the drug.

Side-effects: mild spinning sensation, tiredness, nausea and abdominal cramping. It may aggravate the symptoms of ONCHOCERCIASIS in patients who have that. The drug may interfere with anesthesia for 48 hours after it is taken. Inform the physician or anesthetist.

Dosage: SCHISTOSOMIASIS HEMATOBIUM: 500 mg (adults) or 7.5–10 mg/kg (children), one dose every 2 weeks for three doses. Give as many of these 3 doses as possible; 1 or 2 doses are also helpful, although not as good as three.

FILARIASIS: 10–15 mg/kg, one dose, every 14 days for 5–16 doses.

METRONIDAZOLE

Anti-protozoa, antibiotic

Includes: benzyl metronidazole

Safety class: 1   Stability: C, dark   Pregnancy: B[1]

Brand names: Arilin, Clont, Danizol, Flagyl, Gineflavir, Klion, Orvagil, Trichocide, Vagilen and others.

Generic drug is available. Supplied as 250 mg tablets or capsules. Entamizole is the combination of this drug with DILOXANIDE FUROATE. A liquid form, benzoyl metronidazole, is available in some countries for children.

Indications: ABSCESS with foul-smelling pus, ACUTE ABDOMEN, AMEBIASIS, CANCRUM ORIS, CHOLERA, ENTERIC FEVER, GIARDIASIS, LARVA MIGRANS (in Asia), PELVIC INFECTION, PEPTIC ULCER, PNEUMONIA, TETANUS, TROPICAL ULCER, VAGINITIS.

Also TURISTA, gas, GUINEA WORM, MALABSORPTION.

Used with other drugs in SEPSIS, TETANUS, for wounds with foul-smelling pus, for tooth infections in third molars.

Contraindications: ALLERGY to this drug, some kinds of blood diseases, concurrent or anticipated use of alcohol. It should not be used in a patient who has SEIZURES or in one who has numbness and tingling. Do not give this to a patient who has PORPHYRIA (a hereditary disease).

Precautions: the patient must not drink ALCOHOL while on this drug or for 3 days after taking the last dose. If he does, he will get a severe reaction. There is alcohol in sprays, most liquid medicines and in culinary products such as vanilla extract. Even rubbing alcohol or hand cream on the skin can cause a reaction. Discontinue the drug if dizziness or incoordination occur. If you use this medication in a child with ATTENTION DEFICIT DISORDER, he may temporarily become extremely hyperactive.

---

1 Metronidazole and TINIDAZOLE are used for the same purposes. TINIDAZOLE is pregnancy category C, so it is better to use metronidazole in pregnant women.

Side-effects: nausea, vomiting, abdominal pain, sleepiness, headache and dark urine occur in only a small percentage of patients. Avoid using this the first three months of pregnancy unless the situation is life-threatening.

Overdose and prolonged usage: LIVER FAILURE; see Protocol B.7.

Dosage: reduce the dose with LIVER DISEASE. The following are adult doses; reduce dose according to weight for children. The drug is absorbed well rectally; give it this way if your patient is vomiting, or he has an ACUTE ABDOMEN; the adult dose by rectum is 1000 mg every 8 hours.

ABSCESS: same as CANCRUM ORIS.

AMEBIASIS: 750 mg three times a day for 10 days until cured plus one week; for 10 days for dysentery only.

CANCRUM ORIS: 15 mg/kg IV initially, then 7.5 mg/kg every 6 hours, IV or orally.

CHOLERA: same as CANCRUM ORIS

ENTERIC FEVER: 500 mg 3 times daily for 10 days.

Gas: same as TURISTA.

GIARDIASIS: 250 mg three times daily for 5 days. An alternative dose is 2000 mg daily for 3 days.

GUINEA WORM: 400–500 mg three times a day for 5 days.

LARVA MIGRANS in Asia: 400 mg 3 times daily for 3 weeks.

MALABSORPTION: same as TURISTA.

PELVIC INFECTION: 500 mg twice daily for 14 days, to be used with OFLOXACIN.

PEPTIC ULCER: 500 mg every 8 hours for 14 days, with other medication listed.

PNEUMONIA: same as ACUTE ABDOMEN.

SEPSIS: same as ACUTE ABDOMEN.

TETANUS: 500 mg orally every 6 hours or 1000 mg by rectum every 8 hours, for 10 days.

Tooth infections, third molars: 250–500 mg three times a day until the swelling is down; then take the tooth out.

TROPICAL ULCER: 250 mg three times a day until healed.

TURISTA: 250 mg three times a day for 5 days.

VAGINITIS: bacterial or Trichomonas: 2000 mg, one dose. If this doesn't work, then 500 mg daily for 7 days; then try 2 grams daily for 5 days. Treat both partners at the same time.

Wound infections: like TROPICAL ULCER.

Alternatives: TINIDAZOLE. NITAZOXANIDE is a new antibiotic that has many of the same uses as metronidazole. Seek recent information concerning it.

MICONAZOLE

Anti-fungal

Safety class: 1(cream)   Stability: C   Pregnancy: no adverse events have been reported.

Brand names: Monistat, Daktarin.

Indications: CANDIDA, VAGINITIS, some MYCETOMA, TINEA.

Contraindications: ALLERGY to this drug or any –azole drug. Do not use in or around the eyes.

Side-effects: none when used in a cream form; do not use the injectable—it is dangerous.

Dosage: use sparingly twice a day for 2–4 weeks.

MILK OF MAGNESIA

Laxative

Safety class: 1   Stability: A

Synonym: magnesium sulfate, oral form.[2]

Indications: constipation, used to cause diarrhea. Used for INTESTINAL FLUKE.

Contraindications: ACUTE ABDOMEN, ENTERIC FEVER, KIDNEY DISEASE.

Side-effects: abdominal pain, cramping.

Dosage: 30 ml of 50% solution for adults, every four hours until bowel contents move. For children, 10–30 ml as above.

MILTEFOSINE

Anti-Leishmania drug

Safety class: ?2   Stability unknown

Pregnancy: X: confirm lack of pregnancy before starting and use reliable contraception while taking the drug and for 3 months thereafter. Condoms are not reliable.

Synonym: hexadecylphosphocholine

Brand name: Impavido.

Indications: CUTANEOUS LEISHMANIASIS, VISCERAL LEISHMANIASIS, PKDL (a complication of VL).

Contraindications: pregnancy, ALLERGY to this drug, KIDNEY DISEASE.

Precautions: largely unknown, but there are no problems with anti-HIV drugs. It should be taken after a meal.

Side-effects: nausea, vomiting, diarrhea, KIDNEY DISEASE, possibly infertility, HEPATITIS.

Dosage: the usual adult dose in VISCERAL LEISHMANIASIS is 100 mg/day or 2 mg/kg/day for 4 weeks. Reduce the dose according to weight for children. It may be used down to 2 years of age. The dose may be increased up to 2.5 mg/kg/day for 4–6 weeks. For PKDL, the adult dose is 50 mg twice a day for 12 weeks.

---

2 This is the same chemical as the drug listed as magnesium sulfate. However, the oral form (milk of magnesia) and the IV form (magnesium sulfate) act entirely differently. The oral form stays in the bowel, and has only a bowel effect, whereas the IV form has a whole-body effect. The IV form may be used orally, but the oral form may not be given IV.

MINOCYCLINE

Antibiotic, Gram-negative, similar to DOXYCYCLINE.

Safety class: 2   Stability: A, dark   Pregnancy: D

Brand names: Minocin, Acnamino, Sebomin.

Indications: BRUCELLOSIS and indications the same as DOXYCYCLINE. It might be useful for CHANCROID and LEPROSY. It may be useful as a shotgun treatment for ARTHRITIS.

Contraindications: ALLERGY to any DOXYCYCLINE-type drug. Do not use after the expiration date. Observe the contraindications under DOXYCYCLINE. Do not use this with oral anticoagulants (blood thinners) or with ANTACID.

Precautions: like DOXYCYCLINE, this causes sun sensitivity so patients burn easily. It makes patients prone to CANDIDIASIS, masks the signs and symptoms of appendicitis and causes dark staining of teeth in children under 7 and the offspring of pregnant women who take the drug. The latter effect, however, is not common, and it is questionable if it occurs at all. Stop the drug if the patient develops HEPATITIS or a DYSENTERY-type diarrhea.

Side-effects: abdominal pains, nausea, vomiting, diarrhea, sun-sensitivity.

Dosage: reduce the dose in the presence of KIDNEY DISEASE.

ACTINOMYCOSIS: 1000 mg every 12 hours for 12 months.

ANTHRAX exposure: 100 mg twice daily for 60 days plus immediate immunization.

ARTHRITIS: 100 mg twice daily, duration known

BRUCELLOSIS: 200 mg twice daily; used with other drugs.

CHOLERA: 300 mg, single dose.

LEPROSY: if there is one skin lesion only, it can be used as the sole drug: 100 mg every 12 hours for 6 months. Otherwise combine this with other drugs; the precise dosage is not available.

MALARIA prevention: 100 mg twice daily.

PLAGUE exposure: 100 mg every 12 hours for two days.

Other diseases: 100 mg twice daily for the same duration as DOXYCYCLINE would be given.

MOXIDECT

This is a medication still under development, related to IVERMECTIN. Seek recent information.

MULTIVITAMINS

Safety class: 1   Stability: variable

Indications: deficiency of a vitamin, inability to eat a balanced diet, ALCOHOLISM, MALNUTRITION, MENINGITIS, PLANT POISONING due to argemone oil or lathyrism, pregnancy, SICKLE CELL DISEASE, TROPICAL ULCER, TUBERCULOSIS, wounds that will not heal easily. It may be helpful in PERTUSSIS. It is useful for keeping people from buying and consuming harmful folk medicines.

Contraindications: ALLERGY to the particular brand.

Dosage: 1 to 4 non-prescription tablets daily for adult; reduce maximum dose according to weight for children; follow the instructions for your particular preparation.

NALBUPHINE

Narcotic and narcotic antagonist

Safety class: 1   Stability: A   Pregnancy: C

Brand name: Nubain. Generic product is available. Comes in vials of 10 mg or 20 mg. **It is a controlled substance.**

Indications: pain not due to head injury. It is particularly useful for HEART ATTACK, MIGRAINE and PLEURISY.

Contraindications: head injury, shortness of breath, ALLERGY to this drug, DYSENTERY due to antibiotic usage, any kind of PLANT POISONING or FOOD POISONING. Don't use in a patient with ADDICTION to downers or current usage of DIAZEPAM.

Side-effects: nausea, vomiting, abdominal pain; the patient may have a sensation of numbness from the neck down; this is normal, and it will pass. The patient may become agitated or sedated. He may become constipated.

Precautions: warn the patient not to engage in hazardous activity while taking this drug.

Dosage: the usual adult dose for severe pain is 10 mg IM every 4 hours. Reduce the dose for less severe pain and according to weight for children.

NARCOTICS

This is a drug class. Examples: CODEINE, meperidine, morphine. See specific drugs. CODEINE is the safest, medically and legally and the medication which will least likely be stolen. TRAMADOL, NALBUPHINE and butorphanol are potent pain relievers, related to the narcotics. Do not use any of these drugs in POLIO or for someone short of breath. They decrease the urge to breathe. Warn patients not to engage in hazardous activities while taking any drug of this class.

NELFINAVIR

This is an anti-HIV drug.

NEMA WORM CAPSULE

Veterinary TETRACHLOROETHYLENE; may be used for humans. See TETRACHLOROETHYLENE.

NEOSPORIN

Antibiotic

Safety class: 1   Stability: A

Supplied in oral form and in ointments. (For the ointment form see ANTIBIOTIC OINTMENT.)

Indications: persistent diarrhea; used in ANTIBIOTIC OINTMENTs.

Contraindications: KIDNEY DISEASE when used orally.

Dosage: diarrhea: adult dose is 1000 mg every 6 hours; reduce dose according to weight for children.

NEVIRAPINE

Anti-HIV; nonnucleoside reverse transcriptase inhibitor

Safety class: 3   Stability: C   Pregnancy: B

Brand name: Viramune; comes in 100, 200, 400 mg tablets and liquid with 50 mg/5ml.

Indications: HIV INFECTION

Contraindications: ALLERGY to this drug.

Precautions: RIFAMPIN and RIFABUTIN decrease the effectiveness of this drug.

Side-effects: headache, nausea, vomiting, diarrhea

Dosage: Adult slow-release dose is 200 mg daily for the first 2 weeks, then 400 mg daily, one every 12 hours.

NIACIN

B vitamin, vitamin B_3

Synonyms: niacinamide, nicotinamide

Safety class: 1 oral   Stability: A   Pregnancy: C

Safety class: 3 injectable

Indications: MALNUTRITION, PELLAGRA.

Contraindications: prior ALLERGY to the particular form, GALLBLADDER DISEASE, LIVER DISEASE, PEPTIC ULCER, any bleeding problem. Don't use it in the presence of GLAUCOMA, DIABETES or GOUT.

Precautions: this drug interferes with lab tests for glucose and one test for a hormone.

Side-effects: flushing, nausea, vomiting, itching. The drug appears in breast milk, but this should not be a problem.

Dosage: initially 50 mg oral 10 times a day; reduce to once a day after the symptoms disappear. The injectable form must be given IV, not IM, and it may cause ANAPHYLAXIS. The dose is 25 mg three times a day.

NICLOSAMIDE

Dewormer, anthelmintic

Safety class: 2   Stability: C   Pregnancy: B

Brand names: Cestocide, Devermin, Fenasal, Lintex, Mansonil, Niclocide, Radeverm, Sagimid, Vermitin, Yomesan. Supplied as a chewable, 500 mg tablet.

Indications: INTESTINAL FLUKE, TAPEWORM.

Contraindications: this drug can be used in sick and pregnant patients (i.e. other illness and pregnancy are not contraindications). If you intend to use this for pork TAPEWORM, it is essential that the person not vomit and that you give something to cause diarrhea after the treatment. Otherwise do not use it. It is not very safe for INTESTINAL FLUKE. PRAZIQUANTEL is safer but more expensive.

Side-effects: occasionally nausea, vomiting, diarrhea, abdominal pain.

Dosage: give the drug in the morning on an empty stomach. Have the patient thoroughly chew and swallow the tablets with minimum water. Give something such as MILK OF MAGNESIA to cause diarrhea immediately after the drug, especially with pork TAPEWORM. Dispose of this stool very carefully in a septic system or by burying it deeply. Wash your hands carefully. Adults and children over 8 y.o.: 1000 mg hourly for 2 doses. Children 2–8 years old: 500 mg hourly for 2 doses. Children under 2: 250 mg hourly for 2 doses. For dwarf or rat TAPEWORM, use the two daily doses for 5–7 days. For everything else it is used one day only.

NICOTINIC ACID

This is another form of NIACIN except that patients experience flushing, dizziness, heart fluttering and general itching as a side-effect of the drug. It is not as safe.

NIFEDIPINE

Calcium channel blocker; anti-hypertensive; anti-migraine

Safety class: 2.5   Stability: C   Pregnancy: C

Brand names: Adalat, Afed-tab, Procardia. It comes in immediate release and slow-release forms; each tablet contains 5 mg, 10 mg, 20 mg, 30 mg or 60 mg of drug, the larger tablets being slow-release and the smaller, immediate release.

Indications: HYPERTENSION, TOXEMIA, MIGRAINE

Contraindications: ALLERGY to the drug, low blood pressure, recent HEART ATTACK, PORPHYRIA

Precautions: this may retard labor, but severe TOXEMIA with very high blood pressure probably overrides this consideration. Don't use it for MIGRAINE in the last month of pregnancy.

Side-effects: dizziness, headache, flushing, weakness, nausea, trembling, cramps, cough, wheezing. With the immediate-release forms there may be a sudden and too great a fall in blood pressure and a too-rapid pulse. Watch for this and reduce the dose or withdraw the medication if this happens.

Dosage: immediate release tablets: 5 mg–20 mg three times daily, starting at the lower dosage and working upward until the effect is attained. For slow-release tablets, the dose is daily, starting at 10 mg and working up to the desired effect, the maximum being 90 mg.

NIFURTIMOX

Antichagastic

Safety class: 3   Stability: A   Pregnancy: in animals may cause growth retardation, but not deformities.

Brand names: Bayer 2502; Lampit. The drug is oral. It comes in tablets of 120 mg. It is available in Chile.

Indications: CHAGA'S DISEASE, AFRICAN SLEEPING SICKNESS.

TOC SYMPTOMS DIFFERENTIALS CONDITIONS **DRUG INDEX** REGIONAL NOTES INX

Contraindications: any severe previous reactions to the drug.

Precautions: allergic reactions are common. (See ALLERGY.) Give the drug with ANTACID to avoid stomach upset. Numbness, tingling and weakness may occur. The patient may become very excited and have uncontrolled behavior. Do not use ALCOHOL while taking this drug. The drug is dangerous.

It is very important to treat for the entire duration. Do not under-treat; it is better not to treat at all!

Dosage:

CHAGA'S DISEASE: 2–3 mg/kg 3 or 4 times a day for 90 days; continue treatment for 120 days total if the disease was long-lasting before you began.

AFRICAN SLEEPING SICKNESS: 5 mg/kg every 8 hours for 7 days, used with EFLORNITHINE.

NIRIDAZOLE

Dewormer, anthelmintic

Safety class: 3   Stability: unknown

Brand names: Ambilhar, Bulgarstan. Supplied as 100 mg and 500 mg tablets. It is available in Kenya.

Caution: ordinarily, this drug should not be used. It is included here because it still is available and used in some places.

Indications: SCHISTOSOMIASIS HEMATOBIUM, SCHISTOSOMIASIS MANSONI, occasionally GUINEA WORM and SCHISTOSOMIASIS JAPONICUM. Sometimes used for amebic DYSENTERY, but it does not work well for this. Formerly used for AFRICAN SLEEPING SICKNESS.

Contraindications: LIVER FAILURE, HEART FAILURE, severe MALNUTRITION, severe ANEMIA, current use of ISONIAZID. You should be extremely reluctant to use this if the patient has a history of MENTAL ILLNESS or SEIZURES.

Precautions: the drug usually causes nausea and vomiting; give PROMETHAZINE or another anti-nausea medication 1/2 hour before each dose.

Side-effects: severe side-effects are more frequent in people who have LIVER DISEASE, whatever the cause. It may cause a crisis in those with G6PD DEFICIENCY: Irish and persons of Mediterranean or Hispanic ancestry.

Check the urine just before the first dose and again just before the second dose. If the urobilinogen has definitely increased, do not give the second and subsequent doses. This drug turns urine dark and causes an unpleasant body odor. Be careful about the dose. Too much drug causes a change in mood, confusion, hallucinations, SEIZURES and a rapid pulse. If this happens, decrease the dose. Other side-effects are abdominal cramps, diarrhea, headache and loss of appetite.

Dosage:

GUINEA WORM: 25 mg/kg daily for 10 days.

SCHISTOSOMIASIS: 25 mg/kg to maximum of 1500 mg daily. May be given in one daily dose, but better to give half this dose twice each day.

S. HEMATOBIUM: 5 days.

S. MANSONI: 10 days.

S. JAPONICUM requires three treatments of 10 days each in three consecutive months. The treatment of S. JAPONICUM must be supervised by a physician.

Alternatives: PRAZIQUANTEL is a better drug for all diseases.

NITAZOXANIDE

Antibiotic

Safety class: 3   Stability: C
Pregnancy: reportedly it is okay to use after 3 months.

Brand name: Alinia. Available as a suspension of 20 mg/ml and in tablets of 500 mg.

Indications: many of the same uses as METRONIDAZOLE (which is safer). It is also useful for LIVER FLUKE (fasciola type), in place of CLOXACILLIN for ABSCESS and related conditions and when METRONIDAZOLE does not work for PEPTIC ULCER, and/or GASTRITIS. It is used for CRYPTOSPORIDIOSIS and CYCLOSPORIASIS, also GIARDIASIS and TAPEWORM. It is being developed for HYDATID DISEASE, TUBERCULOSIS and HEPATITIS.

Contraindications: prior ALLERGY to this or related drugs.

Precautions: this interacts badly with a variety of other drugs, causing toxicity. Take it with food. It only works well for CRYPTOSPORIDIOSIS in patients who have good immunity. Don't use it in HIV+ patients or the elderly, newborns, chronically ill or those with CANCER.

Side-effects: nausea, vomiting, diarrhea, abdominal pain.

Dosage: the drug should be given with food.

CRYPTOSPORIDIOSIS: 500 mg twice daily for 3 days in previously healthy patients. Double the dose and prolong the duration in patients with AIDS.

CYCLOSPORIASIS: 500[1] mg twice daily for 7–10 days.

GIARDIASIS: 500 mg twice daily for 3 days.

LIVER FLUKE, fasciola: 7.5 mg/kg twice daily for 7 days.

WORMS: ASCARIASIS, HOOKWORM, STRONGYLOIDIASIS, TAPEWORM, TRICHURIASIS: like CYCLOSPORIASIS.

NORFLOXACIN

Brand name: Utinor

See CIPROFLOXACIN or OFLOXACIN and the package insert. This is used for bacterial DYSENTERY, the usual dose being 800 mg, single dose. It can also be used for ENTERIC FEVER in which case it need only be used for 7 days.

---

1 200 mg ages 4–12 years old; 100 mg ages 1–3

NYSTATIN

Anti-fungal

Safety class: 1 usually   Stability: C   Pregnancy: ?

Brand names: Mycostatin, Nystan, others.

Indications: CANDIDIASIS, TINEA, VAGINITIS.

Contraindications: prior ALLERGY to this drug.

Side-effects: the taste is vile. Occasionally there is nausea, vomiting and diarrhea. If the patient develops EXFOLIATIVE DERMATITIS, stop the drug immediately.

Dosage:

Vaginal tablets or suppositories: 1–2 a day for 7 days.

Cream or ointment: smear sparingly on the affected skin after washing and drying well, twice a day until the rash is cleared plus 2 more days.

Mouth wash: nystatin 100,000 units per ml; place 1 ml in the mouth and hold it there for as long as possible in the area of the white spots. Do this 4 times a day until the problem is resolved.

Alternatives: MICONAZOLE; sun bathe the affected skin areas 15 minutes daily, use yogurt douches for vaginal candidiasis.

OFLOXACIN

Antibiotic, Gram-negative and anti-mycobacterial.

Safety class: 3   Stability ?   Pregnancy: C

Brand names: Floxin, Tarivid,

Indications: Gram-negative infections, CELLULITIS, CHLAMYDIA, GONORRHEA, KIDNEY INFECTION, LEPROSY, LYMPHOGRANULOMA VENEREUM, PELVIC INFECTION, PNEUMONIA, PROSTATITIS, SEPSIS, TUBERCULOSIS, URETHRITIS, URINARY INFECTION. It works much the same as CIPROFLOXACIN.

Contraindications: ALLERGY to any –oxacin antibiotic; age < 18 y.o.; pregnant women. Do not give this together with ANTACIDs. Do not give it to breastfeeding women. It should not be used in those with a history of MENTAL ILLNESS. Do not use this in the presence of LIVER DISEASE or KIDNEY DISEASE without independent professional confirmation. Do not give this to anyone with numbness or weakness.

Precautions: warn the patient against engaging in hazardous activities when starting on this drug, until the side-effects are known for him. Diabetics may lose control of their blood sugar. Elderly may develop tendinitis. Adequate water intake is very important; watch for DEHYDRATION.

Side-effects: headaches, dizziness, insomnia, sun sensitivity, SEIZURES (stop the drug), EXFOLIATIVE DERMATITIS (stop the drug). There may be alterations in pulse and blood pressure, possibly leading to fainting. There may be psychiatric problems such as overt craziness or difficulty moving or feeling.

Dosage: reduce the dose in the presence of KIDNEY DISEASE. Doses are all oral unless specified otherwise.

Most Gram-negative infections: 200 mg twice a day until the patient is better, plus 2 more days.

CHLAMYDIA, 400 mg twice a day for 7 days.

ENTERIC FEVER, 15 mg/kg/day for 2 days or 10 mg/kg/day for 3 days

GONORRHEA: a single dose of 400mg.

KIDNEY INFECTION: 200–400 mg twice daily for 7–14 days.

LEPROSY: 600 mg daily for 8 months. PB leprosy can be treated with 1 month of daily RIFAMPIN plus 400 mg daily ofloxacin.

LYMPHOGRANULOMA VENEREUM: unknown

PELVIC INFECTION: 400 mg twice a day for 14 days; use this with METRONIDAZOLE.

PNEUMONIA: 400 mg twice daily for 10 days.

PROSTATITIS: 200 mg twice a day for 28 days.

SEPSIS: 200 mg IV twice daily.

TUBERCULOSIS: 800 mg daily.

URETHRITIS, URINARY INFECTION: 200–400 mg twice a day for 7 days.

OLTIPRAZ

An older worm medication, no longer in use because of bad side-effects.

ORAL CONTRACEPTIVES

See BIRTH CONTROL PILLS.

ORNIDAZOLE

See TINIDAZOLE; the drug is similar. Check the package insert for dosage.

ORS

Safety class: 1   Stability: A

Synonym: oral rehydration solution.

Brand names: Pedialyte, Ricalyte, Diocalm Junior, Dioralyte, Electrolade, Rehidrat; usually generic product in developing areas.

Recipes to make ORS:

See also Appendix 1, Procedure 2, in Volume 1.

(1) Coconut water, used just as it is, works well or add 1 teaspoon of baking soda to each liter. Do not use this in the presence of KIDNEY DISEASE.

TOC

SYMPTOMS

DIFFERENTIALS

CONDITIONS

DRUG INDEX

REGIONAL NOTES

INX

(2) Dissolve the following in 1.0 liter of drinking water:

Ingredient	Grams	Volume
Glucose	20 grams	4 tsp/ 20 ml
Salt	3.5 grams	1/2 tsp/2.5 ml
Baking soda	2.5 grams	1/2 tsp/2.5 ml
Salt substitute or KCl	1.5 grams	1/4 tsp/1.25 ml

Notes:

Glucose is also called dextrose. If unavailable, you may substitute 30 grams of ordinary sugar (1/8 cup) or 50 grams uncooked rice powder (1/4 cup) (which should be cooked in some of the water before the other ingredients are added to make one liter of ORS).

Baking soda is sodium bicarbonate, $NaHCO_3$. It is not the same as baking powder. (Some commercial ORS preparations use sodium citrate.)

KCl[1] is commonly available as "salt substitute". It is okay to omit this if it is unavailable. As the patient recovers, citrus fruits, bananas and potatoes can supply this element.

Relationships: 3 teaspoons = 1 tablespoon; 4 tablespoons = 1/4 cup; 1 teaspoon = 5 ml.

Use the cleanest water you can conveniently find; speed is most important. Do not heat or boil the solution once it is made up.

Indications: CHOLERA, DEHYDRATION, TURISTA, other diarrhea, DYSENTERY, GASTROENTERITIS, GIARDIASIS, HEAT ILLNESS.

Contraindications: DIABETES,[2] HEART FAILURE, KIDNEY DISEASE. There are no allergic reactions.

Precautions: this is frequently supplied as packets of powder that must be added to water. If too little water is used the resulting strong salt solution will be deadly. If too much water is used it will work just fine.

Dosage: it is important to give enough; too much is never a problem. Dehydrated adults (see DEHYDRATION) get a minimum of 3 liters daily; school aged children, 2 liters; preschoolers 1 liter plus another 1/4 liter of plain water. After this minimum, continue giving it until the top of the patient's tongue is still moist 20 minutes after his last drink. Give POTASSIUM additionally unless the patient has KIDNEY DISEASE. In children under 6 months old, give an equal amount of clean, plain water in addition to the ORS and nourishment. An alternative to ORS is alternating a cup of chicken broth with 1.5 cups of apple juice or orange juice.

OXAMNIQUINE

Anti-schistosome, anthelmintic

Safety class: 2–3   Stability: unknown   Pregnancy: C

Brand names: Mansil, Vansil. Available in 250 mg tablets or 50 mg/ml liquid for children. It is available in Brazil.

Indications: SCHISTOSOMIASIS MANSONI at any stage.

Contraindications: ALLERGY to the drug. Do not use this in patients who have SEIZURES.

Precautions: warn the patient against engaging in hazardous activities until he knows what side-effects he will have from this drug.

Side-effects: drowsiness, dizziness, maybe SEIZURES. These effects occur in only a small percentage of patients. The urine may turn orange-red because of the drug. If used excessively, the drug can destroy the bone marrow.

Dosage: do not give this with food.

In the Americas and East Africa: 10 mg/kg twice a day for one day only.

In other locations: 15 mg/kg for 2 doses, given twice in one day or once a day for 2 days.

For treating a whole village or area: treat everyone every 6 months.

PAIN MEDICINES

See Chapter 8 in Volume 1 and NARCOTICS (this index).

PARA-AMINOSALICYLIC ACID

Anti-tuberculosis

Safety class: 3   Stability: unstable; must refrigerate

Synonym: PAS   Pregnancy: C

Brand name: Paser; also supplied as generic drug.

Indication: TUBERCULOSIS

Contraindications: ALLERGY to this drug, drug that has turned brown or purple, HEART FAILURE.

Side-effects: nausea, vomiting, diarrhea, fever, rash, HEPATITIS, susceptibility to other infections, similar to CHLORAMPHENICOL. Children seem to have much less problem with side-effects than adults. At any rate, these severe side-effects are not common.

Precaution: getting patients to take this is a challenge. The quantity of daily medicine and 3 times a day is a problem.

Dosage: 50 mg/kg three times a day. The usual adult dose is 2.5–4 grams a dose.

---

1 *In the States KCl can be bought in some grocery stores. The brand name is No Salt, in a white container.*

2 *In diabetes, any fluid with sugar in it will make the patient more dehydrated. It is best to rehydrate with a plain solution of 1.0 teaspoon (7 g) or 5 ml of salt per liter of water.*

PARALDEHYDE

Anti-seizure drug, sedative, muscle relaxant

Safety class: 2 by rectum or oral; 3 if IM

Stability: C   Keep below 25°C / 68°F in dark.

Brand name: Paral; it is a liquid chemical. It is an old drug, hard to find, but useful if you can obtain it.

Indications: treatment of muscle spasms in TETANUS; treatment of SEIZURES that will not stop, as in HEAT ILLNESS, MALARIA, MENINGITIS, SEPSIS. Occasionally useful as a sedative and for PERTUSSIS.

Contraindications: do not use drug that is old or discolored or that comes from partially used containers!!! Bad drug is a corrosive, strong acid. It is brownish or cloudy. It burns if a drop is placed on the skin. Good drug is clear and watery. It does not burn on the skin. Do not use this during pregnancy or breastfeeding unless the patient's situation is desperate and there are no alternatives.

Precautions: be sure to observe requirements for safe storage. Give IM only in an emergency and then only in the buttocks, remembering to stay in the upper-outer quadrant. Put your needle in deeply. You should use a glass syringe; this drug will dissolve plastic syringes unless you draw up the drug and give it very quickly. Avoid letting the drug contact rubber or plastic.

Warn your patient against engaging in hazardous activities while he is taking it. He should not drive.

Side-effects: this drug has an awful smell and so will your patient. This is expected. Your patient will be lethargic or unconscious for a longer time after his seizure than he would be otherwise. Pay special attention to his airway.

Dosage:

Sedative: rectally, give 0.2 ml/kg, mixed in twice this amount of olive or cooking oil. The drug can also be given by mouth if your patient can swallow, same dose as rectally. The IM dose is 0.1 ml/kg, not mixed with oil.

SEIZURES from any cause: rectally, give 0.4 ml/kg, mixed in twice this amount of olive or cooking oil and given as an enema; by injection the dose is 0.2 ml/kg IM to maximum of 10 ml (not mixed with oil).

TETANUS: same as SEIZURES.

PERTUSSIS: same as the sedative dose.

Alternatives: DIAZEPAM, PHENOBARBITAL, PHENYTOIN SODIUM.

PAROMOMYCIN

Aminoglycoside antibiotic, both Gram-negative and Gram-positive; dewormer

Safety class: 1 oral and cream; 3 injectable.

Stability: C   Pregnancy: Oral drug probably safe in pregnancy; seek independent confirmation. Available in India.

Synonym: aminosidine

Brand names: Farmiglucin, Gabbromycin, Gabbroral, Humatin, Maramicina, Pargonyl, Tricardil. Supplied as 250 mg capsules.

Indications: CRYPTOSPORIDIOSIS; DYSENTERY, both bacterial and amebic; TAPEWORM. It might be useful for GIARDIASIS. By injection, used for VISCERAL LEISHMANIASIS; in a cream, for CUTANEOUS LEISHMANIASIS.

Contraindications: prior ALLERGY to the drug, an obstructed bowel (abdominal pains and constipation) and KIDNEY DISEASE.

Precautions: the drug may cause abdominal pain and diarrhea. It is not absorbed from the bowel to any extent when given orally. Thus the oral can be used only for bowel problems. The injected drug may cause deafness and/or KIDNEY DISEASE. Do not use this with any other drugs that are toxic to the kidneys. Do not give this to anyone who has muscle weakness.

Dosage: the following are adult doses. Reduce the dose according to weight for children.

CRYPTOSPORIDIOSIS: 10 mg/kg by mouth three times daily for 28 days, then 500 mg twice a day maintenance.

CUTANEOUS LEISHMANIASIS: follow local advice.

DYSENTERY: 500 mg by mouth every 8 hours for 7 days.

TAPEWORM: adults get 1000 mg (1 gram) by mouth every 15 minutes for 4 doses, a total of 4000 mg (4 grams). May be repeated daily for 5 days, but some authorities say that one day or three days is enough.

VISCERAL LEISHMANIASIS: 20mg/kg injection daily for 21 days.

PEFLOXACIN

This is a Gram-negative antibiotic. It is one of the FLUOROQUINOLONES. Its advantage is that it is eliminated from the body slowly, and it gets into the brain, so it is good for some kinds of MENINGITIS. It is also good for ENTERIC FEVER, ABSCESS due to staph and KIDNEY INFECTIONS. Seek other information as regards dosage and side-effects.

The usual dose in LEPROSY is 400 mg daily for 8 months. It might be useful for TUBERCULOSIS; dosage unknown.

PENICILLIN

Antibiotic (Gram-positive)

Safety class: 2   Pregnancy: B

Stability: see below under forms of penicillin

Brand names: too many to list. Generic human and veterinary drug is available.

Indications: ABSCESS, ANTHRAX, ARTHRITIS, BARTONELLOSIS, CANCRUM ORIS, CELLULITIS, DIPHTHERIA, middle EAR INFECTION, EYE INFECTION, GONORRHEA, IMPETIGO, LEPTOSPIROSIS, LYME DISEASE, MEASLES, MENINGITIS, PELVIC INFECTION, PIG-BEL, PINTA, PNEUMONIA, RAT BITE FEVER, RELAPSING FEVER, RESPIRATORY INFECTION, RHEUMATIC FEVER, SEPSIS, STREP THROAT, SYPHILIS, TETANUS, TREPONARID, TROPICAL ULCER, URETHRITIS, YAWS. This may also be used for infected teeth other than third molars.

Contraindications: symptoms of ALLERGY of any sort after having received penicillin or any "cillin" drug. There is some cross-allergy with CEPHALOSPORIN. It should not be used with certain diuretics (water pills) or with oral contraceptives (the contraceptives might not work). Some sources say it should not be used during breastfeeding

Precautions: keep your patient nearby for 30 minutes after the first dose. Do not use penicillin unless you have EPINEPHRINE available or the condition is life-threatening. Life-threatening conditions are those for which the adult dose is 1000 mg or more. Do not use this at the same time as DOXYCYCLINE or CHLORAMPHENICOL unless directed to do so. This may cause DRUG ERUPTION when used for SYPHILIS.

Forms of Penicillin:

Penicillin G: (benzylpenicillin). Stability: Dry A. Liquid D; refrigerate.

Cheapest injectable penicillin. It does not work well by mouth. It must be injected every 2 to 4 hours. The IM injection is painful. It comes as potassium penicillin G and sodium penicillin G. The usual vial contains one million units. The relationship between mg and units is the same as ordinary penicillin, and the two drugs are interchangeable. In a very sick patient or when a disease has progressed rapidly, it is best to use injected penicillin G for the first few doses.

Penicillin V: (pen VK, penicillin potassium phenoxymethyl). Stability: A. This is the common penicillin taken by mouth. It is a form that is not destroyed by stomach acid. It is cheap. It must be taken every 6 hours. 62.5 mg = 100,000 units; 250 mg = 400,000 units.

Procaine penicillin: stability: dry A. Liquid D; refrigerate.

Longer-acting injectable penicillin. It is injected IM; one injection lasts 12–24 hours so it need be given only once or twice daily. It comes in units; use 3–4 million units daily instead of 500 mg of oral penicillin every 6 hours.

Benzathine penicillin: stability: dry A. Liquid D; refrigerate.

Longest-acting injectable penicillin, it is used for IM injection. One shot lasts for 10 days, so it is ideal for someone who is traveling or who is unreliable. Dosage is one time only unless specified otherwise. 2.4 million units of this replaces [250 mg of oral penicillin every 6 hours for 10 days]. Do not use this for very ill patients or those in whom the disease has progressed rapidly. Quite expensive.

Triple penicillin: a mixture of the above three injectable penicillins: benzyl, procaine, and benzathine.

Dosage:

The usual adult doses for the various penicillins refer to the chart on the following page. Reduce the doses according to weight for children. Reduce the doses in KIDNEY DISEASE and in elderly patients. You may need to increase the dose in otherwise-healthy patients from Western cultures and in areas where there has been Western-type medical care.

ABSCESS: mild to moderate.

ANTHRAX: severe; continue for 60 days.

ARTHRITIS: mild to moderate; you should double the dose in a seriously ill patient from a Western culture.

BARTONELLOSIS: moderate to severe for 7 days.

CANCRUM ORIS: severe.

CELLULITIS: mild to moderate.

DIPHTHERIA: mild to moderate.

Middle EAR INFECTION: mild.

EYE INFECTION with fever: moderate to severe.

GONORRHEA treatment 3500 mg penicillin V by mouth in a single initial dose; then 500 mg every 6 hours for 10 days. Do not use the long-acting forms.

GONORRHEA exposure: 3500 mg penicillin V swallowed as a single dose.

IMPETIGO: mild to moderate for 10 days.

LEPTOSPIROSIS:[1] moderate to severe.

LYME DISEASE: dosage on the right column.

MEASLES: mild to moderate.

MENINGITIS: dosage on the right column.

PELVIC INFECTION: same as GONORRHEA treatment.

PIG-BEL: moderate to severe.

PINTA: mild to moderate.

PNEUMONIA: mild to moderate.

PYOMYOSITIS: severe.

RAT BITE FEVER: mild to moderate.

RELAPSING FEVER: moderate.

RESPIRATORY INFECTION: mild to moderate.

RHEUMATIC FEVER: moderate to severe.

SEPSIS: dosage on right column.

SICKLE CELL DISEASE in children. 125 mg pen V, twice daily, from diagnosis until age 5.

STREP INFECTION: mild.

SYPHILIS, congenital (newborn): 50,000 units/kg of pen G or procaine penicillin IM daily for 10 days.

SYPHILIS, congenital (adult) 2.4 mu benzathine pen weekly x 3 weeks. Reduce the dose according to weight for children.

SYPHILIS, primary and secondary: 1.2 mu of procaine pen daily for 10 days. Or, a single IM injection of 2.4 million units of benzathine penicillin for adults; 1.2 mu for children 6–15 y.o.; 0.6 mu for children under 6 y.o. benzathine penicillin is recommended by the World Health Organization because of the trouble getting patients to comply with the long treatment required with penicillin V.

---

1 *It is useless to give antibiotic for leptospirosis if the patient has been ill for 4 days or more.*

TOC SYMPTOMS DIFFERENTIALS CONDITIONS DRUG INDEX REGIONAL NOTES INX

SYPHILIS, latent (between secondary and tertiary) benzathine penicillin 2.4 mu weekly for 3 doses.

SYPHILIS, tertiary: procaine penicillin 1.2 mu daily for 20 days or penicillin G 4 mu every 6 hours for 10–14 days. Do not use benzathine penicillin if there are any neurological symptoms.

TETANUS: mild to moderate.

Tooth infection: 250–500 mg every 6 hours until the problem is better, plus another two days. The tooth should also be pulled.

TREPONARID: a single dose of benzathine penicillin, 600,000 units in children under 6 years old; 1.2 million units in 6–15 years old and 2.4 million units in adults.

TROPICAL ULCER: mild to moderate until totally healed.

URETHRITIS: same as GONORRHEA treatment.

YAWS: mild to moderate.

Alternatives: CLINDAMYCIN for an abscess with foul-smelling pus. ERYTHROMYCIN in penicillin ALLERGY, but **not** in MENINGITIS, **nor** SEPSIS, **nor** EYE INFECTION with fever; in these cases use CHLORAMPHENICOL alone.

	Mild illness	Moderate illness	Severe illness[1]	MENINGITIS, SYPHILIS, LYME DISEASE involving the brain.
Penicillin G = benzyl penicillin = crystalline penicillin	400,000 units every 4 hours IM or IV.	1 million units every 4 hours IM or IV.	2 million units IM or IV every 2– 4 hours until all better plus 5 days.	1–2 million units IV every 4 hours for 21 days.
Penicillin V, the only oral plain penicillin	250 mg every 6 hours for 10 days with strep, until better plus 3 days otherwise.	500 mg every 6 hours for 10 days with strep, until better plus 3 days other-wise.	500 mg every 6 hours for 10 days with strep, until better plus 5 days otherwise.	Don't use this.
Procaine penicillin, a form that lasts for a whole day.	1.2 million units daily IM.	2.4 million units IM daily.	1.2 million units IM twice daily.	Don't use this unless forced to, then like severe illness.
Benzathine penicillin,[2] a form that lasts for 10 days.	2.4 million units in a single IM injection.	Use procaine pen IM for 2 days, then 2.4 mu in a single IM injection.	Use penicillin G until there is improvement, then procaine pen until the patient is up and around, then 2.4 million units IM every week.	Don't use this ever; it does not get into the brain.
Triple penicillin, a combination of G, procaine and benzathine	Determine the dose by the usual single dose for benzathine penicillin; the other components then should be correct. ABSCESS, ANTHRAX, ARTHRITIS, BARTONELLOSIS, CELLULITIS, DIPHTHERIA, MIDDLE EAR INFECTION, IMPETIGO, MEASLES, PINTA, PNEUMONIA, RAT BITE FEVER, RELAPSING FEVER, RESPIRATORY INFECTION, RHEUMATIC FEVER, STREP INFECTION, TETANUS, TREPONARID, TROPICAL ULCER, URETHRITIS, YAWS.		Don't use this unless there is no other option; then be generous on the dose. BARTONELLOSIS, CANCRUM ORIS, EYE INFECTION with fever, LEPTOSPIROSIS, PIG-BEL, PYOMYOSITIS, SEPSIS.	

1 That is, a severe illness without any signs of MENINGITIS: no stiff neck, paralysis, numbness or tingling, patient not unconscious or crazy.

2 Note that this is not the same as benzyl penicillin.

PENTAMIDINE

Anti-protozoa, some pneumonia

Safety class: 3   Stability: C dark   Pregnancy: C

Brand names: Lomidine, Pentacarinat, Pentam; Pentam 300, Nebupent. Supplied in vials of 300 mg. It is extremely expensive.

Indications: AFRICAN SLEEPING SICKNESS, Gambian type, prevention and treatment; CUTANEOUS LEISHMANIASIS; PNEUMONIA with HIV INFECTION; VISCERAL LEISHMANIASIS.

Contraindications: ALLERGY to the drug. If the patient has KIDNEY DISEASE or DIABETES, the drug must be given only in a hospital with a physician's supervision. Do not use it with any blood disease, with any heart disease, in the presence of DEHYDRATION or together with any other drugs that are toxic for the kidney.

Precautions: if the patient becomes sweaty or shaky, panics or loses consciousness, give him sugar.

Be sure to avoid giving the drug into a vein. It works that way but there are much more serious side-effects.

Warn the patient not to engage in hazardous activities while taking this drug.

This drug interacts badly with many other drugs. It is toxic for liver, kidney, heart and bone marrow. It is likely to cause major problems in DIABETES.

Side-effects: a drop of blood pressure with fainting; a drop in blood sugar, muscle weakness, local irritation where the injection is given, occasionally PANCREATITIS.

Dosage: Reduce the dose with KIDNEY DISEASE.

AFRICAN SLEEPING SICKNESS prevention: adult dose is 300–400 mg IM every 6 months. Children get 4 mg/kg.

AFRICAN SLEEPING SICKNESS treatment 4 mg/kg IM daily or every other day, for 10 doses. This does not work for advanced disease with mental symptoms. If it is going to work, you should see an improvement within 24 hours.

CUTANEOUS LEISHMANIASIS: 3 mg/kg every other day for 4 doses or 2 mg/kg every other day for 7 doses.

PNEUMONIA with HIV: 4 mg/kg IM daily for 12–14 days. Improvement should be evident in 4–6 days.

VISCERAL LEISHMANIASIS: 2–3 mg/kg per dose IM every other day or 3 times weekly for 7 doses. Double the duration in the Indian Subcontinent.

PERMETHRIN

Insecticide

Safety class: 1–2   Stability unknown

The drug is safe in pregnancy.

Supplied as 5% cream and 1% lotion

Indications: SCABIES, LICE

Contraindication: ALLERGY to the drug.

Side-effects: this may cause burning/stinging or an increase in itching.

Dosage:

SCABIES: use the cream; massage it into the skin from the neck on down (not just in the area where there is rash and itching). Leave it on for 12 hours before washing it off. Put clothes and bedding out in the sun.

LICE: wash and dry the area. Put the lotion on for 10 minutes, then rinse it off. Treat clothing also by boiling or ironing.

PHENOBARBITAL

Barbiturate, sedative, anti-seizure drug

Safety class: 2–3   Stability: B   Pregnancy: D

Supplied as generic drug.

Indications: emotional upset, EPILEPSY, SEIZURES, TETANUS, TOXEMIA.

Contraindications: ALLERGY to the drug, breathing problem (such as ASTHMA) unrelated to the indication for the drug, MENTAL ILLNESS, PORPHYRIA. Don't use with other sedatives, in diabetic patients, with birth control pills or with LIVER FAILURE or KIDNEY DISEASE.

Precautions: if someone has taken the drug regularly for more than 2 weeks and it should be stopped, stop the drug slowly, reducing the dosage over 3 weeks or more. It takes 2–3 days for the drug to start or stop acting. This drug is mildly addicting.

Warn the patient not to engage in hazardous activities while taking this drug. The drug may decrease the urge to breathe.

Side-effects: sleepiness in some, hyperactivity in some, agitation and confusion in some elderly people. A rash is the most frequent manifestation of ALLERGY. Newborns of women who have taken the drug during pregnancy sometimes have a problem with bleeding. VITAMIN K is effective for this. **The drug makes any pain worse.**

More serious adverse reactions

SERUM SICKNESS: an illness that begins after 10 days on the drug, with symptoms resembling ANAPHYLAXIS, plus, thereafter, protein in the urine and the development of KIDNEY DISEASE. Stop the drug.

EXFOLIATIVE DERMATITIS (peeling skin): stop the drug.

Dosage

Emotional upset: 15–30 mg every 6–12 hours for adults.

SEIZURES, treatment or prevention: 60 mg twice a day for adults. You may increase the dose if ordered by an M.D. Children get 2 mg/kg every 12 hours, by mouth. The dose may be increased to every 8 hours to prevent seizures.

TETANUS: 60 mg by IM injection every 6 hours. You may increase the dose as necessary for control of spasms. Give the lowest dose that will do the job. Reduce the dose according to weight for children.

TOXEMIA: same as SEIZURES.

Alternatives: PHENYTOIN SODIUM, DIAZEPAM, PARALDEHYDE, others.

PHENYTOIN

Anti-seizure drug

Synonym: phenytoin sodium.

Safety class: 3   Stability: A   Pregnancy: D

Safety class: 1 when used for wounds

Brand name: Dilantin. Generic drug is available. Supplied in capsules of 100 mg and in liquid with 125 mg of drug per 5 ml (1 teaspoon). Slow-release forms may be available.

Indications: EPILEPSY; LEPROSY; SEIZURES; sprinkled in ABSCESSes, TROPICAL ULCERs and wounds to aid healing.

Contraindications: prior ALLERGY to the drug. The other contraindications do not apply to the topical use of the drug for ulcer healing. Given orally: do not give ACETAZOLAMIDE to a patient taking this drug, except at the direction of a physician. Do not give it to someone with any heart disease or any blood disease. The drug interacts badly with many others so it is best not to use it in patients taking any other drug regularly. Do not give this to patients who have PORPHYRIA, a hereditary disease.

Precautions: it is best to take this with or after a meal. Decrease the oral dose if the patient has evidence of LIVER FAILURE. After the patient has been on it for a while, withdraw the drug slowly over a few weeks, or he will have SEIZURES. Minimum length of time on the drug for seizures is a year.

Side-effects: the oral drug normally will make the gums of the mouth swollen; this is of no consequence. It may increase the growth of body hair. An overdose will cause incoordination. It may cause a drop in blood pressure, and the patient may appear to be intoxicated.

Dosage: there are long-acting (slow-release) forms available in which the total daily dose can be taken as a single daily dose. Be sure not to take short-acting forms this way. Reduce the dose in LIVER FAILURE, KIDNEY DISEASE, DIABETES and in the elderly.

SEIZURES, EPILEPSY: if the patient does not have LIVER FAILURE or KIDNEY DISEASE and if he has not taken the drug for the last week, adults get 300 mg three times on that first day only. After that, the average adult gets 100 mg three times daily. This may be increased to a maximum of 200 mg three times daily. Children get 2 mg/kg three times daily. Results: 2 days to 2 weeks.

LEPROSY and wounds, ABSCESSes and wounds: open a 100 mg capsule or crush a tablet, and sprinkle the powder into the skin ulcer, abscess or wound daily before bandaging it.

PILOCARPINE

Eye drops which make the pupil of the eye very small; used in GLAUCOMA; use with the direction of a physician. Do not use this in a red eye (aside from GLAUCOMA) or in the presence of insecticides, anesthetics, ASTHMA or EYE INFECTION. Side-effects are unusual.

PIPERAQUINE

⚠ **Take care to distinguish this from PIPERAZINE, listed below. They are two entirely different drugs!**

Anti-malarial, always combined with dihydroartemisinin (see ARTEMISININ)

Safety class: probably 2   Stability unknown

Pregnancy: used a lot but not before 16 weeks.

Brand names: Artekin, Duo-Cotecxin is piperaquine plus dihydroartemisinin. Artecom is the same plus TRIMETHOPRIM additionally. Some preparations add PRIMAQUINE as well: piperaquine 320 mg + DHA 32 mg + TRIMETHOPRIM 180 mg + PRIMAQUINE 10 mg.

Indication: MALARIA

Contraindication: prior ALLERGY.

Precautions: see the entries for each component drug.

Side-effects: only a rash with piperaquine and that rarely. Check the side-effects of the other components.

Dosage: adult dose: piperaquine 600–640 mg by mouth every 24 hours for 4 doses. If the piperaquine dosage is correct, the dosage of the other components will automatically be correct. Some authorities recommend giving a double dose at the beginning.

PIPERAZINE

⚠ **Take care to distinguish this from PIPERAQUINE, listed above. They are two entirely different drugs.**

Dewormer, anthelmintic

Safety class: 2   Stability: A   Pregnancy: B

Brand names: Antepar, Entacyl, Multifuge. Parazine, Perin, Piperate, Pipizan, Vermizine, Worm-expel. Generic veterinary drug is available. Different brand names have different last names for the drug. Adipate, Citrate, Hydrate and Phosphate are all acceptable last names. Doses given are for piperazine hydrate. Drug labels will generally give equivalences of a particular dose to piperazine hydrate. Most tablets contain the equivalent of 250 or 500 mg piperazine hydrate. Liquids contain 100 mg/ml.

Indications: ASCARIASIS, ENTEROBIASIS.

Contraindications: ACUTE ABDOMEN, ALLERGY to the drug. Contraindicated also with current use of phenothiazines, (anti-nausea medicines) and in patients with a history of SEIZURES.

TOC   SYMPTOMS   DIFFERENTIALS   CONDITIONS   DRUG INDEX   REGIONAL NOTES   INX

Precautions: do not use this with PYRANTEL PAMOATE. Piperazine is not well absorbed; it merely paralyzes the worms. Because of this, if the patient is developing an ACUTE ABDOMEN type 3 because of a large wad of worms, it may make his situation worse. Hence it is best not to use it with episodic abdominal pains. Warn the patient against engaging in hazardous activities while taking this drug.

Side-effects: nausea, vomiting, diarrhea, abdominal pain, incoordination. If the patient has a SEIZURE, stop the drug.

Dosage: reduce the dose in KIDNEY DISEASE or LIVER FAILURE.

ASCARIASIS: adults: 3500 mg daily for 2 days. Children: 75 mg/kg daily for 2 days to a maximum of 3500 mg daily. Repeat the treatment 2 weeks later, if possible.

ENTEROBIASIS: same dose for 6 days.

Alternatives: BEPHENIUM HYDROXYNAPHTHOATE, ALBENDAZOLE, MEBENDAZOLE, PYRANTEL PAMOATE. It is generally better to use alternative drugs rather than piperazine, although piperazine may be more available.

POTASSIUM

Mineral

Synonyms: potassium chloride, KCl

Safety class: 2   Stability: A

Supplied as potassium chloride in packets of powder or large, dissolving tablets. There are many forms and sizes. Brand name in the States, in grocery stores, is "No Salt." It is generally found with baking supplies.

Indications: to replace lost potassium due to taking FUROSEAMIDE or HYDROCHLOROTHIAZIDE; to replace lost potassium due to severe diarrhea, or vomiting, thus supplementing ORS. It is important in the management of EBOLA VIRUS DISEASE.

Contraindications: KIDNEY DISEASE, patient taking triamterene or spironolactone.

Precautions: some potassium preparations cause stomach pain or upset. Be sure to note that doses are given in meq rather than mg. 75 mg of KCl = 1 meq potassium. Never use injectable potassium. If the patient is very dehydrated, be sure that he is urinating normally before starting this medication.

Dosage: usual adult dose is 20–30 meq 1 to 3 times daily; reduce dose according to weight for children.

Alternatives: any of the following foods (same contraindications): apricots, avocado, bananas, citrus fruits, coconut water, dates, papaya, potatoes, pumpkin, spinach, tomatoes. Salt substitute usually contains potassium chloride. The product labeled "No Salt" is almost pure potassium chloride.

PRAZIQUANTEL

Anthelmintic, dewormer

Safety class: 1, safe for children   Stability: A

Pregnancy: B or C

Brand names: Biltricide, Cesol, Pyquiton. Veterinary brand names: Distocide, Droncit. Human drug is supplied as 600 mg tablets that are scored so as to break easily. The drug is expensive. The drug is stable so you can ignore expiration dates.

Indications: CYSTICERCOSIS, HYDATID DISEASE; INTESTINAL FLUKE, KATAYAMA DISEASE, LIVER FLUKE (Asian only), PARAGONIMIASIS, SCHISTOSOMIASIS HEMATOBIUM, SCHISTOSOMIASIS INTERCALATUM, SCHISTOSOMIASIS JAPONICUM, SCHISTOSOMIASIS MANSONI, SCHISTOSOMIASIS MEKONGI, TAPEWORM.

Contraindications: ALLERGY to this, CYSTICERCOSIS involving the eyes or given without STEROID. Current use of RIFAMPIN. The patient should not take RIFAMPIN for 4 weeks before praziquantel. He may start RIFAMPIN the day after.

Precautions: the drug appears in human milk. Mothers should not nurse for 72 hours after taking the drug. Safety in pregnancy is uncertain. No definite bad effects have been observed. The drug should be used under close physician supervision if it is used with steroids (DEXAMETHASONE, PREDNISONE or PREDNISOLONE) or with anticonvulsants (DIAZEPAM, PHENYTOIN or PHENOBARBITAL). Warn the patient not to engage in hazardous activities after taking this drug. Do not use this drug if the patient may have consumed rare pork. You may be inadvertently treating CYSTICERCOSIS which requires additional drugs; your patient may have a SEIZURE.

Side-effects: occasional tiredness, abdominal pain, nausea, vomiting, loss of appetite, sweating, drowsiness, headache and dizziness. In a patient with KATAYAMA DISEASE, the symptoms may worsen; either give PREDNISONE before the first dose, or wait until the symptoms decrease by themselves before using this drug.

Dosage: reduce the dose in LIVER DISEASE.

CYSTICERCOSIS: 30 mg/kg every 8 hours for 1 day, followed by 15 mg/kg every 8 hours for 2–4 weeks. Use PREDNISONE and CIMETIDINE also from the day before treatment through day 4 after treatment, possibly anti-seizure drugs also. Seek advice.

HYDATID DISEASE: 50 mg/kg daily x 2 weeks minimum, given along with ALBENDAZOLE until the cysts have disappeared. It is sometimes given only weekly, same dose.

INTESTINAL FLUKE: 25 mg/kg every 8 hours for 3 doses.

LIVER FLUKE: 25 mg/kg every 8 hours for 2 days.

PARAGONIMIASIS: 25 mg/kg 3 times a day for 2 days.

SCHISTOSOMIASIS treatment (all types): 20 mg/kg 3 times in one day after 3 days on PREDNISONE or a similar drug. If the patient has weakness or numbness, then give an initial dose of 40–60 mg/kg along with high-dose HYDROCORTISONE. In this case repeat the treatment in 10 days and again in 3 weeks.

SCHISTOSOMIASIS prevention: single dose of 20 mg/kg, after 3 weeks post-exposure. Before 3 weeks use ARTEMISININ. Use both weekly for continual exposures.

TAPEWORM: fish: 10 mg/kg one dose only. Beef: 5 mg/kg (one dose). Pork: 5 mg/kg (one dose). Dwarf and rat: 25 mg/kg (one dose).

Alternatives: NIRIDAZOLE, but it has bad side-effects and is not safe when used for SCHISTOSOMIASIS JAPONICUM or SCHISTOSOMIASIS MEKONGI. NICLOSAMIDE may be used for TAPEWORM. ALBENDAZOLE works just as well as this for CYSTICERCOSIS.

PREDNISOLONE EYE DROPS

Steroid

Safety class: 3   Stability: A

Brand name: Blephamide ophthalmic. Supplied as a 1% ophthalmic solution or suspension.

Indications: ALLERGY (vernal conjunctivitis); IRITIS; KERATITIS due to SYPHILIS or ONCHOCERCIASIS; TUBERCULOSIS that affects the eye; LEPROSY reaction.

Contraindications: uncertainty of the diagnosis and GLAUCOMA. When used in a patient who has KERATITIS due to HERPES, this drug as eye drops will cause blindness! If you are not able to stain the eyes with fluorescein to check for HERPES, then do not use these drops. When used for longer than 2 weeks, it is likely to cause CATARACT or GLAUCOMA.

Dosage: one drop 2–4 times daily, depending on the severity of the condition. Do not use these drops for more than 2 weeks.

Result should be evident in less than 24 hours.

PREDNISOLONE

See PREDNISONE. The indications, contraindications and doses are all the same. The two drugs can be used interchangeably.

PREDNISONE

Corticosteroid

Safety class: 3   Stability: C   Pregnancy: C or D

Brand names: Deltasone, Orasone. Supplied as 5 mg tablets, sometimes larger tablets with as much as 40 mg.

Indications: AFRICAN SLEEPING SICKNESS (Gambian type); ALLERGY; ANAPHYLAXIS; ASTHMA; CONTACT DERMATITIS; CYSTICERCOSIS; ECZEMA; ENTERIC FEVER; EXFOLIATIVE DERMATITIS; FILARIASIS; KATAYAMA DISEASE; KIDNEY DISEASE; LEPROSY reactions; MALARIA (post-malaria neuro syndrome); some MENINGITIS; ONCHOCERCIASIS; PERICARDITIS; PERTUSSIS; PLANT POISONING, manicheel; RESPIRATORY INFECTION, chronic; spider bites; TRICHINOSIS; TUBERCULOSIS; TYPHUS.

Possible indications: may be useful for ANTHRAX. Used with DEC (drug). Used with PRAZIQUANTEL for SCHISTOSOMIASIS MANSONI or SCHISTOSOMIASIS JAPONICUM.

Contraindications: used in a patient with STRONGYLOIDIASIS it may cause SEPSIS and death. If this is a possibility, treat for STRONGYLOIDIASIS before using this drug.

Probably should not be used in pregnancy, because it may cause cleft palate in the baby.

The drug may activate dormant TUBERCULOSIS. With a history of TB or in an area where TB is common, the drug should be used only with a physician's supervision.

Do not use in the presence of CHAGA'S DISEASE; HEPATITIS B or C or PORPHYRIA.

Do not use this with untreated fungal infections or with myasthenia gravis.

Do not give this in HIV INFECTION, heart disease, disease involving the bowel or eye diseases.

Don't give it the same time as any vaccines (the vaccines won't work) or with diuretics (water pills).

Precautions: it is very important not to use this drug for more than 5 days before stopping it for at least a week, unless there are specific directions to the contrary. If used longer, it needs to be stopped gradually, over weeks, reducing the dose every other day. If the patient has an emotional breakdown, stop the drug gradually if he has been taking it for more than 5 days. The drug may activate a problem with AMEBIASIS, causing complications. Regard any diarrhea side-effect as amebic DYSENTERY, in areas where amebae are common. Have the patient wear a medical ID bracelet if he travels while taking the drug.

Side-effects: the drug decreases immunity (patients are likely to get something else), and it masks fever (the patient won't have a fever with a disease that ordinarily causes a fever) which makes diagnosis very difficult. Additionally, there are bad long-term side-effects of the drug: muscle weakness, brittle bones, PEPTIC ULCER, DIABETES, SHOCK, death, to name a few. These do not generally occur if the drug is used for 5 days or less. The dose of the drug is not as critical as the length of time it is used.

Dosage: the adult doses are given. Reduce the dose according to weight for children.

AFRICAN SLEEPING SICKNESS: for Gambian type, give 1 mg/kg/day up to 40 mg, for the duration of the treatment, then gradually reduce the dose over about 3–4 weeks.

ALLERGY: 10 mg daily for 1–2 days, may extend to 5 days.

ANAPHYLAXIS: 40 mg, usually one dose but you may give this daily for 2 days.

ANTHRAX: 10 mg daily for 5 days.

ASTHMA: same as ALLERGY.

CONTACT DERMATITIS: 10 mg daily for 2–3 days.

CYSTICERCOSIS: 40 mg daily for 5 days, beginning the day before treatment with PRAZIQUANTEL.

Given with DEC: same as ANTHRAX.

ECZEMA: same as ANTHRAX.

ENTERIC FEVER: 40 mg immediately, then 20 mg every 6 hours for 2 more doses.

EXFOLIATIVE DERMATITIS: same as ENTERIC FEVER.

FILARIASIS: same as ANTHRAX.

KATAYAMA DISEASE: same as ANAPHYLAXIS.

KIDNEY DISEASE: use 40 mg daily to begin with; this will have to be continued under a physician's supervision as it will probably need to be continued beyond 5 days.

LEPROSY reactions: 40 mg daily for 5 days.

MALARIA (post malaria neuro syndrome): unknown.

MENINGITIS: same as ANTHRAX

ONCHOCERCIASIS: same as ANTHRAX.

PERICARDITIS: same as ANTHRAX.

PERTUSSIS: same as ANTHRAX.

PLANT POISONING, manicheel: same as ANAPHYLAXIS.

RESPIRATORY INFECTION: same as ANTHRAX.

SCHISTOSOMIASIS: same as ANTHRAX.

Spider bites: 20 mg daily for 2 days.

TRICHINOSIS: same as ANTHRAX.

TUBERCULOSIS: 60 mg daily for 4 weeks, then decrease gradually over 3 months.

TYPHUS: same as ENTERIC FEVER.

Results: it takes about 6 hours for the drug to have any effect.

Alternatives:

Drug	Equivalent dosages	
Prednisone	5 mg	40 mg
Dexamethasone	0.75 mg	6 mg
Hydrocortisone	20 mg	160 mg

PRIMAQUINE

Malaria preventive.

Safety class: 1   Stability: C   Pregnancy: D

The drug is very toxic in overdose for children; a small overdose can kill.

Supplied as generic drug in 7.5 and 15 mg tablets.

Indications: radical cure of MALARIA to be taken when leaving a malarious area for an extended period of time. It is also good to use as a single dose at the end of any malarial treatment; it prevents the spread of malaria within the community.

Contraindications: pregnancy, ALLERGY to the drug, allergy to quinacrine, allergy to iodoquinol (a related drug).

G6PD DEFICIENCY which is most common in persons of Mediterranean descent. Do not give this to persons of Mediterranean (or Irish) descent unless they have been tested for G6PD DEFICIENCY. Do not give it at the same time as the drug quinicrine.

Precautions: watch for urobilinogen in the urine of people taking this drug, and stop the drug if you find it, more than 1+. urobilinogen 1+ is normal.

Side-effects: abdominal cramps, nausea, mild ANEMIA. These effects occur in only a small percentage of patients.

Dosage: at the end of a malaria treatment 30[1] mg, single dose. For a radical cure: 30 mg daily for 14 days; should be taken with food. For persons of Mediterranean heritage (with a mild G6PD DEFICIENCY), give 45 mg once each week to a total of 420 mg, as long as there are no problems. In either case, the critical factor in preventing relapse is the total amount of drug taken. This should be 420 mg.

PROBENECID

Adjunct medication to take with PENICILLIN and some CEPHALOSPORINs.

Safety class: 2   Stability: C, protect from light.

Pregnancy: B

Supplied in tablets of 500 mg

Indications: used with some antibiotics in order to increase the amount in the blood stream. It also increases the effect of the anesthetic KETAMINE. It is used in the prevention of GOUT and with cidofovir in HIV infection.

Contraindications: blood disorders, KIDNEY STONES, KIDNEY DISEASE, PEPTIC ULCER, G6PD DEFICIENCY, GOUT, current use of ASPIRIN.

Precautions: be sure the patient drinks 2–3 liters of water a day, that he does not become dehydrated.

Side-effects: headache, stomach distress, LIVER DISEASE, KIDNEY STONES, various skin problems. Stop the drug if these are severe.

Dosage: usual adult dose is 250 mg twice a day, increasing to 500 mg four times a day. With antibiotics, the dose is 500 mg four times a day. Reduce the dose for the elderly. Reduce the dose according to weight for children.

GOUT: 250 mg twice a day, increasing to 500 mg twice a day.

---

1 *The dose used to be 15 mg daily. This may still be sufficient for small adults. Use 30 mg in large adults.*

PROCHLORPERAZINE

Phenothiazine, sedative, anti-nausea

Safety class: 2   Stability: B, dark   Pregnancy: C

Brand name: Compazine. Generic drug is available. Supplied as 5 mg and 10 mg tablets, 10 mg and 25 mg suppositories.

Indications: nausea, vomiting, emotional upset.

Contraindications: HEART FAILURE, LIVER DISEASE, some blood diseases, lethargic or unconscious patient, children less than 20 lb (10 kg), children who are quite ill or who have DEHYDRATION which is not yet corrected or who have severe HEPATITIS. If you are desperate to get fluids or medicines down a small or ill child, you may use the drug, once or twice only. Do not use in breastfeeding women.

Precautions: occasionally patients get facial muscle spasms as a side-effect. This is harmless but terrifying. Treat them with DIPHENHYDRAMINE IM; it is best not to give this unless you have DIPHENHYDRAMINE available.

Patients become sleepy. Warn the patient not to engage in hazardous activities while taking this drug.

The drug interferes with many different lab tests. Don't believe lab results on blood drawn while the person is taking this.

Watch for NEUROLEPTIC MALIGNANT SYNDROME.

Side-effects: the most common one is a fall in blood pressure when the patient suddenly stands up. Other effects are worsening of GLAUCOMA, constipation, inability to pass urine (especially in older men), susceptibility to HEAT ILLNESS, dry mouth, decrease in sweating, rapid pulse, sensitivity to light, blurred vision. These effects occur in only a small percentage of patients. The drug causes sun sensitivity: easy burning with minimum exposure to light. Routine long-term usage of this drug may cause PARKINSON'S DISEASE.

Dosage: reduce the dose for the elderly. The dose by mouth and by IM injection is the same. By suppository more drug is given since less is absorbed.

Nausea: adults: 5–10 mg orally every 3 hours as needed for nausea and vomiting. Rectal suppository dose is 25 mg every 6 hours.

Children 20–40 kg (44–88 lb): 2.5–5 mg oral every 6 hours.

Children 15–20 kg (33–44 lb): 2.5 mg oral every 6 hours.

Children 10–15 kg (22–33 lb): 2.5 mg oral every 8 hours.

Emotional upset: adults get 10–20 mg orally once, then 5–10 mg every 6 hours. Children get the same dose as for nausea.

Alternatives: PROMETHAZINE is a cheaper and safer alternative. Other alternatives are CHLORPROMAZINE, Mellaril, Sparine, Stelazine. Dosages vary; indications, contraindications, precautions, etc. are similar. Check the package insert and follow instructions for your product. You may use PHENOBARBITAL as a sedative.

PROGUANIL

Malaria preventive

Safety class: 1   Stability: A   Pregnancy: C

Brand name: Paludrine.

Equivalent drug: Chloroguanide. ATOVAQUONE plus proguanil combination brand name is Malarone.

Indications: MALARIA prevention, enlarged spleen with SICKLE CELL DISEASE, TROPICAL SPLENOMEGALY, MALARIA prevention, MALARIA treatment, used with ATOVAQUONE.

Contraindications: ALLERGY to the drug. Don't take this with HIV medicines, with ANTACIDs or with FANSIDAR.

Precautions: in some areas MALARIA is resistant to this. If the patient is in very early pregnancy, she should take FOLINIC ACID with this; it is not otherwise contraindicated in pregnancy. If this is taken at the same time as the oral typhoid immunization the immunization might not take effect. Try to avoid this.

Side-effects: occasionally nausea and loss of appetite occur. These decrease with continued usage.

Dosage: 200 mg daily, adult dose, for MALARIA prevention and for the large spleen of SICKLE CELL DISEASE.

MALARIA treatment 400 mg daily for 3 days, together with ATOVAQUONE. There is a combination drug: ARTEMISININ (artesunate) 4 mg/kg plus DAPSONE 2.5 mg/kg plus proguanil 8 mg/kg all daily for 3 days.

PROMETHAZINE

Anti-nausea, sedative

Safety class: 1   Stability: A, dark   Pregnancy: C

Brand name: Phenergan; generic drug is available. Supplied as 25 and 50 mg tablets. Suppositories, 12.5, 25 and 50 mg available (same dosage). Injectable drug is available (same dosage).

Indications: nausea, vomiting, emotional upset from any cause. It is used in many illnesses.

Contraindications: prior ALLERGY to the drug; age under 2 years, possibly GLAUCOMA or ACUTE ABDOMEN. The drug should not be used with other sedatives or in a hot climate. It should not be used in women who are breastfeeding.

Precautions: since the drug is sedative, do not give it to someone who has to drive, work machinery or stay awake. Do not use this drug for PERTUSSIS. The patient should not drink ALCOHOL while taking this. The drug causes sun sensitivity: burning with minimum exposure. Watch for NEUROLEPTIC MALIGNANT SYNDROME.

Side-effects: the most common one is a fall in blood pressure when the patient stands up. Other effects are worsening of GLAUCOMA, constipation, inability to pass urine (especially in older men), susceptibility to HEAT ILLNESS, dry mouth, decrease in sweating, rapid pulse, sensitivity to light, blurred vision. These effects occur in only a small percentage of patients. Long-term use can lead to PARKINSON'S DISEASE.

TOC   SYMPTOMS   DIFFERENTIALS   CONDITIONS   **DRUG INDEX**   REGIONAL NOTES   INX

Dosage: reduce the dose for the elderly.

Adults get 50 mg every 6 hours as needed. This may be increased to 75 or 100 mg if necessary.

Children get 1 mg/kg every 6 hours as needed. The dose is the same by mouth, by suppository or by IM injection.

Alternatives: CHLORPROMAZINE (Largactil), PROCHLORPERAZINE.

PROPRANOLOL

Beta blocker, antihypertensive, anti-migraine

Safety class: 2   Stability: A, dark   Pregnancy: C

Brand name: Inderal. Supplied as 10, 20, 40, 60 and 80 mg tablets. Long-acting forms are available which may be taken only twice daily. Do not use injectable.

Indications: HEART FAILURE, hypertrophic kind; HYPERTENSION; MIGRAINE HEADACHE; sometimes a rapid pulse; a physician might use it for ANGINA but you should not; advanced liver disease due to SCHISTOSOMIASIS MANSONI or SCHISTOSOMIASIS JAPONICUM; possibly other LIVER DISEASE.

Contraindications: ASTHMA, chronic RESPIRATORY INFECTION, other kinds of HEART FAILURE, pulse less than 60, DIABETES. Do not give this at the same time as anti-depressant medication. Do not give it to alcoholics.

Precautions: if HEART FAILURE develops, withdraw the drug. In a patient with heart trouble, the drug must be stopped gradually, not suddenly.

Those of African genetic heritage may be resistant to propranolol; it may not adequately lower blood pressure.

Warn the patient against engaging in hazardous activities while taking this drug, until he discovers how he tolerates it.

Side-effects: nausea, vomiting, diarrhea or constipation. These effects occur in only a small percentage of patients.

Rarely there is insomnia, bad dreams or dizziness. Depression and fatigue are relatively common. There may be decreased sexual functioning.

Dosage: 10–40 mg by mouth every 6–8 hours. Sometimes slow-release forms are available, which can be taken less frequently. In general this must be maintained indefinitely. Seek professional advice for the dosage in SCHISTOSOMIASIS.

PSEUDOEPHEDRINE

Decongestant

Safety class: 1   Stability: A   Pregnancy: B

Brand names: Sudafed, Galpseud. Also comes under a variety of names as an ingredient in cold tablets. It is frequently combined with antihistamines. See DIPHENHYDRAMINE for a description of what antihistamines do. Comes as 30 mg and 60 mg tablets and 120 mg sustained release tablets.

Indications: stuffy nose due to a RESPIRATORY INFECTION.

Contraindications: HYPERTENSION, ANGINA, some kinds of HEART FAILURE. Do not give this at the same time as anti-depressant medication. Check that the patient's blood pressure is not high before giving this.

Precautions: may make the patient shaky; it is a mild stimulant. In rare cases it might cause SEIZURES and an irregular pulse.

Dosage: 30 or 60 mg by mouth every 4 hours as needed. Sustained release tablets are taken as 120 mg every 12 hours. Use this for a maximum of 5 days.

PYRANTEL PAMOATE

Dewormer; anthelmintic

Safety class: 1   Stability: A   Pregnancy: C

Brand names: Antiminth, Combantrin, Felex, Helmex, Imathal, Nemex, Piranver, Pyraminth, Strongit T. Supplied as 125 mg (base) tablets and as a liquid suspension for children, 250 mg base per 5 ml. In the States this is only available as veterinary drug.

Indications: ASCARIASIS, ENTEROBIASIS, HOOKWORM, possibly STRONGYLOIDIASIS. Used for TURISTA, other diarrhea or MALABSORPTION not responsive to other treatments. This is also a good drug for routine deworming.

Contraindications: ALLERGY to the drug. The drug is not absorbed to any extent, and therefore is safe in pregnancy. Do not use this with PIPERAZINE. Do not use it in children less than 2 years old.

Precautions: might cause some abdominal pain. Before using this, at least partially treat DEHYDRATION, ANEMIA, and/or MALNUTRITION if the patient has one or more of these. Do not use this medicine on an extremely ill, nearly dying patient. The drug will increase blood levels of THEOPHYLLIN, possibly causing toxicity.

Side-effects: nausea, vomiting, diarrhea, abdominal pains, headache, dizziness or fever. These effects occur in only a small percentage of patients. If used excessively it can destroy the bone marrow.

Dosage: you may need to decrease the dosage in LIVER DISEASE, ANEMIA, and/or MALNUTRITION. Otherwise start with an initial doses of 1 or 2 mg/kg; then give 11 mg/kg, maximum of 1000 mg, single dose.

Alternatives: ALBENDAZOLE, BEPHENIUM HYDROXYNAPHTHOATE, MEBENDAZOLE, PIPERAZINE.

PYRAZINAMIDE

Anti-tuberculous

Safety class: 2   Stability: C   Pregnancy: C

Supplied as generic 500 mg tablets.

Indications: TUBERCULOSIS; particularly valuable if the patient has TB MENINGITIS or cavities in his lungs (abnormal lung sounds).

Contraindications: LIVER FAILURE, HEPATITIS. Do not give in the presence of GOUT, DIABETES or PORPHYRIA. The drug appears in breast milk, but that is probably harmless, since it is sometimes prescribed for babies.

Side-effects: sore joints, nausea, vomiting, loss of appetite, fatigue, fevers, flushing. This may cause HEPATITIS, especially at higher doses; stop the drug for this. Also it may cause an attack of GOUT in someone predisposed. It tastes terrible.

Overdose and prolonged usage: LIVER FAILURE see Protocol B.7.

Dosage: reduce the dose in KIDNEY DISEASE and in LIVER DISEASE.

Daily Dosage: 30 mg/kg: 4 tablets for a mid-size adult.

Thrice weekly dosage	
6–8 kg	3/4 of a 500 mg tablet
9–15 kg	1.25 of 500 mg tablets
16–21 kg	Two 500 mg tablets
22–28 kg	2.5
29–34 kg	3
35–44 kg	4
> 45 kg	5
Twice weekly dosage	
3–5 kg	1/2 of a 500 mg tablet
6–8 kg	1
9–15 kg	2
16–21 kg	3
22–28 kg	4
29–34 kg	5
35–44 kg	6
> 45 kg	7

PYRIDOXINE

B vitamin; vitamin B_6

Safety class: 1   Stability: A

Indications: Prevention of side-effects of ISONIAZID, (used in the treatment of TUBERCULOSIS). May be used for the vomiting of pregnancy.

Contraindications: none

Dosage: 25 mg a couple times a week is probably more than enough for an adult. Reduce dose according to weight for children, but just to conserve drug. Pyridoxine is non-toxic. For the vomiting of pregnancy use 25 mg three times daily.

Alternatives: most multivitamins don't contain pyridoxine. Sweet bananas contain quite a bit of pyridoxine, as do peanuts and meat.

PYRIMETHAMINE

Antimalarial

Safety class: 1   Stability: B, dark   Pregnancy: C

Brand names: Daraprim, Malocide; combined with sulfadoxine in FANSIDAR. Supplied in tablet form as 25 mg of base per tablet and as a liquid with 7.8 mg per 5 ml (1 teaspoon).

Indications: prevention of MALARIA; used with SULFADIAZINE in the treatment of TOXOPLASMOSIS; used with sulfadoxine (as in FANSIDAR) in the prevention and treatment of MALARIA. It should not be used in some people with ANEMIA.

Contraindications: ALLERGY to the drug. Do not use it with FANSIDAR. Do not give it to patients with PORPHYRIA.

Precautions: best not to use in reproductive women or during early pregnancy for preventing MALARIA if there are other alternatives. Do not use this alone for MALARIA prevention in children; there have been reports of fatal MALARIA in children so treated. If used at all during very early pregnancy, give FOLINIC ACID. Not recommended for malaria prevention by some government agencies because of rare fatalities attributed to it. If there is new-onset ANEMIA stop the drug.

Side-effects: nausea, vomiting, diarrhea, loss of appetite.

Dosage:

MALARIA prevention not recommended: expatriate adults get 50 mg weekly. Expatriate children get 50 mg on entering the area, then 25 mg per week. Nationals get the same dose once a month at first; if this is inadequate protection, increase to every 3 or 2 weeks. It is best to give CHLOROQUINE also with this.

TOXOPLASMOSIS: adults with AIDS: 100–200 mg daily. Adults without AIDS: 25–50 mg three times a day for 2–5 days, then 25–50 mg daily for 3–4 weeks. The children's dose is 2 mg/kg, given according to the same schedule. This must always be given along with SULFADIAZINE or CLINDAMYCIN.

Alternative: CHLOROQUINE in areas where MALARIA is sensitive to that drug.

PYRONARIDINE

Antimalarial, always combined with ARTEMISININ

Safety class: 2   Stability: unknown   Pregnancy: unknown
Supplied as 100 mg tablets.

Brand names: Malaridine, Pyramax

Indications: MALARIA

Contraindications: ALLERGY to the drug, possibly pregnancy.

Side-effects: abdominal pain and nausea, headache, diarrhea, not severe.

Dosage: for adults: day 1: 8mg/kg every 12 hours for 2 doses; Days 2 and 3: 8mg/kg single dose daily.

TOC SYMPTOMS DIFFERENTIALS CONDITIONS **DRUG INDEX** REGIONAL NOTES INX

QUINIDINE

Antimalarial; anti-arrhythmic heart drug.

Safety class: 3   Stability: C   Pregnancy: C[1]

Brand names: Cardioquin, Duraquin, Quinaglute, Quinalan, Quinidex. Generic drug is available. Supplied as injectable and as tablets of various sizes.

Indications: severe MALARIA, when QUININE either is not available or does not work; occasionally for abnormal heart rhythms, when prescribed by a physician.

Contraindications: ALLERGY to this drug, some kinds of heart disease, an irregular pulse. Those with severe G6PD DEFICIENCY should not take this drug.

Precautions: if this is taken at the same time as grapefruit or its juice, the drug may reach toxic levels, causing life-threatening or sight-threatening side-effects.

This is ordinarily a heart medicine. It can cause blindness or sudden death. It interacts badly with many other medications and thus should only be used on a physician's recommendation. In particular, avoid using it with MEFLOQUIN, QUININE, ACETAZOLAMIDE, any other heart medicines, with myasthenia gravis and with any diuretics (water pills).

The drug should not be combined with other drugs that cause abnormal heart rhythms. The medical jargon is that it prolongs the QT interval. See the back cover.

When given IV, it should be used in an intensive care unit, with heart monitoring and sugar water running in IV. Where heart monitoring is not available, it must be used in life-threatening circumstances only, when there is no other alternative. If there are problems obtaining it in the States, help may be obtained from the Eli Lilly Company: 800-821-0538 or from the CDC malaria hotline: 770-488-7788.

If given orally and "gluconate" is the last name, the drug is absorbed slowly. "Sulfate" is a better last name when rapid action is desirable. Other precautions are the same as for QUININE, with the additional provision that you should watch for a drop in blood pressure.

Side-effects: headache, drop in blood pressure, ringing in the ears, nausea, vomiting, diarrhea, abdominal pains.

Dosage: reduce the dose with KIDNEY DISEASE, LIVER FAILURE (see Protocol B.7), HEART FAILURE and in the elderly. Skip the loading dose if the patient has recently taken this or any -quine or related drug.

MALARIA: 8 mg/kg of base orally every 8 hours for 7 days. The dose for quinidine gluconate[2] IV is 10 mg salt/kg to a maximum of 600 mg, loading dose infused slowly over 1–2 hours, followed by 0.02 mg/kg/minute continuously until able to take oral therapy.

QUININE

Antimalarial

Synonym: quinine sulfate.

Safety class: 2 oral, 3 IV   Stability: C

Pregnancy: occasionally causes miscarriage or premature birth, but malaria is more likely to do this.

Brand names: Aristochin, Dentojel, Quinate, Quinsan, Quiphile, others. Generic drug also available. Supplied as 100, 130, 195, 260, 300 and 325 mg tablets and capsules and as injectable. Sometimes quinine is combined with antibiotics. If you use these combinations, pay careful attention to the dose of quinine, since this is more toxic in overdose than the antibiotics with which it is combined.

Indications: severe MALARIA; sometimes muscle cramps at night.

Contraindications: pregnancy if used for muscle cramps; breastfeeding; pre-existing ringing in the ears; a recent, severe illness that resulted in loss of vision; a previous serious reaction to this drug, (ALLERGY or some other reaction). In patients with irregular heart beats, it requires medical supervision.

Do not use this drug with ASPIRIN, nor with aluminum-containing ANTACIDs.

Do not use it in myasthenia gravis patients. (a type of muscle weakness) or in severe G6PD DEFICIENCY.

Do not use the drug in diabetics except with physician supervision.

Precautions: never give quinine IM.[3] Quinine occasionally causes miscarriage but untreated MALARIA is much more likely to cause miscarriage.

The drug causes HYPOGLYCEMIA which can lead to SEIZURES, BRAIN DAMAGE and death. Be sure to give sugar along with the drug. Pregnant women and children are particularly vulnerable to low blood sugar.

Occasionally a patient will develop swelling around his face and neck; stop the drug.

The drug may cause abnormal heart rhythms. Thus this should not be combined with other such drugs. The medical jargon is that it prolongs the QT interval. See the back cover.

Side-effects: occasionally a patient will experience flushing, itching, rash, fever, belly pain, ringing in the ears, decreased vision. Stop the drug if this occurs soon after you start it. Reduce the dose if it happens after a couple of hours, then stop the drug if symptoms do not disappear within 6 hours or if it happens with the next (reduced) dose.

---

1 This rarely causes miscarriage, but malaria is much more likely than the drug to cause miscarriage.

2 In 10 mg of quinidine gluconate there are 8 mg of quinidine base. So the two dosages are the same.

---

3 It must not be injected IM, since it damages the muscle, and it is dangerous used that way. It is absorbed into the blood stream erratically so the patient may get none at first and then get an overdose the next time it is given, killing him or making him blind.

TOC · SYMPTOMS · DIFFERENTIALS · CONDITIONS · DRUG INDEX · REGIONAL NOTES · INX

Stop the drug for loss of vision that lasts more than an hour. Most vision loss is reversible when the drug is stopped, but there may be permanent blindness.

Reduce the dose of the drug if the pulse becomes excessively fast, slow or irregular.

Try to use another antimalarial drug along with this, to discourage the development of resistance.

Overdose: permanent blindness (large pupils).

Prolonged usage: LIVER FAILURE (see Protocol B.7).

Dosage: reduce the dose with KIDNEY DISEASE or with LIVER FAILURE.

Doses are given orally; use a stomach tube if the patient cannot swallow or is unconscious; see Volume 1, Appendix 1. The drug can be given rectally. The rectal dose is 1.5 times the oral dose if the liquid injectable form is used.

Skip the loading dose if the patient has recently taken QUINIDINE or any –quine drug, including MEFLOQUINE.

MALARIA, severe: initially 20 mg/kg for first (loading) dose only, given IV over 4 hours; thereafter 10 mg/kg IV or orally every 8 hours for 7–14 days for adults. Change from IV to oral medicines when the patient can swallow. Children's dose is 10 mg/kg every 8 hours. Quinimax is a liquid mixture of quinine-like drugs. It may be given IV at 8 mg/kg every 8 hours. It may also be given by rectum (enema) at 20 mg/kg initially followed by 15 mg/kg every 8 hours for a total of 3 days.

MALARIA responds well to AZITHROMYCIN plus quinine, both every 8 hours for 3 days.

Leg cramps: 200–300 mg at night before retiring.

Alternatives: CHLOROQUINE used together with CHLORPHENIRAMINE in the Eastern Hemisphere. Totoquine is a cheap mixture of quinine and related compounds. It is used exactly the same as quinine, same doses, same precautions. QUINIDINE can likewise be used; see previous entry. It works better than quinine in some areas of the world.

QUINOLONES

This is a class of antibiotics; CIPROFLOXACIN, NORFLOXACIN, OFLOXACIN and PEFLOXACIN are examples. They are useful for infections that do not respond to other antibiotics, such as CHANCROID, KIDNEY INFECTION, PNEUMONIA, TYPHOID FEVER, bacterial DYSENTERY, BRUCELLOSIS and SPOTTED FEVER. The last two drugs have been found to successfully treat LEPROSY. Other antibiotics in this class all end in "-oxacin". These drugs may (rarely) cause dizziness, confusion, hallucinations, seizures and sensory changes. These may damage cartilage in growing children. Elderly patients may develop tendinitis or tendon rupture due to these drugs. CIPROFLOXACIN 500 mg is roughly equivalent to NORFLOXACIN 400 mg or OFLOXACIN 300 mg. Resistance to one drug in this group does not necessarily imply resistance to the other drugs.

RANITIDINE

Histamine receptor antagonist

Safety class: 2   Stability: A   Pregnancy: B

Brand name: Zantac.

Indications: GASTRITIS, PEPTIC ULCER, ANAPHYLAXIS.

Contraindications: prior ALLERGY to this drug.

Precautions: stomach acid serves a useful function to kill bacteria taken in by mouth. When acid is neutralized or eliminated by antacids or drugs like this one, it leaves the patient vulnerable. Hence special attention should be paid to food sanitation. Patients become vulnerable to TUBERCULOSIS. There is an increased risk of PNEUMONIA.

This drug interacts badly with quite a number of other drugs, especially KETOCONAZOLE.

If the pulse increases or decreases, then stop the drug

Avoid using this in patients with PORPHYRIA.

Dosage: reduce the dose to ½ of that prescribed in the presence of KIDNEY DISEASE. Reduce the dose somewhat with LIVER FAILURE. Reduce dose according to weight for children.

ANAPHYLAXIS: 500 mg IV, IM or orally every 6 hours for 3 days.

Other indications: adults: 150 mg twice daily or 300 mg at night only.

RIBAVIRIN

Antiviral

Safety class: 3   Pregnancy: X[1]

Stability: C dry. Liquid, use within 24 hrs.

Brand names: Tibavirin, Virazole, Ribasphere.

Indications: some ARBOVIRAL FEVER, some HEPATITIS, LASSA FEVER, any HEMORRHAGIC FEVER caused by a virus except it is not used for EBOLA VIRUS DISEASE.

Contraindications: ALLERGY to the drug, patient taking DIGOXIN currently, pregnancy. This drug causes harm to the fetus in all animals tested. However, if the mother and child will both die anyway if the drug is not given (for example, severe LASSA FEVER) it may be worthwhile to use it. It is contraindicated in males who may impregnate their partners. Pregnancy must be avoided for 6 months. It must not be used with HIV medicines or in patients less than 3 years old.

Precautions: may cause ANEMIA, usually slight; may cause a headache or aggravate shortness of breath in someone with RESPIRATORY INFECTION.

Dosage: adult dose is 30 mg/kg up to a maximum of 2000 mg by mouth initially followed by 16 mg/kg up to 1000 mg maximum every 6 hours for 4 days. Follow this with 8 mg/kg every 8 hours for 6 days. In very ill patients, use 2000 mg IV initially, then 1000 mg IV or orally every 8 hours for 4 days.

---

1 Not only is it contraindicated for pregnant women, but pregnant medical staff should not handle the drug, nor should a pregnant woman be in the room where it is used.

TOC   SYMPTOMS   DIFFERENTIALS   CONDITIONS   **DRUG INDEX**   REGIONAL NOTES   INX

TOC

SYMPTOMS

DIFFERENTIALS

CONDITIONS

DRUG INDEX

REGIONAL NOTES

INX

RIFABUTIN

Pregnancy: B

Brand name: Mycobutin.

This is an antibiotic/anti-tuberculous medication, related to RIFAMPIN, same indications, contraindications and precautions with one exception. This may be used in patients who are taking anti-HIV drugs. There is cross-allergy with RIFAMPIN in causing allergic rashes. There are no other cross-allergies. The usual dosage is about half that of RIFAMPIN, and consequently the adverse side-effects are much less common and less severe. In some cases it will work for TB that is resistant to RIFAMPIN. Like RIFAMPIN, it should not be used by non-professionals in patients who are under treatment for HIV INFECTION.

RIFAMIXIN

Brand name: Xifaxin

This is an antibiotic that is not absorbed from the bowel into the blood stream. It is used for bacterial infections of the bowel, in particular for TURISTA (traveler's diarrhea). The usual dose is 200 mg three times daily. Seek independent information before using this.

RIFAMPIN

Antibiotic, anti-tuberculous

Safety class: 1   Stability: C, dark   Pregnancy: C

Synonym: rifampicin

Brand names: Rifadin, Rifobac, Rimactane. Supplied as 150 and 300 mg tablets or capsules.

Indications: ABSCESS, ANTHRAX, BARTONELLOSIS, BRUCELLOSIS, BURULI ULCER, FILARIASIS, LEPROSY, MENINGITIS prevention, some MYCETOMA, OSTEOMYELITIS, PYOMYOSITIS, Q FEVER, some SPOTTED FEVER, TRENCH FEVER, TUBERCULOSIS, itching due to JAUNDICE.

Contraindications: ALLERGY to the drug; HEPATITIS, but an M.D. may overrule this, ALCOHOLISM. Current usage of drugs for HIV INFECTION.

Precautions: oral contraceptives may not work well when a patient is on this. You may need to increase the dose of some other drugs which the body eliminates more rapidly in patients taking rifampin. The drug appears in breast milk but this is probably harmless because it is, at times, prescribed for infants. Since it is expensive it is frequently counterfeit. It is the drug itself that is an orange/brown color. You can tell the difference between good and counterfeit drug by the intensity of the color.

Side-effects: this turns urine, sweat, breast milk and tears orange. If the urine is not orange, the person has not taken it, or he has taken counterfeit drug. It will turn soft contact lenses orange.

Other effects are abdominal pains, nausea, vomiting, diarrhea, fatigue, headache, itchiness, dizziness and drunken behavior. ALLERGY may also occur. These effects occur in only a small percentage of patients. They can be managed by giving the medication last thing at night.

An unusual but not serious side-effect of intermittent treatment is a feeling of having the "flu": fever, chills, headache, aching bones.

Rare, serious side-effects are RESPIRATORY FAILURE, abnormal bleeding, sudden-onset ANEMIA, HEPATITIS, LIVER FAILURE (see Protocol B.7) or KIDNEY DISEASE. The drug must be stopped for any of these. Sometimes it may be started again after the liver is back to normal.

Dosage: this drug, when used for TB, must be given with other drugs, because resistance develops rapidly.

All doses are adult and oral unless stated otherwise. Reduce the dose according to weight for children. The drug should be taken on an empty stomach. Reduce the dose with any LIVER DISEASE.

ANTHRAX: 300 mg IV every 12 hours

BARTONELLOSIS: 600 mg daily for 14 days; used in the Verruga phase of the disease.

BRUCELLOSIS: 900 mg each morning for 21 days; used with DOXYCYCLINE.

BURULI ULCER: 10 mg/kg daily for 8 weeks, given along with STREPTOMYCIN.

FILARIASIS: this is used as an alternative to DOXYCYCLINE for children. Recommended dose is unknown.

Itching due to JAUNDICE: 10 mg/kg/day

LEPROSY: 600 mg once a month on an empty stomach, to be taken with other medicines. This may be given as the only drug if there is one skin spot only. For PB leprosy, take 600 mg daily along with OFLOXACIN, both for one month.

MENINGITIS prevention: 600 mg daily for 3 days.

MYCETOMA: seek advice from an M.D.

OSTEOMYELITIS: 600 mg daily for 6 weeks.

PYOMYOSITIS: 600–900 mg daily for 6 weeks.

Q FEVER: 600 mg daily for 15 days.

SPOTTED FEVER: 600 mg daily x 7–14 days, shorter if not so ill, 14 days if very ill.

TRENCH FEVER: 600 mg daily for 6 weeks.

TUBERCULOSIS: see the chart on the next page

Alternatives: ISONIAZID, ETHAMBUTOL, STREPTOMYCIN, RIFABUTIN, PAS for TUBERCULOSIS.

Daily dosage	
4–7 kg	1/4 of a 300 mg tablet
7–15 kg	1/2
16–30 kg	1
31–44 lg	1.5
>45 kg	2
Twice or thrice weekly dosage	
4–7 kg	1/4 of a 300 mg tablet
7–15 kg	3/4
16–30 kg	1.25
31–44 kg	2
45-55 kg	2.5
> 55 kg	3

RIFAPENTINE

Pregnancy: C

This is a drug related to RIFAMPIN but longer-lasting. It should not be used in patients with lung cavities on chest x-ray. It is not approved for use in non-lung TB. It should not be used in children, in breastfeeding women or in HIV-positive patients. It discolors body fluids, contact lenses and dentures, just like RIFAMPIN.

The usual adult dose is 600 mg once or twice weekly. It is usually active against all the same organisms as RIFAMPIN. It should be taken with fatty food. It should not be taken with ANTACIDs. You may need to reduce the dose or stop the drug in the presence of LIVER DISEASE. Other precautions, side-effects, etc. are like RIFAMPIN.

RITONAVIR

This is an anti-HIV drug.

SAQUINAVIR

This is an anti-HIV drug.

SECNIDAZOLE

Available in Central and South America.

A drug similar to METRONIDAZOLE and TINIDAZOLE but not yet approved for humans. Reportedly 1500 mg daily for 5 days cures AMEBIASIS. The dose for amebic DYSENTERY is a single dose of 2000 mg or two doses of 1000 mg each, 4 hours apart. The dose for GIARDIASIS is 30 mg/kg in one single dose. The dose for PELVIC INFECTION is 2 grams, single dose.

SILVER SULFADIAZINE

Antibacterial, burn ointment.

Pregnancy: B

Brand names: Silvadene, Flamazine.

This is an antibacterial skin cream that is used especially for burns. It is contraindicated in LIVER FAILURE, KIDNEY DISEASE, pregnancy, breast feeding mothers, newborns, people with PORPHYRIA and patients with ALLERGY to SULFA drugs. It interacts badly with many other drugs. EXFOLIATIVE DERMATITIS, HEPATITIS or a newly developing ANEMIA are reasons to stop the drug. It should be applied sparingly, daily, after washing.

SITAMAQUINE

Anti-Leishmania

Safety class: unknown   Stability: unknown
Pregnancy: unknown

Indications: CUTANEOUS LEISHMANIASIS and VISCERAL LEISHMANIASIS

Contraindications: probably KIDNEY DISEASE.

Side-effects: abdominal pain and headache.

Precautions: it occasionally causes KIDNEY DISEASE. It should be combined with MILTEFOSINE or STIBOGLUCONATE.

Dosage: 2–3 mg/kg daily x 28 days. It does not matter if the patient eats food with this.

SPECTINOMYCIN

Antibiotic, aminoglycoside, Gram-negative

Safety class: 2   Pregnancy: unknown

Stability: dry C, use liquid within 24 hours.

Brand names: Nebcin, Tobricin.

Indications: GONORRHEA; PELVIC INFECTION in those with an ALLERGY to PENICILLIN or when penicillin-type drugs do not work; URETHRITIS. It is not a reliable treatment for CHANCROID, but it may work.

Contraindications: ALLERGY to this drug or any related drug, such as GENTAMYCIN; KIDNEY DISEASE, probably pregnancy. Do not use this in the presence of CIRRHOSIS or LIVER FAILURE.

Precautions: be careful not to exceed the recommended dosage; the drug may cause KIDNEY DISEASE, deafness or both; it occasionally causes this even at recommended doses. Safety in pregnancy is unknown. If you use this, be sure to check the patient in a week or two.

Dosage: adult dose is 2000 mg (2 grams) IM in a single dose except for GONORRHEA which has spread to become a whole-body infection. In that case the dose is 2 grams IM twice daily for 7 days.

TOC   SYMPTOMS   DIFFERENTIALS   CONDITIONS   **DRUG INDEX**   REGIONAL NOTES   INX

SPIRAMYCIN

Anti-toxoplasmosis drug

Brand name: Rovamycine

Safety class: 2   Stability: A
Pregnancy: reportedly okay, the drug of choice

This is not available in the USA; it is available in Europe, the Mediterranean/Middle East and parts of Asia.

Indication: TOXOPLASMOSIS

Contraindication: ALLERGY to this drug

Precautions: take on an empty stomach; stop for abnormal bruising or for LIVER DISEASE.

Side-effects: vomiting, diarrhea, abdominal pain.

Dosage: 1000 mg three times daily for 3 weeks, then discontinue for 2 weeks, then give for another 3 weeks. Continue these 5-week cycles throughout pregnancy.

STEROID

A class of drugs, of which PREDNISONE, HYDROCORTISONE and DEXAMETHASONE are the most common. These drugs reduce inflammation and decrease immunity. They are commonly abused, because they make people feel better fast. However, they also make one more susceptible to infection, cause weight gain, brittle bones and DIABETES. They will cause latent TB to become active (although they are useful for treating some types of TB). They tend to make CHAGA'S DISEASE worse. If someone takes them for more than a week and then stops abruptly, he can develop SHOCK and die. They should not be used in patients with PORPHYRIA. Equivalent doses are 20 mg HYDROCORTISONE, 5 mg PREDNISONE or PREDNISOLONE and 0.75 mg of DEXAMETHASONE.

STIBOGLUCONATE

Antimony compound, anti-Leishmaniasis

Safety class: 3   Stability: unknown

Synonym: pentavalent antimony

Brand names: Pentostam, Glucantime. Supplied as injectable drug; no oral form available. Two forms of the drugs are sodium stibogluconate and meglumine antimoniate—comparable to each other, different geographic availability; neither works well in India.

Indications: CUTANEOUS LEISHMANIASIS, PKDL, VISCERAL LEISHMANIASIS.

Contraindications: breast-feeding mothers, ALLERGY to the drug, KIDNEY DISEASE, pregnancy.

Side-effects: fever, fatigue, diarrhea, ACUTE ABDOMEN, PANCREATITIS, HEPATITIS, nausea, pains. If these occur, stop the drug and do not restart it. Pain may occur at the injection site. It may cause stiff joints.

Precautions: do not give to obese patients without independent advice. The drug prolongs the QT interval of the heart and thus should not be given along with other drugs which bear the same warning. See the back cover. IV drug should not be used by the inexperienced.

Dosage:

This varies from one region to another; follow local advice if it is available. Otherwise:

CUTANEOUS LEISHMANIASIS: Pentostam 20 mg/kg IM daily for 20–28 consecutive days. If this is used with PAROMOMYCIN cream, then just a week might be enough.[1]

PKDL: 20 mg/kg daily until healed; most are healed in 120 days but it may take up to 200 days.

VISCERAL LEISHMANIASIS: 20mg/kg/day for 20–28 days. The spleen size shrinks rapidly, over the first few days, but the drug needs to be given for the entire time.

STREPTOMYCIN

Antibiotic (Gram-negative), aminoglycoside, anti-tuberculous

Safety class: 2   Pregnancy: D
Stability: dry: A; wet & warm 2 days; wet & cold: 4 weeks.

Supplied as generic drug. Veterinary drug is available. This drug is injectable only, never oral.

Indications: BARTONELLOSIS, BRUCELLOSIS, BURULI ULCER, DONOVANOSIS, some MYCETOMA, PLAGUE, RAT BITE FEVER, TUBERCULOSIS, TULAREMIA, sometimes other infections.

Contraindications: ALLERGY to the drug, HEART FAILURE, protein in urine unless an M.D. overrules this, pregnancy unless the problem is life-threatening and there are no other options. Don't use this along with other drugs that are toxic to the kidneys; don't use it in KIDNEY DISEASE. Don't use it with any muscle weakness or in patients who are hard of hearing. Don't use this in the presence of CIRRHOSIS or LIVER FAILURE.

Precautions: this drug may cause deafness or fever and rash. Be careful not to overdose. Check hearing every couple of days; stop the drug if hearing difficulty or fever and rash develop.

If the person begins to be dizzy, stop the drug immediately. Warn him not to engage in hazardous activities when he is taking this.

Do not give it to a patient suffering from DEHYDRATION.

It may on occasion cause SEIZURES or MENTAL ILLNESS.

Side-effects: the site of the IM injection may become excessively painful.

Overdose and prolonged use: KIDNEY DISEASE, deafness.

---

1   *Don't cut the course short if your patient has one of the forms that might later develop MCL—the form that affects the pink, moist areas of the body, and/or the outer ear. This form is mainly in the Americas.*

Dosage: the following doses for those over 50 kg must be reduced according to weight for small adults and children. Reduce the dose to 750 mg for those over 50 years old.

BARTONELLOSIS: 1000 mg (1 gm) IM daily for 5 days.

BRUCELLOSIS: 1000 mg (1 gm) IM daily, used with other medications, for at least the first 2 weeks of the 6-week treatment.

BURULI ULCER: 1000 mg IM daily, along with RIFAMPIN.

DONOVANOSIS: 1000 mg (1 gm) IM daily until totally healed plus another week, used with DOXYCYCLINE.

MYCETOMA: 1000 mg (1 gm) IM daily for 30 days, then on alternate days until healed. Use this with CO-TRIMOXAZOLE or DAPSONE.

PLAGUE: 1000 mg IV or IM twice daily until improved. Then give it daily for 7 more days.

RAT BITE FEVER: 1000 mg (1 gm) IM daily for 14 days.

TUBERCULOSIS daily dosage:

Under 50 years old/over 50 kg: 1000 mg IM

Under 50 kg: 750 mg IM

Over 50 years old: 750 mg IM

Children's dose: 20 mg/kg IM to a maximum of 1000 mg

TULAREMIA: same dose as PLAGUE; continue this for 14 days.

Other infections: 1000 mg (1 gm) IM daily until entirely better plus 2 more days.

Alternatives: other antibiotics.

SULFA

Sulfa drugs, antibiotic, Gram-negative.

Safety class: 2   Stability: A, dark   Pregnancy: C

Specific names included in this: sulfadiazine, sulfisoxazole, sulfamethoxazole, triple sulfa. Use this description for any of the sulfa drugs above. Do not use for sulfapyridine and sulfacytine. Sulfatrim is the same as CO-TRIMOXAZOLE.

Brand names: too many to list. Generic human and veterinary drug is available. Supplied as 500 mg tablets; also supplied as liquid.

Indications: ABSCESS, CHOLERA, ordinary diarrhea, middle EAR INFECTION, EPIDIDYMITIS, KIDNEY INFECTION, RESPIRATORY INFECTION, TOXOPLASMOSIS, TRACHOMA, TURISTA, URETHRITIS, URINARY INFECTION, VAGINITIS. Sulfadiazine ophthalmic ointment may be useful for KERATITIS due to a fungus. See ANTIBIOTIC EYE OINTMENT.

Contraindications: do not give to pregnant women about to deliver (first 8 months are okay), to nursing mothers or to babies under 2 months of age or ill or premature. Do not give any sulfa drug to anyone who has had a previous allergy to any sulfa drug. It is not to be used with G6PD DEFICIENCY or with PORPHYRIA (a hereditary disease). It interacts badly with quite a few other drugs and thus its usage should be supervised.

Precautions: the patient must drink much water, 2–3 liters a day; he must not become or remain dehydrated (see DEHYDRATION) while on this drug.

The drug makes fair skin sensitive to sunburn. It occasionally causes nausea and vomiting. If a red rash resembling a burn or skin peeling develops while the patient is on the drug, stop the drug immediately (see EXFOLIATIVE DERMATITIS).

Stop the drug if the patient develops a new HEPATITIS or ANEMIA.

Side-effects: loss of appetite, nausea, vomiting. These effects are less when the drug is taken with food.

Overdose or prolonged usage: HEPATITIS, LIVER FAILURE.

Dosage: the following are adult doses; reduce dose according to weight for children. Reduce the dose in the presence of KIDNEY DISEASE.

KIDNEY INFECTION: 1000 mg (1 gram) every 6 hours for 5 days

TRACHOMA: 1000 mg (1 gram) every 6 hours for 21 days.

TOXOPLASMOSIS: 1000 mg (1 gram) every 6 hours for 4 weeks; use sulfadiazine, not the other forms.

URINARY INFECTION: same as KIDNEY INFECTION.

Everything else: 1000 mg (1 gm) every 6 hours until the patient recovers and then for 2 more days.

Alternatives: AMPICILLIN, CHLORAMPHENICOL, TETRACYCLINE, STREPTOMYCIN, CO-TRIMOXAZOLE. For CHANCROID use ERYTHROMYCIN.

SULFUR

Elemental sulfur

This is different from the drug SULFA. It is a yellowish powder, one of the chemical elements. It is useful as a body insecticide when mixed into petroleum jelly (Vaseline): 30 grams per 500 gm of petroleum jelly. It is particularly useful for SCABIES. The UK has taken it off the market.

SURAMIN

Safety class: 3   Stability: unknown   Pregnancy: unknown

Supplied as 1-gram vials of powder, add water for injection.

Brand names: Metaret, Germanin, is available in South Africa.

Indications: AFRICAN SLEEPING SICKNESS in the early stages.

Contraindication: ALLERGY to this drug in response to the initial test dose; allergy with prior use.

Precaution: this does not work if the organism has already entered the brain.

Side-effects: painful palms or soles, sharp-shooting pains, may cause KIDNEY DISEASE or LIVER FAILURE (see Protocol B.7) or loss of vision.

Dosage: first give a 100–200 mg test dose to check for ALLERGY. Then, if there is no allergic reaction, give 1000 mg IV on days 1,3,7,14,and 21 for adults. For children the schedule is the same, using 20 mg/kg.

TOC

SYMPTOMS

DIFFERENTIALS

CONDITIONS

DRUG INDEX

REGIONAL NOTES

INX

TAFENOQUINE

This is a drug for both malaria and VISCERAL LEISHMANIASIS. It may also be useful for CHAGA'S DISEASE. It may work for VISCERAL LEISHMANIASIS that is resistant to other drugs. Reportedly the dose for VL in animals is 1.2 to 3.5 mg/kg for 5 days.

The usual adult dose in malaria is 200 mg base per day for 3 days, then 200 mg base weekly for 8 weeks. It has been tested mostly for non-falciparum malaria but might also be useful for falciparum. One study has shown that it is both safe and effective to use as a malaria preventive.

TETANUS IMMUNE GLOBULIN

Synonym: TIG

This is an injectable blood product used to protect against TETANUS in an unimmunized patient with a wound or to treat for the disease.

TETRACHLOROETHYLENE

Dewormer; anthelmintic

Safety class: 2   Stability: D   Pregnancy: B

Brand names: Didakene, Miranon, Nema, Terit, Tetracap. The drug is a liquid. It is supplied as 3 ml of drug in 45 ml of flavored water, also supplied as 1 ml capsules.

Indications: HOOKWORM, INTESTINAL FLUKE.

Contraindications: ALLERGY to the drug, constipation or JAUNDICE. Do not give in the presence of ASCARIASIS or if ASCARIASIS is present in your area, unless you kill the ASCARIS first; otherwise this drug might cause ACUTE ABDOMEN, Type 3. Do not give this to patients with severe MALNUTRITION, severe ANEMIA or those who are very ill.

Do not use this in the presence of obvious LIVER DISEASE, LIVER FAILURE, or HEART FAILURE. Do not use this at the same time as or right after the patient has taken medication that causes a rapid pulse.

Precautions: this may cause burning pain, nausea, vomiting and drunken behavior. There is no harm in this; you should anticipate it. Avoid ALCOHOL and fatty food for one day before and for 3 days after the treatment. The patient may eat 4 hours after the treatment.

Dosage: after a light meal the previous evening, in the morning give the drug 0.12 ml/kg by mouth to a maximum of 5 ml. or according to the following table:

Repeat every 4 hours for 3 or 4 doses. If treating for INTESTINAL FLUKE, it is essential to purge 4–5 hours later; give MILK OF MAGNESIA, castor oil, papaya seeds or anything else that causes diarrhea.

Alternatives: ALBENDAZOLE, BEPHENIUM HYDROXYNAPHTHOATE, MEBENDAZOLE, PYRANTEL PAMOATE

Table of tetrachloroethylene dosages

Kg	3 ml in 45 ml	1 ml capsule
8	no	1 capsule
16	no	2
24	1 unit	3
32	1 unit + 1 capsule	4
40	1.7 units or 1 unit + 2 capsules	5
48	2 units	5
56	2 units	5

TETRACYCLINE

Antibiotic, Gram-negative

Safety class: 1   Stability: B   Pregnancy: D

This is an old drug which has been almost entirely replaced with DOXYCYCLINE.

Related drugs: oxytetracycline (Terramycin), Chlortetracycline (Aureomycin), MINOCYCLINE.

Brand names: Achromycin, Ambramycin, Partrex, Quartex, Sumycin, Tetracyn, Totomycin, Unimycin, Upcyclin, many others. Veterinary drug is available. Supplied as 250 and 500 mg capsules. The drug is a gold color. Brown drug is bad drug. Oxytetracycline is used interchangeably with plain tetracycline.

Indications: same as DOXYCYCLINE.

Contraindications: ALLERGY to the drug, outdated or brown-colored drug, CHAGA'S DISEASE, PORPHYRIA (a hereditary disease). It is contraindicated in KIDNEY DISEASE, but then DOXYCYCLINE may be used.

Precautions: pay special attention to expiration dates; using outdated drug is dangerous. This drug will stain children's teeth permanently when given to pregnant or nursing mothers, or children under 7 y.o. If the patient consumes milk, milk products or ANTACID with the drug, the drug will not work. It will be just like not taking that dose. Occasionally this drug will cause abdominal distress. It may also cause a black, fuzzy tongue (no problem) and may give a false positive or false negative test for sugar in the urine. Fair skin becomes susceptible to sunburn.

If the patient develops a DYSENTERY-type diarrhea while on the drug, stop it immediately.

With BRUCELLOSIS, RELAPSING FEVER, LEPTOSPIROSIS and SYPHILIS the patient may become much sicker for a few hours after the first dose before starting to improve. Do not withdraw the drug for this.

Birth control pills might not work with this drug.

Dosage: reduce the dose in KIDNEY DISEASE. See DOXYCYCLINE and calculate comparable doses. Dosage equivalents with DOXYCYCLINE:

DOXYCYLINE 100 mg daily = Tetracycline 250 mg four times a day.

DOXYCYCLINE 100 mg twice daily = TETRACYLINE 500 mg four times a day.

THEOPHYLLINE

Bronchodilator

Safety class: 2–3   Stability: A, dark   Pregnancy: C

Related drug: aminophylline,[1] aminophyline (British).

Brand names: Accurbron, Quibron, Theo-Dur, Theolair, Nuelin, Lasma. Supplied in many sizes, frequently 200 or 300 mg per tablet and 100 mg per 5 ml (1 teaspoon) liquid. Other sizes may be available. Generic drug is available.

Indications: shortness of breath when it is harder to breathe out than breathe in; prolonged expiration with wheezing from any cause, usually ASTHMA; sometimes ALTITUDE SICKNESS, HAPE; HEART FAILURE; RESPIRATORY INFECTION; SMOKE INHALATION; TUBERCULOSIS. Sometimes it is used for ATTENTION DEFICIT DISORDER, but that is not an approved usage.

Contraindications: previous bad experience with this medication, some kinds of heart disease, HYPERTENSION, prostrate problems. Do not give this with LIVER DISEASE or THYROID TROUBLE of the high-thyroid sort. This interacts badly with many other drugs, so you should seek confirmation of its use if the patient is on anything else.

Precautions: this drug has a narrow margin of safety; the minimally effective dose is not much less than the toxic dose. A mild overdose will cause nausea and vomiting. Reduce the dose if this happens, even if the patient is taking a low dose for his size.

The drug may cause an irregular heart rate causing the patient to complain of palpitations. Frequently patients become nervous when taking the drug. They may have to urinate a lot.

The drug makes people sensitive to the stimulant effect of caffeine, causing insomnia.

This should not be used in persons with a family history of PORPHYRIA.

The drug interferes with laboratory determinations of uric acid. Other drugs interfere with laboratory determinations of the theophyllin level.

Overdose: this is very toxic in overdose; it is a potent agent for suicide.

Dosage: decrease the dose for the elderly. Increase the dose in those taking PHENOBARBITAL and in smokers. Do not crush the long-acting forms or they will not be long-acting; the patient may overdose. The usual dose is 200–300 mg every 8 hours for adults. Children: 5 mg/kg every 8 hours. Long-acting theophylline is used in the same dose every 12 hours. Response: 45 minutes.

Alternatives: ALBUTEROL, METAPROTERENOL. For severe ASTHMA, use EPINEPHRINE; you may use both EPINEPHRINE and theophylline in full doses.

THIABENDAZOLE

Dewormer, anthelmintic

Safety class: 1   Stability: A   Pregnancy: C

Brand names: Bovizole, Coglazol, Equizole, Helmintazole, Hyozole, Mintezol, Nemapan, Omnizole, Polival, Soldrin, TBZ, Thibenzole. Veterinary generic drug is available. Supplied as 500 mg chewable tablets and 100 mg/ml liquid.

Indications: ASCARIASIS, CAPILLARIASIS, ENTEROBIASIS, GUINEA WORM, KERATITIS due to a fungus, STRONGYLOIDIASIS. It may work for some LARVA MIGRANS of the skin type. Not useful for TRICHURIASIS.

Contraindications: ALLERGY to the drug, LIVER FAILURE, KIDNEY DISEASE. Do not give this together with THEOPHYLLINE.

Precautions: discontinue this drug if the patient develops a rash while he is on it.

Side-effects: nausea, vomiting, diarrhea, loss of appetite, dizziness, headache, ringing in the ears and stinky urine. Occasionally causes itching. These effects may occur in up to half of the patients. A less frequent side-effect is a new mental disorder.

Dosage: 25 mg/kg by mouth every 12 hours to a maximum of 1500 mg per dose.

ASCARIASIS: 2 days.

CAPILLARIASIS: seek local advice.

ENTEROBIASIS: 1 day.

GUINEA WORM: 3 days.

KERATITIS due to fungus: half the dose above, given until the problem is completely cleared plus another 3 days.

STRONGYLOIDIASIS: 3 days or same dose by rectum for 14 days.

LARVA MIGRANS: make a cream, mixing 1500 mg of the drug in 15 ml (1 tablespoon) of any skin cream. Apply to the area every 4 hours and leave on until the problem is resolved.

Alternatives: for STRONGYLOIDIASIS, try IVERMECTIN. For other worms, try MEBENDAZOLE or ALBENDAZOLE.

---

1 *Aminophillin might be either oral or injectable. Theophyllin is always oral. The dose is the same.*

THIACETAZONE

Anti-tuberculous

Note that this is not readily available as it has been taken off the market in many places, because of safety issues.

Safety class: 3   Stability: A

Brand name: Thiazina if combined with ISONIAZID.

Indications: TUBERCULOSIS.

Contraindications: East Asian genetic heritage; possibly European genetic heritage; previous ALLERGY or any bad reaction to this drug; currently ill with HIV INFECTION; possibly HIV-positive but not currently ill.

Side-effects: nausea, vomiting, rash, fever, skin color changes, itching, skin peeling off (see EXFOLIATIVE DERMATITIS). Stop the drug for skin redness or peeling! This may also cause bone marrow problems like CHLORAMPHENICOL. The drug must be given daily, not less often. It may cause LIVER DISEASE (see Protocol B.7).

Dosage: usually this is combined with ISONIAZID in the proper proportions; in this case, just give the proper tablet dosage of ISONIAZID and the dosage of thiacetazone will automatically be correct. The table below is for thiacetazone alone.

Daily thiacetazone

Kg body weight	Dosage
< 6 kg	1/2 of a 50 mg tablet
6–12 kg	One 50 mg tablet
13–29 kg	1/2 of a 150 mg tablet
30–50 kg	One 150 mg tablet

THIAMINE

B vitamin; vitamin B_1

Safety class: 1   Stability: A, dark

Brand names: Albafort, Benerva; generic available.

Indications: BERIBERI, burning pains in hands and/or feet.

Contraindications: ALLERGY to the drug.

Dosage: by mouth or IM injection: 200 mg initially, then 100 mg every 8 hours until all symptoms are gone; then give weekly. Improvement within a day; healing slow thereafter.

THIAMPHENICOL

This is a form of CHLORAMPHENICOL which works particularly well for GONORRHEA and some MENINGITIS. It works, but not as well, for the other diseases that CHLORAMPHENICOL is used for. See CHLORAMPHENICOL for specifics.

TIABENDAZOLE

See THIABENDAZOLE, above.

TINIDAZOLE

Antimicrobial, anti-protozoa

Safety class: 1   Stability: C   Pregnancy: C[1]

Brand names: Fasigyn, Pletil, Simplotan, Sorquetan, Tricolam. Supplied as 500 mg tablets.

Indications: ACUTE ABDOMEN, AMEBIASIS, amebic DYSENTERY, GIARDIASIS, PELVIC INFECTION, PEPTIC ULCER, PNEUMONIA, TROPICAL ULCER, VAGINITIS.

Sometimes TURISTA, gas, GUINEA WORM, MALABSORPTION, with other drugs in SEPSIS, TETANUS, for wounds with foul-smelling pus. It may be used for tooth infections in third molars.

Contraindications: ALLERGY to the drug, breastfeeding.

Precautions: the patient must not drink alcohol nor allow any alcohol on his skin while taking the drug or for 3 days afterward. Almost all liquid and cream-type medicines have alcohol in them. Culinary products such as vanilla extract contain alcohol. Most sprays contain alcohol.

Avoid using tinidazole during the first 3 months of pregnancy, except for life-threatening illness.

Side-effects: nausea, vomiting, abdominal pain, sleepiness, headache, dark urine. These effects occur in only a small percentage of patients.

Dosage: the drug is absorbed well rectally; give it this way if your patient is vomiting; the adult dose by rectum is 1000 mg every 8 hours; reduce the dose according to weight for children.

The following are adult doses by mouth unless stated otherwise; reduce dose according to weight for children.

ACUTE ABDOMEN: 1000 mg three times a day for 5 days, given by rectum, not orally.

AMEBIASIS: 2 g daily until cured plus 7 days for liver; intestinal 2 g daily x 3 days

DYSENTERY: 750 mg three times a day for 3 days or else 2000 mg, single dose, followed by another (same) dose a week later.

Gas: same as TURISTA.

GIARDIASIS: 2000 mg, single dose.

GUINEA WORM: 400–500 mg three times a day for 5 days.

MALABSORPTION: same as TURISTA.

PELVIC INFECTION: 500 mg every 8 hours for 10 days.

PEPTIC ULCER: 500 mg every 8 hours for 14 days, with other medication listed.

PNEUMONIA: same as ACUTE ABDOMEN.

SEPSIS: same as ACUTE ABDOMEN.

TETANUS: 500 mg orally every 6 hours or 1000 mg by rectum every 8 hours, for 10 days.

TROPICAL ULCER: 250 mg three times a day until healed.

---

1 METRONIDAZOLE which is used for mostly the same purposes is pregnancy category B and thus preferable to use in pregnant patients.

TURISTA: 250 mg three times a day for 3 days.

VAGINITIS: bacterial: 500 mg three times a day for 7 days;
Trichomonas: 2000 mg, one dose; if this doesn't work, then
2000 mg daily for 5 days. Treat both partners in all cases.

Wounds with foul-smelling pus: 500 mg three times a day
until healed plus another 2 days.

Tooth infections: 500 mg three times a day until the swelling
is down; then pull the tooth.

TOLNAFTATE

Anti-fungal

Safety class: 1   Stability: unknown

Brand names: Aftate, Tinactin.

Usually supplied as a powder.

Indications: TINEA. Not useful for CANDIDIASIS.

Contraindications: ALLERGY to the drug. Do not use by the eyes.

Dosage: apply every 12 hours for 2–4 weeks.

TRAMADOL

Pain medication for moderate to severe pain

Safety class: 3   Stability: C   Pregnancy: C

Brand names: Dromadol; Larapam; Mabron; Zamadol Zydol.
Supplied as oral, injectable and suppository. This is a narcotic-
like drug but not tightly controlled in some countries. It comes
as immediate release and extended release.

Indications: moderate to severe pain, not relieved by
cheaper and safer medications.

Contraindications: any difficulty breathing, head injury,
current use of DIAZEPAM or other sedatives.

Side-effects & Precautions: nausea, vomiting, constipation,
drowsiness. This makes a person breathe less. It interacts
badly with many different drugs.

Dosage: adult dose is 50–100 mg, not more often than every
4 hours, same dose oral, IM and IV.

TRIBENDIMIDINE

An anti-liver-fluke medication, to be used for the kinds of
flukes present in Southeast Asia and the Asian Arctic. It is
available in China, not in the West.

Indications: LIVER FLUKE, chlonorchis and opisthorcis kinds,
maybe STRONGYLOIDIASIS and TAPEWORM, ordinary worms
such as ASCARIASIS (good), PINWORM and HOOKWORM.

Contraindications: allergy to the drug.

Side-effects: reportedly not significant. Seek additional
information elsewhere.

Dosage: 200 mg in children age 5–14; 400 mg in those older,
single dose. Adding KETOCONAZOLE helps the cure rate.

TRICLABENDAZOLE

Brand name: Fasinex.

This is not available in the USA. Veterinary product is
available in Europe, Australia and South Africa.

Indications: LIVER FLUKE due to fascioliasis;
PARAGONIMIASIS.

Contraindications: allergy to the drug. Do not use this for
LIVER FLUKE in the Arctic, Southeast Asia or East Asia.

Side-effects: nausea, vomiting, abdominal pains are side-
effects of the drug itself; dying worms may cause dizziness,
headache and HIVES, sometimes temporary GALLBLADDER
DISEASE symptoms and JAUNDICE.

Dosage: LIVER FLUKE: 10 m/kg body weight taken with fatty
food. Repeat this in 24 hours and again in 3 months. If not
entirely better, repeat this at double the dose.

PARAGONIMIASIS: same dose daily x 3 days.

TROPICAMIDE

Eye dilator

Safety class: 2   Stability: C–D   Pregnancy: C

Brand name: Mydriacyl. Supplied as a 1% solution for eyes
(labeled ophthalmic).

Indications: KERATITIS, IRITIS, for pain relief after an eye injury.

Contraindications: GLAUCOMA. Do not use in patients
with any kind of spastic weakness or in those with DOWN
SYNDROME.

Precautions: this normally burns as it goes into the eye.
Tell the patient to blink but not to squeeze his eye shut.
It will make the eye very sensitive to light; he should wear
sunglasses that eliminate UV light. The eye should be
patched or the patient should stay in a dark room until the
effects are worn off. Vision will be temporarily blurred after
the drops are put in.

Dosage: one drop initially and one drop 5 minutes later.
This will give an effect lasting for at least 6–12 hours.
The medication can be renewed as it wears off.

VALACICLOVIR

Brand name: Valtrex.

This is an anti-HERPES drug, similar to ACYCLOVIR.
You should seek independent information concerning it.

Dosage: 1 gram twice a day for 7 days.

TOC

SYMPTOMS

DIFFERENTIALS

CONDITIONS

DRUG INDEX

REGIONAL NOTES

INX

VERAPAMIL

Calcium antagonist

Safety class: 3   Stability: C   Pregnancy: C

Brand names: Berkatens, Calan, Cordilox, Isoptin, Securon.

Indications: HYPERTENSION, MIGRAINE HEADACHE. Possibly for VISCERAL LEISHMANIASIS. It may be used for a rapid pulse that must be slowed; this must be supervised by a physician.

Contraindications: previous ALLERGY to this drug; a slow pulse; current or recent use of PROPRANOLOL or a similar drug; HEART FAILURE; a low blood pressure; current or recent use of DIGOXIN or a similar medication, any muscle weakness.

Side-effects: headache, dizziness, constipation, a red rash, swelling of the feet, a very slow pulse, a very low blood pressure with fainting. These effects occur in only a small percentage of patients.

Dosage: begin with 120 mg once daily. The usual daily dose is 240 mg once daily, but it is better to start with the lower dose to minimize the chance of an adverse reaction. When stopping the drug it should be stopped slowly. For VISCERAL LEISHMANIASIS the dose should be determined by a physician.

VITAMIN A

Safety class: 2   Stability: A

Synonyms: retinol, retinaldehyde.

Brand name: Aquasol A. Generic drug is available. Supplied as a liquid with 5,000 units of vitamin A per drop (0.1 ml) and as capsules with 25,000 or 50,000 or 200,000 units per capsule. Some capsules have nipples on the ends. The nipples must be cut off and the liquid inside the capsules squirted into the mouth.

Indications: a diet deficient in vitamin A. A high incidence of blindness in the community due to XEROPHTHALMIA indicates that all patients should have the vitamin. In particular, it should be used in all MALNUTRITION before beginning refeeding and in patients with MEASLES at the beginning of the treatment.

Precautions: do not give large doses in pregnancy. High doses over long periods of time are toxic. A single overdose is probably harmless. ZINC is necessary to process vitamin A. Hence it is good to add ZINC.

Dosage: reduce the dose according to weight for children.

Adults get 100,000 units daily for 3 days, then 50,000 units daily for 2 weeks.

In severe cases, children may not be able to absorb the oral form. In that case give an initial injection of vitamin A as retinyl palmitate; adult dose by injection is 100,000 IU (International units), reduce dose according to weight. Give it IM.

Alternatives: a diet high in vitamin A. (See XEROPHTHALMIA in the Condition Index.)

VITAMIN B₁₂

Safety class: 1   Stability: C   Pregnancy: C

Synonyms: hydroxocobalamin, cyanocobalamin, cobalamin.

Brand name: Cobalin-H.

Indications: SPRUE, some ANEMIA, possibly PLANT POISONING due to cassava or tobacco-cow's urine, a vegan diet, COBALAMIN DEFICIENCY.

Contraindications: ALLERGY to this drug.

Dosage: 1 mg IM every 2–3 days for 5 doses, then 1 mg every month. Lesser doses may still be helpful.

VITAMIN C

Safety class: 1   Stability: A

Synonym: ascorbic acid.

Indications: RESPIRATORY INFECTION, SCURVY, HEMOCHROMATOSIS. Sometimes used to make urine more acid.

Contraindication: ALLERGY to this drug.

Dosage: 250–500 mg daily; the drug is not toxic.

VITAMIN D

Safety class: 2   Stability: C

Synonym: calciferol.

Indication: RICKETS.

Contraindication: ALLERGY to the drug.

Precautions: overdose is possible with continued usage of very high doses. Give milk, milk products or rhubarb to provide calcium when giving this drug.

Dosage: the dose varies with the product. Follow the directions which come with your product.

Alternative: sun exposure on the skin without intervening glass.

VITAMIN K

Safety class: 1   Stability: A, dark

Brand name: Aquamephyton. Generic forms may be available.

Indications: bleeding in a newborn, HEMORRHAGIC FEVER, HEPATITIS, YELLOW FEVER, LIVER FAILURE, CIRRHOSIS.

Contraindications: ALLERGY to this drug. This drug might not be tolerated in G6PD DEFICIENCY.

Precautions: be sure not to give this IV.

Dosage: by IM or SQ injection: newborn: 0.5 to 1 mg; adult: 10 mg.

WHITFIELD OINTMENT

Safety class: 1–2   Stability: A

Indication: TINEA.

Contraindication: ALLERGY to this.

Precautions: do not use over more than 1/4 of the body surface at a time. Irritation will occur at the site of application; stop the drug and then, after clearing, resume using it in smaller amounts and less frequently.

Dosage: wash the patient and dry him well twice a day. Then apply the ointment. Do this until the problem is resolved.

YOGURT

This is made by bringing milk to a boil, cooling it, then adding some active yogurt culture and letting the mixture stand in a slightly warm place for 12 hours. The ideal temperature is 110°F (or 43°C). At temperatures cooler than that, the brew cultivates yeast and becomes bubbly. Active yogurt culture can be found in some store-bought yogurt and also in powdered form in health-food stores in Western countries. Yogurt is a good form of milk to use in MILK INTOLERANCE. It works as a vaginal douche for VAGINITIS due to CANDIDIASIS. It may be helpful in GIARDIASIS. It may be helpful in treating ordinary diarrhea, TURISTA.

ZIDOVUDINE

Brand name: Retrovir

Safety class: 2–3   Stability: C   Pregnancy: B

Indications: HIV INFECTION, sometimes bleeding problems caused by HIV, prevention of HIV INFECTION.

Contraindications: ALLERGY to this drug. Current usage of RIFAMPIN and similar drugs.

Precautions: ACETAMINOPHEN decreases the amount in the blood. Do not give with AMPHOTERCIN, CO-TRIMOXAZOLE, CIMETIDINE, SULFADIAZINE, ASPIRIN, ACYCLOVIR, DAPSONE, RIBAVIRIN, GANCICLOVIR, ATOVAQUONE or PENTAMIDINE except on physician advice.

Seek advice before using this in patients with LIVER DISEASE or KIDNEY DISEASE. Stop the drug if the patient develops abnormal bleeding or new or worsening ANEMIA.

Side-effects: nausea, vomiting, abdominal pains, ANEMIA, muscle aching, fatigue, headache. The drug may cause fat accumulation around the waist and in back of the shoulders.

Dosage: decrease the dose in patients with LIVER DISEASE or KIDNEY DISEASE. Stop if LIVER DISEASE develops or for new or worsening ANEMIA.

Adult dose: 100 mg by mouth every 4 hours while awake (500 mg daily) for HIV INFECTION without symptoms. For a bleeding problem due to HIV INFECTION, give 200–400 mg by mouth two or three times a day—only on physician recommendation after a blood test in a higher-level laboratory. For HIV prevention, 300 mg every 12 hours or 200 mg every 9 hours, beginning as soon as possible after the exposure, preferably within 4 hours.

Child dose: seek independent information; in case of child rape, the protocol is given in Volume 1, Appendix 14.

ZINC

Safety class: 1   Stability: A

Supplied as generic drug; 125 mg zinc sulfate monohydrate contains 45 mg of zinc.

Brand names: Solvazinc, Zincomed, Z Span.

Indications: general fatigue in someone not accustomed to the tropics, skin ulcers of any sort, ordinary diarrhea, CUTANEOUS LEISHMANIASIS, HEAT ILLNESS, LEPROSY, SICKLE CELL DISEASE, THALLASEMIA, TROPICAL ULCER, TURISTA, ZINC DEFICIENCY. Given together with VITAMIN A for XEROPHTHALMIA, MALNUTRITION and MEASLES.

Contraindication: ALLERGY to the drug.

Dosage: the following are adult doses; reduce dose according to weight for children. The doses are not precise.

Acclimatizing to the tropics, HEAT ILLNESS, diarrhea: 45 mg zinc daily.

CUTANEOUS LEISHMANIASIS: 5–10 mg/kg zinc sulfate daily (might or might not work).

LEPROSY: 45 mg zinc daily.

SICKLE CELL DISEASE: 45 mg zinc three times a day initially; reduce dose to once daily as the patient improves.

THALLASEMIA: same as SICKLE CELL DISEASE.

TROPICAL ULCER and skin ulcers: zinc from crushed tablets combined with ANTIBIOTIC OINTMENT may help. Commercial zinc paste or tape may be available.

ZINC DEFICIENCY: same as SICKLE CELL DISEASE.

REGIONAL NOTES

TOC   SYMPTOMS   DIFFERENTIALS   CONDITIONS   DRUG INDEX   **REGIONAL NOTES**   INX

INDEX E: EASTERN EUROPE, WESTERN ASIA NOTES

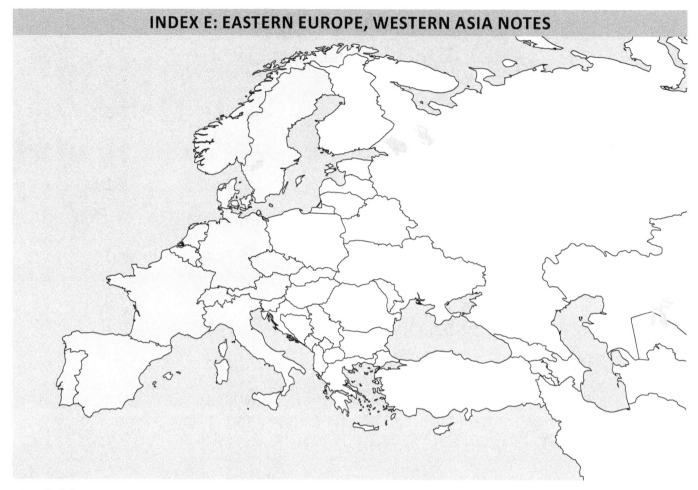

Map disclaimers

- Read the captions carefully. They are not all the same.

- Maps are notoriously unreliable. Conditions may be found in areas not shaded; conditions may be absent in areas that are shaded. Usually a disease is present only in spotty areas within the shaded region. A diagnosis is possible if there is shading anywhere around your location or if your patient has traveled through a shaded area.

- There is lack of shading both where there are no data and also where data exists indicating that the condition is absent. Lack of shading more often indicates lack of data than credible evidence that the condition is absent.

- Epidemiologists and government health officers survey in easy locations, near major roads. If you are in a remote, difficult location the maps may not reflect the reality that you see.

- Beware of shading that stops at political boundaries; germs don't respect border controls.

- Beware of areas that are unshaded for a variety of diseases. It may be because no one educated has ever entered that area and made it out alive. It may also be because intelligent people know enough not to go there.

- At times of civil unrest, natural disaster and migrations, the distribution of diseases changes unpredictably and rapidly. With biological warfare, this problem will be compounded.

TOC
SYMPTOMS
DIFFERENTIALS
CONDITIONS
DRUG INDEX
REGIONAL NOTES
INX

AMEBIASIS

This occurs in the Caucasus region, maybe elsewhere.

ANTHRAX

This is common in the Slavic countries and in Russia.

ARBOVIRAL FEVER

SANDFLY FEVER occurs in this area. A full description is in the Condition Index. The local SANDFLY FEVER geography is in its own entry below.

CRIMEAN-CONGO HEMORRHAGIC FEVER and some ENCEPHALITIS occur.

Similar conditions: see the diseases listed in the chart in Protocol B.2.

BELL'S PALSY

In eastern Europe a common cause is LYME DISEASE. The palsy is frequently present on both sides.

BRUCELLOSIS

Similar regional disease: TULAREMIA.

Brucellosis is common in a broad band across southern Europe and Asia, including Spain, southern France, Italy, Turkey, the Balkans and eastward to the Caspian and Aral Seas.

CANCER

Skin cancer, blood cancer (leukemia) and thyroid cancer are the result of radiation exposure. Bone cancer may be from ingesting radioactive substances in food and water. See RADIATION ILLNESS in the Condition Index. Skin cancer occurs on the eyelids in fair-skinned people in the desert areas of the southern CIS republics.

CHOLERA

This occurs in Russia, Romania and the Ukraine.

CRIMEAN-CONGO HEMORRHAGIC FEVER

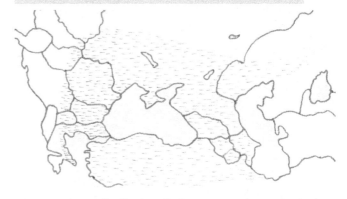

The approximate distribution of Crimean Congo hemorrhagic fever in this area. It may occur elsewhere.

CUTANEOUS LEISHMANIASIS

There are many cases in southern Europe. In urban areas of Asia the skin sores look dry and crusted over; the disease occurs in dogs as well as humans.

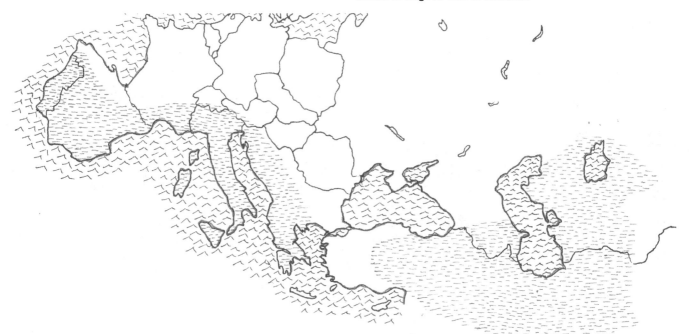

The shaded areas are where cutaneous Leishmaniasis is most likely to occur. Information taken in part from Pro-med Mail.

TOC SYMPTOMS DIFFERENTIALS CONDITIONS DRUG INDEX **REGIONAL NOTES** INX

TOC SYMPTOMS DIFFERENTIALS CONDITIONS DRUG INDEX REGIONAL NOTES INX

DIPHTHERIA

This occurs and is common in the former USSR. It is especially common in Georgia and the Caucasus.

DYSENTERY

The type due to amebae occurs in the Caucasus area.

ENCEPHALITIS

There is a tick-borne encephalitis in eastern Europe/Russia. Immunization should be obtained in Europe for those who will be traveling. Avoid tick bites.

Anti-viral medication at a hospital might help if it is given during the first week of illness.

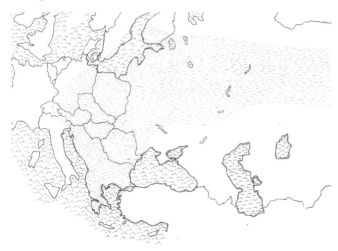

The shaded areas show both European and Russian encephalitis. For your purposes these are indistinguishable.

ENTERIC FEVER

This occurs in Russia and southern Europe, but is very rare in the rest of Eastern Europe.

ENTEROBIASIS

This occurs in Hungary and Armenia and probably the rest of eastern Europe and western Asia, since it tends to spread within temperate climates.

G6PD DEFICIENCY

This is common throughout southern Europe, but there is not much malaria there, so it is not a problem. It is a problem for southern Europeans living in the tropics.

GIARDIASIS

This is common throughout this area. The city water in St. Petersburg is particularly notorious for transmitting giardiasis. It is found even in the Arctic.

HEMORRHAGIC FEVER

In this area the most common form is CRIMEAN-CONGO HEMORRHAGIC FEVER; see the map on the previous page. It is transmitted by ticks and infects a variety of wild and domestic animals in addition to humans. However, it is not a common disease.

HEPATITIS

Hepatitis E is common in the former USSR and Lithuania. A kind of hepatitis that is due to Q FEVER is common in Spain and adjacent areas.

HIV INFECTION

This is common amongst the homosexuals of Moscow. It is common in France, Spain and Italy. In Spain intravenous drug users with AIDS commonly get VISCERAL LEISHMANIASIS.

HYDATID DISEASE

This is particularly common in Eastern Europe and throughout Russia. Both kinds are found in this area. It primarily affects the liver, but it spreads from there to other organs and is very aggressive, like a cancer. It requires sophisticated facilities for laboratory diagnosis and surgical treatment.

HYPERTENSION

This is common in Bulgaria, Hungary, Romania, Russia and Yugoslavia.

INFLUENZA

Similar regional diseases: ARBOVIRAL FEVER, LEPTOSPIROSIS, TULAREMIA, SPOTTED FEVER. See Protocol B.2.

INTESTINAL FLUKE

Metagonimiasis from fish occurs in Russia, Spain and eastern Europe. The only symptom is a mild diarrhea.

Heterophyiasis from fish occurs in Turkey.

LARVA MIGRANS

The deep type (acquired from dogs and cats) occurs throughout the southern two thirds of the former USSR.

LEPROSY

This is relatively common in Romania and in the areas of the southern former USSR adjacent to Iran and Turkey.

LEPTOSPIROSIS

The disease occurs in Germany, associated with field work and the presence of rodents.

LIVER FLUKE

Liver fluke (fascioliasis) is present in some areas only, mainly those that raise sheep or cattle. It occurs in Georgia, Poland and possibly elsewhere. Opisthorchiasis is found in Eastern Europe. It is specifically prevalent in Moscow and the Vlodimir region.

LYME DISEASE

LYME DISEASE occurs east of Berlin, west of Samara and north of the Black Sea, extending north into Finland. It also occurs in Croatia and in Scotland. It commonly presents with BELL'S PALSY and/or with RADICULOPATHY. There is less ARTHRITIS than in the west, but there may be double vision, paralysis of facial muscles, dizziness, deafness, inability to understand and symptoms of MENINGITIS. Regional similar disease: ENCEPHALITIS

MALARIA

Falciparum malaria is reportedly not found in this area at all. Non-falciparum malaria iis found in Turkey.

Similar regional diseases: TULAREMIA, SPOTTED FEVER.

MEASLES

This is common in Poland, Russia and Yugoslavia where few children are immunized.

MENINGITIS

This occurs throughout the area, but it is not common.

PELLAGRA

This used to be common in this area; it may still occur.

PELVIC INFECTION

CHLAMYDIA is a common cause.

PERTUSSIS

This occurs in Hungary, but is not common. It is common in the former USSR and the Ukraine where few children are immunized.

PLAGUE

Plague occurs in the former USSR. It occurs east of the Caspian Sea. It may occur anywhere.

Similar regional diseases: TULAREMIA, SPOTTED FEVER.

PNEUMONIA

In this area, especially in Spain and adjacent areas of south-western Europe, this may be due to Q FEVER, especially likely if the patient had recent contact with newborn animals.

Q FEVER

Q occurs in this entire area, especially south of a line from northern Spain to the north border of Kazakhstan. It has also occurred in the Netherlands.

RADIATION ILLNESS

This is common in this area because of contamination of the environment. CANCER is a complication of such exposure.

RELAPSING FEVER

This occurs in central Germany and east of there. In most places it is a mild disease, but a severe form occurs in the Caucasus area, carried by ticks.

RHEUMATIC FEVER

It is especially common in Russia, Byelorussia, the Ukraine and Bulgaria.

SANDFLY FEVER

This occurs in the Balkan Peninsula and in a large area east of the Caspian Sea. It does not occur in the north, since the flies do not tolerate cold. The description is in the Condition Index.

Similar conditions: see the diseases listed in the chart in Protocol B.2.

SPOTTED FEVER

This occurs commonly in Astrakhan, Russia in the summer time, transmitted by dog ticks in rural areas. A similar regional disease is TULAREMIA. Flea-borne spotted fever occurs also.

STRONGYLOIDIASIS

This is common in the eastern half of the former USSR and in Bulgaria, Hungary and Romania.

SYPHILIS

This is common in the former USSR; it is common in newborns.

TAPEWORM

Fish tapeworm occurs in the indigenous people of the former USSR, in the Volga area, in the Baltic region, in the Danube area of Romania and in the Masurian Lakes area of Poland. Reportedly it causes ANEMIA only in Scandinavia. Pork tapeworm occurs in the southern republics of the former USSR and also in the western republics. It is particularly common in the Slavic areas of Europe.

Rat and dwarf tapeworm occur, but they are rare.

TETANUS

This occurs in Poland, Romania, Hungary, Russia, the Ukraine and Yugoslavia where few children are immunized. It can occur anywhere.

TRENCH FEVER

This is common among the urban poor and homeless.

TRICHINOSIS

This occurs throughout the area.

TRICHURIASIS

This occurs in the Caucasus area, Romania, Hungary and Yugoslavia.

TUBERCULOSIS

Tuberculosis is common in Russia, Hungary and the Ukraine. There are many cases of antibiotic-resistant TB in the newly independent states of the former Soviet Union. One factor was crowded housing. Another factor was medication that was hard to take and lack of patient supervision, so the patients could throw the detestable tablets rather than swallow them. The government erratically supplied TB drugs, so treatment centers commonly ran out. HIV entered the picture in the 1990's, making the situation worse. One needs a cure rate of at least 60% in order to interrupt the transmission of resistant TB.

TURISTA

A form that responds to ERYTHROMYCIN occurs around Moscow, in the Czech Republic and in Slovakia. A viral form causing MALNUTRITION occurs in Tibilisi and the surrounding areas.

TYPHUS

Flea-borne (murine) typhus occurs in Portugal and in Southeast Europe: Yugoslavia, Albania and Romania. It may occur elsewhere also.

Louse-borne typhus occurs in Yugoslavia. Historically it has been prevalent in Europe at times of war, famine and disaster.

Similar regional conditions: TULAREMIA, SPOTTED FEVER, PLAGUE.

VISCERAL LEISHMANIASIS

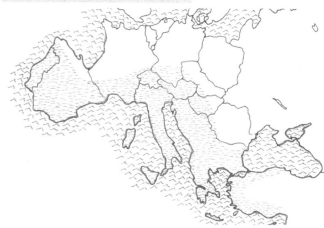

The known distribution of visceral Leishmaniasis. It may also manifest with skin symptoms. See cutaneous Leishmaniasis.

In Spain it is commonly associated with AIDS, especially in intravenous drug users.

In Albania it always causes a large liver and spleen, a fever and weight loss.

In some areas STIBOGLUCONATE is useless; in other areas it works fine.

It tends to be of sudden onset and rapid progression in those who are HIV-positive, whether or not they have full-blown AIDS. The prognosis is poor.

INDEX F: AFRICA NOTES

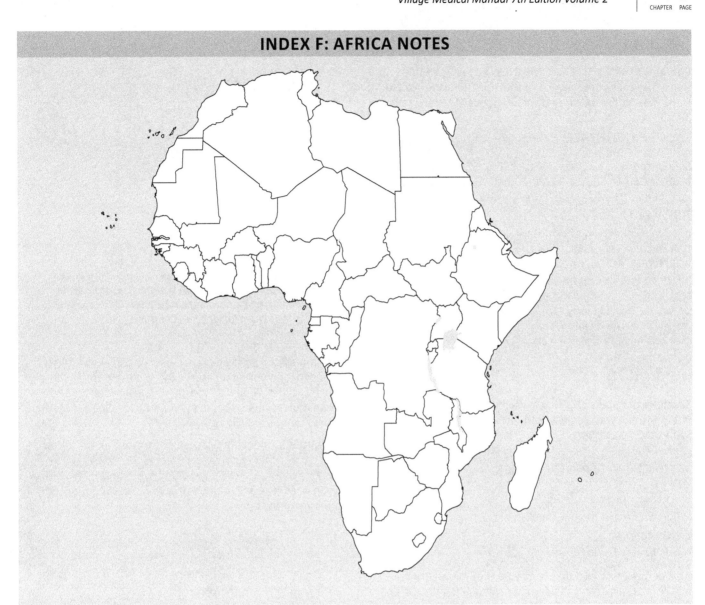

Map disclaimers

- Read the captions carefully. They are not all the same.

- Maps are notoriously unreliable. Conditions may be found in areas not shaded; conditions may be absent in areas that are shaded. Usually a disease is present only in spotty areas within the shaded region. A diagnosis is possible if there is shading anywhere around your location or if your patient has traveled through a shaded area.

- There is lack of shading both where there are no data and also where data exists indicating that the condition is absent. Lack of shading more often indicates lack of data rather than credible evidence that the condition is absent.

- Epidemiologists and government health officers survey in easy locations, near major roads. If you are in a remote, difficult location the maps may not reflect the reality that you see.

- Beware of shading that stops at political boundaries; germs don't respect border controls.

- Beware of areas that are unshaded for a variety of diseases. It may be because no one educated has ever entered that area and made it out alive. It may also be because intelligent people know enough not to go there.

- At times of civil unrest, natural disaster and migrations, the distribution of diseases changes unpredictably and rapidly. With biological warfare, this problem will be compounded.

TOC SYMPTOMS DIFFERENTIALS CONDITIONS DRUG INDEX REGIONAL NOTES INX

ABORTION

Consider AFRICAN SLEEPING SICKNESS and LASSA FEVER, as these may cause both fever and abortion. However, MALARIA is the most common cause of spontaneous abortion.

ACUTE ABDOMEN

Similar regional diseases: SICKLE CELL DISEASE may resemble acute abdomen but the whites of the eyes are yellow, the patient has ANEMIA, and a urine dipstick shows urobilinogen. Treat the SICKLE CELL DISEASE.

In Ethiopia and in South Africa there is a hereditary disease that can look very similar to acute abdomen. It is called PORPHYRIA. Ask your patient if other members of his family have had frequent abdominal pains. If he says "yes", then take some of his urine and set it in the sunlight. If he has porphyria, it will quickly turn a dark color. If that happens, just give pain medication. The patient does not need to be sent to a hospital unless he says, "this time it is different."

ADDICTION

Examples of uppers are: khat in the horn of Africa and betel nut in South Asian women, both recreational drugs. See PLANT POISONING.

AFRICAN SLEEPING SICKNESS

Entry category: two overlapping diseases
Synonym: African trypanosomiasis
Cause: protozoa
Mildly to very ill; class 3–4.

Age: any, but rare in children; may be transmitted from mother to fetus across the placenta. **Who**: bitten by tsetse flies which tend to attack moving targets aggressively. It is more common in nationals than in expatriates. There are two forms of the disease: Gambian or West African and Rhodesian or East African.

In the Gambian form, (West Africa) the flies prefer human hosts; they live in places where people congregate, attacking them as they gather. They are aggressive biters, dive-bombing those walking or driving through their areas, especially at the end of the dry season. They may be plentiful in one area of several acres and totally absent in adjacent areas. Both sexes are affected equally. The Gambian form has been found in urban areas in the Democratic Republic of Congo.

In the Rhodesian form in East Africa, the flies prefer domestic or wild animal blood; they live in trees in savannah. Males are affected most, especially hunters and fishermen, when they happen to go through tsetse-infested areas. Some of the eastern tsetse flies enter villages, causing severe epidemics, but accidental encounters are more the norm.

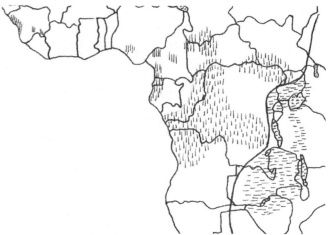

The vertical shading depicts Gambian sleeping sickness; the horizontal shading depicts Rhodesian. The heavy line is the approximate border between the two. Information taken from PLoS Negl Trop Dis 6(10): 2011 and ProMED-mail.

Onset

Gambian sleeping sickness has a very gradual onset; after an incubation period measured in weeks symptoms come and go at first. Then they mostly disappear for a second incubation period measured in months to years before the mental symptoms begin.

In Rhodesian sleeping sickness, the onset is more sudden; death may occur within a few months. The initial skin swelling occurs in 5–15 days. Other symptoms begin with a fever, headache and joint pains within less than 3 weeks from the time of the bite.

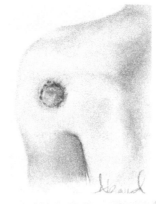

This is the initial reaction to the bite of an infected tsetse fly. Some people skip this stage, moving on directly to the next skin or general manifestation of the illness. AB

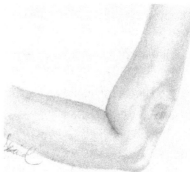

Either with or without the initial bump reaction to the fly bite, this kind of target lesion may develop. A similar pattern might be caused by LYME DISEASE. AB

In both forms, expatriates tend to have a more rapid onset, more fevers and more severe disease. The temperature may be normal in the morning, with fevers only in the evenings.

CLINICAL GAMBIAN

Necessary: slow onset of symptoms which initially come and go; there are large lymph nodes (at first soft, not tender but moveable, not stuck to the skin or underlying muscle) in the back of the neck; fatigue; general muscle pains. After the disease has been present for some time there are mental changes such as sleep problems, incoordination, dizziness, personality changes[1] or trouble thinking.

Usually: no or mild fever, and fever is usually higher evenings than mornings. There is painful swelling of the eyelids, face, neck, abdomen, penis; headache; big spleen; fast pulse; impotence; no menstruation; a flat rash which looks like red rings on white skin (more visible when the skin is warm). There may be ANEMIA.

Maybe: expatriates may have an initial reaction to the bite, like a flu, along with HIVES and itching. The patient may have painful and swollen testicles; a sensation of insects crawling in the skin or general whole-body itching; irregular pulse; weight loss. Symptoms during the early stage are more common in females than in males and in expatriates than nationals.

Miscarriages, stillbirths and newborn deaths are common. Children have delayed mental and sexual development.

Summary

1. Residence in an affected area

2. Headache, fever or both

3. Slow onset

4. Sleep problem, movement/sensation problem or both.

5. Weight loss

6. Swelling or a history of swelling

CLINICAL RHODESIAN

Necessary: [history of the fly bite with subsequent swelling] or [history of episodic high fevers with headaches and joint pains] or both.

Usually: there are skin changes similar to the initial stage of Gambian. The swelling goes away in about two weeks.

Maybe: there may be swollen lymph nodes in the armpit or in the groin. They are not painful and are not matted. The patient's spleen and possibly his liver are enlarged. He may develop JAUNDICE, HEART FAILURE, KIDNEY DISEASE or itching all over. The late stages described below occur within a few months unless the patient dies of HEART FAILURE first.

BOTH TYPES TERMINAL EVENTS

Nationals may have no fever before sleeping, but Europeans always do. There are always trembling and insomnia as initial symptoms of the terminal state. Late sleeping sickness is best described by a quotation from Patrick Manson, the author of early editions of Manson's Tropical Diseases.

"There is a disinclination to exertion; slow, shuffling gait; morose mask-like vacant expression; relaxation of features; hanging of the lower lip; puffiness and drooping of the eyelids; tendency to lapse into sleep or a condition simulating sleep..during the daytime contrasting with restlessness at night; slowness in answering questions; shirking of the day's task. Dull headache is generally present. He will walk, if forced to do so, with unsteady and swaying gait. His speech is difficult to follow. He never spontaneously engages in conversation or even asks for food.. He forgets even to chew his food, falling asleep perhaps in the act of conveying it to his mouth or with the half-masticated bolus still in his cheek.. The habits usually become bestial, and he becomes a drooling, dribbling and drowsy idIOT."

Intolerable itching is common, as are BEDSORES and severe weight loss. In expatriates at least one of the following is always present in the final stages of this disease: excessive sleep, trembling, bizzare behavior, abnormal eye movements.

Complications: HYPOGLYCEMIA, HEART FAILURE, ANEMIA, IRITIS, BRAIN DAMAGE or abnormal bleeding. There is a deficiency in thyroid hormone in many patients in the Congo. This may apply elsewhere, also. It is something to check at a hospital and treat if necessary.

Similar diseases: see Protocols B.2, B.3, B.7, B.10 and B.12. MALARIA may be indistinguishable especially in the early Rhodesian form in expatriates. Sleeping sickness may cause a rapid diagnostic malaria test to be false positive.

The disease's non-response to QUININE and the history of the fly bite are distinctive. There are many causes of large neck lymph nodes. It resembles STROKE and cerebral MALARIA in the later stages, but the onset of coma in sleeping sickness is much slower, over days rather than over minutes to hours. It may be virtually indistinguishable from the late stages of SYPHILIS.

Bush laboratory; a sedimentation rate[2] under 90 is highly unlikely in a patient with sleeping sickness; the test is sensitive but not specific.[3]

Treatment

Prevention: eliminate tsetse flies. In the Gambian form, dogs, pigs and sheep may have the disease in their blood without becoming ill. They pass it on to flies which then transmit it to humans. These animals should not be housed near human dwellings. In western Africa and in Ethiopia, one of the flies that transmits this disease can be eliminated by feeding IVERMECTIN to pigs in the area (dosage unknown; seek other information). The flies feed on pig blood and take in the drug which kills the male flies and keeps the females from breeding. Since the flies that carry this breed in coffee, banana and lantana trees, separating these from the houses might be helpful.

---

1 This may be apathy, irritability or maniacal episodes.

2 See Volume 1, Appendix 2.

3 Sensitive means that if a person has sleeping sickness, his sedimentation rate will certainly be abnormally high. However, there are many other diseases beside sleeping sickness that increase the sedimentation rate. Therefore a normal sedimentation rate is most significant since it tells you that the patient does not have the disease. An elevated rate tells you that the patient is sick, which you knew already before you did the test.

Referrals: laboratory: in the early stage, before mental symptoms start, a thick blood smear stained with Field's stain may show the organisms. This is more sensitive in Rhodesian than Gambian illness. In Gambian illness if the patient has a large lymph node in the back of his neck, a physician or technician might put a needle in it and examine the fluid under a microscope. It must be examined within 15 minutes to show the organisms.

When the mental symptoms begin, the organisms leave the blood and can be found only in spinal fluid obtained by a spinal tap.[1] Many times the parasites are hard to find. A well-equipped lab may be able to spin blood to concentrate the organisms and thus to detect them more readily. Before mental symptoms, the organisms only show up in the blood; after the mental problems begin, they only show up in the spinal fluid.

There are various tests that show antibodies to the sleeping sickness germs, but they should not be the sole basis for treatment; the drugs are toxic. It is imperative to find the sleeping sickness organism in the patient's body. The antibody tests are totally useless for the Rhodesian type of the disease.

Facilities: In the mental stage, imaging with CT or MRI might be helpful.

Practitioners: this being a tropical disease with a very restricted distribution, don't even think of getting care anywhere other than a specialty hospital in Africa or else London. See Volume 1 Appendix 13.

Patient care: this is essential as, once the patient develops mental symptoms, the death rate is 100% without proper treatment. With appropriate treatment, the patient in coma should start to wake up within 72 hours. PENTAMIDINE is useful to prevent the Gambian form of the disease after a bite or in the early stages. Once mental symptoms start treatment is complicated. Two drugs that might be used are SURAMIN and/or MELASOPROL. Both are toxic and require physician supervision. NIRIDAZOLE is a drug that was formerly used, but it is very toxic and should not be used anymore.

Meanwhile

- Be sure he takes in enough food and liquid to stay well-nourished and well-hydrated. Place a stomach tube if necessary, keeping the patient lying on one side once it is in. Use no ASPIRIN. Give plenty of starch and sugar; low blood sugar is a common complication.

- Turn the patient from one side to the other every two hours during the day. Move his arms and legs as far as they will go in each direction at least four times a day. See Appendix 8, Volume 1.

- Treat the patient for SEIZURES if necessary.

- EFLORNITHINE is a drug that works well for Gambian but it only works for about 50% of Rhodesian cases. It is usually given IV at first and then orally later. If your patient is not very ill, you can try to give it orally from the beginning. In most cases of Rhodesian SS one of the older drugs must be used additionally. Below is a list of possibilities:

- If you are forced to use toxic drugs, giving PREDNISONE initially might decrease the side effects.

- The patient must have a spinal tap (lumbar puncture) after treatment is done and then every 6 months for two years thereafter, to be sure there are no more parasites.

- Fexinidazole is a drug under development.

AFRICAN TICK BITE FEVER, AFRICAN TICK TYPHUS

See SPOTTED FEVER in the Condition Index. This is transmitted by cattle ticks. There are frequently multiple eschars (little black scabs) rather than only one. There may be none. The disease is frequently fatal.

AMEBIASIS

Surveys show this to be particularly common in Central African Republic, Ethiopia, Gabon, Gambia, Niger, Rwanda, Somalia, D. R. Congo, in urban areas and the Jos Plateau of Nigeria; rural South Africa, Tanzania and Sudan. It is rare in the desert areas of SW Africa.

In Niger and surrounding areas, those areas that are hot and humid tend to have amebic liver disease. The hot and dry areas tend to have just the DYSENTERY without the liver's being infected.

This disease is a problem in Burundi; it can look just like HEPATITIS or ACUTE ABDOMEN.

ANEMIA

This is common all over Africa except in cultures that consume animal blood, use iron pots for brewing beer or cooking or are pastoral at high-altitudes.

In Chad, most anemia in pregnancy and half of all other anemias are due to IRON deficiency.

In The Gambia, much of the anemia is due to vitamin deficiency from lack of FOLIC ACID or VITAMIN B_{12}.

---

1 *The spinal fluid must be examined immediately after it is taken; the parasites will be destroyed in 20 minutes. If parasites are found in the blood, any abnormality of the spinal fluid indicates the disease is in the late stage.*

ANTHRAX

This is common in Zimbabwe, along the Rift Valley in Ethiopia, in southern Kenya amongst the Maasai, the northern and western parts of the continent and around Lake Victoria. In Zimbabwe it is associated with wild game meat, especially hippopotamus. It may appear similar to CUTANEOUS LEISHMANIASIS or to TUBERCULOSIS of the skin, but its onset is more rapid.

It occurs generally in western Africa and also in Tanzania, frequently in epidemics and many times with multiple cases within families. In about 90% of the cases, the person can trace the disease to some contact with a sick animal.

ARBOVIRAL FEVER

This is a group of diseases, not a single disease. In most areas these diseases are carried by mosquitoes. Two that are listed separately in these notes because of public health concerns are EBOLA VIRUS DISEASE and LASSA FEVER. See Protocol B.2.

RIFT VALLEY FEVER

This occurs mainly in East Africa, south and east of a line between Alexandria, Egypt and Nouamrhar, Mauritania. Reportedly it has been absent from the West African countries that border the Gulf of Guinea (the southern coast of West Africa). This is carried by mosquitoes. Incubation period is 2–7 days. It tends to occur in epidemics at the end of the rainy season in Zambia (Lusaka and Mazabuka), Burkina Faso and Central African Republic (around Bangui). There have been outbreaks in northern Kenya. In many areas of east Africa, RVF affects only cattle; however, in northern Kenya and southern Somalia, there are also human cases and significant numbers of deaths, particularly at times of flooding. This may be contagious. See Protocol B.2. All suspected cases had fever; 89% had ENCEPHALITIS, 10%, hemorrhage and 3%, loss of vision. A total of 169 (55%) of the 309 confirmed or probable cases were also positive for malaria as detected by blood smear. Contact with sick animals and animal products, including blood, meat and milk, were identified as risk factors.

WEST NILE VIRUS

This is a kind of arboviral fever, indistinguishable from HEPATITIS. It occurs occasionally in Central African Republic. It is considered a potential bioterrorist weapon. The incubation is 3–6 days.

IGBO ORA VIRUS

This is found in the rural areas of Ivory Coast. It produces joint pains, but no long-term disabilities and no deaths. It is carried by mosquito; it has an incubation period of 3–12 days.

CRIMEAN-CONGO HEMORRHAGIC FEVER

See the separate entry.

Similar regional diseases: AFRICAN SLEEPING SICKNESS which causes a fever that is either not high or is high only off and on, not continually. LASSA FEVER has a sudden onset of fever; the patient has red eyes and chest pains. Also consider EBOLA VIRUS DISEASE.

ARTHRITIS

Similar regional diseases: SICKLE CELL DISEASE also involves joint pains, but there is either a family history of ANEMIA, episodic abdominal pain or both. In western and central Africa, consider MANSONELLOSIS PERSTANS. In expatriates consider ONCHOCERCIASIS. In East Africa consider HIV INFECTION which causes a symmetrical arthritis of large joints with sparing of the small joints. FILARIASIS can cause an arthritis of the knees which responds readily to DEC.

ASCARIASIS

This is extremely common in SW and central Cameroon; Bauchi, Oyo and Ogun States in Nigeria; amongst the pygmies of D. R. Congo and Rwanda; around Kinshasa, D. R. Congo; and near Entebbe, Uganda.

ASTHMA

The association of asthma and allergies to tiny insects living in dust has been shown for the following areas: Zambia, Zimbabwe and South Africa. It may also occur in other areas. Consider MANSONELLOSIS PERSTANS or FILARIASIS.

BELL'S PALSY

Regional Cause: SICKLE CELL DISEASE

BERIBERI

Cause: thiamine deficiency

There have been outbreaks in western Africa where milled rice has replaced traditional grains and cereals. It occurs in all forms, most commonly in September and October. It seems to affect productive, working males first and most severely. This is also common amongst the Bushmen in the northern Kalahari.

BLADDER STONE

This is common in Niamey. Most (94%) of the patients are male.

BRAIN DAMAGE

This may be caused by AFRICAN SLEEPING SICKNESS, ENCEPHALITIS, MALARIA, and, less commonly, SCHISTOSOMIASIS (any type).

TOC   SYMPTOMS   DIFFERENTIALS   CONDITIONS   DRUG INDEX   REGIONAL NOTES   INX

BRUCELLOSIS

This is especially common north of the equator and in Tanzania. In western Nigeria, about 1/2 of the adults have had this disease at some time. In Mali, about 1/4 of the adults have had this disease.

Brucellosis in Africa tends to invade bones, mainly the spine and the hip, but occasionally the knee(s) and rarely other bones. Mental changes from the disease are also common.

BURKITT LYMPHOMA

This is especially prevalent in the West Nile district of Uganda and in Nigeria. In some areas it may be as common as TUBERCULOSIS. The tumors are most often initially on the jaw bone. In western Cameroon it affects adults also and more often begins in the abdomen.

BURULI ULCER

This is common in Benin and Ghana where it can cause significant disability, compromising the patient's prosperity. In Benin it occurs mostly in those under 15 y.o. and over 50 y.o.

CANCER

Stomach cancer is common near the southern Kenyan border, in Rwanda and Burundi and in adjacent areas of D. R. Congo and Uganda.

Breast cancer in Nigeria tends to affect younger women than in Western countries. When it is diagnosed during pregnancy or nursing, the prognosis is poor.

Bladder cancer is common wherever there is SCHISTOSOMIASIS HEMATOBIUM.

Cancer of the male genitals is particularly common in some areas of Uganda in uncircumcised men. TUBERCULOSIS may look similar.

Cancer of the esophagus occurs mainly in eastern and south-eastern Africa.

Liver cancer is common in Africans, more in humid than dry areas. In Nigeria, liver cancer is the most common kind of cancer. It may affect young people. It is also common in Niger.

Cancer of the nose and throat is common in the South Asian population of Africa.

Kaposi's sarcoma is a skin cancer that is associated with HIV INFECTION, occurring mainly in males. It looks like huge, reddish or bluish WARTS. It is very common in Central African Republic and the Lake Victoria area. It may be symmetrical.

Melanoma is a very aggressive type of skin cancer. It is usually a dark color. It occurs on fair skin, including palms and soles of Africans.

CATARACT

This is very common in the Sahel and Ethiopia.

CELLULITIS

A kind of cellulitis common amongst the pygmies responds to CO-TRIMOXAZOLE.

CEREBRAL PALSY

ARBOVIRAL FEVERs and AFRICAN SLEEPING SICKNESS are regional causes of this.

CHICKEN POX

Similar regional disease: MONKEYPOX is similar but is found almost exclusively in northern D. R. Congo and southern Central African Republic; occasional cases are seen in western Africa. With MONKEYPOX, the lymph nodes are large and the rash breaks out all at once rather than spreading from one part of the skin to another over several days. Also, with MONKEYPOX the patient is moderately to very ill whereas in chicken pox the child is only mildly ill (although an adult with chicken pox may be very ill).

CHOLERA

Cholera outbreaks occur in Cameroon, Sierra Leone, Uganda, Congo, Chad, Tanzania, Mozambique, Liberia, Kenya, Togo, D. R. Congo, Comoro Islands, Somalia. It may occur anywhere. There tends to be more cholera in NE Africa during years of heavy rainfall. In parts of East Africa, it may be resistant to DOXYCYCLINE and CO-TRIMOXAZOLE.

CIRRHOSIS

This may be due to SIDEROSIS.

CRETINISM

The second kind described in the Condition Index is the one that affects most cretins in Africa.

CRIMEAN-CONGO HEMORRHAGIC FEVER

CCHF, EBOLA and Marburg (listed with EBOLA VIRUS DISEASE) are indistinguishable. Any or all of these may occur throughout Africa south of the Sahara except for the Kalahari Desert. CCHF may be prevalent in the eastern portion of southern Africa. See Protocol B.2 and the Condition Index.

CUTANEOUS LEISHMANIASIS

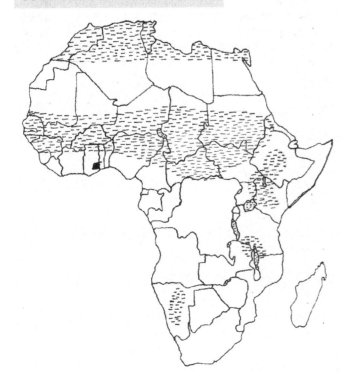

The shaded areas are where cutaneous Leishmaniasis is most likely to occur. Darker shaded areas show the locations of outbreaks. Information taken in part from Pro-med Mail.

It is very common around Ouagadougou, Burkina Faso, the Ho municipality of the Volta region of Ghana and around Khartoum, Sudan. KETOCONAZOLE treatment reportedly works well in Sudan.

CYSTICERCOSIS

This is common in South Africa, Togo, Reunion Island and Madagascar. It is found in areas where pigs are raised in such a way that they come into contact with human waste.

DENGUE FEVER

This is present mostly in the western and eastern coastal areas. It occurs in the Comoro Islands. The mosquito that carries the disease is present inland also, so there is potential for the disease to spread inland. It has been found in Djibouti, Sudan, Kenya, Ivory Coast, Egypt and Burkina Faso.

DEPRESSION

Physiological causes in Africa include DENGUE FEVER, AFRICAN SLEEPING SICKNESS, EBOLA VIRUS DISEASE and Marburg fever (listed with EBOLA VIRUS DISEASE).

DIABETES

SIDEROSIS is a regional cause, mainly in southern Africa. PANCREATITIS is a cause in eastern and western Africa.

DIPHTHERIA

This is known to be common in Algeria and Senegal; it may occur anywhere. Skin diphtheria is common in central Africa. In general diphtheria is not as common in tropical Africa as in other tropics.

DONOVANOSIS

This occurs but is not common in Africa except for South Africa, Zambia and Zimbabwe. The cases that occur are mostly in seaports, along transportation corridors, and large urban areas.

DYSENTERY

Bacterial dysentery is especially common in the lakes region: D. R. Congo, western Uganda, Rwanda and Burundi, especially where there is crowding. In these areas outbreaks are apt to happen in times of drought. It is also extremely common in Ethiopia, Sudan, Chad, Mali and Mauritania. It is usually sensitive to CHLORAMPHENICOL, CO-TRIMOXAZOLE and GENTAMYCIN (any one of these).

Amebic dysentery is common throughout Africa south of the Sahara, except for the Kalahari. In Niger, hot and dry regions tend to have amebic dysentery.

EBOLA VIRUS DISEASE

Cause: virus

This is a specific type of HEMORRHAGIC FEVER. The entry includes Marburg fever which is rare.

Very ill; class 1 or 4; contagious; usually fatal but intensive care might be life-saving.

This occurred originally in the tropical rainforests of Central Africa. It has also occurred in West Africa and Zimbabwe. There are two main types: Sudan and Zaire strains. The Zaire strain is more severe. The Sudan strain occurs in southern Sudan (also adjacent countries), but the Zaire strain is more widespread. Cases have been reported from near the Kenya–Uganda border, from Ivory Coast and various locations in West Africa. The disease has spread widely and may continue to do so.

Age: any, more adults than children. **Who:** it affects pygmies, young adults and farmers preferentially. First cases acquire the disease from unknown sources, possibly bats and/or dogs. Subsequent cases in an epidemic are usually relatives or medical care-givers of initial cases. It appears that those who handle bodies right after death are most susceptible. **Onset:** sudden, over a day or so, after a 3 to 21-day incubation period.

Clinical

Necessary: sudden onset of fever, back pain, red eyes, weakness, loss of appetite, nausea, vomiting, diarrhea and general aching.

Sometimes: subsequently abdominal pain and jaundice may develop. He may develop a rash, beginning on the chest. He may have a sore throat, a cough, trouble swallowing or hiccups. His body may swell.

Finally: some (20%) patients start bleeding all over: nosebleeds, vomiting blood, bloody diarrhea and bleeding from needle sticks. He may bleed from his eyes or ears. The patient at this point is either in a coma or appears "spacy" or "not there". Either with or without bleeding, death ensues.

Case definition: 1. a link with a known case plus a generalized illness OR 2. a fever and generalized illness in the context of an outbreak OR 3. fever and unexplained bleeding.

Similar diseases: see Protocol B.2. (This is one type of arboviral fever.) Also consider other types of HEMORRHAGIC FEVER. Marburg fever is similar but it causes a deep red coloring of the roof of the mouth, starting in the back and moving forward. It also destroys the testicles and can cause long-term emotional changes.

Treatment

Prevention: recently dead corpses are contagious. Protective clothing is essential. Transport should be a towed trailer. Bleach kills the virus. Immunization is available.

Patient care: the usual anti-viral drugs do not work. Curative drugs that are specific for Ebola are being developed and tested. Seek recent information about the best curative drugs and supportive care. Fluid resuscitation (ORS in particular) is most important. IP fluids may be necessary. With good supportive care survivals are not rare. Previously healthy older children and young adults are most likely to survive. *Results:* recovery takes months during which time the patient's semen remains infective.

ENCEPHALITIS

Rift Valley fever, a type of ARBOVIRAL FEVER, is a regional cause of this, as is AFRICAN SLEEPING SICKNESS.

ENTERIC FEVER

Typhoid fever is common all over. *Paratyphoid fever* is uncommon. Typhoid is vastly overdiagnosed all over Africa. Essential features are abdominal complaints, a sustained fever, step-wise progression over days and mental changes.

In The Gambia and Central African Republic in children there is no progressive rise in fever and no relatively slow pulse. It causes mainly abdominal complaints in about 67% and mainly PNEUMONIA in most of the rest. Occasionally it presents like a KIDNEY INFECTION, and occasionally there is no fever at all. It should be suspected in any seriously ill child. This is a common cause of death in patients with HIV INFECTION.

ENTEROBIASIS

This is common all over the world. It has been noted to be especially common near the northern Central African Republic/Cameroon border.

EPILEPSY

Additional causes in Africa are AFRICAN SLEEPING SICKNESS and ONCHOCERCIASIS.

FILARIASIS

Synonym: elephantiasis, non-endemic.

The filariasis in Africa is all of the Bancroftian type. It is commonly an urban problem, related to poverty and poor sanitation in all major cities in the affected areas. It is common in the Nile delta. MANSONELLOSIS PERSTANS is a form of filariasis listed separately.

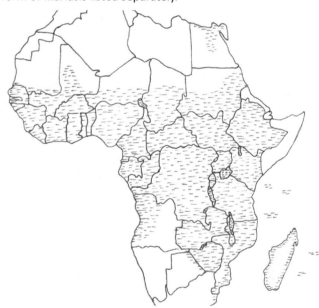

The approximate distribution of filariasis in Africa. It is all Bancroftian filariasis. Note that in Madagascar only the coastal areas are affected. Information taken from PLoS ONE 7(2): 2012 and ProMED-mail.

FLUOROSIS

It is most common in Ethiopia in the Wonji-Shoa, Alem-Tena, Sami-Beta areas and throughout the Rift Valley. It may occur in other areas.

G6PD DEFICIENCY

This is a genetic variant which makes a patient vulnerable to severe reactions to certain drugs. It is very problematic with the anti-malarial drug PRIMAQUINE.

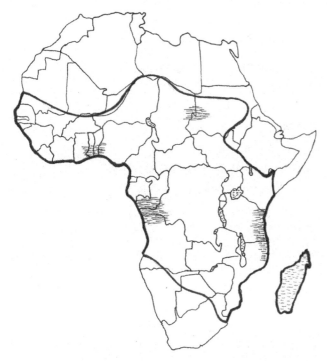

The heavy black lines outline where the problem is common; the shaded areas show where it is very common. Consider the origin of the patient, not his current location. Information derived from PLoS Med 9(11): 2012

GALLBLADDER DISEASE

This is not common in Africans except with SICKLE CELL DISEASE and THALLASEMIA.

GASTROENTERITIS

Similar regional disease: PLANT POISONING due to lolism.

GIARDIASIS

It is found all over Africa, but is especially common around Kinshasa, D. R. Congo and in central Uganda. It is uncommon amongst the pygmies of Rwanda and in Ogun State, Nigeria. It is common in Ethiopia.

GLAUCOMA

Acute glaucoma is rare in Africans. Chronic glaucoma is common in Africans.

GOITER

This is common in the Wedya District of Zimbabwe, but CRETINISM occurs rarely. It is common in the Man Region of Ivory Coast and around Bulape, D. R. Congo. In southern Africa it tends to be common at an altitude over 1000 meters (3300 ft.) and 15 km (9 mi.) or more from the sea. It is common in the central highlands of Ethiopia.

GONORRHEA

In some areas of Kenya, PENICILLIN, DOXYCYCLINE and some CEPHALOSPORINs no longer work. SPECTINOMYCIN and CHLORAMPHENICOL are still useful. Seek local advice.

GUINEA WORM

Synonyms: dracontiasis, dracunculiasis

Mildly to moderately ill; class 1; regional, in rural agricultural areas where water is obtained from wells into which people step. There has been a big WHO effort to eliminate the disease which is changing its distribution. It is not found south of the equator. In Ethiopia it used to be in the Gambella region and in the South Omo area. It has reappeared in Chad.

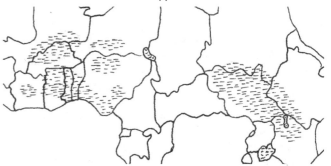

The shading shows where guinea worms have been reported in recent years. They may be eliminated from these areas. They may occur in other areas.

Age: any. **Who:** those who drink water contaminated with microscopic larvae. **Onset:** variable; usually about 1 year after drinking infected water.

Clinical

Necessary: a small bump forms on the skin, usually on the leg, but it may be anywhere. This enlarges to become a blister. It is itchy and frequently burning; the pain is relieved by cold. When the blister breaks, one can see the end of the worm. There is only one worm per bump and each worm is 30–70 cm (12–28 in.) long. An incredibly painful sore forms in place of the blister.

TOC   SYMPTOMS   DIFFERENTIALS   CONDITIONS   DRUG INDEX   REGIONAL NOTES   INX

Maybe: the worm will discharge a milky fluid.

Complications: severe infections may develop because of the open wounds. When parents are infected, their children tend to suffer from MALNUTRITION because of loss of income and lack of care.

Bush laboratory: there is no test for this, but the disease is so distinctive that no lab is required.

Similar diseases: MYIASIS is a skin ulcer with many short, fat "worms". The disease may initially cause KATAYAMA DISEASE. The very painful bump which becomes an ulcer may resemble skin DIPHTHERIA.

Treatment

Prevention: encourage the design of wells which eliminate the possibility of stepping into them. A simple sand filter works well to eliminate parasites from contaminated water, or you can use Temphos (Abate) to treat affected water.

Patient care: the best treatment is for the worm to be surgically removed before the blister forms. This is a relatively easy procedure; it can be done at a level 2 or 3 facility. It reduces the period of disability from weeks to two days. If you already know how to suture wounds, you can do it if shown.

Once the blister forms: immerse the blister or sore in cold water. This makes the worm limp. IBUPROFEN helps to hasten this process. Wind the worm on a small clean stick, a few centimeters a day, not so tightly that the worm breaks. (If it breaks give the patient one of the drugs listed below.) This will gradually draw the worm out. If the patient is bedridden anyway, keeping the area continually wet will draw the worm out faster (in 2 weeks rather than 8–12 weeks). Otherwise keep the area clean and dressed with ANTIBIOTIC OINTMENT to prevent secondary infection. A number of different drugs are also useful, such as METRONIDAZOLE, TINIDAZOLE, MEBENDAZOLE and THIABENDAZOLE. NIRIDAZOLE is an old dangerous drug that should no longer be used.

HEART FAILURE

The restrictive type occurs with LASSA FEVER. It may also occur for no known reason in children with MALNUTRITION in eastern Africa. It is called endomyocardial fibrosis, and it is fatal.

The dilated type occurs with AFRICAN SLEEPING SICKNESS, BERIBERI, some viruses and with pregnancy.

The hypertrophic type occurs in patients with HYPERTENSION.

The valvular type is most common in Africa. It is usually because of RHEUMATIC FEVER.

Regional causative diseases are AFRICAN SLEEPING SICKNESS, LASSA FEVER and SIDEROSIS.

HEMORRHAGIC FEVER

MOST COMMON CAUSATIVE DISEASES

- Algid MALARIA
- EBOLA VIRUS DISEASE: listed separately, these notes.
- YELLOW FEVER: listed separately, these notes.
- LASSA FEVER: listed separately, these notes.

LESS LIKELY CAUSATIVE DISEASES

- CRIMEAN-CONGO HEMORRHAGIC FEVER, described in the Condition Index.
- Rift Valley fever is described under ARBOVIRAL FEVER, these notes.

LEAST COMMON CAUSATIVE DISEASE

- DENGUE FEVER: listed in the Condition Index.

Dengue causes hemorrhagic fever in Asia; it is not directly contagious. Lassa, Ebola, Crimean-Congo and Rift Valley fevers can be directly transmitted from patients to bystanders. Hospital treatment is worthwhile, as it can make a big difference in the chances for survival. Ground transport to a higher-level facility must be in a towed trailer. In all of these cases antibiotics do no good whatsoever.

The geographic distribution of these diseases is changing by the day and week. The web site Pro-MED mail keeps track of the distributions.

HEPATITIS

In Ivory Coast, about 1/3 is hepatitis B, 1/3 is hepatitis E and 1/3 is hepatitis A or other viruses.

Hepatitis B transmission from mother to child is not common in this area except in southern Africa where it is readily transmitted from person to person within households. There is some soft evidence that one means of this transmission is bedbugs.

In the Gezira Region of Sudan, hepatitis B is more common in areas that are crowded and in people who have tattoos. 88% of those over 50 y.o. have had the disease.

In Niger, 100% of the people have had hepatitis B before 40 y.o; 29% carry an associated virus (hepatitis D) that causes liver CANCER.

In southern Africa, 5.5–14% of the people surveyed have had hepatitis B; the percentage was larger near the coast than inland.

In Mali, 42% of reproductive women have had hepatitis B.

In Lagos, half the cases of hepatitis are hepatitis B.

Hepatitis C is most common in Egypt, Libya and D. R. Congo.

Hepatitis E is a common problem all over Africa, especially Algeria, Chad, Ethiopia, Gambia, Kenya, Nigeria and Somalia. Hepatitis E epidemics occur in Somalia mid-May to mid-June. The incubation is about 40 days. Whole-body itching is common.

Similar regional diseases: YELLOW FEVER, LASSA FEVER and PNEUMONIA in Africans. There is protein in the urine with YELLOW FEVER.

In Central African Republic, an ARBOVIRAL FEVER, West Nile virus, may be indistinguishable.

In the Burundi area AMEBIASIS can look very similar; a trial treatment with METRONIDAZOLE might be useful.

If the patient has had recent close contact with newborn animals, he may have Q FEVER which responds to DOXYCYCLINE.

HERNIA

This is common in the groins of Africans; In the Kauta, D. R. Congo area, about 1/4 of the population have groin hernias. UMBILICAL HERNIA is extremely common in African children.

HIV INFECTION

The areas where HIV INFECTION is most prevalent in this region are: Botswana, Burundi, Central African Republic, Ivory Coast, Kenya, Mali, Mozambique, Namibia, Rwanda, South Africa, Zambia and Zimbabwe. TUBERCULOSIS and HIV INFECTION overlap so much that the WHO definition is not very helpful where both are common. In Uganda (where it is a rural as much as an urban disease), it is spread more by sex than blood.

There is usually about a 3–4 month interval between becoming infected and converting the blood test from negative to positive. The disease is very contagious in this stage.

Clinical

SHINGLES is commonly the first problem when a patient gets sick. Over 90% of patients with SHINGLES also have HIV.

In Central African Republic, the disease commonly presents with BELL'S PALSY; CANDIDIASIS and skin CANCER are common complications.

There is a peculiar rash that is common. It consists of little bumps, like soft warts, mainly on the hairy surfaces of the forearms, hands and feet. These bumps itch and, when they are scratched, they break open and release a small drop of clear liquid. Then they heal with a dark scar. The disease progresses during pregnancy.

Africa-specific parameters: PNEUMONIA must be treated with both CHLORAMPHENICOL and AMPICILLIN or else one of the CEPHALOSPORINs. In areas with SCHISTOSOMIASIS, treat all HIV-positive patients with PRAZIQUANTEL.

Schistosomiasis accelerates the progression of HIV infection.

About 33% of patients with respiratory symptoms have TUBERCULOSIS. Their skin tests and their sputum smears are both likely to be negative in spite of their having active disease. Non-lung TB is more common in AIDS patients than the general population. Lung TB in the presence of AIDS frequently affects the lower rather than the upper lung.

Resistance to drugs is developing in Uganda.

HOOKWORM

This is extremely common in central, NE and SW Cameroon; in Chad; in the Bushmen of Namibia; in the Pygmies of Rwanda and the Ituri region of D. R. Congo; on the Jos Plateau and in the Bauchi and Oyo States of Nigeria; and around Bangui, Central African Republic. It is common in central Burkina Faso; around Kinshasa, D. R. Congo; and in the Ogun State of Nigeria. In Ethiopia it is common only where there is agriculture and the altitude is less than 2000 meters (6600 ft.) though it occurs at higher altitudes.

HYDATID DISEASE

This is very common in arid northern Africa, especially along the Niger delta and Libya. It is also very prevalent amongst the people (especially Turkana) in northern Kenya, amongst the Toposa of southern Sudan, the Dassenach, Nyangatom, Hamar and Boran of SW Ethiopia and northern Kenya and amongst the Maasai of Tanzania. It occurs in arable southern Africa also. Where it is common it may be seen in children as well as adults though it affects mostly young to middle-aged adults.

HYPERTENSION

This is common in Africa, with complications being more common in Africans than in Europeans. Africans may be resistant to PROPRANOLOL.

Treatment

Mainly salt restriction, no smoking, weight control and no birth control pills for females, with available medications added as necessary.

HYPOGLYCEMIA

Other causes in Africa are AFRICAN SLEEPING SICKNESS and PLANT POISONING from unripe ackee. With ackee there is a rapid onset of symptoms. With AFRICAN SLEEPING SICKNESS the onset is gradual; nourishment should be provided with the treatment.

HYPOTHERMIA

This is a problem in the Sahara desert and at high elevations. (In the Sahara it gets very cold at night since the sand does not hold the heat well.)

INTESTINAL FLUKE

Heterophyiasis is a type of intestinal fluke that comes from eating raw fish in Egypt.

IRITIS

Regional causes are AFRICAN SLEEPING SICKNESS and LOIASIS.

IRRITABLE BOWEL

Similar regional disease: LIVER FLUKE.

JAUNDICE

Regional causes include YELLOW FEVER. The most common causes are HEPATITIS and MALARIA.

KATAYAMA DISEASE

In Africa, this refers to the initial stage of SCHISTOSOMIASIS (any kind), LOIASIS, GUINEA WORM or HYDATID DISEASE. Sometimes LASSA FEVER can cause a similar problem. It is more common with SCHISTOSOMIASIS MANSONI than SCHISTOSOMIASIS HEMATOBIUM. It is more common in expatriates than nationals.

KIDNEY DISEASE

Nephrotic kidney disease can also be caused by SICKLE CELL DISEASE, SCHISTOSOMIASIS HEMATOBIUM and PLANT POISONING due to impila. The most common causes in Africa are HEPATITIS B, MALARIA, SYPHILIS and SCHISTOSOMIASIS MANSONI. The prognosis is good if the cause is treated.

Regional causes

- Nephritic failure—SICKLE CELL DISEASE.
- Obstructive failure—SCHISTOSOMIASIS HEMATOBIUM.
- Infective failure—AFRICAN SLEEPING SICKNESS.
- Hemolytic failure—SICKLE CELL DISEASE.

KIDNEY INFECTION

Similar regional diseases: SCHISTOSOMIASIS HEMATOBIUM.

KIDNEY STONE

Similar regional disease: SCHISTOSOMIASIS HEMATOBIUM.

LARVA MIGRANS

The skin type is common in the Niger delta. One deep type can be caused by the bite of a fly in humid areas of central Africa (see LOIASIS). LOIASIS causes itching, pain and blindness.

Other types of larva migrans may (in the absence of laboratory facilities) be indistinguishable from LOIASIS. One of these is caused by a worm whose larval form is present in giant snails in Madagascar and Mauritius. When people eat the raw snails, they can acquire the parasite.

LASSA FEVER

Synonym: African hemorrhagic fever (which may also refer to other diseases peculiar to Africa, such as EBOLA VIRUS DISEASE and Marburg).

Mildly to severely ill; class 2–4; contagious; regional

The disease is present in West Africa, south and west of the Chad/Sudan/CAR border point. It is also present in SE Africa, the Lake Nyasa area and south of there to the SA border.

Age: any. **Who:** anyone who has not had that kind of fever. Medical care-givers, especially midwives who have delivered an infected woman, are particularly susceptible. **Onset:** usually over days.

Clinical

Necessary: a high fever with weakness and general body pains.

Usually: the patient has a headache, sore throat or chest pain. The chest pain is a kind of PERICARDITIS.

Occasionally: other symptoms are cough, pain with urination, abdominal pain, vomiting, red eyes, abnormal bleeding and a swollen face. Diarrhea occurs rarely.

The death rate is high, especially in pregnant women, those who have just delivered, in children under 12 y.o. and in babies born to infected mothers.

Complications: PERICARDITIS, HEMORRHAGIC FEVER, BRAIN DAMAGE, HEART FAILURE, KIDNEY DISEASE, SHOCK. When HEMORRHAGIC FEVER develops, there is a sudden drop in blood pressure on the seventh day of illness. With Lassa fever, about 1/4 will become deaf on the average, but the probability varies from one community to the next. Convalescence takes 2–4 weeks. The patient may become bald, but hair will grow back.

Similar diseases: see the list in ARBOVIRAL FEVERs; also YELLOW FEVER (bilirubin in urine), DENGUE FEVER (bone pain is worse), MALARIA (chest pain is unusual), SEPSIS.

There is a similar disease, O'nyong-nyong, in the Uganda/Rwanda/Tanzania area. It is carried by anopheles mosquitoes; see Volume 1 Appendix 10. The difference is that O'nyong-nyong has a severe arthritis connected to it, and it does not cause hemorrhage or death. Recovery is complete and spontaneous, but after a long time.

Bush laboratory: there may be protein in the urine.

TOC SYMPTOMS DIFFERENTIALS CONDITIONS DRUG INDEX REGIONAL NOTES INX

Treatment

Prevention: wear gloves and mask when caring for patients. Only transport the patient in a towed trailer. A vaccine is being developed.

Referrals. Laboratory: very sophisticated hospital laboratories can do blood tests for this. Facilities: intensive care unit, at least level 3. Practitioner: hematologist, infectious disease specialist, and/or someone with prior experience managing this disease.

Patient care: sitting up will minimize his pain. It is desirable to send out any patient who is more than five months pregnant; these women have a very high death rate. Lassa fever responds well to RIBAVIRIN, and immune serum from recovered patients can also be used. Therefore it is worthwhile to transport to a hospital. Neither the drug nor the serum should be used in the village situation.

LEPROSY

This is extremely common in the Sahel and less common, though not rare, in western and central Africa. Africans tend to get the indeterminate and tuberculoid types; less than 10% of their leprosy is lepromatous except for in Ethiopia where lepromatous is more common. Fair Caucasians get the borderline and lepromatous kinds. In Africa the distribution of leprosy is very patchy. If there is a tribal-language word for the disease, probably it was common in the past and still occurs. The countries where it is most common are, in order, Madagascar, Guinea, Niger, Ethiopia, Sudan, DR Congo, Nigeria. Other endemic countries: Benin, Burkina Faso, Chad, Ivory coast, Egypt, Mali, Mozambique, Senegal, Zambia.

In Chad a program of teaching patients about the disease and how to treat it and then letting them treat themselves, was extremely successful, resulting in good compliance.

LEPTOSPIROSIS

This is common in Ethiopia, the Comoros, Somalia, Reunion Island, Nigeria and probably elsewhere. It is mostly a rural disease which occurs during the rainy season.

Similar regional disease: YELLOW FEVER. If in doubt, treat for both.

LIVER FAILURE

The most common causes in this area are HEPATITIS, ALCOHOLISM, SCHISTOSOMIASIS MANSONI and SICKLE CELL DISEASE (mainly in West Africa).

Also consider SIDEROSIS and YELLOW FEVER.

LIVER FLUKE

Liver flukes are present only in some areas, mainly those that raise sheep or cattle. The are in Egypt, Madagascar, Uganda, Kenya and Malawi, possibly elsewhere. Only fascioliasis is present in this region.

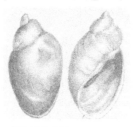

This is the kind of snail that carries Fasciola hepatica. Note the relatively large hole. The height of the snail is 1.4–2.5 cm. AB

LOIASIS

Cause: worm
Synonyms: loa-loa, eye worm, Calabar swellings.

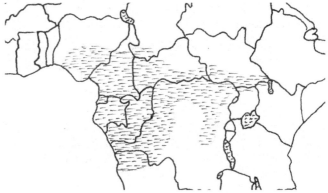

Loiasis occurs in humid central and west Africa. The shading shows the approximate distribution. PLoS Negl Trop Dis 5(6): 2011

Mildly to very ill; class 3; regional, humid areas, in and near rubber plantations and forested areas; never in urban areas. In the Congo it is most common south and central and more common amongst the Bantus than the Pygmies. About 50% of adults in some areas have or have had the problem, and it is one of the commonest medical complaints. In Uganda where the jungle has moved into previously arable areas, LOIASIS has come with it.

Age: any. **Who:** bitten by Chrysops flies. These usually bite below the knees. They prefer bare skin but can bite through socks. **Onset:** about 1 year after the bite.

Clinical

Necessary: the patient has one or more of the following symptoms.

- Small egg-sized lumps, painless or painful, appear on the hands and forearms, sometimes elsewhere on the body. They develop suddenly and last for 3–7 days only, then disappear gradually.
- There is general swelling without a definite lump.
- Worms are seen or felt moving underneath the skin or crossing the whites of the eyes. They are 2.5–7.5 cm (1–3 inches) long.

TOC SYMPTOMS DIFFERENTIALS CONDITIONS DRUG INDEX REGIONAL NOTES INX

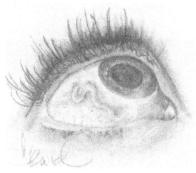

This is the appearance of a worm in a patient's eye. It may be smaller or larger than this. AB

Usually: the worm seeks soft, loose skin: breast, under the front of the tongue, the throat, penis, eyelids and eyes, scrotum. Warmth draws the worm to the surface; cold makes it dive for cover. When worms move under the skin, they cause numbness and tingling or pricking, itching, creeping sensations; occasionally shooting pains or weakness may develop. When they cross the eye, the patient complains first of itching, then of the sensation of having been punched in the eye. The eyes may swell, become red and the patient may have loss of vision.

Sometimes: expatriates have an immediate reaction to the bite. After the incubation period, in expatriates, symptoms of KATAYAMA DISEASE may occur first. Expatriates are more likely to have allergic reactions but negative blood tests (for the larvae) whereas nationals tend to have positive blood tests but few or no symptoms.

Complications: ENCEPHALITIS, blindness, STROKE, HEART FAILURE, KIDNEY DISEASE; PNEUMONIA when the worms first enter the body and migrate through the lungs.

Similar diseases: see Protocols B.6 and B.8. Other types of LARVA MIGRANS (of which this is one kind) may be indistinguishable.

Bush laboratory: the disease may cause protein, blood or both in the urine. Other diseases also cause this.

Treatment

Prevention: control flies, wear long trousers, use screens on houses. Light-colored clothing helps, since the flies are attracted to dark clothing.

Referrals: hospital labs can do blood tests; blood for the tests must be taken between 10 A.M. & 4 P.M.; sometimes several samples must be taken before one is positive. This disease may cause increased eosinophils in the blood count (other diseases may also). You should rely on history rather than lab for treatment, because the history is distinctive and the blood test is not sensitive In particular, never believe a negative test in an expatriate. National Institutes of Health in the States has a good blood test.

Patient care: In the past, IVERMECTIN was used, but there have been major problems with that; it is probably still safe in very mild cases. ALBENDAZOLE is probably safer. DIETHYLCARBAMAZINE might be useful. There can be major problems with any treatment. Check for ONCHOCERCIASIS with eye involvement. Check for FILARIASIS. In these cases, if you treat with DIETHYLCARBAMAZINE, the drug must be started slowly. Reactions to DEC or IVERMECTIN can be dangerous. Seek local advice. Normally DEC reactions are treated as ordinary ALLERGY, but they do not always respond to these medicines.

MALABSORPTION

The most common regional causes: SCHISTOSOMIASIS MANSONI and SPRUE (rarely).

MALARIA

In urban areas with major air pollution there will be no disease transmission. No transmission in these parts.

> Zimbabwe: Harare
>
> Mauritania: parts of the north.
>
> Ethiopia: Addis Ababa.
>
> Kenya: Nairobi—transmission is rare.

Since the mid-1990's, malaria has been moving to progressively higher altitudes. There is transmission up to 2500 meters or 8000 feet. Most of the malaria at the higher altitude is non-falciparum.

Cerebral malaria accounts for about 50% of all pediatric hospital admissions in some parts of Africa. It is a common cause of disability and death.

CHLOROQUINE resistance is present in Africa. In most areas the disease responds well to CHLOROQUINE plus CHLORPHENIRAMINE. In parts of eastern Sudan there is some QUININE resistance. ARTEMISININ eliminates the symptoms the soonest. The artemisia plant grows well in the highlands of central Ethiopia. A helpful website is www.anamed.net.

There is resistance to many drugs in Liberia; this is also a problem in Senegal and Guinea.

The percentage of malaria that is falciparum: Juba, Sudan: 84%; northern Cameroon: nearly 100%; Ituri region of D. R. Congo: 50%; over 50% in Rwanda. In parts of East Africa falciparum malaria is resistant to MEFLOQUINE.

A common complaint is pain in a band around the center back: "waist pain". In East Africa, there is frequently also pain in a band across the back of the shoulders. African children with malaria usually have vomiting and diarrhea. Chronic malaria causes TROPICAL SPLENOMEGALY, mainly in Uganda and Ethiopia.

Similar regional diseases: severe SICKLE CELL DISEASE may be confusing. In expatriates in East Africa, AFRICAN SLEEPING SICKNESS may be very similar. Look for and ask about the initial skin swelling in response to the fly bite.

MALNUTRITION

This is common throughout Africa. ANEMIA and XEROPHTHALMIA are common consequences. African children may have swellings in front of their ears as a consequence of poor nutrition. Camel's milk has more vitamin C than milk from other sources; it should be pasteurized.

Regional diseases associated with this are SICKLE CELL DISEASE, MEASLES, MONKEYPOX and (rarely) SPRUE.

MANSONELLOSIS PERSTANS

Cause: worm larva
Mildly ill; class 1–2; regional;

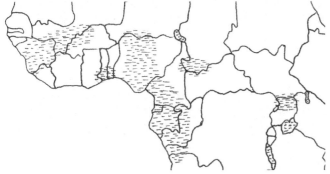

The shading shows where Mansonella perstans has been reported recently. It may occur elsewhere; older maps show a larger distribution. Information derived from Downes and Jacobsen Afr. J. Infect. Dis. (2010) 4(1): 7–14

Age: any, usually adults. **Who:** bitten by culicoides (see Volume 1 Appendix 10. **Onset:** gradual.

Clinical

Necessary: general joint pains without fever.

Usual in expatriates, *common* in nationals: shortness of breath, trouble breathing out, wheezing, itching. Other symptoms of ASTHMA or ALLERGY might also be present.

Sometimes: abdominal pain, especially the right upper abdomen. There may be chronic fatigue over a long time.

Similar diseases Joint pains without high fevers: ARTHRITIS, BRUCELLOSIS; Wheezing: ALLERGY, HEART FAILURE, TUBERCULOSIS; Abdominal pain: PEPTIC ULCER, AMEBIC LIVER DISEASE, GALLBLADDER DISEASE, IRRITABLE BOWEL.

Treatment

Prevention: culicoides are the same as "no-see-ems", tiny insects. See Volume 1 Appendix 10 for instructions as to how to deal with them. One can prevent the disease by taking IVERMECTIN every 3 months.

Referrals: laboratory: there may be an increased eosinophil count. The worm larvae might be seen in a blood smear. Unlike LOIASIS and FILARIASIS, they might be found any time of day or night.

Patient care: traditionally people have used MEBENDAZOLE or else ALBENDAZOLE. DOXYCYCLINE works well by killing the bacteria associated with the parasite. DEC may also be used.

Results: within 1–2 weeks.

MEASLES

Most cases occur in children less than 5 y.o. in unimmunized areas and in 6–12 month-olds in immunized areas. MALNUTRITION in older children and DEHYDRATION in babies, are common causes of death with measles. In all age groups, many deaths are caused by PNEUMONIA. A lack of VITAMIN A in the diet (yellow and orange produce) is associated with both blindness and a higher death rate in several areas. Measles is usually more severe in older children and adults than in babies.

MENINGITIS

Meningitis belt epidemics are caused by meningococcus group A. There have been major epidemics in Kenya and Uganda, including the southern parts of these countries and also in Angola which is well outside the meningitis belt. Reportedly the meningitis belt is expanding because of deforestation; the disease tends to spread rapidly in hot, dry areas. Yearly epidemics occur in the Sahel meningitis belt, February to April.

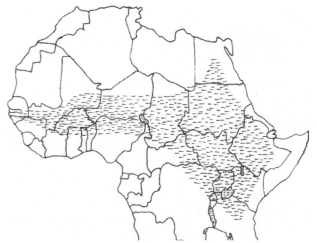

The shaded area is the traditional location of the meningitis belt. Meningitis can occur anywhere.

Similar regional disease: AFRICAN SLEEPING SICKNESS can appear similar.

TOC   SYMPTOMS   DIFFERENTIALS   CONDITIONS   DRUG INDEX   REGIONAL NOTES   INX

MENOPAUSE

African women seldom complain of these symptoms.

MIGRAINE HEADACHE

AFRICAN SLEEPING SICKNESS may appear similar.

MONKEYPOX

Regional: the vast majority of monkeypox cases have been from D. R. Congo.

Cause: virus

Moderately to severely ill; class 1–3; contagious, slightly; .

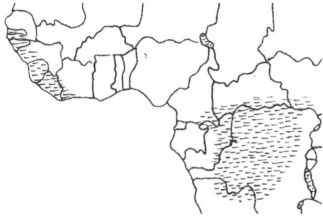

The shading shows the known distribution of monkeypox. Derived from ProMED-mail.

Age: any, mostly less than 15 y.o. **Who:** mostly from towns with a population less than 5000. Most patients report contact with monkeys or small rodents; males more than females. **Onset:** gradually after 7–17 days incubation; begins over 1–3 days, with illness before blisters.

Clinical

The clinical illness is less severe with merely touching or being near, more severe with a bite or scratch from an animal. It infects prairie dogs.

Necessary: fever, headache, backache, sick in bed. Lymph nodes are very large, differentiating this from CHICKEN POX. A fever occurs first. Thereafter, sometime during the first 4 days, a rash of tiny blisters begins on the face and rapidly spreads from there to the rest of the body.[1] The rash is heaviest on the face and limbs. There may be swelling of the skin with the blisters. It is very dense on the hands. It affects the palms and soles in 70% of cases and the mouth in more than half.

Sometimes: if it involves the eyes, the patient may develop KERATITIS. The fever may drop when the rash starts. The patient probably has swollen eyelids. About 1/2 have sore throats and 1/4 have painful skin blisters in the genital area.

In 1/3 there is a second fever, at which time the blister contents change from watery to milky. The rash is usually healed or healing by 4 weeks. The skin spots darken first, then lighten, then the color becomes normal.

Complications: pitting scars, IMPETIGO, PNEUMONIA, DEHYDRATION, MALNUTRITION, EYE INFECTION, SEPSIS, ENCEPHALITIS, BRAIN DAMAGE, death. The death rate is 10% to 30% and occurs almost entirely in young children.

Similar diseases: see Protocol B.13: Fever And Back Pain. Only in monkeypox and smallpox does blistering rash break out over the whole body at once. Before the rash the disease may resemble those listed in Protocol B.2; CHICKENPOX is similar and occurs worldwide. With monkeypox, the lymph nodes are large and the rash breaks out within hours rather than spreading from one part of the skin to another over days. Also, with monkeypox the patient is moderately to very ill whereas in CHICKENPOX a child is only mildly ill (although an adult with CHICKEN POX may be very ill.)

Treatment

Prevention: immunization for smallpox also prevents monkeypox. This immunization is contraindicated in HIV-positive people.

Referrals: laboratory; a very sophisticated hospital lab can do a blood test for this. This kind of facility is likely to be found only in Western countries and the results, in any case, will not influence the management of the disease.

Patient care: cidofovir is an antiviral medication that might be helpful, but generally the treatment is merely supportive. Prevent DEHYDRATION and MALNUTRITION with water and food. PROMETHAZINE may be used for vomiting. Use ACETAMINOPHEN for fevers. Milk from a nursing woman who has had the disease (look for the pitting scars) may be helpful for children. Keep the skin and bedding clean. Use antibiotic or antiseptic ointment on broken blisters.

MONONUCLEOSIS

Children in Ethiopia develop the disease and immunity to it before 10 y.o.; therefore one would not likely see the illness in teens and adults.

Similar regional diseases: LASSA FEVER, BURKITT LYMPHOMA, TOXOPLASMOSIS, TUBERCULOSIS. AFRICAN SLEEPING SICKNESS (the kind found in West Africa) might cause large lymph nodes in the back of the neck.

MOSSY FOOT

The following areas reportedly have mossy foot: Cameroon highlands; Morocco; the entire Rift Valley and particularly the Wolaitta area of southern Ethiopia.

---

1 Rarely the rash might begin on the limbs and spread to the center of the body.

MYCETOMA

This is especially common in Sudan and Niger. In Nigeria among the Igbos, it affects the nose. It is uncommon in Central African Republic and in the highlands of central Ethiopia.

A related disease, chromoblastomycosis, is common in Madagascar, most common in barefoot males in rural areas. It gives the appearance of giant WARTS, covering whole areas of skin. It is treatable only with drugs that must be used by a physician in a hospital setting. Surgery can also help.

In Mali, the most common form in the south, (south of a line between Bamako and Gao) that which causes yellow grains, can be treated as follows: DAPSONE plus CO-TRIMOXAZOLE, both for 6–9 months. You may substitute STREPTOMYCIN for either one of these medicines, using the other oral medicine in addition. If this does not work, surgery may be necessary.

If the mycetoma has black grains, it most likely needs surgery, but MICONAZOLE may help.

There are no reliable maps.

MYIASIS

The Tumbu fly maggot and the Zaire floor maggot are common and peculiar to Africa. Other types of myiasis may also occur.

TUMBU FLY MAGGOT

This is also known as putsi fly or ver du cayor. It is found in scattered areas south of the Sahara. The fly lays its eggs early in the morning, late in the afternoon or in the shade; they are never laid under the noon sun. The egg is laid on wet clothing; when the clothing is worn, the larva burrows into the skin, causing swelling and a small ulcer.

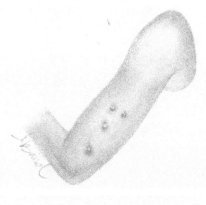

The appearance of tumbu fly lesions on an arm. AB

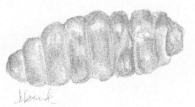

The appearance of a tumbu fly maggot, magnified, looking down from above. Note the segments and the proportions. AB

Treat by putting petroleum jelly on the holes, then squeeze or pick the larva out. This also helps with the diagnosis, because the critter's attempts to breathe cause little bubbles to come up and out through the petroleum jelly. Prevent the problem by totally drying or ironing clothing before wearing.

ZAIRE FLOOR MAGGOT

This is found from northern Nigeria and southern Sudan south to Natal, from sea level to 2250 meters (7500 feet), in arid and humid areas both. The larva is off-white, resembling the tumbu fly larva. It becomes red after sucking the blood of a sleeping victim. When it is full, it drops off the person and hides in the floor near the sleeping mat. The bite is painless. Prevention lies in the use of sleeping surfaces up off the floor.

Similar regional diseases: LOIASIS.

NAIROBI EYE

This is eye pain caused by a flying insect in East Africa. The insect is brown and orange, about 1 cm long and 3 mm wide. They are present in large numbers certain times of year. They tend to fly to the eyes. They cause severe, burning pain of the eyelids, possibly with swelling. The eyeballs are unaffected. The pain responds well to CORTISONE CREAM or any other corticosteroid cream, rubbed on the lids. Do not get these creams into the eye!

ONCHOCERCIASIS

Synonym: sowda.

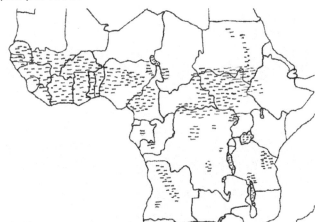

The shaded areas are where the disease has historically been found. Reportedly its distribution has changed drastically due to public health measures. It has been eliminated from some areas, but it has appeared in others.

TOC SYMPTOMS DIFFERENTIALS CONDITIONS DRUG INDEX REGIONAL NOTES INX

Persons with HIV INFECTION tend to have fewer symptoms than those with good immunity.

Sowda is a form that is found in northern Sudan and northern Nigeria. The skin becomes swollen and covered with scaly bumps. There is marked swelling of the lymph nodes, usually in the groins.

In areas where LOIASIS and onchocerciasis coexist, IVERMECTIN should not be used for mass treatment: southeastern Nigeria, southern and central Cameroon, southern Central African Republic, Equatorial Guinea, Gabon, the northern and western portions of D. R. Congo.

ONYALAI

This is a type of HEMORRHAGIC FEVER. The patient develops fever, red eyes, mouth pain, abnormal bleeding (nosebleed, heavy menses, bloody urine or stool, bleeding from minor wounds) that will not stop. There may be large blood blisters. It must be treated at a hospital. SCURVY may appear similar.

PANCREATITIS

A recurrent form of this that results in MALABSORPTION and DIABETES is common in eastern and western Africa.

PARAGONIMIASIS

This occurs in Cameroon, the Congo valley and The Gambia. In Nigeria it is found in the areas surrounding Okigwi, southwest of Enugu. It is also in the Bong area of Liberia. It is not generally common.

PARKINSON'S DISEASE

Similar regional diseases: ENTERIC FEVER in Nigeria; lathyrism (see PLANT POISONING). AFRICAN SLEEPING SICKNESS, appearing similar, must be diagnosed by a spinal tap at a hospital; the parasites will not be in the blood at the stage of trembling.

PELVIC INFECTION

Other causes are TUBERCULOSIS and GONORRHEA. *Similar regional disease:* SCHISTOSOMIASIS HEMATOBIUM.

PEPTIC ULCER

This is particularly common in northern Ethiopia, West African coastal countries, central D. R. Congo, great lakes area of east central Africa, Nairobi area. Frequently it is responsive to a combination of antibiotics and BISMUTH SUBSALICYLATE.

PERICARDITIS

This may occur with LASSA FEVER. Pericarditis is similar to endomyocardial fibrosis, a form of HEART FAILURE (restrictive type) found in east Africa, but pericarditis is curable.

PERTUSSIS

This is especially common in Ethiopia, D. R. Congo, Senegal, Benin, Chad, Congo, Guinea, Liberia, Mali, Mauritania, Togo, Uganda and Burkina Faso.

PHIMOSIS

Similar regional disease: SCHISTOSOMIASIS HEMATOBIUM.

PIG-BEL

Pig-bel occurs in Uganda.

PLAGUE

There is risk of plague in Madagascar, many areas; Malawi southern region; Mozambique, Tete Province; Tanzania, Tanga region; Uganda, Western Region and by Lake Victoria; D. R. Congo, Haut Zaire Province; Zambia, Southern Province; and Zimbabwe, Matabeleland North. It occurs in Western Sahara and in the Kalahari Desert area. In Tanzania and D. R. Congo, it occurs mostly January to March.

PLANT POISONING

See the Condition Index for types of plant poisoning that occur in multiple regions and for the general treatment of plant poisoning. The types listed below occur in some parts of Africa.

Ackee; argemone oil; impila; khasari, khat, konzo, lolism, mantakassa, miraa, miscara, muiragi, tobacco-cow's urine.

PNEUMONIA

In The Gambia, a single injection of triple PENICILLIN worked well for pneumonia in previously healthy people. In Zimbabwe, CO-TRIMOXAZOLE worked just as well as PENICILLIN.

PNEUMOTHORAX

This is rare in Africans and common in Asians.

POLIO

The incidence of polio is decreasing, due to public health campaigns. It occurs wherever local religious or government leaders oppose immunization. It will probably be found in areas of civil unrest, where government workers and health professionals are reluctant to go.

PROCTITIS

The most likely causes are the SEXUALLY TRANSMITTED DISEASEs. This may be due to SCHISTOSOMIASIS MANSONI, SCHISTOSOMIASIS HEMATOBIUM or SCHISTOSOMIASIS INTERCALATUM in areas where these are common.

PROSTATITIS

This may be caused by or mimic or SCHISTOSOMIASIS HEMATOBIUM as well as the worldwide similar diseases.

PYOMYOSITIS

This is more common in the rainy season in eastern Africa, but there is no seasonality in Nigeria. It is almost always caused by staph; drugs that are specifically meant for staph are best, but they are expensive and may not be available. The best common treatment is a combination of CHLORAMPHENICOL plus ERYTHROMYCIN or else CO-TRIMOXAZOLE plus ERYTHROMYCIN. RIFAMPIN, a drug that is usually used for tuberculosis, is also active against staph. It is expensive. A similar condition in West Africa is SICKLE CELL DISEASE.

Q FEVER

This is found throughout Africa except for the Sahara and the Kalahari deserts. It is found throughout Madagascar It is particularly common in northern Tanzania.

RABIES

It is a major problem in Nigeria, Ethiopia and probably in other parts of Africa as well. It does not occur on the Azores, Canary and Madeira islands. It occurs in Mozambique but is not common. The paralytic form is quite common in West Africa.

RELAPSING FEVER

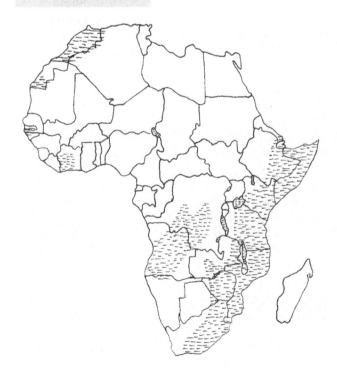

The known distribution of tick-borne relapsing fever The disease tends to be present for a while and generally devastating, then disappear.

In Morroco, southern Mali and in west and central Africa, this is associated with small mammals. It is common. In East Africa there is only human to tick to human transmission. Therefore it is not as common, since it is not maintained in wild animals.

In East Africa, in addition to the other symptoms, there are also red eyes and red-orange urine. The initial fever lasts between 12 hours and 17 days, with the intervening fever-free period being between 1 day and 2 months. When the fever falls it does so rapidly, with drenching sweats. When pregnant women get the disease they commonly die within the first 48 hours if they are not treated. Those who survive frequently give birth prematurely, and commonly their infants die.

Similar regional diseases: YELLOW FEVER shows protein in the urine.

RHEUMATIC FEVER

This is more common in northern and southern Africa than in central and western. It tends to be severe and nearly always involves the heart. The most common age is 6–10 y.o. in central and eastern Africa, but teens and young adults in the Sudan. The rash is rare in any case and impossible to see on black skin. Check for warmth.

RHINITIS

In Western countries this refers to the runny nose caused by ALLERGY or a RESPIRATORY INFECTION (a cold). In southern Africa there is a peculiar form in people with large noses who live in dry areas such as the highveld in Transvaal. The patient complains of an obstructed nose and a loss of smell; his nose is full of fermenting, dried secretions. Relatives and friends complain of the foul, rotten odor of the patient's breath.

Treatment Clean out the nose with a pair of forceps. Then rinse it three times a day with 5 ml (1 teaspoon) of baking soda dissolved in a cup of water. Send the patient home with glycerin nose drops which will keep the nose moist and prevent the problem from recurring.

RUBELLA

This may resemble AFRICAN SLEEPING SICKNESS with large nodes in the back of the neck along with general aching and fever.

SANDFLY FEVER

SANDFLY FEVER is a type of arboviral fever carried by sand flies along the Nile and in northern Africa. The description is in the Condition Index.

SCABIES

A common complication of scabies is IMPETIGO caused by strep; this may cause KIDNEY DISEASE of the nephritic type.

SCHISTOSOMIASIS HEMATOBIUM

Cause: worm

Synonyms: urinary bilharziasis, snail fever, bilharziasis.

Not ill to very ill; class 2; regional. It is especially frequent where there are dams and irrigation canals. Over half the population may be affected.

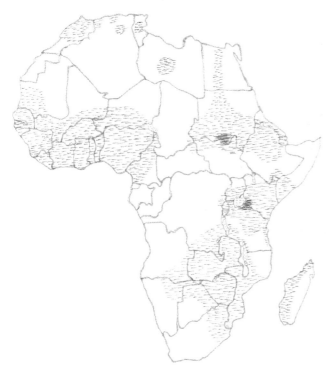

The known distribution of schistosomiasis hematobium. There is a spotty distribution within the shaded area.

Age: any, but especially boys 5–15 y.o. who like to swim.
Who: skin exposed to water in which infected snails live.
Onset: 10–12 weeks after exposure, then over days to weeks.

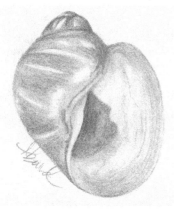

The kinds of snails that transmit this disease. Note that the hole is more than half the height of the snail and there are only 3–4 swirls. The snail is very small, total height 0.7 to 1.5 cm. AB

Initial clinical:

There may be itching of the skin for 2–3 days. Expatriates may begin with KATAYAMA DISEASE: fevers, low abdominal pain, fatigue and symptoms of ALLERGY.

Later clinical:

Necessary: the patient develops bloody urine. Blood may be visible only or mainly at the end of urination. A urine dipstick will demonstrate that it is present.

Usually: there is frequent urination and pain with urination. Nationals may just have bloody urine without other symptoms. Genital symptoms may begin in little girls before puberty: wounds, bleeding, pain and discharge. Women commonly have pelvic discomfort, VAGINITIS symptoms and itching.

Maybe: there is kidney pain resembling KIDNEY STONE and leading to KIDNEY DISEASE. There may be swelling of the end of the penis and possibly bloody semen. This may swell the kidney(s).

Still later clinical:

Maybe: the patient may have to urinate frequently and may dribble, because the bladder becomes rigid; it cannot enlarge to hold its usual volume of urine. Schistosomiasis in returning travelers is mostly without symptoms. However, spinal cord invasion, which is usually a late complication, may appear early.

Complications: ANEMIA and weight loss. The disease contributes to MALNUTRITION. Bladder CANCER may occur, as may KIDNEY INFECTION, inability to urinate, sores and growths on the penis or in the vagina, PELVIC INFECTION and sterility in females, KIDNEY DISEASE, URETHRAL STRICTURE and occasionally RESPIRATORY INFECTION from migrating worms. This disease increases the transmission of HIV INFECTION because it, like SEXUALLY TRANSMITTED DISEASES disrupts the pink moist surfaces.

Either sex may develop thinning and weakening of the bones, resulting in fractures from minor injuries. Sometimes, after years, the worms invade the lungs, causing RESPIRATORY FAILURE and HEART FAILURE. An occasional complication in males is a BLADDER STONE; men with stones cannot urinate unless they jump up and down. Their urine may be bloody during the day and normal at night. In Sudan, one usually does not see the severe bladder problems in older people that are found in some other areas of Africa.

Sometimes this causes problems with the spinal cord: back pain, sharp shooting limb pains, weakness, numbness and tingling and inability to initiate urination. Spinal cord schistosomiasis must be treated promptly with PRAZIQUANTEL and PREDNISONE, not waiting for lab results which may be falsely negative—do this with anyone who has had a prior exposure at any time in his/her life. Higher level imaging (MRI) is helpful.

Similar diseases: SCHISTOSOMIASIS MANSONI (may be indistinguishable); SEXUALLY TRANSMITTED DISEASES; URETHRITIS (visible pus from penis or female urethra); KIDNEY INFECTION (also nitrites and/or leukocytes in urine); KIDNEY DISEASE of other causes; ALLERGY (hives) from other causes; PROSTATITIS (usually men over 50 y.o. only); TB of the genitals; FILARIASIS. This disease may cause VAGINITIS-type symptoms.

Bush laboratory: it is possible to hatch the worm eggs with simple equipment and see the larvae; see Appendix 2 in Volume 1. Provided this is done carefully, it is more sensitive (but less specific) than looking for worm eggs under a microscope.

Treatment

Prevention: avoid physical contact with water in lakes and streams that may have schistosomiasis snails. Use latrines; eliminate snails. Let a bucket of water without snails stand overnight before using it for washing. Reportedly ARTEMISININ works to prevent the disease if taken at the time of exposure. MEFLOQUINE is reportedly helpful also.

Referrals: laboratory: afternoon urine contains blood and protein when checked by dipstick. Laboratories can examine urine under a microscope to see worm eggs. There may be increased eosinophils in a blood count early in the infection, especially in expatriates, but they may be absent later on. Facilities: advanced imaging such as CT and MRI might be helpful, as well as biopsies.

Patient care: PRAZIQUANTEL; METRIFONATE is a cheaper alternative for widespread use. PREDNISONE or PREDNISOLONE might be helpful additionally. Seek medical advice. NIRIDAZOLE is an old, dangerous drug that should no longer be used. The anti-malarial ARTEMISININ-type drugs with MEFLOQUINE are reportedly effective in about 60% of the cases.

Results: improvement starting one month from the PRAZIQUANTEL treatment, complete (if it ever will be) in 6 months. You should do lab determinations to evaluate the effect of the treatment 3 and 6 months after the drug is given.

SCHISTOSOMIASIS INTERCALATUM

Cause: worm

Synonym: bilharzia

Not ill to moderately ill; class 2; regional in western equatorial Africa.

In Port Harcourt, Nigeria, 6% of the children checked had the problem; there was no other kind of schistosomiasis in the area. It is common in equatorial Guinea, in a suburb of Bata. It occurs in Cameroon, Gabon and in an area near Kinshasa, D. R. Congo. It also may occur in Chad, Central African Republic and Congo.

There is a very heavily infected area in Cameroon, department of Mungo and town of Loum. It does not cause human liver disease. It is otherwise the same as SCHISTOSOMIASIS MANSONI.

Age: mostly children. **Who:** those exposed to water containing infected snails. **Onset:** slowly, over weeks to months.

Clinical

This is cattle schistosomiasis that infects humans in central Africa. It causes pain in the left-lower abdomen which increases before each episode of diarrhea. The diarrhea may be bloody.

Similar diseases: DYSENTERY due to amebae; also see listing under SCHISTOSOMIASIS MANSONI in the Condition Index.

Treatment

PRAZIQUANTEL. PREDNISONE or PREDNISOLONE along with the PRAZIQUANTEL might be helpful. Seek medical advice.

SCHISTOSOMIASIS MANSONI

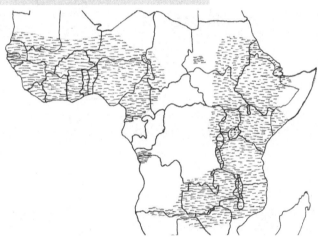

The known distribution of schistosomiasis Mansoni and intercalatum. The two are indistinguishable for your purposes. The distribution is spotty within the shaded areas.

In South Sudan the disease has a more rapid onset than in the north, and it tends to be more severe.

Treatment PRAZIQUANTEL. In D. R. Congo sometimes this drug causes abdominal pain and bloody diarrhea within 30 minutes of the first dose. Do not to stop the drug for this.

SCURVY

Patients with SIDEROSIS are also susceptible to this. It occurs in refugee camps since most relief foods are not fresh. It develops within a few weeks on relief foods. Older females are usually the first affected.

TOC   SYMPTOMS   DIFFERENTIALS   CONDITIONS   DRUG INDEX   REGIONAL NOTES   INX

SEIZURES

Regional disease that may cause seizures AFRICAN SLEEPING SICKNESS, ENCEPHALITIS, ONCHOCERCIASIS.

SEPSIS

Patients with TROPICAL SPLENOMEGALY are very susceptible.

SEXUALLY TRANSMITTED DISEASE

SYPHILIS and HIV INFECTION are most common in urban areas, except for Uganda and Central African Republic, where they are also common in the rural areas. Lower socio-economic prostitutes in Nairobi almost all have at least one SEXUALLY TRANSMITTED DISEASE; CHANCROID is by far the most common and SYPHILIS is second. In Zulus in South Africa all the STD's occur, including DONOVANOSIS. SYPHILIS positivity is about 40%.

SICKLE CELL DISEASE

This generally occurs in persons whose genetic origins are from the countries of west and central Africa that border on the Atlantic.

This is quite rare in Burkina Faso and in East Africa. In Kenya most cases are along the eastern coast and along the southwest border with Uganda. It occurs in Uganda.

SPOTTED FEVER tick typhus

This occurs in three areas.
- Southeast of a line between Bur Sudan (on the Red Sea coast) and the westernmost Namibia/South Africa border. It is common in northern Tanzania and commonly fatal
- Along the Mediterranean coast.
- A few scattered areas of West Africa.

Synonyms in this area: African tick typhus, African tick bite fever.

The African form of spotted fever, is especially common in Rwanda, in arid East Africa north of the equator, in arable and coastal southeast and southern Africa and in the forested areas of coastal western Africa.

It is transmitted by cattle ticks. If you are considering this diagnosis, a valuable clue is finding a tiny black scab or scabs with red halo(s). There are frequently multiple scabs, but there may be none.

The rash associated with African tick typhus shows fairly large (1 cm diameter), pinkish or reddened, flat or slightly raised areas on white skin, possibly with a little blistering, a countable number, probably less than 20, easily missed.

The disease can be rapidly fatal. Treat it on the mere suspicion. Antibiotics should be given until there have been at least two days with no fevers whatsoever.

SPRUE

This occurs rarely in Nigeria, Sudan and Uganda. It is common in dark-skinned nationals in southern Africa. It does not cause ANEMIA in this area.

STREP INFECTION

This is the most frequent cause of sore throat; it must be treated adequately to avoid RHEUMATIC FEVER which is common.

STROKE

This is not uncommon in Uganda. It is most often due to HYPERTENSION. Other common causes of stroke are SICKLE CELL DISEASE, SEPSIS, TOXEMIA, HEART FAILURE, RHEUMATIC FEVER, SYPHILIS and ARBOVIRAL FEVER. In affected areas, it may be due to SCHISTOSOMIASIS (either S. Mansoni or S. hematobium), but only rarely.

Similar regional diseases: AFRICAN SLEEPING SICKNESS (slower onset), SICKLE CELL DISEASE, LASSA FEVER (fever) and HYDATID DISEASE.

STRONGYLOIDIASIS

This is especially common in southwest Cameroon, in the area of Kinshasa, D. R. Congo and in children of the Bushmen of Namibia. It is common in Ogum, Oyo and Bauchi States, Nigeria; Congo; Guinea-Bissau; Central African Republic; and Somalia. It is also common amongst pygmies of D. R. Congo and Rwanda.

Other diseases that decrease natural immunity and thus cause the complication of SEPSIS with this are TROPICAL SPLENOMEGALY and AFRICAN SLEEPING SICKNESS.

SYPHILIS

The rash of secondary syphilis may itch in black Africans. Incoordination is a rare symptom in tertiary syphilis in Africans. In Uganda 33% of adults have positive blood tests for syphilis; in Rwanda, 2%–28%; in Tanzania, Congo, Gabon, Central African Republic and Ethiopia about 17%; and in Burundi, 7.8%. Syphilis of newborns is very common in Mozambique. National physicians are likely to not recognize syphilis. The reason is that medical textbooks are written in the West where the disease has been largely eliminated since the 1940's through mandatory testing of pregnant women. Authors don't write about conditions they never see.

Those with positive blood tests for syphilis are also more likely than others to be infected with HIV. In northern Mauritania and Burkina Faso, much of the syphilis is really TREPONARID, the kind that is not a venereal disease but is transmitted by flies and direct contact. This is probably also true in the rest of arid Africa.

TAPEWORM

Fish tapeworm occurs in Madagascar, Madeira Islands and Central African Republic. Beef and/or pork tapeworms are common in Ethiopia, Kenya and Bauchi State, Nigeria; they occur but are not common in Kavango Territory, Namibia. Rat and beef tapeworms are both common in central Burkina Faso and amongst the pygmies of Rwanda.

TETANUS

This is very common in newborns in Somalia, Nigeria and Ivory Coast. In Ethiopia, it accounts for about 10% of all the deaths in newborns. Some newborns of immunized African mothers may have the disease. Hand-washing by midwives has proved to be a very good preventive in Senegal.

THALLASEMIA

This is very common, but in Africans it is usually a form that is not severe. Indians, Arabs and persons from northern Africa may have a severe form of the disease. In southern Africa ONYALAI may appear similar.

TINEA

Similar regional diseases: AFRICAN SLEEPING SICKNESS rash in Whites, YAWS, TREPONARID, ONCHOCERCIASIS, VITILIGO.

TOXEMIA

This is by far the most common cause of coma in pregnant women in most parts of Africa.

TOXOPLASMOSIS

This is common in Africa (especially in humid areas), but you may not recognize it, because most cases have no symptoms at all. It is particularly important for pregnant women to avoid the infection.

TRACHOMA

This is not a major problem in Liberia or D. R. Congo, but it is in most of the rest of Africa. It used to be very common in northern Nigeria, but it is becoming rare there.

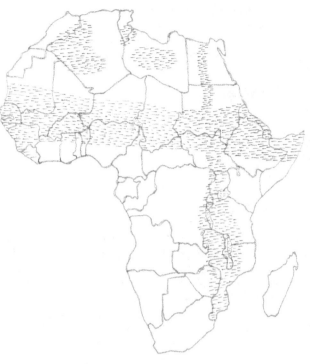

Trachoma occurs all over the world. The shaded areas are those where it is most common.

TREPONARID

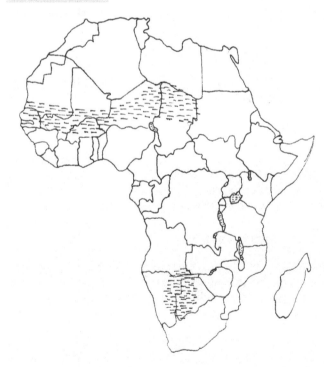

The known distribution of treponarid; it may occur in any hot, dry area with poor sanitation.

Though it is found only in dry areas, it is more common during the rainy season. In Burkina Faso, this is very common amongst the Touareg, Peul and Deon peoples. It occurs in western, northern and southern South Sudan, not in the east so far.

TRICHINOSIS

This is known to occur in West Africa, from Nigeria to Ivory Coast and in the lakes region of East Africa.

Similar regional diseases: AFRICAN SLEEPING SICKNESS, LASSA FEVER.

TRICHURIASIS

This is very common in Africa. In southwest and south central Cameroon, in the Pygmies of Ituri region, D. R. Congo and Rwanda. It is also common in Bauchi State, Oyo State and Ogun State, Nigeria and amongst the adult bushmen of Namibia. It is uncommon in central Burkina Faso; in Calabar, Nigeria; and near the northern Central African Republic/ Cameroon border.

TROPICAL SPASTIC PARAPARESIS

In Ivory Coast, 7.4% of the prostitutes are affected, as well as 13.7% of those with LEPROSY. It is a common cause of difficulty walking. It may occur in the absence of HIV INFECTION. A local similar disease is PLANT POISONING due to lathyrism.

TROPICAL SPLENOMEGALY

Found mainly and commonly in Nigeria, Sudan, Uganda, Zambia, Ethiopia and D. R. Congo.

TROPICAL ULCER

This may be caused by SICKLE CELL DISEASE, CUTANEOUS LEISHMANIASIS and GUINEA WORM may be nearly indistinguishable. In Zimbabwe, it is most common in the rainy months and in teens or younger children.

TUBAL PREGNANCY

The most likely cause is a SEXUALLY TRANSMITTED DISEASE such as CHLAMYDIA or GONORRHEA. SCHISTOSOMIASIS HEMATOBIUM, SCHISTOSOMIASIS MANSONI and TUBERCULOSIS may also contribute to this.

TUBERCULOSIS

In most of Africa it is very common, especially in crowded urban areas and amongst the poor and malnourished. The following countries report many cases: Swaziland, Comoros, Lesotho, Somalia, D. R. Congo, Ethiopia and Reunion Island. In Mauritania there is much drug-resistant tuberculosis.

A peculiar manifestation of TB is the slow growth of hard, painless swellings in the hands and feet. There is no effect on the skin in these cases and these areas do not become ABSCESSes.

Skin TB is particularly common in Ghana, Nigeria, Uganda, South Sudan and Mozambique. In children this may cause large, tender lumps on the shins and the hairy forearms. It is treated like ordinary TB. Surgery may be helpful.

Abdominal TB is common in Africans. It causes diarrhea, burning abdominal pain, lumps in the abdomen, fluid in the abdomen and ACUTE ABDOMEN Type 3, in that order of frequency.

Bone TB affecting the spine is common in Africa; it accounts for about 6% of all TB cases in Burkina Faso, being particularly common there.

PERICARDITIS is commonly caused by TB in southern Africa

Similar regional diseases: with TB in Africans, facial skin will be lighter than the skin of others of the same ethnic group and a little yellowish. HIV INFECTION is indistinguishable in most areas of Africa. PARAGONIMIASIS causes similar symptoms as lung TB, but the patient does not lose weight or feel ill.

About 1/3 of HIV INFECTION patients with respiratory symptoms have TUBERCULOSIS. They tend to respond well to treatment temporarily, but are more likely than others to relapse. They remain contagious for a very long time.

In Malawi, 1/3 of the patients with TB have clubbed finger tips, similar to people with long-standing RESPIRATORY INFECTIONs.

TURISTA

This is frequently responsive to ERYTHROMYCIN.

Diarrhea with blood may be caused by SCHISTOSOMIASIS (any kind).

Over 90% of Bantus have chronic diarrhea when they consume milk, due to LACTOSE INTOLERANCE.

In Zaria, northern Nigeria, severe diarrhea in children under 12 y.o. usually has a bacterial cause. The bacteria usually respond to ERYTHROMYCIN. Those over 12 y.o. more often have diarrhea caused by WORMS, GIARDIASIS or SCHISTOSOMIASIS MANSONI. ROTAVIRUS is a common virus that causes diarrhea and vomiting; the problem lasts for long enough to cause or exacerbate MALNUTRITION.

TOC   SYMPTOMS   DIFFERENTIALS   CONDITIONS   DRUG INDEX   REGIONAL NOTES   INX

It occurs mostly in infants and mostly during the dry season all over Africa. Children should be fed extra when they recover enough to tolerate food.

Campylobacter, a bacterial cause of diarrhea, likewise occurs mostly in the dry season in Africa. Untreated, it lasts over 8 days, is associated with MALNUTRITION and responds to ERYTHROMYCIN. Animals of all sorts may harbor the germ, and it is carried to humans by flies. It is common around Bangui, Central African Republic; and Kivu Province, D. R. Congo.

TYPHUS

There have been major outbreaks during civil unrest .

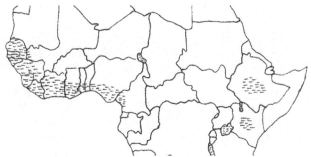

The known distribution of murine typhus. It may occur anywhere rats are plentiful.

URETHRAL STRICTURE

This may also be caused by SCHISTOSOMIASIS HEMATOBIUM or SCHISTOSOMIASIS MANSONI.

URINARY OBSTRUCTION

This may also be caused by SCHISTOSOMIASIS HEMATOBIUM or SCHISTOSOMIASIS MANSONI.

VAGINITIS

This may also be caused by SCHISTOSOMIASIS HEMATOBIUM or SCHISTOSOMIASIS MANSONI.

VISCERAL LEISHMANIASIS

CLINICAL

Sudanese patients frequently have generally enlarged lymph nodes. Africans tend to have large lymph nodes in their groins. Local lore is helpful since symptoms differ according to area. After the illness Africans may have decreased black skin pigmentation and a dry, non-shiny skin texture.

This occurs in Gedaref State, Sudan. In Sudan there may be symptoms of burning feet or GALLBLADDER DISEASE. More than 50% of the patients get PKDL, the skin condition that resembles LEPROSY.

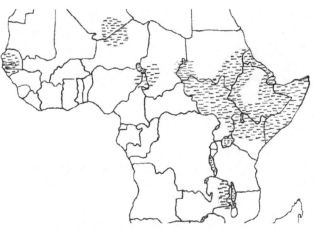

The known distribution of visceral Leishmaniasis. The sandflies that carry it are widely distributed, so it has potential of appearing in many other places. It is common in Somalia. For the north coast of Africa see the R Notes.

VITILIGO

Similar regional disease: ONCHOCERCIASIS may look quite similar, but the history of itching and eye changes should make you suspect that.

WARTS

The rash of HIV INFECTION looks just like this, but it is itchy and there is a drop of water in each bump which is released when it is scratched open.

XEROPHTHALMIA

Pygmies are particularly susceptible. In Tanzania, children who develop this have low-protein diets with mostly starches and few vegetables. It is neither common nor rare in Chad. It occurs in Ethiopia, in Burkina Faso and elsewhere.

YAWS

Synonym: siti (in the Gambia)

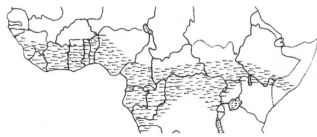

The known distribution of yaws. It may occur in any hot, humid climate where sanitation is poor.

Yaws occurs across all southern South Sudan except for the north and west where there is TREPONARID only.

Similar regional diseases: CUTANEOUS LEISHMANIASIS can appear similar. Swollen fingers resemble SICKLE CELL DISEASE.

YELLOW FEVER

Cause: virus
Moderately to very ill; class 2–4; regional

Epidemics occur during the rainy season. There are epidemics from time to time in west-central Kenya (Rift Valley), Nigeria, Ghana, Senegal, Dafur Sudan, adjacent Chad and probably elsewhere. It occurs in southern Ethiopia.

Age: any, but the majority of cases have been in children. **Who:** unimmunized; frequently in epidemics, transmitted by mosquitoes that bite during the day. **Onset:** over a day or two after an incubation of 3–6 days.

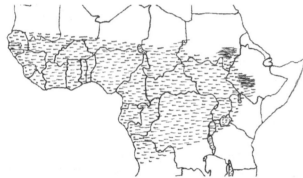

The known distribution of the mosquitoes that carry yellow fever. It occurs in spotty locations within the shaded areas.

Clinical

The WHO definition for yellow fever is as follows: fever plus JAUNDICE plus one or more of the following:
- a slow pulse relative to the fever.
- abnormal bleeding.
- upper abdominal pain.
- protein in urine.
- decreased amount of urine.

Necessary: the patient has fever, nausea and aching all over, especially in the back, the waist area and the limbs. JAUNDICE develops only after several days of illness. The spleen is not enlarged.

Usually: there is a severe headache and eye pain. The pulse is initially rapid, but by day 3 or 4, the pulse slows and may become slow relative to the fever. The mind is clear; the patient does not act intoxicated like he does with TYPHUS, unless he is about to die.

Frequently: there is a day of recovery before the disease starts a second time.

Sometimes: the yellow color of the whites of the eyes may be quite indistinct. It becomes worse gradually, if at all. The face may be swollen. There may be severe bone and joint pains. Vomiting may occur early, as may insomnia, and a tender but non-swollen liver. The vomit is probably mucus at first, turning to black or bloody later on. The patient may have a body odor resembling a butcher shop.

Complications: LIVER FAILURE, KIDNEY DISEASE. Mental symptoms start late and indicate a poor prognosis. An occasional complication is HEMORRHAGIC FEVER: nosebleeds; bleeding gums; bloody stool, urine or vomit; heavy menstruation; major bleeding from minor wounds. There is a high death rate during epidemics.

Similar diseases: Protocols B.2, B.5 and B.9. MALARIA with jaundice is different in that the jaundice appears the first day or two. The pulse in malaria is normal or rapid relative to the fever.

Bush laboratory: bilirubin in the urine is quite common. There is almost always protein in the urine by the second day of illness. There may be blood in the urine on the third or fourth day. Sophisticated hospital laboratories can do blood tests or liver biopsies.

Treatment

Prevention: immunize. Excellent immunization is available. Immunity starts about 10 days after the injection. Persons should be re-immunized every 10 years. Care for patients under a mosquito net to avoid transmitting the disease to others.

Referrals: laboratory and facilities: at least a level 4.

Patient care: same as HEPATITIS and, if necessary, HEMORRHAGIC FEVER. VITAMIN K injections may be helpful.

Results: at least half the patients who develop severe symptoms die. Those who recover have a very long convalescence.

INDEX I: INDIAN SUBCONTINENT NOTES

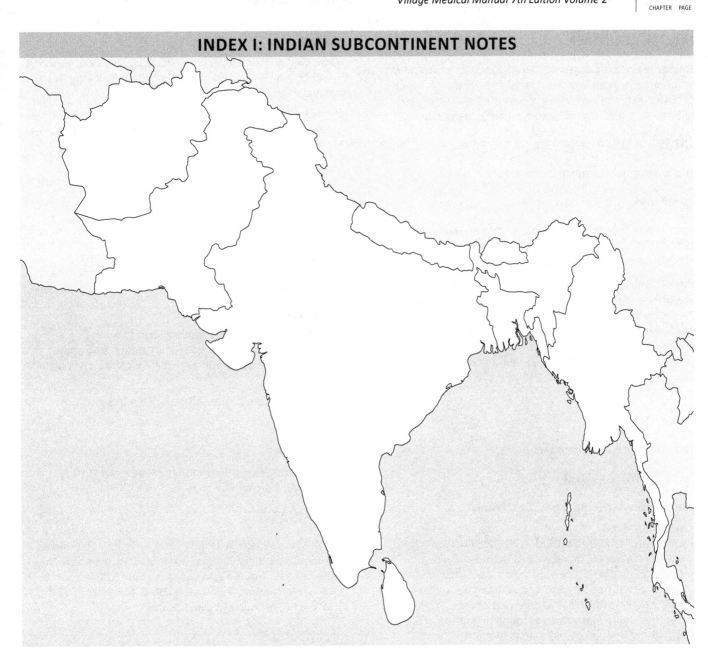

Map disclaimers

- Read the captions carefully. They are not all the same.

- Maps are notoriously unreliable. Conditions may be found in areas not shaded; conditions may be absent in areas that are shaded. Usually a disease is present only in spotty areas within the shaded region. A diagnosis is possible if there is shading anywhere around your location or if your patient has traveled through a shaded area.

- There is lack of shading both where there are no data and also where data exists indicating that the condition is absent. Lack of shading more often indicates lack of data than absence of the condition.

- Epidemiologists and government health officers survey in easy locations, near major roads. If you are in a remote, difficult location the maps may not reflect the reality that you see.

- Beware of shading that stops at political boundaries; germs don't respect border controls.

- Beware of areas that are unshaded for a variety of diseases. It may be because no one educated has ever entered that area and made it out alive. It may also be because intelligent people know enough not to go there.

- At times of civil unrest, natural disaster and migrations, the distribution of diseases changes unpredictably and rapidly. With biological warfare, this problem will be compounded.

ACUTE ABDOMEN

Similar regional diseases: ASCARIASIS, being very common in this area, is a cause of this as well as a mimic. With SICKLE CELL DISEASE, the whites of the eyes are yellow, the patient has ANEMIA, and urobilinogen is found in the urine.

AMEBIASIS

This is extremely common in this area.

ANEMIA

Anemia due to red cell destruction or due to vitamin deficiency can be caused by SICKLE CELL DISEASE which is relatively rare in India, occurring in certain ethnic groups only.

Anemia due to vitamin deficiency may occur in persons who are strict vegans, not eating animal products of any sort. (Vegetarians are those who eat milk and eggs as well as plant products. They are not prone to this.) Vegans develop anemia due to COBALAMIN DEFICIENCY after 3 years on a strict vegan diet. It is important not to treat these people with FOLATE or FOLIC ACID alone; also give milk or eggs in the diet or VITAMIN B$_{12}$.[1]

ANTHRAX

This is common in Afghanistan.

ARBOVIRAL FEVER

The following types are present in this area:

- DENGUE FEVER.
- CRIMEAN-CONGO HEMORRHAGIC FEVER occurs in the western half of India and west of there.
- CHIKUNGUNYA FEVER which is mostly an urban disease in this area. It is rapidly spreading, so maps are useless. In the past it was mostly in the eastern part of India. It occurs in outbreaks with many cases at the same time.
- Kyasanur Forest disease is described below.

Kyasanur Forest disease

Cause: virus
Synonym: monkey fever

Moderately ill to very ill; class 2; regional; mainly in India, rarely in Saudi Arabia. It occurs in India south of Ahmadabad and west of Bangalore. There is potential of its spreading throughout southern India, since the ticks are present through this wider area.

Age: any. **Who:** those bitten by ticks. The disease occurs in monkeys, rats, lemurs and other wild animals. Those living in areas where monkeys are dying are prone to get the disease. **Onset:** very sudden, over hours, with an incubation of 4–12 days.

Clinical

Necessary: an initial fever with headache, eye pain, vomiting and general muscle pains. It is uncertain how long this initial phase lasts.

Usually: the patient's eyes are red, the face is flushed and the patient avoids light and eye movement, because it causes more pain.

Commonly: the liver, spleen and lymph nodes are large. HEMORRHAGIC FEVER, RESPIRATORY FAILURE and KIDNEY DISEASE may develop.

Sometimes: after apparent recovery lasting 1–3 weeks, the patient develops ENCEPHALITIS due to this virus.

Similar diseases: see Protocol B.2 and other relevant protocols. LEPTOSPIROSIS is indistinguishable. Therefore, if there is flooding, use DOXYCYCLINE to cover that possibility.

Treatment

Keep the patient hydrated and well fed. Use ACETAMINOPHEN only for pain. The disease is possibly contagious, so sending out for higher-level care must be in a towed trailer.

Results: death rate 5–10%. KIDNEY DISEASE is a common complication.

ARTHRITIS

RHEUMATIC FEVER, CHIKUNGUNYA FEVER and REITER SYNDROME are common causes.

ASCARIASIS

This is very common in Kashmir, Bangladesh, central India and southwest India. In many areas of India, especially the south, over 90% of the population harbor these worms. Ascariasis commonly mimics GALLBLADDER DISEASE and ACUTE ABDOMEN; it can cause both.

BELL'S PALSY

This may be caused by SICKLE CELL DISEASE.

BERIBERI

This is common in the area.

BLADDER STONE

Bladder stones are common in coastal Andhra Pradesh.

BRAIN DAMAGE

The most common local causes are HIV INFECTION and Japanese ENCEPHALITIS.

---

1 *An alternative is ground, raw liver. This is unsafe because it carries some diseases, but the risk may be worth it if the patient is desperate. Be sure the liver is from a healthy animal.*

BRUCELLOSIS

The problem occurs in the Rajasthan, Punjab and Haryana areas and probably elsewhere. It is a disease of pastoralists. Those who consume unpasteurized dairy products are most at risk.

CANCER

In India, about 1/2 of all cancers are cancers of the mouth, in contrast to 1–3% in the rest of the world. It is found mostly in the poor and is related to chewing "pan" or to smoking "chutta" or "bidis". Look for a painless lump or thickening; an abnormally colored area of the pink moist part; a sore that does not heal; trouble opening the mouth; or trouble swallowing. Hindus in India have a fairly high frequency of cancer of the penis. In women cancer of the cervix and cancer of the breast are most common.

CANCRUM ORIS

This is frequently a complication of VISCERAL LEISHMANIASIS.

CEREBRAL PALSY

An important cause in this area is Japanese ENCEPHALITIS.

CHICKEN POX

In India much of the adult population is not immune to chicken pox. In teen-agers and young adults there can be very serious complications, e.g. ENCEPHALITIS. Also chicken pox is very serious in pregnancy and amongst HIV-infected patients. When and if immunization is available, urge all acquaintances to be immunized.

CHOLERA

In this area it routinely accounts for a small percent of all diarrhea. Areas where the problem is common are those with stagnant or sluggish water, frequent flooding and less than 100 meters elevation. This is mainly in coastal areas near the mouths of major rivers. It is also common in Nepal, mainly during the summer months. There have been outbreaks in Afghanistan. Cholera is becoming resistant to CIPROFLOXACIN in India.

CIRRHOSIS

INDIAN CHILDHOOD CIRRHOSIS is the most common regional cause of cirrhosis in children.

CRETINISM

In the Himalayan area, cretinism is common. About half have the first kind and half, the second. In the rest of south Asia, most cretins are of the first kind.

CRYPTOSPORIDIOSIS

In Bangladesh this is very common in children under 5 years old. In older children GIARDIASIS and AMEBIASIS are more common.

CUTANEOUS LEISHMANIASIS

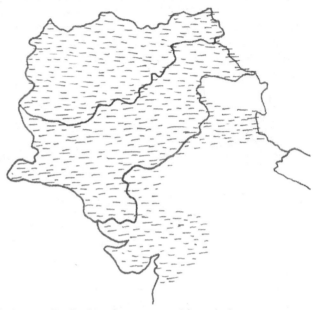

The known distribution of cutaneous Leishmaniasis.

It may also occur elsewhere. It may manifest like visceral Leishmaniasis, especially in those with poor immunity. It is particularly common in Afghanistan and Pakistan, extending northward.

CYSTICERCOSIS

This is found only in areas where pigs are raised in such a way that they come in contact with human waste. It may occur in vegetarians who consume unsanitary food and water. It is a common cause of EPILEPSY amongst the Gurkhas of Nepal.

DENGUE FEVER

This is quite common in urban and semi-urban areas. HEMORRHAGIC FEVER as a complication has not been common. It occurs in Sri Lanka, New Delhi, Vellore, Madras, Bangladesh and in the Maldives.

DIABETES

This is commonly associated with PANCREATITIS in southern India.

DIPHTHERIA

This is very common and occurs mostly in the rainy season. Deaths are from HEART FAILURE. Deaths are almost all in the unimmunized. In Bangladesh this is mostly a disease of the middle and upper classes

DONOVANOSIS

This is common along the southeast coast of India.

DYSENTERY

Bacterial dysentery occurs off and on all over this area. Usually there are blood and mucus in the stool from the beginning; sometimes there is watery diarrhea at first which changes to dysentery in 1–2 days. There is usually a high fever and severe abdominal pain, but rarely DEHYDRATION. One complication is SEPSIS which is common in India and Bangladesh in children under 4 years old and especially in those less than 1 year old. Up to 15% of the patients die. Another complication is REITER SYNDROME. In some areas bacterial DYSENTERY is resistant to CO-TRIMOXAZOLE.

Amebic dysentery is uncommon in urban areas of Bangldesh; It is common in children 0–2 y.o. in southern India.

ENCEPHALITIS

Japanese encephalitis (JE) occurs in Nepal and in nearby adjacent areas of India. There is potential of its occurring south of the 30th parallel and as far west as Pakistan. Thousands of cases of JE have been recorded from west Bengal, with a 35% death rate and substantial long-term disabilities in survivors. There is less problem in Calcutta than in the surrounding rural areas. Pigs and water buffalo harbor the virus without becoming ill, and mosquitoes pass it from them to human beings.

Patients are mostly well-nourished; almost all have a depressed level of consciousness, paralysis and seizures; following a 2–10-day initial illness of headache, fever and vomiting.

An immunization for JE is available. Vaccinate for long-term residency, for rural sojourns, and/or agricultural areas.

RIBAVIRIN does no good whatsoever for treatment.

Encephalitis may also result from CHICKEN POX. See the note above under CHICKEN POX.

Kyasanur Forest disease, another form of encephalitis, is described under ARBOVIRAL FEVER in this Index.

ENTERIC FEVER

Synonyms: typhoid fever, paratyphoid fever

This is extremely common in Nepal, associated with poor sanitation. Clinically enteric fever and murine TYPHUS cannot be distinguished; treat for both if you suspect either, but don't use CIPROFLOXACIN which tends to make TYPHUS worse.

Paratyphoid occurs in the India area. It is mainly from unsanitary food.

Enteric fever is extremely variable by region and by patient. In India it frequently begins with a fever that rises and falls before it finally rises and stays there. In Nepal the chief complaint is usually a sustained, high fever. Other symptoms, if they occur, are similar to those in the rest of the world, but STROKE or paralysis is an occasional complication.

Treatment

Afghanistan, Pakistan and India report typhoid that is resistant to CHLORAMPHENICOL, AMPICILLIN and CO-TRIMOXAZOLE. Use one of the CEPHALOSPORINs in these cases. Much of the enteric fever in India is resistant to CIPROFLOXACIN.

FILARIASIS

Synonym: elephantiasis, non-endemic.

Two types of filariasis are Bancroftian and Brugian.

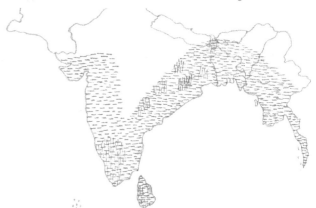

The horizontal shading shows the area of Bancroftian filariasis; the vertical shading shows Brugian filariasis. Bull. Wid Hlth OSragnt.eJ} 1962, 27, 529–541

Bancroftian filariasis

This often affects legs and the male genitals. It occurs all along the west coast of India and also east of Bangalore and south of the 28th parallel. It also occurs in the Maldives and Sri Lanka.

Brugian filariasis

This causes attacks that come and go, usually lasting just 4 days at a time. It often affects arms and breasts as well as legs but only rarely the genitals. It occurs in the area around Bangalore and west of there to the coast.

TOC   SYMPTOMS   DIFFERENTIALS   CONDITIONS   DRUG INDEX   REGIONAL NOTES   INX

G6PD DEFICIENCY

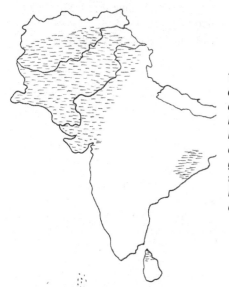

The shaded areas are where this condition is most likely to be found. It may occur anywhere. The genetic heritage of the patient is important, not his current location.

GALLBLADDER DISEASE

Persons with SICKLE CELL DISEASE or THALLASEMIA are particularly prone to this, and it is common in northern India.

GIARDIASIS

This is particularly common in urban Bangladesh. It also occurs commonly in southern India.

GOITER

This is especially common in inland and high-altitude areas. It may also occur in frequently flooded river deltas near the ocean, where iodine is continually washed out of the soil.

GUINEA WORM

Synonym: dracunculiasis

This used to be reported from this area, from locations in eastern India, south-eastern Pakistan and north-central Pakistan. The World Health Organization states that it has been eradicated. The condition is described in the F regional notes.

HEART FAILURE

In the Kerala area, restrictive failure develops for no known reason. It usually affects poor people with poor nutrition, mostly young males and older females. It develops over months to years. There is no known cure; it is inevitably fatal. Valvular heart failure is usually due to RHEUMATIC FEVER which is very common, especially in northern India.

HEMORRHAGIC FEVER

In this area, this may (rarely) be associated with DENGUE FEVER as well as (more commonly) various ARBOVIRAL FEVERs. See Protocol B.2.

HEPATITIS

Hepatitis A, B, C and E are all common in Afghanistan.

Hepatitis B is uncommon in mountainous Nepal. Most epidemics in the area occur during the rainy season and are due to hepatitis E, the kind that is dangerous during pregnancy. Non-pregnant patients do not become desperately ill from it, but it requires a very long convalescence. In India about 1/2 of all hepatitis is hepatitis A; 1/4 is hepatitis B and 1/4 is hepatitis E. Yearly epidemics are common. There is another, unidentified water-borne hepatitis also. Hepatitis D is common in India.

If the patient had recent contact with newborn animals, he might have Q FEVER, a kind of bacterial hepatitis. This occurs in Afghanistan as well as elsewhere. It responds to antibiotics.

HERPES

This is very common in India.

HIV INFECTION

The spread of HIV INFECTION in India has been along the major transport routes. The most common symptoms are fever, weight loss, loss of appetite, large lymph nodes and general body weakness. It is also very common in Burma.

Similar regional diseases: VISCERAL LEISHMANIASIS mainly affects the 2–15 y.o. population which is largely spared from HIV.

HOOKWORM

There is a very high frequency of hookworm in the south of India; it is a major cause of ANEMIA there.

HYDATID DISEASE

It occurs, but is not common, in this area. It occurs in central India, northern Pakistan, Afghanistan and northward from there. In these areas it is alveolar hydatid disease, caused by eating food contaminated by wild animal stool as well as from dogs living close to people. It is a very aggressive disease that behaves like CANCER. It more often affects the abdomen than the lungs. In some areas ALBENDAZOLE works well, and in other areas it does not.

INTESTINAL FLUKE

Fasciolopsiasis is found in India and Bangladesh. It is prevalent in Maharashtra State of India, in northwest India, Bangladesh and Burma. It is most common on the banks of large lakes with lotus plants and snails where there is sewage contamination of the water. In such areas, 15% to 22% of the population may be infected.

TOC

SYMPTOMS

DIFFERENTIALS

CONDITIONS

DRUG INDEX

REGIONAL NOTES

INX

IRRITABLE BOWEL

Similar regional diseases: LIVER FLUKE, INTESTINAL FLUKE.

KATAYAMA DISEASE

In this area, usually this is the initial stage of HYDATID DISEASE, usually in expatriates. It is rare.

KIDNEY DISEASE

In India 40% of the kidney disease is nephritic, mostly due to skin infections; 40%, nephrotic due to multiple causes including PLANT POISONING from argemone oil; 8% hemolytic failure due to bacterial DYSENTERY; and 12% slow failure due to unknown causes. SICKLE CELL DISEASE is a cause of hemolytic, nephritic or nephrotic kidney disease. KYASANUR FOREST DISEASE is a cause of this condition.

KYASANUR FOREST DISEASE

This is described under ARBOVIRAL FEVER in this index.

LARVA MIGRANS

A very severe deep type, gnathostomiasis, from handling raw meat with bare hands, occurs in Burma and in the Bengal area of India. Use rubber gloves when handling raw meat!

LEPROSY

This is very common in this area. India alone contains 76% of the world's leprosy patients. The disease is also very common in Bangladesh.

Similar regional diseases: PKDL, a complication of VISCERAL LEISHMANIASIS.

LEPTOSPIROSIS

This occurs mostly in Afghanistan and the eastern part of India and Nepal, most frequently during the yearly monsoons. It occurs but is not common in Madras. The death rate is 36%, usually from LIVER FAILURE. In this area the disease resembles MENINGITIS with a stiff neck being very common. The eyes may not be red.

LICE

Similar regional diseases; a similar disease is a fungal infection of the hair which causes white or black bumps on the hairs. This fungal infection is common in southern India. Wash the hair with commercial shampoo and apply 1% CLOTRIMAZOLE lotion daily. Results in 4 weeks.

LIVER FLUKE

This is present in some areas only, mainly those that raise sheep or cattle. It reportedly occurs in some areas of Afghanistan and India. It is probably mostly fascioliasis.

MALABSORPTION

The most common causes in this area are PANCREATITIS in southern India, SPRUE and GIARDIASIS throughout the area.

MALARIA

The following areas reportedly have no malaria transmission, but you should seek local information. Malaria is reportedly present at least up to 2500 meters, although the malaria at higher elevations is almost all non-falciparum. These are the areas reportedly free of transmission:

- Afghanistan: Kabul.
- Bangladesh: Dhaka.
- Burma: urban areas.
- Nepal: urban areas and above 2500 meters.

In India malaria has been entering urban areas; the mosquitoes are adapting to air pollution, and they are becoming resistant to insecticides. At least 50% of the malaria is falciparum.

There has been an increase in the number of malaria cases in Afghanistan, particularly the north. The disease is most prevalent during the summer months, the peak being in August. It is about 98–99% non-falciparum malaria from April to September and mostly falciparum during September to November. It occurs mainly along the north and south borders of the country and in a north-south swathe near the eastern half of the country. Falciparum is common in Kabul province.

The malaria in Bangladesh and Bhutan is at least 1/3 falciparum. In Bangladesh, falciparum is especially common in the Chittagong Division.

In Burma, amodiaquine-artesunate is not a good treatment.

MALNUTRITION

The northern half of India is a kwashiorkor area. All over India general malnutrition, iron deficiency, xerophthalmia and iodine deficiency are common.

MEASLES

In this area it is the fourth most common cause of death in children. In urban areas, it occurs mainly in children between 1 and 2 y.o. and always under 5 y.o.; in rural areas it affects children in all age groups in a village at once, in epidemics which occur every couple of years. In small towns the pattern is something between urban and rural patterns. There are complications in about 50% of all cases.

The most common complication is PNEUMONIA which may respond to PENICILLIN, CEPHALOSPORIN or CLOXACILLIN.

MENINGITIS

There have been epidemics of meningococcal meningitis in India and Nepal. This is the kind that has a very rapid onset and spreads rapidly in the community. In this area LEPTOSPIROSIS can be very similar.

MONKEY FEVER

See Kyasanur Forest disease described under ARBOVIRAL FEVER, this index.

MOSSY FOOT

Mossy foot occurs in parts of India and Sri Lanka.

MYCETOMA

In this area mycetoma is especially common in arid areas where there are thorny plants. It is almost all due to bacteria except in West Bengal, India where there are a variety of types.

PANCREATITIS

This is a cause of MALABSORPTION and DIABETES in southern and eastern India.

PARAGONIMIASIS

This occurs only in India and Sri Lanka. It is common in eastern India.

PARKINSON'S DISEASE

Similar regional diseases: PLANT POISONING: lathyrism.

PELLAGRA

It occurs especially in northern India and Pakistan and with BERIBERI in Madras state.

PLAGUE

This occurs in the northern parts of this area, including Afghanistan and in Burma. It has occurred in northern Pakistan, northern India and Nepal. It occurs sporadically and also in epidemics. It may occur anywhere.

POLIO

Polio had been common in Bhutan, Burma, India and Bangladesh; at present Pakistan and Afghanistan are the only countries listed as having it.

Q FEVER

This occurs throughout this area except for the Himalayas and eastern Burma.

RABIES

This is a major problem in parts of India, especially West Bengal and in Afghanistan.

RAT BITE FEVER

This is very common around Mombay.

RELAPSING FEVER

Tick-borne relapsing fever is present in this area north of the 30th parallel. It occurs in Afghanistan, Pakistan, northern India, east into western China.

Louse-borne relapsing fever is present throughout this area.

RESPIRATORY INFECTION

A regional cause is PARAGONIMIASIS. Croup is common in this area.

RHEUMATIC FEVER

This is more common in the Indian area than the rest of the developing world. Sri Lanka has the most in the world, and it is very common in northern India and in Nepal. If you suspect this, give the patient monthly injections of benzathine PENICILLIN.

RICKETS

This is particularly common in Muslim cultures and around Mombay.

SANDFLY FEVER

This is present throughout Pakistan, Afghanistan, Iran and north of these areas. It is present in India north of the 20th parallel (Mumbai on the west coast). It reportedly does not occur in Bangladesh or Nepal. Its description is in the Condition Index.

SCABIES

This is probably the most common skin problem in India. An ethnic cure is a neem: turmeric paste, 4:1 by weight, rubbed on the skin daily for 15 days or until the patient is cured, whichever is sooner.

SCHISTOSOMIASIS

Schistosomiasis reportedly is absent in this area.

SCRUB TYPHUS

Scrub typhus is present throughout the Indian subcontinent and Asia, as far north as the northern border of Mongolia. It is mostly resistant to DOXYCYCLINE. Use AZITHROMYCIN or RIFAMPIN. It is common in Sri Lanka and may be indistinguishable there from SPOTTED FEVER.

SCURVY

This occurs, but is not common in the area.

SEIZURES

Common causes are FEBRILE SEIZURES, cerebral MALARIA and Japanese ENCEPHALITIS. PLANT POISONING due to margosa oil may also cause seizures.

SEPSIS

This is most commonly related to TROPICAL SPLENOMEGALY, VISCERAL LEISHMANIASIS or bacterial DYSENTERY. Melioidosis is a form of SEPSIS that occurs in rural areas in India and Sri Lanka.

There are some nasty bacteria in this area that cause sepsis only responsive to two unusual drugs: tigamycin and colistin. They are resistant to everything else.

SEXUALLY TRANSMITTED DISEASE

The most common types of SEXUALLY TRANSMITTED DISEASEs are HERPES, SYPHILIS and HIV INFECTION. In southern India the most common diseases are SYPHILIS in males and VAGINITIS due to trichomonas in females. GONORRHEA occurs commonly in both.

CHANCROID, DONOVANOSIS and LYMPHOGRANULOMA VENEREUM occur, but are not as common except DONOVANOSIS in south-eastern coastal India.

SICKLE CELL DISEASE

This occurs in the Tharu people of southern Nepal, in Orissa and Madhya Pradesh states of India amongst certain tribal groups, and in some tribal groups west, north-west and southwest of Mysore, India.

SPOTTED FEVER

Synonym: tick typhus

This occurs in various areas of India, Pakistan and Nepal. It is the same kind as Mediterranean tick typhus. There is almost always an eschar—a tiny scab where the organism entered the body. Search for it. If you don't find it, the diagnosis is unlikely. The disease is generally milder than the African form, but there are occasional severe complications. It is common in Sri Lanka and may be indistinguishable from SCRUB TYPHUS.

SPRUE

This is more common in South Asia than in other areas of the developing world. It usually starts between March and September. It may affect children in southern India, and these cases are quite unresponsive to treatment. In this region it does not usually cause ANEMIA.

In the Vellore, India area the problem tends to be sudden in onset. About half of the patients have fever. It may occur in epidemics.

STREP INFECTION

This is common, as is RHEUMATIC FEVER, in northern India and in Sri Lanka. In these areas, treat any sore throat as strep throat. Be sure to treat for the entire 10 days.

STRONGYLOIDIASIS

This worm occurs commonly near Mysore, India. When this occurs along with TROPICAL SPLENOMEGALY, SEPSIS may result.

SYPHILIS

This is very common in southern India.

TAPEWORM

Rat tapeworm is common around Madras, India. Pork tapeworm occurs in India. Fish tapeworm occurs in Bangladesh.

TETANUS

Neonatal tetanus is very common in India and Bangladesh, affecting up to 7% of all live births.

THALLASEMIA

This is very common in Maldivia. In the Delhi area of India most families with this problem were originally Pakistani.

TINEA

This is very common in Maldivia and the Madras area of India.

TOXEMIA

In southern India this is especially common during the hot dry season.

TOXOPLASMOSIS

Those with TROPICAL SPLENOMEGALY are especially vulnerable to becoming ill with this.

TOC · SYMPTOMS · DIFFERENTIALS · CONDITIONS · DRUG INDEX · REGIONAL NOTES · INX

TRACHOMA

This is especially common in northern India, in Nepal and in relatively arid central Burma.

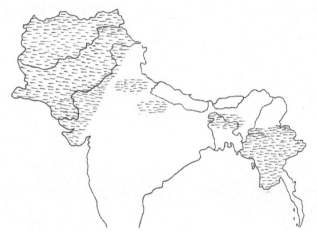

The shaded areas are where trachoma is most common. It occurs everywhere.

TRICHINOSIS

This is rare in this area except for northern India.

TRICHURIASIS

This is very common in southern India, with over 95% of children infected; it is less common in central India. It is common in urban Bangladesh, north-eastern India and in Sri Lanka.

TROPICAL SPASTIC PARAPARESIS

This is common in southern India.

TROPICAL SPLENOMEGALY

This is present in Bangladesh and in India.

TROPICAL ULCER

In India this is an urban problem; in other areas it is mostly rural.

TUBERCULOSIS

Maldivia, Pakistan, Afghanistan, India and Sri Lanka have very many cases. Skin tests in nationals are almost all positive by age 20. TB that affects the abdomen commonly causes ACUTE ABDOMEN, Type 3. Multiple drug-resistant TB occurs.

TUNGIASIS

This occurs in Pakistan and the west coast of India.

TURISTA

Watery diarrhea in the north of India is mostly due to a virus in the winter months; antibiotics do no good. In Maldivia, diarrhea is usually due to TRICHURIASIS or GIARDIASIS.

In Bangladesh, GIARDIASIS is common, as is a peculiar form of diarrhea that is curable with ERYTHROMYCIN. Diarrhea that responds to DOXYCYCLINE is common in both India and Bangladesh. In India, SEPSIS is a common complication of diarrhea; when this occurs, the patient may have urobilinogen in his urine so the disease resembles MALARIA. In and near Nepal consider CYCLOSPORIASIS.

TYPHUS

Louse-borne typhus is found in the northern highlands of India, Pakistan and Afghanistan and also in the Himalayas. It occurs wherever there are body lice.

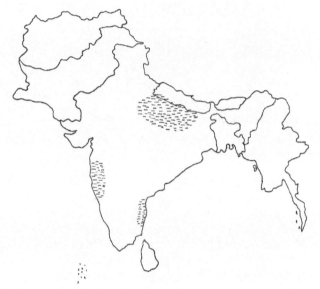

The known distribution of murine typhus. It may occur anywhere.

Murine typhus is also common in Burma, especially coastal areas, especially summer and autumn. It may occur wherever there are rats. In this area it may be indistinguishable from ENTERIC FEVER; treat for both if you treat for either. Avoid using CIPROFLOXACIN.

VISCERAL LEISHMANIASIS

A large percentage of the worldwide VL is found in the Indian subcontinent. In India it is mostly in 5–15 year olds, more male than female, more rural and uneducated. The spleen is larger than the liver. Most patients have a fever. It may be totally without symptoms in the Bojar area.

There is a lot of resistance to STIBOGLUCONATE. PKDL occurs in less than 20% of the patients in this area.

It is prevalent in eastern Nepal, Dharan town area.

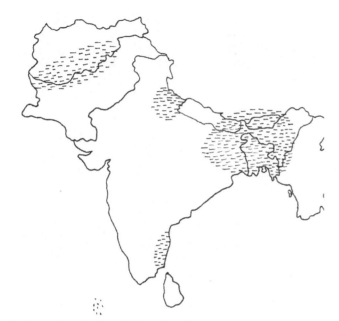

The known distribution of visceral Leishmaniasis.

YAWS

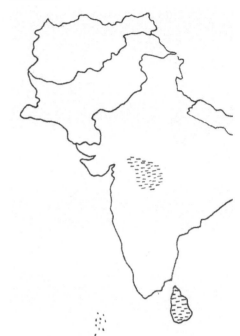

The known distribution of yaws. It may occur in any hot, humid environment.

XEROPHTHALMIA

This is found especially in remote rural areas of the southern half of India, in Bangladesh, Nepal and Bhutan. It occurs, but is less of a problem, in the far northern states of India. In most of Asia there is a very high mortality rate for blind children, up to 75% in the first 3 months of blindness. This is due to infection, because the VITAMIN A deficiency that causes the xerophthalmia also decreases immunity. Small weekly doses of VITAMIN A will cut the death rate to half.

INDEX K: CENTRAL ASIAN REPUBLICS NOTES

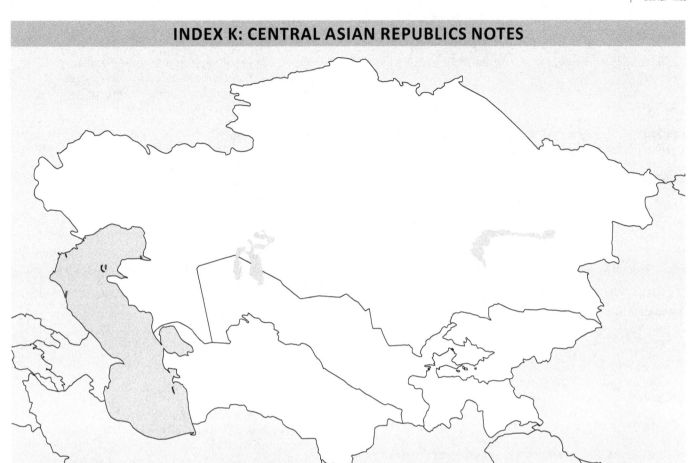

TOC

SYMPTOMS

DIFFERENTIALS

CONDITIONS

DRUG INDEX

REGIONAL NOTES

INX

TOC SYMPTOMS DIFFERENTIALS CONDITIONS DRUG INDEX REGIONAL NOTES INX

AMEBIASIS

Amebiasis occurs in this area; the extent and distribution are unknown.

ANTHRAX

Outbreaks in Kyrgyzstan are associated with sick cattle being slaughtered for human consumption.

ARBOVIRAL FEVER

CRIMEAN-CONGO HEMORRHAGIC FEVER occurs in the southwest portion of this area; the extent and distribution are unknown.

ASCARIASIS

Infection with ascaris is common in this area, especially amongst school children.

BRUCELLOSIS

Brucellosis occurs in this area; the extent and distribution are unknown. Reportedly it is generally common. It is common in Kyrgyzstan.

CANCER

The prevalent types of cancer are unknown, except that cancer of the gallbladder is associated with the liver fluke, Opisthorcus felineus, which comes from eating raw or pickled fish.

CRYPTOSPORIDIOSIS

This is a cause of diarrhea that is common in this area.

CUTANEOUS LEISHMANIASIS

This is mostly caused by Leishmania major; it is prevalent in throughout the –stan republics and may be very aggressive. Other than that, its prevalence is unknown. It is associated with wild gerbils.

DIPHTHERIA

Outbreaks have occurred with the social upheavals that accompanied the breakup of the Soviet Union and the subsequent lack of routine immunizations.

ENCEPHALITIS

Japanese encephalitis does not occur in this area. Russian spring summer encephalitis does occur.

ENTEROBIASIS

This is prevalent in this area, especially where there are shared beds. It tends to be more of a temperate than a tropical disease.

HEPATITIS

Hepatitis B used to be very common, but mandatory immunization of all newborns has drastically decreased its prevalence. Hepatitis E is common in the former USSR, especially Turkmenia and Kirghiz.

HIV INFECTION

There has been a tremendous upsurge in cases of HIV infection, along with the opportunistic infections that accompany this, especially TB.

HYDATID DISEASE

This is very common in the area, both from contact with dogs and from eating plants that may be contaminated with wild animal stool. It may affect even children.

LARVA MIGRANS

This occurs in the area, due to a worm that normally affects dogs.

LIVER FLUKE

The most prevalent kind is Opisthorcus felineus, indistinguishable with your facilities from Opisthorcus viverni which occurs in Southeast Asia. It is transmitted by uncooked fish known as stroganima. It is common in Kazakhstan and Ukraine. Fasciola hepatica also occurs in this area. It comes from eating water plants.

LYME DISEASE

This is present in an east-west swathe throughout central Asia. It extends fairly far north. It is similar to the disease in Europe, causing BELL'S PALSY and RADICULOPATHY. There is less ARTHRITIS than in the West, but there may be double vision, paralysis of facial muscles, dizziness, deafness, inability to understand and symptoms of MENINGITIS.

MALARIA

In this area almost all the malaria is vivax, and there is not much of that. Several areas have been declared free of it in the past, but with human migrations it will always come back. It is, in any case, not very prevalent. There is probably no falciparum malaria in this area. Kazakhstan is reportedly free of malaria and always has been.

PLAGUE

Plague occurs in the area, just east of the Caspian sea and in southern Kazakhstan; it may occur elsewhere.

POLIO

Polio has again become common because of the lack of routine immunization.

Q FEVER

Q fever occurs in this area, the extent and distribution unknown.

RELAPSING FEVER

Tick borne relapsing fever occurs in this area, transmitted by soft ticks which bite at night without the subject being aware of it. The disease is associated with camping and poor housing.

RHEUMATIC FEVER

This is common in this area.

SANDFLY FEVER

This is common in the southern portions of this region but not in the far north.

SPOTTED FEVER

Tick borne spotted fever occurs in this area, probably the Mediterranean variety.

SYPHILIS

This has become common with the disruption of routine health services, with the HIV infection epidemic, and in common with other sexually transmitted diseases.

TAPEWORM

Rat tapeworm is common, especially in children. Beef tapeworm is also common in this area.

TOXOPLASMOSIS

This is reportedly common in rural Kazakhstan and even more common in urban areas.

TREPONARID

This is common in the arid parts of this area, more to the west than the east.

TRICHINOSIS

This is common in this area, associated with insufficiently cooked meat from wild animals or pigs.

TUBERCULOSIS

This problem has mushroomed, and much of it is drug-resistant.

TULAREMIA

This occurs in this area commonly, associated with small animals.

VISCERAL LEISHMANIASIS

The type that is present in this area is caused by *Leishmania infantum*, the same kind that is prevalent in the Mediterranean area. It affects mostly babies and young children.

INDEX M: AMERICAS NOTES

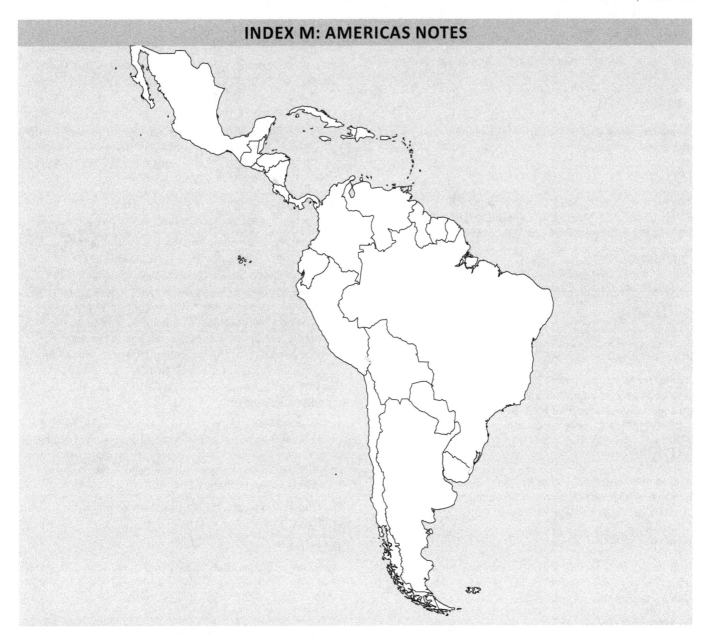

Map disclaimers

- Read the captions carefully. They are not all the same.

- Maps are notoriously unreliable. Conditions may be found in areas not shaded; conditions may be absent in areas that are shaded. Usually a disease is present only in spotty areas within the shaded region. A diagnosis is possible if there is shading anywhere around your location or if your patient has traveled through a shaded area.

- There is lack of shading both where there are no data and also where data exists indicating that the condition is absent. Lack of shading more often indicates lack of data than absence of the condition.

- Epidemiologists and government health officers survey in easy locations, near major roads. If you are in a remote, difficult location the maps may not reflect the reality that you see.

- Beware of shading that stops at political boundaries; germs don't respect border controls.

- Beware of areas that are unshaded for a variety of diseases. It may be because no one educated has ever entered that area and made it out alive. It may also be because intelligent people know enough not to go there.

- At times of civil unrest, natural disaster and migrations, the distribution of diseases changes unpredictably and rapidly. With biological warfare, this problem will be compounded.

AMEBIASIS

This is especially common in Mexico, Colombia and eastern South America.

ANAPHYLAXIS

Similar regional diseases: PLANT POISONING due to atriplicism or manicheel.

ANEMIA

Anemia due to red cell destruction occurs with SCHISTOSOMIASIS MANSONI, VISCERAL LEISHMANIASIS, BARTONELLOSIS and SICKLE CELL DISEASE.

ANTHRAX

It is especially in Haiti, Central America and Chile.

ARTHRITIS

This occurs with COCCIDIOMYCOSIS, BARTONELLOSIS and CHIKUNGUNYA.

Similar regional diseases: SICKLE CELL DISEASE (in Africans) also involves joint pains, but there is either ANEMIA, episodic abdominal pain or both. In expatriates consider ONCHOCERCIASIS; see the map in these notes.

ASTHMA

In Colombia, Brazil, Argentina and Venezuela, this may be due to a small insect that lives in house dust. Where this occurs, occasional spraying with insecticide may be helpful.

BURULI ULCER

BURULI ULCER occurs in Mexico, especially in areas that are marshy or have frequent floods, as well as in Cuba, Dominican Republic, Bolivia and French Guiana.

BARTONELLOSIS

Cause: bacteria

Synonyms: Oroya Fever, Verruga Fever, Guaitara Fever, Carrion's disease.

Mildly to severely ill; class 1–3; present in Peru and the adjacent countries, on the west side of the Andes, between 800 and 3000 meters (2500 and 9500 feet) elevation.

Age: any. **Who:** bitten by sand flies which bite at night, especially January to April. **Onset:** Oroya fever incubation 2 weeks to 4 months, slow onset. Verruga fever occurs 2–3 months after the Oroya stage or possibly without Oroya.

Clinical

There are two forms: Oroya fever and Verruga fever. Some patients have a mixture of the two types.

Oroya fever

First there is marked fatigue, then an up and down fever and rapidly developing ANEMIA (shortness of breath, paleness, fatigue) and JAUNDICE. There is headache and severe joint and deep bone pain. The pain over the center front of the chest is the worst. The patient may be irrational (hyperactive and/or bizarre). There may be a large spleen and large lymph nodes. The liver may also be enlarged and tender. In severe cases HEMORRHAGIC FEVER may develop. Death usually occurs in 2–3 weeks in untreated cases.

Verruga fever:

Initially there is a fever, usually low, plus severe joint pains.

After that there are bumps on the skin; with the bumps, the fever drops. The bumps form in crops. They are most often small (2–4 mm) but sometimes large (up to 4 cm). The smaller bumps are most common on the face and on the hairy surfaces of the limbs. The larger bumps are mostly on the non-hairy surfaces of the limbs, near or on the larger joints. Larger bumps do not form in the mouth or in the genital area. The larger bumps tend to kill the flesh, change into ulcers or cause GANGRENE. ENTERIC FEVER is frequently present along with Bartonellosis; this causes additional symptoms.

Similar conditions: see Protocols B.2, B.3, B.5, B.6 and B.11. Oroya fever may be virtually indistinguishable from ordinary or cerebral MALARIA. Verruga fever may be quite similar to DENGUE FEVER, but dengue does not cause skin bumps. The disease may resemble HEPATITIS.

Bush laboratory: urine may test positive for blood, urobilinogen or both.

Treatment

Prevention: eliminate sand flies; avoid bites. Sand flies are weak fliers; a fan is helpful. Spray clothing, and use fine-mesh mosquito nets with insect repellent or insecticide.

Referrals: laboratory; a medical laboratory can do a blood smear which is reliable. Facilities; a level 3 hospital will have IV antibiotics; surgery might be necessary.

Patient care: current recommendations: for Oroya phase, either CIPROFLOXACIN or else [CHLORAMPHENICOL plus PENICILLIN]. For the Verruga phase, RIFAMPIN, AZITHROMYCIN or ERYTHROMYCIN. FOLATE is helpful for ANEMIA.

Previous recommendations: CHLORAMPHENICOL and AMPICILLIN are best as they are also useful for ENTERIC FEVER. PENICILLIN, STREPTOMYCIN and DOXYCYCLINE work for BARTONELLOSIS, but do not touch ENTERIC FEVER.

BRUCELLOSIS

This occurs in the western and northern portions of South America, in the Caribbean and in Mexico. It is very common in Argentina, Peru and the Minas Gerais area of Brazil.

BURKITT LYMPHOMA

In this area it initially affects mostly the nose, mouth and jaw, occasionally the abdomen in females.

CANCER

Cancer of the cervix is common in some countries of South America and in Costa Rica.

Stomach cancer is common in Costa Rica.

Cancer of the penis may be locally common.

Liver cancer is less common than in some parts of the tropics, but more common than in temperate, Western countries.

CHAGA'S DISEASE

Cause: protozoa

Synonym: South American trypanosomiasis

Mildly to very ill; class 3–4; regional; it does not occur in the Caribbean. The distribution is between the 41st parallel south and the northern border of Mexico, but the Amazon basin is largely free of the disease.

Age: any, especially children. **Who:** bitten by reduviid or vinchuca bugs, usually near the eye. After the bug bites it defecates, and the organisms in the stool enter the small break in the skin. They also can enter pink, moist surfaces (like the eye and mouth), but they cannot enter intact skin. Once the feces are dry they are not infective. Many people have the organism in their bodies but are perfectly healthy. They become ill when their immunity wanes because of old age, CANCER or HIV INFECTION. Infants of infected mothers may have the disease. There is also oral transmission from eating food contaminated with the stool of the bug. Some claim that bedbugs can transmit the disease. **Onset:** swelling develops around the site of the bug bite. In 14 days a rash develops and the generalized body problems follow up to 4–6 weeks later according to some authorities but years later according to others.

Clinical

Symptoms may vary by geographic area and by altitude.

Usually: the initial stage is without symptoms.

Sometimes: initially there is swelling at the site of the bite, usually the eye. The swelling lasts for weeks, in contrast to a simple bug bite in which the swelling lasts for days. The swelling is painless and non-pitting. There may be a rough, discolored area on the skin.

Maybe: swelling may appear elsewhere in the body also. The skin may look red or bruised. There may be fever, aching all over and evidence of an EYE INFECTION, a problem with which this is easily confused. The lymph nodes may be large. The cheeks may be swollen as in MUMPS.

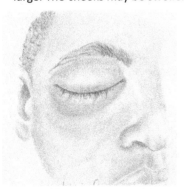

This eye is swollen shut, and it has been that way for most of a week. Ordinary insect bites look similar, but the swelling clears within a day or so. AB

Occasionally: the patient may develop the more advanced form of the disease: HEART FAILURE, a heart murmur, a very slow, fast or irregular pulse, but usually no shortness of breath. There may be sudden death. The person may have an enlarged liver and spleen; he may develop constipation and difficulty swallowing. These late changes may result in death.

Finally: about 5/8 of those infected have no long-term symptoms, 1/4 have heart problems and 1/8 have swallowing, bowel or nerve problems. The north has mostly HEART FAILURE. In the south swallowing and bowel problems are common All patients with swallowing or bowel problems also have HEART FAILURE.

Any swallowing or bowel problem without HEART FAILURE is not due to Chaga's. The disease is rapidly fatal in those who have full-blown AIDS.

The history of the swelling around the eye and the presence of any two of the following constitute sufficient grounds for diagnosis in an area where the disease is common:
- large liver.
- large spleen.
- fever without another cause.
- swollen feet.

In some areas chest pains, abnormal pulse and heart murmurs may be diagnostic also.

Complications: MENINGITIS, ENCEPHALITIS.

Similar conditions: EYE INFECTION and HEART FAILURE from other causes may have similar symptoms. INFLUENZA may look similar. See Protocols B.6. B.7, B.8 and B.12.

Treatment

Prevention: all mammals are susceptible to the organism; one should avoid eating raw or rare mammal meat. Infected mammals keep the bugs infected. Armadillos and opossums are the most important creatures to carry the organism. The main way to discourage the disease is to make houses inhospitable to the bugs by plastering walls and spraying with residual insecticides. Systems have been developed for ridding whole communities of the bugs.

Referrals: laboratory: there is no lab that you can do, but hospitals can do serology. The serology is sensitive but not specific. The organisms are sometimes found in a blood smear; the test is specific but not sensitive. Another technique is to have bugs feed on the patient and then sacrifice the bugs to look for the organism. Facilities: the drugs to treat this are toxic, and the complications are numerous, so referral is highly desirable. *Patient care:* NIFURTAMOX and BENZNIDAZOLE are the two drugs that are most often used. They must be used in a hospital setting. In the meantime, avoid using DOXYCYCLINE, PREDNISONE and related drugs, as they tend to make the disease worse.

TOC

SYMPTOMS

DIFFERENTIALS

CONDITIONS

DRUG INDEX

REGIONAL NOTES

INX

CHIKUNGUNYA FEVER

This occurs in outbreaks in this area, especially the Caribbean. The distribution is changing rapidly.

CHOLERA

There have been epidemics in this area. The overwhelming majority of cases have been in Haiti, Peru. Brazil, Colombia, Ecuador, Guatemala, Mexico and Panama.

COCCIDIOMYCOSIS

Cause: fungus

Synonyms: coccidioidal granuloma, desert fever, desert rheumatism, valley fever.

Mildly to severely ill; class 3; Arid areas only, low elevation, between 40° north and 40° south. Onset is mostly late summer and early fall.

Age: any. **Who:** those exposed to dust. The overwhelming, fatal form is most common in those of African genetic heritage, Asians, native Americans, Mexicans and pregnant women. **Onset:** variable; incubation is 10–14 days.

Clinical

Symptoms are variable, ranging from a mild, flu-like illness to an overwhelming, fatal PNEUMONIA. Typically the patient has fever, cough, chest pain and fatigue, lasting from 3 days to 2 weeks. This may go away, or it may become a chronic illness, resembling TUBERCULOSIS. There may be large lymph nodes which break open and drain. ERYTHEMA NODOSUM develops in 25% of the patients.

Similar conditions: see Protocols B.4 and B.12.

Treatment

Laboratory: there are blood tests and sputum tests to confirm the diagnosis. This is really necessary, because it looks just like TUBERCULOSIS, but it is treated entirely differently. *Facilities:* imaging might be helpful. MRI is better than CT for this.

Patient care: the drug of choice is AMPHOTERICIN B. It is a dangerous drug which should not be used by the medically untrained. Send the patient out for treatment. FLUCONAZOLE or ITRACONAZOLE might be helpful.

CRETINISM

In the Americas, the first kind of cretinism affects 90% of the cretins. (See CRETINISM in the Condition Index)

CRYPTOSPORIDIOSIS

This is very common in northeast Brazil.

CUTANEOUS LEISHMANIASIS

Synonym: chiclero ulcer

The high-risk period for acquiring this disease is the end of the dry season. In the RioGrande area you should watch for the complication of mucocutaneous Leishmaniasis and treat it aggressively.

Leishmania Mexicana extends from the 15th parallel south up past the Mexico/Texas border. It is also present in Hispaniola.

Leishmania Viannia occurs from the Tropic of Capricorn in the south up to and including the Yukatan Peninsula in the north.

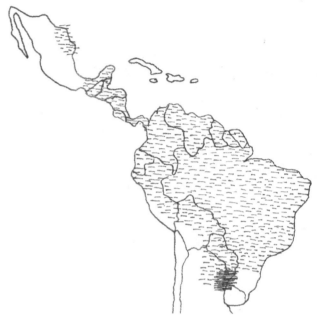

The shaded areas are where cutaneous Leishmaniasis is most likely to occur. Darker shaded areas show the locations of outbreaks. Information taken in part from ProMed-mail.

It may manifest like visceral Leishmaniasis, especially in those with poor immunity. In some areas of Bolivia the disease responds well to oral MILTEFOSINE. In other areas this is not true. Local lore is indispensable in choosing treatments.

CYSTICERCOSIS

This is the most common cause of adult-onset EPILEPSY in this area. It is found where pigs are raised in such a way that they come into contact with human waste. It is particularly common in Mexico.

DENGUE FEVER

In this region it is found in Central America, South America north of Argentina and in the Caribbean. There have been epidemics with HEMORRHAGIC FEVER, resulting in deaths. Those who die do so about the sixth day of illness. Many of them had ASTHMA or SICKLE CELL DISEASE before becoming ill with this. About half have itching and about 1 in 7 have a visible rash. If a person lives past the seventh day of illness, he usually recovers.

DIPHTHERIA

This is found especially in Barbados and the Dominican Republic.

DONOVANOSIS

In this area it is found mostly in the Caribbean and along the northern coast of South America.

DYSENTERY

Amebic dysentery is particularly common in Mexico, Brazil (especially the Amazon) and Chile.

ENCEPHALITIS

The most common kind is Venezuelan equine encephalitis, found in Venezuela and adjacent countries. Other less common kinds occur in Central America and in the Caribbean. Rocio encephalitis occurs in a small area south of Santos, Sao Paulo State, Brazil. The disease may occur anywhere. A similar regional disease is Rocky Mountain SPOTTED FEVER.

ENTERIC FEVER

This is common in the Caribbean, Mexico, Venezuela, Chile and Peru. Paratyphoid occurs mainly on the north coast of South America.

EYE INFECTION

Similar regional disease: CHAGA'S DISEASE.

FILARIASIS

Synonym: elephantiasis, non-endemic.

The filarasis in this area is all of the ordinary (Bancroftian) type.

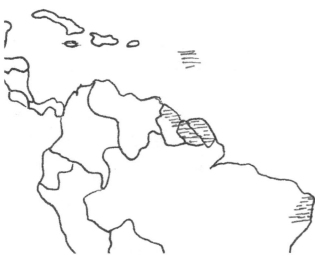

The known distribution of filariasis. PLoS Negl Trop Dis 5(2): e964.

G6PD DEFICIENCY

This is common in the area, but the distribution is such that it is impossible to make a meaningful map.

HEART FAILURE

Restrictive heart failure of unknown cause occurs in Mexico, Colombia, Venezuela and possibly Brazil.

Regional causes of heart failure are SCHISTOSOMIASIS MANSONI and CHAGA'S DISEASE.

HEMORRHAGIC FEVER

Hemorrhagic fever due to DENGUE FEVER occurs in the Dominican Republic, El Salvador, Nicaragua, St. Lucia, Colombia and possibly elsewhere. A regional cause of hemorrhagic fever is YELLOW FEVER. Aside from YELLOW FEVER and DENGUE FEVER which are listed separately, the most common types are Argentine hemorrhagic fever with epidemics every January to August and Bolivian hemorrhagic fever. These are both carried by rodents. Venezuelan HF is similar to LASSA FEVER (see F Notes); it is probably contagious. There are yearly outbreaks in the states of Portuguesa and Barinas, especially during November to January, involving mostly agricultural workers. About one third of the patients die.

HEPATITIS

Hepatitis B is very common in the Amazon Basin, moderately common in the Caribbean, Central America, the Andes and Brazil, and relatively uncommon in Mexico and in temperate South America.

Hepatitis E reportedly occurs in Mexico.

Q FEVER which responds well to DOXYCYCLINE or RIFAMPIN causes a hepatitis in people who handle newborn animals.

Similar regional diseases: BARTONELLOSIS.

HERNIA

This is particularly common in those of African genetic heritage.

HIV INFECTION

This is very common in the Caribbean. It is most common in Bermuda, the Bahamas, Barbados, Trinidad and Tobago. It is more heterosexually than homosexually transmitted, with about half the cases being in the 25–35 y.o. age range. In areas with SCHISTOSOMIASIS MANSONI you should treat all HIV infected patients with PRAZIQUANTEL. SCHISTOSOMIASIS accelerates the progression of HIV.

HOOKWORM

This is common in the Caribbean. In South America, give a second treatment a week after the first.

HYDATID DISEASE

This is particularly common in Argentina, Uruguay, southern Brazil and Chile in sheep- and cattle-raising areas; it is transmitted by dogs.

HYPOGLYCEMIA

This may be caused by PLANT POISONING: ackee, in which case it is of sudden onset and requires immediate treatment.

INTESTINAL FLUKE

Only one kind is found in this region, Gastrodisciasis. It is found only in Guyana, and it causes diarrhea only.

IRRITABLE BOWEL

Similar regional diseases: CHAGA'S DISEASE.

JAUNDICE

Regional causes are YELLOW FEVER and BARTONELLOSIS.

KIDNEY DISEASE

Nephritic failure is common in Trinidad, West Indies. Preschoolers usually survive it well with treatment, but adolescents do not do as well.

Regional causes of *hemolytic failure* are SICKLE CELL DISEASE (African genetic heritage only) and BARTONELLOSIS (Peru and adjacent countries only).

LEPROSY

The countries in this region where it is common, from the most common on down are: Brazil, Paraguay, Venezuela, Dominican Republic, Colombia, Guyana, Cuba, Trinidad and Tobago, Argentina, Ecuador, Mexico. Reportedly it is absent from Chile.

LEPTOSPIROSIS

This is common in Belize, Barbados, Nicaragua and urban Brazil. It occurs all over Latin America. If the patient has respiratory symptoms his prognosis is poor.

LIVER FAILURE

Add the following regional causes:

PLANT POISONING from akee may cause liver failure, as may YELLOW FEVER, both being regional causes.

LIVER FLUKE

Fascioliasis is present in some areas, mainly those that raise sheep or cattle. There is an area with much liver fluke in Asillo zone, Puno Region, Peru. It occurs in Argentina, Brazil, Bolivia, Central America, Chile, Colombia, Cuba, Mexico, Peru, Puerto Rico, Uruguay. Mass treatment of children with TRICLABENDAZOLE is safe and effective.

MALARIA

In some parts of the world malaria is spreading to previously malaria-free areas. Hence the information below might change over time. The following areas reportedly have no malaria transmission, but you should seek locally current information.
- Bolivia: urban areas and above 2500 m (8250 ft.).
- Brazil: some urban areas.
- Colombia: urban areas and above 2500 m.
- Ecuador: Galapagos islands and above 1500 m (5000 ft.).
- Guyana: central Georgetown.
- Mexico: urban areas; rural areas above 2500 m.
- Panama: urban areas.
- Peru: urban areas.
- Surinam: Paramaribo; interior over 2500 m.
- Venezuela: urban areas.

In the Amazon area of Brazil, it is useless to try to eradicate malaria by treating those who are ill, since many people have the disease without feeling sick at all.

There reportedly is much FANSIDAR resistance all over South America, but FANSIDAR works well in Peru. There is reportedly no CHLOROQUINE resistance in Haiti, the Dominican Republic, in Central America north of the Panama Canal or in the northern 1/5 of Argentina. This may change.

MANSONELLOSIS PERSTANS

Cause: worm larva

Age: any, usually adults. **Who:** bitten by culicoides (see the section on insects, Volume 1, Appendix 10). **Onset:** gradual.

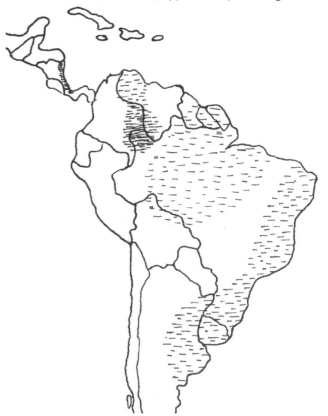

The known distribution of Mansonellosis perstans.

TOC   SYMPTOMS   DIFFERENTIALS   CONDITIONS   DRUG INDEX   REGIONAL NOTES   INX

Clinical

Necessary: general joint pains without fever.

Usual in expatriates, common in nationals: shortness of breath, trouble breathing out, wheezing, itching. Other symptoms of ASTHMA or ALLERGY might also be present.

Sometimes: abdominal pain, especially the right upper abdomen. It may cause chronic fatigue.

Similar conditions: *joint pains without fevers*: ARTHRITIS and similar diseases. *Wheezing and itching resemble* ALLERGY of other causes. *Abdominal pain* is similar to PEPTIC ULCER, AMEBIC LIVER DISEASE, GALLBLADDER DISEASE, LIVER FLUKE or IRRITABLE BOWEL.

Treatment

Prevention: deal with culicoides—see Volume 1, Appendix 10.

Referrals: laboratory: there is always an increased eosinophil count. The worm larvae might be seen in a blood smear. Unlike FILARIASIS, they might be found any time of day or night.

Patient care: DOXYCYCLINE works the best by killing bacteria on which the worms depend. MEBENDAZOLE or ALBENDAZOLE was previously used, but they did not work well. One can prevent the disease by taking IVERMECTIN every 3 months.

Results: within 1–2 weeks.

MOSSY FOOT

Mossy foot has been reported from Ecuador, Guatemala, Mexico and Peru.

MYCETOMA

A local form of this, Lobo's disease, occurs in the Amazon Basin, Costa Rica and Panama. Lumps the size of small bird eggs form on the skin. The skin on top is red and shiny. The disease progresses slowly. There is no treatment.

Similar condition: tertiary SYPHILIS.

MYIASIS

Forms that occur worldwide are particularly common in Paraguay.

A local form of skin myiasis is the macaw worm, the larval form of bot flies. The eggs are carried on other insects and deposited on the skin. The larvae are shaped like little gourds. They may be removed by stretching the hole and popping them out. The larvae are acquired along paths and the edges of forested areas.

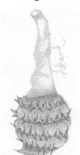

A macaw worm larva, greatly magnified; note the spiny ball and the stem. AB

ONCHOCERCIASIS

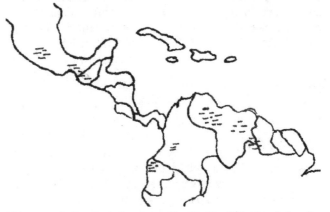

This occurs in the shaded areas and by the Brazil/Venezuela border area. Information derived in part from PLoS Negl Trop Dis 5(2): 2011

The flies that carry onchocerciasis have a much more extensive range than the disease. Hence there is much potential for the spread of the disease. There have been public health campaigns against the disease; thus it has been virtually eliminated in some areas.

PARAGONIMIASIS

This occurs in Colombia, Costa Rica, Mexico, Peru.
It is present to some extent from Peru up to Canada.

PINTA

Cause: spirochete

Synonyms: endemic treponematosis, endemic syphilis.

Mildly to moderately ill; class 1–2; regional: in the past it has been in Cuba, Dominican Republic, Guadaloupe and Haiti. It is less common now than previously, due to public health campaigns. Its present distribution is uncertain.

Age: any, mainly in children and young adults. **Who:** those living near others who have the disease. It is not extremely common anywhere, but it is mostly in poor rural areas that are over-crowded. It is more common in arid than in humid areas. **Onset:** incubation 7–20 days, then within hours to days. The numbers of spots may increase slowly over months.

Clinical

Primary and secondary: at first there is one, then many red bumps on parts of the skin not covered with clothing. These grow over months to flat, scaly, irregular areas. They do not turn into ulcers. At first these areas are darker than normal skin, but with time they become lighter than normal skin or they may be various abnormal colors. The colors vary on each person and also from person to person. They also vary in size. They are symmetrical in 1/3, scaling in 1/3 and itchy in 1/4 of the patients. These areas persist for years and finally heal with significant scarring. The spots occur mostly on the front of the lower leg and on the top of the foot. Lymph nodes near the skin areas may become enlarged, but there is no other general body illness.

Tertiary: in tertiary disease, the skin is whitish and dry with much thickening and many folds. There do not appear to be whole-body symptoms like tertiary SYPHILIS or related diseases.

Similar conditions: flat, scaly, irregular areas might resemble LEPROSY (never itchy), TINEA (indistinguishable), CUTANEOUS LEISHMANIASIS (usually not flat), YAWS (no need to distinguish). The thick, swollen skin might resemble FILARIASIS or MOSSY FOOT.

Treatment

Prevention: general sanitation; early treatment of known cases.

Referrals: laboratory: all blood tests for SYPHILIS will be positive.

Patient care: use PENICILLIN, DOXYCYCLINE or ERYTHROMYCIN.

Results: some results in 48 hours; complete in one week in primary and secondary; healing may take weeks with tertiary, and it may never be complete.

PLAGUE

Plague occurs in Bolivia, LaPaz Department; Brazil, Bahia and Paraiba States; Ecuador, Chimborazo Province; Peru, many areas, northern Argentina. It has not been reported from Central America or the Caribbean.

Since it occurs in the south-western States, it may also be found in northern Mexico. It may occur anywhere.

PNEUMONIA

This might be caused by Rocky Mountain SPOTTED FEVER.

Similar regional diseases: PARAGONIMIASIS, COCCIDIOMYCOSIS.

PNEUMOTHORAX

This is rare in those of African genetic heritage and common in Asians.

PYOMYOSITIS

This is common in the indigenous peoples of eastern tropical Ecuador.

RECTAL PROLAPSE

This may be due to SCHISTOSOMIASIS MANSONI.

RELAPSING FEVER

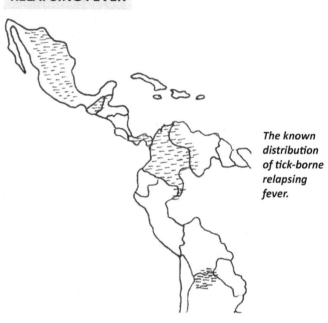

The known distribution of tick-borne relapsing fever.

RESPIRATORY INFECTION

Similar regional diseases: COCCIDIOMYCOSIS, PARAGONIMIASIS.

RHEUMATIC FEVER

This is very common in Chile, affecting 5–20 y.o. people almost exclusively. The death rate is high. It is also very common in Mexico City.

RICKETTSIOSIS

This is a general term that includes Rocky Mountain SPOTTED FEVER.

SCABIES

This is very common in the Caribbean with epidemics occurring.

SCHISTOSOMIASIS MANSONI

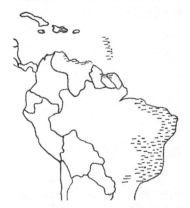

The known distribution of schistosomiasis Mansoni. PLoS Negl Trop Dis 5(2): e964.

SEXUALLY TRANSMITTED DISEASE

GONORRHEA is very common all over, especially in Jamaica; CHANCROID is common and is increasing in El Salvador. DONOVANOSIS occurs in the Caribbean.

SICKLE CELL DISEASE

This occurs only in those of African descent.

SPOTTED FEVER,[1] African tick typhus

See the F regional notes. Reportedly this is present in the French West Indies. Reportedly there are no fatalities, but the same disease is commonly fatal in Africa.

SPOTTED FEVER[1], ROCKY MOUNTAIN

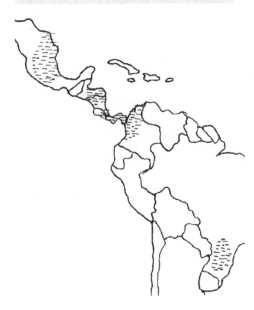

RMSF is found in the shaded areas. It is also found in almost all the States, especially the south-central and southeast, not just the Rocky Mountains. It is particularly common in the south-eastern States. It is prevalent in western Canada.

Cause: Rickettsiae, an intermediate organism

Synonyms: Rickettsiosis, Rocky Mountain spotted fever.[2]

Moderately to very ill; class 2–3, depending on how ill.

Age: any. **Who:** tick-bitten. Susceptible patients are those who spend time outdoors or who have dogs that run freely outside and bring ticks home. People who have G6PD DEFICIENCY and the elderly are generally sicker. It affects those of African descent more than Europeans and males more than females. **Onset:** sudden; incubation 6 to 10 days.

Clinical

Necessary: fever, chills, headache, fatigue, joint and muscle pains (especially in the larger joints), nausea, vomiting and loss of appetite. The spleen is large, tender and firm.

Usually: there is a small scar from the tick bite. The rash appears between days 2 and 5, sometimes as early as day 1 and sometimes not at all. (Older folks and Africans are likely to skip the rash.) It occurs first on the forehead, ankles, wrists and forearms and then on the trunk, palms and soles. At first the spots are red and they blanch with pressure; later they become little black-and-blue spots. It can cause symptoms of PNEUMONIA, ENCEPHALITIS or KIDNEY DISEASE. If the patient dies, it is usually between days 8 and 15. Death is particularly common in males of African or Mediterranean (Hispanic, Italian, Greek, Jewish, Irish, Arab) descent. A rapid pulse and respiratory rate indicates a bad prognosis. Untreated, the fever drops over days during the third week. The skin may peel off.

Other symptoms: there may be mental clouding after a few days. There is swelling around the eyes and possibly swelling of the hands and feet. The neck may be stiff. Muscles are very tender; gentle squeezing will cause severe pain. The patient may have a big liver. He may have genital pain, and his genitals may be destroyed with GANGRENE.

Complications: blindness, deafness, HEART FAILURE, BRAIN DAMAGE, death.

Similar conditions: see Protocols B.2 and B.11.

Typhus is similar except that the rash starts on the trunk and moves to the limbs. VINCENT STOMATITIS may cause similar mouth lesions. LEPTOSPIROSIS may be indistinguishable.

Bush laboratory: the patient may have bilirubin in his urine.

Treatment

Prevention: avoid tick bites: exclude dogs from houses; protect arms and legs when pushing through brush; do not sleep on the ground. Remove ticks immediately after they attach.

---

1 *See the Powerpoint lecture entitled Intermediate Organisms.*

2 *In this region almost all spotted fever is Rocky Mountain spotted fever rather than the more mild African tick typhus. Therefore it is important to use this description rather than the description in the main Condition Index.*

TOC SYMPTOMS DIFFERENTIALS CONDITIONS DRUG INDEX REGIONAL NOTES INX

Referrals: laboratory; a blood test, the Felix-Weil, is useless. In larger hospitals, more advanced tests may be available. With the usual tests, the disease must be present for 6 days before they turn positive. **It is important not to wait for a positive lab test before starting treatment. If you think of the diagnosis, treat it.**

Patient care: CHLORAMPHENICOL, DOXYCYCLINE. For this disease DOXYCYCLINE can be used at any age. The risk from it is less than the risk from CHLORAMPHENICOL, and there are currently no other proven options. Do not use CHLORAMPHENICOL alone; use it with DOXYCYCLINE. CIPROFLOXACIN works in the laboratory, but it is not reliable for treating patients. The patient must be treated until he has been without a fever for a full two days. CO-TRIMOXAZOLE and other sulfa drugs tend to make the disease worse. RIFAMPIN might work; give it for 7–14 days, the shorter time if the patient is not so sick and for 14 days if he/she is very sick. Some patients respond slowly; you might not see any improvement for the first 7 days.

STRONGYLOIDIASIS

This is particularly common in Brazil, the Caribbean, Ecuador, Costa Rica, Panama and Colombia. It is less common but still not rare in Venezuela and in Bolivia.

VISCERAL LEISHMANIASIS and HIV decrease natural immunity. When either of these occurs along with strongyloidiasis, SEPSIS may result.

SYPHILIS

This is very common in Trinidad and presumably in the rest of the Caribbean.

TAPEWORM

Fish tapeworm is especially found in Argentina, southern Chile and the coast of Peru. Pork tapeworm is especially found in Mexico, Central America and Peru.

THALLASEMIA

In the Western Hemisphere it is present to a significant extent only in ethnic groups from Europe, Africa or Asia. In persons of Hispanic ancestry, this may cause severe problems similar to those of the Arabs, Jews and others of Mediterranean genetic origin.

Similar regional diseases: SICKLE CELL DISEASE, BARTONELLOSIS, TROPICAL SPLENOMEGALY, VISCERAL LEISHMANIASIS.

TINEA

Tinea imbricata occurs in Central and South America.

TOXOPLASMOSIS

This is extremely common in Brazil, more so than anywhere else in the world. Try to protect pregnant women.

TRACHOMA

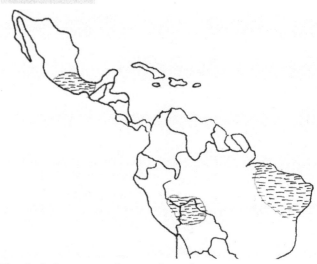

The shaded areas are where trachoma is most common. It occurs worldwide. It is known to be common in Brazil.

TREPONARID

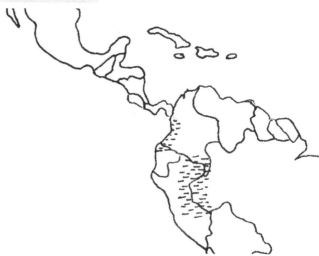

The known distribution of treponarid. It may occur anywhere that is hot and dry, with poor sanitation.

TRICHINOSIS

This is known to occur in eastern Brazil, in Chile and in Mexico.

TRICHURIASIS

This is very common in the Caribbean.

TROPICAL SPASTIC PARAPARESIS

This is common in the Americas, particularly Jamaica; Colombia; and Martinique, French West Indies. In the Caribbean area 90% of the cases are females.

TROPICAL SPLENOMEGALY

This occurs in the Amazon area. In Venezuela, it is most common in the Amazonas Territory where it affects 44% of the inhabitants over 10 y.o.

TUBERCULOSIS

This is very common in the Caribbean and in Bolivia, Peru, Chile and Panama. Multiple drug-resistant TB is common in Bolivia.

TUNGIASIS

This occurs in all of Central America, Mexico and the northern 3/4 of South America.

TURISTA

In Venezuela, about 60% of the diarrheas in children should respond to DOXYCYCLINE.

TYPHUS

Louse-borne typhus occurs in central Mexico, the Andes and western Bolivia.

Murine typhus occurs also in entire Central America, up to the Rio Grande River and beyond into the States. It is carried there by cat and opossum fleas. It also occurs in Colombia; it is more common in coastal areas than further inland.

VISCERAL LEISHMANIASIS

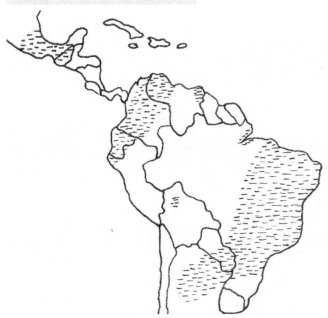

The known distribution of visceral Leishmaniasis.

This occurs in dry or only moderately humid mountainous areas below 800 m (2500 ft.). It is mainly rural. Epidemics are more likely after a drought. In addition to the areas shown, it occurs in the Caribbean in south-western Guadaloupe and in central Martinique. It occurs both in NW and NE Argentina and in Chiapas, SE Mexico.

Age: in Brazil, most patients are less than 5 y.o.; everywhere else most patients are under 20 y.o.

VITILIGO

Similar regional diseases: ONCHOCERCIASIS

WARTS

Similar regional disease: BARTONELLOSIS.

XEROPHTHALMIA

This is known to occur in Haiti and Brazil

YAWS

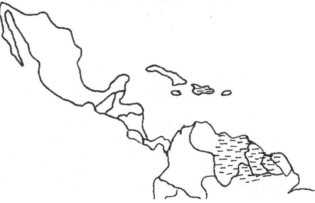

The known distribution of yaws. It may occur in any hot, humid climate.

YELLOW FEVER

Cause: virus

Moderately to very ill; class 2–4; regional

Epidemics occur during the rainy season.

Age: any but the majority of cases have been in children. **Who:** unimmunized; frequently in epidemics, transmitted by mosquitoes that bite during the day. **Onset:** over a day or two after an incubation of 3–6 days.

Clinical

The WHO definition for yellow fever: fever plus bilirubin in the urine plus one or more of the following:
• a slow pulse relative to the fever.
• abnormal bleeding.
• upper abdominal pain.
• protein in urine.
• decreased amount of urine.

TOC   SYMPTOMS   DIFFERENTIALS   CONDITIONS   DRUG INDEX   REGIONAL NOTES   INX

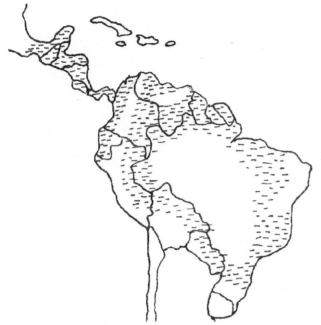

The known distribution of yellow fever. The mosquitoes that carry this are widespread, so the disease may also spread.

Clinical

Necessary: the patient has fever, nausea and aching all over, especially in the back, the waist area and the limbs. JAUNDICE develops only after several days of illness. The spleen is not enlarged.

Usually: there is a severe headache and eye pain. The pulse is initially rapid, but by day 3 or 4, the pulse slows and may become slow relative to the fever. The mind is clear; the patient does not act intoxicated like he does with TYPHUS unless he is about to die.

Frequently: there is a day of recovery before the disease starts a second time.

Sometimes: the yellow color of the whites of the eyes may be quite indistinct. It becomes worse gradually, if at all. The face may be swollen. There may be severe general bone and joint pains. Vomiting may occur early, as may insomnia and a tender but non-swollen liver. The vomit is probably mucus at first, turning to black or bloody later on. The patient may have a body odor resembling a butcher shop.

Complications: LIVER FAILURE, KIDNEY DISEASE. Mental symptoms start late and indicate a poor prognosis. An occasional complication is HEMORRHAGIC FEVER: nosebleeds; bleeding gums; bloody stool, urine or vomit; heavy menstruation; major bleeding from minor wounds. There is a high death rate during epidemics.

Similar diseases: Protocols B.2, B.5 and B.9. MALARIA with jaundice is different in that the jaundice appears the first day or two. The pulse in malaria is normal or rapid relative to the fever.

Bush laboratory: bilirubin in the urine is quite common. There is almost always protein in the urine by the second day of illness. There may be blood in the urine on the third or fourth day. Sophisticated hospital laboratories can do blood tests or liver biopsies.

Treatment

Prevention: immunize. Excellent immunization is available. Immunity starts about 10 days after the injection. Persons should be re-immunized every 10 years. Be sure to care for patients under a mosquito net to avoid transmitting the disease to others.

Referrals: laboratory: this requires a level 4 lab at least. Facilities: at least a level 4.

Patient care: same as HEPATITIS and, if necessary, HEMORRHAGIC FEVER. VITAMIN K injections may be helpful.

Results: at least half the patients who develop severe symptoms die. Those who recover have a very long convalescence.

INDEX N: ARCTIC NOTES

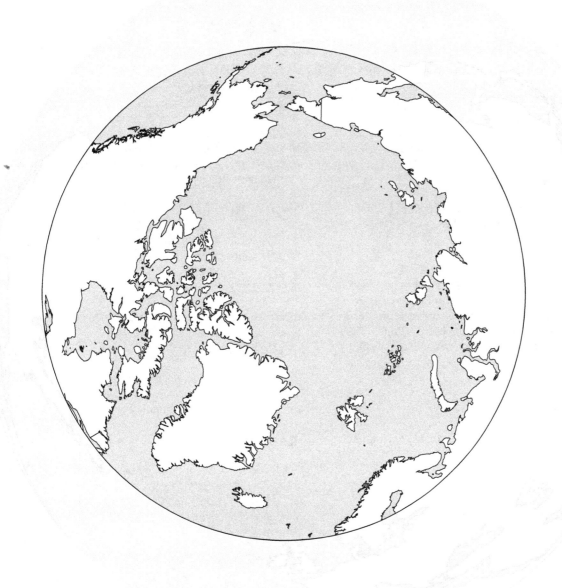

TOC

SYMPTOMS

DIFFERENTIALS

CONDITIONS

DRUG INDEX

REGIONAL NOTES

INX

ANEMIA

In the Arctic this is commonly due to iron deficiency; peptic ulcer and consequent bleeding is frequently the underlying cause. It occurs in spite of a high meat consumption. If the person eats poorly cooked fresh water fish, then treat for fish TAPEWORM which is also a common cause of anemia in this area.

BRUCELLOSIS

This occurs in this area, acquired through both reindeer and caribou.

CRYPTOSPORIDIOSIS

In northern Quebec it is associated with seals.

EAR INFECTION, MIDDLE

Use amoxicillin under age 6; use penicillin over age 6; ear infections are especially common in Alaskan native children.

ENCEPHALITIS

Tick borne encephalitis and Siberian encephalitis both occur in the Asian Arctic extending south near the eastern coast, to Vladivostok. They can be transmitted by the consumption of unpasteurized dairy products as well as by insect bites. They are most common in the spring and summer. Immunization is available in Europe. Treatment is only supportive; provide food, water, treatment of symptoms and sanitation.

FOOD POISONING

Botulism occurs when meats are left out to age or cure and then eaten. Polar bear liver is toxic.

GIARDIASIS

Giardiasis is related to contact with water where seals have been, as well as other mammals.

HEPATITIS

Hepatitis A is unusual in the Arctic. He*patitis B* is common, a frequent cause of LIVER FAILURE in Alaska. He*patitis E* is related to caribou meat in the Canadian Inuit and in Siberia.

HYDATID DISEASE

Cystic: this is common in the Asian arctic where dogs live close to people. It may affect any organ.

Alveolar: occurs in western Alaska and Russia; don't eat food gathered from the wild without cooking it first. This may also be transmitted by dog contact.

LIVER FLUKE

A kind of liver fluke, *Opisthorcis felineus*, occurs in Russia and Siberia. It is indistinguishable from *Opisthorcis viverni* which is prevalent in Thailand. The symptoms mimic GALLBLADDER DISEASE. The parasite can cause CANCER. It comes from eating insufficiently cooked fish.

LYME DISEASE

This occurs in eastern Russia.

MALNUTRITION

Vitamin D deficiency is very common in this area, but sea mammals, fish and whale blubber contain the vitamin. All pregnant women need vitamin D supplementation, as do infants who are fed formula. Formula is not sufficiently fortified with vitamin D.

PEPTIC ULCER

In the Arctic a bacterial cause is common, especially in Canadian aboriginals.

PERTUSSIS

This is very common where there is no immunization.

PNEUMONIA

This is very common in northern Quebec. It is common throughout the Arctic. Many of the bacteria are resistant to antibiotics because of antibiotic abuse.

RABIES

This is common in non-human mammals except in northern Scandinavia. It is carried by the Arctic fox. Dogs may have rabies but still appear healthy for a long time. Most of the rabies is paralytic rather than furious. Rabies is rare in humans.

RHEUMATIC FEVER

Rheumatic fever is common amongst the Yakut of eastern Siberia.

RICKETS

Vitamin D deficiency is very common in this area, but sea mammals, fish and whale blubber contain the vitamin. All pregnant women need vitamin D supplementation, as do infants who are fed formula. Formula is not sufficiently fortified with vitamin D.

SCURVY

This is common in the Arctic, due to lack of fresh fruits and vegetables.

SEPSIS

Greenland: use Gram-positive and Gram-negative antibiotics both and also cover staph. The best oral drugs for staph are either CLOXACILLIN or [RIFAMPIN plus CO-TRIMOXAZOLE].

SEXUALLY TRANSMITTED DISEASES

All sexually transmitted diseases are many times more prevalent in the Arctic than in more temperate and tropical climates. They are found more in females than males, more in the native population than in those of European descent.

SPOTTED FEVER

Spotted fever occurs in Mongolia and Siberia only. Another name is Siberian tick typhus.

TAPEWORM

Fish tapeworm is common; it requires cold fresh water. Be sure fresh water fish are well cooked. Pickling is not sufficient to kill the cysts.

TOXOPLASMOSIS

This is common in northern Canada. It is related to caribou and seal meat and to contaminated drinking water.

TRICHINOSIS

This is especially common in northern Canada. It may be caused by a unique species associated with polar bear, seal and walrus meat. It withstands freezing temperatures for long periods of time. Thorough cooking is necessary to prevent the disease. Smoking, salting and drying are not good enough. The first episode is the same as ordinary trichinosis; subsequent episodes are associated with prolonged diarrhea without fever after an episode of muscle weakness.

TUBERCULOSIS

This is common.

Arctic houses are frequently crowded and bathing is a luxury. Hence lice thrive. Many of the diseases and conditions that are labeled "tropical" are actually conditions that are associated with poverty rather than a warm climate per se. Many of them occur in impoverished cold climates. This is particularly true for louse-borne diseases: typhus, trench fever, relapsing fever. The following are diseases, often thought of as tropical, which are found in the Arctic region:

BRUCELLOSIS	CRYPTOSPORIDIOSIS	MEDITERRANEAN SPOTTED FEVER
CELLULITIS	GIARDIASIS	RELAPSING FEVER
CHOLERA	LYME DISEASE	STRONGYLOIDIASIS

In the *North American* Arctic the main problems are: BRUCELLOSIS, TOXOPLASMOSIS, TRICHINOSIS, GIARDIASIS, CRYPTOSPORIDIOSIS, ECHINOCOCCOSIS, RABIES and TULAREMIA.

In the *Russian* Arctic the main problems are: TUBERCULOSIS, ENCEPHALITIS, TULAREMIA, BRUCELLOSIS, LEPTOSPIROSIS, RABIES, ANTHRAX, LYME DISEASE.

The following are truly tropical diseases which will not ordinarily be found in the Arctic:

Arboviral fever	Dengue fever	Malaria	Tropical ulcer
Chikungunya	Filariasis	Schistosomiasis	Visceral Leishmaniasis
Ascariasis	Hemorrhagic fever	Spotted fever	Yaws
Cutaneous Leishmaniasis	Hookworm	Trichuriasis	Yellow fever

INDEX O: EAST ASIA NOTES

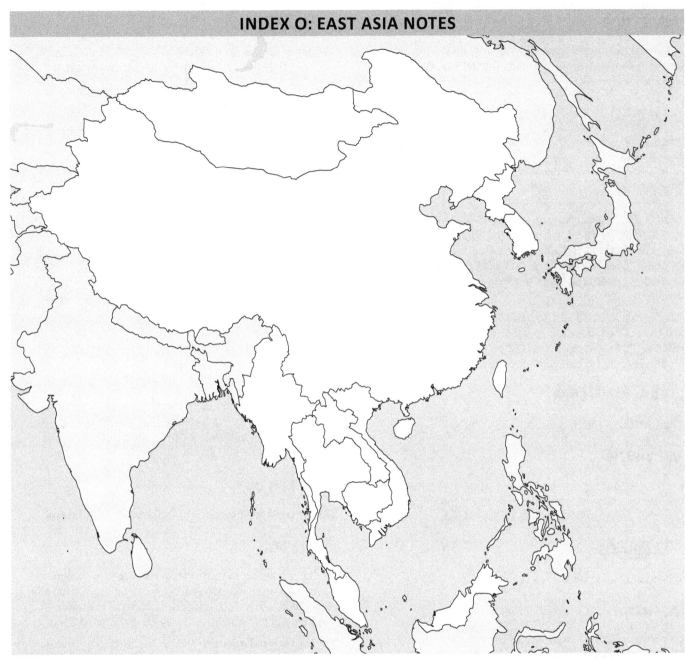

Map disclaimers

- Read the captions carefully. They are not all the same.

- Maps are notoriously unreliable. Conditions may be found in areas not shaded; conditions may be absent in areas that are shaded. Usually a disease is present only in spotty areas within the shaded region. A diagnosis is possible if there is shading anywhere around your location or if your patient has traveled through a shaded area.

- There is lack of shading both where there are no data and also where data exists indicating that the condition is absent. Lack of shading more often indicates lack of data than absence of the condition.

- Epidemiologists and government health officers survey in easy locations, near major roads. If you are in a remote, difficult location the maps may not reflect the reality that you see.

- Beware of shading that stops at political boundaries; germs don't respect border controls.

- Beware of areas that are unshaded for a variety of diseases. It may be because no one educated has ever entered that area and made it out alive. It may also be because intelligent people know enough not to go there.

- At times of civil unrest, natural disaster and migrations, the distribution of diseases changes unpredictably and rapidly. With biological warfare, this problem will be compounded.

TOC SYMPTOMS DIFFERENTIALS CONDITIONS DRUG INDEX **REGIONAL NOTES** INX

ADDICTION

A regional example of uppers is miang which is used in northern Thailand. Betel nut (under PLANT POISONING) is also used regionally.

AMEBIASIS

This is especially common in Taiwan, China and Thailand. It is not common in Laos.

ANEMIA

Anemia due to red cell destruction, while most often due to MALARIA, may be due to THALLASEMIA in persons from northeast Thailand and adjacent areas. It may also be due to OVALOCYTOSIS in Malaysians. TROPICAL SPLENOMEGALY may cause this in scattered areas, and VISCERAL LEISHMANIASIS in China.

Anemia due to blood loss: if the stool is positive for blood and the problem does not respond to treatment for HOOKWORM, consider SCHISTOSOMIASIS JAPONICUM in areas where that is prevalent. See the map.

ARBOVIRAL FEVER

CHIKUNGUNYA FEVER has spread into China.

ARTHRITIS

In China, RICKETS is a common and RHEUMATIC FEVER, an uncommon cause of arthritis; in Indochina, the situation is reversed. Suspect RICKETS in Muslim women.

ASCARIASIS

This is common in Laos.

ASTHMA

This is especially common in Indochina. The kind caused by little insects living in dust is common in China and Taiwan. It may be common elsewhere also.

BERIBERI

This is common in agricultural workers in Malaysia.

BLADDER STONE

This occurs in this area.

BRAIN DAMAGE

Regional causes are Japanese ENCEPHALITIS and SCHISTOSOMIASIS JAPONICUM.

BRUCELLOSIS

This is a problem in some areas of China.

CANCER

Cancer of the mouth is caused by the use of betel nut or miang (northern Thailand). (See PLANT POISONING.)

Cancer of the nose and throat is more common than average in this area, due to a virus.

Cancer of the stomach is quite common in the easternmost areas, but the cause is uncertain.

Cancer of the bile duct (gallbladder area) is common in areas with LIVER FLUKE, especially in northeast Thailand.

Cancer of the liver is very prevalent in this area. It appears to be related to HEPATITIS B as well as PLANT POISONING (aflatoxin) due to sausage and moldy peanuts.

CANCRUM ORIS

This is rare in the region, except for areas of China with VISCERAL LEISHMANIASIS.

CHANCROID

This is particularly common in Korea and in Indochina. In Southeast Asia many strains of this are resistant to DOXYCYCLINE, SULFA and CO-TRIMOXAZOLE. Most strains are sensitive to ERYTHROMYCIN, CHLORAMPHENICOL, ceftriaxone (see CEPHALOSPORIN), CIPROFLOXACIN and other -oxacins.

CHICKEN POX

Similar regional disease: SPOTTED FEVER, Rickettsial pox.

CHOLERA

This occurs mainly in epidemics in times of war, drought or flood, although single cases occur here and there in Indochina. It is common in Malaysia but does not occur in Taiwan. It occurs from time to time in Korea and mainland China.

Similar regional disease: FOOD POISONING from rice.

CIRRHOSIS

Regional causes are SCHISTOSOMIASIS JAPONICUM (particularly in China) and INDIAN CHILDHOOD CIRRHOSIS.

CRETINISM

The first kind of cretinism[1] affects most cretins in Asia except for the Himalayan area where it affects only 50%. The second kind affects 50% of the cretins in the Himalayan area and rare cretins elsewhere in Asia.

CYSTICERCOSIS

It is very common in Korea and in China.

---

1 *This refers to the description in the Condition Index.*

DENGUE FEVER

In Indochina this is very common. There are yearly epidemics in urban areas during the rainy season. The mosquitoes that carry the disease breed in house plants. In China there are also epidemics, especially in the south. DENGUE HEMORRHAGIC FEVER occurs throughout this area. See HEMORRHAGIC FEVER also.

DEPRESSION

This may be caused by LIVER FLUKE.

DIPHTHERIA

This is not common but it does occur sometimes in the crowded slum areas of Thailand and presumably other Asian countries. In Burma SCRUB TYPHUS may appear similar.

DONOVANOSIS

It is not common, but it does occur in this region.

DYSENTERY

Amebic dysentery is generally very common in Indochina, but relatively uncommon in mainland China.
Bacterial dysentery is common throughout Indochina.

Similar regional diseases: SCHISTOSOMIASIS JAPONICUM and PIG-BEL (uncommon).

ENCEPHALITIS

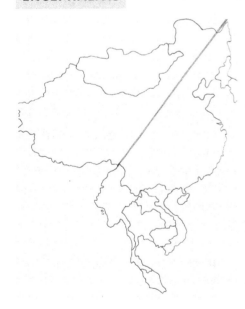

The known distribution of Japanese encephalitis. It occurs southeast of this line and throughout Indochina. The disease occurs but is not so common in the rest of the area. About 40% of those who get the disease die from it, and most of the rest have long-term disability.

The only common kind of encephalitis in the southern part of this area is Japanese encephalitis. It occurs south and east of a line drawn between the China-Burma-India border point and Khabarovsk, Russia. It also occurs throughout Southeast Asia. There are yearly epidemics in Indochina, especially in northern Thailand, with most cases in July; it is carried by evening-biting mosquitoes.

Prevention: there is a good immunization available for JE. Patients should be cared for under mosquito nets to avoid infecting the local mosquitoes and thus transmitting the disease. RIBAVIRIN does absolutely no good for treatment.

ENTERIC FEVER

Typhoid fever occurs mainly from June to September in Korea. It occurs all year in Indochina.

Paratyphoid is mainly from unsanitary food; it is not common in this area.

Similar regional disease: the second phase of SCHISTOSOMIASIS JAPONICUM, about 30-90 days after exposure, may resemble this. Consider this carefully, as the treatments are quite different.

FILARIASIS

Synonym: elephantiasis, non-endemic.

This occurs in eastern China. There are two types of filariasis: Brugian and Bancroftian:

Bancroftian filariasis often affects legs and the male genitals. It seldom or never affects breasts and arms. It is found in the southeast of China and as far north along the coast as Qingdao. It is also found throughout Vietnam and on the island of Hainan.

Brugian filariasis often affects the breasts and arms.

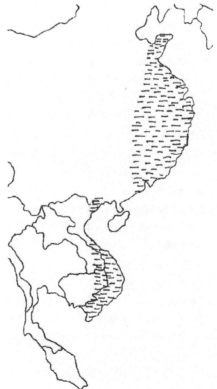

The known distribution of Bancroftian filariasis. Additionally, Brugian filariasis is found throughout the Malaysian peninsula.

FOOD POISONING

Gallbladder of raw fish: see separate entry below.

There are two kinds of food poisons that are peculiar to this area:

rice that has stood at room temperature for a day or two grows bacteria that cause severe, watery diarrhea.

raw shellfish (mussels, clams and oysters) concentrate a toxin which causes symptoms within 30 minutes. It starts with tingling and numbness around the mouth first and then the limbs. Later, vomiting and incoordination occur. Death is not uncommon. It initially appears similar to HYPERVENTILATION.

G6PD DEFICIENCY

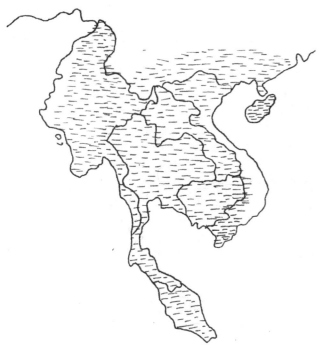

These are the areas at greatest risk for this condition. The area of the patient's genetic heritage is important, not his current location. Information derived from PLoS Med 9(11): 2012

GALLBLADDER DISEASE

This is particularly associated with OVALOCYTOSIS (Malaysia), THALLASEMIA (northeast Thailand and adjacent areas) and LIVER FLUKE (northeast Thailand and the Far East). It is a common cause of ACUTE ABDOMEN in eastern Asia.

GALLBLADDER OF RAW FISH

This is from carp, which is a bottom feeder—caught with hooks or nets that have heavy weights. It is poisonous even after it is cooked. It is used in Asia as a Chinese traditional medicine for poor eyesight. It causes nausea, vomiting, diarrhea, abdominal pain, LIVER FAILURE and KIDNEY DISEASE. For similar conditions see Protocol B.7.

Treatment: not feasible in the village situation.

GIARDIASIS

In mainland China it is not common, but when it occurs symptoms tend to be severe.

GOITER

Regional, especially in lowland river deltas, inland and high-altitude areas; rare to very common.

In Burma it is common both in lowland and hilly areas. It is also common amongst the Penans (Malaysia).

In mainland China, goiter due to IODINE excess occurs in the Kuitun-usum area and also in sea-coastal areas where people consume kelp salt and pickled vegetables.

HEART ATTACK

This is common in mainland China.

HEART FAILURE

This is common in mainland China. Regional diseases that are associated with it are SCHISTOSOMIASIS JAPONICUM and KESHAN DISEASE.

HEMORRHAGIC FEVER

In Indochina the most common cause is DENGUE FEVER in children and expatriate adults. In the easternmost areas (the eastern parts of China, in Japan and Korea) it may be caused by an ARBOVIRAL FEVER associated with KIDNEY DISEASE; it is usually fatal. Hemorrhagic fever occurs in Xinjiang Province, NW China.

HEPATITIS

Most local people have been exposed to hepatitis B prenatally or during childhood; it is a common problem in expatriates. It may be food- or water-borne in this area. Epidemics affecting nationals are usually water-borne hepatitis E in Burma, Thailand, southern China and Malaysia. In Mongolia hepatitis A is very common but hepatitis E is rare.

Similar regional diseases: SCHISTOSOMIASIS JAPONICUM and LIVER FLUKE. LEPTOSPIROSIS (common in Malaysia and central Thailand) may be indistinguishable.

HIV INFECTION

This is very common in Thailand. There is also a focus on the Thai-Burmese border, the "Golden Triangle".

HOOKWORM

This is common throughout this area. It is very common amongst agricultural workers, amongst the Ibans of Malaysia and in Anhui Province of mainland China. In Cambodia, about 50% of the population are infected.

TOC

SYMPTOMS

DIFFERENTIALS

CONDITIONS

DRUG INDEX

REGIONAL NOTES

INX

HYDATID DISEASE

Both kinds occur in Mongolia and also in north and north-west China: Gansu, Ningxia Hui, Qinghai, Sichuan and Xingjiang; these are high-altitude areas in the Liupan mountains. Red foxes and small mammals are the hosts for the type transmitted by wild animal stool. This kind may also be transmitted by dogs who live close to people. It is not common, but when it occurs it is very aggressive. Ordinary hydatid disease is passed between domestic dogs and sheep. Risk factors are poor hygiene, female gender, low income, limited education, dog ownership, and lack of well water.

This is not common, but it may occur in Indochina (Laos and Vietnam) and in the Himalaya area.

HYPERVENTILATION

Similar regional disease: FOOD POISONING. See the entry in this index.

INTESTINAL FLUKE

One kind is echinostomiasis which occurs in Taiwan, and has minimal symptoms. It comes from eating inadequately cooked tadpoles, snails, fish and frogs.

A second kind is metagonimiasis which is from eating raw fish. It is especially common in Korea. It provokes a high eosinophil count (hospital lab) and may result in HEART FAILURE. It may also invade the brain or spinal cord like SCHISTOSOMIASIS.

Another kind, fasciolopsiasis, is particularly common in Thailand amongst children who eat fresh-water plants. It is also common in Taiwan and the Far East generally. It is very common on the banks of large lakes with lotus plants and snails where there is sewage contamination of the water. In such areas up to 25% of the population may be infected.

JAUNDICE

The most common causes in this area are HEPATITIS, MALARIA, LEPTOSPIROSIS, AMEBIASIS. Less common causes are LIVER FLUKE, INDIAN CHILDHOOD CIRRHOSIS, liver CANCER and SCHISTOSOMIASIS JAPONICUM.

KATAYAMA DISEASE

This refers to the initial stage of SCHISTOSOMIASIS JAPONICUM (common) or HYDATID DISEASE (rare).

KESHAN DISEASE

Cause: selenium deficiency

Very ill; class 3; mainland China

Age: adolescents and adults. **Who:** those eating a diet low in selenium (one of the minerals) **Onset:** very sudden.

Clinical

This is a type of sudden, severe, HEART FAILURE (floppy type). It is almost invariably fatal.

Treatment

Prevention: use selenium supplements in the diet.

Patient care: this should be done at a hospital, but the patient will probably die in any case. Treating it like ordinary HEART FAILURE might help temporarily.

KIDNEY DISEASE

Nephritic kidney disease is very common in Indochina.

Infective/toxic type of kidney disease is caused by a kind of ARBOVIRAL FEVER which can become HEMORRHAGIC FEVER in the Far East.

Hemolytic type may be caused by OVALOCYTOSIS in Malaysia.

LARVA MIGRANS

In Sarawak (Borneo) and Thailand eating raw snail is a common source; in central and northern Thailand it comes from handling raw meat without gloves. This kind of deep larva migrans is called gnathostomiasis. It can cause very serious problems, including blindness. Handle raw meat only with gloves or tongs.

Similar regional diseases: deep larva migrans, if it is in the liver, may mimic LIVER FLUKE. In China, PARAGONIMIASIS may cause symptoms resembling skin-type larva migrans.

LEPROSY

This is very common throughout this area.

LEPTOSPIROSIS

This may occur in epidemics. It is common in Indochina and Korea. It occurs in mainland China and in Thailand. In Malaysia it is common in oil palm and rubber workers, but not common in rice farmers.

LIVER FAILURE

Add the following regional causes:
   SCHISTOSOMIASIS JAPONICUM.
   LIVER FLUKE.

LIVER FLUKE

Synonyms: Chinese liver fluke, chlonorchiasis, opisthorchiasis (this is the kind that occurs in Thailand and other parts of Indochina).

This is present in the eastern 1/3 of China, all the way north into Siberia and throughout Indochina. In Laos, 36% of the population is infected.

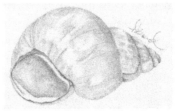

A magnified snail that carries the liver fluke; actual lengths are 1–1.5 cm. Note the many swirls and the relatively small hole. AB

LYME DISEASE

This is known to occur in NE China.

MALABSORPTION

SCHISTOSOMIASIS JAPONICUM is a regional cause;
See Protocol B.14 for other causes.

MALARIA

The following areas have no malaria transmission at all: Brunei, Korea (N & S), Hong Kong, Japan, Macao, Mongolia, Singapore, Taiwan. Also reportedly there is no malaria transmission in the following areas, but check local information. Malaria has been moving to higher elevations in many parts of the world, up to 2500 meters (8000 feet).

- Cambodia: above 1500 m (5000 ft.).
- China: the north of the country, urban areas and the south above 1500 m (5000 ft.).
- Laos: Vientiane.
- Thailand: Bangkok and suburbs, Pattaya, Phuket.
- Vietnam: above 1500 m (5000 ft.); the Red and Mekong deltas.
- One should keep in mind that, worldwide, malaria is entering areas where it previously was not transmitted. Therefore the areas listed above might be newly endemic. Seek local lore.
- Knowlesi malaria is spreading throughout Southeast Asia.

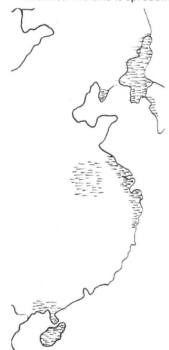

The shaded areas are where vivax malaria is known to occur in China and North Korea.

In the following areas, malaria is extremely common: Sarawak, Sabah, hilly border areas of Malaysia and of Thailand and the southern half of China. Vivax malaria extends quite far north in eastern China.

In southern China almost all the malaria is non-falciparum; in Indochina it is almost all falciparum. In Thailand it is almost all resistant to CHLOROQUINE and FANSIDAR. It is partly resistant to QUININE, and there is some MEFLOQUINE resistance.

In Malaysia rural aboriginals are quite immune to falciparum after age 20, while town dwellers are more vulnerable in adulthood.

MALNUTRITION

Kwashiorkor occurs in the northern half of China. In Malaysia, marasmus is more common. Patients who have VISCERAL LEISHMANIASIS or SCHISTOSOMIASIS JAPONICUM are likely to have more problems with malnutrition.

MELIOIDOSIS

See SEPSIS. This is a form of SEPSIS that occurs in rural Indochina.

MENINGITIS

There have been meningococcal meningitis epidemics in Mongolia. This is the kind of meningitis with rapid onset and rapid spread throughout the community.

PARAGONIMIASIS

This is generally common throughout the area.

PELLAGRA

This is common in corn-growing parts of China.

PIG-BEL

This is not common but might occur in rural Asia.

PLAGUE

This is known to occur in Vietnam, Burma, Mongolia and central China.

PLANT POISONING

Atriplicism occurs in China.

PNEUMOTHORAX

This is common in Asians.

POLIO

This had been common in Indochina, especially Laos. It has reportedly been eliminated.

RABIES

This is a major problem in Thailand due to lack of routine immunization of dogs.

RELAPSING FEVER

This occurs anywhere there is crowding and body lice. Reportedly it is uncommon and occurs on the Asian mainland only, not on islands. It might spread.

RHEUMATIC FEVER

This is very common in Thailand and Mongolia; less so in mainland China and Taiwan.

RICKETS

This is particularly common in females and babies in Muslim cultures and in China.

SCHISTOSOMIASIS JAPONICUM

Cause: worm

Synonyms: bilharzia, snail fever, Japonicum.

Mildly ill to very ill; class 2; regional; this is particularly common in Fujian Province of China and generally in southern China, south of the Yangtze River and along both banks of the river. This description also applies to SCHISTOSOMIASIS MEKONGI; the two diseases are indistinguishable for your purposes.

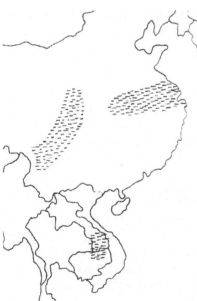

The known distribution of schistosomiasis Japonicum and schistosomiasis Mekongi. There is a spotty distribution within the shaded area.

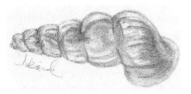

The type of snail that carries schistosomiasis Japonicum, enlarged. Note the small hole and many swirls. Some have stripes and some do not. The actual length is about 0.7–1 cm. AB

Age: any. **Who**: skin exposed to water with infected snails.
Onset: beginning 3–7 weeks after exposure.

Clinical

Initially: in Westerners this frequently starts as KATAYAMA DISEASE. Nationals skip this stage.

30 to 90 days after exposure: the patient may have lower-right abdominal pains with fevers, diarrhea or DYSENTERY and cough. The DYSENTERY may be profuse. This stage can look just like ENTERIC FEVER. The patient is probably unable to work.

Three to five years later: the person has LIVER FAILURE with a large liver, large spleen and an abdomen full of fluid so he looks pregnant. The liver enlarges before the spleen, the opposite of MALARIA. Frequently it is the left lobe which enlarges; this may be confused with splenic enlargement. The patient will have a decreased appetite and weight loss. Children grow poorly, and they may have delayed sexual maturity. Alternatively, the patient may have chronic diarrhea, DYSENTERY and MALABSORPTION (prompt, watery diarrhea whenever he eats anything).

Complications: it may cause CANCER of the rectum. The organism may invade the brain, causing paralysis, SEIZURES, bizzare behavior, blindness and possibly coma. This is called neuro-schistosomiasis. It may invade the lung, causing RESPIRATORY INFECTION and HEART FAILURE. These symptoms must be treated promptly on mere suspicion in anyone who has had any exposure during his or her lifetime. Be sure to use PREDNISONE as well as PRAZIQUANTEL.

Similar Conditions: *fever and fatigue*: in the early stage resembles ENTERIC FEVER and SERUM SICKNESS. (KATAYAMA DISEASE is a type of SERUM SICKNESS). *Later stages* are difficult to distinguish from LIVER FAILURE and MALABSORPTION from other causes; See Protocols B.7 and B.14. *Brain effects* sometimes resemble POLIO (paralysis), STROKE (paralysis), ENCEPHALITIS (seizures, bizzare behavior), CYSTICERCOSIS (seizures).

Bush laboratory: one can hatch the worm eggs and see the larvae using simple equipment. See Appendix 2 in Volume 1. This is more sensitive (more likely will be positive in the presence of the disease) than an egg search in a higher-level laboratory.

Treatment

Prevention: use latrines; avoid exposure of skin to contaminated water; let a bucket of water without snails stand overnight before washing with it. Use ARTEMISININ for the first 21 days after exposure; use PRAZIQUANTEL after 21 days and again after 6–12 weeks. Persons, such as fishermen, who are repeatedly exposed should take both ARTEMISININ and PRAZIQUANTEL weekly.

TOC

SYMPTOMS

DIFFERENTIALS

CONDITIONS

DRUG INDEX

REGIONAL NOTES

INX

Referrals: laboratory: the worm eggs can be found in the stool during the second stage of the disease. (Stool may be negative for eggs during the KATAYAMA phase.) The blood count may show increased eosinophils during the first and second stages only, in about 1/2 of the expatriates who get the disease.

Patient care: PRAZIQUANTEL. It is effective and safe enough to use even if you are not certain of the diagnosis. Occasionally patients get a severe allergic response (see ALLERGY) to the first dose of the drug. This is treated like any other ALLERGY, but do not stop the drug. It is due to dead and dying worms and will not recur as severely with subsequent doses.

If there are neurological symptoms (seizures, paralysis, loss of sensation, altered mental status), additionally use DEXAMETHASONE, PREDNISONE or PREDNISOLONE, as you would for MENINGITIS due to TB. With neuro-schistosomiasis it is necessary to give the patient a second treatment with PRAZIQUANTEL 4–6 weeks later.

If you don't have PRAZIQUANTEL, reportedly MEFLOQUINE plus ARTEMISININ (as artesunate) works almost as well as PRAZIQUANTEL. Seek recent information.

In advanced liver disease PROPRANOLOL might be helpful. In either case seek professional medical advice. NIRIDAZOLE is an old, dangerous drug that should no longer be used. During the KATAYAMA phase it is essential to use PREDNISONE also. See the Drug Index.

Results: you should do repeat lab at 1, 3 and 6 months. When schistosomiasis and HEPATITIS occur together, the prognosis is very poor.

SCHISTOSOMIASIS MEKONGI

Synonyms: bilharzia, snail fever.

See SCHISTOSOMIASIS JAPONICUM. This disease is indistinguishable and the treatment is the same. The distinction is only academic. Schistosomiasis Mekongi is found on Khong Island in southern Laos, in fishermen on house boats near Kratie, east Kampuchea and amongst the Orang Asli in Pahang and Perak States in Malaysia.

SCRUB TYPHUS

This occurs in the rural Asian and Pacific areas below 3800 m (12,500 ft.); it is most common in palm oil workers. It occurs throughout Asia between the north coast of Australia and the northern border of Mongolia, and also throughout the Indian subcontinent. A form of scrub typhus found in Burma causes huge node swelling in the neck, resembling DIPHTHERIA.

SEIZURES

Regional causative diseases are PARAGONIMIASIS and SCHISTOSOMIASIS JAPONICUM.

SEPSIS

Melioidosis is a form of this that occurs in rural Indochina. There is a high death rate, especially in those with DIABETES or KIDNEY DISEASE.

SPOTTED FEVER (TICK TYPHUS)

Rickettsial pox may occur in Korea. In eastern Mongolia the problem is very common.

SPRUE

This occurs in the entire area except for western China and Korea.

STROKE

Regional causes are SCHISTOSOMIASIS JAPONICUM and PARAGONIMIASIS. In China the problem is common and is usually due to HYPERTENSION.

STRONGYLOIDIASIS

This is very common in Indochina. The disease tends to persist in those who have had it; worms can be detected 30 years after the patient's last exposure.

Similar regional disease: SCHISTOSOMIASIS JAPONICUM in its initial stages.

SYPHILIS

In Thailand and in Mongolia syphilis is common. Congenital syphilis is common in newborns.

TAPEWORM

The dwarf and rat tapeworms are common in Asia. Pork tapeworm is common in China. In Mongolia there is only beef tapeworm.

THALLASEMIA

In southern China, northeastern Thailand and the surrounding areas this is quite common.

Similar regional diseases: VISCERAL LEISHMANIASIS, OVALOCYTOSIS.

TINEA

Tinea imbricata occurs in some coastal areas.

TOXEMIA

This is very common in China. In Malaysia it is more common amongst the Indians than Malays or Chinese, probably because of their depressed economic status.

TOXOPLASMOSIS

This is not common in China or Malaysia. There is a small risk in Thailand.

TRACHOMA

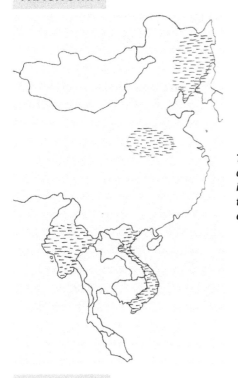

The shaded areas are where trachoma is most common in this region. It may occur anywhere.

TREPONARID

This is found only in western China in this region.

TRICHINOSIS

This is common in mainland China. There have been small outbreaks in northern Thailand. It is rare in Muslim areas where pork is not used, but it does occur.

TRICHURIASIS

This is very common in Laos, amongst agricultural workers, in Ibans and in urban slums of Malaysia. In many areas of China most people have this.

TROPICAL SPLENOMEGALY

According to some sources this occurs in parts of China; according to others it does not occur at all in this area.

TUBERCULOSIS

This is known to be common in Burma, Cambodia, Laos, Sabah, Vietnam, Sarawak and West Malaysia. In the Far East it is most common in Macau, Korea, Hong Kong, Japan and Taiwan. Skin TB occurs in Malaysia. Multiple drug-resistant TB is common in Korea.

TYPHUS

SCRUB TYPHUS is listed separately in the Condition Index. Tick typhus and Rickettsial pox are listed under SPOTTED FEVER.

Louse-borne typhus occurs in northern China and near the Himalaya area.

Murine typhus is common in China, Korea and Thailand. It is most common in coastal areas, more during the summer than the winter.

VISCERAL LEISHMANIASIS

In China Gansu Province it may be found up to 1000 meters (3300 ft.). It does not occur in Indochina.

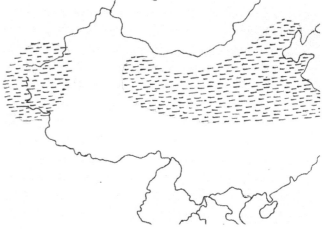

The known distribution of visceral Leishmaniasis. Information from Parasites & Vectors 2012, 5:31

Age: most less than 10 y.o.; in northwest China 95% are less than 5 years old; in the North Tarim River Valley most are less than 2 years old although parents may also be infected.

Clinical

In China, some patients have darkening of their skin, HEART FAILURE and nosebleeds. Their lymph nodes may be generally enlarged, but their livers and spleens may be of normal size. In the North Tarim River Valley patients get bumps on their skin. The death rate is high.

XEROPHTHALMIA

This is widespread in the rice-eating areas of Asia. In Thailand it is a rural problem. In most of Asia there is a very high mortality rate for children who are blinded by this—up to 75% in the first 3 months after loss of vision. The deaths are mostly from infections because of the loss of immunity with this illness.

YAWS

Reportedly this does not occur in the Far East, and it is uncommon in Indochina, occurring only in humid areas with grossly inadequate medical care.

INDEX R: MEDITERRANEAN AND MIDDLE EAST NOTES

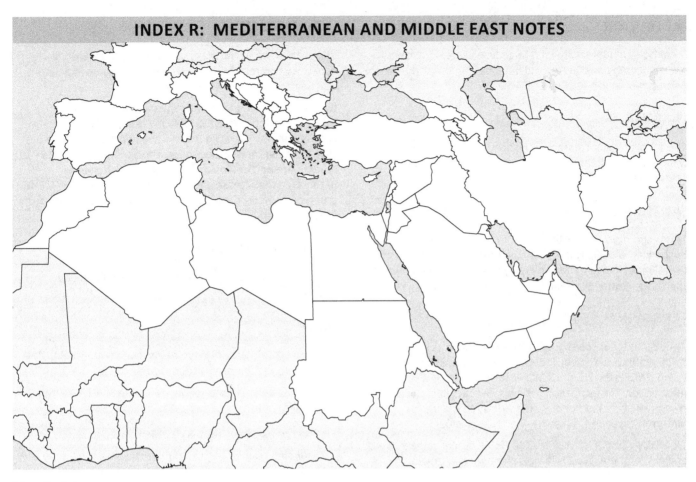

Map disclaimers

- Read the captions carefully. They are not all the same.

- Maps are notoriously unreliable. Conditions may be found in areas not shaded; conditions may be absent in areas that are shaded. Usually a disease is present only in spotty areas within the shaded region. A diagnosis is possible if there is shading anywhere around your location or if your patient has traveled through a shaded area.

- There is lack of shading both where there are no data and also where data exists indicating that that condition is absent. Lack of shading more often indicates lack of data than absence of the condition.

- Beware of shading that stops at political boundaries; germs don't respect border controls.

- Beware of areas that are unshaded for a variety of diseases. It may be because no one educated has ever entered that area and made it out alive. It may also be because intelligent people know enough not to go there.

- At times of civil unrest, natural disaster and migrations, the distribution of diseases changes unpredictably and rapidly. With biological warfare, this problem will be compounded.

TOC   SYMPTOMS   DIFFERENTIALS   CONDITIONS   DRUG INDEX   REGIONAL NOTES   INX

ADDICTION

Local types of uppers are khat (mainly in eastern Ethiopia and adjacent Somali areas) and betel nut (amongst the South Asian population.) See PLANT POISONING.

AMEBIASIS

This is particularly common in Algeria, Egypt and in the Middle East south and east of Turkey. It is less common in southern Europe.

ANTHRAX

This is common in the Middle East in areas of animal husbandry, especially Iran, Iraq and northern Africa. It is most prevalent in late dry and early rainy seasons, in areas where the soil is neutral or alkaline.

ARBOVIRAL FEVER

Although it is not common, Rift Valley fever occurs in Egypt, Saudi Arabia and Yemen, It occasionally results in loss of vision, ENCEPHALITIS, or HEMORRHAGIC FEVER. It is carried by mosquitoes. The incubation period is 2–7 days. It is particularly common in times of flooding. The virus is considered a bioterrorist weapon. It may be directly contagious.

CRIMEAN-CONGO HEMORRHAGIC FEVER occurs in the Balkans and east of there. West Nile virus is common in Israel.

ASCARIASIS

This may exist, but is not likely to be a big public health problem in areas with less than 1200 mm rainfall per year. This includes most of this area.

BELL'S PALSY

A regional cause of this is tick-borne RELAPSING FEVER, which is common throughout this area.

BERIBERI

This is very common in eastern Afghanistan but not common in Syria or the rest of the Middle East.

BLADDER STONE

This occurs, especially in areas with SCHISTOSOMIASIS HEMATOBIUM.

BRAIN DAMAGE

The most likely local causes are HEAT ILLNESS and possibly SCHISTOSOMIASIS MANSONI.

BRUCELLOSIS

This is common in North Africa and the Middle East. It is especially common in Iran, Iraq, Kuwait, Jordan, Israel, the Red Sea area and the Mediterranean rim.

It is very common in the Van region of Turkey. In this area of the world it is related to milk and buttermilk more than cheese and raw liver. It is more prevalent in sheep and goats than in camels and cattle. Those who assist in the delivery of animals are particularly prone to getting the disease.
In this area the disease affects children, causing MENINGITIS, paralysis or incoordination. In Jordan this occurs mostly from May to September.

BURKITT LYMPHOMA

This is rare if it occurs at all in the Mediterranean and Middle East.

CANCER

The cancers that are common in most developing countries are common in this area also. In addition:

bladder cancer is common in areas with SCHISTOSOMIASIS HEMATOBIUM.

cancer of the esophagus is common throughout this area.

lymphoma (cancer of the lymph nodes) may be locally common. It starts with large painless lymph nodes, similar to TUBERCULOSIS.

skin cancer of the eyelids occurs in fair-skinned people in the desert areas in this region.

CAPILLARIASIS

This occurs in Egypt; a closely related disease occurs in Iran to some extent.

CHOLERA

Cholera occurs in Iraq and Iran only, mainly in epidemics in times of drought or flood.

CIRRHOSIS

This may be due to drinking too much ALCOHOL, to SCHISTOSOMIASIS MANSONI, HEMOCHROMATOSIS or other diseases. It is worse with poor nutrition. See INDIAN CHILDHOOD CIRRHOSIS if the patient is a child of that ethnic origin.

CUTANEOUS LEISHMANIASIS

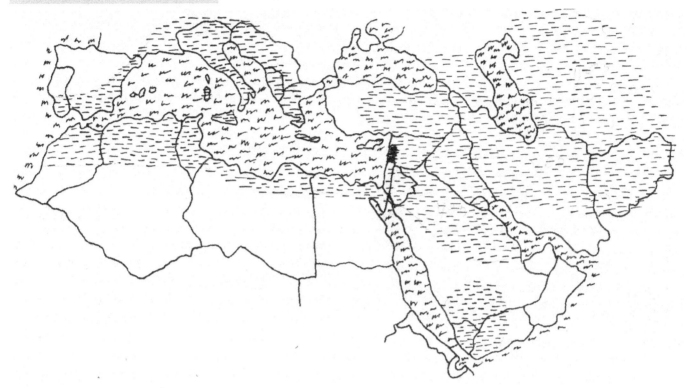

The shaded areas are where cutaneous Leishmaniasis is most likely to occur. Darker shaded areas show the locations of recent outbreaks. Information taken in part from ProMED-mail.

It may manifest like VISCERAL LEISHMANIASIS in those with poor immunity.

In the Arabian Peninsula and along the north coast of Africa, it is almost all *L. major*. In Turkey and the Balkans, it is almost all *L. tropica*. In Israel, it is present along the Jordan River from the Dead Sea north for about 25 miles, about 5 miles on both sides of the river. In this area gerbils harbor the disease and the sand flies that breed in their burrows pass it on to humans. In rural desert areas the disease is maintained in the rodent population, and the skin sores tend to be large and wet. In urban areas the sores are dry and crusted over; the disease is maintained in dogs and humans.

Treatment

Prevention: avoid contact with dogs; use insect repellents when such contact is unavoidable. Bednets may be helpful.

Patient care: in Saudi Arabia add ZINC to the treatment and use it for 4 months.

CYSTICERCOSIS

Although pork is not raised or consumed much in this area, there are a lot of household servants who come from pork tapeworm-endemic areas. So cysticercosis is not as unusual as one might suppose it is.

DENGUE FEVER

This is a disease that is present almost worldwide, but it reportedly is not found in this area. The mosquitoes that transmit it are widespread, so the disease may occur.

DYSENTERY

Amebic dysentery is common in Algiers and is uncommon in Saudi Arabia.

ENCEPHALITIS

Tick-borne encephalitis is found on the Balkan Peninsula and adjacent areas of Italy; it may also be found in other areas.

ENTERIC FEVER

Typhoid fever that is resistant to multiple drugs is now common in Egypt.

Paratyphoid fever occurs in the Mediterranean area. In this area, there usually is fever plus some abdominal symptoms. However, it may present as fever and cough, resembling BRONCHITIS or PNEUMONIA. It may resemble MENINGITIS or ENCEPHALITIS, or it may cause just fever and bizzare behavior.

Treatment In this area where there is resistance to antibiotics, use second- or third-generation CEPHALOSPORINs or CIPROFLOXACIN.

TOC

SYMPTOMS

DIFFERENTIALS

CONDITIONS

DRUG INDEX

REGIONAL NOTES

INX

EPILEPSY

In this area it may be caused by ONCHOCERCIASIS.

FAVUS

Cause: fungus

This is a fungal infection of the scalp which is common in the Middle East and the Mediterranean area. Initially it looks like TINEA. With time, round, bald patches develop and then yellow crusts appear on the scalp. The hair never grows back.

Treatment GRISEOFULVIN. On day 1, shave the head and start the GRISEOFULVIN. On day 25 shave the head again. On day 31, the drug may be stopped. This should cure the problem. Check the person again on day 42. If there is any sign of the disease at that time, repeat the treatment.

FILARIASIS

Synonym: elephantiasis, non-endemic.

This disease is present almost worldwide but it has, in the past, not been found in the Middle East and the Mediterranean areas except in eastern coastal Yemen and in coastal Turkey, opposite Cyprus. Recently it has been reported to be common in the southern Nile delta area of Egypt. It is carried there by Culex mosquitoes. See Volume 1, Appendix 10.

G6PD DEFICIENCY

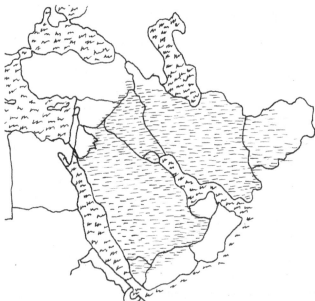

The shaded areas are where this problem is most common. The relevant area is that of the patient's genetic heritage, not his current location. Information derived from PLoS Med 9(11): 2012

GASTROENTERITIS

Similar regional diseases: PLANT POISONING due to lolism.

GIARDIASIS

This is very common in the Middle East, especially in Algiers, Saudi Arabia and Yemen in areas of poor sanitation.

GOITER

This is due to IODINE deficiency in mountainous areas of the eastern Mediterranean and southern Egypt.

GUINEA WORM

Cause: worm

Synonyms: dracontiasis, dracunculiasis.

Mildly to moderately ill; class 1; regional: occured in Saudi Arabia and possibly in areas of Afghanistan adjacent to Pakistan, where water was obtained from wells into which people step. The distribution is presently unknown because of conflict in the region.

Age: any. **Who:** those who drink water contaminated with microscopic larvae. **Onset**: variable; usually about 1 year after drinking infected water.

Clinical

Necessary: a small bump forms, usually on the leg, but it may be elsewhere, particularly skin that is exposed to water. This enlarges to become a blister. It is itchy and frequently burning; the pain is relieved by cold. When the blister breaks, one can see the end of the worm. A painful open sore forms in place of the blister. There is only one worm per blister or sore, and each worm is 30-70 cm (12-28 in.) long.

Maybe: the worm will discharge a milky fluid.

Complications: secondary wound infection, OSTEOMYELITIS.

Similar conditions: none except possibly in the very early stages.

Treatment

Prevention: encourage design of wells that eliminates the possibility of people climbing down into them. A simple sand filter works well to eliminate parasites from contaminated water. Use temphos (Abate) to treat affected water supplies.

Patient care: the best treatment is for the worm to be surgically removed before the blister forms. This is a relatively easy procedure. It reduces the period of disability from weeks to two days. If you already know how to suture wounds, it would be feasible for you to learn how to do the procedure.

Once the blister forms: immerse the blister or sore in cold water. This makes the worm limp. Having the patient take IBUPROFEN helps also. Wind the worm on a small clean stick, a few centimeters a day, not so tightly that the worm breaks. This will gradually draw the worm out. (If the worm breaks, treat promptly with one of the medications listed below.) If the patient is bedridden anyway, keeping the area continually moist will hasten the worm expulsion (2 weeks vs. 2-3 months). Otherwise keep the area clean and dressed with ANTIBIOTIC OINTMENT to prevent infection. A number of different drugs are also useful, such as METRONIDAZOLE, TINIDAZOLE, MEBENDAZOLE and THIABENDAZOLE.

HEMORRHAGIC FEVER

This occurs in Greece as well as other parts of the Mediterranean; it is not common. KIDNEY DISEASE is an occasional complication. It must be treated in a hospital.

CRIMEAN-CONGO HEMORRHAGIC FEVER is a local form that is most common in northern Iraq and amongst Kuwaiti Bedouins. It also occurs in the Western Province of Saudi Arabia, the Mecca area. It is carried by ticks which live on domestic animals and bite humans who rest in shaded areas. It is also contagious, being directly transmitted from patients to healthy people. Most cases occur from June to September. It looks very similar, in its early stages, to ARBOVIRAL FEVER caused by sand flies in this area. It can be distinguished by the fact that it has a slow pulse relative to the fever and by the presence of protein and blood in the urine. It is potentially a bioterrorist weapon.

Treatment: RIBAVIRIN, with hospitalization. However, evacuation is not advisable; better to let the patient die than to start a worldwide epidemic.

HEPATITIS

Almost everyone has been exposed to hepatitis A in childhood and is immune by adulthood. Hepatitis B is more prevalent in Saudi Arabia than in any other part of the world, according to a Saudi medical journal. Hepatitis C is most common in Turkey and in non-Bedouin Saudi Arabs. Hepatitis is also common in Egypt, especially hepatitis B and hepatitis E. Gamma globulin from the States does not protect against hepatitis E, but that from France does. Reportedly hepatitis E does not frequently cause LIVER FAILURE in pregnancy in Egypt as it does elsewhere. Many cases are entirely without symptoms.

HIV INFECTION

It is reportedly very common amongst prostitutes in Djibouti. It is mostly an urban problem which is spreading to rural areas.

HYDATID DISEASE

This is very common in the Middle East and arid northern Africa. Females are affected more than males, and most are 50-60 years old. The liver is the most common organ affected, followed by lung, kidney and spleen.

INTESTINAL FLUKE

In this area, this is heterophyiasis which is prevalent in the Nile delta, Israel, Tunisia, Turkey and the Port Said areas. It causes a high eosinophil count (hospital lab) but other diseases do also.

Complications: HEART FAILURE or damage to the brain or spinal cord, similar to SCHISTOSOMIASIS.

IRITIS

This may be associated with ONCHOCERCIASIS on the Arabian Peninsula.

KATAYAMA DISEASE

Cause: allergy/worm

This refers to the initial stage of SCHISTOSOMIASIS (either kind), GUINEA WORM or HYDATID DISEASE. It is common with SCHISTOSOMIASIS MANSONI but rare with SCHISTOSOMIASIS HEMATOBIUM and the other diseases.

KIDNEY DISEASE

Nephritic type is extremely common in the Middle East. It usually follows STREP THROAT.

Obstructive type: SCHISTOSOMIASIS HEMATOBIUM.

Hemolytic type: SICKLE CELL DISEASE.

KIDNEY INFECTION

Similar regional diseases: SCHISTOSOMIASIS HEMATOBIUM, SCHISTOSOMIASIS MANSONI.

KIDNEY STONE

Similar regional disease: SCHISTOSOMIASIS HEMATOBIUM.

LARVA MIGRANS

The deep type occurs in Israel, especially in the humid areas and in the Mosul area of Iraq.

LEPROSY

This occurs in the area, but according to WHO statistics, it is not common in the region as a whole. Among these countries, it occurs mainly in Yemen and Egypt.

LEPTOSPIROSIS

This is not common in the Middle East. In Portugal, cattle get the disease as well as persons handling infected animals. It commonly results in a MENINGITIS-type illness which should be treated with antibiotics to cover both this and ordinary MENINGITIS.

LIVER FLUKE

Fascioliasis is present in some areas only, mainly those that raise sheep or cattle. It is particularly common in the Nile Delta. It also occurs in Algeria, Morocco, Tunisia, Turkey, Iran, Iraq, Yemen and Afghanistan.

LYME DISEASE

Lyme disease occurs in this area.

LYMPHOGRANULOMA VENEREUM

This is particularly common in northern Africa.

MALARIA

CHLOROQUINE-sensitive malaria occurs in Turkey, Iraq, Saudi Arabia, Egypt and the islands of the Mediterranean. CHLOROQUINE-resistant malaria occurs in Iran and Afghanistan; it may spread.

There has been a rapid increase in the amount of malaria in northern Afghanistan. This may spill over into Iran. In Afghanistan most malaria is falciparum from September to November, and most is non-falciparum from April to September. The following areas reportedly have no malaria transmission at all: Bahrain, Cyprus, Israel, Jordan, Kuwait, Lebanon, Qatar, Maldives. In Turkey and Iraq, there is no falciparum malaria. The malaria in Oman, Saudi Arabia and Yemen is mostly falciparum. That in Iran and United Arab Emirates is about 1/4 falciparum. In the rest of the Middle East falciparum malaria is rare.

Also reportedly free of malaria transmission are:

- Afghanistan: Kabul.
- Iran: areas in the northern part of the country above 1500 m (5000 ft.).
- Iraq: over 1500 m (5000 ft.).
- Oman: central area.
- Saudi Arabia: western part above 2000 m (6600 ft.).

One should note that the geographical extent of malaria transmission is expanding worldwide, and it is occurring at progressively higher elevations, in many areas up to 2500 meters (8000 feet). Seek local lore.

MALNUTRITION

Kwashiorkor is generally common in north Africa and the Middle East. In refeeding, one should note that camel milk has more vitamin C than milk of other sources.

MENINGITIS

In Kuwait this is not common; about 75% of the cases that occur in children are treatable with AMPICILLIN and CHLORAMPHENICOL. There have been meningococcal epidemics in Saudi Arabia. This is the form of meningitis with very rapid onset and rapid spread within the community.

Similar regional diseases: LEPTOSPIROSIS, BRUCELLOSIS, especially in children.

MONONUCLEOSIS

A very similar disease is a form of VISCERAL LEISHMANIASIS which occurs in Saudi Arabia. See VISCERAL LEISHMANIASIS in these notes.

MOSSY FOOT

Mossy foot occurs in Morocco and perhaps elsewhere.

MYCETOMA

This is common in Sudan.

MYIASIS

The Tumbu fly occurs in southwestern Saudi Arabia.

ONCHOCERCIASIS

This is present in Yemen at an altitude of 300–1200 m (1000-4000 ft.); in wadis, Ghayl, Rasyan, Zabid, Rima, Surdud and possibly Siham and Harad; in Saudi Arabia near the wadis in the Asir region. Eye symptoms are rare in the Middle East, but the skin symptoms are usually severe enough to prevent working. Sowda is a form that is found in Yemen and northern Sudan. The skin becomes swollen and covered with scaly bumps. There is swelling of the lymph nodes, usually in the groin.

PELLAGRA

This occurs in the Black Sea area of Turkey and the corn-growing areas of Iran. It reportedly does not occur in Lebanon, Syria or Iraq.

PELVIC INFECTION

Similar regional diseases: SCHISTOSOMIASIS HEMATOBIUM, SCHISTOSOMIASIS MANSONI.

PHIMOSIS

Similar regional disease: SCHISTOSOMIASIS HEMATOBIUM.

PLAGUE

This has been reported from Libya, Iran, northern Iraq, Asir area of Saudi Arabia, NW Yemen and Western Sahara. There is a focus of infection in the Oran area of northern Algeria. It may occur elsewhere.

PLANT POISONING

Regional types are khat and lolism.

PNEUMONIA

There is a nasty pneumonia in the Middle East called MERS-CoV, transmitted by camels. It is viral; antibiotics are useless. It tends to kill those with other medical issues, mostly the elderly. It may be more widespread than currently realized. Supportive care at a level 4-5 hospital is helpful.

POLIO

This was very common in Afghanistan, Yemen, Iraq, Egypt, Lebanon, Pakistan and Oman. Recent worldwide immunization programs may have changed this. It is reportedly still common in areas of Iran and in the Iraq/Turkey border area. You can expect to see it wherever WHO personnel have not been welcomed.

PROCTITIS

Regional causes are SCHISTOSOMIASIS MANSONI and SCHISTOSOMIASIS HEMATOBIUM.

PROSTATITIS

Similar regional diseases: SCHISTOSOMIASIS MANSONI and SCHISTOSOMIASIS HEMATOBIUM

Q FEVER

This is common throughout the area but reportedly not in the southeastern portion of the Arabian peninsula; it occurs worldwide except for New Zealand. It presents differently in different areas. In Greece it is 95% pneumonia. In Iran it is about half hepatitis and half pneumonia. There it is associated with herds of goats. There was an outbreak in Israel, due to the germs in an air conditioner. It may present like an ordinary flu.

RELAPSING FEVER

Reportedly this is common in Morocco, maintained in small mammals and transmitted by ticks.

RHEUMATIC FEVER

This is common in Algeria, Egypt, Morocco, Iran, Cyprus and Kuwait.

RICKETS

This is particularly common in Muslim cultures, especially among women and babies, due to lack of skin exposure to the sun. It is widespread in the Middle East in Lebanon, Syria, Iraq, Saudi Arabia, Turkey and Iran.

SANDFLY FEVER

This is common throughout Egypt, Iran, Iraq and western Saudi Arabia, mainly June to August.

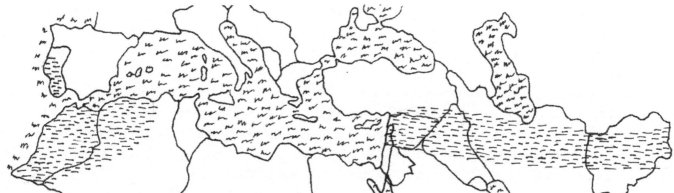

The known distribution of tick-borne relapsing fever.

TOC

SYMPTOMS

DIFFERENTIALS

CONDITIONS

DRUG INDEX

REGIONAL NOTES

INX

SCHISTOSOMIASIS HEMATOBIUM

Cause: worm

Synonyms: urinary bilharziasis, snail fever, bilharzia.

Not ill to very ill; class 2; regional; this is especially frequent where there are dams and irrigation canals.

In the Taiz province of Yemen, up to 90% of the people are infected in the western, southern and northern parts of the province. All ages and both sexes are affected. The problem is less common, however, at higher than at lower altitudes.

Age: any, but especially boys 5–15 y.o. who like to swim.
Who: skin exposed to water in which infected snails live.
Onset: 10–12 weeks after exposure, then over days to weeks.

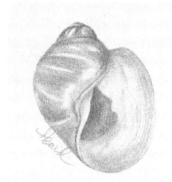

The kind of snail that carries schistosomiasis hematobium. Note the large hole and only 3 or 4 swirls. The length is about 0.7–1.0 cm. AB

Clinical initially

Immediately after the exposure to contaminated water, mainly in expatriates, there may be itching of the skin for 2-3 days. After the incubation period, Caucasians usually begin with KATAYAMA DISEASE: fevers, low abdominal pain, fatigue and symptoms of ALLERGY. Nationals may skip these symptoms.

Clinical later

Necessary: the patient develops bloody urine. Blood may be visible only or mainly at the end of urination. If it is not visible a urine dipstick will demonstrate that it is present, at least sometimes.

Usually: there is frequent urination and pain with urination. Nationals may just have bloody urine without other symptoms. Genital symptoms may begin in little girls before puberty: wounds, bleeding, pain and discharge. Women commonly have pelvic discomfort, VAGINITIS symptoms and itching.

Maybe: there is kidney pain resembling KIDNEY STONE and leading to KIDNEY DISEASE. There may be swelling of the end of the penis and possibly bloody semen. Women may have pain with intercourse or infertility. This may cause a very large kidney or kidneys.

Occasionally: it can cause PROCTITIS or symptoms resembling SCHISTOSOMIASIS MANSONI.

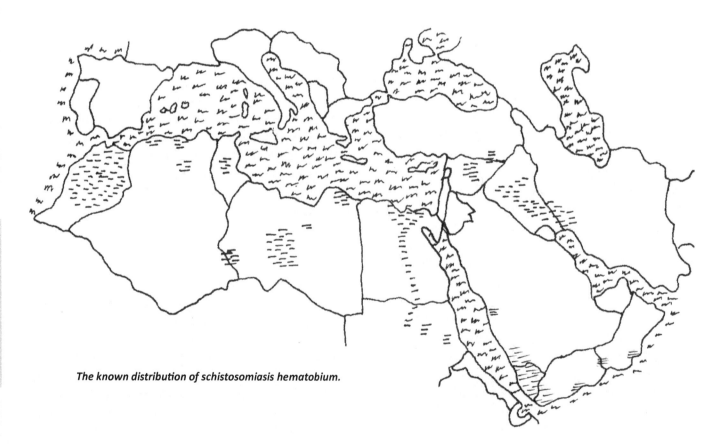

The known distribution of schistosomiasis hematobium.

Clinical still later

The patient may have to urinate frequently and may dribble because the bladder becomes rigid; it cannot enlarge to hold its usual volume of urine.

Complications: sometimes this causes problems with the spinal cord: sharp, shooting pains, weakness, numbness and tingling, inability to start urinating. This is called neuro-schistosomiasis.

It must be treated promptly with PRAZIQUANTEL and PREDNISONE, not waiting for lab results which may be falsely negative—do this with anyone who has had a prior exposure at any time in his/her life. High-tech imaging (MRI) is most helpful, but do not delay treatment.

ANEMIA and weight loss are likely. The disease evidently contributes to MALNUTRITION, since children show a growth spurt after treatment. Other complications are: VAGINITIS-type symptoms, bladder CANCER, KIDNEY INFECTION, inability to urinate, sores and growths on penis or in vagina, sterility in females, KIDNEY DISEASE, URETHRAL STRICTURE and occasionally RESPIRATORY INFECTION from migrating worms. The bones may become thin and weak, so fractures occur with minor injuries. Sometimes, after years, the worms invade the lungs, causing RESPIRATORY FAILURE and HEART FAILURE.

Females may develop PELVIC INFECTION or CANCER. In both sexes the infection promotes the transmission of the HIV virus. In males an occasional complication is a BLADDER STONE; men with stones cannot urinate unless they jump up and down. Their urine may be bloody during the day and normal at night.

Similar Conditions: SEXUALLY TRANSMITTED DISEASES are the main point of confusion. URETHRITIS (visible pus from penis or female urethra), KIDNEY INFECTION (also nitrites and/or leukocytes in urine), KIDNEY DISEASE of other causes, ALLERGY (hives) from other causes, PROSTATITIS (usually men over 50 y.o. only), TUBERCULOSIS of the genitals, FILARIASIS.

Bush laboratory: afternoon urine will test positive for blood (and protein) with a urine dipstick. It helps to have the patient exercise before urinating and examine the last few drops. One can hatch the worm eggs and see the larvae using simple equipment. See Appendix 2 in Volume 1.

Treatment

Prevention: use latrines, eliminate snails, avoid water exposure. Let a bucket of water stand overnight before using it for washing; be sure there are no snails in the water. Use ARTEMISININ for the first 21 days after exposure; use PRAZIQUANTEL after 21 days and again after 6–12 weeks. Persons, such as fishermen, who are repeatedly exposed should take both ARTEMISININ and PRAZIQUANTEL weekly.

Referrals: laboratory: eggs can be found with a microscope. The blood count may show increased eosinophils early in the disease, especially in expatriates; they may be absent later on. Facilities: if there are any complications a level 4 or 5 facility is appropriate. In advanced disease biopsy, CT or MRI might be helpful.

Patient care: PRAZIQUANTEL; PREDNISONE or PREDNISOLONE along with the PRAZIQUANTEL might be helpful. It is essential with neuro-schistosomiasis. With neuro-schistosomiasis a second treatment is required, 4–6 weeks after the first treatment.

METRIFONATE is a cheaper alternative for widespread use. NIRIDAZOLE is an old, dangerous drug that should no longer be used. MEFLOQUINE plus ARTEMISININ (as artesunate) reportedly works almost as well as PRAZIQUANTEL. Seek recent information.

Results: these should be evaluated at 3 and 6 months after treatment. Improvement starts after about one month.

SCHISTOSOMIASIS MANSONI

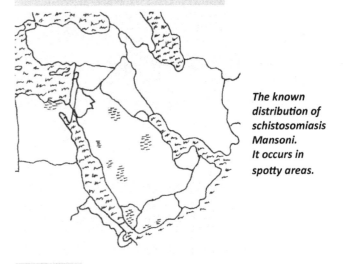

The known distribution of schistosomiasis Mansoni. It occurs in spotty areas.

SCURVY

This is especially common in the Middle East in Lebanon, Syria, Iraq, Saudi Arabia, Iran and northeast Turkey.

SEPSIS

This may be related to VISCERAL LEISHMANIASIS.

SICKLE CELL DISEASE

This occurs mainly in scattered areas near the Persian Gulf. There are not the severe symptoms of the African disease. In Saudi Arabia it occurs mostly in the Shi'i Muslims of the Qatif and Al-Hasa Oases; the ANEMIA is mild to moderate, leg ulcers are rare, and the spleen is large in adults. There is a form of severe sickle cell disease in Jizan, Quamfeda, Fayfa and NW of Jeda, Saudi Arabia.

SPOTTED FEVER

Tick typhus occurs in areas adjacent to the Mediterranean, Black and Caspian Seas. Other forms of the disease reportedly are not found in this region. In Israel, spotted fever is almost always found in teens or younger children. The best drugs in this area are: DOXYCYCLINE, CHLORAMPHENICOL, [RIFAMPIN plus ERYTHROMYCIN] and possibly CLARITHROMYCIN. In any case it is important to treat until the fever has been absent for 3 days.

SPRUE

This is particularly common in the eastern coastal Mediterranean area and in Syria.

STROKE

This may be caused by SICKLE CELL DISEASE, SCHISTOSOMIASIS MANSONI and SCHISTOSOMIASIS HEMATOBIUM, though rarely.

STRONGYLOIDIASIS

This is particularly common in Turkey and Iran.

Similar regional diseases: SCHISTOSOMIASIS MANSONI.

SYPHILIS

This is common in the nomads of the desert areas of the Middle East.

TAPEWORM

Beef tapeworm occurs in Lebanon and *fish tapeworm* occurs in Israel.

TETANUS

Tetanus in newborns is very common in Iraq; there are many home births, and immunization is uncommon.

TINEA

See FAVUS in this index for a form of tinea that is peculiar to the Mediterranean and Middle East. Ordinary tinea also occurs in this area.

TOXOPLASMOSIS

This is a problem in Libya and in the mountainous areas of Iran.

TRACHOMA

This is common all over the Middle East, especially northern Africa and Saudi Arabia; more in low-income areas with dirt, flies and overcrowding. It is less common amongst nomads and in sparsely populated areas.

TREPONARID

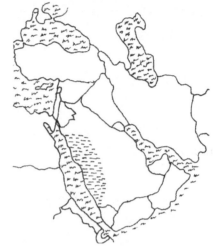

The known distribution of treponarid. It may occur in any hot dry location where sanitation is poor.

TRICHINOSIS

This is rare to unknown in Jewish and Muslim areas where pork is prohibited.

TRICHURIASIS

This occurs in Yemen Arab Republic.

TROPICAL SPLENOMEGALY

Some sources say that it does not occur in the Middle East and other sources say that it does occur. It is rare if it occurs at all.

TROPICAL ULCER

Regional associated diseases are SICKLE CELL DISEASE and CUTANEOUS LEISHMANIASIS.

TUBAL PREGNANCY

This may be caused by SCHISTOSOMIASIS MANSONI or SCHISTOSOMIASIS HEMATOBIUM.

TUBERCULOSIS

This is quite common in Iraq. In Israel (and presumably elsewhere) a large percentage of TB involves the urinary system, lymph nodes and bones. See the description under CANCER (in this index) of a form of cancer that can mimic lymph node tuberculosis. Also consider that in Saudi Arabia there is a form of VISCERAL LEISHMANIASIS that can mimic both MONONUCLEOSIS and lymph node tuberculosis.

TURISTA

In Egypt it is most serious and prevalent in children below 24 months in the summer and autumn of the year. In Saudi Arabia, most diarrhea in children is due to a virus; it does not respond to antibiotics. If it continues in spite of ORS, ERYTHROMYCIN is the antibiotic most likely to succeed.

TYPHUS

Louse-borne typhus is at higher and cooler areas in Africa, Iraq and Kuwait where there are crowding and body LICE. It occurs at some locations within the Balkan Peninsula and in northern Algeria.

Murine typhus is common amongst garbage collectors and others exposed to garbage in Egypt. There have been outbreaks in Kuwait. It occurs in Tunisia, Algeria and Morocco, as well as the Balkan Peninsula, Israel and the Sinai (and adjacent) areas.

URETHRAL STRICTURE

This may be caused by SCHISTOSOMIASIS MANSONI or SCHISTOSOMIASIS HEMATOBIUM.

URINARY OBSTRUCTION

This may be caused by SCHISTOSOMIASIS MANSONI or SCHISTOSOMIASIS HEMATOBIUM.

VAGINITIS

This may be caused by SCHISTOSOMIASIS MANSONI or SCHISTOSOMIASIS HEMATOBIUM.

VISCERAL LEISHMANIASIS

L. Donovani which affects both children and adults occurs throughout this area. L. infantum, which affects mostly babies, occurs only along the Mediterranean rim in and west of the Balkans. It is more common in southern Europe than in North Africa. The affected areas are constantly changing. In Israel where dogs harbor the disease, sand flies carry it from the dogs to humans. In this area tender spleens are common.

It may manifest with skin symptoms in some people.

The parasite that usually causes CUTANEOUS LEISHMANIASIS will occasionally cause visceral Leishmaniasis in Westerners in Saudi Arabia and Iraq. It causes fatigue, fever, diarrhea, abdominal pains and large lymph nodes.

In Israel most visceral Leishmaniasis occurs in children under 6 years old, not in HIV-positive adults.

Visceral Leishmaniasis in the presence of HIV INFECTION may be of sudden onset and rapid progression, with a very bad prognosis.

This is an urban problem in Tbilisi, Georgia; it affects both dogs and humans there. This may also apply to areas adjacent to Georgia.

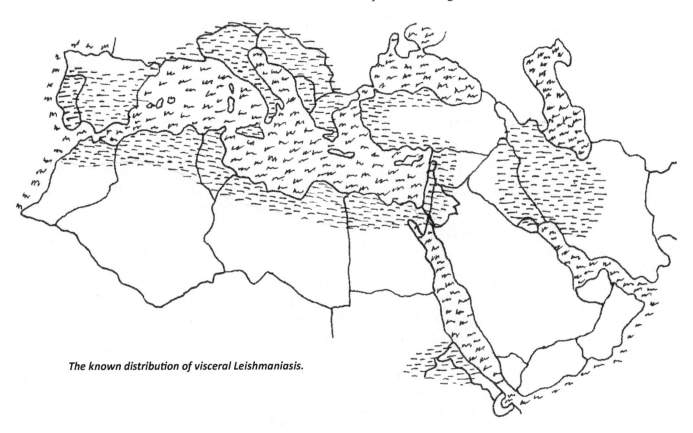

The known distribution of visceral Leishmaniasis.

XEROPHTHALMIA

This occurs in the Nile Valley, along the northwest coast of Africa, along the southeast coast of the Red Sea, in Syria, Iraq, Saudi Arabia, Turkey and Iran.

YAWS

This is a disease closely related to TREPONARID. It occurs mainly in the humid tropics; thus it is probably rare if it exists at all in the Middle East. At any rate, it is nearly indistinguishable from TREPONARID and is treated similarly.

INDEX S: SOUTHEAST ASIA NOTES

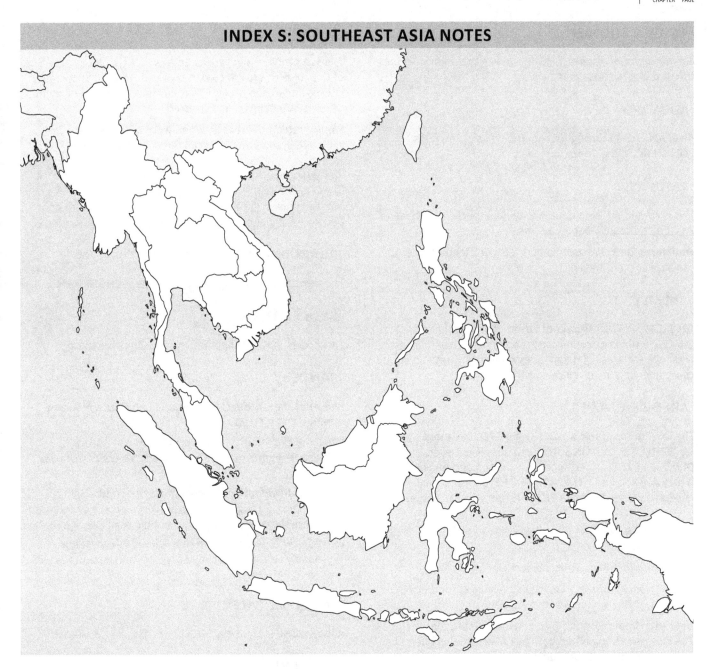

TOC

SYMPTOMS

DIFFERENTIALS

CONDITIONS

DRUG INDEX

REGIONAL NOTES

INX

Map disclaimers

- Read the captions carefully. They are not all the same.

- Maps are notoriously unreliable. Conditions may be found in areas not shaded; conditions may be absent in areas that are shaded. Usually a disease is present only in spotty areas within the shaded region. A diagnosis is possible if there is shading anywhere around your location or if your patient has traveled through a shaded area.

- There is lack of shading both where there are no data and also where data exists indicating that that condition is absent. Lack of shading more often indicates lack of data than absence of the condition.

- Beware of shading that stops at political boundaries; germs don't respect border controls.

- Beware of areas that are unshaded for a variety of diseases. It may be because no one educated has ever entered that area and made it out alive. It may also be because intelligent people know enough not to go there.

- At times of civil unrest, natural disaster and migrations, the distribution of diseases changes unpredictably and rapidly. With biological warfare, this problem will be compounded.

TOC

SYMPTOMS

DIFFERENTIALS

CONDITIONS

DRUG INDEX

REGIONAL NOTES

INX

ACUTE ABDOMEN

Similar regional diseases: PIG-BEL may either mimic or cause this, but it is rare except in Papua.

ADDICTION

Betel nut is used throughout Southeast Asia. See PLANT POISONING in the Condition Index.

AMEBIASIS

This is common throughout Indochina, especially in Thailand. It is not common in Papua or Laos.

Similar regional diseases: in northeast Thailand LIVER FLUKE can appear quite similar.

ANEMIA

TROPICAL SPLENOMEGALY occurs in Vietnam and Papua. THALLASEMIA is extremely common in northeast Thailand and adjacent areas of neighboring countries. These both cause anemia due to red cell destruction.

ARBOVIRAL FEVER

The local forms of this are DENGUE FEVER, Japanese ENCEPHALITIS, CHIKUNGUNYA and Ross River fever. DENGUE FEVER is listed separately in the Condition Index; it may develop into HEMORRHAGIC FEVER. For Japanese encephalitis, see the ENCEPHALITIS entry in these notes.

ROSS RIVER FEVER
Cause: virus

Synonyms: Ross River virus, epidemic polyarthritis.

Mildly to very ill; class 2; regional: it occurs in southern Vietnam, in the Mollucas and in Papua.

Age: any. **Who:** mosquito-bitten, females more than males. The disease is transmitted both by Culex (evening biters) and Aedes (day biters). **Onset:** unknown.

Clinical

This causes a high fever with a severe ARTHRITIS that lasts for a long time (months to years) but eventually goes away. It is not known to cause problems in unborn babies.

Similar Conditions: see Protocol B.2.

Treatment

Prevention: since this is transmitted mostly by day and evening-biting mosquitoes, insect repellent during the day is helpful, but bed nets at night do not help to prevent the disease except perhaps for those who go to bed very early.

Patient care: ASPIRIN, ACETAMINOPHEN or IBUPROFEN for the pain and fever. Antibiotics do no good at all. Keep the patient under a mosquito net or covered in repellant, to avoid transmitting the disease.

ASCARIASIS

This is a problem all over the Southeast Asian area. Over 1/3 of the children are affected in Java and Floros. It is common in Laos and in peninsular Malaysia amongst Indian oil palm workers, affecting mainly children.

Similar regional diseases: when worms invade the gallbladder, the symptoms can mimic LIVER FLUKE.

BERIBERI

This is common in peninsular Malaysia and anywhere poor people eat a diet of white rice with little else.

BRAIN DAMAGE

The most common local cause is Japanese ENCEPHALITIS.

BRUCELLOSIS

This occurs in the Philippines and possibly elsewhere.

CANCER

Cancer of the bile ducts is common in northeast Thailand where LIVER FLUKE occurs.

Cancer of the mouth is relatively common in northern Thailand where miang is chewed and where betel nut is used.

Cancer of the mouth and nose affects the South Asian population throughout this area. Also persons of southern Chinese descent are more susceptible than average to this.

Liver cancer is very common throughout this area; it is probably related to spoilage of grains and peanuts as well as to HEPATITIS B.

CEREBRAL PALSY

A local cause is Japanese ENCEPHALITIS.

CHANCROID

Many cases in this area are resistant to DOXYCYCLINE and CO-TRIMOXAZOLE. They usually respond to ERYTHROMYCIN, CHLORAMPHENICOL, ceftriaxone (CEPHALOSPORIN) and CIPROFLOXACIN (and other -oxacin drugs).

CHICKEN POX

In Southeast Asia, much of the adult population is not immune to chicken pox. In teenagers and young adults there can be very serious complications, e.g. ENCEPHALITIS. Also chicken pox is very serious in pregnancy and amongst HIV-infected patients. Reportedly in the Philippines facial blisters are prominent.

CHOLERA

This occurs mainly in epidemics in times of drought or flood, except in Indonesia where it accounts for up to 50% of all diarrhea cases in hospitals. It is relatively common all over Southeast Asia. The most common areas affected are Indonesia, Burma. Cambodia and Malaysia.

CIRRHOSIS

Regional causes of this are SCHISTOSOMIASIS JAPONICUM and INDIAN CHILDHOOD CIRRHOSIS; also consider the worldwide causes.

CRETINISM

Of the two kinds of cretinism listed, it is the first kind which affects most cretins in this area.

CYSTICERCOSIS

This is very common in Papua and in Bali. STRONGYLOIDIASIS is also common in some areas there, so the treatment is quite problematic.

DENGUE FEVER

This is present throughout Southeast Asia. The distribution of the disease varies from year to year. It is especially common in Papua, and it occurs regularly in other parts of Indonesia. It is common in Jakarta. In Sarawak it is common inland but not on the coast. It occurs most commonly in July in Thailand and in November in the Philippines. HEMORRHAGIC FEVER is a common complication. In Cambodia, dengue and dengue hemorrhagic fever are reported from all areas. Malaysia reports yearly epidemics in all areas and the Federal Territory, Selangor and Johor are most affected. In Vietnam dengue is a major public health problem with most cases occurring in June.

DIABETES

This occurs as a complication of chronic PANCREATITIS in Indonesia.

DIPHTHERIA

This occurs throughout this area in the unimmunized, mostly with groups of cases appearing in crowded inner-city areas. In Burma a form of SCRUB TYPHUS looks just like diphtheria with massive swelling of the neck.

DONOVANOSIS

This is very common in Papua.

DYSENTERY

In Chiang Mai Province, Thailand, both types occur but bacterial is more common. Both kinds are common in Flores and central Java, Indonesia. In Thailand dysentery due to shigella is resistant to most antibiotics. (Symptoms are a high fever, prostration and very many very small diarrhea movements that look like plain blood.) Seek professional care early.

Similar regional diseases: PIG-BEL in Papua. In other areas, consider PARAGONIMIASIS or SCHISTOSOMIASIS JAPONICUM.

ENCEPHALITIS

Japanese encephalitis (JE) is the most common local cause of encephalitis. It occurs throughout this area, but it is less common in southern than in northern Thailand. An immunization is available in Bangkok. RIBAVIRIN does absolutely no good for treatment.

JE is carried by Culex mosquitoes (see Appendix 10.) There is a 40% death rate with JE, and most of the survivors have significant long-term disabilities.

In certain areas SCHISTOSOMIASIS JAPONICUM may also cause encephalitis.

ENTERIC FEVER

This is quite common in all Indochina. It is particularly common in Jayapura. There are some abdominal symptoms present in almost all patients: nausea and vomiting; constipation; diarrhea; or abdominal cramps; occasionally it may cause isolated, sustained fever without other symptoms.

Similar regional diseases: see Protocols B.2 and B.9.

FILARIASIS

Synonym: elephantiasis, non-endemic.

In this area, there are two types of filariasis: Bancroftian and Brugian.

Bancrofian filariasis swells the legs and genitals. A scrotum may be so large that it has to be carried in a wheelbarrow.

Brugian filariasis often affects arms and breasts as well as the legs, but rarely the genitals.

TOC
SYMPTOMS
DIFFERENTIALS
CONDITIONS
DRUG INDEX
REGIONAL NOTES
INX

TOC

SYMPTOMS

DIFFERENTIALS

CONDITIONS

DRUG INDEX

REGIONAL NOTES

INX

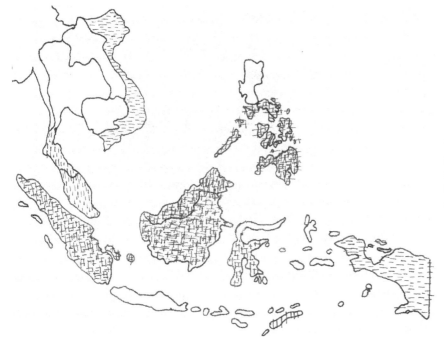

The known distribution of filariasis. The vertical lines indicate Brugian filariasis; the horizontal lines indicate Bancroftian filariasis. The areas with +'s have both kinds. Bull. Wld Hlth Org 1962, 27, 529-541

FOOD POISONING

There are three kinds that are peculiar to this area:

rice that has stood at room temperature for a day or two grows bacteria that cause severe, watery diarrhea.

raw shellfish (mussels, clams and oysters) concentrate a toxin which causes symptoms within 30 minutes. It starts with tingling and numbness around the mouth first and then the limbs. Later, vomiting and incoordination occur. Death is not uncommon. It may appear similar to HYPERVENTILATION.

gallbladder of raw fish: see the separate entry below.

G6PD DEFICIENCY

This is a genetic variation that causes problems when affected patients take certain medications. See the map below for where it is most common. It may occur anywhere.

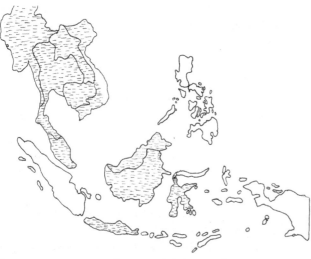

The most common areas for G6PD deficiency. Information derived from PLoS Med 9(11): 2012

GALLBLADDER DISEASE

Similar regional disease: LIVER FLUKE.

GALLBLADDER OF RAW FISH

This is from carp which is a bottom feeder, caught with heavy weights on lines or nets. It is still poisonous if and when it is cooked. It is used in Asia as a Chinese traditional medicine for poor eyesight, it causes nausea, vomiting, diarrhea, abdominal pain, LIVER FAILURE and KIDNEY DISEASE.

Treatment is not feasible in the village situation. Send out.

GASTROENTERITIS

Similar regional diseases: PIG-BEL (mostly Papua), CAPILLARIASIS (mostly the Philippines).

GIARDIASIS

This is generally common in Southeast Asia. In Chiang Mai Province, Thailand, it affects mainly younger children.

GOITER

This is common in the Penans of Sarawak. It generally occurs in lowland river deltas, in inland areas and at higher altitudes. It is very common in the highlands of Papua.

HEART FAILURE

The most common regional causes are THALLASEMIA, RHEUMATIC FEVER, SCHISTOSOMIASIS JAPONICUM and Beriberi.

HEMORRHAGIC FEVER

This is almost all caused by DENGUE FEVER.

HEPATITIS

Hepatitis B is especially common in Indonesia where almost everyone has had the disease before 5 years of age. It may be transmitted prenatally from mother to baby.

Hepatitis D is common also.

Similar regional diseases: see the note under SPOTTED FEVER in this index. LEPTOSPIROSIS is as common as hepatitis in Malaysia. Also consider SCHISTOSOMIASIS JAPONICUM, THALLASEMIA.

In some areas, hepatitis might be caused by Q FEVER rather than a virus. In this case the patient probably had close contact with newborn animals. Antibiotics, then, may be helpful.

HIV INFECTION

This has become epidemic in Thailand, along the Thai-Burmese border area and in Burma and Cambodia.

HOOKWORM

This is especially common in Sumatra and Java, Indonesia. About 50% of Cambodians are infected. It is also common in Chiang Mai Province, Thailand, affecting mainly 10-15 y.o. children. It is common in peninsular Malaysia amongst Indian oil palm workers, affecting mainly children. In Papua, hookworm is found everywhere, but the infection is usually with only a few worms rather than many.

HYDATID DISEASE

This does not occur in the islands of Southeast Asia but may rarely occur in mainland Indochina.

INTESTINAL FLUKE

Echinostomiasis occurs in Indonesia, Philippines and Thailand, and has minimal symptoms. It comes from eating inadequately cooked tadpoles, snails, fish and frogs.

Fasciolopsiasis, is particularly common in Kalimantan, Sumatra and Indochina. It is found on the banks of large lakes with lotus plants and snails where there is sewage contamination of the water. In such areas up to 25% of the population may be infected. The most commonly affected plants are the water chestnut, water caltrop and water hyacinth.

Similar conditions: also consider CAPILLARIASIS in the Philippines.

JAUNDICE

The most common regional causes are HEPATITIS, LEPTOSPIROSIS, LIVER FLUKE (in northeastern Thailand) and SCHISTOSOMIASIS JAPONICUM.

KATAYAMA DISEASE

In this area this is almost always due to the initial stage of SCHISTOSOMIASIS JAPONICUM.

KIDNEY DISEASE

The most common causes in this region are MALARIA, LEPTOSPIROSIS and THALLASEMIA. OVALOCYTOSIS, in eastern Papua, causes kidney disease due to destruction of red blood cells.

LARVA MIGRANS

In this area the deep type, gnathostomiasis, is caused by eating or handling raw or rare tadpoles, frogs, snakes, fish, chicken, slugs or snails. Avoiding such infections involves using rubber gloves or tongs whenever handling raw meat. Such meats must be well cooked before they are eaten. These are very serious infections which must be treated by a physician. They are most common in Thailand.

LEPROSY

Leprosy is most common in Indonesia, Burma and Nepal; Thailand, Vietnam, Cambodia and the Philippines have many patients also.

LEPTOSPIROSIS

This is generally common in this region, particularly in Jayapura. In Malaysia it is common around oil palm and rubber estates. It is not common on rice farms.

LIVER FAILURE

The most common causes are MALARIA, LEPTOSPIROSIS, HEPATITIS, ALCOHOLISM and AMEBIASIS. In Indian children, consider INDIAN CHILDHOOD CIRRHOSIS.

LIVER FLUKE

Synonym for the local form: opisthorchiasis

This is common in Indonesia, NE Thailand and Laos.

In Thailand, symptoms of GALLBLADDER DISEASE are common. (See the illustration of the pain pattern in the main Condition Index under GALLBLADDER DISEASE.)

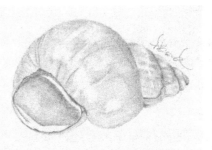

This is a magnified view of the snail that carries the larva of the liver fluke; the actual height is about 1.5 cm. Note the relatively small hole and the few swirls.

AB

TOC   SYMPTOMS   DIFFERENTIALS   CONDITIONS   DRUG INDEX   REGIONAL NOTES   INX

MALABSORPTION

The most common regional causes are GIARDIASIS and SPRUE. CAPILLARIASIS is a common cause in the northern coastal Philippines and northern Mindanao. Consider also INTESTINAL FLUKE. Also see Protocol B.14.

MALARIA

The following areas reportedly have no malaria transmission. However, malaria has been moving to progressively higher elevations in recent years, in many areas as high as 2500 meters (8000 feet). Seek current information.

- Indonesia: urban areas except for Papua.
- Laos: Vientiane.
- Philippines: urban areas and areas above 1500 m (5000 ft.).
- Thailand: Bangkok and its suburbs; Pataya, Phuket.
- Vietnam: above 1500 m (5000 ft.); the Red and Mekong deltas.
- Cambodia: above 1500 m (5000 ft.).

Over all, about 1/2 to 2/3 of the malaria in this area is falciparum, and it is almost all resistant to CHLOROQUINE and FANSIDAR. Non-falciparum malaria is becoming resistant to CHLOROQUINE, particularly in Indonesia and Burma. Knowlesi malaria is becoming is becoming prevalent throughout Malaysia and in adjacent areas of Indonesia and Thailand; it may spread. It accounts for about a third of the total malaria cases. It tends to cause rapid-onset RESPIRATORY FAILURE. It is sensitive to CHLOROQUINE and ARTEMISININ, resistant to MEFLOQUINE. It must be treated quickly; even a short delay may be fatal.

Thailand: most falciparum malaria is resistant to CHLOROQUINE, FANSIDAR and MEFLOQUINE; 85% of malaria is falciparum. There is some resistance to QUININE, but ARTEMISININ and QUINIDINE are very useful. HALOFANTRINE is dangerous. Daily DOXYCYCLINE works for prevention.

Near the Thai-Burma border there is a form of malaria that causes KIDNEY DISEASE of the nephrotic type. That kind of malaria is sensitive to CHLOROQUINE.

Burma: the amodiaquine-artesunate combination is not good for treatment.

Malaysia: resistance of falciparum to CHLOROQUINE is common, but less than half of the malaria is falciparum. All malaria in this area should be treated with CHLOROQUINE; add another drug for falciparum.

Indonesia: about 40% of the malaria is falciparum and resistance is common. CHLOROQUINE-resistant vivax malaria also is common in this area. Some vivax malaria is resistant to ARTEMISININ combination drugs also.

Philippines: about 60% of the malaria is falciparum and resistance is common.

Thailand/Vietnam/Laos border area there is resistance to ARTEMISININ.

MALNUTRITION

This is particularly common in refugee camps where there is general malnutrition as well as specific vitamin deficiency diseases.

MEASLES

In fair skin the rash is red spotted; in black skin it is sandpapery; in Asians it has an intermediate appearance.

MELIOIDOSIS

See SEPSIS. This is a form of very serious SEPSIS found in Indochina and the Pacific. It frequently presents as PNEUMONIA in someone who is in ill health.

MOSSY FOOT

Java, Indonesia reportedly has an area with mossy foot.

PARAGONIMIASIS

This occurs in some areas of Southeast Asia, distribution unknown. It is common in the Philippines.

PERTUSSIS

This is extremely common in the Philippines.

PIG-BEL

This is very common in Papua.

PLAGUE

This occurs in many areas of Vietnam, mostly January to April, and in Burma. There are occasional worldwide epidemics. It may occur anywhere.

PLANT POISONING

A regional form is djenkol bean.

PNEUMONIA

Very common in children, it accounts for about 50% of all infant deaths in the Philippines and Thailand. Also see the note under SPOTTED FEVER in these notes. Consider MELIOIDOSIS in someone who has been chronically ill or is an alcoholic.

PNEUMOTHORAX

This is a common problem in Asians.

POLIO

This was previously common in the Philippines, Indonesia, Burma, Laos, Vietnam. Reportedly it has been eliminated.

Q FEVER

Reportedly this is common in the western third of Burma.

RABIES

This is not present in Papua, on Timor, Indonesia or on Palawan, Philippines. It is a major problem in Thailand.

RHEUMATIC FEVER

This is very common in the Philippines.

RICKETS

This is particularly common in Muslim cultures.

RICKETTSIOSIS

This is a term that covers SPOTTED FEVER and TYPHUS. These diseases are common in Jayapura.

RUBELLA

There have been outbreaks in this area.

SCHISTOSOMIASIS JAPONICUM

Cause: worm

Synonyms: bilharzia, snail fever

Mildly ill to very ill; class 2; regional; it occurs in scattred portions of the shaded area on the map.

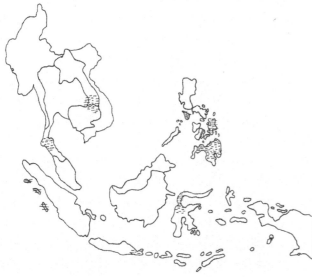

The known distribution of schistosomiasis Japonicum and schistosomiasis Mekongi; the two are indistinguishable for your purposes. In Sulawesi it is only in the Napu and Lindu valleys.

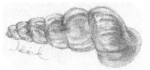

A magnified view of the snail that carries schistosomiasis japonicum. Note the small hole and many swirls. Some have stripes and some do not. Actual lengths are 0.5-1.0 cm. AB

Age: any. **Who:** skin exposed to water with infected snails. **Onset:** beginning 3–7 weeks after exposure.

Clinical initially

Initially: in Westerners this frequently starts as KATAYAMA DISEASE. Nationals may skip this stage.

Clinical 30—90 days after exposure

The patient may have lower-right abdominal pains with fever, diarrhea or DYSENTERY and cough. The DYSENTERY may be profuse. This stage can look just like ENTERIC FEVER. The patient is probably unable to work.

Clinical 3—5 years later

The person has LIVER FAILURE with a large liver, large spleen and an abdomen full of fluid so he looks pregnant. The liver enlarges before the spleen (the opposite of MALARIA) and frequently involves the left lobe of the liver which can mimic spleen enlargement. The liver will decrease in size, but the spleen remains large. The patient will have a decreased appetite and weight loss.

Children grow poorly, and they may have delayed sexual maturity. Alternatively, the patient may have chronic diarrhea, DYSENTERY and MALABSORPTION. The organism may invade the brain, causing SEIZURES, bizzare behavior, paralysis, blindness and possibly coma. This is known as neuro-schistosomiasis. It must be treated promptly on mere suspicion in anyone who has had any exposure during his, or her lifetime. Be sure to use PREDNISONE as well as PRAZIQUANTEL.

Complication: CANCER of the rectum, LIVER FAILURE, HEART FAILURE, RESPIRATORY FAILURE.

Similar Conditions: *fever and fatigue:* in the early stage resembles ENTERIC FEVER and SERUM SICKNESS. Later stages are difficult to distinguish from LIVER FAILURE and MALABSORPTION from other causes; see Protocol B.14. *Brain effects* sometimes resemble POLIO (paralysis), STROKE (paralysis), ENCEPHALITIS (seizures, bizzare behavior), CYSTICERCOSIS (seizures).

Bush laboratory: it is possible to hatch the eggs to see larvae that emerge, using simple equipment, Appendix 2, Volume 1. The hatching test is sensitive; it will most likely be positive in the presence of the disease. Take the stool sample between 10 AM and 2 PM.

Treatment

Prevention: use latrines; avoid exposure of skin to contaminated water; let a bucket of water without snails stand overnight before washing with it. Use ARTEMISININ for the first 21 days after exposure; use PRAZIQUANTEL after 21 days and again after 6–12 weeks. Persons such as fishermen, who are repeatedly exposed, should take both ARTEMISININ and PRAZIQUANTEL weekly.

Referrals: laboratory: the worm eggs may be found in the stool, beginning sometime in the KATAYAMA phase and lasting into the full-blown disease. After the disease has become chronic, the eggs may be absent. A blood count may show many eosinophils early in the disease, but it might not later on. There are also antibody tests; you can believe a positive result, but not a negative one. Facilities: if there are any complications it is important to send out to a level 4 or 5 facility with tropical medicine expertise.

Patient care: PRAZIQUANTEL is effective and safe enough to use even if you are not certain of the diagnosis. For severe KATAYAMA, give PREDNISONE on days 1-5. Start PRAZIQUANTEL on day 3. This will prevent worsening of the KATAYAMA DISEASE. Occasionally patients get a severe allergic response (see ALLERGY) to the first dose of the drug. This is treated like any other ALLERGY, but do not stop the drug. It is due to dead and dying worms, and it will not recur as severely, if at all, with subsequent doses. PREDNISONE or PREDNISOLONE along with the PRAZIQUANTEL might be helpful. In advanced liver disease PROPRANOLOL might be helpful. In either case seek professional medical advice. NIRIDAZOLE is an old, dangerous drug that should no longer be used. MEFLOQUINE plus ARTEMISININ (as artesunate) might be effective. This is one of the ACT drugs.

If there are neurological symptoms (seizures, paralysis, loss of sensation, altered mental status), use DEXAMETHASONE or another corticosteroid, as you would for MENINGITIS due to TUBERCULOSIS, preferably by injection and use PRAZIQUANTEL. In this case it is essential to give another treatment 4–6 weeks later, since the first treatment may not have killed all the developing worms.

Results: you should evaluate the results of the treatment at 1, 3 and 6 months after giving the drug.

SCHISTOSOMIASIS MEKONGI

This disease is nearly identical to SCHISTOSOMIASIS JAPONICUM, the differences being merely academic. It occurs in Cambodia, in two areas along the Mekong River. The symptoms and treatment are the same.

SCRUB TYPHUS

This is present throughout the Asia-Pacific area, from the north coast of Australia north to the northern border of Mongolia and the entire Indian subcontinent. Previous distribution maps are now known to be in error.

This is most common in palm oil workers. It is rare in Sabah. Amongst the Khmer refugees in Thailand, it is the most common cause of general illness with fevers. In Malaysia 20% of all fevers are due to scrub typhus.

Reportedly scrub typhus in Burma can cause huge lymph nodes so the entire neck is twice its normal diameter and the condition looks like the bull neck of DIPHTHERIA. In northern Thailand and possibly some other areas, it is resistant to DOXYCYCLINE and CHLORAMPHENICOL, so you should use RIFAMPIN or AZITHROMYCIN

SEIZURES

Regional causes of seizures include Japanese ENCEPHALITIS, PARAGONIMIASIS and SCHISTOSOMIASIS JAPONICUM.

SEPSIS

Patients with TROPICAL SPLENOMEGALY in Vietnam are particularly susceptible to sepsis.

Melioidosis is a peculiar form of this which occurs in rural areas of Indochina. The incubation period can be very long, a matter of years. It usually affects those in ill health otherwise: patients with DIABETES, CIRRHOSIS, KIDNEY DISEASE or other chronic diseases. Most infections occur within 2 weeks of the onset of heavy rain or else through exposure to water per occupation or recreation. Melioidosis in someone with DIABETES or KIDNEY DISEASE frequently is fatal.

SPOTTED FEVER

This probably does not occur in this area; at any rate it does not cause severe illness. A similar bacterial disease, Q FEVER, is present in this area. It causes a severe "flu," PNEUMONIA, or HEPATITIS.

SPRUE

This is most common in Indochina, Indonesia and the Philippines.

STROKE

This may be caused by SCHISTOSOMIASIS JAPONICUM.

STRONGYLOIDIASIS

This may cause SEPSIS in the presence of TROPICAL SPLENOMEGALY. It is common in Chiang Mai Province, Thailand, affecting mainly 10-15 y.o. children. It is relatively common all over Southeast Asia, especially Cambodia.

SYPHILIS

This is especially common in Thailand. Many Thai newborns have congenital syphilis.

TETANUS

This is a common cause of death in newborns in Indonesia.

THALLASEMIA

This is common throughout Indochina, mostly in people of Chinese and Malay origins. It is very common in NE Thailand and in refugees from neighboring areas. OVALOCYTOSIS, similar but less serious, is found mainly in Malaysia and in eastern Papua.

TINEA

Tinea imbricata occurs especially in Papua.

TOXOPLASMOSIS

This is generally not prevalent in arid regions, at high elevation and in Malaysia. There is a small risk of acquiring it in Thailand. TROPICAL SPLENOMEGALY makes a person prone to developing the disease.

TRACHOMA

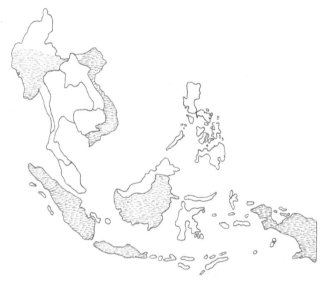

This is the area where trachoma is most common. It occurs worldwide and may be found anywhere.

TRICHINOSIS

Generally not common in Indochina, but there are occasional outbreaks of the disease in northern Thailand. It has not been reported to occur in the Asian islands.

TRICHURIASIS

This is extremely common throughout this area, with more than 50% of the population affected in most of Laos, Indonesia, Malaysia and the Philippines.

TROPICAL SPLENOMEGALY

This occurs mainly in Papua at 280-500 meters (900-1600 ft.). It also occurs in the Philippines and Vietnam.

TROPICAL ULCER

This is very common in the highlands of Papua.

TUBERCULOSIS

This is very common throughout this area; it affects about 10% of Cambodians. Reportedly, BCG immunization gives 83% protection against the disease in this area.

Similar regional disease: PARAGONIMIASIS

TURISTA

If diarrhea is severe see CHOLERA which is common.

TYPHUS

See TYPHUS or SCRUB TYPHUS in the main Condition Index. Both *louse-borne* and *murine* typhus occur in this area. In Malaysia 20%-50% of all illnesses with fevers are due to murine typhus.

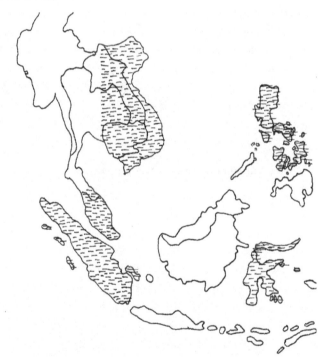

The known distribution of murine typhus; it may occur elsewhere.

XEROPHTHALMIA

This is especially common in rural peninsular Malaysia. In Thailand it is a rural, not an urban problem. In most of Asia there is a very high mortality rate for children who are blinded by this-up to 75% in the first 3 months. They die from infections due to the decreased immunity caused by the disease.

TOC   SYMPTOMS   DIFFERENTIALS   CONDITIONS   DRUG INDEX   REGIONAL NOTES   INX

YAWS

In this area it is most prevalent in Cambodia, Indonesia, rural Kalimantan, on Sumatra, in the Moluccas, on Timor and especially in Papua. In Papua it is most common in the lower altitude highlands.

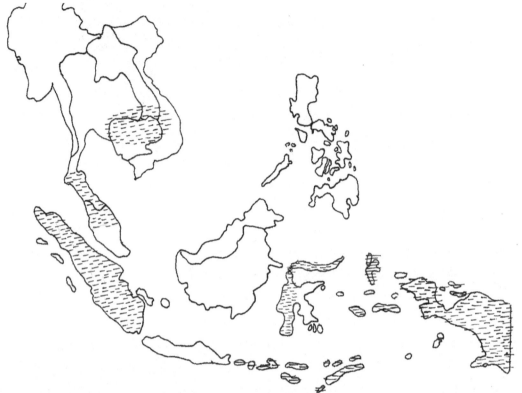

The known distribution of yaws. It may occur wherever there is poor sanitation.

TOC   SYMPTOMS   DIFFERENTIALS   CONDITIONS   DRUG INDEX   REGIONAL NOTES   INX

INDEX U: SOUTH PACIFIC NOTES

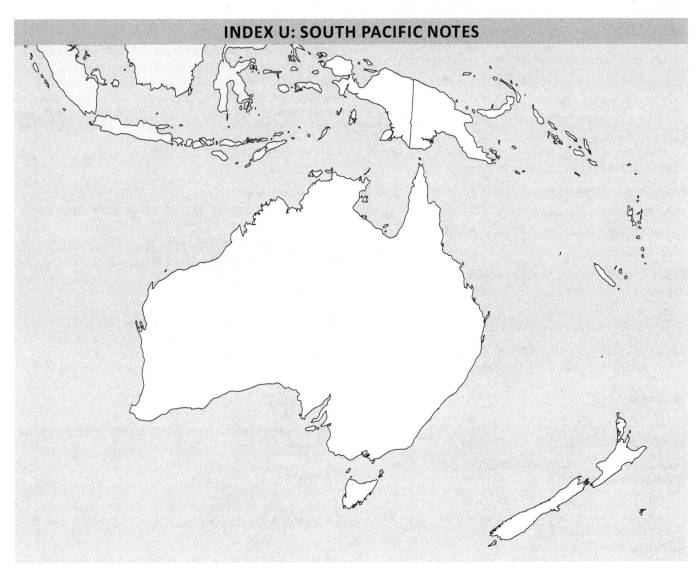

TOC

SYMPTOMS

DIFFERENTIALS

CONDITIONS

DRUG INDEX

REGIONAL NOTES

INX

Map disclaimers

- Read the captions carefully. They are not all the same.

- Maps are notoriously unreliable. Conditions may be found in areas not shaded; conditions may be absent in areas that are shaded. Usually a disease is present only in spotty areas within the shaded region. A diagnosis is possible if there is shading anywhere around your location or if your patient has traveled through a shaded area.

- There is lack of shading both where there are no data and also where data exists indicating that the condition is absent. Lack of shading more often indicates lack of data than absence of the condition.

- Epidemiologists and government health officers survey in easy locations, near major roads. If you are in a remote, difficult location the maps may not reflect the reality that you see.

- Beware of shading that stops at political boundaries; germs don't respect border controls.

- Beware of areas that are unshaded for a variety of diseases. It may be because no one educated has ever entered that area and made it out alive. It may also be because intelligent people know enough not to go there.

- At times of civil unrest, natural disaster and migrations, the distribution of diseases changes unpredictably and rapidly. With biological warfare, this problem will be compounded.

ADDICTION

Uppers: local examples are:

betel nut is described under PLANT POISONING in the Condition Index.

pituri, used by Australian aboriginals, has the effects of both uppers and outers. It is made from the stems and leaves of an eect shrub, 3–4 meters (9–12 ft.) tall, which is treated with ash. The drug causes hallucinations.

Downers: local examples are:

kava (also known as yanonga).

ALCOHOL is commonly abused by the Australian aborigines (amongst others).

Outers: the only example peculiar to the area is pituri, described above.

AMEBIASIS

This is particularly common in Tutelle, Tuvalu, Wallis and Futuna Islands, New Caledonia and Gilbert Island.

ANEMIA

Much of the anemia in pregnancy is due to MALARIA; it causes small babies but not premature births.

Anemia due to red cell destruction may be caused by the following diseases in this area:

- MALARIA.
- OVALOCYTOSIS, along the north shore of New Guinea and in the central highlands.
- TROPICAL SPLENOMEGALY.
- THALLASEMIA, common in New Guinea.

ANTHRAX

This is found in Australia, New Guinea and Polynesia.

ARBOVIRAL FEVER

DENGUE FEVER, the most common, is listed separately in this Index and the Condition Index.

Murray Valley fever occurs in eastern Australia and on the island of New Guinea; it is a kind of ENCEPHALITIS and/or HEMORRHAGIC FEVER. (See the Condition Index.)

Ross River fever is also common and is described below.

ROSS RIVER FEVER

Cause: virus

Synonyms: Ross River virus, epidemic polyarthritis.

Mildly to very ill; class 2; regional; it occurs throughout this area except for the northern half of Western Australia.

Age: any. **Who:** mosquito-bitten. This is transmitted by both Culex (night-biters) and Aedes (day biters) **Onset:** unknown.

Clinical

This causes a high fever with a severe ARTHRITIS that lasts for a long time (months to years) but eventually goes away. The arthritis is symmetrical, involving at least 2 of the following pairs of joints: wrist, elbow, knee, ankle. It may also involve the small joints. There is a rash in 50%, but a true fever in less than half. It is not known to cause problems in unborn babies.

Similar conditions: see Protocol B.6.A.

Treatment

Prevention: since this is transmitted mostly by mosquitoes, insect repellent during the day is helpful and also bed nets at night.

Patient care: ASPIRIN, ACETAMINOPHEN or IBUPROFEN for the pain and fever. Antibiotics do no good at all.

ARTHRITIS

A common local cause is Ross River fever, a form of ARBOVIRAL FEVER. There is also a hereditary arthritis that occurs in this area. It affects few joints, usually asymmetrically. GOUT is common in some Pacific islands.

ASCARIASIS

This is common in New Guinea, and in many areas infections are heavy.

ASTHMA

In New Guinea and Australia this is commonly caused by an insect that lives in house dust.

BRAIN DAMAGE

In this area, the most likely causes are cerebral MALARIA and Murray Valley fever (See ENCEPHALITIS).

BRUCELLOSIS

This occurs in Australia, New Zealand and the Solomon Islands.

BURKITT LYMPHOMA

This occurs in New Guinea near the equator. It presents mostly with tumors of the jaw.

BURULI ULCER

BURULI ULCERs are common in the Kumusi River area and in central Australia, but they occur throughout the region.

CANCER

BURKITT LYMPHOMA is a common type of childhood cancer.

Breast cancer is uncommon; it occurs more in the islands than elsewhere.

Cervical cancer is the most common cancer in females.

Liver cancer is the most common cancer in males.

Thyroid cancer is the second most common cancer in both sexes in Vanuatu. It is common throughout the Pacific area.

CHAGA'S DISEASE

The bugs that transmit this are present in Australia, but it has not yet been known to occur. It is a disease of the Western Hemisphere.

CHANCROID

This is common in all tropical parts of the Pacific area.

CHIKUNGUNYA

This is common in New Caledonia.

CHOLERA

This is generally common in Indonesia where it accounts for up to 50% of all diarrhea that is severe enough to send the patient to the hospital. It occurs in the Caroline Islands.

CRETINISM

This is particularly common in the central highlands of New Guinea.

CYSTICERCOSIS

This is very common in the highlands of New Guinea. It is the most common cause of SEIZURES that start during adult life.

DENGUE FEVER

This is common throughout most of the South Pacific, especially New Guinea. In Australia it is found mainly in North Queensland, also in the Torres strain area. It occurs in Fiji and New Caledonia. In Tonga and Vanuatu dengue is reportedly not common.

DIABETES

This is very common in the aboriginals in the Kimberly area.

DIPHTHERIA

Skin infections with diphtheria occur in the islands of the Pacific.

DONOVANOSIS

This is very prevalent in New Guinea, New Britain and in Australia amongst the aboriginal population. In many areas it is the most common sexually transmitted disease.

DYSENTERY

Bacterial dysentery is particularly common in Australia.

The southern coastal areas of New Guinea and surrounding islands have much amebic dysentery.

Similar regional disease: PIG-BEL.

EAR INFECTION, MIDDLE

Aboriginals in the Kimberly area frequently develop chronic middle ear infections caused by a peculiar germ that can be treated with SULFA, CO-TRIMOXAZOLE, DOXYCYCLINE or ERYTHROMYCIN. It does not respond to other drugs.

In central Australia, the common germ responds well to AMPICILLIN and CO-TRIMOXAZOLE. The HIB immunization prevents it.

ENCEPHALITIS

Japanese encephalitis occurs in Australia (Torres Strait and Cape York Peninsula), Papua New Guinea and throughout the Pacific Islands. RIBAVIRIN does absolutely no good for treatment.

Murray Valley fever is a local form of encephalitis; see ARBOVIRAL FEVER and also the Condition Index.

ENTERIC FEVER

In Papua New Guinea there are frequent complications as this affects the brain: deafness, incoordination and weakness that ascends from the feet upward. Seek professional medical care early.

ENTEROBIASIS

This is common in the area, with about half the adults infected.

FILARIASIS

Synonym: elephantiasis, non-endemic.

Only the Bancroftian form is found in this area.

The disease occurs mostly below 1200 meters (4000 ft.), mostly during the rainy season, mostly in heavily populated areas. It is present in most of the Pacific islands other than Australia and New Zealand. It is uncommon but not absent from American Samoa.

In French Polynesia it is very prevalent on Bora Bora, Maupiti, Kauehi, Kaukura, Taipivai and Puamau. It is not common but it exists in New Caledonia. In Vanuatu, it is carried by the same species of mosquito that carries MALARIA. The disease is particularly common in the central and northern islands, especially the Torres Islands and the Cook Islands.

TOC   SYMPTOMS   DIFFERENTIALS   CONDITIONS   DRUG INDEX   REGIONAL NOTES   INX

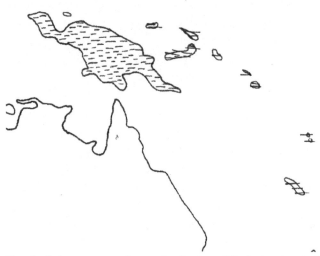

The shaded areas approximate distribution of filariasis. Historically it was rampant throughout the Pacific islands. Because of public health initiatives, its extent is somewhat decreased. BMC Infectious Diseases 2009, 9:92

Prevention: IVERMECTIN is not quite as good as DEC for prevention, but it is adequate if given twice a year.

FOOD POISONING

A form found in New Caledonia, New Zealand and Polynesia is due to Ciguatera fish, causing vomiting and diarrhea as well as strange sensations (numbness and tingling), weakness and possibly itching of the palms and soles.

Treatment: the same as general treatment for PLANT POISONING.

G6PD DEFICIENCY

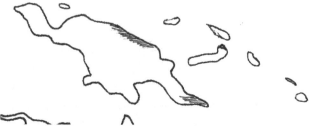

The shaded areas show the greatest prevalence of the condition. It may occur anywhere, particularly with migrations. Pay attention to the patient's origin, not to his present location.

GALLBLADDER DISEASE

This may be caused by OVALOCYTOSIS.

GIARDIASIS

This is very common in Australian aboriginals.

GOITER

One finds this especially in inland and high-altitude areas. It occurs in southeast Australia. Scattered areas on the island of New Guinea are affected, as well as parts of New Britain and the northern portion of the Solomon Islands.

GONORRHEA

In this area there is much resistance to quinolones: CIPROFLOXACIN and related antibiotics. Do not use them.

HEART FAILURE

Valvular failure is common in Tonga, as a result of RHEUMATIC FEVER and birth defects.

HEMORRHAGIC FEVER

This disease occurs, but is not common, in French Polynesia. When it occurs it is usually due to DENGUE FEVER or ARBOVIRAL FEVER (Murray Valley fever).

HEPATITIS

This is extremely common in the South Pacific area. Almost all children have had hepatitis B before 10 years of age in Tonga and the aboriginal areas of Australia. It may be transmitted prenatally from mother to baby. Chronic hepatitis from this is common in Kiribati. Hepatitis B and D are more common in Nauru than anywhere else in the world. Hepatitis E is presently not known to occur here, but it will probably appear in time.

HIV INFECTION

This occurs in Australia. In Papua New Guinea there are many cases of (probably) falsely positive HIV tests. (This means that the blood test indicates the person has the disease when he really does not.) In comparison to the rest of the world, this region has the lowest HIV-positive rate.

HOOKWORM

This is uncommon above 2000 meters (6600 ft.) elevation and in areas too dry for agriculture. It is common in New Guinea, but people are not usually very sick with it. In Australia it occurs to a significant extent only in the Kimberly area.

HYDATID DISEASE

This is common in the Collie area of SW Australia and in New Zealand. It does not occur in Tasmania. In this area only the kind transmitted by dogs occurs. You should suspect the problem where dogs are allowed to lick children's faces. Usually these are arid areas.

HYPERTENSION

This is especially common amongst aboriginals.

IMPETIGO

This is especially common in Australian aboriginals.

JAUNDICE

The most common regional causes are LEPTOSPIROSIS, HEPATITIS, MALARIA, THALLASEMIA, OVALOCYTOSIS.

KIDNEY DISEASE

Nephritic kidney disease is common in aboriginals, usually from CELLULITIS.

Hemolytic kidney disease may result from OVALOCYTOSIS.

LARVA MIGRANS

The deep type, acquired from eating raw snails, occurs in New Britain, Port Moresby, Lae, New Ireland, Bougainville Island and the highlands of New Guinea. It may cause ENCEPHALITIS. It should be treated in a hospital.

LEPROSY

It is common in New Guinea, in all the Pacific islands and amongst aboriginal Australians in the North Territory. It is particularly common in French Polynesia, especially Gambier and the Southern Marquesas. About 60% is indeterminate or tuberculoid and about 40% lepromatous.

In this area leprosy might be acquired from using woven mats that have been used by leprous patients. The fine, rough strands inoculate the leprosy germ into the skin of the user. Presumably wearing thick clothing would prevent this.

Treatment: in Vanuatu and possibly surrounding islands, nationals have a very high rate (11%) of adverse reactions to DAPSONE. Their skin peels off, and there is a high death rate. This occurs at 3-7 weeks after the beginning of treatment. Don't use DAPSONE in this area.

LEPTOSPIROSIS

This occurs in Australia. It is common in New Zealand. It is extremely common on Tahiti Island in French Polynesia and in New Caledonia. It especially affects middle-aged farmers between March and May. In this area, about 1 in 4 cases is very serious, complicated by JAUNDICE and sometimes LIVER FAILURE, resulting in some deaths. If you suspect it treat it promptly.

LIVER FAILURE

The most common regional causes are LEPTOSPIROSIS, HEPATITIS, ALCOHOLISM and MALARIA.

LIVER FLUKE

Probably this cannot be acquired in the area. The few cases that have been reported have been from Australia, in persons who acquired the worm elsewhere.

LYME DISEASE

This is known to occur in Australia, along the sea coast north of Sydney.

LYMPHOGRANULOMA VENEREUM

This occurs in warmer areas of the Pacific.

MALABSORPTION

The most common regional causes are GIARDIASIS, TRICHURIASIS, PIG-BEL and STRONGYLOIDIASIS.

MALARIA

This is widespread in this area; about 2/3 to 3/4 of the malaria being falciparum. In west-central Papua, over 50% of children less than 10 years old are affected. Those surviving to adulthood are immune to it.

Some of the non-falciparum (as well as falciparum) malaria is resistant to CHLOROQUINE, particularly in Papua. Patients infected in areas with chloroquine-resistant vivax malaria (particularly Indonesia) should be treated with ATOVAQUONE-PROGUANIL, MEFLOQUINE or [QUININE plus DOXYCYCLINE]. They should then receive PRIMAQUINE for 14 days to prevent relapse. Resistance to some ACTs is an increasing problem.

Reportedly there is no malaria transmission in Australia. Other areas reportedly free of malaria transmission are:

- New Zealand entirely.
- Vanuatu, Futuna Island.

Malaria had not been transmitted at high-altitudes, but it is now occurring at progressively higher elevations, in areas previously free of it. Resistance to FANSIDAR is widespread.

The best recent information may be obtained from the British Embassy. Also the Worldwide Antimalarial Resistance Network has developed an online database of malaria resistance.

MALNUTRITION

Kwashiorkor is common in New Guinea; Australian aboriginals have stunted growth rather than skinny arms when they are malnourished. The BMI is useless for them. Measure their height and compare it to that of normally nourished children of the same age and ethnic origin. When you are first in an area, measure the height of well-nourished children (as determined by normal hair color) of various ages to establish a standard.

Complications: PIG-BEL is a common complication of refeeding.

MEASLES

In PNG, measles accounts for about 1/3 of deaths in children in hospitals. Children should be immunized at 6 months of age.

MELIOIDOSIS

In Australia skin melioidosis presents as pustules or little spontaneous skin ulcers in those not otherwise sick. There are usually less than 10. People who are very sick may have pustules all over.

PARAGONIMIASIS

This occurs in some areas of Papua New Guinea, the Solomon Islands, Western Samoa and American Samoa.

PEPTIC ULCER

Similar regional diseases: PIG-BEL.

PERTUSSIS

This is very common in the South Pacific.

PIG-BEL

This is very common in New Guinea, especially the southern highlands.

PLAGUE

This is not known to occur in this area. However, if there were a worldwide epidemic, there is nothing to prevent its occurrence.

PLANT POISONING

Plant poisoning due to argemone oil occurs in the Pacific islands.

PNEUMONIA

This is by far the most common cause of death in New Guinea. A pneumonia that responds to AMPICILLIN but not PENICILLIN is common in aboriginal central Australia.

POLIO

This was particularly common on Wallis and Futuna Islands. It reportedly has been eliminated.

PYOMYOSITIS

This might be in the shoulder, arm or back. It usually responds to ERYTHROMYCIN.

Q FEVER

This occurs worldwide except for New Zealand. In Australia it occurs east of a line drawn between Wellesley Island and Point Fowler.

RABIES

This is present nearly worldwide, but reportedly does not occur on the island of New Guinea or in Australia.

RHEUMATIC FEVER

This is particularly common amongst aboriginal Australians, on the Cook Islands, in French Polynesia, on the Torres Straits Islands, in the Maoris of New Zealand and in Tonga.

SCABIES

This is present worldwide, common everywhere, but especially in aboriginal Australia and highland New Guinea.

SCRUB TYPHUS

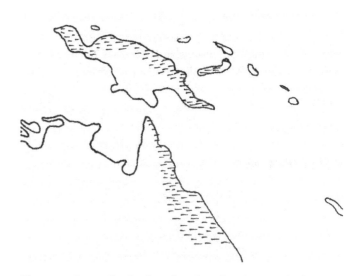

The approximate distribution of scrub typhus. It occurs in the eastern Solomon Islands and in Vanuatu.

SEIZURES

In New Guinea, the most common cause of adult-onset seizures is CYSTICERCOSIS.

SEPSIS

Patients with TROPICAL SPLENOMEGALY are prone to this. A form of STRONGYLOIDIASIS in New Guinea causes overwhelming sepsis in babies. Melioidosis is a peculiar form of sepsis which occurs in rural areas of Indochina as well as in northern Australia, around Darwin, in the aboriginal population, north of 20° latitude. Most infections occur within 2 weeks of the onset of heavy rains or at other times with water exposure. The incubation period can be very long, a matter of years. It usually affects those in ill health otherwise: patients with DIABETES, CIRRHOSIS, KIDNEY DISEASE or other chronic diseases. It frequently results in death.

SPOTTED FEVER

Tick typhus occurs in Queensland. It is usually a mild disease but might cause KIDNEY DISEASE, RESPIRATORY FAILURE or GANGRENE. It is occasionally fatal.

SPRUE

This might occur in northern Australia and possibly Papua, New Guinea.

STRONGYLOIDIASIS

Synonym: swollen baby syndrome

On the island of New Guinea, this is very common in the southern half of the island, from sea level to 1500 meters (5000 ft.). It causes an overwhelming infection (see SEPSIS) and death in children in the Gulf Provinces, known as swollen baby syndrome. It is also common in aboriginals of the Kimberly area. It is particularly likely to cause SEPSIS in those who also have TROPICAL SPLENOMEGALY.

SYPHILIS

This is reportedly common in Fiji. All blood tests for syphilis will be positive in YAWS which is very common in the island of New Guinea and in TREPONARID which occurs in central Australia.

TAPEWORM

Rat or dwarf tapeworm is common among the aboriginals of the Kimberly area and the highlands of Papua New Guinea. *Fish tapeworm* occurs in Australia and New Guinea.

THALLASEMIA

This is very common all over the island of New Guinea.

TINEA

Synonym: kaskad.

This is common in Australian aboriginals. Tinea imbricata (kaskad) is very common below 1500 meters (5000 ft.) on the island of New Guinea.

TOXOPLASMOSIS

TROPICAL SPLENOMEGALY causes one to be more prone to this. In the Pacific area, it is very common in those who live with cats, and it occurs, though less commonly, in those who live apart from cats.

TRACHOMA

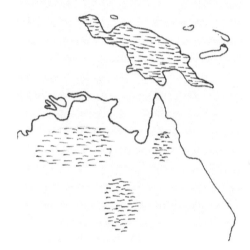

This occurs throughout the area, but it is most common in the shaded areas. AR

TREPONARID

This is found in central Australia. Though it is found only in dry areas, it is more common during the rainy season.

TRICHINOSIS

This is rare to non-existent in this area.

TRICHURIASIS

This is very common in Queensland but not in western Australia. It is common in New Guinea and may be very severe in some areas.

TROPICAL SPASTIC PARAPARESIS

This occurs on the Solomon Islands.

TROPICAL SPLENOMEGALY

This is common in New Guinea, especially in the upper Watut Valley, Morobe Province.

TROPICAL ULCER

This is common throughout the island of New Guinea.

TUBERCULOSIS

This is common in the Pacific area except for Australia, New Zealand, Niue and Guam.

TURISTA

In southwest Australia, GIARDIASIS and diarrhea responsive to ERYTHROMYCIN are common. In urban areas, a viral diarrhea that causes MALNUTRITION is common.

TYPHUS

Tick typhus is listed under SPOTTED FEVER; murine typhus and louse-borne typhus are described in the Condition Index.

SCRUB TYPHUS is a separate entry in this Index.

Murine typhus occurs along the east coast of Australia and in the area around Perth.

YANONGA

See ADDICTION due to kava, in this Index. This is an alternative name.

YAWS

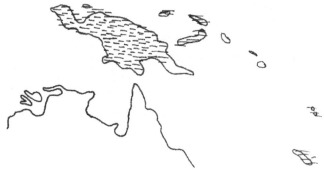

The known distribution of yaws. Additionally, it is common in aboriginal Australians.

In ethnic groups where there is much promiscuity, you should be reluctant to treat many people for yaws. If you do so, the group, over time, will become vulnerable to SYPHILIS which has worse long term consequences.

NAVIGATING THE INDEX

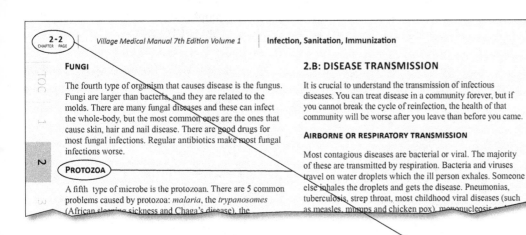

Number prefixes denote entries found in **Volume 1** (chapter-page.)

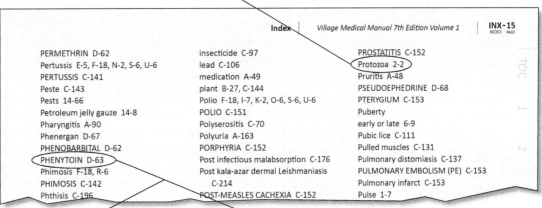

UPPER CASE entries denote the main information on the subject.

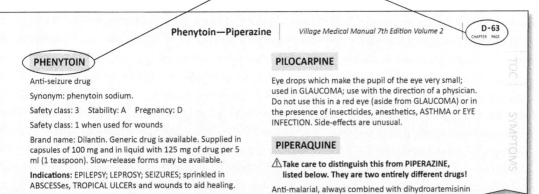

Letter prefixes denote entries found in **Volume 2** (section-page.)

Within Volume 2—

A	=	Symptom Index
B	=	Differential Index
C	=	Condition Index
D	=	Drug Index
E–U	=	Regional Indices

Within the Regional Indicies, the following letter designations are for these specific regions:

E	=	Eastern Europe and western Asia	N	=	Arctic
F	=	Africa south of the Sahara	O	=	Eastern Asia
I	=	Indian subcontinent	R	=	Mediterranean and Middle East
K	=	Central Asian Republics	S	=	Southeast Asia
M	=	Americas	U	=	Pacific

TOC   SYMPTOMS   DIFFERENTIALS   CONDITIONS   DRUG INDEX   REGIONAL NOTES

INX

TOC   SYMPTOMS   DIFFERENTIALS   CONDITIONS   DRUG INDEX   REGIONAL NOTES   INX

TOC   SYMPTOMS   DIFFERENTIALS   CONDITIONS   DRUG INDEX   REGIONAL NOTES

INX

P

TOC SYMPTOMS DIFFERENTIALS CONDITIONS DRUG INDEX REGIONAL NOTES INX

SYMPTOMS | DIFFERENTIALS | CONDITIONS | DRUG INDEX | REGIONAL NOTES

TOC

INX

TOC

SYMPTOMS

DIFFERENTIALS

CONDITIONS

DRUG INDEX

REGIONAL NOTES

INX

CPSIA information can be obtained
at www.ICGtesting.com
Printed in the USA
BVHW090501140120
569235BV00005B/9/P